Tarascon Pocket Pharmacopoeia®

2015 Professional Desk Reference Edition

16TH EDITION

"Desire to take medicines ... distinguishes man from animals."
—Sir William Osler

Editor-in-Chief
Richard J. Hamilton, MD, FAAEM, FACMT, FACEP
Professor and Chair, Department of Emergency Medicine
Drexel University College of Medicine
Philadelphia, PA

JONES & BARTLETT
LEARNING

DC metformin if Cr 1.4 or greater

World Headquarters
Jones & Bartlett Learning
5 Wall Street
Burlington, MA 01803
978-443-5000
info@jblearning.com
www.jblearning.com

Jones & Bartlett Learning books and products are available through most bookstores and online booksellers. To contact Jones & Bartlett Learning directly, call 800-832-0034, fax 978-443-8000, or visit our website www.jblearning.com.

Substantial discounts on bulk quantities of Jones & Bartlett Learning publications are available to corporations, professional associations, and other qualified organizations. For details and specific discount information, contact the special sales department at Jones & Bartlett Learning via the above contact information or send an email to specialsales@jblearning.com.

Copyright © 2015 by Jones & Bartlett Learning, LLC, an Ascend Learning Company
All rights reserved. No part of the material protected by this copyright may be reproduced or utilized in any form, electronic or mechanical, including photocopying, recording, or by any information storage and retrieval system, without written permission from the copyright owner.

The information in the *Pocket Pharmacopoeia* is compiled from sources believed to be reliable, and exhaustive efforts have been put forth to make the book as accurate as possible. The *Pocket Pharmacopoeia* is edited by a panel of drug information experts with extensive peer review and input from more than 50 practicing clinicians of multiple specialties. Our goal is to provide health professionals focused, core prescribing information in a convenient, organized, and concise fashion. We include FDA-approved dosing indications and those off-label uses that have a reasonable basis to support their use. *However, the accuracy and completeness of this work cannot be guaranteed.* Despite our best efforts this book may contain typographical errors and omissions. The *Pocket Pharmacopoeia* is intended as a quick and convenient reminder of information you have already learned elsewhere. The contents are to be used as a guide only, and healthcare professionals should use sound clinical judgment and individualize therapy to each specific patient care situation. This book is not meant to be a replacement for training, experience, continuing medical education, or studying the latest drug prescribing literature. This book is sold without warranties of any kind, expressed or implied, and the publisher and editors disclaim any liability, loss, or damage caused by the contents. Although drug companies purchase and distribute our books as promotional items, the Tarascon editorial staff alone determines all book content.

Production Credits
Chief Executive Officer: Ty Field
President: James Homer
V.P., Design and Production: Anne Spencer
V.P., Manufacturing and Inventory Control:
 Therese Connell
Manufacturing and Inventory Control Supervisor:
 Amy Bacus
Executive Editor: Nancy Anastasi Duffy
Production Editor: Daniel Stone
Digital Marketing Manager: Jennifer Sharp
Composition: Cenveo
Text and Cover Design: Anne Spencer
Printing and Binding: Edward Brothers Malloy
Cover Printing: Edward Brothers Malloy

The cover woodcut is *The Apothecary* by Jost Amman, Frankfurt, 1574.

ISSN: 1945-9084
ISBN: 978-1-284-07508-3

6048
Printed in the United States of America
19 18 17 16 15 10 9 8 7 6 5 4 3 2

You no doubt spent many hours contemplating the front cover and *The Apothecary* by Jost Amman. Did you solve the problem of the apothecary's balance scale and weights and the minimum number and size of weights (in ounces) necessary to weigh all integer ounces from 1 to 121? There is more than a little mathematics to the solution. With a balance scale there are three places for the weight — off the scale, on the left, or on the right. That means for n weights there are 3n possible arrangements. Since one of those choices is no weights on the scale (measuring nothing) we can eliminate one of these arrangements. Also we can eliminate the mirror image arrangements (where we have the same weights just on opposite sides). This means that for n weights we can measure $(3n - 1)/2$ integer weights. Hence 5 weights will get us 121 ounces, 4 weights gets 40 ounces, etc. The weights each weigh 1, 3, 9, 27, and 81 ounces. Claude Bachet first solved this problem for 4 weights. Interestingly, it was in Claude Bachet's translation of Diophantus Arithmetica, that Fermat scribbled his claim that he had a proof that no three positive integers a, b, and c can satisfy the equation an + bn = cn for any integer value of n greater than two (also known as Fermat's Last Theorem).

This year's puzzler is fairly simple and cryptographic. Two physicians need a way to securely send medical records to each other. Unfortunately their computerized systems are all down and they need to send the paper records via the mail. Dr. Ron has an empty lockable box with a padlock of which only he knows the combination. Dr. Adi has the medical records and a padlock and only he knows the combination to this lock. How can Dr. Adi send the records to Dr. Ron? The combination to the locks cannot be shared between the two physicians in any way. When the records are in the box they must be locked at all times until Dr. Ron has them. The padlocks also cannot be shipped unlocked (or else they could be intercepted and replaced).

TARASCON POCKET PHARMACOPOEIA EDITORIAL STAFF*

EDITOR IN CHIEF
Richard J. Hamilton, MD, FAAEM, FACMT, FACEP, Professor and Chair, Department of Emergency Medicine, Drexel University College of Medicine, Philadelphia, PA

ASSOCIATE EDITORS
Jill E. Allen, PharmD, BCPS, Pin Oak Associates, Drug Information Consultant, Salt Lake City, UT

Kim K. Birtcher, MS, PharmD, BCPS, Clinical Professor, University of Houston College of Pharmacy, Houston, TX

Jill S. Borchert, PharmD, BCPS, Professor, Pharmacy Practice, Director, PGY1 Residency Program, Midwestern University Chicago College of Pharmacy, Downers Grove, IL

Marie Cottman, PharmD, Owner, Pacific Compounding Pharmacy and Consultations, Inc., Lecturer, Department of Pharmaceutics and Medicinal Chemistry at Thomas J. Long School of Pharmacy and Health Sciences, University of the Pacific, Stockton, CA

Deborah Hass, PharmD, BCOP, BCPS, Investigational Drug Pharmacist, Pharmacy Department, Dana Farber Cancer Institute, Boston, MA

William A. Kehoe, PharmD, MA, BCPS, Professor of Pharmacy Practice and Psychology, University of the Pacific, Stockton, CA

Neeta Bahal O'Mara, PharmD, BCPS, Coldstream Consulting LLC, Skillman, NJ

Jeffrey T. Sherer, MPH, PharmD, BCPS, Clinical Associate Professor, University of Houston College of Pharmacy, Houston, TX

William Terneus Jr, PharmD, BCPS, Martin Health System, Tradition Medical Center, Stuart, FL

EDITORIAL BOARD
Steven R. Abel, PharmD, FASHP, Associate Dean for Clinical Programs, Bucke Professor and Head, Department of Pharmacy Practice , Purdue University College of Pharmacy, West Lafayette, IN

David R. Adams, MD, PharmD, Department of Dermatology, Penn State College of Medicine, Penn State Milton S. Hershey Medical Center, Hershey, PA

Heath P. Adams, PharmD, Department of Pharmacy, Trover Health Systems Regional Medical Center, Madisonville, KY

Giovannina M. Anthony, MD, Obstetrics and Gynecology, Women's Health Center of Jackson, Jackson, WY

Ouida Antle, PharmD, Carewest, Calgary, Alberta, Canada

Bruce Barrett, MD, PhD, Associate Professor of Family Medicine, University of Wisconsin, Madison, WI

Sandra Harley Counts, PharmD, AHEC Associate Professor of Family Medicine (Anderson), AnMed Health Family Medicine Residency Program, Anderson, SC

Gary E. Davis, PharmD, Neuroscience Clinical Coordinator, Adjunct Assistant Professor, University of Utah Hospital and Clinics, Department of Pharmacy Services, Salt Lake City, UT

*Affiliations are given for information purposes only, and no affiliation sponsorship is claimed.

EDITORIAL BOARD, cont.

Lori M. Dickerson, PharmD, Professor of Family Medicine, Medical University of South Carolina, Charleston, SC

Joseph S. Esherick, MD, FAAFP, Family Medicine, Ventura County Medical Center, Ventura, CA

Randall L. Goodman, MD, FACS, Opthalmology, Shepard Eye Center, Santa Maria, CA

David Greenes, MD, Division of Emergency Medicine, Children's Hospital, Boston, MA

James R. Herman, MD, PhD, FACS, Urology Associates of Kingsport, Kingsport, TN

Jeffrey Jacobson, MD, Chief, Division of Infectious Disease and HIV Medicine, Drexel University College of Medicine, Philadelphia, PA

Arlyn J. LaBair, MD, Family Medicine, Denver, CO

Marc J. Laufgraben, MD, MBA, Endocrinology, Clinical Associate Professor of Medicine, Brown University, Providence, RI

Allen E. Lavee, MD, Anesthesiology, San Francisco, CA

Lawrence Loo, MD, Internal Medicine, Professor of Medicine, Department of Medicine, Loma Linda University School of Medicine, Loma Linda, CA

Yun Lu, PharmD, MS, BCPS, Clinical Associate Professor, University of Minnesota, Hennepin County Medical Center, Minneapolis, MN

Andrea Luisi, PharmD, BCPS, Cumberland, RI

Ian R. McNicholl, PharmD, BCPS (AQ – Infectious Diseases), AAHIVE, Associate Clinical Professor, Clinical Pharmacy Specialist, UCSF Positive Health Program, Editor, UCSF Center for HIV Information, Drug Interaction Database, San Francisco, CA

Susan M. Miller, PharmD, BCPS, Pharmacy Clinic Coordinator, Cape Fear Valley Health System, Fayetteville, NC

Melissa J. Nirenberg, MD, PhD, Associate Professor of Neurology, NYU School of Medicine, New York, NY

John Noviasky, PharmD, BCPS, Associate Director of Pharmacy-Clinical Services, Upstate University Hospital, Syracuse, NY

Mary Ellis Pickett, MD, Associate Professor of Medicine, Oregon Health and Science University, Portland, OR

Joseph Saseen, PharmD, BCPS, CLS, Professor, University of Colorado, Schools of Pharmacy and Medicine, Aurora, CO

Timothy W. Smith, D.Phil, MD, Associate Professor of Medicine, Washington University School of Medicine, St. Louis, MO

Ronald L. Swaab, MD, Hematology and Oncology, Pottstown Memorial Regional Cancer Center, Pottstown, PA

Andrew E. Thompson, MD, Rheumatology, Assistant Professor of Medicine, University of Western Ontario, Canada

Kristin Walter, MD, Pulmonary and Critical Care Medicine, St. Joseph Hospital, Chicago, IL

Izak F. Wessels, M.Med, FRCSE, FRCOphth, FACS, Allied Eye Associates, Chattanooga, TN; and Clinical Associate Professor of Ophthalmology, Loma Linda University, Loma Linda, CA

Robert M. Wood, MD, Family Medicine, Santa Maria, CA; In Honor of Robert L. Wood, MD.

CONTENTS

PAGE INDEX FOR TABLES

PREFACE TO THE TARASCON POCKET PHARMACOPOEIA®

The *Tarascon Pocket Pharmacopoeia®* arranges drugs by clinical class with a comprehensive index in the back. Trade names are italicized and capitalized. Drug doses shown in mg/kg are generally intended for children, while fixed doses represent typical adult recommendations. Brackets indicate currently available formulations, although not all pharmacies stock all formulations. The availability of generic, over-the-counter, and scored formulations is mentioned. We have set the disease or indication in red for the pharmaceutical agent. It is meant to function as an aid to find information quickly. Codes are as follows:

▶ **METABOLISM & EXCRETION:** **L** = primarily liver, **K** = primarily kidney, **LK** = both, but liver > kidney, **KL** = both, but kidney > liver.

⚲ **SAFETY IN PREGNANCY:** **A** = Safety established using human studies, **B** = Presumed safety based on animal studies, **C** = Uncertain safety; no human studies and animal studies show an adverse effect, **D** = Unsafe - evidence of risk that may in certain clinical circumstances be justifiable, **X** = Highly unsafe - risk of use outweighs any possible benefit. For drugs that have not been assigned a category: **+** Generally accepted as safe, **?** Safety unknown or controversial, **−** Generally regarded as unsafe.

▶ **SAFETY IN LACTATION:** **+** Generally accepted as safe, **?** Safety unknown or controversial, **−** Generally regarded as unsafe. Many of our "**+**" listings are from the AAP policy "The Transfer of Drugs and Other Chemicals Into Human Milk" (see www.aap.org) and may differ from those recommended by the manufacturer.

© **DEA CONTROLLED SUBSTANCES:** **I** = High abuse potential, no accepted use (eg, heroin, marijuana), **II** = High abuse potential and severe dependence liability (eg, morphine, codeine, hydromorphone, cocaine, amphetamines, methylphenidate, secobarbital). Some states require triplicates. **III** = Moderate dependence liability (eg, *Tylenol #3, Vicodin*), **IV** = Limited dependence liability (benzodiazepines, propoxyphene, phentermine), **V** = Limited abuse potential (eg, *Lomotil*).

$ **RELATIVE COST:** Cost codes used are "per month" of maintenance therapy (eg, antihypertensives) or "per course" of short-term therapy (eg, antibiotics). Codes are calculated using average wholesale prices (at press time in US dollars) for the most common indication and route of each drug at a typical adult dosage. For maintenance therapy, costs are calculated based upon a 30-day supply or the quantity that might typically be used in a given month. For short-term therapy (ie, 10 days or less), costs are calculated on a single treatment course. When multiple forms are available (eg, generics), these codes reflect the least expensive generally available product. When drugs don't neatly fit into the classification scheme above, we have assigned codes based upon the relative cost of other similar drugs. *These codes should be used as a rough guide only*, as (1) they reflect cost, not charges, (2) pricing often varies substantially from location to location and time to time, and (3) HMOs, Medicaid, and buying groups often negotiate quite different pricing. Check with your local pharmacy if you have any questions.

Code	Cost
$	< $25
$$	$25 to $49
$$$	$50 to $99
$$$$	$100 to $199
$$$$$	≥ $200

🍁 CANADIAN TRADE NAMES: Unique common Canadian trade names not used in the US are listed after a maple leaf symbol. Trade names used in both nations or only in the US are displayed without such notation.

ABBREVIATIONS IN TEXT

AAP	American Academy of Pediatrics	kg	kilogram
ACCP	American College of Chest Physicians	lbs	pounds
ACR	American College of Rheumatology	LFT	liver function test
ACT	activated clotting time	LV	left ventricular
ADHD	attention deficit hyperactivity disorder	LVEF	left ventricular ejection fraction
AHA	American Heart Association	m^2	square meters
Al	aluminum	MAOI	monoamine oxidase inhibitor
ANC	absolute neutrophil count	mcg	microgram
ASA	aspirin	MDI	metered dose inhaler
BP	blood pressure	mEq	milliequivalent
BPH	benign prostatic hyperplasia	mg	milligram
BUN	blood urea nitrogen	Mg	magnesium
Ca	calcium	MI	myocardial infarction
CAD	coronary artery disease	min	minute
cap	capsule	mL	milliliter
cm	centimeter	mo	months old
CMV	cytomegalovirus	MRSA	methicillin-resistant *Staphylococcus aureus*
CNS	central nervous system	ng	nanogram
COPD	chronic obstructive pulmonary disease	NHLBI	National Heart, Lung, and Blood Institute
CrCl	creatinine clearance	NPH	neutral protamine hagedorn
CVA	stroke	NS	normal saline
CYP	cytochrome P450	N/V	nausea/vomiting
D5W	5% dextrose	NYHA	New York Heart Association
dL	deciliter	OA	osteoarthritis
DM	diabetes mellitus	oz	ounces
DMARD	disease-modifying drug	pc	after meals
DPI	dry powder inhaler	PO	by mouth
DRESS	drug rash eosinophilia and systemic symptoms	PR	by rectum
ECG	electrocardiogram	prn	as needed
EPS	extrapyramidal symptoms	PTT	partial thromboplastin time
ET	endotracheal	q	every
g	gram	RA	rheumatoid arthritis
GERD	gastroesophageal reflux disease	RSV	respiratory syncytial virus
gtts	drops	SC	subcutaneous
GU	genitourinary	sec	second
h	hour	soln	solution
HAART	highly active antiretroviral therapy	supp	suppository
Hb	hemoglobin	susp	suspension
HCTZ	hydrochlorothiazide	tab	tablet
HIT	heparin-induced thrombocytopenia	TB	tuberculosis
HSV	herpes simplex virus	TCA	tricyclic antidepressant
HTN	hypertension	TNF	tumor necrosis factor
IM	intramuscular	TPN	total parenteral nutrition
INR	international normalized ratio	UTI	urinary tract infection
IU	international units	wt	weight
IV	intravenous	y	year
JIA	juvenile idiopathic arthritis	yo	years old

THERAPEUTIC DRUG LEVELS

Drug	Level	Optimal Timing
amikacin peak	20–35 mcg/mL	30 minutes after infusion
amikacin trough	<5 mcg/mL	Just prior to next dose
carbamazepine trough	4–12 mcg/mL	Just prior to next dose
cyclosporine trough	50–300 ng/mL	Just prior to next dose
digoxin	0.8–2.0 ng/mL	Just prior to next dose
ethosuximide trough	40–100 mcg/mL	Just prior to next dose
gentamicin peak	5–10 mcg/mL	30 minutes after infusion
gentamicin trough	<2 mcg/mL	Just prior to next dose
lidocaine	1.5–5 mcg/mL	12–24 hours after start of infusion
lithium trough	0.6–1.2 meq/l	Just prior to first morning dose
NAPA	10–30 mcg/mL	Just prior to next procainamide dose
phenobarbital trough	15–40 mcg/mL	Just prior to next dose
phenytoin trough	10–20 mcg/mL	Just prior to next dose
primidone trough	5–12 mcg/mL	Just prior to next dose
procainamide	4–10 mcg/mL	Just prior to next dose
quinidine	2–5 mcg/mL	Just prior to next dose
theophylline	5–15 mcg/mL	8–12 hours after once daily dose
tobramycin peak	5–10 mcg/mL	30 minutes after infusion
tobramycin trough	<2 mcg/mL	Just prior to next dose
valproate trough (epilepsy)	50–100 mcg/mL	Just prior to next dose
valproate trough (mania)	45–125 mcg/mL	Just prior to next dose
vancomycin trough[1]	10–20 mg/L	Just prior to next dose
zonisamide[2]	10–40 mcg/mL	Just prior to dose

[1]Maintain trough >10 mg/L to avoid resistance; optimal trough for complicated infections is 15–20 mg/L
[2]Ranges not firmly established but supported by clinical trial results

PEDIATRIC DRUGS	strength	freq	2mo	4mo	6mo	9mo	12mo	15mo	2yo	3yo	5yo
Age		*Kg*	5	6½	8	9	10	11	13	15	19
		lbs	11	15	17	20	22	24	28	33	42
med	*strength*	*freq*	*teaspoons of liquid per dose (1 tsp = 5 mL)*								
Tylenol (mg)		q4h	80	80	120	120	160	160	200	240	280
Tylenol (tsp)	160/t	q4h	½	½	¾	¾	1	1	1¼	1½	1¾
ibuprofen (mg)		q6h	--	--	75†	75†	100	100	125	150	175
ibuprofen (tsp)	100/t	q6h	--	--	¾t	¾t	1	1	1¼	1½	1¾
amoxicillin or	125/t	bid	1	1¼	1½	1¾	1¾	2	2¼	2¾	3½
Augmentin	200/t	bid	½	¾	1	1	1¼	1¼	1½	1¾	2¼
(not otitis media)	250/t	bid	½	½	¾	¾	1	1	1¼	1¼	1¾
	400/t	bid	¼	½	½	½	¾	¾	¾	1	1
amoxicillin,	200/t	bid	1	1¼	1¾	2	2	2¼	2¾	3	4
(otitis media)‡	250/t	bid	¾	1¼	1½	1½	1¾	1¾	2¼	2½	3¼
	400/t	bid	½	¾	¾	1	1	1¼	1½	1½	2
Augmentin ES‡	600/t	bid	?	½	½	¾	¾	¾	1	1¼	1½
azithromycin*§	100/t	qd	¼†	½†	½	½	½	½	¾	¾	1
(5-day Rx)	200/t	qd	--	¼†	¼	¼	¼	¼	½	½	½
Bactrim/Septra	---	bid	½	¾	1	1	1	1¼	1½	1½	2
cefaclor*	125/t	bid	1	1	1¼	1½	1½	1¾	2	2½	3
"	250/t	bid	½	½	¾	¾	¾	1	1	1¼	1½
cefadroxil	125/t	bid	½	¾	1	1	1¼	1¼	1½	1¾	2¼
"	250/t	bid	¼	½	½	½	¾	¾	¾	1	1
cefdinir	125/t	qd	--	¾†	1	1	1	1¼	1½	1¾	2
Cefixime	100/t	qd	½	½	¾	¾	¾	1	1	1¼	1½
cefprozil*	125/t	bid	--	¾†	1	1	1¼	1½	1½	2	2¼
"	250/t	bid	--	½†	½	½	¾	¾	¾	1	1¼
cefuroxime	125/t	bid	--	¾	¾	1	1	1	1½	1¾	2¼
cephalexin	125/t	qid	--	½	¾	¾	1	1	1¼	1½	1¾
"	250/t	qid	--	¼	¼	½	½	½	¾	¾	1
clarithromycin	125/t	bid	½†	½	½	½	¾	¾	¾	1	1¼
"	250/t	bid	--	--	--	¼	½	½	½	½	¾
dicloxacillin	62½/t	qid	½	¾	1	1	1¼	1¼	1½	1¾	2
nitrofurantoin	25/t	qid	¼	½	½	½	½	¾	¾	¾	1
Pediazole	---	tid	½	½	¾	¾	1	1	1	1¼	1½
penicillin V**	250/t	bid-tid	--	1	1	1	1	1	1	1	1
cetirizine	5/t	qd	--	--	½	½	½	½	½	½	½
Benadryl	12.5/t	q6h	½	½	¾	¾	1	1	1¼	1½	2
prednisolone	15/t	qd	¼	½	½	¾	¾	¾	1	1	1¼
prednisone	5/t	qd	1	1¼	1½	1¾	2	2¼	2½	3	3¾
Robitussin	---	q4h	--	--	¼†	¼†	½	½	¾	¾	1
Tylenol w/ codeine		q4h	--	--	--	--	--	--	--	1	1

* Dose shown is for otitis media only; see dosing in text for alternative indications.
† Dosing at this age/weight not recommended by manufacturer.
‡ AAP now recommends high dose (80-90 mg/kg/d) for all otitis media in children; with Augmentin used as ES only.
§ Give a double dose of azithromycin the first day.
**AHA dosing for streptococcal pharyngitis. Treat for 10 days.
tsp/t = teaspoon; q = every; h = hour; kg = kilogram; Lbs = pounds; ml = mililiter; bid = two times per day; qd = every day; qid = four times per day; tid = three times per day

PEDIATRIC VITAL SIGNS AND INTRAVENOUS DRUGS

Age		Pre-matr	New-born	2m	4m	6m	9m	12m	15m	2y	3y	5y
Weight	(kg)	2	3½	5	6½	8	9	10	11	13	15	19
	(lbs)	4¼	7½	11	15	17	20	22	24	28	33	42
Maint fluids	(mL/h)	8	14	20	26	32	36	40	42	46	50	58
ET tube	(mm)	2½	3/3½	3½	3½	3½	4	4	4½	4½	4½	5
Defib	(Joules)	4	7	10	13	16	18	20	22	26	30	38
Systolic BP	(high)	70	80	85	90	95	100	103	104	106	109	114
	(low)	40	60	70	70	70	70	70	70	75	75	80
Pulse rate	(high)	145	145	180	180	180	160	160	160	150	150	135
	(low)	100	100	110	110	110	100	100	100	90	90	65
Resp rate	(high)	60	60	50	50	50	46	46	30	30	25	25
	(low)	35	30	30	30	24	24	20	20	20	20	20
adenosine	(mg)	0.2	0.3	0.5	0.6	0.8	0.9	1	1.1	1.3	1.5	1.9
atropine	(mg)	0.1	0.1	0.1	0.13	0.16	0.18	0.2	0.22	0.26	0.30	0.38
Benadryl	(mg)	-	-	5	6½	8	9	10	11	13	15	19
bicarbonate	(meq)	2	3½	5	6½	8	9	10	11	13	15	19
dextrose	(g)	1	2	5	6½	8	9	10	11	13	15	19
epinephrine	(mg)	.02	.04	.05	.07	.08	.09	0.1	0.11	0.13	0.15	0.19
lidocaine	(mg)	2	3½	5	6½	8	9	10	11	13	15	19
morphine	(mg)	0.2	0.3	0.5	0.6	0.8	0.9	1	1.1	1.3	1.5	1.9
mannitol	(g)	2	3½	5	6½	8	9	10	11	13	15	19
naloxone	(mg)	.02	.04	.05	.07	.08	.09	0.1	0.11	0.13	0.15	0.19
diazepam	(mg)	0.6	1	1.5	2	2.5	2.7	3	3.3	3.9	4.5	5
fosphenytoin*	(PE)	40	70	100	130	160	180	200	220	260	300	380
lorazepam	(mg)	0.1	0.2	0.3	0.35	0.4	0.5	0.5	0.6	0.7	0.8	1.0
phenobarb	(mg)	30	60	75	100	125	125	150	175	200	225	275
phenytoin*	(mg)	40	70	100	130	160	180	200	220	260	300	380
ampicillin	(mg)	100	175	250	325	400	450	500	550	650	750	1000
ceftriaxone	(mg)	-	-	250	325	400	450	500	550	650	750	1000
cefotaxime	(mg)	100	175	250	325	400	450	500	550	650	750	1000
gentamicin	(mg)	5	8	12	16	20	22	25	27	32	37	47

*Loading doses; fosphenytoin dosed in "phenytoin equivalents."

CONVERSIONS	Liquid:	Weight:
Temperature:	1 fluid ounce = 30 mL	1 kilogram = 2.2 lbs
F = (1.8) C + 32	1 teaspoon = 5 mL	1 ounce = 30 g
C = (F − 32)/1.8	1 tablespoon = 15 mL	1 grain = 65 mg

INHIBITORS, INDUCERS, AND SUBSTRATES OF CYTOCHROME P450 ISOZYMES

The cytochrome P450 (CYP) inhibitors and inducers below do not necessarily cause clinically important interactions with substrates listed. We exclude in vitro data, which can be inaccurate. Refer to other resources for more information if an interaction is suspected based on this chart. A drug that inhibits CYP subfamily activity can block the metabolism of substrates of that enzyme, and substrate accumulation and toxicity may result. CYP inhibitors are classified by how much they increase the area-under-the-curve (AUC) of a substrate: weak (1.25- to 2-fold), moderate (2- to 5-fold), or strong (≥5 fold). A drug that induces CYP subfamily activity increases substrate metabolism and reduced substrate efficacy may result. CYP inducers are classified by how much they decrease the AUC of a substrate: weak (20 to 50%), moderate (50 to 80%) and strong (>80%). A drug is considered a sensitive substrate if a CYP inhibitor increases the AUC of that drug by ≥5-fold. While AUC increases of >50% often do not affect patient response, smaller increases can be important if the therapeutic range is narrow (e.g., theophylline, warfarin, cyclosporine). This table may be incomplete since new evidence about drug interactions is continually being identified.

CYP1A2

Inhibitors. *Strong*: ciprofloxacin, fluvoxamine. *Moderate*: methoxalan, mexiletine, oral contraceptives, phenylpropanolamine, vemurafenib, zileuton. *Weak*: acyclovir, allopurinol, caffeine, cimetidine, disulfiram, echinacea, famotidine, propafenone, propranolol, simeprevir, terbinafine, ticlopidine, verapamil. *Unclassified*: amiodarone, atazanavir, citalopram, clarithromycin, deferasirox, estradiol, isoniazid, peginterferon alfa-2a.
Inducers. *Moderate*: montelukast, phenytoin, smoking. *Weak*: omeprazole, phenobarbital. *Unclassified*: carbamazepine, charcoal-broiled foods, rifampin, ritonavir, tipranavir-ritonavir.
Substrates. *Sensitive*: caffeine, duloxetine, melatonin, rameltion, tacrine, tizanidine. *Unclassified*: acetaminophen, amitriptyline, asenapine, bendamustine, cinacalcet, clomipramine, clozapine, cyclobenzaprine, erlotinib, estradiol, fluvoxamine, haloperidol, imipramine, loxapine, mexiletine, mirtazapine, naproxen, olanzapine, ondansetron, pomalidomide, propranolol, rasagiline, riluzole, roflumilast, ropinirole, ropivacaine, R-warfarin, tasimelteon, theophylline, zileuton, zolmitriptan.

CYP2B6

Inhibitors. *Weak*: clopidogrel, prasugrel, ticlopidine.
Inducers. *Moderate*: efavirenz, rifampin. *Weak*: nevirapine, artemether (in *Coartem*). *Unclassified*: baicalin (in *Limbrel*), ritonavir.
Substrates. *Sensitive*: bupropion, efavirenz. *Unclassified*: cyclophosphamide, ketamine, meperidine, methadone, nevirapine, prasugrel, propofol.

CYP2C8

Inhibitors. *Strong*: clopidogrel, gemfibrozil. *Moderate*: deferasirox. *Weak*: fluvoxamine, ketoconazole, trimethoprim.
Inducers. *Moderate*: rifampin. *Unclassified*: barbiturates, carbamazepine, rifabutin.
Substrates. *Sensitive*: repaglinide. *Unclassified*: amiodarone, carbamazepine, dabrafenib, ibuprofen, imatinib, isotretinoin, loperamide, montelukast, paclitaxel, pioglitazone, rosiglitazone, treprostinil.

CYP2C9

Inhibitors. *Moderate*: amiodarone, fluconazole, miconazole, oxandrolone. *Weak*: capecitabine, cotrimoxazole, etravirine, fluvastatin, fluvoxamine, metronidazole, oritavancin, sulfinpyrazone, tigecycline, voriconazole, zafirlukast. *Unclassified*: cimetidine, fenofibrate, fenofibric acid, fluorouracil, imatinib, isoniazid, leflunomide, ritonavir.
Inducers. *Moderate*: carbamazepine, rifampin. *Weak*: aprepitant, bosentan, elvitegravir, phenobarbital, St. John's wort. *Unclassified*: rifapentine.
Substrates. *Sensitive*: celecoxib. *Unclassified*: azilsartan, bosentan, chlorpropamide, diclofenac, etravirine, fluoxetine, flurbiprofen, fluvastatin, formoterol, glimepiride, glipizide, glyburide, ibuprofen, irbesartan, losartan, mefenamic acid, meloxicam, montelukast, naproxen, nateglinide, ospemifene, phenytoin, piroxicam, ramelteon, sildenafil, tolbutamide, torsemide, vardenafil, voriconazole, S-warfarin, zafirlukast, zileuton.

CYP2C19

Inhibitors. *Strong*: fluconazole, fluvoxamine, ticlopidine. *Moderate*: esomeprazole, fluoxetine, moclobemide, omeprazole, voriconazole. *Weak*: armodafinil, carbamazepine, cimetidine, etravirine, felbamate, human growth hormone, ketoconazole, oral contraceptives, oritavancin. *Unclassified*: chloramphenicol, eslicarbazepine, isoniazid, modafinil, oxcarbazepine .
Inducers. *Moderate*: rifampin. *Unclassified*: efavirenz, St. John's wort.
Substrates. *Sensitive*: lansoprazole, omeprazole. *Unclassified*: amitriptyline, bortezomib, carisoprodol, cilostazol, citalopram, clobazam, clomipramine, clopidogrel, clozapine, cyclophosphamide, desipramine, dexlansoprazole, diazepam, escitalopram, esomeprazole, etravirine, formoterol, imipramine, lacosamide, methadone, moclobamide, nelfinavir, pantoprazole, phenytoin, progesterone, proguanil, propranolol, rabeprazole, sertraline, tofacitinib, voriconazole, R-warfarin.

(cont.)

INHIBITORS, INDUCERS, AND SUBSTRATES OF CYTOCHROME P450 ISOZYMES (Continued)

CYP2D6

Inhibitors. *Strong*: bupropion, fluoxetine, paroxetine, quinidine.
Moderate: cinacalcet, dronedarone, duloxetine, mirabegron, terbinafine.
Weak: amiodarone, asenapine, celecoxib, cimetidine, desvenlafaxine, diltiazem, diphenhydramine, echinacea, escitalopram, febuxostat, gefitinib, hydralazine, hydroxychloroquine, imitinib, methadone, oral contraceptives, propafenone, ranitidine, ritonavir, sertraline, telithromycin, venlafaxine, vemurafenib, verapamil. *Unclassified*: abiraterone, chloroquine, clobazam, clomipramine, cobicistat, fluphenazine, haloperidol, lorcaserin, lumefantrine (in *Coartem*), metoclopramide, moclobamide, perphenazine, quinine, ranolazine, thioridazine.
Inducers. None known.
Substrates. *Sensitive*: atomoxetine, desipramine, dextromethorphan, metoprolol, nebivolol, perphenazine, tolterodine, venlafaxine. *Unclassified*: amitriptyline, aripiprazole, carvedilol, cevimeline, chlorpheniramine, chlorpromazine, cinacalcet, clomipramine, codeine*, darifenacin, dihydrocodeine, dolasetron, donepezil, doxepin, duloxetine, fesoterodine, flecainide, fluoxetine, formoterol, galantamine, haloperidol, hydrocodone, iloperidone, imipramine, loratadine, loxapine, maprotiline, methadone, methamphetamine, metoclopramide, meclizine, mexiletine, mirtazapine, morphine, nortriptyline, ondansetron, paroxetine, promethazine, propafenone, propranolol, quetiapine, risperidone, ritonavir, tamoxifen, tamsulosin, tetrabenazine, thioridazine, timolol, tramadol*, trazodone, vortioxetine.
* Metabolism by CYP2D6 required to convert to active analgesic metabolite; analgesia may be impaired by CYP2D6 inhibitors.

CYP3A4

Inhibitors. *Strong*: boceprevir, clarithromycin, cobicistat, conivaptan, indinavir, itraconazole, ketoconazole, lopinavir-ritonavir, nefazodone, nelfi navir, posaconazole, ritonavir, saquinavir, telithromycin, voriconazole.
Moderate: aprepitant, atazanavir, ciprofloxacin, crizotinib, darunavir-ritonavir, diltiazem, dronedarone, erythromycin, fluconazole, fosamprenavir, grapefruit juice (variable), imatinib, verapamil. *Weak*: alprazolam, amiodarone, amlodipine, atorvastatin, bicalutamide, cilostazol, cimetidine, cyclosporine, everolimus, fluoxetine, fluvoxamine, ginko, goldenseal, isoniazid, ivacaftor, lapatinib, lomitapide, nilotinib, oral contraceptives, ranitidine, ranolazine, simeprevir, ticagrelor, tipranavir-ritonavir, zileuton. *Unclassified*: danazol, miconazole, quinine, quinupristin-dalfopristin, sertraline.
Inducers. *Strong*: carbamazepine, mitotane, phenytoin, rifampin, rifapentine, St. Johns wort. *Moderate*: bosentan, efavirenz, etravirine, modafinil, nafcillin. *Weak:* aprepitant, armodafinil, clobazam, echinacea, fosamprenavir, oritavancin, pioglitazone, rufinamide. *Unclassified:* artemether (in *Coartem*), barbiturates, dabrafenib, dexamethasone, eslicarbazepine, ethosuximide, griseovulvin, nevirapine, oxcarbazepine, primidone, rifabutin, ritonavir, tocilizumab, vemurafenib.
Substrates. *Sensitive:* alfentanil, aprepitant, budesonide, buspirone, conivaptan, darifenacin, darunavir, dasatinib, dronedarone, eletriptan, eplerenone, everolimus, felodipine, fluticasone, ibrutinib, indinavir, ivacaftor, lomitapide, lopinavir (in *Kaletra*), lovastatin, lurasidone, maraviroc, midazolam, nisoldipine, quetiapine, saquinavir, sildenafil, simvastatin, sirolimus, tipranavir, tolvaptan, triazolam, vardenafil. *Unclassified:* alfuzosin, aliskiren, almotriptan, alprazolam, amiodarone, amlodipine, apixaban, apremilast, aripiprazole, armodafinil, artemether (in *Coartem*), atazanavir, atorvastatin, avanafil, axitinib, bedaquiline, boceprevir, bortezomib, bosentan, bosutinib, brentuximab, bromocriptine, buprenorphine, cabozantinib, carbamazepine, ceritinib, cevimeline, cilostazol, cinacalcet, cisapride, citalopram, clarithromycin, clomipramine, clonazepam, clopidogrel, clobazam, clozapine, cobicistat, colchicine, corticosteroids, crizotinib, cyclophosphamide, cyclosporine, dabrafenib, dapsone, desogestrel, desvenlafaxine, dexamethasone, dexlansoprazole, diazepam, dihydroergotamine, diltiazem, disopyramide, docetaxel, dofetilide, dolasetron, domperidone, donepezil, doxorubicin, dutasteride, efavirenz, elvitegravir, ergotamine, erlotinib, erythromycin, escitalopram, esomeprazole, eszopiclone, ethinyl estradiol, etoposide, etravirine, fentanyl, fesoterodine, finasteride, fosamprenavir, fosaprepitant, galantamine, gefitinib, guanfacine, haloperidol, hydrocodone, ifosfamide, iloperidone, imatinib, imipramine, irinotecan, isradipine, itraconazole, ixabepilone, ketamine, ketoconazole, lansoprazole, lapatinib, letrozole, lidocaine, loratadine, loxapine, lumefantrine (in *Coartem*), macitentan, methylergonovine, mifepristone, mirtazapine, modafinil, mometasone, nateglinide, nefazodone, nelfi navir, nevirapine, nicardipine, nifedipine, nilotinib, nimodipine, ondansetron, ospemifene, oxybutynin, oxycodone, paclitaxel, pantoprazole, pazopanib, pimozide, pioglitazone, pomalidomide, ponatinib, prasugrel, praziquantel, quinidine, quinine, rabeprazole, ramelteon, ranolazine, regorafenib, repaglinide, rifabutin, rifampin, ritonavir, rivaroxaban, roflumilast, romidepsin, ruxolitinib, saxagliptin, sertraline, silodosin, solifenacin, sufentanil, sunitinib, tacrolimus, tadalafil, tamoxifen, tamsulosin, tasimelteon, telaprevir, telithromycin, temsirolimus, testosterone, tiagabine, ticagrelor, tinidazole, tofacitinib, tolterodine, tramadol, trazodone, verapamil, vilazodone, vinblastine, vincristine, vinorelbine, vorapaxar, voriconazole, R-warfarin, zaleplon, ziprasidone, zolpidem, zonisamide.

INHIBITORS, INDUCERS, AND SUBSTRATES OF P-GLYCOPROTEIN

The p-glycoprotein (P-gp) inhibitors and inducers listed below do not necessarily cause clinically important interactions with P-gp substrates. We attempt to exclude in vitro data which can be inaccurate. Refer to other resources for more information if an interaction is suspected based on this chart. P-gp is an efflux transporter that pumps drugs out of cells. In the gut, P-gp reduces drug absorption by pumping drugs into the gut lumen. In the kidney, it increases drug excretion by pumping drugs into urine. P-gp inhibitors can increase exposure to P-gp substrates, potentially increasing their risk of toxicity. P-gp inducers can reduce exposure to P-gp substrates, increasing the risk of treatment failure. Some drugs are dual inhibitors of P-gp and CYP 3A4 (e.g., clarithromycin, dronedarone, erythromycin, itraconazole, ketoconazole, verapamil), while others are dual inducers of P-gp and CYP 3A4 (e.g., carbamazepine, phenytoin, rifampin, St. John's wort). Potent p-gp inhibitors are defined here as drugs that increase the area-under-the-curve (AUC) of a p-gp substrate (digoxin or fexofenadine) by ≥1.5-fold. This table may be incomplete since new evidence about drug interactions is continually being identified.

Inhibitors. *Potent:* amiodarone, clarithromycin, cyclosporine, dronedarone, itraconazole, lapatinib, lopinavir-ritonavir, ranolazine, ritonavir, verapamil. *Unclassified:* atorvastatin, azithromycin, captopril, carvedilol, cobicistat, conivaptan, darunavir-ritonavir, diltiazem, dipyridamole, erythromycin, etravirine, everolimus, felodipine, indinavir, isradipine, ketoconazole, lomitapide, naproxen, nifedipine, nilotinib, posaconazole, quinidine, saquinavir-ritonavir, simeprevir, telmisartan, ticagrelor.

Inducers: carbamazepine, fosamprenavir, phenytoin, rifampin, St. John's wort, tipranavir-ritonavir*.

*Tipranavir induces CYP3A4 and P-gp, while ritonavir inhibits both pathways. This makes it difficult to predict the effect of ritonavir-boosted tipranavir on substrates of P-gp.

Substrates: aliskiren, ambrisentan, apixaban, boceprevir, ceritinib, clobazam, clopidogrel, colchicine, cyclosporine, dabigatran, digoxin, diltiazem, docetaxel, dolutegravir, etoposide, everolimus, fexofenadine, fosamprenavir, imatinib, indinavir, lapatinib, linagliptin, loperamide, lovastatin, maraviroc, morphine, nadolol, nilotinib, paclitaxel, paliperidone, pomalidomide, posaconazole, pravastatin, propranolol, quinidine, ranolazine, rifaximin, rivaroxaban, romidepsin, saquinavir, saxagliptin, silodosin, simeprevir, sirolimus, sitagliptin, sofosbuvir, tacrolimus, telaprevir, tenofovir, tolvaptan, topotecan, vinblastine, vincristine.

CORONARY ARTERY DISEASE 10-YEAR RISK

Framingham model for calculating 10–year risk for coronary artery disease (CAD) in patients without diabetes or clinically evident CAD. Diabetes is considered a CAD risk "equivalent", i.e., the prospective risk of CAD in diabetics is similar to those with established CAD. Automated calculator available at: http://hin.nhlbi.nih.gov/atpiii/calculator.asp?usertype=prof (NCEP, JAMA 2001; 285:2497)

MEN

Age	Points	Age	Points
20–34	-9	55–59	8
35–39	-4	60–64	10
40–44	0	65–69	11
45–49	3	70–74	12
50–54	6	75–79	13

Choles-terol*	Age (years)				
	20–39	40–49	50–59	60–69	70–79
<160	0	0	0	0	0
160–199	4	3	2	1	0
200–239	7	5	3	1	0
240–279	9	6	4	2	1
280+	11	8	5	3	1

*Total in mg/dL

Age (years)	20–39	40–49	50–59	60–69	70–79
Nonsmoker	0	0	0	0	0
Smoker	8	5	3	1	1

HDLmg/dL	Points	HDLmg/dL	Points
60+	-1	40–49	1
50–59	0	<40	2

Systolic BP	If Untreated	If Treated
<120mmHg	0	0
120–129 mmHg	0	1
130–139 mmHg	1	2
140–159 mmHg	1	2
160+ mmHg	2	3

Point Total	10–Year Risk	Point Total	10–Year Risk
0	1%	9	5%
1	1%	10	6%
2	1%	11	8%
3	1%	12	10%
4	1%	13	12%
5	2%	14	16%
6	2%	15	20%
7	3%	16	25%
8	4%	17+	30+%

WOMEN

Age	Points	Age	Points
20–34	-7	55–59	8
35–39	-3	60–64	10
40–44	0	65–69	12
45–49	3	70–74	14
50–54	6	75–79	16

Choles-terol*	Age (years)				
	20–39	40–49	50–59	60–69	70–79
<160	0	0	0	0	0
160–199	4	3	2	1	1
200–239	8	6	4	2	1
240–279	11	8	5	3	2
280+	13	10	7	4	2

Age (years)	20–39	40–49	50–59	60–69	70–79
Nonsmoker	0	0	0	0	0
Smoker	9	7	4	2	1

HDLmg/dL	Points	HDLmg/dL	Points
60+	-1	40–49	1
50–59	0	<40	2

Systolic BP	If Untreated	If Treated
<120 mmHg	0	0
120–129 mmHg	1	3
130–139 mmHg	2	4
140–159 mmHg	3	5
160+ mmHg	4	6

Point Total	10–Year Risk	Point Total	10–Year Risk
<9	<1%	17	5%
9	1%	18	6%
10	1%	19	8%
11	1%	20	11%
12	1%	21	14%
13	2%	22	17%
14	2%	23	22%
15	3%	24	27%
16	4%	25+	30+%

DRUG THERAPY REFERENCE WEBSITES (selected)

Professional societies or governmental agencies with drug therapy guidelines		
AAP	American Academy of Pediatrics	www.aap.org
ACC	American College of Cardiology	www.acc.org
ACCP	American College of Chest Physicians	www.chestnet.org
ACCP	American College of Clinical Pharmacy	www.accp.com
ADA	American Diabetes Association	www.diabetes.org
AHA	American Heart Association	www.heart.org
AHRQ	Agency for Healthcare Research and Quality	www.ahcpr.gov
AIDSinfo	HIV Treatment, Prevention, and Research	www.aidsinfo.nih.gov
AMA	American Medical Association	www.ama-assn.org
APA	American Psychiatric Association	www.psych.org
APA	American Psychological Association	www.apa.org
ASHP	Amer. Society Health-Systems Pharmacists	
	Drug Shortages Resource Center	www.ashp.org/shortages
ATS	American Thoracic Society	www.thoracic.org
CDC	Centers for Disease Control and Prevention	www.cdc.gov
CDC	CDC bioterrorism and radiation exposures	www.bt.cdc.gov
IDSA	Infectious Diseases Society of America	www.idsociety.org
MHA	Malignant Hyperthermia Association	www.mhaus.org

Other therapy reference sites	
Cochrane library	www.cochrane.org
Emergency Contraception Website	www.not-2-late.com
Immunization Action Coalition	www.immunize.org
QTDrug lists	www.crediblemeds.org/
Managing Contraception	www.managingcontraception.com

ANALGESICS

OPIOID EQUIVALENCY*

Opioid	PO	IV/SC/IM	Opioid	PO	IV/SC/IM
buprenorphine	n/a	0.3–0.4 mg	meperidine	300 mg	75 mg
butorphanol	n/a	2 mg	methadone	5–15 mg	2.5–10 mg
codeine	130 mg	75 mg	morphine	30 mg	10 mg
fentanyl	?	0.1 mg	nalbuphine	n/a	10 mg
hydrocodone	20 mg	n/a	oxycodone	20 mg	n/a
hydromorphone	7.5 mg	1.5 mg	oxymorphone	10 mg	1 mg
levorphanol	4 mg	2 mg	pentazocine	50 mg	30 mg

*Approximate equianalgesic doses as adapted from the 2003 American Pain Society (www.ampainsoc.org) guidelines and the 1992 AHCPR guidelines. Not available = "n/a." See drug entries themselves for starting doses. Many recommend initially using lower than equivalent doses when switching between different opioids. IV doses should be titrated slowly with appropriate monitoring. All PO dosing is with immediate-release preparations. Individualize all dosing, especially in the elderly, children, and in those with chronic pain, opioid naïve, or hepatic/renal insufficiency.

ANALGESICS: Muscle Relaxants

NOTE: May cause drowsiness and/or sedation, which may be enhanced by alcohol and other CNS depressants.

BACLOFEN (*Lioresal, *Lioresal, Lioresal D.S.*) ▶K ♀C ▶+ $
WARNING — Abrupt discontinuation of intrathecal baclofen has been associated with life-threatening sequelae and/or death.
ADULT — Spasticity related to MS or spinal cord disease/injury: 5 mg PO three times per day for 3 days, 10 mg PO three times per day for 3 days, 15 mg PO three times per day for 3 days, then 20 mg PO three times per day for 3 days. Max dose: 20 mg PO four times per day. Spasticity related to spinal cord disease/injury, unresponsive to oral therapy: Specialized dosing via implantable intrathecal pump.
PEDS — Spasticity related to spinal cord disease/injury: Specialized dosing via implantable intrathecal pump.
UNAPPROVED ADULT — Trigeminal neuralgia: 30 to 80 mg/day PO divided three to four times per day. Tardive dyskinesia: 40 to 60 mg/day PO divided three to four times per day. Intractable hiccups: 15 to 45 mg PO divided three times per day.
UNAPPROVED PEDS — Spasticity age 2 yo or order: 10 to 15 mg/day PO divided q 8 h. Max doses 40 mg/day for age 2 to 7 yo, 60 mg/day for age 8 yo or older.
FORMS — Generic only: Tabs 10, 20 mg.
NOTES — Hallucinations and seizures with abrupt withdrawal. Administer with caution if impaired renal function. Efficacy not established for rheumatic disorders, CVA, cerebral palsy, or Parkinson's disease.
MOA — Skeletal muscle relaxant.
ADVERSE EFFECTS — Serious: Hallucinations and seizures with abrupt withdrawal. Frequent: Hypotonia, somnolence, dizziness.

CARISOPRODOL (*Soma*) ▶LK ♀? ▶– ©IV $
ADULT — Acute musculoskeletal pain: 350 mg PO three to four times per day with meals and at bedtime.
PEDS — Not approved in children.
FORMS — Generic/Trade: Tabs 350 mg. Trade only: Tabs 250 mg.
NOTES — Contraindicated in porphyria, caution in renal or hepatic insufficiency. Abuse potential. Use with caution if addiction-prone. Withdrawal and possible seizures with abrupt discontinuation. Sedative effects can result in impaired driving.
MOA — Skeletal muscle relaxant.
ADVERSE EFFECTS — Serious: Idiosyncratic reaction with angioedema, hypotension, and anaphylactoid shock. Frequent: Dizziness and drowsiness.

CHLORZOXAZONE (*Parafon Forte DSC, Lorzone, Remular-S*) ▶LK ♀C ▶? $
WARNING — If signs/symptoms of liver dysfunction are observed, discontinue use.
ADULT — Musculoskeletal pain: Start 500 mg PO three to four times per day, increase prn to 750 mg three to four times per day. After clinical improvement, decrease to 250 mg PO three to four times per day.
PEDS — Not approved in children.
UNAPPROVED PEDS — Musculoskeletal pain: 125 to 500 mg PO three to four times per day or 20 mg/kg/day divided three to four times per day depending on age and wt.
FORMS — Generic/Trade: Tabs 500 mg (Parafon Forte DSC 500 mg tabs, scored). Trade only : Tabs 250 mg (Remular-S), Tabs 375 , 750mg (Lorzone)
NOTES — Use with caution in patients with history of drug allergies. Discontinue if allergic drug reactions occur or for signs/symptoms of liver dysfunction. May turn urine orange or purple-red.
MOA — Skeletal muscle relaxant.
ADVERSE EFFECTS — Serious: Hypersensitivity, hepatotoxicity. Frequent: Dizziness and drowsiness.

CYCLOBENZAPRINE (*Amrix, Flexeril, Fexmid*) ▶LK ♀B ▶? $

ADULT — Musculoskeletal pain: 5 to 10 mg PO three times per day up to max dose of 30 mg/day or 15 to 30 mg (extended release) PO daily. Not recommended in elderly or for use longer than 2 to 3 weeks.

PEDS — Not approved in children.

FORMS — Generic/Trade: Tab 5, 7.5, 10 mg. Extended-release caps 15, 30 mg ($$$$$).

NOTES — Contraindicated with recent or concomitant MAOI use, immediately post MI, in patients with arrhythmias, conduction disturbances, heart failure, and hyperthyroidism. Not effective for cerebral or spinal cord disease or in children with cerebral palsy. May have similar adverse effects and drug interactions as TCAs. Caution with urinary retention, angle-closure glaucoma, increased intraocular pressure.

MOA — Skeletal muscle relaxant.

ADVERSE EFFECTS — Serious: Arrhythmia. Frequent: Drowsiness, dizziness, dry mouth, blurred vision.

DANTROLENE (*Dantrium*) ▶LK ♀C ▶– $$$$

WARNING — Hepatotoxicity, monitor LFTs. Use the lowest possible effective dose.

ADULT — Chronic spasticity related to spinal cord injury, CVA, cerebral palsy, MS: 25 mg PO daily to start, increase to 25 mg two to four times per day, then by 25 mg up to max of 100 mg two to four times per day if necessary. Maintain each dosage level for 4 to 7 days to determine response. Use the lowest possible effective dose. Malignant hyperthermia: 2.5 mg/kg rapid IV push q 5 to 10 min continuing until symptoms subside or to a max 10 mg/kg/dose. Doses of up to 40 mg/kg have been used. Follow with 4 to 8 mg/kg/day PO divided three to four times per day for 1 to 3 days to prevent recurrence.

PEDS — Chronic spasticity: 0.5 mg/kg PO two times per day to start; increase to 0.5 mg/kg three to four times per day, then by increments of 0.5 mg/kg up to 3 mg/kg two to four times per day. Max dose 100 mg PO four times per day. Malignant hyperthermia: Use adult dose.

UNAPPROVED ADULT — Neuroleptic malignant syndrome, heat stroke: 1 to 3 mg/kg/day PO/IV divided four times per day.

FORMS — Generic/Trade: Caps 25, 50, 100 mg.

NOTES — Photosensitization may occur. Warfarin may decrease protein binding of dantrolene and increase dantrolene's effect. Hyperkalemia and cardiovascular collapse have been reported with concomitant calcium channel blockers such as verapamil. The following website may be useful for malignant hyperthermia: www.mhaus.org.

MOA — Skeletal muscle relaxant.

ADVERSE EFFECTS — Serious: Hepatotoxicity. Frequent: Drowsiness, dizziness and weakness.

METAXALONE (*Skelaxin*) ▶LK ♀? ▶? $$$$

ADULT — Musculoskeletal pain: 800 mg PO three to four times per day.

PEDS — Use adult dose for age older than 12 yo.

FORMS — Generic/Trade: Tabs 800 mg, scored.

NOTES — Contraindicated in serious renal or hepatic insufficiency or history of drug-induced hemolytic or other anemia. Beware of hypersensitivity reactions, leukopenia, hemolytic anemia, and jaundice. Monitor LFTs. Coadministration with food, especially a high-fat meal, enhances absorption significantly and may increase CNS depression.

MOA — Skeletal muscle relaxant.

ADVERSE EFFECTS — Serious: Hypersensitivity, jaundice. Frequent: Drowsiness, dizziness, nausea.

METHOCARBAMOL (*Robaxin, Robaxin-750*) ▶LK ♀C ▶? $

ADULT — Musculoskeletal pain, acute relief: 1500 mg PO four times per day or 1000 mg IM/IV three times per day for 48 to 72 h. Maintenance: 1000 mg PO four times per day, 750 mg PO q 4 h, or 1500 mg PO three times per day. Tetanus: Specialized dosing.

PEDS — Tetanus: Specialized dosing.

FORMS — Generic/Trade: Tabs 500 and 750 mg. OTC in Canada.

NOTES — Max IV rate of undiluted drug 3 mL/min to avoid syncope, hypotension, and bradycardia. Total parenteral dosage should not exceed 3 g/day for more than 3 consecutive days, except in the treatment of tetanus. Urine may turn brown, black, or green.

MOA — Skeletal muscle relaxant.

ADVERSE EFFECTS — Serious: Syncope, hypotension. Frequent: Drowsiness, dizziness, discolored urine (brown, black, green).

ORPHENADRINE (*Norflex*) ▶LK ♀C ▶? $$

ADULT — Musculoskeletal pain: 100 mg PO two times per day. 60 mg IV/IM two times per day.

PEDS — Not approved in children.

UNAPPROVED ADULT — Leg cramps: 100 mg PO at bedtime.

FORMS — Generic only: 100 mg extended-release. OTC in Canada.

NOTES — Contraindicated in glaucoma, pyloric or duodenal obstruction, BPH, and myasthenia gravis. Some products contain sulfites, which may cause allergic reactions. May increase anticholinergic effects of amantadine and decrease therapeutic effects of phenothiazines. Side effects include dry mouth, urinary retention and hesitancy, constipation, headache, and GI upset.

MOA — Skeletal muscle relaxant.

ADVERSE EFFECTS — Serious: Hypersensitivity, syncope. Frequent: Dry mouth, dizziness, constipation.

TIZANIDINE (*Zanaflex*) ▶LK ♀C ▶? $$$$

ADULT — Muscle spasticity due to MS or spinal cord injury: 4 to 8 mg PO q 6 to 8 h prn, max dose 36 mg/day.

PEDS — Not approved in children.

FORMS — Generic/Trade: Tabs 4 mg, scored. Caps 2, 4, 6 mg. Generic only: Tabs 2 mg.

NOTES — Monitor LFTs. Avoid in hepatic or renal insufficiency. Alcohol, oral contraceptives, fluvoxamine, and ciprofloxacin increase tizanidine levels; may cause significant decreases in BP and increased drowsiness and psychomotor impairment.

(cont.)

TIZANIDINE (*cont.*)

Concurrent antihypertensives may exacerbate hypotension. Dry mouth, somnolence, sedation, asthenia, and dizziness most common side effects.

MOA — Skeletal muscle relaxant.
ADVERSE EFFECTS — Serious: Hypotension, hepatotoxicity. Frequent: Dry mouth, somnolence, asthenia, and dizziness.

ANALGESICS: Non-Opioid Analgesic Combinations

NOTE: Refer to individual components for further information. Carisoprodol and butalbital may be habit-forming; butalbital contraindicated with porphyria. May cause drowsiness and/or sedation, which may be enhanced by alcohol and other CNS depressants. Avoid exceeding 4 g/day of acetaminophen in combination products. Caution people who drink 3 or more alcoholic drinks/day to limit acetaminophen use to 2.5 g/day due to additive liver toxicity.

ASCRIPTIN (acetylsalicylic acid + aluminum hydroxide + magnesium hydroxide + calcium carbonate) ▶K ♀D ▶? $
WARNING — Multiple strengths; see FORMS.
ADULT — Pain: 1 to 2 tabs PO q 4 h.
PEDS — Not approved in children.
FORMS — OTC Trade only: Tabs 325 mg aspirin/50 mg magnesium hydroxide/50 mg Al hydroxide/50 mg Ca carbonate (Ascriptin and Aspir-Mox). 500 mg aspirin/33 mg magnesium hydroxide/33 mg Al hydroxide/237 mg Ca carbonate (Ascriptin Maximum Strength).
NOTES — See NSAIDs—Salicylic Acid subclass warning.
MOA — Anti-inflammatory, analgesic.
ADVERSE EFFECTS — Serious: Hypersensitivity, Reye's syndrome, GI bleeding, nephrotoxicity. Frequent: Nausea, dyspepsia.

BUFFERIN (acetylsalicylic acid + calcium carbonate + magnesium oxide + magnesium carbonate) ▶K ♀D ▶? $
ADULT — Pain: 1 to 2 tabs/caps PO q 4 h while symptoms persist. Max 12 in 24 h.
PEDS — Not approved in children.
FORMS — OTC Trade only: Tabs/caps 325 mg aspirin/158 mg Ca carbonate/63 mg of magnesium oxide/34 mg of magnesium carbonate. Bufferin ES: 500 mg aspirin/222.3 mg Ca carbonate/88.9 mg of magnesium oxide/55.6 mg of Mg carbonate.
NOTES — See NSAIDs—Salicylic Acid subclass warning.
MOA — Anti-inflammatory, analgesic.
ADVERSE EFFECTS — Serious: Hypersensitivity, Reye's syndrome, GI bleeding, nephrotoxicity. Frequent: Nausea, dyspepsia.

ESGIC (acetaminophen + butalbital + caffeine) ▶LK ♀C ▶? $
WARNING — Multiple strengths; see FORMS and write specific product on Rx.
ADULT — Tension or muscle contraction headache: 1 to 2 tabs or caps PO q 4 h. Max 6 in 24 h.
PEDS — Not approved in children.
FORMS — Generic only: Tabs/caps, 325 mg acetaminophen/50 mg butalbital/40 mg caffeine. Oral soln 325/50/40 mg per 15 mL. Generic/Trade: Tabs, Esgic Plus is 500/50/40 mg.
MOA — Serious: Hepatotoxicity. Frequent: Drowsiness and dizziness.

EXCEDRIN MIGRAINE (acetaminophen + acetylsalicylic acid + caffeine) ▶LK ♀D ▶? $
ADULT — Migraine headache: 2 tabs/caps/geltabs PO q 6 h while symptoms persist. Max 8 in 24 h.

PEDS — Use adult dose for age 12 or older.
FORMS — OTC Generic/Trade: Tabs/caps/geltabs 250 mg acetaminophen/250 mg aspirin/65 mg caffeine.
NOTES — See NSAIDs—Salicylic Acid subclass warning. Avoid concomitant use of other acetaminophen-containing products.
MOA — Combination analgesic.
ADVERSE EFFECTS — Serious: Hepatotoxicity, hypersensitivity, Reye's syndrome, GI bleeding, nephrotoxicity. Frequent: Dyspepsia, nervousness, insomnia.

FIORICET (acetaminophen + butalbital + caffeine) ▶LK ♀C ▶? $
ADULT — Tension or muscle contraction headache: 1 to 2 tabs PO q 4 h. Max 6 in 24 h.
PEDS — Not approved in children.
FORMS — Generic/Trade: Tabs 325 mg acetaminophen/50 mg butalbital/40 mg caffeine.
MOA — Serious: Hepatotoxicity. Frequent: Drowsiness and dizziness.

FIORINAL (acetylsalicylic acid + butalbital + caffeine, ✚*Trianal*) ▶KL ♀D ▶– ©III $$
ADULT — Tension or muscle contraction headache: 1 to 2 tabs PO q 4 h. Max 6 tabs in 24 h.
PEDS — Not approved in children.
FORMS — Generic/Trade: Caps 325 mg aspirin/ 50 mg butalbital/40 mg caffeine.
NOTES — See NSAIDs—Salicylic Acid subclass warning.
MOA — Combination analgesic.
ADVERSE EFFECTS — Serious: Hypersensitivity, Reye's syndrome, GI bleeding, nephrotoxicity. Frequent: Drowsiness and dizziness.

GOODY'S EXTRA STRENGTH HEADACHE POWDER (acetaminophen + acetylsalicylic acid + caffeine) ▶LK ♀D ▶? $
ADULT — Headache: Place 1 powder on tongue and follow with liquid, or stir powder into a glass of water or other liquid. Repeat in 4 to 6 h prn. Max 4 powders in 24 h.
PEDS — Use adult dose for age 12 yo or older.
FORMS — OTC trade only: 260 mg acetaminophen/520 mg aspirin/32.5 mg caffeine per powder paper.
NOTES — See NSAIDs—Salicylic Acid subclass warning.
MOA — Combination analgesic.
ADVERSE EFFECTS — Serious: Hepatotoxicity, hypersensitivity, Reye's syndrome, GI bleeding, nephrotoxicity. Frequent: Dyspepsia.

NORGESIC (orphenadrine + acetylsalicylic acid + caffeine) ▶KL ♀D ▶? $$$
WARNING — Multiple strengths; see FORMS and write specific product on Rx.
ADULT — Musculoskeletal pain: Norgesic: 1 to 2 tabs PO three to four times per day. Norgesic Forte: 1 tab PO three to four times per day.
PEDS — Not approved in children.
FORMS — Generic only: Tabs 25 mg orphenadrine/385 mg aspirin/30 mg caffeine (Norgesic). Tabs 50/770/60 mg (Norgesic Forte).
NOTES — See NSAIDs—Salicylic Acid subclass warning.
MOA — Combination analgesic/muscle relaxant.
ADVERSE EFFECTS — Serious: Hypersensitivity, Reye's syndrome, GI bleeding, nephrotoxicity, syncope. Frequent: Dry mouth, dizziness, constipation.

PHRENILIN (acetaminophen + butalbital) ▶LK ♀C ▶? $
WARNING — Multiple strengths; see FORMS and write specific product on Rx.
ADULT — Tension or muscle contraction headache: Phrenilin: 1 to 2 tabs PO q 4 h. Phrenilin Forte: 1 cap PO q 4 h. Max 6 in 24 h.
PEDS — Not approved in children.
FORMS — Generic/Trade: Tabs, 325 mg acetaminophen/50 mg butalbital (Phrenilin). Caps, 650/50 mg (Phrenilin Forte).
MOA — Serious: Hepatotoxicity. Frequent: Drowsiness and dizziness.

SEDAPAP (acetaminophen + butalbital) ▶LK ♀C ▶? $
ADULT — Tension or muscle contraction headache: 1 to 2 tabs PO q 4 h. Max 6 tabs in 24 h.
PEDS — Not approved in children.
FORMS — Generic only: Tabs 650 mg acetaminophen/50 mg butalbital.
MOA — Serious: Hepatotoxicity. Frequent: Drowsiness and dizziness.

SOMA COMPOUND (carisoprodol + acetylsalicylic acid) ▶LK ♀D ▶– ©IV $$$
ADULT — Musculoskeletal pain: 1 to 2 tabs PO four times per day.
PEDS — Not approved in children.
FORMS — Generic only: Tabs 200 mg carisoprodol/325 mg aspirin.
NOTES — See NSAIDs—Salicylic Acid subclass warning. Carisoprodol may be habit-forming. Withdrawal with abrupt discontinuation.
MOA — Combination analgesic/muscle relaxant.
ADVERSE EFFECTS — Serious: Hypersensitivity, Reye's syndrome, GI bleeding, nephrotoxicity. Idiosyncratic reaction with angioedema, hypotension and anaphylactoid shock. Frequent: Dizziness and drowsiness.

ULTRACET (tramadol + acetaminophen, ✱*Tramacet*) ▶KL ♀C ▶– ©IV $$
ADULT — Acute pain: 2 tabs PO q 4 to 6 h prn, (up to 8 tabs/day for no more than 5 days). If CrCl is less than 30 mL/min, increase the dosing interval to 12 h. Consider a similar adjustment in elderly patients and in cirrhosis.
PEDS — Not approved in children.
FORMS — Generic/Trade: Tabs 37.5 mg tramadol/325 mg acetaminophen.
NOTES — Do not use with other acetaminophen-containing drugs due to potential for hepatotoxicity. Contraindicated in acute intoxication with alcohol, hypnotics, centrally acting analgesics, opioids, or psychotropic drugs. Seizures may occur with concurrent antidepressants or with seizure disorder. Use with great caution with MAOIs or in combination with SSRIs due to potential for serotonin syndrome; dose adjustment may be needed. Withdrawal symptoms may occur in patients dependent on opioids or with abrupt discontinuation. Overdose treated with naloxone may increase seizure risk. The most frequent side effects are somnolence and constipation.
MOA — Combination analgesic.
ADVERSE EFFECTS — Serious: Seizures, anaphylactoid reactions, hepatotoxicity. Frequent: Constipation, somnolence.

ANALGESICS: Non-Steroidal Anti-Inflammatories—COX-2 Inhibitors

NOTE: The risk of serious cardiovascular events and GI bleeding may be increased in patients taking long-term, high-dose NSAIDs, COX-2 inhibitors, and non-selective agents. All NSAIDs and COX-2 inhibitors are contraindicated immediately post-CABG surgery. The FDA advises evaluating alternative therapy or using the lowest effective dose of these drugs. Fewer GI side effects than 1st-generation NSAIDs and no effect on platelets, but other NSAID-related side effects (renal dysfunction, fluid retention, CNS) are possible. May cause fluid retention or exacerbate heart failure. May elevate BP or blunt effects of antihypertensives and loop diuretics. Not substitutes for aspirin for cardiovascular prophylaxis due to lack of antiplatelet effects. Monitor INR with warfarin. May increase lithium levels. Caution in aspirin-sensitive asthma. Use around the time of conception appears to increase the risk of miscarriage (use acetaminophen instead).

CELECOXIB (*Celebrex*) ▶L ♀C (D in 3rd trimester) ▶? $$$$$
WARNING — Increases the risk of serious cardiovascular events and GI bleeding. Contraindicated immediately post-CABG surgery.
ADULT — OA, ankylosing spondylitis: 200 mg PO daily or 100 mg PO two times per day. RA: 100 to 200 mg PO two times per day. Familial adenomatous polyposis (FAP), as an adjunct to usual care: 400 mg PO two times per day with food. Acute pain, dysmenorrhea: 400 mg once, then 200 mg PO two times per day. May take an additional 200 mg on day 1.
PEDS — JRA: Give 50 mg PO two times per day for age 2 to 17 yo and wt 10 to 25 kg, give 100 mg PO two times per day for wt greater than 25 kg.

(cont.)

CELECOXIB (*cont.*)
FORMS — Trade only: Caps 50, 100, 200, 400 mg.
NOTES — Contraindicated in sulfonamide allergy. Decrease dose by 50% in hepatic dysfunction. Caps may be opened and sprinkled into 1 teaspoon of apple sauce and taken immediately with water.

Drugs that inhibit CYP2C9, such as fluconazole, increase concentrations. Lithium concentrations increased.
MOA — Anti-inflammatory, analgesic.
ADVERSE EFFECTS — Serious: Nephrotoxicity, hepatotoxicity, SJS. Frequent: Fluid retention.

ANALGESICS: Non-Steroidal Anti-Inflammatories—Salicylic Acid Derivatives

NOTE: The risk of serious cardiovascular events and GI bleeding may be increased in patients taking long-term, high-dose NSAIDs, both COX-2 inhibitors as well as non-selective agents (excluding aspirin). All NSAIDs and COX-2 inhibitors are contraindicated immediately post CABG surgery. The FDA advises evaluating alternative therapy or using the lowest effective dose of these drugs. Avoid in aspirin allergy and in children younger than 17 yo with chickenpox or flu due to association with Reye’s syndrome. May potentiate warfarin, heparin, valproic acid, methotrexate. Unlike aspirin, derivatives may have less GI toxicity and negligible effects on platelet aggregation and renal prostaglandins. Caution in aspirin-sensitive asthma. Ibuprofen and possibly other NSAIDs may antagonize antiplatelet effects of aspirin if given simultaneously. Use around the time of conception appears to increase the risk of miscarriage (use acetaminophen instead).

ACETYLSALICYLIC ACID (*Ecotrin, Empirin, Halfprin, Bayer, Anacin, Zorprin, Aspirin, ✷Asaphen, Entrophen, Novasen*) ▶K ♀D ▶? $
ADULT — Mild to moderate pain, fever: 325 to 650 mg PO/PR q 4 h prn. Acute rheumatic fever: 5 to 8 g/day, initially. RA/OA: 3.2 to 6 g/day in divided doses. Platelet aggregation inhibition: 81 to 325 mg PO daily.
PEDS — Mild to moderate pain, fever: 10 to 15 mg/kg/dose PO q 4 to 6 h not to exceed 60 to 80 mg/kg/day. JRA: 60 to 100 mg/kg/day PO divided q 6 to 8 h. Acute rheumatic fever: 100 mg/kg/day PO/PR for 2 weeks, then 75 mg/kg/day for 4 to 6 weeks. Kawasaki disease: 80 to 100 mg/kg/day divided four times per day PO/PR until fever resolves, then 3 to 5 mg/kg/day PO q am for 7 weeks or longer if there is ECG evidence of coronary artery abnormalities.
UNAPPROVED ADULT — Primary prevention of cardiovascular events (10-year CHD risk more than 6 to 10% based on Framingham risk scoring): 75 to 325 mg PO daily. Post ST-elevation MI: 162 to 325 mg PO on day 1, continue indefinitely at 75 to 162 mg/day. Post non-ST-elevation MI: 162 to 325 mg PO on day 1, continue indefinitely at 75 to 162 mg/day. Long-term antithrombotic therapy for chronic atrial fib/flutter in patients with low to moderate risk of CVA (age younger than 75 yo without risk factors): 325 mg PO daily. Percutaneous coronary intervention pretreatment: Already taking daily aspirin therapy: 75 to 325 mg PO before procedure. Not already taking daily aspirin therapy: 300 to 325 mg PO at least 2 to 24 h before procedure. Post-percutaneous coronary intervention: 325 mg daily in combination with clopidogrel for at least 1 month after bare metal stent placement, at least 3 to 6 months after drug-eluting stent placement; then 75 to 162 mg PO daily indefinitely. Post-percutaneous coronary brachytherapy: 75 to 325 mg daily in combination with clopidogrel indefinitely.
FORMS — Generic/Trade (OTC): Tabs, 325, 500 mg; chewable 81 mg; enteric-coated 81, 162 mg

(Halfprin), 81, 325, 500 mg (Ecotrin), 650, 975 mg. Trade only: Tabs, controlled-release 650, 800 mg (ZORprin, Rx). Generic only (OTC): Supps 60, 120, 200, 300, 600 mg.
NOTES — Consider discontinuation 1 week prior to surgery (except coronary bypass or in 1st year post-coronary stent implantation) because of the possibility of postop bleeding. Aspirin intolerance occurs in 4% to 19% of asthmatics. Use caution in liver damage, renal insufficiency, peptic ulcer, or bleeding tendencies. Crush or chew tabs (including enteric-coated products) in 1st dose with acute MI. Higher doses of aspirin (1.3 g/day) have not been shown to be superior to low doses in preventing TIAs and CVAs.
MOA — Anti-inflammatory, antipyretic, analgesic. Inhibits prostaglandin synthesis and platelet aggregation by inactivating the enzyme cyclooxygenase.
ADVERSE EFFECTS — Serious: Hypersensitivity, Reye's syndrome, GI bleeding, nephrotoxicity. Frequent: Nausea, dyspepsia, tinnitus (large doses), dizziness (large doses).
CHOLINE MAGNESIUM TRISALICYLATE (*Trilisate*) ▶K ♀C (D in 3rd trimester) ▶? $$
ADULT — RA/OA: 1500 mg PO two times per day. Mild to moderate pain, fever: 1000 to 1500 mg PO two times per day.
PEDS — RA, mild to moderate pain: 50 mg/kg/day (up to 37 kg) PO divided two times per day.
FORMS — Generic only: Tabs 500, 750, 1000 mg. Soln 500 mg/5 mL.
MOA — Serious: Hypersensitivity, Reye's syndrome, GI bleeding, nephrotoxicity. Frequent: Nausea, dyspepsia.
DIFLUNISAL (*Dolobid*) ▶K ♀C (D in 3rd trimester) ▶– $$$
ADULT — Mild to moderate pain: Initially: 500 mg to 1 g PO, then 250 to 500 mg PO q 8 to 12 h. RA/OA: 500 mg to 1 g PO divided two times per day. Max dose 1.5 g/day.

(cont.)

DIFLUNISAL (cont.)
PEDS — Not approved in children.
FORMS — Generic only: Tabs 500 mg.
NOTES — Do not crush or chew tabs. Increases acetaminophen levels.
MOA — Anti-inflammatory, analgesic.
ADVERSE EFFECTS — Serious: Hypersensitivity, Reye's syndrome, GI bleeding, nephrotoxicity. Frequent: Nausea, dyspepsia.

SALSALATE (Salflex, Disalcid, Amigesic) ▶K ♀C (D in 3rd trimester) ▶? $$
ADULT — RA/OA: 3000 mg/day PO divided q 8 to 12 h.
PEDS — Not approved in children.
FORMS — Generic only: Tabs 500, 750 mg, scored.
MOA — Serious: Hypersensitivity, Reye's syndrome, GI bleeding, nephrotoxicity. Frequent: Nausea, dyspepsia.

ANALGESICS—NSAIDS

Salicylic acid derivatives	ASA, diflunisal, salsalate, Trilisate
Propionic acids	flurbiprofen, ibuprofen, ketoprofen, naproxen, oxaprozin
Acetic acids	diclofenac, etodolac, indomethacin, ketorolac, nabumetone, sulindac, tolmetin
Fenamates	meclofenamate
Oxicams	meloxicam, piroxicam
COX-2 inhibitors	celecoxib

Note: If one class fails, consider another.

ANALGESICS: Non-Steroidal Anti-Inflammatories—Other

NOTE: The risk of serious cardiovascular events and GI bleeding may be increased in patients taking long-term, high-dose NSAIDs, both COX-2 inhibitors as well as non-selective agents. All NSAIDs and COX-2 inhibitors are contraindicated immediately post-CABG surgery. The FDA advises evaluating alternative therapy or using the lowest effective dose of these drugs. Chronic use associated with renal insufficiency, gastritis, peptic ulcer disease, GI bleeds. Caution in liver disease. May cause fluid retention or exacerbate heart failure. May elevate BP or blunt effects of antihypertensives and loop diuretics. May increase levels of methotrexate, lithium, phenytoin, digoxin, and cyclosporine. May potentiate warfarin. Caution in aspirin-sensitive asthma. Ibuprofen or other NSAIDs may antagonize antiplatelet effects of aspirin if given simultaneously. Use around the time of conception appears to increase the risk of miscarriage (use acetaminophen instead).

ARTHROTEC (diclofenac + misoprostol) ▶LK ♀X ▶– $$$$$
WARNING — Because of the abortifacient property of the misoprostol component, it is contraindicated in women who are pregnant. Caution in women with childbearing potential; effective contraception is essential.
ADULT — OA: One 50/200 PO three times per day. RA: One 50/200 PO three to four times per day. If intolerant, may use 50/200 or 75/200 PO two times per day.
PEDS — Not approved in children.
FORMS — Generic/Trade: Tabs 50 mg/200 mcg, 75 mg/200 mcg, diclofenac/misoprostol.
NOTES — Refer to individual components. Abdominal pain and diarrhea may occur. Check LFTs at baseline, within 4 to 8 weeks of initiation, then periodically. Do not crush or chew tabs.
MOA — Anti-inflammatory/mucosal protectant, analgesic.
ADVERSE EFFECTS — Serious: Fetal death, nephrotoxicity, gastritis, peptic ulcer disease, GI bleeds. Frequent: Diarrhea, abdominal pain, nausea, dyspepsia.

DICLOFENAC (Voltaren, Voltaren XR, Cataflam, Flector, Zipsor, Cambia, Zorvolex, ✤Voltaren Rapide) ▶L ♀B (D in 3rd trimester) ▶– $$$
WARNING — Multiple strengths; see FORMS and write specific product on Rx.
ADULT — OA: Immediate- or delayed-release: 50 mg PO two to three times per day or 75 mg two times per day. Extended-release 100 mg PO daily. Gel: Apply 4 g to knees or 2 g to hands four times per day using enclosed dosing card. RA: Immediate- or delayed-release 50 mg PO three to four times per day or 75 mg two times per day. Extended-release 100 mg PO one to two times per day. Ankylosing spondylitis: Immediate- or delayed-release 25 mg PO four times per day and at bedtime. Analgesia and primary dysmenorrhea: Immediate- or delayed-release 50 mg PO three times per day. Acute pain of strains, sprains, or contusions: Apply 1 patch to painful area two times per day. Acute migraine with or without aura: 50 mg single dose (Cambia), mix packet with 30 to 60 mL water.
PEDS — Not approved in children.

ANALGESICS: Non-Steroidal Anti-Inflammatories 7

DICLOFENAC (*cont.*)

UNAPPROVED PEDS — JRA: 2 to 3 mg/kg/day PO.

FORMS — Generic/Trade: Tabs, immediate-release (Cataflam) 50 mg, extended-release (Voltaren XR) 100 mg. Generic only: Tabs, delayed-release 25, 50, 75 mg. Trade only: Patch (Flector) 1.3% diclofenac epolamine. Topical gel (Voltaren) 1% 100 g tube. Trade only: Caps, liquid-filled (Zipsor) 25 mg. Caps, (Zorvolex) 18, 35 mg. Trade only: Powder for oral soln (Cambia) 50 mg.

NOTES — Check LFTs at baseline, within 4 to 8 weeks of initiation, then periodically. Do not apply patch to damaged or nonintact skin. Wash hands and avoid eye contact when handling the patch. Do not wear patch while bathing or showering.

MOA — Anti-inflammatory, analgesic.

ADVERSE EFFECTS — Serious: Hypersensitivity, GI bleeding, hepato/nephrotoxicity. Frequent: Nausea, dyspepsia, pruritus and dermatitis with patch and gel.

ETODOLAC ▶L ♀C (D in 3rd trimester) ▶– $

WARNING — Multiple strengths; write specific product on Rx.

ADULT — OA: 400 mg PO two to three times per day. 300 mg PO two to three times per day. 200 mg PO three to four times per day. Extended release 400 to 1200 mg PO daily. Mild to moderate pain: 200 to 400 mg q 6 to 8 h. (Up to 1200 mg/day or if wt 60 kg or less, 20 mg/kg/day).

PEDS — Not approved in children.

UNAPPROVED ADULT — RA, ankylosing spondylitis: 300 to 400 mg PO two times per day. Tendinitis, bursitis, and acute gout: 300 to 400 mg PO two to four times per day, then taper.

FORMS — Generic only: Caps, immediate-release: 200, 300 mg. Tabs, immediate-release: 400, 500 mg. Tabs, extended-release: 400, 500, 600 mg.

NOTES — Brand name Lodine no longer marketed.

MOA — Anti-inflammatory, analgesic.

ADVERSE EFFECTS — Serious: Hypersensitivity, GI bleeding, nephrotoxicity, toxic epidermal necrolysis. Frequent: Nausea, dyspepsia.

FENOPROFEN (*Nalfon*) ▶L ♀C (D in 3rd trimester) ▶– $$$

WARNING — Appears to represent a greater nephrotoxicity risk than other NSAIDs.

ADULT — RA/OA: 300 to 600 mg PO three to four times per day. Max dose: 3200 mg/day. Mild to moderate pain: 200 mg PO q 4 to 6 h prn.

PEDS — Not approved in children.

FORMS — Generic Only: Tab 600 mg. Trade Only: Caps 200 and 400 mg.

MOA — Anti-inflammatory, analgesic.

ADVERSE EFFECTS — Serious: Hypersensitivity, GI bleeding, nephrotoxicity. Frequent: Nausea, dyspepsia.

FLURBIPROFEN (*Ansaid*) ▶L ♀B (D in 3rd trimester) ▶+ $$$

ADULT — RA/OA: 200 to 300 mg/day PO divided two to four times per day. Max single dose 100 mg.

PEDS — Not approved in children.

UNAPPROVED ADULT — Ankylosing spondylitis: 150 to 300 mg/day PO divided two to four times per day. Mild to moderate pain: 50 mg PO q 6 h. Primary dysmenorrhea: 50 mg PO daily at onset, discontinue when pain subsides. Tendinitis, bursitis, acute gout, acute migraine: 100 mg PO at onset, then 50 mg PO four times per day, then taper.

UNAPPROVED PEDS — JRA: 4 mg/kg/day PO.

FORMS — Generic/Trade: Tabs, immediate-release 50, 100 mg.

MOA — Serious: Hypersensitivity, GI bleeding, nephrotoxicity. Frequent: Nausea, dyspepsia.

IBUPROFEN (*Motrin, Advil, Nuprin, Rufen, NeoProfen, Caldolor*) ▶L ♀B (D in 3rd trimester) ▶+ $

ADULT — RA/OA, gout: 200 to 800 mg PO three to four times per day. Mild to moderate pain: 400 mg PO q 4 to 6 h. 400 to 800 mg IV (Caldolor) q 6 h prn. 400 mg IV (Caldolor) q 4 to 6 h or 100 to 200 mg q 4 h prn. Primary dysmenorrhea: 400 mg PO q 4 h prn. Fever: 200 mg PO q 4 to 6 h prn. Migraine pain: 200 to 400 mg PO not to exceed 400 mg in 24 h unless directed by a physician (OTC dosing). Max dose 3.2 g/day.

PEDS — JRA: 30 to 50 mg/kg/day PO divided q 6 h. Max dose 2400 mg/24 h. 20 mg/kg/day may be adequate for milder disease. Analgesic/antipyretic age older than 6 mo: 5 to 10 mg/kg PO q 6 to 8 h, prn. Max dose 40 mg/kg/day. Patent ductus arteriosus in neonates age 32 weeks gestational age or younger weighing 500 to 1500 g (NeoProfen): Specialized dosing.

FORMS — OTC: Caps/Liqui-Gel Caps 200 mg. Tabs 100, 200 mg. Chewable tabs 100 mg. Susp (infant gtts) 50 mg/1.25 mL (with calibrated dropper), 100 mg/5 mL. Rx Generic/Trade: Tabs 400, 600, 800 mg.

NOTES — May antagonize antiplatelet effects of aspirin if given simultaneously. Take aspirin 2 h prior to ibuprofen. Administer IV (Caldolor) over at least 30 min; hydration important.

MOA — Anti-inflammatory/antipyretic, analgesic.

ADVERSE EFFECTS — Serious: Hypersensitivity, GI bleeding, nephrotoxicity. Frequent: Nausea, dyspepsia.

INDOMETHACIN (*Indocin, Indocin SR, Indocin IV*) ▶L ♀B (D in 3rd trimester) ▶+ $

WARNING — Multiple strengths; see FORMS and write specific product on Rx. Use during labor increases risk of fetal and maternal complications: Premature closure of the ductus arteriosus, fetal pulmonary HTN, oligohydramnios, higher rate of postpartum hemorrhage.

ADULT — RA/OA, ankylosing spondylitis: 25 mg PO two to three times per day to start. Increase incrementally to a total daily dose of 150 to 200 mg. Bursitis/tendinitis: 75 to 150 mg/day PO divided three to four times per day. Acute gout: 50 mg PO three times per day until pain tolerable, rapidly taper dose to discontinue. Sustained-release: 75 mg PO one to two times per day.

PEDS — Closure of patent ductus arteriosus in neonates: Initial dose 0.2 mg/kg IV, if additional doses

(cont.)

INDOMETHACIN (*cont.*)

necessary, dose and frequency (q 12 h or q 24 h) based on neonate's age and urine output.

UNAPPROVED ADULT — Primary dysmenorrhea: 25 mg PO three to four times per day. Cluster headache: 75 to 150 mg SR PO daily. Polyhydramnios: 2.2 to 3 mg/kg/day PO based on maternal wt; premature closure of the ductus arteriosus has been reported. Preterm labor: Initial 50 to 100 mg PO followed by 25 mg PO q 6 to 12 h up to 48 h.

UNAPPROVED PEDS — JRA: 1 to 3 mg/kg/day three to four times per day to start. Increase prn to max dose of 4 mg/kg/day or 200 mg/day, whichever is less.

FORMS — Generic only: Caps, immediate-release 25, 50 mg. Caps, sustained-release 75 mg. Trade only: Suppository 50 mg. Oral susp 25 mg/5 mL (237 mL)

NOTES — May aggravate depression or other psychiatric disturbances. Do not crush sustained-release cap.

MOA — Anti-inflammatory, analgesic. Prostaglandin inhibition leads to closure of a patent ductus arteriosus. Tocolytic.

ADVERSE EFFECTS — Serious: Hypersensitivity, GI bleeding, nephrotoxicity. During labor: Premature closure of the ductus arteriosus and fetal pulmonary hypertension, oligohydramnios, postpartum hemorrhage. Frequent: Nausea, dyspepsia, dizziness, drowsiness.

KETOPROFEN (*Orudis, Orudis KT, Actron, Oruvail*) ▶L ♀B (D in 3rd trimester) ▶– $$$

ADULT — RA/OA: 75 mg PO three times per day or 50 mg PO four times per day. Extended-release 200 mg PO daily. Mild to moderate pain, primary dysmenorrhea: 25 to 50 mg PO q 6 to 8 h prn.

PEDS — Not approved in children.

UNAPPROVED PEDS — JRA: 100 to 200 mg/m²/day PO. Max dose 320 mg/day.

FORMS — Rx Generic only: Caps, extended-release 200 mg. Caps, immediate-release 50, 75 mg.

MOA — Serious: Hypersensitivity, GI bleeding, nephrotoxicity. Frequent: Nausea, dyspepsia.

KETOROLAC (*Toradol*) ▶L ♀C (D in 3rd trimester) ▶+ $

WARNING — Indicated for short-term (up to 5 days) therapy only. Ketorolac is a potent NSAID and can cause serious GI and renal adverse effects. It may also increase the risk of bleeding by inhibiting platelet function. Contraindicated in patients with active peptic ulcer disease, recent GI bleeding or perforation, a history of peptic ulcer disease or GI bleeding, or advanced renal impairment.

ADULT — Moderately severe, acute pain, single-dose treatment: 30 to 60 mg IM or 15 to 30 mg IV. Multiple-dose treatment: 15 to 30 mg IV/IM q 6 h. IV/IM doses are not to exceed 60 mg/day for age 65 yo or older, wt less than 50 kg, and patients with moderately elevated serum creatinine. Oral continuation therapy: 10 mg PO q 4 to 6 h prn, max dose 40 mg/day. Combined duration IV/IM and PO is not to exceed 5 days.

PEDS — Not approved in children.

UNAPPROVED PEDS — Pain: 0.5 mg/kg/dose IM/IV q 6 h (up to 30 mg q 6 h or 120 mg/day), give 10 mg PO q 6 h prn (up to 40 mg/day) for wt greater than 50 kg.

FORMS — Generic only: Tabs 10 mg.

MOA — Serious: Hypersensitivity, GI bleeding, nephrotoxicity. Frequent: Nausea, dyspepsia.

MECLOFENAMATE ▶L ♀B (D in 3rd trimester) ▶– $$$

ADULT — Mild to moderate pain: 50 mg PO q 4 to 6 h prn. Max dose 400 mg/day. Menorrhagia and primary dysmenorrhea: 100 mg PO three times per day for up to 6 days. RA/OA: 200 to 400 mg/day PO divided three to four times per day.

PEDS — Not approved in children.

UNAPPROVED PEDS — JRA: 3 to 7.5 mg/kg/day PO. Max dose 300 mg/day.

FORMS — Generic only: Caps 50, 100 mg.

NOTES — Reversible autoimmune hemolytic anemia with use for longer than 12 months.

MOA — Anti-inflammatory, analgesic.

ADVERSE EFFECTS — Serious: Hypersensitivity, GI bleeding, nephrotoxicity, autoimmune hemolytic anemia. Frequent: Nausea, dyspepsia.

MEFENAMIC ACID (*Ponstel, ✴Ponstan*) ▶L ♀D ▶– $$$$$

ADULT — Mild to moderate pain, primary dysmenorrhea: 500 mg PO initially, then 250 mg PO q 6 h prn for up to 1 week.

PEDS — Use adult dose for age older than 14 yo.

FORMS — Generic/Trade: Caps 250 mg.

MOA — Serious: Hypersensitivity, GI bleeding, nephrotoxicity, autoimmune hemolytic anemia. Frequent: Nausea, dyspepsia.

MELOXICAM (*Mobic, ✴Mobicox*) ▶L ♀C (D in 3rd trimester) ▶? $

ADULT — RA/OA: 7.5 mg PO daily. Max dose 15 mg/day.

PEDS — JRA: age 2 yo or older: 0.125 mg/kg PO daily to max of 7.5 mg.

FORMS — Generic/Trade: Tabs 7.5, 15 mg. Susp 7.5 mg/5 mL (1.5 mg/mL).

NOTES — Shake susp gently before using. This is not a selective COX-2 inhibitor.

MOA — Anti-inflammatory, analgesic.

ADVERSE EFFECTS — Serious: Hypersensitivity, GI bleeding, nephrotoxicity. Frequent: Nausea, dyspepsia.

NABUMETONE (*Relafen*) ▶L ♀C (D in 3rd trimester) ▶– $$

ADULT — RA/OA: Initial: Two 500 mg tabs (1000 mg) PO daily. May increase to 1500 to 2000 mg PO daily or divided two times per day. Dosages more than 2000 mg/day have not been studied.

PEDS — Not approved in children.

FORMS — Generic only: Tabs 500, 750 mg.

MOA — Serious: Hypersensitivity, GI bleeding, nephrotoxicity, hepatotoxicity, Stevens-Johnson syndrome, erythema multiforme, toxic epidermal necrolysis, eosinophilic pneumonia. Frequent: Nausea, dyspepsia.

NAPROXEN (*Naprosyn, Aleve, Anaprox, EC-Naprosyn, Naprelan, Prevacid NapraPac*) ▶L ♀B (D in 3rd trimester) ▶+ $$$

WARNING — Multiple strengths; see FORMS and write specific product on Rx.

NAPROXEN (*cont.*)

ADULT — RA/OA, ankylosing spondylitis, pain, dysmenorrhea, acute tendinitis and bursitis, fever: 250 to 500 mg PO two times per day. Delayed-release: 375 to 500 mg PO two times per day (do not crush or chew). Controlled-release: 750 to 1000 mg PO daily. Acute gout: 750 mg PO once, then 250 mg PO q 8 h until the attack subsides. Controlled-release: 1000 to 1500 mg PO once, then 1000 mg PO daily until the attack subsides.

PEDS — JRA: 10 to 20 mg/kg/day PO divided two times per day (up to 1250 mg/24 h). Pain for age older than 2 yo: 5 to 7 mg/kg/dose PO q 8 to 12 h.

UNAPPROVED ADULT — Acute migraine: 750 mg PO once, then 250 to 500 mg PO prn. Migraine prophylaxis, menstrual migraine: 500 mg PO two times per day beginning 1 day prior to onset of menses and ending on last day of period.

FORMS — OTC Generic/Trade (Aleve): Tabs, immediate-release 200 mg. OTC Trade only (Aleve): Caps, Gelcaps, immediate-release 200 mg. Rx Generic/Trade: Tabs, immediate-release (Naprosyn) 250, 375, 500 mg. (Anaprox) 275, 550 mg. Tabs, delayed-release enteric coated (EC-Naprosyn) 375, 500 mg. Tabs, controlled-release (Naprelan) 375, 500, 750 mg. Susp (Naprosyn) 125 mg/5 mL. Prevacid NapraPAC: 7 lansoprazole 15 mg caps packaged with 14 naproxen tabs 375 mg or 500 mg.

NOTES — All dosing is based on naproxen content; 500 mg naproxen is equivalent to 550 mg naproxen sodium.

MOA — Anti-inflammatory, analgesic.

ADVERSE EFFECTS — Serious: Hypersensitivity, GI bleeding, nephrotoxicity. Frequent: Nausea, dyspepsia.

OXAPROZIN (*Daypro*) ▶L ♀C (D in 3rd trimester) ▶– $$$

ADULT — RA/OA: 1200 mg PO daily. Max dose 1800 mg/day or 26 mg/kg/day, whichever is lower.

PEDS — Not approved in children.

FORMS — Generic/Trade: Tabs 600 mg, trade scored.

MOA — Serious: Hypersensitivity, GI bleeding, nephrotoxicity. Frequent: Nausea, dyspepsia.

PIROXICAM (*Feldene, Fexicam*) ▶L ♀B (D in 3rd trimester) ▶+ $$$

ADULT — RA/OA: 20 mg PO daily or divided two times per day.

PEDS — Not approved in children.

UNAPPROVED ADULT — Primary dysmenorrhea: 20 to 40 mg PO daily for 3 days.

FORMS — Generic/Trade: Caps 10, 20 mg.

MOA — Serious: Hypersensitivity, GI bleeding, nephrotoxicity. Frequent: Nausea, dyspepsia.

SULINDAC (*Clinoril*) ▶L ♀B (D in 3rd trimester) ▶– $

ADULT — RA/OA, ankylosing spondylitis: 150 mg PO two times per day. Bursitis, tendinitis, acute gout: 200 mg PO two times per day, decrease after response. Max dose: 400 mg/day.

PEDS — Not approved in children.

UNAPPROVED PEDS — JRA: 4 mg/kg/day PO divided two times per day.

FORMS — Generic/Trade: Tabs 200 mg. Generic only: Tabs 150 mg.

NOTES — Sulindac-associated pancreatitis and a potentially fatal hypersensitivity syndrome have occurred.

MOA — Anti-inflammatory, analgesic.

ADVERSE EFFECTS — Serious: Hypersensitivity, GI bleeding, nephrotoxicity, pancreatitis. Frequent: Nausea, dyspepsia.

TOLMETIN (*Tolectin*) ▶L ♀C (D in 3rd trimester) ▶+ $$$

ADULT — RA/OA: 400 mg PO three times per day to start. Range 600 to 1800 mg/day PO divided three times per day.

PEDS — JRA age 2 yo or older: 20 mg/kg/day PO divided three to four times per day to start. Range 15 to 30 mg/kg/day divided three to four times per day. Max dose 2 g/24 h.

UNAPPROVED PEDS — Pain age 2 yo or older: 5 to 7 mg/kg/dose PO q 6 to 8 h. Max dose 2 g/24 h.

FORMS — Generic only: Tabs 200 (scored), 600 mg. Caps 400 mg.

NOTES — Rare anaphylaxis.

MOA — Anti-inflammatory, analgesic.

ADVERSE EFFECTS — Serious: Hypersensitivity, GI bleeding, nephrotoxicity. Frequent: Nausea, dyspepsia.

ANALGESICS: Opioid Agonist-Antagonists

NOTE: May cause drowsiness and/or sedation, which may be enhanced by alcohol and other CNS depressants. Opioid agonist-antagonists may result in inadequate pain control and/or withdrawal effects in the opioid-dependent. Reserve IM for when alternative routes are not feasible.

BUPRENORPHINE (*Buprenex, Butrans, Subutex*) ▶L ♀C ▶– ©III $ IV, $$$$$ SL

ADULT — Moderate to severe pain: 0.3 to 0.6 mg IM or slow IV, q 6 h prn. Max single dose 0.6 mg. Treatment of opioid dependence: Induction 8 mg SL on day 1, 16 mg SL on day 2. Maintenance: 16 mg SL daily. Can individualize to range of 4 to 24 mg SL daily. Moderate to severe chronic pain: 5 to 20 mcg/h patch changed q 7 days.

PEDS — Moderate to severe pain: 2 to 12 yo: 2 to 6 mcg/kg/dose IM or slow IV q 4 to 6 h. Max single dose 6 mcg/kg. Patch not approved for use in children.

FORMS — Generic only: SL Tabs 2, 8 mg. Trade only (Butrans): transdermal patches 5, 10, 20 mcg/h.

NOTES — May cause bradycardia, hypotension, and respiratory depression. Concurrent use with diazepam has resulted in respiratory and cardiovascular collapse. For opioid dependence Subutex is preferred over Suboxone for induction. Suboxone preferred for maintenance. Prescribers must complete training and apply for special DEA number. See www.suboxone.com.

MOA — Opioid agonist-antagonist analgesic.

(cont.)

BUPRENORPHINE (*cont.*)

ADVERSE EFFECTS — Serious: Respiratory depression, hepatitis, hypersensitivity. Frequent: Sedation, dizziness, nausea, headache, constipation.

BUTORPHANOL (*Stadol, Stadol NS*) ▶LK ♀C ▶+ ©IV $$$

WARNING — Approved as a nasal spray in 1991 and has been promoted as a safe treatment for migraine headaches. There have been numerous reports of dependence-addiction and major psychological disturbances. These problems have been documented by the FDA. Stadol NS should be used for patients with infrequent but severe migraine attacks for whom all other common abortive treatments have failed. Experts recommend restriction to no more than 2 bottles (30 sprays) per month in patients who are appropriate candidates for this medication.

ADULT — Pain, including postop pain: 0.5 to 2 mg IV q 3 to 4 h prn. 1 to 4 mg IM q 3 to 4 h prn. Obstetric pain during labor: 1 to 2 mg IV/IM at full term in early labor, repeat after 4 h. Last resort for migraine pain: 1 mg nasal spray (1 spray in 1 nostril). If no pain relief in 60 to 90 min, may give a 2nd spray in the other nostril. Additional doses q 3 to 4 h prn.

PEDS — Not approved in children.

FORMS — Generic only: Nasal spray 1 mg/spray, 2.5 mL bottle (14 to 15 doses/bottle).

NOTES — May increase cardiac workload.

MOA — Opioid agonist-antagonist analgesic.

ADVERSE EFFECTS — Serious: Respiratory depression. Frequent: Sedation, dizziness.

NALBUPHINE (*Nubain*) ▶LK ♀? ▶? $

ADULT — Moderate to severe pain including obstetrical analgesia during labor and delivery: 10 to 20 mg SC/IM/IV q 3 to 6 h prn. Max dose 160 mg/day.

PEDS — Not approved in children.

MOA — Serious: Respiratory depression. Frequent: Sedation, dizziness, nausea.

PENTAZOCINE (*Talwin NX*) ▶LK ♀C ▶? ©IV $$$

WARNING — The oral form (Talwin NX) may cause fatal reactions if injected.

ADULT — Moderate to severe pain: Talwin: 30 mg IM/IV q 3 to 4 h prn, max dose 360 mg/day. Talwin NX: 1 tab PO q 3 to 4 h, max 12 tabs/day.

PEDS — Not approved in children.

FORMS — Generic/Trade: Tabs 50 mg with 0.5 mg naloxone, trade scored.

NOTES — Rotate injection sites. Can cause hallucinations, disorientation, and seizures. Concomitant sibutramine may precipitate serotonin syndrome.

MOA — Opioid agonist-antagonist analgesic.

ADVERSE EFFECTS — Serious: Respiratory depression, seizures, hallucinations, hypersensitivity. Frequent: Sedation, dizziness, nausea.

ANALGESICS: Opioid Agonists

FENTANYL TRANSDERMALDOSE (Dosing based on ongoing morphine requirement.)

Morphine* (IV/IM)	Morphine* (PO)	Transdermal fentanyl*
10–22 mg/d	60–134 mg/d	25 mcg/h
23–37 mg/d	135–224 mg/d	50 mcg/h
38–52 mg/d	225–314 mg/d	75 mcg/h
53–67 mg/d	315–404 mg/d	100 mcg/h

*For higher morphine doses, see product insert for transdermal fentanyl equivalencies.

NOTE: May cause life-threatening respiratory depression. May cause drowsiness and/or sedation, which may be enhanced by alcohol and other CNS depressants. Patients with chronic pain may require more frequent and higher dosing. Opioids commonly cause constipation. All opioids are pregnancy class D if used for prolonged periods or in high doses at term.

CODEINE ▶LK ♀C ▶– ©II $

WARNING — Do not use IV in children due to large histamine-release and cardiovascular effects. Use in nursing mothers has led to infant death.

ADULT — Mild to moderate pain: 15 to 60 mg PO/IM/IV/SC q 4 to 6 h. Max dose 360 mg in 24 h. Antitussive: 10 to 20 mg PO q 4 to 6 h prn. Max dose 120 mg in 24 h.

PEDS — Mild to moderate pain in age 1 yo or older: 0.5 to 1 mg/kg PO/SC/IM q 4 to 6 h, max dose 60 mg/dose. Antitussive: Give 2.5 to 5 mg PO q 4 to 6 h prn (up to 30 mg/day) for age 2 to 5 yo, give 5 to 10 mg PO q 4 to 6 h prn (up to 60 mg/day) for age 6 to 12 yo.

FORMS — Generic only: Tabs 15, 30, 60 mg. Oral soln: 30 mg/5 mL.

MOA — Opioid agonist analgesic.

ADVERSE EFFECTS — Serious: Respiratory depression/arrest. Frequent: N/V, constipation, sedation.

FENTANYL (*Duragesic, Actiq, Fentora, Sublimaze, Abstral, Subsys, Lazanda, Onsolis*) ▶L ♀C ▶+ ©II $ - varies by therapy

WARNING — Duragesic patches, Actiq, Fentora, Abstral, Subsys, and Lazanda are contraindicated in the management of acute or postop pain due to potentially life-threatening respiratory depression in opioid non-tolerant patients. Instruct patients and their caregivers that even used patches/lozenges on a stick can be fatal to a child or pet. Dispose via toilet. Actiq and Fentora are not interchangeable. IONSYS: For hospital use only; remove prior to discharge. Can cause life-threatening respiratory depression.

ADULT — Duragesic Patches: Chronic pain: 12 to 100 mcg/h patch q 72 h. Titrate dose to the needs of the patient. Some patients require q 48 h dosing. May wear more than 1 patch to achieve the correct analgesic effect. Actiq: Breakthrough cancer pain: 200 to 1600 mcg sucked over 15 min, if 200 mcg ineffective for 6 units use higher strength. Goal is 4 lozenges on a stick/day in conjunction with long-acting opioid. Buccal tab (Fentora) for breakthrough cancer pain: 100 to 800 mcg, titrated to pain relief; may repeat once after 30 min during single episode of breakthrough pain. See prescribing information for dose conversion from transmucosal lozenges. Buccal soluble film (Onsolis) for breakthrough cancer pain: 200 to 1200 mcg, titrated to pain relief; no more than 4 doses/day separated by at least 2 h. Postop analgesia: 50 to 100 mcg IM; repeat in 1 to 2 h prn. Sublingual tab (Abstral) for breakthrough cancer pain: 100 mcg, may repeat once after 30 minutes. Specialized titration. Sublingual spray (Subsys) for breakthrough cancer pain: 100 mcg, may repeat once after 30 minutes. Specialized titration. Nasal spray (Lazanda) for breakthrough cancer pain: 100 mcg. Specialized titration. IONSYS: Acute postop pain: Specialized dosing.

PEDS — Transdermal (Duragesic): Not approved in children younger than 2 yo or in opioid-naive. Use adult dosing for age older than 2 yo. Children converting to a 25 mcg patch should be receiving 45 mg or more oral morphine equivalents/day. Actiq: Not approved for age younger than 16 yo. IONSYS not approved in children. Abstral, Subsys, and Lazanda: Not approved for age younger than 18.

UNAPPROVED ADULT — Analgesia/procedural sedation/labor analgesia: 50 to 100 mcg IV or IM q 1 to 2 h prn.

UNAPPROVED PEDS — Analgesia: 1 to 2 mcg/kg/dose IV/IM q 30 to 60 min prn or continuous IV infusion 1 to 3 mcg/kg/h (not to exceed adult dosing). Procedural sedation: 2 to 3 mcg/kg/dose for age 1 to 3 yo; 1 to 2 mcg/kg/dose for age 3 to 12 yo, 0.5 to 1 mcg/kg/dose (not to exceed adult dosing) for age older than 12 yo, procedural sedation doses may repeated q 30 to 60 min prn.

FORMS — Generic/Trade: Transdermal patches 12, 25, 50, 75, 100 mcg/h. Actiq lozenges on a stick, berry flavored 200, 400, 600, 800, 1200, 1600 mcg. Trade only: (Fentora) buccal tab 100, 200, 400, 600, 800 mcg, packs of 4 or 28 tabs. Trade only: (Onsolis) buccal soluble film 200, 400, 600, 800, 1200 mcg in child-resistant, protective foil, packs of 30 films. Trade only: (Abstral) sublingual tab: 100, 200, 300, 400, 600, 800 mcg, packs of 4 or 32 tabs. Trade only: (Subsys) sublingual spray: 100, 200, 400, 600, 800, 1200, 1600 mcg blister packs in cartons of 10 and 30 (30 only for for 1200 and 1600 mcg). Trade only: (Lazanda) nasal spray: 100, 400 mcg/spray, 8 sprays/bottle.

NOTES — Do not use patches for acute pain or in opioid-naive patients. Oral transmucosal fentanyl doses of 5 mcg/kg provide effects similar to 0.75 to 1.25 mcg/kg of fentanyl IM. Lozenges on a stick should be sucked, not chewed. Flush lozenge remnants (without stick) down the toilet. For transdermal systems: Apply patch to non-hairy skin. Clip (not shave) hair if you have to apply to hairy area. Fever or external heat sources may increase fentanyl released from patch. Patch should be removed prior to MRI and reapplied after the test. Dispose of a used patch by folding with the adhesive side of the patch adhering to itself, then flush it down the toilet immediately. Do not cut the patch in half. For Duragesic patches and Actiq lozenges on a stick: Titrate dose as high as necessary to relieve cancer or nonmalignant pain where chronic opioids are necessary. Do not suck, chew, or swallow buccal tab. IONSYS: Apply to intact skin on the chest or upper arm. Each dose, activated by the patient, is delivered over a 10-min period. Remove prior to hospital discharge. Do not allow gel to touch mucous membranes. Dispose using gloves. Keep all forms of fentanyl out of the reach of children or pets. Concomitant use with potent CYP3A4 inhibitors such as ritonavir, ketoconazole, itraconazole, troleandomycin, clarithromycin, nelfinavir, and nefazodone may result in an increase in fentanyl plasma concentrations, which could increase or prolong adverse drug effects and may cause potentially fatal respiratory depression. ONSOLIS is available only through the FOCUS Program and requires prescriber, pharmacy, and patient enrollment. Used films should be discarded into toilet. Abstral, Subsys, and Lazanda: outpatients, prescribers, pharmacies, and distributors must be enrolled in TIRF REMS Access program before patient may receive medication.

MOA — Opioid agonist analgesic.

ADVERSE EFFECTS — Serious: Respiratory depression/arrest, chest wall rigidity. Frequent: N/V, constipation, sedation, skin irritation, dental decay with Actiq.

HYDROMORPHONE (*Dilaudid, Exalgo, ✦Hydromorph Contin*) ▶L ♀C ▶? ©II $$

ADULT — Moderate to severe pain: 2 to 4 mg PO q 4 to 6 h. Initial dose (opioid-naive) 0.5 to 2 mg SC/IM or slow IV q 4 to 6 h prn. 3 mg PR q 6 to 8 h. Controlled-release tabs: 8 to 64 mg daily.

(cont.)

HYDROMORPHONE (*cont.*)

PEDS — Not approved in children.
UNAPPROVED PEDS — Pain age 12 yo or younger: 0.03 to 0.08 mg/kg PO q 4 to 6 h prn. 0.015 mg/kg/dose IV q 4 to 6 h prn, use adult dose for older than 12 yo.
FORMS — Generic/Trade: Tabs 2, 4, 8 mg (8 mg trade scored). Oral soln 5 mg/5 mL. Controlled-release tabs (Exalgo): 8, 12, 16, 32 mg.
NOTES — In opioid-naive patients, consider an initial dose of 0.5 mg or less IM/SC/IV. SC/IM/IV doses after initial dose should be individualized. May be given by slow IV injection over 2 to 5 min. Titrate dose as high as necessary to relieve cancer or nonmalignant pain where chronic opioids are necessary. 1.5 mg IV = 7.5 mg PO. Exalgo intended for opioid-tolerant patients only.
MOA — Opioid agonist analgesic.
ADVERSE EFFECTS — Serious: Respiratory depression/arrest. Frequent: N/V, constipation, sedation.

LEVORPHANOL (*Levo-Dromoran*) ▶L ♀C ▶? ©II $$$$
ADULT — Moderate to severe pain: 2 mg PO q 6 to 8 h prn. Increase to 4 mg if necessary.
PEDS — Not approved in children.
FORMS — Generic only: Tabs 2 mg, scored.
MOA — Serious: Respiratory depression/arrest. Frequent: N/V, constipation, sedation.
ADVERSE EFFECTS — TAB001,TAB002

MEPERIDINE (*Demerol, pethidine*) ▶LK ♀C but + ▶+ ©II $$
ADULT — Moderate to severe pain: 50 to 150 mg IM/SC/PO q 3 to 4 h prn. OB analgesia: When pains become regular, 50 to 100 mg IM/SC q 1 to 3 h. May also be given slow IV diluted to 10 mg/mL, or by continuous IV infusion diluted to 1 mg/mL.
PEDS — Moderate to severe pain: 1 to 1.8 mg/kg IM/SC/PO or slow IV (see adult dosing) up to adult dose, q 3 to 4 h prn.
FORMS — Generic/Trade: Tabs 50 (trade scored), 100 mg. Generic only: Syrup 50 mg/5 mL.
NOTES — Avoid in renal insufficiency and in elderly due to risk of metabolite accumulation and increased risk of CNS disturbance and seizures. Multiple drug interactions including MAOIs and SSRIs. Poor oral absorption/efficacy. 75 mg meperidine IV/IM/SC = 300 mg meperidine PO. Take syrup with ½ glass (4 oz) water. Due to the risk of seizures at high doses, meperidine is not a good choice for treatment of chronic pain. Not recommended in children.
MOA — Opioid agonist analgesic.
ADVERSE EFFECTS — Serious: Respiratory depression/arrest, seizures, anaphylaxis. Frequent: N/V, constipation, sedation.

METHADONE (*Diskets, Dolophine, Methadose, ✦Metadol*) ▶L ♀C ▶? ©II $
WARNING — High doses (mean approximately 200 mg/day) have been inconclusively associated with arrhythmia (torsade de pointes), particularly in those with preexisting risk factors. Caution in opioid-naive patients. Elimination half-life (8 to 59

h) far longer than its duration of analgesic action (4 to 8 h); monitor for respiratory depression and titrate accordingly. Use caution with escalating doses.
ADULT — Severe pain in opioid-tolerant patients: Initial dose is 2.5 mg IM/SC/PO q 8 to 12 h prn. Titrate up by 2.5 mg per dose every 5 to 7 days as necessary to relieve cancer or nonmalignant pain where chronic opioids are necessary. May start as high as 10 mg per dose if opioid dependent patient and dosing is managed by experienced practitioner using an opioid converson formula. Opioid dependence: Typical dose to prevent withdrawal is 20 mg PO daily but must be managed by an experienced practitioner. Treatment longer than 3 weeks is maintenance and only permitted in approved treatment programs. Opioid-naive patients: Not recommended in opioid naive patients, as first line treatment of acute pain, mild chronic pain, postoperative pain, or as a PRN medication.
PEDS — Not approved in children.
UNAPPROVED PEDS — Pain age 12 yo or younger: 0.7 mg/kg/24 h divided q 4 to 6 h PO/SC/IM/IV prn. Max 10 mg/dose.
FORMS — Generic/Trade: Tabs 5, 10 mg. Dispersible tabs 40 mg (for opioid dependence only). Oral concentrate (Intensol): 10 mg/mL. Generic only: Oral soln 5, 10 mg/5 mL.
NOTES — Titrate dose as high as necessary to relieve cancer or nonmalignant pain where chronic opioids are necessary. Every 8 to 12 h dosing may decrease the risk of drug accumulation and overdose. Treatment for opioid dependence longer than 3 weeks is maintenance and only permitted in approved treatment programs. Drug interactions leading to decreased methadone levels with enzyme-inducing HIV drugs (e.g., efavirenz, nevirapine) and other potent inducers such as rifampin. Monitor for opiate withdrawal symptoms and increase methadone if necessary. Rapid metabolizers may require more frequent daily dosing.
MOA — Opioid agonist analgesic.
ADVERSE EFFECTS — Serious: Respiratory depression/cardiorespiratory arrest, dependence, withdrawal, seizures, bradycardia. Frequent: N/V, constipation, sedation, dry mouth, urinary retention, rash.

MORPHINE (*MS Contin, Kadian, Avinza, Roxanol, Oramorph SR, MSIR, DepoDur, ✦Statex, M.O.S., Doloral, M-Eslon*) ▶LK ♀C ▶+ ©II varies by therapy
WARNING — Multiple strengths; see FORMS and write specific product on Rx. Drinking alcohol while taking Avinza may result in a rapid release of a potentially fatal dose of morphine.
ADULT — Moderate to severe pain: 10 to 30 mg PO q 4 h (immediate-release tabs, or oral soln). Controlled-release (MS Contin, Oramorph SR): 30 mg PO q 8 to 12 h. (Kadian): 20 mg PO q 12 to 24 h. Extended-release caps (Avinza): 30 mg PO daily. 10 mg q 4 h IM/SC. 2.5 to 15 mg/70 kg IV over 4 to 5 min. 10 to 20 mg PR q 4 h. Pain with

MORPHINE (*cont.*)

major surgery (DepoDur): 10 to 15 mg once epidurally at the lumbar level prior to surgery (max dose 20 mg), or 10 mg epidurally after clamping of the umbilical cord with cesarean section.

PEDS — Moderate to severe pain: 0.1 to 0.2 mg/kg up to 15 mg IM/SC/IV q 2 to 4 h.

UNAPPROVED PEDS — Moderate to severe pain: 0.2 to 0.5 mg/kg/dose PO (immediate-release) q 4 to 6 h. 0.3 to 0.6 mg/kg/dose PO (controlled-release) q 12 h.

FORMS — Generic only: Tabs, immediate-release 15, 30 mg ($). Oral soln: 10 mg/5 mL, 20 mg/5 mL, 20 mg/mL (concentrate). Rectal supps 5, 10, 20, 30 mg. Generic/Trade: Controlled-release tabs (MS Contin) 15, 30, 60, 100, 200 mg ($$$$). Controlled-release caps (Kadian) 20, 30, 50, 60, 80, 100 mg ($$$$$). Trade only: Controlled-release caps (Kadian) 10, 40, 70, 130, 150, 200 mg. Extended-release caps (Avinza) 30, 45, 60, 75, 90, 120 mg.

NOTES — Titrate dose as high as necessary to relieve cancer or nonmalignant pain where chronic opioids are necessary. The active metabolites may accumulate in hepatic/renal insufficiency and the elderly leading to increased analgesic and sedative effects. Do not break, chew, or crush MS Contin or Oramorph SR. Kadian and Avinza caps may be opened and sprinkled in applesauce for easier administration; however, the pellets should not be crushed or chewed. Doses more than 1600 mg/day of Avinza contain a potentially nephrotoxic quantity of fumaric acid. Do not mix DepoDur with other medications; do not administer any other medications into epidural space for for at least 48 h. Severe opiate overdose with respiratory depression has occurred with intrathecal leakage of DepoDur.

MOA — Opioid agonist analgesic.

ADVERSE EFFECTS — Serious: Respiratory depression/arrest. Frequent: N/V, constipation, sedation, hypotension.

OXYCODONE (*Roxicodone, OxyContin, Percolone, OxyIR, OxyFAST, Oxecta, ✦Endocodone, Supeudol, OxyNEO*) ▶L ♀B ▶– ©II $ - varies by therapy

WARNING — Do not prescribe OxyContin tabs on a prn basis. 80 mg tabs for use in opioid-tolerant patients only. Multiple strengths; see FORMS and write specific product on Rx. Do not break, chew, or crush controlled-release preparations.

ADULT — Moderate to severe pain: 5 mg PO q 4 to 6 h prn. Controlled-release tabs: 10 to 40 mg PO q 12 h (no supporting data for shorter dosing intervals for controlled-release tabs).

PEDS — Not approved in children.

UNAPPROVED PEDS — Pain age 12 yo or younger: 0.05 to 0.3 mg/kg/dose q 4 to 6 h PO prn to max of 10 mg/dose.

FORMS — Generic only: Immediate-release: Tabs 5, 10, 20 mg. Caps 5 mg. Oral soln 5 mg/5 mL. Generic/Trade: Tab 15, 30 mg. Oral concentrate 20 mg/mL. Trade only: Immediate-release abuse deterrent tabs (Oxecta): 5, 7.5 mg. Controlled-release tabs: 10, 15, 20, 30, 40, 60, 80 mg ($$$$$).

NOTES — Titrate dose as high as necessary to relieve cancer or nonmalignant pain where chronic opioids are necessary.

MOA — Opioid agonist analgesic.

ADVERSE EFFECTS — Serious: Respiratory depression/arrest. Frequent: N/V, constipation, sedation.

OXYMORPHONE (*Opana, Opana ER*) ▶L ♀C ▶? ©II $$$$$

WARNING — Do not break, chew, dissolve, or crush extended-release tabs due to a rapid release and absorption of a potentially fatal dose of oxymorphone.

ADULT — Moderate to severe pain: 10 to 20 mg PO q 4 to 6 h (immediate-release) or 5 mg q 12 h (extended-release) 1 h before or 2 h after meals. Titrate q 3 to 7 days until adequate pain relief. 1 to 1.5 mg IM/SC q 4 to 6 h prn. 0.5 mg IV initial dose in healthy patients then q 4 to 6 h prn, increase dose until pain adequately controlled.

PEDS — Not approved in children.

FORMS — Generic/Trade: immediate-release (IR) tabs 5, 10 mg. Extended-release tabs (ER) 5, 7.5, 10, 15, 20, 30, 40 mg. Trade only: Injection 1 mg/mL.

NOTES — Contraindicated in moderate to severe hepatic dysfunction. Decrease dose in elderly and with CrCl < 50 mL/min. Avoid alcohol.

MOA — Opioid agonist analgesic.

ADVERSE EFFECTS — Serious: Respiratory depression/arrest. Frequent: N/V, constipation, sedation.

ANALGESICS: Opioid Analgesic Combinations

NOTE: Refer to individual components for further information. May cause drowsiness and/or sedation, which may be enhanced by alcohol and other CNS depressants. Opioids, carisoprodol, and butalbital may be habit-forming. Avoid exceeding 4 g/day of acetaminophen in combination products. Caution people who drink 3 or more alcoholic drinks/day to limit acetaminophen use to 2.5 g/day due to additive liver toxicity. Opioids commonly cause constipation; concurrent laxatives are recommended. All opioids are pregnancy class D if used for prolonged periods or in high doses at term.

ANEXSIA (hydrocodone + acetaminophen) ▶LK ♀C ▶– ©II $

WARNING — Multiple strengths; see FORMS and write specific product on Rx.

ADULT — Moderate pain: 1 tab PO q 4 to 6 h prn.

PEDS — Not approved in children.

FORMS — Generic only: Tabs 5/325, 7.5/325, 10/325 mg hydrocodone/mg acetaminophen, scored.

MOA — Serious: Respiratory depression/arrest, hepatotoxicity. Frequent: N/V, constipation, sedation.

ADVERSE EFFECTS — TAB003

CAPITAL WITH CODEINE SUSPENSION (acetaminophen + codeine) ►LK ♀C ▶? ©V $
ADULT — Moderate pain: 15 mL PO q 4 h prn.
PEDS — Moderate pain: Give 5 mL PO q 4 to 6 h prn for age 3 to 6 yo, give 10 mL PO q 4 to 6 h prn for age 7 to 12 yo, use adult dose for age older than 12 yo.
FORMS — Generic only: Soln, 120 mg/5 mL and 12 mg/5 mL (APAP/Codeine).Trade only: Suspension, 120 mg/5 mL and 12 mg/5 mL (APAP/Codeine).
MOA — Serious: Respiratory depression/arrest, hepatotoxicity. Frequent: N/V, constipation, sedation.
ADVERSE EFFECTS — TAB003

COMBUNOX (oxycodone + ibuprofen) ►L ♀C (D in 3rd trimester) ▶? ©II $$$
ADULT — Moderate to severe pain: 1 tab PO q 6 h prn for no more than 7 days. Max dose 4 tabs/24 h.
PEDS — Moderate to severe pain for age 14 yo or older: Use adult dose.
FORMS — Generic only: Tabs 5 mg oxycodone/ 400 mg ibuprofen.
NOTES — For short-term (no more than 7 days) management of pain. See NSAIDs—Other subclass warning and individual components.
MOA — Combination analgesic.
ADVERSE EFFECTS — Serious: Respiratory depression/arrest, hypersensitivity, GI bleeding, nephrotoxicity. Frequent: N/V, constipation, dyspepsia, sedation.

EMPIRIN WITH CODEINE (acetylsalicylic acid + codeine, ✱292 tab) ►LK ♀D ▶– ©III $
WARNING — Multiple strengths; see FORMS and write specific product on Rx.
ADULT — Moderate pain: 1 to 2 tabs PO q 4 h prn.
PEDS — Not approved in children.
FORMS — Generic/Trade: No US formulation available. Tabs 325/30, 325/60 mg aspirin/mg codeine
MOA — Serious: Respiratory depression/arrest, hypersensitivity, Reye's syndrome, GI bleeding, nephrotoxicity. Frequent: N/V, dyspepsia, constipation, sedation.
ADVERSE EFFECTS — TAB003

FIORICET WITH CODEINE (acetaminophen + butalbital + caffeine + codeine) ►LK ♀C ▶– ©III $$$
ADULT — Moderate pain: 1 to 2 caps PO q 4 h prn, max dose 6 caps/day.
PEDS — Not approved in children.
FORMS — Generic/Trade: Caps 325 mg acetaminophen/50 mg butalbital/40 mg caffeine/ 30 mg codeine.
MOA — Serious: Respiratory depression/arrest, hepatotoxicity. Frequent: N/V, constipation, sedation.
ADVERSE EFFECTS — TAB003

FIORINAL WITH CODEINE (acetylsalicylic acid + butalbital + caffeine + codeine, ✱Fiorinal C-1/4, Fiorinal C-1/2, Trianal C-1/4, Trianal C-1/2) ►LK ♀D ▶– ©III $$$
ADULT — Moderate pain: 1 to 2 caps PO q 4 h prn, max dose 6 caps/day.
PEDS — Not approved in children.
FORMS — Generic/Trade: Caps 325 mg aspirin/50 mg butalbital/40 mg caffeine/30 mg codeine.
MOA — Serious: Respiratory depression/arrest, hypersensitivity, Reye's syndrome, GI bleeding,

nephrotoxicity. Frequent: N/V, dyspepsia, constipation, sedation.
ADVERSE EFFECTS — TAB003

IBUDONEREPREXAIN (hydrocodone + ibuprofen) ►LK ♀– ▶? ©II $$
ADULT — Moderate pain: 1 tab PO q 4 to 6 h prn, max dose 5 tabs/day.
PEDS — Not approved in children.
FORMS — Generic/Trade: Tabs 2.5/200, 5/200, and 10/200 mg hydrocodone/ibuprofen.
NOTES — See NSAIDs—Other subclass warning.
MOA — Combination analgesic.
ADVERSE EFFECTS — Serious: Respiratory depression/arrest, hypersensitivity, GI bleeding, nephrotoxicity. Frequent: N/V, constipation, dyspepsia, sedation.

LORCET (hydrocodone + acetaminophen) ►LK ♀C ▶– ©II $$
WARNING — Multiple strengths; see FORMS and write specific product on Rx.
ADULT — Moderate pain: 1 to 2 caps (5/325) PO q 4 to 6 h prn, max dose 8 caps/day. 1 tab PO q 4 to 6 h prn (7.5/325 and 10/325), max dose 6 tabs/day.
PEDS — Not approved in children.
FORMS — Generic/Trade: Tabs 5/325, 7.5/325, 10/325 mg hydrocodone/acetaminophen.
MOA — Serious: Respiratory depression/arrest, hepatotoxicity. Frequent: N/V, constipation, sedation.
ADVERSE EFFECTS — TAB003

LORTAB (hydrocodone + acetaminophen) ►LK ♀C ▶– ©II $
WARNING — Multiple strengths; see FORMS and write specific product on Rx.
ADULT — Moderate pain: 1 to 2 tabs 2.5/325 and 5/325 PO q 4 to 6 h prn, max dose 8 tabs/day. 1 tab 7.5/325 and 10/325 PO q 4 to 6 h prn, max dose 5 tabs/day.
PEDS — Not approved in children.
FORMS — Generic/Trade: Lortab 5/325 (scored), Lortab 7.5/325 (trade scored), Lortab 10/325 mg hydrocodone/mg acetaminophen. Generic only: Tabs 2.5/325 mg.
MOA — Serious: Respiratory depression/arrest, hepatotoxicity. Frequent: N/V, constipation, sedation.
ADVERSE EFFECTS — TAB003

MERSYNDOL WITH CODEINE (acetaminophen + codeine + doxylamine) ►LK ♀C ▶? $
ADULT — Canada only. Headaches, cold symptoms, muscle aches, neuralgia: 1 to 2 tabs PO q 4 to 6 h prn. Maximum 12 tabs/24 h.
PEDS — Not approved in children.
FORMS — Canada Trade only: OTC tab 325 mg acetaminophen/8 mg codeine phosphate/5 mg doxylamine.
NOTES — May be habit-forming. Hepatotoxicity may be increased with acetaminophen overdose and may be enhanced with concomitant chronic alcohol ingestion.
MOA — Combination analgesic.
ADVERSE EFFECTS — See components.

NORCO (hydrocodone + acetaminophen) ▶L ♀C ▶? ©II $$
WARNING — Multiple strengths; see FORMS and write specific product on Rx.
ADULT — Moderate to severe pain: 1 to 2 tabs PO q 4 to 6 h prn (5/325), max dose 12 tabs/day. 1 tab (7.5/325 and 10/325) PO q 4 to 6 h prn, max dose 8 and 6 tabs/day, respectively.
PEDS — Not approved in children.
FORMS — Generic/Trade: Tabs 5/325, 7.5/325, 10/325 mg hydrocodone/acetaminophen, scored. Generic only: solution 7.5/325 mg per 15 mL.
MOA — Serious: Respiratory depression/arrest, hepatotoxicity. Frequent: N/V, constipation, sedation.
ADVERSE EFFECTS — TAB003

PERCOCET (oxycodone + acetaminophen, ✸*Percocet-demi, Oxycocet, Endocet*) ▶L ♀C ▶– ©II $
WARNING — Multiple strengths; see FORMS and write specific product on Rx.
ADULT — Moderate to severe pain: 1 to 2 tabs PO q 4 to 6 h prn (2.5/325 and 5/325 mg). 1 tab PO q 4 to 6 h prn (7.5/325 and 10/325 mg).
PEDS — Not approved in children.
FORMS — Generic/Trade: oxycodone/acetaminophen Tabs 2.5/325, 5/325, 7.5/325, 10/325 mg. Trade Only: (Primlev) tabs 2.5/300, 5/300, 7.5/300, 10/300 mg. Generic Only: 10/325 mg.
MOA — Serious: Respiratory depression/arrest, hepatotoxicity. Frequent: N/V, constipation, sedation.
ADVERSE EFFECTS — TAB003

PERCODAN (oxycodone + acetylsalicylic acid, ✸*Oxycodan*) ▶LK ♀D ▶– ©II $$
ADULT — Moderate to severe pain: 1 tab PO q 6 h prn.
PEDS — Not approved in children.
FORMS — Generic/Trade: Tabs 4.88/325 mg oxycodone/aspirin (trade scored).
MOA — Serious: Respiratory depression/arrest, hypersensitivity, Reye's syndrome, GI bleeding, nephrotoxicity. Frequent: N/V, dyspepsia, constipation, sedation.
ADVERSE EFFECTS — TAB003

ROXICET (oxycodone + acetaminophen) ▶L ♀C ▶– ©II $
WARNING — Multiple strengths; see FORMS and write specific product on Rx.
ADULT — Moderate to severe pain: 1 tab PO q 6 h prn. Oral soln: 5 mL PO q 6 h prn.
PEDS — Not approved in children.
FORMS — Generic/Trade: Tabs 5/325 mg. Caps/Caplets 5/325 mg. Soln 5/325 per 5 mL, mg oxycodone/acetaminophen.
MOA — Serious: Respiratory depression/arrest, hepatotoxicity. Frequent: N/V, constipation, sedation.
ADVERSE EFFECTS — TAB003

SOMA COMPOUND WITH CODEINE (carisoprodol + acetylsalicylic acid + codeine) ▶L ♀D ▶– ©III $$$$
ADULT — Moderate to severe musculoskeletal pain: 1 to 2 tabs PO four times per day prn.
PEDS — Not approved in children.
FORMS — Generic only: Tabs 200 mg carisoprodol/ 325 mg aspirin/16 mg codeine.

NOTES — Refer to individual components. Withdrawal with abrupt discontinuation.
MOA — Combination analgesic.
ADVERSE EFFECTS — Serious: Respiratory depression/arrest, hypersensitivity, Reye's syndrome, GI bleeding, nephrotoxicity, idiosyncratic reaction with angioedema, hypotension, and anaphylactoid shock. Frequent: N/V, dyspepsia, constipation, sedation.

SYNALGOS-DC (dihydrocodeine + acetylsalicylic acid + caffeine) ▶L ♀C ▶– ©III $$$
WARNING — Case reports of prolonged erections when taken concomitantly with sildenafil.
ADULT — Moderate to severe pain: 2 caps PO q 4 h prn.
PEDS — Not approved in children.
FORMS — Generic/Trade: Caps 16 mg dihydrocodeine/ 356.4 mg aspirin/30 mg caffeine.
NOTES — Most common use is dental pain. Refer to individual components.
MOA — Combination analgesic.
ADVERSE EFFECTS — Serious: Respiratory depression/arrest. Frequent: N/V, constipation, sedation.

TYLENOL WITH CODEINE (codeine + acetaminophen, ✸*Tylenol #1, Tylenol # 2, Tylenol # 3, Tylenol # 4, Atasol 8, Atasol 15, Atasol 30*) ▶LK ♀C ▶? ©III $
WARNING — Multiple strengths; see FORMS and write specific product on Rx.
ADULT — Moderate pain: 1 to 2 tabs PO q 4 h prn.
PEDS — Moderate pain: Elixir: Give 5 mL q 4 to 6 h prn for age 3 to 6 yo, give 10 mL q 4 to 6 h prn for age 7 to 12 yo, use adult dose for age older than 12 yo.
FORMS — Generic only: Tabs Tylenol #2 (15/300). Tylenol with Codeine Elixir/Susp/Soln 12/120 per 5 mL, mg codeine/mg acetaminophen. Generic/Trade: Tabs Tylenol #3 (30/300), Tylenol #4 (60/300).
MOA — Serious: Respiratory depression/arrest, hepatotoxicity. Frequent: N/V, constipation, sedation.
ADVERSE EFFECTS — TAB003

VICODIN (hydrocodone + acetaminophen) ▶LK ♀C ▶? ©II $$$
WARNING — Multiple strengths; see FORMS and write specific product on Rx.
ADULT — Moderate pain: 5/300 mg (max dose 8 tabs/day) and 7.5/300 mg (max dose of 6 tabs/day): 1 to 2 tabs PO q 4 to 6 h prn. 10/300 mg: 1 tab PO q 4 to 6 h prn (max of 6 tabs/day).
PEDS — Not approved in children.
FORMS — Generic/Trade: Tabs Vicodin (5/300), Vicodin ES (7.5/300), Vicodin HP (10/300), scored, mg hydrocodone/mg acetaminophen.
MOA — Serious: Respiratory depression/arrest, hepatotoxicity. Frequent: N/V, constipation, sedation.
ADVERSE EFFECTS — TAB003

VICOPROFEN (hydrocodone + ibuprofen) ▶LK ♀– ▶? ©II $$
ADULT — Moderate pain: 1 tab PO q 4 to 6 h prn, max dose 5 tabs/day.
PEDS — Not approved in children.

VICOPROFEN (cont.)

FORMS — Generic/Trade: Tabs 7.5/200 mg hydroco-done/ibuprofen. Generic only: Tabs 2.5/200, 5/200, 10/200 mg.

NOTES — See NSAIDs—Other subclass warning.

MOA — Combination analgesic.

ADVERSE EFFECTS — Serious: Respiratory depression/arrest, hypersensitivity, GI bleeding, nephrotoxicity. Frequent: N/V, constipation, dyspepsia, sedation.

XODOL (hydrocodone + acetaminophen) ▶LK ♀C ▶– ©II $$$

ADULT — Moderate pain: 1 tab PO q 4 to 6 h prn, max 6 doses/day.

PEDS — Not approved in children.

FORMS — Generic/Trade only: Tabs 5/300, 7.5/300, 10/300 mg hydrocodone/acetaminophen.

MOA — Serious: Respiratory depression/arrest, hepatotoxicity. Frequent: N/V, constipation, sedation.

ADVERSE EFFECTS — TAB003

ANALGESICS: Opioid Antagonists

NOTE: May result in withdrawal in the opioid-dependent, including life-threatening withdrawal if administered to neonates born to opioid-dependent mothers. Rare pulmonary edema, cardiovascular instability, hypotension, HTN, ventricular tachycardia, and ventricular fibrillation have been reported in connection with opioid reversal.

NALOXONE (*Narcan*) ▶LK ♀B ▶? $

ADULT — Management of opioid overdose: 0.4 to 2 mg IV. May repeat IV at 2 to 3 min intervals up to 10 mg. Use IM/SC/ET if IV not available. IV infusion: 2 mg in 500 mL D5W or NS (0.004 mg/mL); titrate according to response. Partial postop opioid reversal: 0.1 to 0.2 mg IV at 2 to 3 min intervals; repeat IM doses may be required at 1 to 2 h intervals.

PEDS — Management of opioid overdose: 0.01 mg/kg IV. Give a subsequent dose of 0.1 mg/kg if inadequate response. Use IM/SC/ET if IV not available. Partial postop opioid reversal: 0.005 to 0.01 mg IV at 2 to 3 min intervals.

NOTES — Watch patients for re-emergence of opioid effects.

MOA — Opioid antagonist.

ADVERSE EFFECTS — Serious: Pulmonary edema, cardiovascular instability, hypo/hypertension, ventricular tachycardia and fibrillation, opioid withdrawal. Frequent: Nausea and tachycardia.

ANALGESICS: Other Analgesics

ACETAMINOPHEN (*Tylenol, Panadol, Tempra, Ofirmev, paracetamol, ✚Abenol, Atasol, Pediatrix*) ▶LK ♀B ▶+ $

ADULT — Analgesic/antipyretic: 325 to 1000 mg PO q 4 to 6 h prn. 650 mg PR q 4 to 6 h prn. Max dose 4 g/day. OA: Extended-release: 2 caps PO q 8 h around the clock. Max dose 6 caps/day.

PEDS — Analgesic/antipyretic: 10 to 15 mg/kg q 4 to 6 h PO/PR prn. Max 5 doses/day.

UNAPPROVED ADULT — OA: 1000 mg PO 4 times per day.

FORMS — OTC: Tabs 325, 500, 650 mg. Chewable Tabs 80 mg. Oral disintegrating Tabs 80, 160 mg. Caps/Gelcaps 500 mg. Extended-release caplets 650 mg. Liquid 160 mg/5 mL, 500 mg/15 mL. Supps 80, 120, 325, 650 mg.

NOTES — Risk of hepatotoxicity with chronic use, especially in alcoholics. Caution in those who drink 3 or more drinks/day. Rectal administration may produce lower/less reliable plasma levels.

MOA — Analgesic/antipyretic.

ADVERSE EFFECTS — Serious: Hepatotoxicity. Frequent: None.

CANNIBIS SATIVA L. EXTRACT (✚*Sativex*) ▶LK ♀X ▶– $$$$

ADULT — Canada only. Adjunctive treatment for the symptomatic relief of neuropathic pain in multiple sclerosis: Start: 1 spray q 4 h (max 4 times per day), and titrated upwards as tolerated. Limited experience with more than 12 sprays/day.

PEDS — Not approved in children.

FORMS — Canada Trade only: Buccal spray, 27 mg/mL delta-9-tetrahydrocannabinol and 25 mg/mL cannabidiol, delivers 100 mcL per actuation, 5.5 mL vials containing up to 51 actuations per vial.

NOTES — Contraindicated in pregnancy, childbearing potential without birth control, history of psychosis, serious heart disease. Contains ethanol. Use cautiously if history of substance abuse.

MOA — Acts at cannabinoid receptors in the CNS and peripheral tissues to mediate cannabinoid-induced analgesia.

ADVERSE EFFECTS — Serious: orthostatic hypotension, syncope. Frequent: Administration site irritation, headache, depression, dizziness.

CLONIDINE—EPIDURAL (*Duraclon*) ▶LK ♀C ▶– $$$$$

WARNING — Not recommended for obstetrical, post-partum or perioperative pain management due to hypotension and bradycardia. Abrupt discontinuation may result in a rapid BP rise.

ADULT — Severe cancer pain in combination with opioids: Specialized epidural dosing.

PEDS — Severe cancer pain in combination with opioids: Specialized epidural dosing.

NOTES — Bradycardia and hypotension common. May be exacerbated by beta-blockers, certain calcium channel blockers, and digoxin.

MOA — Central analgesic - prevents pain signal transmission to the brain.

ADVERSE EFFECTS — Serious: Bradycardia, hypotension. Frequent: Hypotension, sedation, dry mouth.

MIDOL TEEN FORMULA (acetaminophen + pamabrom) ►LK ♀B ►+ $
ADULT — Menstrual cramps: 2 caps PO q 4 to 6 h.
PEDS — Use adult dose for age older than 12 yo.
FORMS — Generic/Trade OTC: Caps 325 mg acetaminophen/25 mg pamabrom (diuretic).
NOTES — Hepatotoxicity with chronic use, especially in alcoholics.
MOA — Analgesic/diuretic.
ADVERSE EFFECTS — Serious: Hepatotoxicity. Frequent: None.

TAPENTADOL (*Nucynta, Nucynta ER*) ►LK ♀C ►– ©II $$$$
WARNING — Abuse potential.
ADULT — Moderate to severe acute pain: Immediate release: 50 to 100 mg PO q 4 to 6 h prn. Max dose 600 mg/day. If moderate hepatic impairment, decrease dose to 50 mg PO q 8 h. Moderate to severe chronic pain: Extended release: 50 to 250 mg PO twice daily. Start at 50 mg PO twice daily if patient not currently taking opioids. Do not use in severe renal or hepatic impairment.
PEDS — Not approved in children younger than 18 yo.
FORMS — Trade only: Immediate-release ($$$$): Tabs 50, 75, 100 mg. Extended-release ($$$$$): Tabs 50, 100, 150, 200, 250 mg.
NOTES — When switching from immediate release to extended release form, use same total daily dose. Contraindicated in acute intoxication with alcohol, hypnotics, centrally acting analgesics, opioids, or psychotropic drugs and with respiratory depression. Use with caution in patients with known seizure disorders. Seizures and/or serotonin syndrome may occur with concurrent antidepressants, triptans, linezolid, lithium, St. John's wort.
MOA — Opioid agonist/norepinephrine reuptake inhibitor.
ADVERSE EFFECTS — Serious: Seizures, anaphylactoid reactions, respiratory depression. Frequent: Nausea, dizziness, vomiting, somnolence.

TRAMADOL (*Ultram, Ultram ER, Ryzolt, Conzip, Rybix ODT, ✱Zytram XL, Tridural, Ralivia*) ►KL ♀C ►– ©IV $$$
ADULT — Moderate to moderately severe pain: 50 to 100 mg PO q 4 to 6 h prn. Max dose 400 mg/day. If older than 75 yo, use less than 300 mg/day PO in divided doses. If CrCl less than 30 mL/min, increase the dosing interval to 12 h. If cirrhosis, decrease dose to 50 mg PO q 12 h. Chronic pain, extended-release: 100 to 300 mg PO daily. Do not use if CrCl less than 30 mL/min or with severe hepatic dysfunction.
PEDS — Not approved in children younger than 16 yo.
FORMS — Generic/Trade: Tabs, immediate-release 50 mg. Extended-release tabs 100, 200, 300 mg. Trade Only: (Conzip) Extended-release caps 100, 150, 200, 300 mg. (Rybix) ODT 50 mg
NOTES — Contraindicated in acute intoxication with alcohol, hypnotics, centrally acting analgesics, opioids, or psychotropic drugs. Seizures and/or serotonin syndrome may occur with concurrent antidepressants, triptans, linezolid, lithium, St. John's wort, or enzyme-inducing drugs such as ketoconazole and erythromycin; use with caution and adjust dose. Withdrawal symptoms may occur in patients dependent on opioids or with abrupt discontinuation. Overdose treated with naloxone may increase seizures. Carbamazepine decreases tramadol levels. The most frequent side effects are nausea and constipation. ER tabs cannot be crushed, chewed, or split.
MOA — Opioid agonist/norepinephrine and serotonin reuptake inhibitor.
ADVERSE EFFECTS — Serious: Seizures, anaphylactoid reactions. Frequent: Constipation, nausea, somnolence.

ZICONOTIDE (*Prialt*) ►Plasma ♀C ►? $$$$$
WARNING — Severe psychiatric and neurologic impairment may occur. Monitor for mood changes, hallucinations, or cognitive changes. Contraindicated if history of psychosis.
ADULT — Severe intractable chronic pain: Specialized intrathecal dosing.
PEDS — Not approved in children younger than 16 yo.
NOTES — Contraindicated in patients with history of psychosis, uncontrolled bleeding, spinal canal obstruction or infection at the infusion site. Does not prevent opioid withdrawal; gradually taper while instituting ziconotide therapy. Monitor CK periodically.
MOA — Blocks N-type calcium channels on nociceptive afferent nerves.
ADVERSE EFFECTS — Serious: Hallucinations, cognitive impairment, meningitis, myopathy, rhabdomyolysis and renal failure. Frequent: Dizziness, nausea, confusion, headache, somnolence, nystagmus, asthenia, pain, increased serum CK levels.

ANESTHESIA

ANESTHESIA: Anesthetics and Sedatives

ALFENTANIL (Alfenta) ▶L ♀C ▶? ©II $
ADULT — IV general anesthesia adjunct; specialized dosing.
PEDS — Not approved in children.
MOA — Serious: Respiratory depression, hypotension, bradycardia, chest wall rigidity, increased intracranial pressure, opiate dependence, hypersensitivity. Frequent: Sedation, N/V.

DESFLURANE (Suprane) ▶Respiratory ♀B ▶+ Varies
ADULT — General anesthetic gas; specialized dosing.
PEDS — Not recommended for induction due to high rate of laryngospasm.
NOTES — Minimum Alveolar Concentration (MAC) 6.0%. Known trigger of malignant hyperthermia; see mhaus.org.
MOA — CNS depressant
ADVERSE EFFECTS — Serious: Apnea, malignant hyperthermia. Frequent: Recovery N/V.

DEXMEDETOMIDINE (Precedex) ▶LK ♀C ▶? $$$$$
ADULT — ICU sedation less than 24 h: Load 1 mcg/kg over 10 min followed by infusion 0.2 to 0.7 mcg/kg/h titrated to desired sedation endpoint.
PEDS — Not recommended age younger than 18 yo.
NOTES — Alpha-2-adrenergic agonist with sedative properties. Beware of bradycardia and hypotension. Avoid in advanced heart block.
MOA — Alpha-2 adrenergic agonist with sedative properties.
ADVERSE EFFECTS — Serious: Bradycardia, heart block, hypotension. Frequent: Sedation.

ENFLURANE (Ethrane) ▶Respiratory/L ♀B ▶? Varies
ADULT — Rarely used general anesthetic gas; specialized dosing.
PEDS — Age younger than 5 yo: Rarely used general anesthetic gas; specialized dosing.
NOTES — Minimum Alveolar Concentration (MAC) 1.68%. Known trigger of malignant hyperthermia; see mhaus.org.
MOA — CNS depressant
ADVERSE EFFECTS — Serious: Apnea, malignant hyperthermia, nephrotoxicity. Frequent: Recovery N/V.

ETOMIDATE (Amidate) ▶L ♀C ▶? $
ADULT — Anesthesia induction/rapid sequence intubation: 0.3 mg/kg IV.
PEDS — Age younger than 10 yo: Not approved. Age 10 yo or older: Use adult dosing.
UNAPPROVED PEDS — Anesthesia induction/rapid sequence intubation: 0.3 mg/kg IV.
NOTES — Adrenocortical suppression, but rarely of clinical significance.
MOA — Nonbarbiturate hypnotic without analgesic properties.
ADVERSE EFFECTS — Serious: Respiratory depression, hypotension, adrenal suppression. Frequent: Myoclonus, N/V.

HALOTHANE (Fluothane) ▶Respiratory/L ♀C ▶? Varies
ADULT — Rarely used general anesthetic gas; specialized dosing.
PEDS — Rarely used general anesthetic gas; specialized dosing.
NOTES — Minimum Alveolar Concentration (MAC) 0.77%. Known trigger of malignant hyperthermia; see mhaus.org.
MOA — CNS depressant
ADVERSE EFFECTS — Serious: Apnea, malignant hyperthermia, hepatitis. Frequent: Recovery N/V.

ISOFLURANE (Forane) ▶Respiratory ♀C ▶? Varies
ADULT — General anesthetic gas; specialized dosing.
PEDS — General anesthetic gas; specialized dosing.
NOTES — Minimum Alveolar Concentration (MAC) 1.15%. Known trigger of malignant hyperthermia; see mhaus.org.
MOA — CNS depressant
ADVERSE EFFECTS — Serious: Apnea, malignant hyperthermia. Frequent: Recovery N/V.

KETAMINE (Ketalar) ▶L ♀? ▶? ©III $
WARNING — Postanesthetic emergence reactions up to 24 hours later manifested as dreamlike state, vivid imagery, hallucinations, and delirium reported in about 12% of cases. Incidence reduced when 1) age less than 15 yo or greater than 65 yo, 2) concommitant use of benzodiazepines, lower dose, or used as induction agent only (because of use of post intubation sedation).
ADULT — Dissociative sedation, Induction: Adult: 1 to 2 mg/kg IV over 1 to 2 min (produces 5 to 10 min dissociative state) or 6.5 to 13 mg/kg IM (produces 10 to 20 min dissociative state). Consider concurrent adminstration of benzodiazepine (minimize emergence) and atropine (minimizes hypersalivation).
PEDS — Dissociative sedation, Induction: Age greater than 3 mo: 1 to 2 mg/kg IV (produces 5 to 10 min dissociative state) over 1 to 2 min or 4 to 5 mg/kg IM (produces 10 to 20 min dissociative state). Not approved for age less than 3 mo. Consider concurrent adminstration of benzodiazepine (minimize emergence) and atropine (minimizes hypersalivation).
FORMS — Generic/Trade: 10 mg/mL, 50 mg/mL, 100 mg/mL
NOTES — Recent evidence suggests no change in intracranial pressure and safe in head injured patients. However, avoid if CAD or HTN. Concurrent atropine minimizes hypersalivation; can be combined in same syringe with ketamine for IM use. Emergence reaction limits value dissociative sedation agent in ages 15 to 65.
MOA — Dissociative agent.

(cont.)

KETAMINE *(cont.)*

ADVERSE EFFECTS — Serious: Laryngospasm, hallucinatory emergence reactions, hypersalivation. Frequent: Nystagmus, hypertension, tachycardia, N/V, muscular hypertonicity, myoclonus.

METHOHEXITAL (*Brevital*) ▶L ♀B ▶? ⓒIV $$
ADULT — Anesthesia induction: 1 to 1.5 mg/kg IV.
PEDS — Anesthesia induction: 6.6 to 10 mg/kg IM or 25 mg/kg PR.
UNAPPROVED PEDS — Sedation for diagnostic imaging: 25 mg/kg PR.
MOA — Serious: Respiratory depression, hypotension, bronchospasm. Frequent: Respiratory depression, hypotension.

MIDAZOLAM (*Versed*) ▶LK ♀D ▶– ⓒIV $
WARNING — Beware of respiratory depression/apnea. Administer with appropriate monitoring.
ADULT — Sedation/anxiolysis: 0.07 to 0.08 mg/kg IM (5 mg in average adult); or 1 mg IV slowly q 2 to 3 min up to 5 mg. Anesthesia induction: 0.3 to 0.35 mg/kg IV over 20 to 30 sec.
PEDS — Sedation/anxiolysis: Oral route 0.25 to 1 mg/kg (0.5 mg/kg most effective) to maximum of 20 mg PO, IM route 0.1 to 0.15 mg/kg IM. IV route initial dose 0.05 to 0.1 mg/kg IV, then titrated to max 0.6 mg/kg for age 6 mo to 5 yo, initial dose 0.025 to 0.05 mg/kg IV, then titrated to max 0.4 mg/kg for age 6 to 12 yo.
UNAPPROVED PEDS — Sedation/anxiolysis: Intranasal 0.2 to 0.4 mg/kg. Rectal: 0.25 to 0.5 mg/kg PR. Status epilepticus: Load 0.15 mg/kg IV followed by infusion 1 mcg/kg/min and titrate dose upward q 5 min prn.
FORMS — Generic only: Injection: 1 mg/mL, 5 mg/mL, Oral liquid 2 mg/mL.
NOTES — Use lower doses in the elderly, chronically ill, and those receiving concurrent CNS depressants.
MOA — Short-acting benzodiazepine sedative.
ADVERSE EFFECTS — Serious: Respiratory depression. Frequent: Sedation.

NITROUS OXIDE (*Entonox*) ▶Respiratory ♀- ▶? Varies
ADULT — General anesthetic gas; specialized dosing.
PEDS — General anesthetic gas; specialized dosing.
NOTES — Always maintain at least 20% oxygen administration.
MOA — CNS depressant
ADVERSE EFFECTS — Serious: Apnea, malignant hyperthermia, pressure accumulation (middle ear, bowel obstruction, pneumothorax), abuse dependence. Frequent: Recovery N/V.

PENTOBARBITAL (*Nembutal*) ▶LK ♀D ▶? ⓒII $$$$$
ADULT — Rarely used; other drugs preferred. Hypnotic: 150 to 200 mg IM or 100 mg IV at a rate of 50 mg/min, maximum dose is 500 mg.
PEDS — FDA approved for active seizing, but other agents preferred.
UNAPPROVED PEDS — Procedural sedation: 1 to 6 mg/kg IV, adjusted in increments of 1 to 2 mg/kg to desired effect, or 2 to 6 mg/kg IM, max 100 mg. Do not exceed 50 mg/min.

MOA — Serious: Respiratory depression, blood dyscrasias, anemia, thrombocytopenia, Stevens-Johnson syndrome, angioedema, dependence, withdrawal reactions. Frequent: Drowsiness, fatigue, N/V bradycardia, paradoxical CNS excitation.

PROPOFOL (*Diprivan*) ▶L ♀B ▶– $
WARNING — Beware of respiratory depression/apnea. Administer with appropriate monitoring.
ADULT — Anesthesia (age younger than 55 yo): 40 mg IV q 10 sec until induction onset (typical 2 to 2.5 mg/kg). Follow with maintenance infusion generally 100 to 200 mcg/kg/min. Lower doses in elderly or for sedation. ICU ventilator sedation: Infusion 5 to 50 mcg/kg/min.
PEDS — Anesthesia age 3 yo or older: 2.5 to 3.5 mg/kg IV over 20 to 30 sec, followed with infusion 125 to 300 mcg/kg/min. Not recommended if age younger than 3 yo or for prolonged ICU use.
UNAPPROVED ADULT — Deep sedation: 1 mg/kg IV over 20 to 30 sec. Repeat 0.5 mg/kg IV prn. Intubation adjunct: 2.0 to 2.5 mg/kg IV.
UNAPPROVED PEDS — Deep sedation: 1 mg/kg IV (max 40 mg) over 20 to 30 sec. Repeat 0.5 mg/kg (max 20 mg) IV prn.
NOTES — Avoid with egg or soy allergies. Prolonged infusions may lead to hypertriglyceridemia. Injection pain can be treated or pretreated with lidocaine 40 to 50 mg IV.
MOA — Nonbarbiturate hypnotic without analgesic properties.
ADVERSE EFFECTS — Serious: Respiratory depression, hypotension, hypersensitivity. Frequent: Injection site pain, sedation.

REMIFENTANIL (*Ultiva*) ▶L ♀C ▶? ⓒII $$
ADULT — IV general anesthesia adjunct; specialized dosing.
PEDS — IV general anesthesia adjunct; specialized dosing.
MOA — Serious: Respiratory depression, hypotension, bradycardia, chest wall rigidity, opiate dependence, hypersensitivity. Frequent: Sedation, N/V.

SEVOFLURANE (*Ultane*, ✱*Sevorane*) ▶Respiratory/L ♀B ▶? Varies
ADULT — General anesthetic gas; specialized dosing.
PEDS — General anesthetic gas; specialized dosing.
NOTES — Minimum Alveolar Concentration (MAC) 2.05%. Known trigger of malignant hyperthermia; see mhaus.org.
MOA — CNS depressant
ADVERSE EFFECTS — Serious: Apnea, malignant hyperthermia. Frequent: Recovery N/V.

SUFENTANIL (*Sufenta*) ▶L ♀C ▶? ⓒII $$
ADULT — IV anesthesia adjunct: Specialized dosing.
PEDS — IV anesthesia adjunct: Specialized dosing.
MOA — Serious: Respiratory depression, hypotension, bradycardia, chest wall rigidity, opiate dependence, hypersensitivity. Frequent: Sedation, N/V.

ANESTHESIA: Local Anesthetics

NOTE: Risk of chondrolysis in patients receiving intra-articular infusions of local anesthetics following arthroscopic and other surgical procedures

ARTICAINE (*Septocaine, Zorcaine*) ▶LK ♀C ▶? $
ADULT — Dental local anesthesia: 4% injection.
PEDS — Dental local anesthesia age 4 yo or older: 4% injection.
FORMS — 4% (includes epinephrine 1:100,000).
NOTES — Do not exceed 7 mg/kg total dose.
MOA — Amide local anesthetic.
ADVERSE EFFECTS — Serious: Seizures, cardiovascular depression, bradycardia, hypersensitivity, methemoglobinemia. Frequent: None.

BUPIVACAINE (*Marcaine, Sensorcaine*) ▶LK ♀C ▶? $
ADULT — Local anesthesia, nerve block: 0.25% injection.
PEDS — Not recommended in children age younger than 12 yo.
FORMS — 0.25%, 0.5%, 0.75%, all with or without epinephrine.
NOTES — Onset 5 min, duration 2 to 4 h (longer with epi). Amide group. Max dose 2.5 mg/kg alone, or 3.0 mg/kg with epinephrine.
MOA — Amide local anesthetic.
ADVERSE EFFECTS — Serious: Seizures, cardiovascular depression, bradycardia, hypersensitivity, methemoglobinemia. Frequent: None.

BUPIVACAINE LIPOSOME (*Exparel*) ▶L - ♀C ▶– $$$$$
ADULT — Bunionectomy: Infiltrate 7 mL of EXPAREL into the tissues surrounding the osteotomy and 1 mL into the subcutaneous tissue for a total of 8 ml (106 mg). Hemorrhoidectomy: Dilute 20 mL (266 mg) of EXPAREL with 10 mL of saline, for a total of 30 mL, and divide the mixture into six 5 mL aliquots. Perform the anal block by visualizing the anal sphincter as a clock face and slowly infiltrating one aliquot to each of the even numbers. Do not inject other local anesthetics into the same site or inject through wet antiseptic on the skin. Dosing forms do not have pharmacologic bioequivalence to plain bupivacaine.
PEDS — Not approved for use age less than 18 yo.
FORMS — 10 and 20 ml single use vial, 1.3% (13.3 mg/mL)
MOA — Suspension of multivesicular liposomes containing bupivacaine that provides up to 72 hours of pain control.
ADVERSE EFFECTS — Significant systemic absorption with CNS and cardiovascular effects. Hypersensitivity. Intra-articular injections have resulted in chondrolysis. Caution for increase drug effect in hepatic and/or renal impairment as it is metabolized by the liver and cleared by the kidneys.

CHLOROPROCAINE (*Nesacaine*) ▶LK ♀C ▶? $
ADULT — Local and regional anesthesia: 1% to 3% injection.
PEDS — Local and regional anesthesia if 3 yo or older: 1% to 3% injection.
FORMS — 1, 2, 3%.
NOTES — Maximum local dose: 11 mg/kg

MOA — Ester local anesthetic
ADVERSE EFFECTS — Serious: Seizures, cardiovascular depression, bradycardia, hypersensitivity, methemoglobinemia. Frequent: None.

LIDOCAINE—LOCAL ANESTHETIC (*Xylocaine*) ▶LK ♀B ▶? $
ADULT — Local anesthesia: 0.5 to 1% injection. Without epinephrine: max dose 4.5 mg/kg not to exceed 300 mg. With epinephrine: max dose 7 mg/kg not exceed 500 mg. Dose for regional block varies by region.
PEDS — Local anesthesia: 0.5 to 1% injection.
FORMS — 0.5, 1, 1.5, 2%. With epi: 0.5, 1, 1.5, 2%.
NOTES — Onset within 2 min, duration 30 to 60 min (longer with epi). Amide group. Use "cardiac lidocaine" (ie, IV formulation) for Bier blocks at maximum dose of 3 mg/kg so that neither epinephrine nor methylparaben are injected IV.
MOA — Amide local anesthetic.
ADVERSE EFFECTS — Serious: Seizures, cardiovascular depression, bradycardia, hypersensitivity, methemoglobinemia. Frequent: None.

MEPIVACAINE (*Carbocaine, Polocaine*) ▶LK ♀C ▶? $
ADULT — Nerve block: 1% to 2% injection.
PEDS — Nerve block: 1% to 2% injection. Use less than 2% concentration if age younger than 3 yo or wt less than 30 pounds.
FORMS — 1, 1.5, 2, 3%.
NOTES — Onset 3 to 5 min, duration 45 to 90 min. Amide group. Max local dose 5 to 6 mg/kg.
MOA — Amide local anesthetic.
ADVERSE EFFECTS — Serious: Seizures, cardiovascular depression, bradycardia, hypersensitivity, methemoglobinemia, nephrotoxicity. Frequent: None.

ORAQIX (prilocaine + lidocaine–local anesthetic) ▶LK ♀B ▶? $
ADULT — Local anesthetic gel applied to periodontal pockets using blunt-tipped applicator: 4% injection.
PEDS — Not approved in children.
FORMS — Gel 2.5% + 2.5% with applicator.
NOTES — Do not exceed maximum dose for lidocaine or prilocaine.
MOA — Amide local anesthetic combination.
ADVERSE EFFECTS — Serious: Seizures, cardiovascular depression, bradycardia, hypersensitivity, methemoglobinemia. Frequent: None.

PRILOCAINE (*Citanest*) ▶LK ♀B ▶? $
ADULT — Nerve block and dental procedures: 4% injection.
PEDS — Nerve block and dental procedures, age older than 9 mo: 4% injection.
FORMS — 4%, 4% with epinephrine
NOTES — Contraindicated if younger than 6 to 9 mo. If younger than 5 yo, maximum local dose is 3 to 4 mg/kg (with or without epinephrine). If 5 yo or older, maximum local dose is 5 mg/kg without epinephrine and 7 mg/kg with epinephrine.

PRILOCAINE (cont.)
MOA — Amide local anesthetic
ADVERSE EFFECTS — Serious: Seizures, cardiovascular depression, bradycardia, hypersensitivity, methemoglobinemia. Frequent: None.
PROCAINE (Novocain) ▶Plasma ♀C ▶? $
ADULT — Local and regional anesthesia: 1% to 2% injection. Spinal anesthesia: 10%.
PEDS — Local and regional anesthesia: 1% to 2% injection. Spinal anesthesia: 10%.
FORMS — 1, 2, 10%.
MOA — Ester local anesthetic
ADVERSE EFFECTS — Serious: Seizures, cardiovascular depression, bradycardia, hypersensitivity, methemoglobinemia. Frequent: None.
ROPIVACAINE (Naropin) ▶LK ♀B ▶? $
WARNING — Inadvertent intravascular injection may result in arrhythmia or cardiac arrest.

ADULT — Local and regional anesthesia: 0.2% to 1% injection.
PEDS — Not approved in children.
FORMS — 0.2, 0.5, 0.75, 1%.
MOA — Amide local anesthetic
ADVERSE EFFECTS — Serious: Seizures, cardiovascular depression, bradycardia, hypersensitivity, methemoglobinemia. Frequent: None.
TETRACAINE (Pontocaine, ✸amethocaine) ▶Plasma ♀C ▶? $
ADULT — Spinal anesthesia.
PEDS — Not approved in children.
FORMS — Injection: 1%
MOA — Ester local anesthetic
ADVERSE EFFECTS — Serious: Seizures, cardiovascular depression, bradycardia, hypersensitivity, methemoglobinemia. Frequent: None.

ANESTHESIA: Neuromuscular Blockade Reversal Agents

NEOSTIGMINE (Bloxiverz) ▶L ♀C ▶? $$$$
ADULT — Reversal of nondepolarizing neuromuscular blocking agents:0.03 to 0.07 mg/kg slow IV (preceded by atropine or glycopyrrolate). Max 0.07 mg/kg or 5 mg whichever is less.
PEDS — Reversal of non depolarizing neuromuscular blocking agents: Use adult dosing.

MOA — Reversible cholinesterase inhibitor.
ADVERSE EFFECTS — Serious: Cholinergic toxicity, respiratory paralysis, bronchospasm, arrhythmias, cardiac arrest, seizures. Frequent: N/V, diarrhea, abdominal cramping, dizziness, headache, muscle cramps/weakness, fasciculations, hypersalivation, increased bronchial secretions, miosis.

ANESTHESIA: Neuromuscular Blockers

NOTE: Should be administered only by those skilled in airway management and respiratory support.

ATRACURIUM (Tracrium) ▶Plasma ♀C ▶? $
ADULT — Paralysis: 0.4 to 0.5 mg/kg IV.
PEDS — Paralysis age 2 yo or older: 0.4 to 0.5 mg/kg IV.
NOTES — Duration 15 to 30 min. Hoffman degradation.
MOA — Nondepolarizing skeletal muscle relaxant.
ADVERSE EFFECTS — Serious: Apnea, bronchospasm, hypersensitivity. Frequent: Apnea, rash.
CISATRACURIUM (Nimbex) ▶Plasma ♀B ▶? $
ADULT — Paralysis: 0.15 to 0.2 mg/kg IV.
PEDS — Paralysis: 0.1 mg/kg IV over 5 to 10 sec.
NOTES — Duration 30 to 60 min. Hoffman degradation.
MOA — Nondepolarizing skeletal muscle relaxant.
ADVERSE EFFECTS — Serious: Apnea, bradycardia, bronchospasm. Frequent: Apnea.
PANCURONIUM (Pavulon) ▶LK ♀C ▶? $
ADULT — Paralysis: 0.04 to 0.1 mg/kg IV.
PEDS — Paralysis (beyond neonatal age): 0.04 to 0.1 mg/kg IV.
NOTES — Duration 45 min. Decrease dose if renal disease.
MOA — Nondepolarizing skeletal muscle relaxant.
ADVERSE EFFECTS — Serious: Apnea, hypersensitivity, bronchospasm. Frequent: Apnea, tachycardia.
ROCURONIUM (Zemuron) ▶L ♀B ▶? $$
ADULT — Paralysis: 0.6 mg/kg IV. Rapid sequence intubation: 0.6 to 1.2 mg/kg IV. Continuous

infusion: 10 to 12 mcg/kg/min; first verify spontaneous recovery from bolus dose.
PEDS — Paralysis (age older than 3 mo): 0.6 mg/kg IV. Continuous infusion: 12 mcg/kg/min; first verify spontaneous recovery from bolus dose.
NOTES — Duration 30 min. Decrease dose if severe liver disease.
MOA — Nondepolarizing skeletal muscle relaxant.
ADVERSE EFFECTS — Serious: Apnea, bronchospasm. Frequent: Apnea.
SUCCINYLCHOLINE (Anectine, Quelicin) ▶Plasma ♀C ▶? $
ADULT — Paralysis : 0.6 to 1.1 mg/kg IV.
PEDS — Paralysis age younger than 5 yo: 2 mg/kg IV. Paralysis age 5 yo or older: 1 mg/kg IV.
NOTES — Avoid in hyperkalemia, myopathies, eye injuries, rhabdomyolysis, subacute burn, and syndromes of denervated or disused musculature (eg, paralysis from spinal cord injury or major CVA). If immediate cardiac arrest and ET tube is in correct place and no tension pneumothorax evident, strongly consider empiric treatment for hyperkalemia. Succinylcholine can trigger malignant hyperthermia; see www.mhaus.org.
MOA — Ultra-short acting depolarizing skeletal muscle relaxant.
ADVERSE EFFECTS — Serious: Apnea, bradycardia, hyperkalemia, malignant hyperthermia. Frequent: Apnea, fasciculations, muscle pain.

VECURONIUM (*Norcuron*) ▶LK ♀C ▶? $

ADULT — Paralysis: 0.08 to 0.1 mg/kg IV bolus. Continuous infusion: 0.8 to 1.2 mcg/kg/min; first verify spontaneous recovery from bolus dose.

PEDS — Age younger than 7 weeks: Safety has not been established. Age 7 weeks to 1 yo: Moderately more sensitive on a mg/kg dose compared to adults and take 1.5 for longer to recover. Age 1 to 10 yo: May require a slightly higher initial dose and may also require supplementation slightly more often than older patients. Paralysis age 10 yo or older: 0.08 to 0.1 mg/kg IV bolus. Continuous infusion: 0.8 to 1.2 mcg/kg/min; first verify spontaneous recovery from bolus dose.

NOTES — Duration 15 to 30 min. Decrease dose in severe liver disease.

MOA — Nondepolarizing skeletal muscle relaxant.

ADVERSE EFFECTS — Serious: Apnea. Frequent: Apnea.

ANTIMICROBIALS

ANTIVIRAL DRUGS FOR INFLUENZA

ANTIVIRAL DRUGS FOR INFLUENZA	Treatment* (Duration of 5 days)	Prevention (Duration of 7 to 10 days post-exposure)[†]
OSELTAMIVIR (*Tamiflu*)		
Adults and adolescents age 13 years and older		
	75 mg PO bid	75 mg PO once daily
Children, 1 year of age and older[‡]		
Body weight ≤15 kg	30 mg PO bid	30 mg PO once daily
Body weight >15 to 23 kg	45 mg PO bid	45 mg PO once daily
Body weight >23 to 40 kg	60 mg PO bid	60 mg PO once daily
Body weight >40 kg	75 mg PO bid	75 mg PO once daily
Infants, newborn to 11 months of age[‡]		
Age 3 to 11 months old[‖]	3 mg/kg/dose PO bid	3 mg/kg/dose PO only daily
Age younger than 3 months old[§]	3 mg/kg/dose PO bid	Not for routine prophylaxis in infants <3 months old
ZANAMIVIR (*Relenza*)**		
Adults and children (age 7 years and older for treatment, age 5 years and older for prophylaxis)		
	10 mg (two 5-mg inhalations) bid	10 mg (two 5-mg inhalations) once daily

(cont.)

ANTIVIRAL DRUGS FOR INFLUENZA (*continued*)

Adapted from http://www.cdc.gov/flu/professionals/antivirals/summary-clinicians.htm.

*Start treatment as soon as possible; benefit is greatest when started within 2 days of symptom onset. Consider longer treatment for patients who remain severely ill after 5 days of treatment.

†Duration is 10 days after household exposure, and 7 days after most recent known exposure in other situations. For long-term care facilities and hospitals, prophylaxis should last a minimum of 14 days and up to 7 days after the most recent known case was identified.

‡Oseltamivir is FDA-approved for treatment of influenza in infants 2 weeks of age and older and prevention of influenza in children 1 year of age and older. Tamiflu prescribing information contains instructions for pharmacists to compound a 6 mg/mL suspension when Tamiflu suspension is not available. Tamiflu suspension is provided with a 10 mL oral dispenser measured in mL. Capsules can be opened and the contents mixed with sweetened fluids to mask bitter taste. Make sure units of measure on dosing instructions match dosing device provided.

¶AAP (http://pediatrics.aappublications.org/content/early/2014/09/17/peds.2014-2413) recommends that infants age 9 to 11 mo receive oseltamivir 3.5 mg/kg/dose PO bid for treatment and 3.5 mg/kg/dose PO once daily for chemoprophylaxis. The recommendation is based on data from the CASG 114 study that suggests a higher dose is necessary to obtain adequate oseltamivir exposure in this age group. There is no evidence to suggest that the higher dose is more effective or causes more adverse effects than the usual dose.

§This dose is not intended for premature infants. Immature renal function may lead to slow clearance and high concentrations of oseltamivir in this age group.

**Zanamivir should not be used by patients with underlying pulmonary disease. Do not attempt to use *Relenza* in a nebulizer or ventilator; lactose in the formulation may cause the device to malfunction.

bid=two times per day.

PROPHYLAXIS FOR BACTERIAL ENDOCARDITIS*

Limited to dental or respiratory tract procedures in patients at highest risk. All regimens are single dose administered 30–60 minutes prior to procedure.	
Standard regimen	Amoxicillin 2 g PO
Unable to take oral meds	Ampicillin 2 g IM/IV; or cefazolin† or ceftriaxone† 1 g IM/IV
Allergic to penicillin	Clindamycin 600 mg PO; or cephalexin† 2 g PO; or azithromycin or clarithromycin 500 mg PO
Allergic to penicillin and unable to take oral meds	Clindamycin 600 mg IM/IV; or cefazolin† or ceftriaxone† 1 g IM/IV
Pediatric drug doses	Pediatric dose should not exceed adult dose. Amoxicillin 50 mg/kg, ampicillin 50 mg/kg, azithromycin 15 mg/kg, cephalexin† 50 mg/kg, cefazolin† 50 mg/kg, ceftriaxone† 50 mg/kg, clarithromycin 15 mg/kg, clindamycin 20 mg/kg.

*For additional details of the 2007 AHA guidelines, see http://www.americanheart.org.

†Avoid cephalosporins if prior penicillin-associated anaphylaxis, angioedema, or urticaria.

OVERVIEW OF BACTERIAL PATHOGENS (Selected)

By bacterial class

<u>Gram-positive aerobic cocci:</u> Staphylococci: *S. epidermidis* (coagulase-negative), *S. aureus* (coagulase-positive); Streptococci: *S.pneumoniae* (*pneumococcus*), *S.pyogenes* (Group A), *S. agalactiae* (Group B), *enterococcus*
<u>Gram-positive aerobic/facultatively anaero bicbacilli:</u> *Bacillus,Corynebacterium diphtheriae, Erysipelothrix rhusiopathiae, Listeria monocytogenes, Nocardia*
<u>Gram-negative aerobic diplococci:</u> *Moraxella catarrhalis, Neisseria gonorrhoeae, Neisseria meningitidis*
<u>Gram-negative aerobic coccobacilli:</u> *Haemophilus ducreyi, H. influenzae*
<u>Gram-negative aerobic bacilli:</u> *Acinetobacter, Bartonella* species, *Bordetell apertussis, Brucella, Burkholderia cepacia, Campylobacter, Francisella tularensis, Helicobacter pylori, Legionella pneumophila, Pseudomonas aeruginosa, Stenotrophomonas maltophilia, Vibrio cholerae, Yersinia*
<u>Gram-negative facultativelyan aerobic bacilli:</u> *Aeromonas hydrophila, Eikenella corrodens, Pasteurella multocida*; Enterobacteriaceae: *E. coli, Citrobacter, Shigella, Salmonella, Klebsiella, Enterobacter, Hafnia, Serratia, Proteus, Providencia*
<u>**Anaerobes:**</u> *Actinomyces, Bacteroides fragilis,Clostridium botulinum,Clostridium difficile, Clostridium perfringens, Clostridium tetani, Fusobacterium, Lactobacillus, Peptostreptococcus*
<u>**Defective Cell Wall Bacteria:**</u> *Chlamydia pneumoniae, Chlamydia psittaci, Chlamydia trachomatis, Coxiella burnetii, Mycoplasma pneumoniae, Rickettsia prowazekii, Rickettsia rickettsii, Rickettsia typhi, Ureaplasma urealyticum*
<u>**Spirochetes:**</u> *Borrelia burgdorferi, Leptospira, Treponema pallidum*
<u>**Mycobacteria:**</u> *M. avium* complex, *M. kansasii, M. leprae, M. tuberculosis*

By bacterial name

Acinetobacter **Gram-negative aerobic bacilli**
Actinomyces **Anaerobes**
Aeromonas hydrophila **Gram-negative facultatively anaerobic bacilli**
Bacillus **Gram-positive aerobic/facultatively anaerobic bacilli**
Bacteroides fragilis **Anaerobes**
Bartonella species **Gram-negative aerobic bacilli**
Bordetella pertussis **Gram-negative aerobic bacilli**
Borrelia burgdorferi **Spirochetes**
Brucella **Gram-negative aerobic bacilli**
Burkholderia cepacia **Gram-negative aerobic bacilli**
Campylobacter **Gram-negative aerobic bacilli**
Chlamydia pneumoniae **Defective cell wall bacteria**
Chlamydia psittaci **Defective cell wall bacteria**
Chlamydia trachomatis **Defective cell wall bacteria**
Citrobacter **Gram-negative facultatively anaerobic bacilli**
Clostridium botulinum **Anaerobes**
Clostridium difficile **Anaerobes**
Clostridium perfringens **Anaerobes**
Clostridium tetani **Anaerobes**

(cont.)

OVERVIEW OF BACTERIAL PATHOGENS (*continued*)

Corynebacterium diphtheriae Gram-positive aerobic/facultatively anaerobicb acilli
Coxiella burnetii Defective cell wal lbacteria
E. coli Gram-negative facultatively anaerobic bacilli
Eikenella corrodens Gram-negative facultatively anaerobic bacilli
Enterobacter Gram-negative facultatively anaerobic bacilli
Enterobacteriaceae Gram-negative facultatively anaerobic bacilli
Enterococcus Gram-positive aerobic cocci
Erysipelothrix rhusiopathiae Gram-positive aerobic/facultatively anaerobic bacilli
Francisella tularensis Gram-negative aerobic bacilli
Fusobacterium Anaerobes
Haemophilus ducreyi Gram-negative aerobic coccobacilli
Haemophilus influenzae Gram-negative aerobic coccobacilli
Hafnia Gram-negative facultatively anaerobic bacilli
Helicobacter pylori Gram-negative aerobic bacilli
Klebsiella Gram-negative facultatively anaerobic bacilli
Lactobacillus Anaerobes
Legionella pneumophila Gram-negative aerobic bacilli
Leptospira Spirochetes
Listeria monocytogenes Gram-positive aerobic/facultatively anaerobic bacilli
M. avium complex Mycobacteria
M. kansasii Mycobacteria
M. leprae Mycobacteria
M. tuberculosis Mycobacteria
Moraxella catarrhalis Gram-negative aerobic diplococci
Myocoplasma pneumoniae Defective cell wall bacteria
Neisseriag onorrhoeae Gram-negative aerobic diplococci
Neisseria meningitidis Gram-negative aerobi cdiplococci
Nocardia Gram-positiv eaerobic/facultatively anaerobic bacilli
Pasteurella multocida Gram-negative facultatively anaerobic bacilli
Peptostreptococcus Anaerobes
Pneumococcus Gram-positive aerobic cocci
Proteus Gram-negative facultatively anaerobic bacilli
Providencia Gram-negativef acultatively anaerobic bacilli
Pseudomonas aeruginosa Gram-negative aerobic bacilli
Rickettsiap rowazekii Defective cell wall bacteria
Rickettsia rickettsii Defective cell wall bacteria
Rickettsia typhi Defective cell wal lbacteria
Salmonella Gram-negative facultatively anaerobic bacilli
Serratia Gram-negative facultatively anaerobic bacilli
Shigella Gram-negative facultatively anaerobic bacilli
Staph aureus (coagulase positive) Gram-positiv eaerobic cocci
Staph epidermidis (coagulasenegative) Gram-positive aerobic cocci
Stenotrophomonas maltophilia Gram-negative aerobic bacilli
Strep agalactiae (Group B) Gram-positive aerobic cocci
Strep pneumoniae (pneumococcus) Gram-positive aerobi ccocci

(cont.)

OVERVIEW OF BACTERIAL PATHOGENS (*continued*)

Strep pyogenes (GroupA) **Gram-positive aerobic cocci**
Streptococci **Gram-positive aerobic cocci**
Treponema pallidum **Spirochetes**
Ureaplasma urealyticum **Defective cell wall bacteria**
Vibrio cholerae **Gram-negative aerobic bacilli**
Yersinia **Gram-negative aerobic bacilli**

ACUTE BACTERIAL SINUSITIS IN ADULTS AND CHILDREN[§] IDSA TREATMENT RECOMMENDATIONS

Initial therapy in patients without risk factors for resistance and infection of mild to moderate severity	
Adults: Amoxicillin-clavulanate 500 mg /125 mg PO three times per day or 875 mg/125 mg PO two times per day for 5 to 7 days	Peds: Amoxicillin-clavulanate§ 45 mg /kg/day PO two times per day for 10 to 14 days
Initial therapy in patients with severe infection, risk factors for resistance,[†] or high endemic rate of invasive penicillin-nonsusceptible *S. pneumoniae* (≥10%)	
Adults: Treat for 5 to 7 days with: 1) Amoxicillin-clavulanate* 2000 mg /125 mg PO two times per day 2) Doxycycline 100 mg PO two times per day or 200 mg PO once daily	Peds: Amoxicillin-clavulanate* 90 mg/kg/day PO two times per day for 10 to 14 days
Beta-lactam allergy	
Adults: Treat for 5 to 7 days with: 1) Doxycycline 100 mg PO two times per day or 200 mg PO once daily 2) Levofloxacin 500 mg PO once daily 3) Moxifloxacin 400 mg PO once daily	Peds, type 1 hypersensitivity: Levofloxacin 10 to 20 mg/kg/day PO divided q 12-24 h for 10 to 14 days Peds, not type 1 hypersensitivity: Clindamycin[‡] 30 to 40 mg/kg/day PO divided three times per day plus cefixime 8 mg/kg/day PO divided two times per day or cefpodoxime 10 mg/kg/day PO divided two times per day for 10 to 14 days
Risk factors for antibiotic resistance[†] or failed first-line therapy	
Adults: Treat for 5 to 7 days with: 1) Amoxicillin-clavulanate* 2000 mg /125 mg PO two times per day 2) Levofloxacin 500 mg PO once daily 3) Moxifloxacin 400 mg PO once daily	Peds: Treat for 10 to 14 days with: 1) Amoxicillin-clavulanate* 90 mg/kg/day PO divided two times per day 2) Clindamycin[‡] 30 to 40 mg/kg/day PO divided three times per day plus cefixime 8 mg/kg/day PO divided two times per day or cefpodoxime 10 mg/kg/day PO divided two times per day 3) Levofloxacin 10 to 20 mg/kg/day PO divided q 12 to 24 h
Severe infection requiring hospitalization	
Adults: 1) Ampicillin-sulbactam 1.5 to 3 g IV q 6 h 2) Levofloxacin 500 mg PO/IV once daily 3) Moxifloxacin 400 mg PO/IV once daily 4) Ceftriaxone 1 to 2 g IV q 12 to 24 h 5) Cefotaxime 2 g IV q 4 to 6 h	Peds: 1) Ampicillin-sulbactam 200 to 400 mg /kg/day IV q 6 h 2) Ceftriaxone 50 mg/kg/day IV q 12 h 3) Cefotaxime 100 to 200 mg/kg/day IV q 6 h 4) Levofloxacin 10 to 20 mg/kg/day IV q 12 to 24 h

Adapted from *Clin Infect Dis* 2012;54(8):e72-ell2. Available online at: http://www.idsociety.org.

(cont.)

ACUTE BACTERIAL SINUSITIS IN ADULTS AND CHILDREN§ IDSA TREATMENT RECOMMENDATIONS (*continued*)

* High-dose amoxicillin-clavulanate recommended for geographic regions with high endemic rates (at least 10%) of invasive penicillin-nonsusceptible *S. pneumoniae*, those with severe infection (e.g., evidence of systemic toxicity with fever of 39°C or higher, and threat of suppurative complications), or risk factors for antibiotic resistance. Use the 14:1 formulation of amoxicillin-clavulanate that provides amoxicillin 90 mg/kg/day and clavulanate 6.4 mg/kg/day. In Canada, the 14:1 formulation of amoxicillin-clavulanate is not available, so it is necessary to give the 7:1 formulation with additional amoxicillin. Do not increase the dose of the 4:1 or 7:1 amoxicillin-clavulanate formulation in order to achieve a higher dose of amoxicillin; this strategy gives an excessive dose of clavulanate which increases the risk of diarrhea.

† Risk factors for antibiotic resistance include attendance at daycare, age younger than 2 yo or older than 65 yo, recent hospitalization, antibiotic use within the past month, or patients who are immunocompromised.

‡ Clindamycin resistance in *S. pneumoniae* is common in some areas of the United States.

§ American Academy of Pediatrics guideline for management of sinusitis in children (*Pediatrics* 2013; 132:e262–e280;available online at: http://pediatrics.aappublications.org) recommends amoxicillin as first-line treatment of uncomplicated acute sinusitis when antimicrobial resistance is not suspected. Amoxicillin 45 mg/kg/day divided two times per day is recommended for mild-moderate sinusitis in children 2 years old or older who do not attend daycare and have not been treated with an antibiotic in the last 4 weeks. Amoxicillin 80 to 90 mg/kg/day divided two times daily (max 2 g/dose) is recommended in communities with a high prevalence of nonsusceptible *S. pneumoniae* (at least 10%). Amoxicillin-clavulanate 80 to 90 mg/kg/day divided two times per day (max 2 g/dose) is an option for moderate-severe sinusitis, and sinusitis in children less than 2 years old, attending daycare, or who have received an antibiotic in the last 4 weeks.

C. difficile Infection (CDI) in Adults: IDSA/SHEA and ACG Treatment Recommendations		
Severity initial episode	**Clinical signs**	**Treatment**
Mild to moderate	IDSA: WBC ≤15,000 AND serum creatinine <1.5 times premorbid level ACG: Diarrhea with signs or symptoms not meeting severe or complicated criteria	Metronidazole 500 mg PO q8h for 10 to 14 days[a] ACG: If unable to take metronidazole, use vancomycin 125 mg PO q6h for 10 days. If no response to metronidazole in 5 to 7 days, consider vancomycin.
Severe[b]	IDSA: WBC ≥15,000 OR serum creatinine ≥1.5 times premorbid level ACG: Serum albumin <3 g/dL plus ONE of the following: • WBC ≥15,000 • Abdominal tenderness	Vancomycin 125 mg PO q6h for 10 to 14 days[a]
Severe and complicated[b]	IDSA: Hypotension or shock, ileus, megacolon ACG: Any of the following attributable to CDI: • ICU admission for CDI • Hypotension +/- required use of vasopressors • Fever ≥38.5°C • Ileus or significant abdominal distention • Mental status changes • WBC ≥35,000 or <2000 • Serum lactate >2.2 mmol/L End organ failure (mechanical ventilation, renal failure, etc)	Vancomycin 500 mg PO/NG q6h plus metronidazole 500 mg IV q8h IDSA: Consider adding vancomycin 500 mg/100 mL[c] normal saline retention enema q6h if complete ileus. ACG: Add vancomycin 500 mg/500 mL[c] normal saline enema q6h if complicated CDI with ileus or toxic colon and/or significant abdominal distention.

ACUTE BACTERIAL SINUSITIS IN ADULTS AND CHILDREN[§] IDSA TREATMENT RECOMMENDATIONS (*continued*)

Recurrent episodes		
First recurrence	---	Same as initial episode, stratified by severity. IDSA: Use vancomycin if WBC ≥15,000 or serum creatinine is increasing.
Second recurrence	---	Vancomycin taper and/or pulsed regimen[d]

Adapted from: *Infect Control Hosp Epidemiol* 2010;31:431. Available online at: http://www.idsociety.org. *Am J Gastroenterol* 2013;108:478–98. Available online at: http://gi.org.

[a]ACG recommends 10 days of therapy on the basis that clinical trials only evaluated 10 days of treatment.

[b]IDSA: Consider colectomy in patients with severe CDI. ACG: Get surgical consultation for patients with complicated CDI. Consider surgery for patients with any of the following attributed to CDI: hypotension requiring vasopressors; clinical signs of sepsis and organ dysfunction (renal and pulmonary); mental status changes; WBC ≥50,000; lactate ≥5 mmol/L; or failure to improve on medical therapy after 5 days.

[c]IDSA recommends diluting vancomycin in 100 mL for administration as enema. ACG recommends diluting vancomycin in a larger volume (500 mL) in order to ensure delivery to ascending and transverse colon.

[d]IDSA taper example: Vancomycin 125 mg PO QID for 10 to 14 days, then 125 mg two times per day for 7 days, then 125 mg once daily for 7 days, then 125 mg every 2 or 3 days for 2 to 8 weeks. ACG proposed pulse regimen: Vancomycin 125 mg PO q6h for 10 days, then 125 mg once every 3 days for 10 doses. Note: If there is a third recurrence after a pulsed vancomycin regimen, ACG recommends considering fecal microbiota transplant.

ACUTE OTITIS MEDIA (AOM) IN CHILDREN: AMERICAN ACADEMY OF PEDIATICS TREATMENT RECOMMENDATIONS

Initial Treatment (immediate or delayed[b])	
First-line	**First-line if penicillin-allergic[d]**
Amoxicillin 80 to 90 mg/kg/day PO divided 2 times per day[a] OR Amoxicillin-clavulanate[c] 90 mg/kg/day PO divided 2 times per day[a]	Cefdinir 14 mg/kg/day PO divided 1 or 2 times per day[a] OR Cefuroxime 30 mg/kg/day PO divided 2 times per day[a] OR Cefpodoxime 10 mg/kg/day PO divided 2 times per day[a] OR Ceftriaxone 50 mg IM/IV once daily for 1 or 3 days
Treatment After First Antibiotic Failure	
If initial treatment was amoxicillin, use amoxicillin-clavulanate[c] 90 mg/kg/day PO divided 2 times per day.[a] If initial treatment was amoxicillin-clavulanate or oral third-generation cephalosporin, use ceftriaxone 50 mg IM/IV once daily for 3 days. Consider clindamycin 30 to 40 mg/kg/day PO divided 3 times per day ± third-generation cephalosporin if penicillin-resistant *S pneumoniae* suspected.[a]	

(cont.)

ACUTE OTITIS MEDIA (AOM) IN CHILDREN: AMERICAN ACADEMY OF PEDIATICS TREATMENT RECOMMENDATIONS (*continued*)

Treatment After Second Antibiotic Failure
Clindamycin 30 to 40 mg/kg/day PO divided 3 times per day + 3rd-generation cephalosporin.[a]   Consider tympanocentesis and consult infectious diseases specialist if multidrug-resistant bacteria detected.

Adapted from *Pediatrics* 2013;131:e964−e999. Available online at: http://pediatrics.aappublications.org.

[a]The duration of oral treatment is 10 days for age <2 yo and children of any age with severe symptoms, 7 days for age 2 to 5 yo with mild to moderate symptoms, and 5 to 7 days for age ≥6 yo with mild to moderate symptoms.

[b]This guideline is for uncomplicated AOM in children age 6 mo to 12 yo. Immediate treatment is recommended for children with otorrhea or severe symptoms (moderate to severe pain, pain for ≥48 h, or temperature ≥39°C), and bilateral AOM in children age 6 to 23 mo. Observation for 48 to 72 h before antibiotic therapy is an option for children age 6 to 23 mo with unilateral AOM and mild symptoms (mild pain for <48 h and temperature <39°C), or children 2 yo and older with unilateral/bilateral AOM and mild symptoms. Observation must have mechanism for follow-up and initiation of antibiotic if child worsens or does not improve within 48 to 72 h of symptom onset. Do not use observation if follow-up is unsure.

[c]Consider in patients who have received amoxicillin in the past 30 days or who have the otitis-conjunctivitis syndrome. Use the 14:1 formulation of amoxicillin-clavulanate that provides amoxicillin 90 mg/kg/day and clavulanate 6.4 mg/kg/day. In Canada, the 14:1 formulation of amoxicillin-clavulanate is not available, so it is necessary to give the 7:1 ratio formulation with additional amoxicillin. Do not increase the dose of a 4:1 or 7:1 amoxicillin-clavulanate formulation in order to achieve a higher dose of amoxicillin; this strategy gives an excessive dose of clavulanate which increases the risk of diarrhea.

[d]Cefdinir, cefuroxime, cefpodoxime, and ceftriaxone are highly unlikely to cross-react with penicillin. Excluding patients with a history of a severe reaction, the reaction rate in patients who have not undergone penicillin skin testing is estimated at 0.1%. A drug allergy practice parameter (*Ann Allergy Asthma Immunol* 2010;105:259−73; available at http://www.allergyparameters.org) recommends that a cephalosporin can be given to patients who do not have a history of a severe and/or recent allergic reaction to penicillin. Options for patients with a history of an IgE-mediated reaction to penicillin include substitution of a non-beta-lactam antibiotic, or the performance of penicillin or cephalosporin skin testing to evaluate the risk of cephalosporin administration.

SEXUALLY TRANSMITTED DISEASES & VAGINITIS*

Bacterial vaginosis	(1) metronidazole 5 g of 0.75% gel intravaginally daily for 5 days OR 500 mg PO two times per day for 7 days; (2) clindamycin 5 g of 2% cream intravaginally at bedtime for 7 days. Alternative: tinidazole 2 g PO once daily for 2 days OR 1 g PO once daily for 5 days. In pregnancy: (1) metronidazole 500 mg PO two times per day for 7 days OR 250 mg PO three times per day for 7 days; (2) clindamycin 300 mg PO two times per day for 7 days.
Candidal vaginitis	(1) intravaginal butoconazole, clotrimazole, miconazole, terconazole, or tioconazole; (2) fluconazole 150 mg PO single dose.
Chancroid	(1) azithromycin 1 g PO single dose; (2) ceftriaxone 250 mg IM single dose; (3) ciprofloxacin 500 mg PO two times per day for 3 days.
Chlamydia	First-line: either azithromycin 1 g PO single dose or doxycycline 100 mg PO two times per day for 7 days. Second-line: fluoroquinolones or erythromycin. In pregnancy: (1) azithromycin 1 g PO single dose; (2) amoxicillin 500 mg PO three times per day for 7 days. Repeat NAAT[†] 3 weeks after treatment in pregnant women.

(cont.)

SEXUALLY TRANSMITTED DISEASES & VAGINITIS* (*continued*)

Epididymitis	(1) ceftriaxone 250 mg IM single dose + doxycycline 100 mg PO two times per day for 10 days; (2) ofloxacin 300 mg PO two times per day or levofloxacin 500 mg PO daily for 10 days if enteric organisms suspected, or negative gonococcal culture or NAAT.[‡]
Gonorrhea	First-line: ceftriaxone 250 mg IM single dose + azithromycin 1 g PO single dose (preferred) or doxycycline 100 mg PO two times per day for 7 days. Second-line, if ceftriaxone is unavailable: cefixime 400 mg PO (not for pharyngeal) + azithromycin (preferred)/doxycycline.[‡] Test-of-cure (culture and sensitivity preferred over NAAT[†]) required for cefixime. Consult infectious diseases expert if severe cephalosporin allergy.
Gonorrhea, disseminated	Initially treat with ceftriaxone 1 g IM/IV q 24 h until 24 to 48 h after improvement. Second-line alternatives: (1) cefotaxime 1 g IV q 8 h; (2) ceftizoxime 1 g IV q 8 h. Complete at least 1 week of treatment with cefixime tabs 400 mg PO two times per day.
Gonorrhea, meningitis	Ceftriaxone 1 to 2 g IV q 12 h for 10 to 14 days.
Gonorrhea, endocarditis	Ceftriaxone 1 to 2 g IV q 12 h for at least 4 weeks.
Granuloma inguinale	Doxycycline 100 mg PO two times per day for at least 3 weeks and until lesions completely healed. Alternative azithromycin 1 g PO once weekly for at least 3 weeks and until lesions completely healed.
Herpes simplex, genital, first episode	(1) acyclovir 400 mg PO three times per day for 7 to 10 days; (2) famciclovir 250 mg PO three times per day for 7 to 10 days; (3) valacyclovir 1 g PO two times per day for 7 to 10 days.
Herpes simplex, genital, recurrent	(1) acyclovir 400 mg PO three times per day for 5 days; (2) acyclovir 800 mg PO three times per day for 2 days or two times per day for 5 days; (3) famciclovir 125 mg PO two times per day for 5 days; (4) famciclovir 1 g PO two times per day for 1 day; (5) famciclovir 500 mg PO for 1 dose, then 250 mg PO two times per day for 2 days; (6) valacyclovir 500 mg PO two times per day for 3 days; (7) valacyclovir 1 g PO daily for 5 days.
Herpes simplex, suppressive therapy	(1) acyclovir 400 mg PO two times per day; (2) famciclovir 250 mg PO two times per day; (3) valacyclovir 500 to 1000 mg PO daily. Valacyclovir 500 mg PO for daily may be less effective than other valacyclovir/acyclovir regimens in patients who have 10 or more recurrences per year.
Herpes simplex, prevention of transmission	For patients with no more than 9 recurrences per year: valacyclovir 500 mg PO daily by source partner, in conjunction with safer sex practices.
Herpes simplex, genital, recurrent in HIV infection	(1) acyclovir 400 mg PO three times per day for 5 to 10 days; (2) famciclovir 500 mg PO two times per day for 5 to 10 days; (3) valacyclovir 1 g PO two times per day for 5 to 10 days.
Herpes, suppressive therapy in HIV infection	(1) acyclovir 400 to 800 mg PO two to three times per day; (2) famciclovir 500 mg PO two times per day; (3) valacyclovir 500 mg PO two times per day.

(cont.)

SEXUALLY TRANSMITTED DISEASES & VAGINITIS* (*continued*)

Lympho-granuloma venereum	(1) doxycycline 100 mg PO two times per day for 21 days. Alternative: erythromycin base 500 mg PO four times per day for 21 days.
Pelvic inflammatory disease (PID), inpatient regimens	(1) cefoxitin 2 g IV q 6 h + doxycycline 100 mg IV/PO q 12 h; (2) clindamycin 900 mg IV q 8 h + gentamicin 2 mg/kg IM/IV loading dose, then 1.5 mg/kg IM/IV q 8 h (can substitute 3 to 5 mg/kg once-daily dosing). Can switch to PO therapy within 24 h of improvement.
Pelvic inflammatory disease (PID), outpatient treatment	Ceftriaxone 250 mg IM single dose + doxycycline 100 mg PO two times per day +/− metronidazole 500 mg PO two times per day for 14 days.
Proctitis, proctocolitis, enteritis	Ceftriaxone 250 mg IM single dose + doxycycline 100 mg PO two times per day for 7 days.
Sexual assault prophylaxis	Ceftriaxone 250 mg IM single dose + metronidazole 2 g PO single dose + azithromycin 1 g PO single dose/doxycycline 100 mg PO two times per day for 7 days.
Syphilis, primary, secondary, or early latent, i.e., duration less than 1 year	(1) benzathine penicillin 2.4 million units IM single dose. (2) doxycycline 100 mg PO two times per day for 2 weeks if penicillin-allergic.
Syphilis, late latent or unknown duration	(1) benzathine penicillin 2.4 million units IM q week for three doses; (2) doxycycline 100 mg PO two times per day for 4 weeks if penicillin-allergic.
Syphilis, tertiary	Benzathine penicillin 2.4 million units IM q week for three doses. Consult infectious disease specialist for management of penicillin-allergic patients.
Syphilis, neuro	(1) penicillin G 18 to 24 million units/day continuous IV infusion or 3 to 4 million units IV q 4 h for 10 to 14 days; (2) if compliance can be ensured, consider procaine penicillin 2.4 million units IM daily + probenecid 500 mg PO four times per day, both for 10 to 14 days.
Syphilis in pregnancy	Treat only with penicillin regimen for stage of syphilis as noted above. For primary, secondary, or early latent syphilis in pregnancy, some experts recommend a second dose of benzathine penicillin 2.4 million units. IM one week after the initial dose. Use penicillin-desensitization protocol if penicillin-allergic.
Trichomoniasis	Metronidazole (can use in pregnancy) or tinidazole, each 2 g PO single dose.
Urethritis, Cervicitis	Test for chlamydia and gonorrhea with NAAT.[†] Treat based on test results or treat presumptively if high risk of infection (chlamydia: age 25 yo or younger, new/multiple sex partners, or unprotected sex; gonorrhea: population prevalence greater than 5%), esp. if NAAT[‡] unavailable or patient unlikely to return for follow-up.

SEXUALLY TRANSMITTED DISEASES & VAGINITIS* (*continued*)

Urethritis, persistent/ recurrent	Metronidazole/tinidazole 2 g PO single dose + azithromycin 1 g PO single dose (if not used in 1st episode).

*MMWR 2010;59:RR-12 or http://www.cdc.gov/STD/treatment/ and *MMWR* 2012;61(31):590. Treat sexual partners for all except herpes, *Candida*, and bacterial vaginosis.

†NAAT = nucleic acid amplification test.

‡There is a growing threat of multidrug-resistant gonorrhea, with high-level azithromycin resistance and reduced cephalosporin susceptibility reported in the US in 2011. Ceftriaxone is the most effective cephalosporin for treatment of gonorrhea. Cefixime is now second-line because of increasing risk of resistance. If cefixime treatment failure occurs, retreat with ceftriaxone 250 mg IM plus azithromycin 2 g PO both single dose and obtain infectious disease consultation. If ceftriaxone treatment failure occurs, consult infectious disease expert and CDC. Do not use azithromycin monotherapy for routine treatment of gonorrhea. If azithromycin is used in patients with cephalosporin allergy, use azithromycin 2 g PO single dose and perform culture (preferred) or NAAT in 1 week. Report treatment failure to state/local health department within 24 h. As of April 2007, the CDC no longer recommends fluoroquinolones for gonorrhea or PID because of high resistance rates. Do not consider fluoroquinolone unless antimicrobial susceptibility can be documented by culture. If parenteral cephalosporin not feasible for PID (and NAAT is negative or culture documents fluoroquinolone susceptibility), can consider levofloxacin 500 mg PO once daily or ofloxacin 400 mg PO two times per day ± metronidazole 500 mg PO two times per day for 14 days.

ANTIMICROBIALS: Aminoglycosides

NOTE: See also Dermatology and Ophthalmology.

AMIKACIN ▸K ♀D ▸? $$
WARNING — Nephrotoxicity, ototoxicity.
ADULT — Gram-negative infections: 15 mg/kg/day (up to 1500 mg/day) IM/IV divided q 8 to 12 h.
PEDS — Gram-negative infections: 15 mg/kg/day (up to 1500 mg/day) IM/IV divided q 8 to 12 h. Neonates: 10 mg/kg load, then 7.5 mg/kg IM/IV q 12 h.
UNAPPROVED ADULT — Once-daily dosing: 15 mg/kg IV q 24 h. Once-daily dosing for cystic fibrosis: 30 to 35 mg/kg IV q 24 h with target peak of 80 to 120 mg/L and trough of <10 mg/L. Adjust dose based on levels; use past effective dose if available. TB (2nd-line treatment): 15 mg/kg (up to 1 g) IM/IV daily; 10 mg/kg (up to 750 mg) IM/IV daily for age older than 59 yo.
UNAPPROVED PEDS — Severe infections: 15 to 22.5 mg/kg/day IV divided q 8 h. Some experts recommend 30 mg/kg/day. Once-daily dosing: 15 to 20 mg/kg IV q 24 h. Once-daily dosing for cystic fibrosis: 30 to 35 mg/kg IV q 24 h with target peak of 80 to 120 mg/L and trough of <10 mg/L. Adjust dose based on levels; use past effective dose if available. TB (2nd-line treatment): 15 to 30 mg/kg (up to 1 g) IM/IV daily.
NOTES — May enhance effects of neuromuscular blockers. Avoid other ototoxic/nephrotoxic drugs. Individualize dose in renal dysfunction, burn patients. Base dose on average of actual and ideal body wt in obesity. Peak 20 to 35 mcg/mL, trough less than 5 mcg/mL.
MOA — Inhibits bacterial protein synthesis by interfering with function of ribosomal 30S subunit. Bactericidal.
ADVERSE EFFECTS — Serious and frequent: Nephrotoxicity, neuromuscular blockade, ototoxicity. Serious and rare: Vestibular toxicity.

GENTAMICIN ▸K ♀D ▸+ $$
WARNING — Nephrotoxicity, ototoxicity.
ADULT — Gram-negative infections: 3 to 5 mg/kg/day IM/IV divided q 8 h. See table for prophylaxis of bacterial endocarditis.
PEDS — Gram-negative infections: 2.5 mg/kg IM/IV q 12 h for age younger than 1 week old and wt greater than 2 kg; 2 to 2.5 mg/kg IM/IV q 8 h for age 1 week old or older and wt greater than 2 kg. Cystic fibrosis: 9 mg/kg/day IV in divided doses with target peak of 8 to 12 mcg/mL.
UNAPPROVED ADULT — Once-daily dosing for Gram-negative infections: 5 to 7 mg/kg IV q 24 h. Endocarditis: 3 mg/kg/day for synergy with another agent. Give once daily for viridans streptococci, 2 to 3 divided doses for staphylococci, 3 divided doses for enterococci.
UNAPPROVED PEDS — Once-daily dosing: 5 to 7 mg/kg IV q 24 h. Give 4 mg/kg IV q 24 h for age younger than 1 week and full-term.
NOTES — May enhance effects of neuromuscular blockers. Avoid other ototoxic/nephrotoxic drugs. Individualize dose in renal dysfunction, burn patients. Base dose on average of actual and ideal body wt in obesity. Peak 5 to 10 mcg/mL, trough less than 2 mcg/mL.
MOA — Inhibits bacterial protein synthesis by interfering with function of ribosomal 30S subunit. Bactericidal.
ADVERSE EFFECTS — Serious and frequent: Nephrotoxicity, neuromuscular blockade, ototoxicity. Serious and rare: Vestibular toxicity.

STREPTOMYCIN ▸K ♀D ▸+ $$$$$
WARNING — Nephrotoxicity, ototoxicity. Monitor audiometry, renal function, and electrolytes.

(cont.)

STREPTOMYCIN (*cont.*)

ADULT — Combined therapy for TB: 15 mg/kg (up to 1 g) IM/IV daily. 10 mg/kg (up to 750 mg) IM/IV daily if age 60 yo or older.

PEDS — Combined therapy for TB: 20 to 40 mg/kg (up to 1 g) IM daily.

UNAPPROVED ADULT — Same IM dosing can be given IV. Streptococcal endocarditis: 7.5 mg/kg IV/IM two times per day. Go to www.americanheart.org for further info.

NOTES — Contraindicated in pregnancy. Obtain baseline audiogram, vestibular, and Romberg testing, and renal function. Monitor renal function and vestibular and auditory symptoms monthly. May enhance effects of neuromuscular blockers. Avoid other ototoxic/nephrotoxic drugs. Individualize dose in renal dysfunction.

MOA — Inhibits bacterial protein synthesis by interfering with function of ribosomal 30S subunit. Bactericidal.

ADVERSE EFFECTS — Serious and frequent: Ototoxicity, vestibular toxicity. Serious and rare: Nephrotoxicity, neuromuscular blockade. Frequent: Circumoral paresthesias immediately after injection.

TOBRAMYCIN (*Tobi, Bethkis*) ▶K ♀D ▶+ $$

WARNING — Nephrotoxicity, ototoxicity.

ADULT — Gram-negative infections: 3 to 5 mg/kg/day IM/IV divided q 8 h. Parenteral for severe cystic fibrosis: Initial dose of 10 mg/kg/day IV divided q 6 h with target peak of 8 to 12 mcg/mL. Adjust dose based on levels; use past effective dose if available. Inhaled for cystic fibrosis: 300 mg nebulized (Tobi, Bethkis) or 4 caps inhaled (Tobi Podhaler) two times per day 28 days on, then 28 days off.

PEDS — Gram-negative infections: 2 to 2.5 mg/kg IV q 8 h or 1.5 to 1.9 mg/kg IV q 6 h. Give 4 mg/kg/day divided q 12 h for premature/full-term neonates age 1 week old or younger. Parenteral for severe cystic fibrosis: Initial dose of 10 mg/kg/day IV divided q 6 h with target peak of 8 to 12 mcg/mL. Adjust dose based on levels; use past effective dose if available. Inhaled for cystic fibrosis age 6 yo or older: 300 mg nebulized (Tobi, Bethkis) or 4 caps inhaled (Tobi Podhaler) two times per day 28 days on, then 28 days off.

UNAPPROVED ADULT — Once-daily dosing: 5 to 7 mg/kg IV q 24 h. Once-daily dosing for cystic fibrosis: 10 to 12 mg/kg IV q 24 h. with target peak of 20 to 30 mg/L and trough of <1 mg/L.

UNAPPROVED PEDS — Once-daily dosing: 5 to 7 mg/kg IV q 24 h. Once-daily dosing for cystic fibrosis: 10 to 12 mg/kg IV q 24 h with target peak of 20 to 30 mg/L and trough of <1 mg/L.

FORMS — Generic/Trade: TOBI 300 mg/5 mL ampules for nebulizer ($$$$$). Trade Only: Bethkis 300 mg/4 mL ampules for nebulizer ($$$$$). TOBI Podhaler 28 mg caps for inhalation ($$$$$).

NOTES — May enhance effects of neuromuscular blockers. Exacerbation of myasthenia gravis. Avoid other ototoxic/nephrotoxic drugs. Individualize dose in renal dysfunction, burn patients. Base dose on average of actual and ideal body wt in obesity. Peak 5 to 10 mcg/mL, trough < 2 mcg/mL. Nebulized/inhaled tobramycin: Routine monitoring of levels not required. Consider audiograms for patients with or at increased risk of auditory dysfunction. Do not coadminister diuretics including IV mannitol. Tobi Podhaler: Do not place caps in podhaler until immediately before inhalation. Make sure each cap is empty after inhalation. If powder is still in cap, repeat inhalation until empty. Patients taking multiple inhaled drugs should take Tobi Podhaler last.

MOA — Inhibits bacterial protein synthesis by interfering with function of ribosomal 30S subunit. Bactericidal.

ADVERSE EFFECTS — Serious and frequent: Nephrotoxicity, neuromuscular blockade, ototoxicity. Serious and rare: Vestibular toxicity. Inhaled tobramycin: Bronchospasm, dysphonia, tinnitus, hearing loss.

ANTIMICROBIALS: Antifungal Agents—Azoles

NOTE: See www.idsociety.org for guidelines on the management of fungal infections. See www.aidsinfo.nih.gov for management of fungal infections in HIV-infected patients.

CLOTRIMAZOLE ▶L ♀C ▶? $$$$

ADULT — Oropharyngeal candidiasis: 1 troche dissolved slowly in mouth 5 times per day for 14 days. Prevention of oropharyngeal candidiasis in immunocompromised patients: 1 troche dissolved slowly in mouth three times per day until end of chemotherapy or high-dose corticosteroids.

PEDS — Oropharyngeal candidiasis, age 3 yo or older: Use adult dose.

FORMS — Generic only: Oral troches 10 mg.

MOA — Serious: None.

FLUCONAZOLE (*Diflucan*, *✦CanesOral*) ▶K ♀C for single-dose treatment of vaginal candidiasis, D for all other indications ▶+ $$$$

ADULT — Vaginal candidiasis: 150 mg PO single dose ($). All other dosing regimens IV/PO. Oropharyngeal candidiasis: 200 mg first day, then 100 mg daily for at least 2 weeks. Esophageal candidiasis: 200 mg first day, then 100 mg daily (up to 400 mg/day) for at least 3 weeks and continuing for 2 weeks past symptom resolution. Systemic candidiasis: Up to 400 mg daily. Candidal UTI, peritonitis: 50 to 200 mg daily. See UNAPPROVED ADULT for IDSA regimens for Candida infections. Cryptococcal meningitis: 400 mg daily until 10 to 12 weeks after cerebrospinal fluid is culture negative (see UNAPPROVED ADULT for first-line regimen). Suppression of cryptococcal meningitis relapse in AIDS: 200 mg daily until immune system reconstitution. Prevention of

FLUCONAZOLE (*cont.*)

candidiasis after bone marrow transplant: 400 mg daily starting several days before neutropenia and continuing until ANC >1000 cells/mm³ for 7 days. Tinea versicolor: 400 mg PO single dose or 300 mg PO once weekly for 2 weeks (2 doses total).
PEDS — All dosing regimens IV/PO. Oropharyngeal candidiasis: 6 mg/kg first day, then 3 mg/kg daily for at least 2 weeks. Esophageal candidiasis: 6 mg/kg first day, then 3 mg/kg daily (up to 12 mg/kg daily) for at least 3 weeks and continuing for 2 weeks past symptom resolution. Systemic candidiasis: 6 to 12 mg/kg daily. See UNAPPROVED PEDS for alternative regimens for Candida infections. Cryptococcal meningitis: 12 mg/kg on first day, then 6 to 12 mg/kg daily until 10 to 12 weeks after cerebrospinal fluid is culture negative. Suppression of cryptococcal meningitis relapse in AIDS: 6 mg/kg daily. Peds/adult dose equivalents: 3 mg/kg peds equivalent to 100 mg adult; 6 mg/kg peds equivalent to 200 mg adult; 12 mg/kg peds equivalent to 400 mg adult; max peds dose is 600 mg/day.
UNAPPROVED ADULT — Onychomycosis, fingernail: 150 to 300 mg PO q week for 3 to 6 months. Onychomycosis, toenail: 150 to 300 mg PO q week for 6 to 12 months. Recurrent vaginal candidiasis: 100 to 200 mg PO q 3rd day for 3 doses, then 100 to 200 mg PO q week for 6 months. Oropharyngeal candidiasis: 100 to 200 mg daily for 7 to 14 days. Esophageal candidiasis: 200 to 400 mg daily for 14 to 21 days. Candidemia: 800 mg first day, then 400 mg once a day. Treat for 14 days after first negative blood culture and resolution of signs/symptoms. Candida pyelonephritis: 200 to 400 mg (3 to 6 mg/kg) daily for 14 days. Prevention of candidal infections in high-risk neutropenic pts: 400 mg/day during period of risk for neutropenia. Cryptococcal meningitis (per IDSA guideline): Amphotericin B preferably in combo with flucytosine for at least 2 weeks (induction), followed by fluconazole 400 mg PO once daily for 8 weeks (consolidation), then chronic suppression with fluconazole 200 mg PO once daily until immune system reconstitution. Treatment/suppression of coccidioidomycosis in HIV infection: 400 mg PO once daily.
UNAPPROVED PEDS — Oropharyngeal candidiasis: 6 mg/kg first day, then 3 mg/kg once daily for 7 to 14 days. Esophageal candidiasis: 12 mg/kg first day, then 6 mg/kg once daily for 14 to 21 days. Systemic Candida infection: 12 mg/kg on first day, then 6 to 12 mg/kg once daily. Cryptococcal meningitis: Amphotericin B preferably in combo with flucytosine for 2 weeks (induction), followed by fluconazole 12 mg/kg on first day, then 6 to 12 mg/kg (max 800 mg) IV/PO once a day for at least 8 weeks (consolidation), then chronic suppression with lower dose of fluconazole.
FORMS — Generic/Trade: Tabs 50, 100, 150, 200 mg. 150 mg tab in single-dose blister pack. Susp 10, 40 mg/mL (35 mL).
NOTES — Inhibitor of CYP2C9 (strong) and CYP3A4 (moderate). Many drug interactions, including increased levels of alfentanil, celecoxib, cyclosporine, fentanyl, flurbiprofen, fluvastatin (limit fluvastatin to 20 mg/day), glyburide, glipizide, losartan, lovastatin, methadone, phenytoin, rifabutin, simvastatin, sirolimus, tacrolimus, theophylline, tofacitinib (reduce tofacitinib dose to 5 mg once daily), tolbutamide, and increased INR with warfarin. Do not coadminister with voriconazole, or drugs that prolong the QT interval and are metabolized by CYP3A4 (e.g. erythromycin, pimozide, quinidine). Dosing in renal dysfunction: Reduce maintenance dose by 50% for CrCl 11 to 50 mL/min. Hemodialysis: Give recommended dose after each dialysis. Single dose during first trimester of pregnancy does not appear to increase risk of congenital birth defects.
MOA — Triazole that inhibits the synthesis of ergosterol (a sterol required for normal fungal cytoplasmic membrane).
ADVERSE EFFECTS — Serious: Hepatotoxicity (rare), anaphylaxis (rare), exfoliative skin disorders (rare). Frequent: Increased transaminase levels. Single-dose for vaginal candidiasis: Headache, nausea, abdominal pain.

ITRACONAZOLE (*Onmel, Sporanox*) ▶L ♀C ▶– $$$$$
WARNING — Strong CYP 3A4 inhibitor. Inhibition of CYP3A4 metabolism by itraconazole can lead to dangerously high levels of some drugs. High levels of some can prolong QT interval (see QT drugs table). Contraindicated with felodipine, dofetilide, ergot alkaloids, lovastatin, PO midazolam, methadone, nisoldipine, pimozide, quinidine, simvastatin, triazolam. Negative inotrope (may be additive with calcium channel blockers); reassess treatment if signs/symptoms of heart failure develop. Not for use in ventricular dysfunction (CHF or history of CHF) unless for life-threatening or serious infection. Do not use caps for onychomycosis in patients with left ventricular dysfunction.
ADULT — Caps: Take caps or tabs with full meal. Onychomycosis, toenails: 200 mg PO daily for 12 weeks. Onychomycosis "pulse dosing" for fingernails: 200 mg PO two times per day for 1st week of month for 2 months. Test nail specimen to confirm diagnosis before prescribing. Aspergillosis in patients intolerant/refractory to amphotericin, blastomycosis, histoplasmosis: 200 mg PO one to two times per day. Treat for at least 3 months. For life-threatening infections, load with 200 mg PO three times per day for 3 days. Oral soln: Swish and swallow in 10 mL increments on empty stomach. Oropharyngeal candidiasis: 200 mg soln PO daily for 1 to 2 weeks. Oropharyngeal candidiasis unresponsive to fluconazole: 100 mg soln PO two times per day. Esophageal candidiasis: 100 to 200 mg soln PO daily for at least 3 weeks and continuing for 2 weeks past symptom resoln.
PEDS — Not approved in children.
UNAPPROVED ADULT — Caps: Onychomycosis "pulse dosing" for toenails: 200 mg PO two times per day for 1st week of month for 3 to 4 months. Confirm

(cont.)

ITRACONAZOLE (*cont.*)

diagnosis with nail specimen lab testing before prescribing. Prevention of histoplasmosis in HIV infection: 200 mg PO once daily. Treatment/suppression of coccidioidomycosis in HIV infection: 200 mg PO two times per day. Fluconazole-refractory oropharyngeal or esophageal candidiasis: 200 mg PO of oral soln daily for 14 to 21 days.

UNAPPROVED PEDS — Oropharyngeal candidiasis, age 5 yo or older: Oral soln 2.5 mg/kg PO two times per day (max 200 to 400 mg/day) for 7 to 14 days. Esophageal candidiasis, age 5 yo or older: Oral soln 2.5 mg/kg PO two times per day or 5 mg/kg PO once daily for minimum of 14 to 21 days. Caps usually ineffective for esophageal candidiasis.

FORMS — Trade only: Tabs 200 mg (Onmel). Oral soln 10 mg/mL (Sporanox-150 mL). Generic/Trade: Caps 100 mg.

NOTES — Hepatotoxicity, even during 1st weeks of therapy. Monitor LFTs if baseline abnormal LFTs or history of drug-induced hepatotoxicity; consider monitoring in all patients. Decreased absorption of itraconazole with antacids, buffered didanosine, H2 blockers, proton pump inhibitors, or achlorhydria. Itraconazole levels reduced by carbamazepine, isoniazid, nevirapine, phenobarbital, phenytoin, rifabutin and rifampin, and potentially efavirenz. Itraconazole strongly inhibits CYP3A4 metabolism of many drugs. May increase adverse effects of trazodone; consider reducing trazodone dose. May increase QT interval with disopyramide. Caps and oral soln not interchangeable. Oral soln may be preferred in serious infections due to greater absorption. Oral soln may not achieve adequate levels in cystic fibrosis patients; consider alternative if no response. Start therapy for onychomycosis on days 1 to 2 of menses in women of childbearing potential and advise against pregnancy until 2 months after therapy ends.

MOA — Triazole that inhibits the synthesis of ergosterol (a sterol required for normal fungal cytoplasmic membrane).

ADVERSE EFFECTS — Serious: Negative inotrope, hepatotoxicity (even early in therapy), hypokalemia (with high doses). Frequent: GI complaints, allergic rash.

KETOCONAZOLE (*Nizoral*) ▶L ♀C ▶?+ $$$

WARNING — Do not use unless other antifungal drugs are unavailable, not tolerated, and benefit of ketoconazole outweighs risk of hepatotoxicity, adrenal insufficiency, and drug interactions. Hepatotoxicity: Inform patients of risk and monitor. Ketoconazole is a strong CYP3A4 inhibitor and can prolong the QT interval. Coadministration with cisapride, disopyramide, dofetilide, dronedarone, methadone, pimozide, ranolazine, and quinidine is contraindicated due to increased risk of QT prolongation and potential for torsades.

ADULT — Blastomycosis, coccidioidomycosis, histoplasmosis, chromomycosis, paracoccidioidomycosis, in patients who failed or did not tolerate other antifungal drugs: 200 to 400 mg PO daily.

PEDS — Blastomycosis, coccidioidomycosis, histoplasmosis, chromomycosis, paracoccidioidomycosis, in patients age 2 yo or older who failed or did not tolerate other antifungal drugs: 3.3 to 6.6 mg/kg PO daily.

FORMS — Generic only: Tabs 200 mg.

NOTES — Hepatotoxicity; obtain baseline LFTs and monitor ALT weekly. Contraindicated if acute/chronic liver disease. Can cause adrenal insufficiency (doses of 400 mg/day or greater); monitor adrenal function in patients with adrenal insufficiency, borderline adrenal function, or prolonged periods of stress. Decreased absorption of ketoconazole by antacids, H2 blockers, proton pump inhibitors, buffered didanosine, and achlorhydria. Ketoconazole levels reduced by isoniazid, rifampin, and potentially efavirenz. Do not exceed 200 mg/day of ketoconazole with ritonavir, saquinavir, or Kaletra. Ketoconazole inhibits CYP3A4 metabolism of many drugs and can prolong the QT interval. Contraindicated with alprazolam, cisapride, colchicine, disopyramide, dofetilide, dronedarone, eplerenone, ergot alkaloids, felodipine, irinotecan, lovastatin, lurasidone, oral midazolam, methadone, nisoldipine, pimozide, ranolazine, salmeterol, simvastatin, quinidine, tolvaptan, triazolam. May increase adverse effects of trazodone; consider reducing trazodone dose.

MOA — Triazole that inhibits the synthesis of ergosterol (a sterol required for normal fungal cytoplasmic membrane). Inhibits adrenal function at doses of 400 mg/day or more. Reduces testosterone levels at doses of 800 to 1600 mg/day.

ADVERSE EFFECTS — Serious: Hepatotoxicity (even early in therapy). Adrenal insufficiency at doses of 400 mg/day or greater. Frequent: Dose-dependent N/V.

MICONAZOLE—BUCCAL (*Oravig*) ▶L ♀C ▶? $$$$$

ADULT — Oropharyngeal candidiasis: Apply 50 mg buccal tab to gums once daily for 14 days. Apply rounded side of tab to upper gum above incisor in the morning after brushing teeth. Hold in place for 30 seconds. Tab can be used if it sticks to cheek, inside of lip, or gum. Apply to new site each day.

PEDS — Not approved in children. Not recommended for younger children due to potential risk of choking.

FORMS — Trade only: Buccal tabs 50 mg.

NOTES — Contraindicated if hypersensitivity to milk protein concentrate. Increased INR with warfarin. Buccal tab is intended to remain in place until it dissolves. If it falls off within 6 hours of application, reposition tab. If it does not stay in place, apply a new tab. If tab is swallowed within first 6 hours, drink a glass of water and apply a new tab. No action is needed if tab falls off or is swallowed after it has been in place for at least 6 hours. Do not chew gum while tab is in place.

MOA — Triazole that inhibits the synthesis of ergosterol (a sterol required for normal fungal cytoplasmic membrane).

ADVERSE EFFECTS — Severe: Hypersensitivity.

POSACONAZOLE (*Noxafil, ✦Posanol*) ▶Glucuronidation ♀C ▶– $$$$$

ADULT — Prevention of invasive Aspergillus or Candida infection: 200 mg (5 mL) susp PO three times per day OR 300 mg delayed-release tabs PO two times per day on the first day, then 300 mg PO once daily OR 300 mg IV two times per day on first day, then 300 mg IV once daily. Duration of treatment based on recovery from neutropenia or level of immunosuppression. Oropharyngeal candidiasis: 100 mg (2.5 mL) PO twice on day 1, then 100 mg PO once daily for 13 days. Oropharyngeal candidiasis resistant to itraconazole/fluconazole: 400 mg (10 mL) PO two times per day; duration of therapy based on severity of underlying disease and clinical response. Take susp during or within 20 min of full meal or liquid nutritional supplement. Take delayed-release tabs with food. IV posaconazole: Can give first dose by peripheral IV infusion over 30 minutes; Infuse additional doses over 90 minutes by central venous line or peripherally inserted central catheter.

PEDS — Prevention of invasive Aspergillus or Candida infection, age 13 yo or older: 200 mg (5 mL) susp PO three times per day OR 300 mg delayed-release tabs two times per day on the first day, then 300 mg once daily. Oropharyngeal candidiasis, age 13 yo or older: 100 mg (2.5 mL) PO twice on day 1, then 100 mg PO once daily for 13 days. Oropharyngeal candidiasis resistant to itraconazole/fluconazole, age 13 yo or older: 400 mg (10 mL) PO two times per day; duration of therapy based on severity of underlying disease and clinical response. Take susp during or within 20 min of full meal or liquid nutritional supplement. Take delayed-release tabs with food. IV posaconazole is not approved for use in children.

UNAPPROVED ADULT — Invasive pulmonary aspergillosis: 200 mg susp PO four times per day, then 400 mg PO two times per day when stable. Treat invasive pulmonary aspergillosis for at least 6 to 12 weeks; treat immunosuppressed patients throughout immunosuppression and until lesions resolved. Fluconazole-refractory oropharyngeal candidiasis: 400 mg susp PO two times per day for 3 days, then 400 mg PO once daily for up to 28 days. Fluconazole-refractory esophageal candidiasis: 400 mg susp PO two times per day for 14 to 21 days.

FORMS — Trade only: Delayed-release tabs 100 mg. Oral susp 40 mg/mL (105 mL).

NOTES — Consider alternative or monitor for breakthrough fungal infection if patient cannot take susp during or within 20 min of a full meal or liquid nutritional supplement. If meal or liquid supplement not tolerated, consider giving with acidic carbonated drink (eg, ginger ale) or switch to delayed-release tab if indicated. Monitor for breakthrough fungal infection if severe vomiting/diarrhea, posaconazole susp is given by NG tube, or proton pump inhibitor or metoclopramide is coadministered with susp. Avoid cimetidine or esomepreazole with posaconazole susp, but not delayed-release tabs. Posaconazole is a strong CYP3A4 inhibitor. Contraindicated with atorvastatin, ergot alkaloids, lovastatin, simvastatin, sirolimus, and CYP3A4 substrates that prolong the QT interval, including pimozide and quinidine. Correct electrolyte imbalances before starting posaconazole. Monitor for adverse effects of atazanavir, ritonavir, alprazolam, midazolam, triazolam. Consider dosage reduction of vinca alkaloids, calcium channel blockers. Reduce cyclosporine dose by 25% and tacrolimus dose by 66% when posaconazole started; monitor levels of cyclosporine, tacrolimus. Posaconazole levels reduced by efavirenz, rifabutin, and phenytoin; phenytoin and rifabutin levels increased by posaconazole. Do not coadminister unless benefit exceeds risk. Monitor for rifabutin adverse effects. Posaconazole levels reduced by fosamprenavir; monitor for breakthrough fungal infection. Do not split, crush, or chew delayed-release tabs. Delayed-release tab and PO susp are not interchangeable. Renal impairment: Monitor for breakthrough fungal infection in patients with renal impairment receiving PO posaconazole. Vehicle for IV posaconazole can accumulate in renal impairment; avoid if eGFR <50 mL/min unless benefit exceeds risk of accumulation. If IV posaconazole is used in renal impairment, monitor serum creatinine and consider other treatment if increase occurs.

MOA — Triazole that inhibits the synthesis of ergosterol (a sterol required for normal fungal cytoplasmic membrane).

ADVERSE EFFECTS — Serious: Possible hepatotoxicity. Torsades de pointes possibly related to drug interactions in which CYP3A4 inhibiton by posaconazole increases exposure of CYP 3A4 substrates that prolong QT interval. Repeat peripheral infusion of IV posaconazole can cause infusion site reactions. Frequent: diarrhea, N/V, fever, headache, cough, hypokalemia.

VORICONAZOLE (*Vfend*) ▶L ♀D ▶? $$$$$

ADULT — Invasive aspergillosis: 6 mg/kg IV q 12 h for 2 doses, then 4 mg/kg IV q 12 h. Systemic candidiasis: 6 mg/kg IV q 12 h for 2 doses, then 3 to 4 mg/kg IV q 12 h. Treat until at least 14 days past resoln of signs/symptoms or last positive blood culture. Maintenance therapy, aspergillosis or candidiasis: 200 mg PO two times per day. For wt less than 40 kg, reduce to 100 mg PO two times per day. See prescribing information for dosage adjustments for poor response/adverse effects. Esophageal candidiasis: 200 mg PO q 12 h for at least 14 days and 7 days past resolution of signs/symptoms. For wt less than 40 kg, reduce to 100 mg PO two times per day. Dosage adjustment for efavirenz: Voriconazole 400 mg PO two times per day with efavirenz 300 mg (use caps) PO once daily. Take tabs or susp 1 h before or after meals.

PEDS — Safety and efficacy not established in children younger than 12 yo. Use adult dose age 12 yo or older.

(cont.)

VORICONAZOLE *(cont.)*

UNAPPROVED ADULT — Fluconazole-refractory oropharyngeal or esophageal candidiasis: 200 mg PO two times per day for 14 to 21 days. For wt less than 40 kg, reduce to 100 mg PO two times per day.

UNAPPROVED PEDS — In children younger than 12 yo, 7 mg/kg IV q 12 h is comparable to 4 mg/kg IV q 12 h in adults. Invasive aspergillosis: 7 mg/kg (max 400 mg) IV q 12 h for 2 doses, then 7 mg/kg (max 200 mg) IV/PO q 12 h. AAP oral regimen for fungal infections: 10 mg/kg PO q 12 h for 2 doses, then 7 mg/kg PO q 12 h.

FORMS — Generic/Trade: Tabs 50, 200 mg (contains lactose). Susp 40 mg/mL (75 mL).

NOTES — Anaphylactoid reactions (IV only), QT interval prolongation, severe skin reactions and photosensitivity, hepatotoxicity rarely. Transient visual disturbances common; advise against hazardous tasks (if vision impaired), night driving and strong, direct sunlight. Monitor visual (if treated for more than 28 days), liver, and renal function. Monitor pancreatic function if at risk for acute pancreatitis (recent chemotherapy/bone marrow transplant). Many drug interactions. Substrate and inhibitor of CYP2C9, 2C19, and 3A4. Do not use with carbamazepine, ergot alkaloids, everolimus, fluconazole, lopinavir-ritonavir (Kaletra), phenobarbital, pimozide, quinidine, rifabutin, rifampin, ritonavir 400 mg two times per day, sirolimus, or St. John's wort. Ritonavir decreases voriconazole levels; avoid coadministration unless benefit exceeds risk. Dosage adjustments for drug interactions with cyclosporine, omeprazole, phenytoin, tacrolimus in prescribing information. Increased INR with warfarin. Could inhibit metabolism of benzodiazepines, calcium channel blockers, fentanyl, ibuprofen, methadone, oxycodone, and statins. When combining voriconazole with oral contraceptives monitor for adverse effects from increased levels of voriconazole, estrogen, and progestin. Dilute IV to 5 mg/mL or less; max infusion rate is 3 mg/kg/h over 1 to 2 h. Do not infuse IV voriconazole at same time as a blood product/concentrated electrolytes even if given by separate IV lines. IV voriconazole can be infused at the same time as non-concentrated electrolytes/total parenteral nutrition if given by separate lines; give TPN by different port if multi-lumen catheter is used. Vehicle in IV form may accumulate in renal impairment; oral preferred if CrCl less than 50 mL/min. Mild/moderate cirrhosis (Child-Pugh class A/B): Same loading dose and reduce maintenance dose by 50%. Oral susp stable for 14 days at room temperature.

MOA — Triazole that inhibits the synthesis of ergosterol (a sterol required for normal fungal cytoplasmic membrane).

ADVERSE EFFECTS — Serious: Anaphylactoid reactions (IV only), QT interval prolongation, hepatotoxicity (rare), severe skin reactions & photosensitivity rarely, pancreatitis. Frequent: Mild transient visual disturbances, rash, elevated LFTs. Other: Hallucinations, confusion.

ANTIMICROBIALS: Antifungal Agents—Echinocandins

NOTE: See www.idsociety.org for guidelines on the management of fungal infections.

ANIDULAFUNGIN *(Eraxis)* ▶Degraded chemically ♀C ▶? $$$$$

ADULT — Candidemia, other systemic candidal infections: 200 mg IV load on day 1, then 100 mg IV once daily until at least 14 days after last positive culture. Esophageal candidiasis: 100 mg IV load on day 1, then 50 mg IV once daily for at least 14 days, and continuing for at least 7 days after symptoms resolved.

PEDS — Not approved in children.

UNAPPROVED PEDS — 0.75 to 1.5 mg/kg IV once daily. Systemic Candida infections, age 2 yo or older: 1.5 mg/kg IV once daily.

NOTES — Can cause anaphylaxis. Max infusion rate of 1.1 mg/min to prevent histamine reactions. Diluent contains dehydrated alcohol.

MOA — Echinocandin that blocks the synthesis of glucan, a fungal cell wall polysaccharide.

ADVERSE EFFECTS — Hepatotoxicity (rare). Anaphylaxis, including shock. Histamine reactions (rash, urticaria, flushing pruritus, dyspnea, hypotension) minimized by infusion rate less than 1.1 mg/min. Diarrhea, hypokalemia, N/V.

CASPOFUNGIN *(Cancidas)* ▶KL ♀C ▶? $$$$$

ADULT — Infuse IV over 1 h. Aspergillosis, candidemia, empiric therapy of fungal infection in febrile neutropenia: 70 mg loading dose on day 1, then 50 mg once daily. Patients taking rifampin: 70 mg once daily. Consider this dose with other enzyme inducers (such as carbamazepine, dexamethasone, efavirenz, nevirapine, phenytoin) or if inadequate response to lower dose in febrile neutropenia or aspergillosis. Esophageal candidiasis: 50 mg daily. Duration of therapy in invasive aspergillosis is based on severity, treatment response, and resolution of immunosuppression. Treat candidal infections for at least 14 days after last positive culture. For empiric therapy of febrile neutropenia, treat until neutropenia resolved. If fungal infection confirmed, treat for at least 14 days and continue treatment for at least 7 days after symptoms and neutropenia resolved.

PEDS — Infuse IV over 1 h. Aspergillosis, candidemia, esophageal candidiasis, empiric therapy of fungal infection in febrile neutropenia, 3 mo to 17 yo: 70 mg/m² loading dose on day 1, then 50 mg/m² once daily. Consider increasing daily dose to 70 mg/m² up to max of 70 mg once daily if coadministered with enzyme inducers (such as carbamazepine, dexamethasone, efavirenz, nevirapine, phenytoin, or rifampin) or if inadequate response to lower dose in febrile neutropenia or aspergillosis. Duration of therapy in invasive aspergillosis is based on

CASPOFUNGIN (*cont.*)

severity, treatment response, and resolution of immunosuppression. Treat Candida infections for at least 14 days after last positive culture. For empiric therapy of febrile neutropenia, treat until neutropenia resolved. If fungal infection confirmed, treat for at least 14 days and continue treatment for at least 7 days after symptoms and neutropenia resolved. If vial strength is available, in order to improve dosing accuracy, use 50 mg vial (5 mg/mL) for pediatric dose less than 50 mg and 70 mg vial (7 mg/mL) for pediatric dose greater than 50 mg.

NOTES — Abnormal LFTs reported; possible risk of hepatitis. Monitor hepatic function if abnormal LFTs. Cyclosporine increases caspofungin levels and hepatic transaminases; risk of concomitant use unclear. Caspofungin decreases tacrolimus levels. Dosage adjustment in adults with moderate liver dysfunction (Child-Pugh score 7 to 9): 35 mg IV daily (after 70 mg loading dose in patients with invasive aspergillosis).

MOA — Echinocandin that blocks the synthesis of glucan, a fungal cell wall polysaccharide.

ADVERSE EFFECTS — Serious: Anaphylaxis (rare). Abnormal LFTs reported; possible risk of hepatitis. Frequent: Fever, rash, N/V, diarrhea, hypokalemia, phlebitis at injection site. Some infusion reactions (like facial flushing, angioedema, bronchospasm) caused by histamine release.

MICAFUNGIN (*Mycamine*) ▶L, feces ♀C ▶? $$$$$
ADULT — Esophageal candidiasis: 150 mg IV once daily. Candidemia, acute disseminated candidiasis,

Candida peritonitis/abscess: 100 mg IV once daily. Prevention of candidal infections in bone marrow transplant patients: 50 mg IV once daily. Infuse over 1 h. Histamine-mediated reactions possible with more rapid infusion. Flush existing IV lines with NS before micafungin infusion.

PEDS — Esophageal candidiasis, age 4 mo and older: 3 mg/kg IV once daily for wt 30 kg or less; 2.5 mg/kg IV up to 150 mg once daily for wt greater than 30 kg. Candidemia, acute disseminated candidiasis, Candida peritonitis/abscess, age 4 mo and older: 2 mg/kg up to 100 mg IV once daily. Prevention of candidal infections in bone marrow transplant patients, age 4 mo and older: 1 mg/kg up to 50 mg IV once daily. Infuse over 1 h. Histamine-mediated reactions possible with more rapid infusion. Infuse concentrations >1.5 mg/mL by central catheter. Flush existing IV lines with NS before micafungin infusion.

UNAPPROVED ADULT — Prophylaxis of invasive aspergillosis: 50 mg IV once daily. Infuse IV over 1 h.

NOTES — Increases levels of sirolimus and nifedipine. Not dialyzed. Protect diluted soln from light. Do not mix with other meds; it may precipitate.

MOA — Echinocandin that blocks the synthesis of glucan, a fungal cell wall polysaccharide.

ADVERSE EFFECTS — Serious: Anaphylaxis/anaphylactoid reactions (rare); renal/hepatic dysfunction; hemolysis/hemolytic anemia. Frequent: Rash. Injection site reactions more common with peripheral infusion.

ANTIMICROBIALS: Antifungal Agents—Polyenes

NOTE: See www.idsociety.org for guidelines on the management of fungal infections.

AMPHOTERICIN B DEOXYCHOLATE ▶Tissues ♀B ▶? $$$$$
WARNING — Do not use IV route for noninvasive fungal infections (oral thrush, vaginal or esophageal candidiasis) in patients with normal neutrophil counts.

ADULT — Life-threatening systemic fungal infections: Test dose 1 mg slow IV. Wait 2 to 4 h, and if tolerated start 0.25 mg/kg IV daily. Advance to 0.5 to 1.5 mg/kg/day depending on fungal type. Maximum dose 1.5 mg/kg/day. Infuse over 2 to 6 h. Hydrate with 500 mL NS before and after infusion to decrease risk of nephrotoxicity.

PEDS — No remaining FDA-approved indications.

UNAPPROVED ADULT — Alternative regimen, life-threatening systemic fungal infections: 1 mg test dose as part of first infusion (no need for separate IV bag); if tolerated continue infusion, giving target dose of 0.5 to 1.5 mg/kg on first day. Candidemia: 0.5 to 1 mg/kg IV daily. Treat until 14 days after first negative blood culture and resolution of signs/symptoms. Symptomatic Candida cystitis: 0.3 to 0.6 mg/kg IV for 1 to 7 days. Candida pyelonephritis: 0.5 to 0.7 mg/kg IV daily (± flucytosine). Cryptococcal meningitis

in HIV infection: 0.7 mg/kg/day IV preferably in combo with flucytosine 25 mg/kg PO q 6 h for 2 weeks. Follow with fluconazole consolidation, then fluconazole chronic suppression until immune reconstitution.

UNAPPROVED PEDS — Systemic life-threatening fungal infections: Test dose 0.1 mg/kg (max of 1 mg) slow IV. Wait 2 to 4 h, and if tolerated start 0.25 mg/kg IV once daily. Advance to 0.5 to 1.5 mg/kg/day depending on fungal type. Maximum dose 1.5 mg/kg/day. Infuse over 2 to 6 h. Hydrate with 10 to 15 mL/kg NS before infusion to decrease risk of nephrotoxicity. Alternative dosing regimen: Give test dose as part of first infusion (separate IV bag not needed); if tolerated continue infusion, giving target dose of 0.5 to 1.5 mg/kg on first day. Cryptococcal infection in HIV-infected patients: 0.7 to 1 mg/kg IV once daily may add flucytosine depending on site and severity of infection.

NOTES — Acute infusion reactions, anaphylaxis, nephrotoxicity, hypokalemia, hypomagnesemia, acidosis, anemia. Monitor renal and hepatic function, CBC, serum electrolytes. Lipid formulations better tolerated, preferred in renal dysfunction.

(cont.)

AMPHOTERICIN B DEOXYCHOLATE (*cont.*)

MOA — Polyene antifungal, Insertion into fungal cytoplasmic membrane increases membrane permeability.

ADVERSE EFFECTS — Serious for IV Fungizone: Anaphylaxis, anemia, nephrotoxicity. Frequent: Acute infusion reactions, nephrotoxicity (hypokalemia, hypomagnesemia, renal tubular acidosis).

AMPHOTERICIN B LIPID FORMULATIONS (*Amphotec, Abelcet, AmBisome*) ▶? ♀B ▶? $$$$$

ADULT — Lipid formulations used primarily in patients refractory/intolerant to amphotericin deoxycholate. Abelcet: Invasive fungal infections: 5 mg/kg/day IV at 2.5 mg/kg/h. Shake infusion bag q 2 h. AmBisome: Infuse IV over 2 h. Empiric therapy of fungal infections in febrile neutropenia: 3 mg/kg/day. Aspergillus, candidal, cryptococcal infections: 3 to 5 mg/kg/day. Visceral leishmaniasis: 3 mg/kg IV on days 1 to 5 and days 14 and 21 for immunocompetent patients; 4 mg/kg IV on days 1 to 5 and days 10, 17, 24, 31 and 38 for immunocompromised patients. Cryptococcal meningitis in HIV infection: 6 mg/kg/day. Amphotec: Aspergillosis: Test dose of 10 mL over 15 to 30 min, observe for 30 min, then 3 to 4 mg/kg/day IV at 1 mg/kg/h.

PEDS — Lipid formulations used primarily in patients refractory/intolerant to amphotericin deoxycholate.

Abelcet: Invasive fungal infections: 5 mg/kg/day IV at 2.5 mg/kg/h. Shake infusion bag q 2 h. AmBisome: Infuse IV over 2 h. Empiric therapy of fungal infections in febrile neutropenia: 3 mg/kg/day. Aspergillus, candidal, cryptococcal infections: 3 to 5 mg/kg/day. Visceral leishmaniasis: 3 mg/kg IV on days 1 to 5 and days 14 and 21 for immunocompetent patients; 4 mg/kg IV on days 1 to 5 and days 10, 17, 24, 31 and 38 for immunocompromised patients. Cryptococcal meningitis in HIV infection: 6 mg/kg/day. Amphotec: Aspergillosis: Test dose of 10 mL over 15 to 30 min, observe for 30 min, then 3 to 4 mg/kg/day IV at 1 mg/kg/h.

NOTES — Acute infusion reactions, anaphylaxis, nephrotoxicity, hypokalemia, hypomagnesemia, acidosis. Lipid formulations better tolerated than amphotericin deoxycholate, preferred in renal dysfunction. Monitor renal and hepatic function, CBC, electrolytes.

MOA — Polyene antifungal, Insertion into fungal cytoplasmic membrane increases membrane permeability.

ADVERSE EFFECTS — Serious: Anaphylaxis. Frequent: Acute infusion reactions, nephrotoxicity (hypokalemia, hypomagnesemia, renal tubular acidosis). Lipid formulations better tolerated than amphotericin deoxycholate.

ANTIMICROBIALS: Antifungal Agents—Other

NOTE: See www.idsociety.org for guidelines on the management of fungal infections.

FLUCYTOSINE (*Ancobon*) ▶K ♀C ▶– $$$$$

WARNING — Extreme caution in renal or bone marrow impairment. Monitor hematologic, hepatic, renal function in all patients.

ADULT — Candidal/cryptococcal infections: 50 to 150 mg/kg/day PO divided four times per day. Candida UTI: 100 mg/kg/day PO divided four times per day for 7 to 10 days for symptomatic cystitis, for 14 days (± amphotericin deoxycholate) for pyelonephritis. Initial therapy for cryptococcal meningitis: 100 mg/kg/day PO divided four times per day.

PEDS — Not approved in children.

UNAPPROVED PEDS — Candidal/cryptococcal infections: 50 to 150 mg/kg/day PO divided four times per day.

FORMS — Generic/Trade: Caps 250, 500 mg.

NOTES — Flucytosine is given with other antifungal agents. Myelosuppression. Reduce nausea by taking caps a few at a time over 15 min. Monitor flucytosine levels with target peak level 2 h after dose of 30 to 80 mcg/mL. Reduce dose in renal dysfunction. Avoid in children with severe renal dysfunction.

MOA — Deaminated to inhibitor of thymidylate synthetase, which interferes with DNA synthesis.

ADVERSE EFFECTS — Serious: Myelosuppression (frequent); anaphylaxis; hepatic, renal, cardiac and CNS toxicity (all rare). Frequent: N/V, diarrhea, rash.

GRISEOFULVIN (*Grifulvin V*) ▶Skin ♀C ▶ $$$$

ADULT — Tinea: 500 mg PO daily for 4 to 6 weeks for capitis, 2 to 4 weeks for corporis, 4 to 8 weeks for

pedis, 4 months for fingernails, 6 months for toenails. Can use 1 g/day for pedis and unguium.

PEDS — Tinea: 11 mg/kg PO daily for 4 to 6 weeks for capitis, 2 to 4 weeks for corporis, 4 to 8 weeks for pedis, 4 months for fingernails, 6 months for toenails.

UNAPPROVED PEDS — Tinea capitis: AAP recommends 10 to 20 mg/kg (max 1 g) PO daily for 4 to 6 weeks, continuing for 2 weeks past symptom resolution. Some infections may require 20 to 25 mg/kg/day or ultramicrosize griseofulvin 5 to 10 mg/kg (max 750 mg) PO daily.

FORMS — Generic/Trade: Susp 125 mg/5 mL (120 mL). Tabs 500 mg. Generic only: Tabs 250 mg.

NOTES — Do not use in liver failure, porphyria. May cause photosensitivity, lupus-like syndrome/exacerbation of lupus. Decreased INR with warfarin, decreased efficacy of oral contraceptives. Ultramicrosize formulations have greater GI absorption, and are available with different strengths and dosing.

MOA — Inhibits fungal mitosis by disrupting mitotic spindle.

ADVERSE EFFECTS — Serious: Photosensitivity, lupus-like syndrome/exacerbation of lupus, increased porphyrins (not for use by patients with porphyria). Frequent: Allergic skin reactions, headache.

GRISEOFULVIN ULTRAMICROSIZE (*Gris-PEG*) ▶Skin ♀C ▶? $$$$$

ADULT — Tinea: 375 mg PO daily for 4 to 6 weeks for capitis, 2 to 4 weeks for corporis, 4 to 8 weeks for

GRISEOFULVIN ULTRAMICROSIZE (cont.)

pedis, 4 months for fingernails, 6 months for toenails. Can use 750 mg/day for pedis and unguium. Best absorption when given after meal containing fat.

PEDS — Tinea, age 2 yo or older: 7.3 mg/kg PO daily for 4 to 6 weeks for capitis, 2 to 4 weeks for corporis, 4 to 8 weeks for pedis, 4 months for fingernails, 6 months for toenails. Give 82.5 to 165 mg PO daily for 13.6 to 22.6 kg. Give 165 to 330 mg for wt greater than 22.6 kg. Tinea capitis: AAP recommends 5 to 15 mg/kg (up to 750 mg) PO daily for 4 to 6 weeks, continuing for 2 weeks past symptom resolution. Best absorption when given after meal containing fat.

FORMS — Generic/Trade: Tabs 125, 250 mg.

NOTES — Do not use in liver failure, porphyria. May cause photosensitivity, lupus-like syndrome/exacerbation of lupus. Decreased INR with warfarin, decreased efficacy of oral contraceptives. Microsize formulations, which have lower GI absorption, are available with different strengths and dosing.

MOA — Inhibits fungal mitosis by disrupting mitotic spindle.

ADVERSE EFFECTS — Serious: Photosensitivity, lupus-like syndrome/exacerbation of lupus, increased porphyrins (not for use by patients with porphyria). Frequent: Allergic skin reactions, headache.

NYSTATIN ▶Not absorbed ♀B ▶+ $

ADULT — Non-esophageal mucus membrane gastrointestinal candidiasis: 1 to 2 tabs PO 3 times per day.

PEDS — Thrush, infants: 2 mL/dose PO with 1 mL in each cheek four times per day. Premature and low wt infants: 0.5 mL PO in each cheek four times per day. Thrush, older children: 4 to 6 mL PO swish and swallow four times per day.

FORMS — Generic only: Susp 100,000 units/mL (60, 480 mL). Film-coated tabs 500,000 units.

MOA — Serious: None. Frequent: None.

TERBINAFINE (Lamisil) ▶LK ♀B ▶– $$$$$

ADULT — Onychomycosis: 250 mg PO daily for 6 weeks for fingernails, for 12 weeks for toenails.

PEDS — Tinea capitis, age 4 yo or older: Give granules once daily with food for 6 weeks: 125 mg for wt less than 25 kg, 187.5 mg for wt 25 to 35 kg, 250 mg for wt greater than 35 kg.

UNAPPROVED PEDS — Onychomycosis: Give PO once daily at dose of 67.5 mg for wt less than 20 kg, 125 mg for wt 20 to 40 kg, 250 mg for wt greater than 40 kg. Treat for 6 weeks for fingernails, for 12 weeks for toenails.

FORMS — Generic/Trade: Tabs 250 mg. Trade only: Oral granules 125, 187.5 mg/packet.

NOTES — Hepatotoxicity; monitor AST and ALT at baseline. Neutropenia; discontinue if neutrophils ≤1000 cells/mm3. May rarely cause or exacerbate lupus. Do not use in liver disease or CrCl <50 mL/min. Test nail specimen to confirm diagnosis before prescribing. Inhibitor of CYP2D6.

MOA — Inhibits squalene epoxidase, an enzyme involved in the synthesis of ergosterol (a sterol required for normal fungal cytoplasmic membrane).

ADVERSE EFFECTS — Serious: Hepatotoxicity, neutropenia, depression, Stevens-Johnson syndrome, toxic epidermal necrolysis, DRESS, taste and smell disturbances (severe, prolonged, or permanent). May rarely cause or exacerbate lupus. Frequent: N/V, rash.

ANTIMICROBIALS: Antimalarials

NOTE: For help treating malaria or getting antimalarials, see www.cdc.gov/malaria or call the "malaria hotline"; (770) 488-7788 Monday-Friday 9:00 am to 5:00 pm EST; after hours/weekend (770) 488-7100. Pediatric doses of antimalarials should never exceed adult doses.

CHLOROQUINE (Aralen) ▶KL ♀C but + ▶+ $

WARNING — Review product labeling for precautions and adverse effects before prescribing.

ADULT — Doses as chloroquine phosphate. Malaria prophylaxis, chloroquine-sensitive areas: 500 mg PO q week from 1 to 2 weeks before exposure to 4 weeks after. Malaria treatment, chloroquine-sensitive areas: 1 g PO once, then 500 mg PO at 6, 24, and 48 h. Total dose is 2.5 g. Extraintestinal amebiasis: 1 g PO daily for 2 days, then 500 mg PO daily for 2 to 3 weeks.

PEDS — Doses as chloroquine phosphate. Malaria prophylaxis, chloroquine-sensitive areas: 8.3 mg/kg (up to 500 mg) PO q week from 1 to 2 weeks before exposure to 4 weeks after. Malaria treatment, chloroquine-sensitive areas: 16.7 mg/kg PO once, then 8.3 mg/kg at 6, 24, and 48 h. Do not exceed adult dose. Chloroquine phosphate 8.3 mg/kg is equivalent to chloroquine base 5 mg/kg.

FORMS — Generic only: Tabs 250 mg. Generic/Trade: Tabs 500 mg (500 mg phosphate equivalent to 300 mg base).

NOTES — Can prolong QT interval and cause torsades. Retinopathy with chronic/high doses; eye exams required. May cause seizures (caution advised if epilepsy); ototoxicity (caution advised if hearing loss); myopathy (discontinue if muscle weakness develops); bone marrow toxicity (monitor CBC if long-term use); exacerbation of psoriasis. Concentrates in liver; caution advised if hepatic disease, alcoholism, or hepatotoxic drugs. Antacids reduce absorption; give at least 4 h apart. May increase cyclosporine levels. As little as 1 g can cause fatal overdose in a child. Fatal malaria reported after chloroquine used as malaria prophylaxis in areas with chloroquine resistance; use only in areas without resistance. Other agents are superior for severe chloroquine-sensitive malaria. Maternal antimalarial prophylaxis doesn't harm breastfed infant or protect infant from

(cont.)

CHLOROQUINE (*cont.*)

malaria. Use with primaquine phosphate for treatment of P. vivax or P. ovale.

MOA — Plasmodicidal mechanism of action unknown, may inhibit heme polymerase or interact with DNA.

ADVERSE EFFECTS — Serious: Retinopathy with chronic/high doses; can cause torsades. Fatal malaria in patients receiving chloroquine prophylaxis in areas with chloroquine resistance.

COARTEM (artemether + lumefantrine) ▶L ♀C ▶? $$$$

ADULT — Uncomplicated malaria, wt 35 kg or greater: 4 tabs PO two times per day for 3 days. On day 1, give 2nd dose 8 h after 1st dose. Take with food.

PEDS — Uncomplicated malaria, wt greater than 5 kg and age 2 mo or older: Take with food two times per day for 3 days. On day 1, give 2nd dose 8 h after 1st dose. Dose based on wt: 1 tab for 5 to 14 kg; 2 tabs for 15 to 24 kg; 3 tabs for 25 to 34 kg; 4 tab for 35 kg or greater.

FORMS — Trade only: Tabs, artemether 20 mg + lumefantrine 120 mg.

NOTES — Can prolong QT interval; avoid using in proarrhythmic conditions or with drugs that prolong QT interval. Monitor ECG if quinine/quinidine or other antimalarial that prolongs QT interval is given soon after Coartem, due to long half-life of lumefantrine. Do not use Coartem and halofantrine within 1 month of each other. Contraindicated with strong CYP3A4 inducers (eg carbamazepine, phenytoin, rifampin, St John's wort). May inhibit CYP2D6; avoid with drugs metabolized by CYP2D6 that have cardiac effects and caution with CYP3A4 inhibitors as both interactions may prolong QT interval. Repeat the dose if vomiting occurs within 1 to 2 h; use another antimalarial if second dose is vomited. Can crush tabs and mix with 1 to 2 tsp water immediately before the dose.

MOA — Artemether and lumefantrine are blood schizonticides.

ADVERSE EFFECTS — Serious: Urticaria/angioedema. Can prolong QT interval. Frequent: Headache, anorexia, dizziness, asthenia in adults. Fever, cough, vomiting, anorexia, headache in children.

MALARONE (atovaquone + proguanil) ▶Feces; LK ♀ C ▶? $$$$$

ADULT — Malaria prophylaxis: 1 adult tab PO once daily from 1 to 2 days before exposure until 7 days after. Malaria treatment: 4 adult tabs PO once daily for 3 days. Take with food/milky drink at same time each day. Repeat dose if vomiting within 1 h after the dose. CDC recommends for presumptive self-treatment of malaria (same dose as for treatment, but not for patients currently taking it for prophylaxis).

PEDS — Safety and efficacy established in children with wt 11 kg or greater for prevention, and 5 kg or greater for treatment. Prevention of malaria: Give following dose based on wt PO once daily from 1 to 2 days before exposure until 7 days after: 1 ped tab for 11 to 20 kg; 2 ped tabs for 21 to 30 kg; 3 ped tabs for 31 to 40 kg; 1 adult tab for greater than 40 kg. Treatment of malaria: Give following dose based on wt PO once daily for 3 days: 2 ped tabs for 5 to 8 kg; 3 ped tabs for 9 to 10 kg; 1 adult tab for 11 to 20 kg; 2 adult tabs for 21 to 30 kg; 3 adult tabs for 31 to 40 kg; 4 adult tabs for greater than 40 kg. Take with food or milky drink at same time each day. Repeat dose if vomiting occurs within 1 h after dose.

UNAPPROVED PEDS — CDC doses for prevention of malaria: Give following dose based on wt PO once daily from 1 to 2 days before exposure until 7 days after: ½ ped tab for 5 to 8 kg; ¾ ped tab for 9 to 10 kg. Not advised for infants less than 5 kg.

FORMS — Generic/Trade: Adult tabs atovaquone 250 mg + proguanil 100 mg. Pediatric tabs 62.5 mg + 25 mg.

NOTES — Vomiting common with malaria treatment doses (consider antiemetic). Monitor parasitemia. Atovaquone levels may be decreased by tetracycline, metoclopramide (use another antiemetic if possible), and rifampin (avoid). Proguanil may increase the INR with warfarin. If CrCl less than 30 mL/min avoid for malaria prophylaxis and use cautiously for treatment. CDC recommends against use by women breastfeeding infant weighing less than 5 kg.

MOA — Atovaquone and proguanil interfere with two different pyrimidine biosynthesis pathways. Atovaquone inhibits parasitic mitochondrial electron transport. A proguanil metabolite, cycloguanil, inhibits dihydrofolate reductase.

ADVERSE EFFECTS — Serious: Hepatitis/increased LFTs, anaphylaxis, Stevens-Johnson syndrome, photosensitivity. Frequent: Vomiting with malaria treatment doses, GI complaints, headache, asthenia, dizziness.

MEFLOQUINE ▶L ♀B ▶? $$

WARNING — Neurologic or psychiatric adverse effects such as dizziness, tinnitus, anxiety, hallucinations, and paranoia may persist.

ADULT — Malaria prophylaxis, chloroquine-resistant areas: 250 mg PO once weekly from 1 week before exposure until 4 weeks after. CDC recommends starting mefloquine prophylaxis at least 2 weeks before exposure. Malaria treatment: 1250 mg PO single dose. Take on full stomach with at least 8 oz water.

PEDS — Malaria treatment: 20 to 25 mg/kg PO; given in 1 to 2 divided doses 6 to 8 h apart to reduce risk of vomiting. Repeat full dose if vomiting within 30 min after dose; repeat ½ dose if vomiting within 30 to 60 min after dose. Experience limited in infants age younger than 3 mo or wt less than 5 kg. Malaria prophylaxis: Give approximately 5 mg/kg PO once weekly starting 1 week before exposure until 4 weeks after. Dose according to wt: ½ tab for 20 to 30 kg; ¾ tab for 30 to 45 kg; 1 tab for greater than 45 kg. Experience limited in patients with wt less than 20 kg. CDC recommends starting mefloquine prophylaxis at least 2 weeks before exposure. Pharmacist can compound small doses. Take on full stomach.

MEFLOQUINE (*cont.*)

UNAPPROVED ADULT — CDC regimen for malaria: 750 mg PO followed by 500 mg PO 6 to 12 h later, for total of 1250 mg. Quinine + doxycycline/tetracycline/clindamycin or atovaquone-proguanil preferred over mefloquine because of high rate of neuropsychiatric adverse effects with malaria treatment doses of mefloquine.

UNAPPROVED PEDS — Malaria prophylaxis, chloroquine-resistant areas: CDC recommends these PO doses once weekly starting at least 2 weeks before exposure until 4 weeks after: 5 mg/kg for wt 9 kg or less; ¼ tab for wt greater than 9 to 19 kg; ½ tab for wt greater than 19 to 30 kg; ¾ tab for wt greater than 30 to 45 kg; 1 tab for wt greater than 45 kg. Malaria treatment for wt less than 45 kg: 15 mg/kg PO, then 10 mg/kg PO given 8 to 12 h after 1st dose. Take on full stomach with at least 8 oz water.

FORMS — Generic only: Tabs 250 mg.

NOTES — Cardiac conduction disturbances. Do not use with ziprasidone. Do not give until 12 h after the last dose of quinidine, quinine, or chloroquine; may cause ECG changes and seizures. Contraindicated for prophylaxis if depression (active/recent), generalized anxiety disorder, psychosis, schizophrenia, other major psychiatric disorder, or history of seizures. Tell patients to discontinue if psychiatric symptoms occur during prophylaxis. May cause drowsiness (warn about hazardous tasks). Can crush tabs and mix with a little water, milk, or other liquid. Pharmacists can put small doses into caps to mask bitter taste. Decreases valproate levels. Rifampin decreases mefloquine levels. Maternal use of antimalarial prophylaxis doesn't harm or protect breastfed infant from malaria.

MOA — Acts as blood schizonticide, exact mechanism of action is unknown.

ADVERSE EFFECTS — Serious: Cardiac conduction disturbances including QT prolongation, psychiatric reactions. Frequent: Dizziness, loss of balance, sleep disturbances (especially early in therapy and in women). Early vomiting in children with malaria treatment dose.

PRIMAQUINE ▶L ♀– ▶– $$$

WARNING — Review product labeling for precautions and adverse effects and document normal G6PD level before prescribing.

ADULT — Prevention of relapse, P. vivax/ovale malaria: 30 mg base PO daily for 14 days.

PEDS — Not approved in children.

UNAPPROVED ADULT — Pneumocystis in patients intolerant to trimethoprim/sulfamethoxazole: 15 to 30 mg primaquine base PO daily plus clindamycin 600 mg IV q 6 h to 900 mg IV q 8 h or 300 mg PO q 6 h or 450 mg PO q 8 h for 21 days. Primary prevention of malaria in special circumstances: 30 mg base PO once daily beginning 1 to 2 days before exposure until 7 days after (consult with malaria expert; contact CDC at 770–488–7788 for info).

UNAPPROVED PEDS — Prevention of relapse, P. vivax/ovale malaria: 0.5 mg/kg (up to 30 mg) base PO once daily for 14 days. Primary prevention of malaria in special circumstances: 0.5 mg/kg (up to 30 mg) base PO once daily beginning 1 to 2 days before exposure until 7 days after (consult with malaria expert; contact CDC at 770-488-7788 for info).

FORMS — Generic only: Tabs 26.3 mg (equiv to 15 mg base).

NOTES — Causes hemolytic anemia in G6PD deficiency, methemoglobinemia in NADH methemoglobin reductase deficiency. Contraindicated in pregnancy and G6PD deficiency; screen for deficiency before prescribing. Stop if dark urine or anemia. Avoid in patients with RA or SLE, recent quinacrine use, or use of other bone marrow suppressants.

MOA — Unknown. May affect mitochondrial electron transport chain or pyrimidine synthesis. Active against all forms of malaria; only drug active against latent parasites in liver.

ADVERSE EFFECTS — Serious: Hemolytic anemia with G6PD deficiency, methemoglobinemia with NADH methemoglobin reductase deficiency.

QUININE (*Qualaquin*) ▶L ♀C ▶+? $$$$$

WARNING — FDA has repeatedly warned that the risks of using quinine for management of nocturnal leg cramps (an unapproved indication) exceed any potential benefit. Risks include life-threatening hematological reactions, especially thrombocytopenia and hemolytic-uremic syndrome/thrombotic thrombocytopenic purpura (HUS/TTP). HUS/TTP can cause chronic renal impairment.

ADULT — Malaria: 648 mg PO three times per day for 3 days (Africa/South America) or 7 days (Southeast Asia). Also give 7-day course of doxycycline, tetracycline, or clindamycin.

PEDS — Not approved in children.

UNAPPROVED ADULT — Nocturnal leg cramps: 260 to 325 mg PO at bedtime. FDA warns that risks outweigh benefits for this indication.

UNAPPROVED PEDS — Malaria: 25 to 30 mg/kg/day (up to 2 g/day) PO divided q 8 h for 3 days (Africa/South America) or 7 days (Southeast Asia). Also give 7-day course of doxycycline, tetracycline, or clindamycin.

FORMS — Generic/Trade: Caps 324 mg.

NOTES — Thrombocytopenia, hemolytic uremic syndrome/thrombotic thrombocytopenic purpura, cinchonism, hemolytic anemia with G6PD deficiency, cardiac conduction disturbances, hearing impairment. Contraindicated if prolonged QT interval, optic neuritis, myasthenia gravis, or hypersensitivity to quinine, quinidine, or mefloquine. Can prolong PR/QRS interval; esp if structural heart disease/pre-existing conduction system abnormalities, elderly with sick sinus syndrome, atrial fibrillation with slow ventricular response, myocardial ischemia, other drugs that prolong PR/QRS interval (flecainide, quinidine). Many drug interactions. Do not use with clarithromycin, erythromycin, rifampin, ritonavir, neuromuscular blockers. May increase

(cont.)

QUININE (cont.)

digoxin levels. Monitor INR with warfarin. Antacids decrease quinine absorption. Rule out G6PD deficiency in breastfed at-risk infant before giving quinine to mother. Use in hepatic impairment: No dosage adjustment for mild/moderate (Child-Pugh A/B) impairment, but monitor for adverse effects. Do not use if severe (Child-Pugh C) impairment.

MOA — Unknown, may have similar mechanism of action as chloroquine.
ADVERSE EFFECTS — Serious: Thrombocytopenia, hemolytic uremic syndrome/thrombotic thrombocytopenic purpura, cinchonism, hemolytic anemia with G6PD deficiency, cardiac conduction disturbances, hearing impairment with high levels, hypoglycemia (especially in pregnant women).

ANTIMICROBIALS: Antimycobacterial Agents

NOTE: Treat active mycobacterial infection with at least 2 drugs. See guidelines at www.thoracic.org/statements/ and www.aidsinfo.nih.gov. Get baseline LFTs, creatinine, and platelet count before treating TB. Evaluate at least monthly for adverse drug reactions. Routine liver and renal function tests not needed unless baseline dysfunction or increased risk of hepatotoxicity.

BEDAQUILINE (Sirturo) ▶L ♀B ▶– $$$$$
WARNING — Higher mortality rate with bedaquiline in a clinical trial; use only when other drugs are ineffective. Can prolong QT interval; may cause additive QT interval prolongation with other drugs that prolong QT interval.
ADULT — Pulmonary multi-drug resistant TB: 400 mg PO once daily for 2 weeks, then 200 mg PO 3 times per week for 22 weeks. Take with food. Intended for directly observed therapy in combo with at least 3 drugs active against patients TB isolate.
PEDS — Safety and efficacy not established in children.
FORMS — Trade Only: 100 mg tab.
NOTES — Can prolong QT interval. Monitor ECG at baseline, and 2, 12, and 24 weeks after starting bedaquiline and if syncope occurs. Monitor electrolytes at baseline (correct if needed) and if QT prolongation detected. Monitor ECG if given with other drugs that prolong QT interval, or patient has history of torsades, congenital long QT syndrome, hypothyroidism and bradyarrhythmias, uncompensated heart failure, or low serum calcium, magnesium, or potassium. Discontinue if significant ventricular arrhythmia or QT interval >500 ms. Increases risk of hepatic adverse events; monitor LFTs and symptoms at baseline, monthly, and as needed. If AST/ALT > 3xULN, repeat test within 48 h, test for viral hepatitis, and discontinue other hepatotoxic drugs. Discontinue bedaquiline if AST/ALT increase plus total bilirubin >2xULN; AST/ALT >8xULN; or AST/ALT elevation for >2 weeks. Avoid hepatotoxic drugs and alcohol during treatment. Avoid coadministration with strong CYP3A4 inducers including rifamycins. Avoid giving strong CYP3A4 inhibitors for more than 14 days if possible. Tell patients to swallow tabs whole with water. No dosage adjustment for mild/moderate hepatic impairment; monitor for increase in adverse events if severe hepatic impairment.
MOA — Diarylquinoline antimycobacterial drug that inhibits mycobacterial ATP-synthase, blocking energy generation in the organism.
ADVERSE EFFECTS — Severe: Increased mortality in a clinical trial, QT interval prolongation, increased risk of hepatic adverse events. Frequent: Nausea, arthralgia, headache, hemoptysis, chest pain.

CLOFAZIMINE ▶feces ♀C ▶?-
ADULT — Approved for leprosy therapy.
PEDS — Not approved in children.
FORMS — Caps 50 mg. For leprosy, contact National Hansen's Disease Program (phone 800–642–2477).
NOTES — Abdominal pain common; rare reports of splenic infarction, bowel obstruction, and GI bleeding. Pink to brownish-black skin pigmentation that may persist for months to years after drug is discontinued. Discoloration of urine, body secretions.
MOA — Unknown.
ADVERSE EFFECTS — Serious: Rare reports of splenic infarction, bowel obstruction, and GI bleeding. Frequent: Abdominal pain, discoloration of urine and body secretions, pink to brownish-black skin pigmentation that may persist for months to years.

DAPSONE (Aczone) ▶LK ♀C ▶– $$$$
ADULT — Leprosy: 100 mg PO daily with rifampin ± clofazimine or ethionamide. Acne (Aczone; $$$$): Apply two times per day.
PEDS — Leprosy: 1 mg/kg (up to 100 mg) PO daily with other antimycobacterial agents. Acne, 12 to 17 yo (Aczone; $$$$$): Apply two times per day.
UNAPPROVED ADULT — Pneumocystis pneumonia prophylaxis: 100 mg PO daily. Pneumocystis pneumonia treatment: 100 mg PO daily with trimethoprim 5 mg/kg PO three times per day for 21 days.
UNAPPROVED PEDS — Pneumocystis pneumonia prophylaxis, age 1 mo or older: 2 mg/kg (up to 100 mg/day) PO once daily or 4 mg/kg/week (up to 200 mg/week) PO once weekly.
FORMS — Generic only: Tabs 25, 100 mg. Trade only (Aczone): Topical gel 5% 30, 60, 90 g.
NOTES — Oral: Blood dyscrasias, severe allergic skin reactions, sulfone syndrome, hemolysis in G6PD deficiency, hepatotoxicity, neuropathy, photosensitivity, leprosy reactional states. Monitor CBC weekly for 4 weeks, then monthly for 6 months, then twice a year. Monitor LFTs.
MOA — Sulfone that inhibits dihydropteroate synthase and prevents bacterial folic acid synthesis.
ADVERSE EFFECTS — Serious: Blood dyscrasias, allergic skin reactions, sulfone syndrome, hemolysis in G6PD deficiency, hepatotoxicity, neuropathy, photosensitivity, leprosy reactional states. Frequent:

DAPSONE (*cont.*)

Rash, headache, GI complaints, mononucleosis-like syndrome. Topical, frequent: dryness, pruritus, erythema, scaling.

ETHAMBUTOL (*Myambutol, ✦Etibi*) ▶LK ♀C but + ▶+ $$$$

ADULT — TB: ATS and CDC recommend 15 to 20 mg/kg PO daily. Dose with whole tabs based on estimated lean body weight: 800 mg PO daily for wt 40 to 55 kg, 1200 mg PO daily for wt 56 to 75 kg, 1600 mg PO daily for wt 76 to 90 kg. Max dose regardless of wt is 1600 mg/day. Consider monitoring blood levels to ensure dose is adequate if weight >90 kg.

PEDS — TB: ATS and CDC recommend 15 to 20 mg/kg (up to 1 g) PO daily. Use cautiously if visual acuity cannot be monitored. Manufacturer recommends against use in children younger than 13 yo.

UNAPPROVED ADULT — Treatment or prevention of recurrent Mycobacterium avium complex disease in HIV infection: 15 to 25 mg/kg (up to 1600 mg) PO daily with clarithromycin/azithromycin ± rifabutin.

UNAPPROVED PEDS — Treatment or prevention of recurrent Mycobacterium avium complex disease in HIV infection: 15 mg/kg (up to 900 mg) PO daily with clarithromycin/azithromycin ± rifabutin.

FORMS — Generic/Trade: Tabs 100, 400 mg.

NOTES — Can cause retrobulbar neuritis. Avoid, if possible, in patients with optic neuritis. Test visual acuity and color discrimination at baseline. Ask about visual disturbances monthly. Monitor visual acuity and color discrimination monthly if dose is greater than 15 to 20 mg/kg, duration is longer than 2 months, or renal dysfunction. Advise patients to report any change in vision immediately; do not use in those who cannot report visual symptoms (e.g., children, unconscious). Do not give aluminum hydroxide antacid until at least 4 h after ethambutol dose. Reduce dose in renal impairment.

MOA — Inhibits arabinosyl transferase enzymes involved in synthesis of mycobacterial cell wall.

ADVERSE EFFECTS — Serious: Retrobulbar neuritis, peripheral neuropathy, anaphylactoid reactions.

ISONIAZID (*INH, ✦Isotamine*) ▶LK ♀C but + ▶+ $

WARNING — Hepatotoxicity. Obtain baseline LFTs. Monitor LFTs monthly in high-risk patients (HIV, signs/history of liver disease, abnormal LFTs at baseline, pregnancy/postpartum, alcoholism/regular alcohol use, some patients older than 35 yo). Tell all patients to stop isoniazid and call at once if hepatotoxicity symptoms develop. Discontinue if ALT at least 3 times the upper limit of normal with hepatotoxicity symptoms or ALT at least 5 times the upper limit of normal without hepatotoxicity symptoms.

ADULT — TB treatment: 5 mg/kg (up to 300 mg) PO daily or 15 mg/kg (up to 900 mg) twice or three times a week. Latent TB: 300 mg PO daily.

PEDS — TB treatment: 10 to 15 mg/kg (up to 300 mg) PO daily. Latent TB: 10 mg/kg (up to 300 mg) PO daily.

UNAPPROVED ADULT — American Thoracic Society regimen, latent TB: 5 mg/kg (up to 300 mg) PO daily for 9 months (6 months adequate if HIV-negative, but less effective than 9 months). Weekly regimen for latent TB: Give once weekly for 12 weeks isoniazid 15 mg/kg PO rounded up to nearest 50 or 100 mg (max 900 mg) + rifapentine 750 mg for wt 32.1 to 49.9 kg or rifapentine 900 mg for wt 50 kg or greater. Regimen intended for directly observed therapy; not recommended for HIV-infected patients treated with antiretrovirals, or for use during pregnancy.

UNAPPROVED PEDS — American Thoracic Society regimen, latent TB: 10 to 20 mg/kg (up to 300 mg) PO daily for 9 months. Weekly regimen for latent TB, age 12 yo or older: Give once weekly for 12 weeks isoniazid 15 mg/kg PO rounded up to nearest 50 or 100 mg (max 900 mg) + rifapentine dosed according to wt. Rifapentine dose is 300 mg for 10 to 14 kg; 450 mg for 14.1 to 25 kg; 600 mg for 25.1 to 32 kg; 750 mg for wt 32.1 to 49.9 kg; 900 mg for wt 50 kg or greater. Regimen intended for directly observed therapy; not recommended for HIV-infected patients treated with antiretrovirals, or use during pregnancy.

FORMS — Generic only: Tabs 100, 300 mg. Syrup 50 mg/5 mL.

NOTES — To reduce risk of peripheral neuropathy, give pyridoxine if alcoholism, diabetes, HIV, uremia, malnutrition, seizure disorder, pregnant/breastfeeding woman, breastfed infant of INH-treated mother. Many drug interactions.

MOA — Inhibits synthesis of mycolic acid, a component of mycobacterial cell walls.

ADVERSE EFFECTS — Serious: Hepatotoxicity, peripheral neuropathy, lupus. Frequent: Increased LFTs, positive ANA.

PYRAZINAMIDE (*PZA, ✦Tebrazid*) ▶LK ♀C ▶? $$$$

WARNING — The ATS and CDC recommend against general use of 2-month regimen of rifampin + pyrazinamide for latent TB due to reports of fatal hepatotoxicity.

ADULT — TB: ATS and CDC recommend 20 to 25 mg/kg PO daily. Dose with whole tabs based on estimated lean body weight: Give 1000 mg PO daily for 40 to 55 kg, 1500 mg daily for 56 to 75 kg, 2000 mg for 76 to 90 kg. Max dose regardless of wt is 2000 mg PO daily. Consider monitoring blood levels to ensure dose is adequate if weight >90 kg.

PEDS — TB: 15 to 30 mg/kg (up to 2000 mg) PO daily.

FORMS — Generic only: Tabs 500 mg.

NOTES — Hepatotoxicity, hyperuricemia (avoid in acute gout). Obtain LFTs at baseline. Monitor periodically in high-risk patients (HIV infection, alcoholism, pregnancy, signs/history of liver disease, abnormal LFTs at baseline). Discontinue if ALT is at least 3 times the upper limit of normal with hepatotoxicity symptoms or ALT is at least 5 times upper limit of normal without hepatotoxicity symptoms. Consider reduced dose in renal dysfunction.

MOA — Unknown.

(cont.)

PYRAZINAMIDE (*cont.*)

ADVERSE EFFECTS — Serious: Hepatotoxicity. Frequent: Hyperuricemia, polyarthralgia, myalgia, mild anorexia, nausea.

RIFABUTIN (*Mycobutin*) ▶L ♀B ▶? $$$$$

ADULT — Prevention of disseminated Mycobacterium avium complex disease in AIDS: 300 mg PO daily; can give 150 mg PO two times per day if GI upset. Per HIV guidelines, reduce rifabutin dose for coadministration with unboosted atazanavir or fosamprenavir; or ritonavir-boosted atazanavir, darunavir, fosamprenavir, lopinavir (Kaletra), saquinavir, or tipranavir: 150 mg PO once daily or 300 mg PO three times per week. For ritonavir-boosted regimens, monitor antimycobacterial activity and consider therapeutic drug monitoring. Reduce dose for nelfinavir (use nelfinavir 1250 mg PO two times per day), unboosted indinavir (increase indinavir to 1000 mg PO q 8 h): 150 mg PO daily. Dosage increase for efavirenz: 450 to 600 mg PO daily or 600 mg PO three times per week. Use standard rifabutin dose with etravirine (without ritonavir-boosted protease inhibitor) or nevirapine. Avoid rifabutin in patients receiving etravirine with a ritonavir-boosted protease inhibitor or rilpivirine. Monitor CBC at least weekly. Consider dosage adjustment based on rifabutin levels for patients receiving antiretroviral drugs.

PEDS — Not approved in children.

UNAPPROVED ADULT — TB or Mycobacterium avium complex disease treatment in AIDS: 300 mg PO daily. Dosage reduction for ritonavir-boosted protease inhibitors: 150 mg PO once daily or 300 mg PO three times per week. For ritonavir-boosted regimens, monitor antimycobacterial activity and consider therapeutic drug monitoring.

UNAPPROVED PEDS — Mycobacterium avium complex disease. Prophylaxis: Give 5 mg/kg (up to 300 mg) PO daily for age younger than 6 yo; give 300 mg PO daily for age 6 yo or older. Treatment: 10 to 20 mg/kg (max 300 mg/day) PO once daily. TB: 10 to 20 mg/kg (up to 300 mg/day) PO once daily.

FORMS — Generic/Trade: Caps 150 mg.

NOTES — Uveitis (with high doses or if metabolism inhibited by other drugs), hepatotoxicity, thrombocytopenia, neutropenia. Obtain CBC and LFTs at baseline. Monitor periodically in high-risk patients (HIV infection, alcoholism, pregnancy, signs/history of liver disease, abnormal LFTs at baseline). May induce liver metabolism of other drugs including oral contraceptives, protease inhibitors, and azole antifungals. Substrate of CYP3A4; azole antifungals, clarithromycin, and protease inhibitors increase rifabutin levels. Urine, body secretion, soft contact lenses may turn orange-brown. Consider dosage reduction for hepatic dysfunction.

MOA — Rifamycin derivative that inhibits bacterial RNA polymerase.

ADVERSE EFFECTS — Serious: Uveitis (with high doses or if metabolism inhibited by other drugs), hepatotoxicity, thrombocytopenia, neutropenia. Frequent: Arthralgia/myalgia; GI upset; increased LFTs; orange-brown discoloration of urine, body secretion, soft contact lenses.

RIFAMATE (isoniazid + rifampin) ▶LK ♀C but + ▶+ $$$$$

WARNING — Hepatotoxicity.

ADULT — TB: 2 caps PO daily on empty stomach.

PEDS — Not approved in children.

FORMS — Trade only: Caps isoniazid 150 mg + rifampin 300 mg.

NOTES — See components. Monitor LFTs at baseline and periodically during therapy.

MOA — See components.

ADVERSE EFFECTS — See components.

RIFAMPIN (*Rifadin,* ❋*Rofact*) ▶L ♀C but + ▶+ $$$$

WARNING — The ATS and CDC recommend against general use of 2-month regimen of rifampin + pyrazinamide for latent TB due to reports of fatal hepatotoxicity.

ADULT — TB: 10 mg/kg (up to 600 mg) PO/IV daily. Neisseria meningitidis carriers: 600 mg PO two times per day for 2 days. Take oral doses on empty stomach. IV and PO doses are the same.

PEDS — TB: 10 to 20 mg/kg (up to 600 mg) PO/IV daily. Neisseria meningitidis carriers: Age younger than 1 mo, 5 mg/kg PO two times per day for 2 days; age 1 mo or older, 10 mg/kg (up to 600 mg) PO two times per day for 2 days. Take oral doses on empty stomach. IV and PO doses are the same.

UNAPPROVED ADULT — Prophylaxis of H. influenzae type b infection: 20 mg/kg (up to 600 mg) PO daily for 4 days. Leprosy: 600 mg PO q month with dapsone. ATS regimen for latent TB: 10 mg/kg up to 600 mg PO daily for 4 months. Staphylococcal prosthetic valve endocarditis: 300 mg PO q 8 h in combination with gentamicin plus nafcillin, oxacillin, or vancomycin. Take on empty stomach.

UNAPPROVED PEDS — Prophylaxis of H. influenzae type b infection: Age younger than 1 mo, 10 mg/kg PO daily for 4 days; age 1 mo or older, 20 mg/kg up to 600 mg PO daily for 4 days. Prophylaxis of invasive meningococcal disease: Age younger than 1 mo, 5 mg/kg PO two times per day for 2 days; age 1 mo or older, 10 mg/kg (up to 600 mg) PO two times per day for 2 days. ATS regimen for latent tuberculosis: 10 to 20 mg/kg (up to 600 mg) PO daily for 4 months. Take on empty stomach.

FORMS — Generic/Trade: Caps 150, 300 mg. Pharmacists can make oral susp.

NOTES — Hepatotoxicity, thrombocytopenia. When treating TB, obtain baseline CBC, LFTs. Monitor periodically in high-risk patients (HIV infection, alcoholism, pregnancy, signs/history of liver disease, abnormal LFTs at baseline). Discontinue if ALT is at least 3 times the upper limit of normal with hepatotoxicity symptoms or ALT is at least 5 times the upper limit of normal without hepatotoxicity symptoms. Avoid interruptions in rifampin therapy; rare renal hypersensitivity reactions can occur after resumption. Induces hepatic metabolism of many drugs; check other sources for dosage adjustments

RIFAMPIN (*cont.*)

before prescribing. If used with rifampin, consider increasing efavirenz to 800 mg once daily at bedtime if wt greater than 60 kg. Do not use rifampin with HIV protease inhibitors, rilpivirine, or Stribild. Decreased efficacy of oral contraceptives; use nonhormonal method. Decreased INR with warfarin; monitor daily or as needed. Adjust dose for hepatic impairment. Colors urine, body secretions, soft contact lenses red-orange. Give prophylactic vitamin K 10 mg IM single dose to newborns of women taking rifampin. IV rifampin is stable for 4 h after dilution in dextrose 5%.

MOA — Rifamycin derivative that inhibits bacterial RNA polymerase.

ADVERSE EFFECTS — Serious: Hepatotoxicity, thrombocytopenia, exacerbation of porphyria, serious skin reactions (rare). Potential risk of hemorrhagic disease in newborns of women taking rifampin; give vitamin K 10 mg IM x 1 to newborn. Frequent: Rash, pruritus, arthralgia/myalgia; orange-brown discoloration of urine, body secretion, soft contact lenses.

RIFAPENTINE (*Priftin, RPT*) ▸Esterases, feces ♀C ▶? $$$$

ADULT — TB: 600 mg PO twice a week for 2 months, then once a week for 4 months. Use only for continuation therapy in selected HIV-negative patients.

PEDS — Not approved in children younger than 12 yo.

UNAPPROVED ADULT — Weekly regimen for latent TB: Give once weekly for 12 weeks isoniazid 15 mg/kg PO rounded up to nearest 50 or 100 mg (max 900 mg) + rifapentine 750 mg for wt 32.1 to 49.9 kg or 900 mg for wt 50 kg or greater. Regimen intended for directly observed therapy; not recommended for HIV-infected patients treated with antiretrovirals, or for use during pregnancy.

UNAPPROVED PEDS — Weekly regimen for latent TB, age 12 yo or older: Give once weekly for 12 weeks isoniazid 15 mg/kg PO rounded up to nearest 50 or 100 mg (max 900 mg) + rifapentine PO dosed according to wt. Rifapentine dose is 300 mg for 10 to 14 kg; 450 mg for 14.1 to 25 kg; 600 mg for 25.1 to 32 kg; 750 mg for wt 32.1 to 49.9 kg; 900 mg for wt 50 kg or greater. Regimen intended for directly observed therapy; not recommended for HIV-infected patients treated with antiretrovirals or for use during pregnancy.

FORMS — Trade only: Tabs 150 mg.

NOTES — Hepatotoxicity, thrombocytopenia, exacerbation of porphyria. Obtain CBC and LFTs at baseline. Monitor LFTs periodically in high-risk patients (alcoholism, pregnancy, signs/history of liver disease, abnormal LFTs at baseline). Do not use in porphyria. Urine, body secretions, contact lenses, and dentures may turn red-orange. May induce liver metabolism of other drugs including oral contraceptives. Advise women taking hormonal contractive to use barrier contraceptive during treatment. Avoid with protease inhibitors, NNRTIs, and maraviroc.

MOA — Long-acting derivative of rifampin, a rifamycin that inhibits bacterial RNA polymerase.

ADVERSE EFFECTS — Serious: Hepatotoxicity, thrombocytopenia, exacerbation of porphyria, neutropenia (rare). Frequent: Hyperuricemia, orange-brown discoloration of urine, body secretion, soft contact lenses.

RIFATER (isoniazid + rifampin + pyrazinamide) ▸LK ♀C ▶? $$$$$

WARNING — Hepatotoxicity.

ADULT — TB, initial 2 months of treatment: 4 tabs daily for wt less than 45 kg, 5 tabs daily for 45 to 54 kg, 6 tabs daily for 55 kg or greater. Additional pyrazinamide tabs required to provide adequate dose for wt greater than 90 kg. Take PO on empty stomach. Can finish treatment with Rifamate.

PEDS — Ratio of formulation may not be appropriate for children younger than 15 yo.

FORMS — Trade only: Tabs isoniazid 50 mg + rifampin 120 mg + pyrazinamide 300 mg.

NOTES — See components. Monitor LFTs at baseline and during therapy. Do not use in patients with renal dysfunction.

MOA — See components.

ADVERSE EFFECTS — See components.

ANTIMICROBIALS: Antiparasitics

ALBENDAZOLE (*Albenza*) ▸L ♀C ▶? $$$$$

ADULT — Hydatid disease, neurocysticercosis: 15 mg/kg/day (up to 800 mg/day) PO divided in two doses for wt less than 60 kg; 400 mg PO two times per day for wt 60 kg or greater. Treatment duration varies. Take with food.

PEDS — Hydatid disease, neurocysticercosis: 15 mg/kg/day (up to 800 mg/day) PO divided in two doses for wt less than 60 kg; 400 mg PO two times per day for wt 60 kg or greater. Treatment duration varies. Take with food.

UNAPPROVED ADULT — Hookworm, whipworm, pinworm, roundworm: 400 mg PO single dose. Repeat in 2 weeks for pinworm. Cutaneous larva migrans: 200 mg PO two times per day for 3 days. Giardia: 400 mg PO daily for 5 days. Intestinal/disseminated microsporidiosis in HIV infection (not for ocular or caused by E. bienuesi/V. corneae): 400 mg PO two times per day until CD4 count higher than 200 for more than 6 months after starting antiretrovirals.

UNAPPROVED PEDS — Roundworm, hookworm, pinworm, whipworm: 400 mg PO single dose. Repeat in 2 weeks for pinworm. Cutaneous larva migrans: 200 mg PO two times per day for 3 days. Giardia: 400 mg PO daily for 5 days.

FORMS — Trade only: Tabs 200 mg.

NOTES — Associated with bone marrow suppression (especially if liver disease), increased LFTs (common with long-term use), and hepatotoxicity (rare). Monitor CBC and LFTs before starting and then q 2 weeks; discontinue if significant changes. Consider corticosteroids and anticonvulsants in

(cont.)

ALBENDAZOLE (*cont.*)

neurocysticercosis. Consider diagnosis of preexisting neurocysticercosis if patient develops neurologic symptoms soon after albendazole treatment for another indication. Get negative pregnancy test before treatment and warn against getting pregnant until 1 month after treatment. Treat close contacts for pinworms. Can crush/chew tabs and swallow with water.

MOA — Anthelmintic that inhibits the formation of microtubules and causes glucose depletion.

ADVERSE EFFECTS — Serious: Nephrotoxicity, bone marrow suppression, hepatotoxicity (usually with long-term use). Increased LFTs increases risk of liver failure or bone marrow suppression. Frequent: Abnormal LFTs, abdominal pain.

ATOVAQUONE (*Mepron*) ▶feces ♀C ▶? $$$$$

ADULT — Pneumocystis pneumonia in patients intolerant to trimethoprim-sulfamethoxazole: Treatment 750 mg PO two times per day for 21 days. Prevention 1500 mg PO daily. Take with meals.

PEDS — Pneumocystis pneumonia in patients intolerant to trimethoprim-sulfamethoxazole, 13 to 16 yo: Treatment, 750 mg PO two times per day for 21 days. Prevention, 1500 mg PO daily. Take with meals.

UNAPPROVED PEDS — Prevention of recurrent Pneumocystis pneumonia in HIV infection: 30 mg/kg PO daily for age 1 to 3 mo; 45 mg/kg PO daily for age 4 to 24 mo; 30 mg/kg PO daily for age 25 mo or older. Take with meals.

FORMS — Generic/Trade: Susp 750 mg/5 mL (210 mL). Trade only: foil pouch 750 mg/5 mL (5 mL).

NOTES — Efficacy of atovaquone may be decreased by rifampin (consider using alternative), rifabutin, or rifapentine.

MOA — Ubiquinone analog that may inhibit nucleic acid and ATP synthesis via effects on mitochondrial electron transport.

ADVERSE EFFECTS — Serious: Hepatotoxicity (rare). Frequent: Rash, nausea, fever, headache, insomnia, increased LFTs.

IODOQUINOL (*Yodoxin, diiodohydroxyquin, ✸Diodoquin*) ▶Not absorbed ♀? ▶? $$$

ADULT — Intestinal amebiasis: 650 mg PO three times per day after meals for 20 days.

PEDS — Intestinal amebiasis: 40 mg/kg/day PO divided three times per day for 20 days. Do not exceed adult dose.

FORMS — Trade only: Tabs 210, 650 mg.

NOTES — Optic neuritis/atrophy, peripheral neuropathy with prolonged high doses. Interference with some thyroid function tests for up to 6 months after treatment.

MOA — Luminal agent, mechanism unknown.

ADVERSE EFFECTS — Serious: Optic neuritis/atrophy, peripheral neuropathy with prolonged high doses. Interference with some thyroid function tests for up to 6 months after treatment.

IVERMECTIN (*Stromectol*) ▶L ♀C ▶+ $$

ADULT — Strongyloidiasis: 200 mcg/kg PO single dose. Onchocerciasis: 150 mcg/kg PO single dose

q 3 to 12 months. Take on empty stomach with water.

PEDS — Strongyloidiasis: 200 mcg/kg PO single dose. Onchocerciasis: 150 mcg/kg PO single dose q 3 to 12 months. Take on empty stomach with water. Safety and efficacy not established in children less than 15 kg.

UNAPPROVED ADULT — Scabies: 200 mcg/kg PO, repeated in 7 to 14 days. Pubic lice: 250 mcg/kg PO repeated in 2 weeks. Cutaneous larva migrans: 150 to 200 mcg/kg PO single dose. Take on empty stomach with water. Head lice (resistant): 200 mcg/kg PO, repeat in 1 week.

UNAPPROVED PEDS — Scabies: 200 mcg/kg PO, repeated at least 7 days later. Head lice: 200 to 400 mcg/kg PO single dose; repeat in 7 days. Cutaneous larva migrans: 150 to 200 mcg/kg PO single dose. Take on empty stomach with water. Not for wt less than 15 kg.

FORMS — Trade only: Tabs 3 mg.

NOTES — Mazzotti and ophthalmic reactions with treatment for onchocerciasis. May need repeat/monthly treatment for strongyloidiasis in immunocompromised/HIV-infected patients. Increased INRs with warfarin reported rarely.

MOA — Binds to glutamate-gated chloride ion channels in invertebrate nerve and muscle cells; this leads to paralysis and death of the parasite.

ADVERSE EFFECTS — Serious: Mazzotti & ophthalmic reactions with treatment for onchocerciasis. Frequent: Nausea.

MILTEFOSINE (*Impavido*) ▶L ♀D ▶-

WARNING — Can cause fetal harm; contraindicated during pregnancy. Obtain pregnancy test before giving miltefosine to women of childbearing potential and advise them to use effective contraception during and for 5 months after miltefosine.

ADULT — Visceral, cutaneous, or mucosal leishmaniasis: 50 mg PO three times per day for 28 days. Give with food to minimize GI adverse effects.

PEDS — Visceral, cutaneous, or mucosal leishmaniasis, age 12 yo and older: 50 mg PO two times per day for 28 days for wt 30 to 44 kg; 50 mg PO three times per day for 28 days for wt 45 kg or greater. Give with food to minimize GI adverse effects.

UNAPPROVED ADULT — Free-living ameba infection: Contact CDC Emergency Operations Center at (770) 488-7100 for guidance on miltefosine treatment of suspected Naegleria fowleri, Balamuthia mandrillaris, Acanthamoeba infection.

UNAPPROVED PEDS — Free-living ameba infection: Contact CDC Emergency Operations Center at (770) 488-7100 for miltefosine to treat suspected Naegleria fowleri, Balamuthia mandrillaris, or Acanthamoeba infection.

FORMS — Trade only: Caps 50 mg. Provided on blister cards with 14 caps per card.

NOTES — Contraindicated in Sjogren-Larsson-Syndrome. Potential reproductive toxicity based on impaired fertility in animal studies. Can increase serum creatinine; monitor renal function weekly

MILTEFOSINE (*cont.*)

and for 4 weeks after treatment. Can increase transaminases; monitor liver function during treatment. Can cause volume depletion due to N/V; encourage fluid intake. Monitor platelet count during therapy for visceral leishmaniasis due to disease-related risk of thrombocyopenia. Advise women of childbearing potential using oral contraceptives to use an additional or alternative contraceptive if they develop N/V or diarrhea with miltefosine. Avoid breastfeeding during and for 5 months after treatment with miltefosine.

MOA — Unknown, but anti-leishmaniasis activity may involve interactions with membrane lipids, inhibition of mitochondrial function, and apoptosis-like cell death.

ADVERSE EFFECTS — Serious: Potential reproductive toxicity based on impaired fertility in animal studies. Volume depletion due to vomiting and diarrhea. Stevens- Johnson syndrome. Frequent: N/V, diarrhea, headache, anorexia, dizziness, abdominal pain, pruritus, somnolence, increased transaminases, increased serum creatinine.

NITAZOXANIDE (*Alinia*) ►L ♀B ▶? $$$$

ADULT — Cryptosporidial or giardial diarrhea: 500 mg PO two times per day with food for 3 days.

PEDS — Cryptosporidial or giardial diarrhea: 100 mg two times per day for 1 to 3 yo; 200 mg two times per day for 4 to 11 yo; 500 mg two times per day for 12 yo or older. Give PO with food for 3 days. Use susp if younger than 12 yo.

UNAPPROVED ADULT — C. difficile–associated diarrhea: 500 mg PO two times per day for 10 days. Cryptosporidiosis in HIV infection (alternative therapy in addition to concurrent HAART): 500 to 1000 mg PO two times per day with food for 14 days.

FORMS — Trade only: Oral susp 100 mg/5 mL (60 mL). Tabs 500 mg.

NOTES — Turns urine bright yellow. Susp contains 1.5 g sucrose/5 mL. Store susp at room temperature for up to 7 days.

MOA — Antiprotozoal agent that interferes with electron transfer reaction required for anaerobic energy metabolism.

ADVERSE EFFECTS — Mild and transient abdominal pain, diarrhea, vomiting, headache. Discolors urine bright yellow.

PAROMOMYCIN ►Not absorbed ♀C ▶? $$$$$

ADULT — Intestinal amebiasis: 25 to 35 mg/kg/day PO divided three times per day with or after meals for 5 to 10 days.

PEDS — Intestinal amebiasis: 25 to 35 mg/kg/day PO divided three times per day with or after meals for 5 to 10 days.

UNAPPROVED ADULT — Giardiasis: 500 mg PO three times per day for 7 days.

UNAPPROVED PEDS — Giardiasis: 25 to 35 mg/kg/day PO divided three times per day with or after meals for 7 days.

FORMS — Generic only: Caps 250 mg.

NOTES — Nephrotoxicity possible in inflammatory bowel disease due to increased systemic absorption. Not effective for extraintestinal amebiasis.

MOA — Aminoglycoside, inhibits parasitic protein synthesis by interfering with function of ribosomal 30S subunit.

ADVERSE EFFECTS — Serious: Nephrotoxicity possible with systemic absorption in inflammatory bowel disease. Frequent: GI distress.

PENTAMIDINE (*Pentam, NebuPent*) ►K ♀C ▶– $$$$

ADULT — Pneumocystis pneumonia treatment: 4 mg/kg IM/IV daily for 21 days. Some experts reduce to 3 mg/kg IM/IV daily if toxicity. IV infused over 60 to 90 min. NebuPent for Pneumocystis pneumonia prevention: 300 mg nebulized q 4 weeks.

PEDS — Pneumocystis pneumonia treatment: 4 mg/kg IM/IV daily for 21 days. NebuPent not approved in children.

UNAPPROVED PEDS — Pneumocystis pneumonia prevention, age 5 yo or older: 300 mg NebuPent nebulized q 4 weeks.

FORMS — Trade only: Aerosol 300 mg.

NOTES — Contraindicated with ziprasidone. Fatalities due to severe hypotension, hypoglycemia, cardiac arrhythmias with IM/IV. Have patient lie down, check BP, and keep resuscitation equipment nearby during IM/IV injection. May cause torsades (IV route only), hyperglycemia, neutropenia, nephrotoxicity, pancreatitis, and hypocalcemia. Monitor BUN, serum creatinine, blood glucose, CBC, LFTs, serum calcium, and ECG. Bronchospasm with inhalation (consider bronchodilator). Reduce IM/IV dose in renal dysfunction.

MOA — Unknown.

ADVERSE EFFECTS — Serious: Fatalities due to severe hypotension, hypoglycemia, cardiac arrhythmias with IM/IV. Extravasation of injection site. Can also cause hyperglycemia, neutropenia (frequent), nephrotoxicity, pancreatitis, torsades (IV route only), & hypocalcemia. Inhaled pentamidine can cause bronchospasm.

PRAZIQUANTEL (*Biltricide*) ►LK ♀B ▶– $$$$

ADULT — Schistosomiasis: 20 mg/kg PO q 4 to 6 h for 3 doses. Liver flukes: 25 mg/kg PO q 4 to 6 h for 3 doses.

PEDS — Schistosomiasis: 20 mg/kg PO q 4 to 6 h for 3 doses. Liver flukes: 25 mg/kg PO q 4 to 6 h for 3 doses.

UNAPPROVED ADULT — Fish, dog, beef, pork intestinal tapeworms: 10 mg/kg PO single dose.

UNAPPROVED PEDS — Fish, dog, beef, pork intestinal tapeworms: 10 mg/kg PO single dose.

FORMS — Trade only: Tabs 600 mg.

NOTES — Contraindicated in ocular cysticercosis. May cause drowsiness; do not drive or operate machinery for 48 h. Phenytoin, carbamazepine, rifampin (contraindicated), and dexamethasone may lower praziquantel levels enough to cause treatment failure. Albendazole is preferred for neurocysticercosis because it avoids these drug interactions. CYP3A4 inhibitors may increase praziquantel exposure.

(cont.)

PRAZIQUANTEL (cont.)

Take with liquids during a meal. Do not chew tabs. Manufacturer advises against breastfeeding until 72 h after treatment.

MOA — Trematodicide that induces rapid contraction of schistosomes by affecting cell membrane permeability.

ADVERSE EFFECTS — Serious: None. Frequent: Drowsiness.

PYRANTEL (Pin-X, Pinworm, ✱Combantrin) ▶Not absorbed ♀– ▶? $

ADULT — Pinworm, roundworm: 11 mg/kg (up to 1 g) PO single dose. Repeat in 2 weeks for pinworm.

PEDS — Pinworm, roundworm: 11 mg/kg (up to 1 g) PO single dose. Repeat in 2 weeks for pinworm.

UNAPPROVED ADULT — Hookworm: 11 mg/kg (up to 1 g) PO daily for 3 days.

UNAPPROVED PEDS — Hookworm: 11 mg/kg (up to 1 g) PO daily for 3 days.

FORMS — OTC Trade only (Pin-X): Susp 144 mg/mL (equivalent to 50 mg/mL of pyrantel base) 30, 60 mL. Tabs 720.5 mg (equivalent to 250 mg of pyrantel base). OTC Generic only: Caps 180 mg (equivalent to 62.5 mg of pyrantel base).

NOTES — Purging not necessary. Treat close contacts for pinworms.

MOA — Acts as agonist at nicotinic acetylcholine receptors of sensitive nematodes, depolarizing neuromuscular blocker that paralyzes the worm.

ADVERSE EFFECTS — Serious: None. Frequent: None.

PYRIMETHAMINE (Daraprim) ▶L ♀C ▶+ $$$$$

ADULT — Toxoplasmosis, immunocompetent patients: 50 to 75 mg PO daily for 1 to 3 weeks, then reduce dose by 50% for 4 to 5 more weeks. Give with leucovorin (10 to 15 mg daily) and sulfadiazine. Reduce initial dose in seizure disorders.

PEDS — Toxoplasmosis: 1 mg/kg/day PO divided two times per day for 2 to 4 days, then reduce by 50% for 1 month. Give with sulfadiazine and leucovorin. Reduce initial dose in seizure disorders.

UNAPPROVED ADULT — See regimen for acute treatment of CNS toxoplasmosis in sulfadiazine entry.

UNAPPROVED PEDS — Acquired toxoplasmosis: 2 mg/kg (up to 50 mg) PO once daily for 3 days, then 1 mg/kg (up to 25 mg) PO once daily + sulfadiazine 25 to 50 mg/kg PO (up to 1 to 1.5 g/dose) PO four times per day. Give leucovorin 10 to 25 mg/day PO. Treat for at least 6 weeks followed by chronic suppressive therapy.

FORMS — Trade only: Tabs 25 mg.

NOTES — Hemolytic anemia in G6PD deficiency, dose-related folate deficiency, hypersensitivity. Monitor CBC.

MOA — Folic acid antagonist.

ADVERSE EFFECTS — Serious: Hemolytic anemia in G6PD deficiency, dose-related folate deficiency, hypersensitivity.

TINIDAZOLE (Tindamax) ▶KL ♀C ▶? ?– $$

WARNING — Metronidazole, a related drug, was carcinogenic in animal studies.

ADULT — Trichomoniasis or giardiasis: 2 g PO single dose. Amebiasis: 2 g PO once daily for 3 days. Bacterial vaginosis: 2 g PO once daily for 2 days or 1 g PO once daily for 5 days. Take with food.

PEDS — Giardiasis, age older than 3 yo: 50 mg/kg (up to 2 g) PO single dose. Amebiasis, age older than 3 yo: 50 mg/kg (up to 2 g) PO once daily for 3 days. Take with food.

UNAPPROVED ADULT — Recurrent/persistent urethritis: 2 g PO single dose.

FORMS — Generic/Trade: Tabs 250, 500 mg. Pharmacists can compound oral susp.

NOTES — Give iodoquinol/paromomycin after treatment for amebic dysentery or liver abscess. Disulfiram reaction; avoid alcohol for at least 3 days after treatment. Can minimize infant exposure by withholding breastfeeding for 3 days after maternal single dose. May increase levels of cyclosporine, fluorouracil, lithium, phenytoin, tacrolimus. May increase INR with warfarin. Do not give at same time as cholestyramine. For patients undergoing hemodialysis: Give supplemental dose after dialysis session.

MOA — 5-Nitroimidazole derivative with amebicidal, Giardiacidal, and trichomonacidal activity.

ADVERSE EFFECTS — Serious: Seizures, peripheral neuropathy. Frequent: Anorexia, headache, dizziness. May be better tolerated than metronidazole. Transient neutropenia, leukopenia.

ANTIMICROBIALS: Antiviral Agents—Anti-CMV

CIDOFOVIR (Vistide) ▶K ♀C ▶– $$$$$

WARNING — Severe nephrotoxicity. Granulocytopenia: Monitor neutrophil counts.

ADULT — CMV retinitis: 5 mg/kg IV weekly for 2 weeks, then 5 mg/kg every other week. Give probenecid 2 g PO 3 h before and 1 g PO 2 h and 8 h after infusion. Give NS with each infusion.

PEDS — Not approved in children.

NOTES — Fanconi-like syndrome. Stop nephrotoxic drugs at least 1 week before cidofovir. Get serum creatinine, urine protein before each dose. See prescribing information for dosage adjustments based on renal function. Do not use if creatinine is greater than 1.5 mg/dL, CrCl 55 mL/min or less, or urine protein 100 mg/dL (2+) or greater. Hold/decrease zidovudine dose by 50% on day cidofovir is given. Tell women not to get pregnant until 1 month after and men to use barrier contraceptive until 3 months after cidofovir. Ocular hypotony: Monitor intraocular pressure.

MOA — Selectively inhibits cytomegalovirus DNA polymerase.

ADVERSE EFFECTS — Serious: Nephrotoxicity (also frequent), Fanconi syndrome, neutropenia (also frequent), metabolic acidosis, iritis/uveitis, ocular hypotony. Frequent: Nausea, fever, alopecia, myalgia.

FOSCARNET (Foscavir) ▶K ♀C ▶? $$$$$

WARNING — Nephrotoxicity; seizures due to mineral/electrolyte imbalance.

FOSCARNET (*cont.*)

ADULT — Hydrate before infusion. CMV retinitis: 60 mg/kg IV (over 1 h) q 8 h or 90 mg/kg IV (over 1.5 to 2 h) q 12 h for 2 to 3 weeks, then 90 to 120 mg/kg IV daily over 2 h. Acyclovir-resistant HSV infection: 40 mg/kg IV (over 1 h) q 8 to 12 h for 2 to 3 weeks or until healed.

PEDS — Not approved in children. Deposits into teeth and bone of young animals.

NOTES — Granulocytopenia, anemia, vein irritation, penile ulcers. Decreased ionized serum calcium, especially with IV pentamidine. Must use IV pump to avoid rapid administration. Monitor renal function, serum calcium, magnesium, phosphate, potassium. Reduce dose in renal impairment. Stop foscarnet if CrCl decreases to less than 0.4 mL/min/kg.

MOA — Direct inhibitor of herpesvirus DNA polymerase.

ADVERSE EFFECTS — Serious: Nephrotoxicity (also frequent), neutropenia, penile ulcers. Electrolyte/mineral disorders. Frequent: Headache, fatigue, nausea, fever.

GANCICLOVIR (*Cytovene*) ▸K ♀C ▶– $$$$$

WARNING — Neutropenia, anemia, thrombocytopenia. Do not use if ANC less than 500/mm^3 or platelets less than 25,000/mm^3.

ADULT — CMV retinitis. Induction: 5 mg/kg IV q 12 h for 14 to 21 days. Maintenance: 6 mg/kg IV daily for 5 days/week or 5 mg/kg IV daily. Prevention of CMV disease after organ transplant: 5 mg/kg IV q 12 h for 7 to 14 days, then 6 mg/kg IV daily for 5 days/week. Give IV infusion over 1 h.

PEDS — Safety and efficacy not established in children; potential carcinogenic or reproductive adverse effects.

UNAPPROVED PEDS — CMV retinitis, age older than 3 mo. Induction: 5 mg/kg IV q 12 h for 14 to 21 days. Maintenance: 5 mg/kg IV daily or 6 mg/kg IV daily for 5 days/weeks. Symptomatic congenital CMV infection: 6 mg/kg IV q 12 h for 6 weeks.

NOTES — Neutropenia (worsened by zidovudine), phlebitis/pain at infusion site, increased seizure risk with imipenem. Monitor CBC, renal function. Reduce dose if CrCl less than 70 mL/min. Adequate hydration required. Potential teratogen. Tell women not to get pregnant during and men to use barrier

contraceptive at least 3 months after treatment. Potential carcinogen. Follow guidelines for handling/disposal of cytotoxic agents.

MOA — Inhibits viral DNA synthesis.

ADVERSE EFFECTS — Serious: Myelosuppression (frequent), fever (frequent), hepatic and renal dysfunction, retinal detachment. Frequent: GI complaints, headache, phlebitis at injection site, rash, confusion.

VALGANCICLOVIR (*Valcyte*) ▸K ♀C ▶– $$$$$

WARNING — Myelosuppression may occur at any time. Monitor CBC and platelet count frequently. Do not use if ANC less than 500/mm^3, platelets less than 25,000/mm^3, hemoglobin less than 8 g/dL.

ADULT — CMV retinitis: 900 mg PO two times per day for 21 days, then 900 mg PO daily. Prevention of CMV disease in high-risk transplant patients: 900 mg PO daily given within 10 days post-transplant until 100 days post-transplant for heart or kidney-pancreas or 200 days for kidney transplant. Give with food.

PEDS — Prevention of CMV disease in high-risk kidney/heart transplant patients 4 months of age and older: Daily dose in mg is 7 × body surface area × CrCl (calculated with modified Schwartz formula). Give PO once daily from within 10 days post-transplant to 100 days post-transplant. Max dose of 900 mg/day. Give with food.

FORMS — Trade only: Tabs 450 mg. Oral soln 50 mg/mL.

NOTES — Contraindicated in ganciclovir allergy. Potential teratogen. Tell women not to get pregnant until 1 month after and men to use barrier contraceptive until at least 3 months after treatment. CNS toxicity; warn against hazardous tasks. May increase serum creatinine; monitor renal function. Reduce dose if CrCl less than 60 mL/min. Use ganciclovir instead in hemodialysis patients. Potential drug interactions with didanosine, mycophenolate, zidovudine. Potential carcinogen. Avoid direct contact with broken/crushed tabs; do not intentionally break/crush tabs. Follow guidelines for handling/disposal of cytotoxic agents.

MOA — Prodrug of ganciclovir.

ADVERSE EFFECTS — Similar to ganciclovir.

ANTIMICROBIALS: Antiviral Agents—Anti-HIV—CCR5 Antagonists

MARAVIROC (*Selzentry, MVC, ✦Celsentri*) ▸LK ♀B ▶– $$$$$

WARNING — Hepatotoxicity with allergic features, including DRESS. May have prodrome of severe rash or systemic allergic reaction. Monitor LFTs at baseline and if rash, allergic reaction, or signs/symptoms of hepatitis. Consider discontinuation if signs/symptoms of hepatitis, or increased LFTs with rash or other systemic symptoms. Caution if baseline liver dysfunction or coinfection with hepatitis B/C.

ADULT — Combination therapy for HIV infection: 150 mg PO two times per day with strong CYP3A4

inhibitors (boceprevir, clarithromycin, itraconazole, ketoconazole, most protease inhibitors including ritonavir-boosted fosamprenavir); 300 mg PO two times per day with drugs that are not strong CYP3A4 inducers/inhibitors (NRTIs, tipranavir-ritonavir, nevirapine, enfuvirtide, raltegravir; rifabutin without a strong CYP3A4 inhibitor or inducer); 600 mg PO two times per day with strong CYP3A4 inducers (efavirenz, etravirine, rifampin, carbamazepine, phenobarbital, phenytoin). Do not give maraviroc with unboosted fosamprenavir. Tropism test before treatment; not for dual/mixed or CXCR4-tropic HIV infection.

(cont.)

MARAVIROC (*cont.*)

PEDS — Not recommended for age younger than 16 yo based on lack of data.

FORMS — Trade only: Tabs 150, 300 mg.

NOTES — Discontinue immediately if signs/sx of severe skin or hypersensitivity reaction. May increase risk of myocardial ischemia or MI. Theoretical risk of infection/malignancy due to effects on immune system. Metabolized by CYP3A4; do not use with St. John's wort. Increased risk of postural hypotension in renal impairment. Contraindicated in patients with CrCl less than 30 mL/min who are taking a strong CYP3A4 inhibitor or inducer. Consider dosage reduction to 150 mg two times per day if postural hypotension occurs in patients with CrCL less than 30 mL/min.

MOA — CCR5 coreceptor antagonist prevents entry of CCR5-tropic HIV into uninfected CD4 T-cells.

ADVERSE EFFECTS — Serious: Hepatotoxicity with allergic features, including DRESS. Severe skin or hypersensitivity reactions. Immune reconstitution syndrome. May increase risk of myocardial ischemia or MI. May cause postural hypotension, esp in patients with impaired renal function. Frequent: Cough, fever, upper respiratory tract infection, rash, joint symptoms, muscle pain, abdominal pain, dizziness, increased AST.

ANTIMICROBIALS: Antiviral Agents—Anti-HIV—Combinations

NOTE: Nucleoside reverse transcriptase inhibitors can cause lactic acidosis and hepatic steatosis.

ATRIPLA (efavirenz + emtricitabine + tenofovir) ▶KL ♀D ▶– $$$$$

WARNING — Tenofovir: Potentially fatal lactic acidosis and hepatosteatosis. Entricitabine and tenofovir: Severe acute exacerbation of hepatitis B after discontinuation in patients coinfected with HIV and hepatitis B.

ADULT — Combination therapy for HIV infection: 1 tab PO once daily on empty stomach, preferably at bedtime. Atripla can be used alone or in combination with other antiretrovirals that are not already in the tab.

PEDS — Consider antihistamine prophylaxis to prevent efavirenz rash before starting Atripla. Combination therapy for HIV infection, age 12 yo or older and wt 40 kg or greater: 1 tab PO once daily on empty stomach, preferably at bedtime. Atripla can be used alone or in combination with other antiretrovirals that are not already in the tab.

FORMS — Trade only: Tabs efavirenz 600 mg + emtricitabine 200 mg + tenofovir 300 mg.

NOTES — See components. Not for CrCl less than 50 mL/min; assess CrCl before treatment. Monitor CrCl, urine glucose, urine protein, serum phosphorus before and during treatment in patients at risk for renal impairment. Do not give Atripla with lamivudine or boceprevir. Efavirenz induces CYP3A4, causing many drug interactions. Coadministration with rifampin: Add 200 mg/day of efavirenz if Atripla is given with rifampin if wt 50 kg or greater.

MOA — Emtricitabine is a nucleoside reverse transcriptase inhibitor structurally related to lamivudine; cross-resistance documented. Tenofovir is a nucleotide reverse transcriptase inhibitor. Emtricitabine and tenofovir have activity against hepatitis B. Efavirenz is a non-nucleoside reverse transcriptase inhibitor.

ADVERSE EFFECTS — Serious: Emtricitabine, tenofovir: Lactic acidosis/hepatic steatosis; severe acute exacerbation of hepatitis B after discontinuing either drug in patients coinfected with HIV and hepatitis B. Efavirenz: Depression, other psychiatric reactions, convulsions, severe rash, Stevens-Johnson syndrome. See components for other adverse effects.

COMBIVIR (lamivudine + zidovudine) ▶LK ♀C ▶– $$$$$

WARNING — Zidovudine: Bone marrow suppression, myopathy. Lamivudine: Severe acute exacerbation of hepatitis B can occur after discontinuation of lamivudine in patients coinfected with HIV + hepatitis B. Monitor closely for at least 2 months after discontinuing lamivudine in such patients; consider treating hepatitis B.

ADULT — Combination therapy for HIV infection: 1 tab PO bid.

PEDS — Combination therapy for HIV infection, wt 30 kg or greater: 1 tab PO bid.

FORMS — Generic/Trade: Tabs lamivudine 150 mg + zidovudine 300 mg.

NOTES — See components. Monitor CBC. Not for wt less than 30 kg, CrCl < 50 mL/min, hepatic dysfunction, or if dosage adjustment required.

MOA — See components.

ADVERSE EFFECTS — Serious: Lactic acidosis/hepatic steatosis; exacerbation of hepatitis B after discontinuation of lamivudine. See components for other adverse effects.

COMPLERA (emtricitabine + rilpivirine + tenofovir) ▶KL ♀B ▶– $$$$$

WARNING — Tenofovir: Potentially fatal lactic acidosis and hepatosteatosis. Emtricitabine and tenofovir: Severe acute exacerbation of hepatitis B after discontinuation in patients coinfected with HIV and hepatitis B.

ADULT — Combination therapy of HIV, treatment-naive adults with baseline HIV RNA ≤100,000 copies/mL: 1 tab PO once daily with food. Also an option for adults with HIV RNA <50 copies/mL for at least 6 months on stable ritonavir-boosted protease inhibitor-containing regimen (no history of virologic failure, on first/second antiretroviral regimen, with no current/past history of resistance to components of Complera). Monitor HIV RNA for virologic failure/rebound after switching to Complera. When coadministered with rifabutin, give 1 tab Complera plus 25 mg rilpivirine PO once daily with a meal.

COMPLERA (cont.)

PEDS — Safety and efficacy not established in children.
FORMS — Trade only: Tabs emtricitabine 200 mg + rilpivirine 25 mg + tenofovir 300 mg.
NOTES — See components. Not for CrCl <50 mL/min; assess CrCl before treatment. Monitor CrCl, urine glucose, urine protein, serum phosphorus before and during treatment in patients at risk for renal impairment. Dosage adjustment not required for mild/moderate hepatic impairment (Child-Pugh Class A/B). Rilpivirine has higher virologic failure rate than efavirenz in patients with baseline HIV RNA >100,000 copies/mL. Rilpivirine resistance rate is increased if baseline CD4+ count <200 cells/mm³. Rilpivirine has higher overall treatment resistance, NNRTI cross-resistance, and tenofovir and lamivudine/emtricitabine resistance than efavirenz. Contraindicated with carbamazepine, dexamethasone (more than a single dose), oxcarbazepine, phenobarbital, phenytoin, proton pump inhibitors, rifampin, rifapentine, St. John's wort.
MOA — Emtricitabine is a nucleoside reverse transcriptase inhibitor structurally related to lamivudine; cross-resistance documented. Tenofovir is a nucleotide reverse transcriptase inhibitor. Emtricitabine and tenofovir have activity against hepatitis B. Rilpivirine is a non-nucleoside reverse transcriptase inhibitor that inhibits HIV reverse transcriptase by different mechanism of action from NRTIs. Cross-resistance possible between rilpivirine and other NNRTIs.
ADVERSE EFFECTS — Serious: Emtricitabine, tenofovir: Lactic acidosis/hepatic steatosis; severe acute exacerbation of hepatitis B after discontinuing either drug in patients coinfected with HIV and hepatitis B. Rilpivirine: Depressive disorders (frequent), fat redistribution (causality unclear), immune reconstitution syndrome, hepatotoxicity. See components for other adverse effects.

EPZICOM (abacavir + lamivudine, ✦*Kivexa*) ▶LK ♀C ▶– $$$$$
WARNING — Abacavir: Potentially fatal hypersensitivity reactions. HLA-B*5701 predisposes to hypersensitivity; screen before starting abacavir and avoid if positive test. Never rechallenge with abacavir after suspected reaction. Abacavir and lamivudine: Lactic acidosis and hepatosteatosis. Lamivudine: Exacerbation of hepatitis B after discontinuation in patients coinfected with HIV and hepatitis B.
ADULT — Combination therapy for HIV infection: 1 tab PO daily.
PEDS — Safety and efficacy not established in children.
FORMS — Trade only: Tabs abacavir 600 mg + lamivudine 300 mg.
NOTES — See components. Not for patients with CrCl less than 50 mL/min, hepatic dysfunction, or if dosage adjustment required.
MOA — See components.

ADVERSE EFFECTS — Serious: Potentially fatal hypersensitivity (abacavir); lactic acidosis/hepatic steatosis (abacavir or lamivudine); exacerbation of hepatitis B after discontinuation in patients co-infected with HIV and hepatitis B (lamivudine). See components for other adverse effects.

STRIBILD (elvitegravir + cobicistat + emtricitabine + tenofovir) ▶KL ♀B ▶– $$$$$
WARNING — Tenofovir: Potentially fatal lactic acidosis and hepatosteatosis. Emtricitabine and tenofovir: Severe acute exacerbation of hepatitis B after discontinuation in patients coinfected with HIV and hepatitis B.
ADULT — HIV infection, treatment-naive: 1 tab PO once daily with food. Do not use Stribild with other antiretroviral drugs.
PEDS — Safety and efficacy not established in children.
FORMS — Trade only: Tabs elvitegravir 150 mg + cobicistat 150 mg + emtricitabine 200 mg + tenofovir 300 mg.
NOTES — See components. Test for hepatitis B infection before treatment. Monitor CrCl, urine glucose, urine protein before and during treatment. Monitor serum phosphorus in patients at risk for renal impairment. Do not start if CrCl <70 mL/min; stop if CrCl declines to <50 mL/min. Many drug interactions. Cobicistat is strong CYP 3A4 inhibitor. Contraindicated with alfuzosin, colchicine in patients with renal/hepatic impairment, ergot alkaloids, lovastatin, oral midazolam, pimozide, rifabutin, rifampin, rifapentine, salmeterol, high-dose sildenafil for pulmonary hypertension, simvastatin, St. John's wort, triazolam. Do not give >200 mg/day of itraconazole/ketoconazole. Reduce clarithromycin dose by 50% if CrCl is 50 to 60 mL/min. Monitor INR with warfarin. Reduce dose of colchicine, bosentan, or high-dose tadalafil for pulmonary hypertension. For erectile dysfunction, reduce to max single doses of sildenafil 25 mg in 48 h, vardenafil 2.5 mg in 72 h, tadalafil 10 mg in 72 h. Monitor levels of cyclosporine, tacrolimus, sirolimus. Use lowest starting dose of atorvastatin. Separate doses of antacids by at least 2 h.
MOA — Elvitegravir is an integrase strand transfer inhibitor. Cobicistat inhibits CYP3A4; it is included in Stribild to increase exposure to elvitegravir. Emtricitabine is a nucleoside reverse transcriptase inhibitor. Tenofovir is a nucleotide reverse transcriptase inhibitor.
ADVERSE EFFECTS — Serious: Lactic acidosis/hepatic steatosis; severe acute exacerbation of hepatitis B; new onset or worsening renal impairment; decreases in bone mineral density; immune reconstitution syndrome. Frequent: nausea, diarrhea.

TRIZIVIR (abacavir + lamivudine + zidovudine) ▶LK ♀C ▶– $$$$$
WARNING — Abacavir: Life-threatening hypersensitivity. HLA-B*5701 predisposes to hypersensitivity; screen before starting abacavir and avoid

(cont.)

TRIZIVIR (cont.)

if positive test. Never rechallenge with abacavir after suspected reaction. Abacavir and lamivudine: Lactic acidosis and hepatosteatosis. Zidovudine: Bone marrow suppression, myopathy.
ADULT — HIV infection, alone (not a preferred regimen) or in combination with other agents: 1 tab PO two times per day.
PEDS — HIV infection in adolescents 40 kg or greater, alone (not a preferred regimen) or in combination with other agents: 1 tab PO two times per day.
FORMS — Generic/Trade: Tabs abacavir 300 mg + lamivudine 150 mg + zidovudine 300 mg.
NOTES — See components. Monitor CBC. Not for wt less than 40 kg, CrCl less than 50 mL/min or if dosage adjustment required.
MOA — See components.
ADVERSE EFFECTS — Serious: Lactic acidosis/ hepatic steatosis, see components for other adverse effects. Frequent: Hypersensitivity, N/V, fever/chills.

TRUVADA (emtricitabine + tenofovir) ▶K ♀B ▶– $$$$$
WARNING — Emtricitabine and tenofovir: Potentially fatal lactic acidosis and hepatosteatosis; severe acute exacerbation of hepatitis B after discontinuation in patients coinfected with HIV and hepatitis B. Confirm HIV-negative status (including acute HIV infection) before using Truvada for pre-exposure prophylaxis of HIV infection.
ADULT — Combination therapy for HIV infection: 1 tab PO daily in combination with other antiretroviral drugs. Pre-exposure prophylaxis (PrEP) of HIV in adults at high risk for sexually-acquired HIV: 1 tab PO once daily. Screen for HIV every 3 months in patients taking it for PrEP.
PEDS — Combination therapy for HIV infection, age 12 yo or older and wt 35 kg or greater: 1 tab PO daily.

UNAPPROVED ADULT — Antiviral-resistant chronic hepatitis B in HIV-coinfected patients: 1 tab PO daily. Pre-exposure prophylaxis (PrEP) of HIV in injecting drug users: 1 tab PO once daily. Screen for HIV every 3 months in patients taking it for PrEP.
FORMS — Trade only: Tabs emtricitabine 200 mg + tenofovir 300 mg.
NOTES — See components. Do not use in a triple nucleoside regimen. Monitor CrCl, urine glucose, urine protein, serum phosphorus before and during treatment in patients with or at risk for renal impairment. Not for HIV-infected patients with CrCl <30 mL/min or hemodialysis; hepatic dysfunction; or if dosage adjustment required. Increase dosing interval to q 48 h if CrCl 30 to 49 mL/min. Do not use for pre-exposure prophylaxis if CrCl <60 mL/min. Use with didanosine cautiously; reduce didanosine dose to 250 mg for adults over 60 kg, monitor for adverse effects and discontinue didanosine if they occur. Dosage adjustment of didanosine unclear if wt less than 60 kg. Give Videx EC + Truvada on empty stomach or with light meal. Give buffered didanosine + Truvada on empty stomach. Atazanavir and lopinavir/ritonavir increase tenofovir levels; monitor and discontinue Truvada if tenofovir adverse effects. Tenofovir decreases atazanavir levels. If atazanavir is used with Truvada, use 300 mg atazanavir + 100 mg ritonavir. Do not use Truvada with lamivudine, adefovir or unboosted atazanavir.
MOA — See components.
ADVERSE EFFECTS — Serious: Lactic acidosis/ hepatic steatosis (emtricitabine and tenofovir); severe acute exacerbation of hepatitis B after discontinuing either drug in patients coinfected with HIV and hepatitis B. See components for other adverse effects. Frequent adverse effects with Truvada for PrEP: headache, abdominal pain, weight loss. Decrease in bone mineral density with Truvada used for PrEP.

ANTIMICROBIALS: Antiviral Agents—Anti-HIV—Fusion Inhibitors

ENFUVIRTIDE (*Fuzeon, T-20*) ▶Serum ♀B ▶– $$$$$
ADULT — Combination therapy for HIV infection: 90 mg SC two times per day. Give each injection at new site in upper arm, anterior thigh, or abdomen, avoiding areas with current injection site reaction.
PEDS — Combination therapy for HIV infection, 6 to 16 yo: 2 mg/kg (up to 90 mg) SC two times per day. Give each injection at new site in upper arm, anterior thigh, or abdomen, avoiding areas with current injection site reaction.
FORMS — 30-day kit with vials, diluent, syringes, alcohol wipes. Single-dose vials contain 108 mg to provide delivery of 90 mg enfuvirtide.
NOTES — Increased risk of bacterial pneumonia; monitor for signs and symptoms of pneumonia. Biojector 2000 can cause bruising/hematoma, and persistent nerve pain if used near large nerves.

Reconstitute with 1.1 mL sterile water for injection. Allow vial to stand until powder dissolves completely (up to 45 min). Do not shake. Inject 1 mL (90 mg) and discard unused soln.
MOA — Peptide that binds with glycoprotein on HIV viral envelope; prevents fusion of virus with CD4+ cells.
ADVERSE EFFECTS — Serious: Increased risk of bacterial pneumonia, hypersensitivity (may include flu-like symptoms, hypotension, increased LFTs), immune reconstitution syndrome, peripheral neuropathy, pancreatitis. Frequent: Injection site reactions (including induration, cysts, nodules), eosinophilia. Biojector 2000 can cause bruising, hematoma, and persistent nerve pain if used near large nerves. Anticoagulants, hemophilia, or other coagulation disorder may increase risk of post-injection bleeding.

ANTIMICROBIALS: Antiviral Agents—Anti-HIV—Integrase Strand Transfer Inhibitor

DOLUTEGRAVIR (*Tivicay*, *DTG*) ▶glucuronidation ♀B ▶– $$$$$
ADULT — Combination therapy of HIV, integrase strand inhibitor (INSTI)-naïve: 50 mg PO once daily; increase to 50 mg PO two times per day if coadministered with efavirenz, fosamprenavir-ritonavir, tipranavir-ritonavir, or rifampin. INSTI-experienced with INSTI resistance substitutions or suspected INSTI resistance: 50 mg PO two times per day.
PEDS — Combination therapy of HIV, age 12 yo or older and wt 40 kg or greater. Integrase strand inhibitor (INSTI)-naïve: 50 mg PO once daily; increase to 50 mg PO two times per day if coadministered with efavirenz, fosamprenavir-ritonavir, tipranavir-ritonavir, or rifampin.
FORMS — Trade only: Tabs 50 mg.
NOTES — Give dolutegravir 2 h before or 6 h after cation-containing antacid/laxative, sucralfate, oral calcium/iron, buffered drugs. Dolutegravir can be given with PO calcium/iron if they are taken with a meal. May increase metformin exposure; monitor closely and consider metformin dosage reduction. Do not give with etravirine unless coadministered with ritonavir-boosted atazanavir or darunavir, or lopinavir-ritonavir. Coadministration with dofetilide contraindicated. Do not coadminister with carbamazepine, oxcarbazepine, phenytoin, phenobarbital, St John's wort.
MOA — Inhibits HIV-1 integrase, an enzyme required for insertion of virus into host genome. Inhibition of integrase prevents viral propagation.
ADVERSE EFFECTS — Serious: Severe hypersensitivity reactions; increased transaminases, esp if coinfected with hepatitis B or C. Frequent: Insomnia, headache.

RALTEGRAVIR (*Isentress, RAL*) ▶Glucuronidation ♀C ▶– $$$$$
WARNING —
ADULT — Combination therapy for HIV infection: 400 mg PO two times per day. Increase to 800 mg PO two times per day if given with rifampin.
PEDS — Combination therapy for HIV infection, 4 weeks of age and older: Film-coated tabs, wt 25 kg or greater: 400 mg PO two times per day. Chew tabs, wt 11 kg or greater: Give PO two times per day at a dose of 75 mg for wt 11 to less than 14 kg; 100 mg for 14 to less than 20 kg; 150 mg for 20 to less than 28 kg; 200 mg for 28 to less than 40 kg; 300 mg for 40 kg or greater. Max dose of chew tabs is 300 mg two times per day. Oral susp, age 4 weeks and older and weight 3 kg to less than 20 kg: Give PO two times per day at a dose of 20 mg for 3 to less than 4 kg; 30 mg for 4 to less than 6 kg; 40 mg for 6 to less than 8 kg; 60 mg for 8 to less than 11 kg; 80 mg for 11 to less than 14 kg; 100 mg for 14 to less than 20 kg. Max dose of oral susp is 100 mg PO two times per day. Pour contents of susp packet into 5 mL of water and mix. Measure dose with syringe and give orally within 30 minutes of mixing. Discard any remaining susp. Wt-based dosing of chew tab and susp is ~6 kg/kg/dose two times per day. Do not substitute chew tabs or oral susp for 400 mg film-coated tabs.
FORMS — Trade only: Film-coated tabs 400 mg. Chewable tabs (contain phenylalanine): 25, 100 mg. Single-use packets of powder for oral susp: 100 mg/5 mL.
NOTES — Myopathy and rhabdomyolysis reported; caution advised for coadministration with drugs that cause myopathy. Can cause severe skin and hypersensitivity reactions including Stevens-Johnson syndrome; stop raltegravir if signs or symptoms occur. Do not give aluminum/magnesium antacids within 2 hours of raltegravir dose; use calcium carbonate antacid instead. Do not cut or crush 400 mg film-coated tabs.
MOA — Inhibits HIV-1 integrase, an enzyme required for insertion of virus into host genome. Inhibition of integrase prevents viral propagation.
ADVERSE EFFECTS — Serious: Myopathy and rhabdomyolysis (causality unclear). Severe skin and hypersensitivity reactions, including Stevens-Johnson syndrome, toxic epidermal necrolysis, and drug rash with eosinophilia and systemic symptoms (DRESS). Immune reconstitution syndrome. Frequent: Insomnia, headache, increased CPK.

ANTIMICROBIALS: Antiviral Agents—Anti-HIV—Non-Nucleoside Reverse Transcriptase Inhibitors

NOTE: Many serious drug interactions - always check before prescribing!

EFAVIRENZ (*Sustiva, EFV*) ▶L ♀D ▶– $$$$$
ADULT — Combination therapy for HIV infection: 600 mg PO once daily. Coadministration with voriconazole: Use voriconazole maintenance dose of 400 mg PO two times per day and reduce efavirenz to 300 mg (use caps) PO once daily. Take on empty stomach, preferably at bedtime.
PEDS — Consider antihistamine prophylaxis to prevent rash before starting. Combination therapy for HIV infection, age 3 mo or older and wt 3.5 kg or greater: Give PO once daily at a dose of 100 mg for 3.5 to less than 5 kg; 150 mg for 5 to less than 7.5 kg; 200 mg for 7.5 to less than 15 kg; 250 mg for 15 to less than 20 kg; 300 mg for 20 to less than 25 kg; 350 mg for 25 to less than 32.5 kg; 400 mg for 32.5 to less than 40 kg; 600 mg for wt 40 kg or greater. Take on empty stomach, preferably at bedtime. Capsule contents can be sprinkled on 1 to 2 teaspoons of food; do not give additional food for 2 h.
FORMS — Trade only: Caps 50, 200 mg. Tabs 600 mg.
NOTES — Psychiatric/CNS reactions (warn about hazardous tasks), rash (stop treatment if severe),

(cont.)

EFAVIRENZ (*cont.*)

increased cholesterol (monitor). False-positive with Microgenics cannabinoid screening test. Monitor LFTs if given with ritonavir, hepatotoxic drugs, or to patients with hepatitis B/C. Induces CYP3A4. Many drug interactions including decreased levels of anticonvulsants, artemether/lumefantrine (Coartem), atorvastatin, bupropion, diltiazem, itraconazole, methadone, posaconazole, pravastatin, simvastatin, and probably cyclosporine, ketoconazole, sirolimus, and tacrolimus. Do not give with boceprevir, ergot alkaloids, other NNRTIs, pimozide, St. John's wort, or triazolam. Do not give with atazanavir to treatment-experienced patients. Midazolam contraindicated in labeling; but can use single dose IV cautiously with monitoring for procedural sedation. If used with rifampin, increase efavirenz to 800 mg once daily at bedtime if wt 50 kg or greater. High risk of rash when taken with clarithromycin; consider alternative antimicrobial. Potentially teratogenic; get negative pregnancy test before use by women of child-bearing potential and recommend barrier contraceptive until 12 weeks after efavirenz is stopped.

MOA — Inhibits HIV reverse transcriptase by different mechanism of action from NRTIs. Cross-resistance possible between efavirenz and nevirapine.

ADVERSE EFFECTS — Serious: Depression and other psychiatric reactions, convulsions, severe rash, Stevens-Johnson syndrome, lipoatrophy, hepatotoxicity (rare), immune reconstitution syndrome. Frequent: Rash (especially in children), CNS symptoms (dizziness, insomnia, vivid dreams, impaired concentration; warn about hazardous tasks).

ETRAVIRINE (*Intelence, ETR*) ▶L ♀B ▶– $$$$$

ADULT — Combination therapy for treatment-resistant HIV infection: 200 mg PO two times per day after meals.

PEDS — Combination therapy for treatment-resistant HIV infection age 6 yo and older: Give PO two times per day after meals at 100 mg per dose for 16 to less than 20 kg; 125 mg per dose for 20 to less than 25 kg; 150 mg per dose for 25 to less than 30 kg; 200 mg per dose for 30 kg or greater.

FORMS — Trade only: Tabs 25, 100, 200 mg.

NOTES — Severe skin reactions, Stevens-Johnson syndrome, hypersensitivity. Induces CYP3A4 and inhibits CYP2C9 and 2C19; substrate of CYP2C9, 2C19, and 3A4. Do not give with carbamazepine, efavirenz, nevirapine, phenobarbital, phenytoin, rifampin, rifapentine, rilpivirine, ritonavir 600 mg two times per day; ritonavir-boosted tipranavir/fosamprenavir/atazanavir; St. John's wort. Give rifabutin 300 mg once daily with etravirine (without ritonavir-boosted protease inhibitor). Avoid rifabutin in patients receiving etravirine with a protease inhibitor. Monitor INR with warfarin. May need dosage reduction of fluvastatin or diazepam. Consider alternative to clarithromycin for Mycobacterium avium complex treatment or prevention. Consider monitoring antiarrhythmic blood levels. May reduce

exposure to Coartem. Can disperse tabs in water and take immediately if swallowing difficulty. Do not disperse tabs in grapefruit juice, or warm or carbonated drinks.

MOA — Inhibits HIV reverse transcriptase by different mechanism of action from NRTIs.

ADVERSE EFFECTS — Serious: Severe rash (rare) including Stevens-Johnson syndrome, toxic epidermal necrolysis, and DRESS. Immune reconstitution syndrome. Frequent: Mild/moderate rash between weeks 2-4 of therapy; nausea.

NEVIRAPINE (*Viramune, Viramune XR, NVP*) ▶LK ♀C ▶– $$$$$

WARNING — Life-threatening skin reactions, hypersensitivity, and hepatotoxicity. Monitor clinical and lab status intensively during first 18 weeks of therapy (risk of rash and/or hepatotoxicity greatest during first 6 weeks of therapy) and frequently thereafter. Consider LFTs at baseline, before and 2 weeks after dose increase, and at least once a month. Rapidly progressive liver failure can occur after only a few weeks of therapy. Stop nevirapine and never rechallenge if clinical hepatitis, severe rash, or rash with constitutional symptoms/increased LFTs. Obtain LFTs if rash occurs. Risk of hepatotoxicity with rash high in women or high CD4 count (women with CD4 count greater than 250 especially high risk, including pregnant women). Do not use if CD4 count greater than 250 in women or greater than 400 in men unless benefit clearly outweighs risk. Elevated LFTs or hepatitis B/C infection at baseline increases risk of hepatotoxicity. Hepatotoxicity not reported after single doses of nevirapine or in children.

ADULT — Combination therapy for HIV infection: 200 mg PO daily for 14 days, then 200 mg PO two times per day or Viramune XR 400 mg PO once daily. Patients maintained on immediate-release tabs can switch directly to Viramune XR. Dose titration reduces risk of rash. If rash develops, do not increase dose until it resolves. If stopped for more than 7 days, restart with initial dose.

PEDS — Combination therapy for HIV infection, age 15 days old or older: 150 mg/m^2 PO once daily for 14 days, then 150 mg/m^2 two times per day (max dose 200 mg two times per day). Dose titration reduces risk of rash. If rash develops, do not increase dose until it resolves. If stopped for more than 7 days, restart with initial dose. Per HIV guidelines, children 8 yo or younger may require up to 200 mg/m^2 PO two times per day (max dose 200 mg two times per day). Viramune XR, age 6 yo and older: 200 mg PO once daily for BSA 0.58 to 0.83 m^2; 300 mg PO once daily for BSA 0.84 to 1.16 m^2; 400 mg PO once daily for BSA ≥1.17 m^2. To reduce risk of rash, patients should receive immediate-release nevirapine 150 mg/m^2 once daily (max 200 mg/day) for at least 14 days before conversion to Viramune XR. Patients already maintained on twice daily immediate-release nevirapine can switch directly to Viramune XR.

NEVIRAPINE (*cont.*)

UNAPPROVED ADULT — Combination therapy for HIV infection: 200 mg PO daily for 14 days, then 400 mg PO daily. Prevention of maternal-fetal HIV transmission, maternal dosing: 200 mg PO single dose at onset of labor. Do not add single-dose nevirapine to standard HIV regimens in pregnant women in the United States.

UNAPPROVED PEDS — Prevention of maternal-fetal HIV transmission, neonatal dose: 2 mg/kg PO single dose within 3 days of birth.

FORMS — Generic/Trade: Tabs 200 mg. Susp 50 mg/5 mL (240 mL). Extended-release tabs 400 mg. Trade only: Extended-release tabs (Viramune XR) 100 mg.

NOTES — CYP3A4 inducer. May require increased methadone dose. Do not give with atazanavir, boceprevir, ketoconazole, hormonal contraceptives, or St. John's wort. Granulocytopenia more common in children receiving zidovudine and nevirapine. Contraindicated if Child-Pugh Class B/C liver failure. Give supplemental dose of 200 mg after dialysis session. Do not use for post-exposure prophylaxis in HIV-uninfected patients. Do not use in infants who have been exposed to nevirapine as part of maternal-infant prophylaxis. Do not chew, crush, or split Viramune XR tabs.

MOA — Inhibits HIV reverse transcriptase by different mechanism of action from NRTIs. Cross-resistance possible between efavirenz and nevirapine.

ADVERSE EFFECTS — Serious: Life-threatening rash (including Stevens-Johnson syndrome, toxic epidermal necrolysis, exfoliative dermatitis), hypersensitivity, hepatotoxicity. Risk of severe rash and/or hepatotoxicity (they can occur together) is greatest in first 6 weeks of therapy and is especially high in women with CD4 count greater than 250. Rhabdomyolysis can occur with skin reaction or hepatotoxicity. Granulocytopenia more common in children receiving zidovudine and nevirapine. Frequent: Increased LFTs, erythema, pruritus, maculopapular rash, dry desquamation.

RILPIVIRINE (*Edurant, RPV*) ▶L ♀B ▶– $$$$$

ADULT — Combination therapy of HIV infection, treatment-naive adults with HIV RNA ≤100,000 copies/mL: 25 mg PO once daily with a meal. Dosage adjustment for rifabutin: Rilpivirine 50 mg PO once daily with a meal.

PEDS — Safety and efficacy not established in children.

FORMS — Trade only: Tabs 25 mg.

NOTES — Rilpivirine has higher virologic failure rate than efavirenz in patients with baseline HIV RNA >100,000 copies/mL. Rilpivirine resistance rate is increased if baseline CD4+ count <200 cells/mm³. Rilpivirine has higher overall treatment resistance, NNRTI cross-resistance, and tenofovir and lamivudine/ emtricitabine resistance than efavirenz. Hepatoxocity/increased LFTs: Monitor LFTs in patients with underlying liver disease or increased LFTs at baseline. Consider monitoring LFTs in all patients. Metabolized by CYP3A4. Contraindicated with carbamazepine, dexamethasone (more than single dose), oxcarbazepine, phenobarbital, phenytoin, proton pump inhibitors, rifampin, rifapentine, St. John's wort. Use cautiously with drugs that cause torsades; supratherapeutic doses of rilpivirine prolonged QT interval. Give antacids at least 2 h before or 4 h after rilpivirine. Give H2 blockers at least 12 h before or 4 h after rilpivirine. Monitor for reduced response to methadone. Store in original bottle to protect from light.

MOA — Inhibits HIV reverse transcriptase by different mechanism of action from NRTIs. Cross-resistance possible between rilpivirine and other NNRTIs.

ADVERSE EFFECTS — Serious: Depressive disorders (frequent), fat redistribution (causality unclear), immune reconstitution syndrome, hepatotoxicity (rare), increased LFTs.

ANTIMICROBIALS: Antiviral Agents—Anti-HIV—Nucleoside/Nucleotide Reverse Transcriptase Inhibitors

NOTE: Can cause lactic acidosis and hepatic steatosis.

ABACAVIR (*Ziagen, ABC*) ▶L ♀C ▶– $$$$$

WARNING — Potentially fatal hypersensitivity (look for fever, rash, GI symptoms, cough, dyspnea, pharyngitis, or other respiratory symptoms). Stop at once and never rechallenge after suspected reaction. Fatal reactions can recur within hours of rechallenge in patients with previously unrecognized reaction. HLA-B*5701 predisposes to hypersensitivity; screen before starting abacavir and avoid if positive test. Label HLA-B*5701-positive patients as abacavir-allergic in medical record.

ADULT — Combination therapy for HIV infection: 300 mg PO two times per day or 600 mg PO daily. Severe hypersensitivity may be more common with single daily dose.

PEDS — Combination therapy for HIV infection. Oral soln, age 3 mo or older: 8 mg/kg (up to 300 mg) PO two times per day. Tabs: 150 mg PO two times per day for wt 14 to 21 kg; 150 mg PO q am and 300 mg PO q pm for wt 22 kg to 29 kg; 300 mg PO two times per day for wt 30 kg or greater.

FORMS — Generic/Trade: Tabs 300 mg scored. Trade only: soln 20 mg/mL (240 mL).

NOTES — Reduce dose for mild hepatic dysfunction (Child-Pugh score 5 to 6): 200 mg (10 mL of oral soln) PO two times per day. FDA safety review did not find increased risk of myocardial infarction with abacavir.

MOA — Reduces HIV replication within infected cells by inhibiting HIV reverse transcriptase.

(cont.)

ABACAVIR (*cont.*)

ADVERSE EFFECTS — Serious: Life-threatening hypersensitivity, lactic acidosis/hepatic steatosis. bone marrow suppression. FDA safety review did not find increased risk of myocardial infarction with abacavir. Frequent: GI complaints.

DIDANOSINE (*Videx, Videx EC, DDI*) ▶LK ♀B ▶– $$$$$

WARNING — Potentially fatal pancreatitis; avoid other drugs that can cause pancreatitis. Avoid didanosine + stavudine in pregnancy due to reports of fatal lactic acidosis with pancreatitis or hepatic steatosis.

ADULT — Combination therapy for HIV infection: Videx EC: 250 mg PO daily for wt less than 60 kg. 400 mg PO daily for wt 60 kg or greater. Take on empty stomach. If taken with tenofovir, reduce dose to 200 mg for wt less than 60 kg and 250 mg for 60 kg or greater. Dosage reduction unclear with tenofovir if CrCl less than 60 mL/min. Give tenofovir + Videx EC on empty stomach or with light meal.

PEDS — Combination therapy for HIV infection: 100 mg/m^2 PO two times per day for age 2 weeks to 8 mo. 120 mg/m^2 PO two times per day for age older than 8 mo (do not exceed adult dose). Videx EC: Give PO once daily 200 mg for wt 20 to 24 kg, 250 mg for wt 25 to 59 kg, 400 mg for wt 60 kg or greater.

FORMS — Generic/Trade: Delayed-release caps (Videx EC): 125, 200, 250, 400 mg. Pediatric powder for oral soln (buffered with antacid) 10 mg/mL. Generic only: Tabs for oral susp (chewable; buffered with antacid) 100, 150, 200 mg.

NOTES — Not recommended as part of an initial HIV treatment regimen, primarily because of toxicity. Peripheral neuropathy (use cautiously with other neurotoxic drugs), retinal changes, optic neuritis, retinal depigmentation in children, hyperuricemia. Risk of lactic acidosis, pancreatitis, and peripheral neuropathy increased by concomitant stavudine. Diarrhea with buffered powder. See prescribing information for reduced dose if CrCl less than 60 mL/min. Do not use with allopurinol. Give some medications at least 1 h (indinavir), 2 h (atazanavir, ciprofloxacin, levofloxacin, norfloxacin, ofloxacin, itraconazole, ketoconazole, ritonavir, dapsone, tetracyclines), or 4 h (moxifloxacin, gatifloxacin) before buffered didanosine. Contraindicated with ribavirin due to risk of didanosine toxicity. Methadone may reduce efficacy of didanosine, especially with buffered pediatric powder; use Videx EC instead of powder with methadone and monitor for reduced didanosine efficacy.

MOA — Reduces HIV replication within infected cells by inhibiting HIV reverse transcriptase.

ADVERSE EFFECTS — Serious: Lactic acidosis/hepatic steatosis, symptomatic hyperlactatemia, fatal lactic acidosis with stavudine plus didanosine in pregnant women (avoid concomitant use), retinal toxicity, pancreatitis (frequent; risk increased by stavudine), peripheral neuropathy (frequent; risk increased by stavudine), non-cirrhotic portal hypertension (rare). Frequent: Fever, GI complaints, headache, rash.

EMTRICITABINE (*Emtriva, FTC*) ▶K ♀B ▶– $$$$$

WARNING — Severe acute exacerbation of hepatitis B can occur after discontinuation in patients coinfected with HIV and hepatitis B. Monitor closely for at least 2 months; consider treating hepatitis B.

ADULT — Combination therapy for HIV infection: 200 mg cap PO daily. Oral soln: 240 mg (24 mL) PO daily.

PEDS — Combination therapy for HIV: Give 3 mg/kg oral soln PO once daily for age birth to 3 mo; 6 mg/kg PO once daily (up to 240 mg) for age older than 3 mo. Give 200 mg cap PO once daily for wt greater than 33 kg.

FORMS — Trade only: Caps 200 mg. Oral soln 10 mg/mL (170 mL).

NOTES — Reduce dose in adults with renal dysfunction. Caps: Give 200 mg PO q 96 h if CrCl less than 15 mL/min or hemodialysis; 200 mg PO q 72 h if CrCl 15 to 29 mL/min; 200 mg PO q 48 h if CrCl 30 to 49 mL/min. Oral soln: 60 mg q 24 h if CrCl less than 15 mL/min or hemodialysis; 80 mg q 24 h if CrCl 15 to 29 mL/min; 120 mg q 24 h if CrCl 30 to 49 mL/min; refrigerate oral soln if possible; stable for 3 months at room temp.

MOA — Reduces HIV replication within infected cells by inhibiting HIV reverse transcriptase. Structurally related to lamivudine; cross-resistance documented. Has activity against hepatitis B.

ADVERSE EFFECTS — Serious: Lactic acidosis/hepatic steatosis. Frequent: Headache, diarrhea, nausea, rash. Other: Hyperpigmentation on palms/soles primarily in non-Caucasians.

LAMIVUDINE (*Epivir, Epivir-HBV, 3TC, ✳Heptovir*) ▶K ♀C ▶– $$$$$

WARNING — Lower dose of lamivudine in Epivir-HBV can cause HIV resistance; test for HIV before prescribing Epivir-HBV. Severe acute exacerbation of hepatitis B can occur after discontinuation of lamivudine in patients coinfected with HIV and hepatitis B. Monitor closely for at least 2 months after discontinuing lamivudine in such patients; consider treating hepatitis B.

ADULT — Epivir for combination therapy for HIV infection: 300 mg PO daily or 150 mg PO two times per day. Epivir-HBV for chronic hepatitis B: 100 mg PO daily. Coinfection with HIV and hepatitis B requires higher dose of lamivudine for HIV infection.

PEDS — Epivir for HIV infection: 3 mo to 16 yo, 4 mg/kg (up to 150 mg) PO two times per day. Epivir tabs: 75 mg two times per day for 14 to 21 kg, 75 mg q am and 150 mg q pm for 22 to 29 kg; 150 mg two times per day for 30 kg or greater; 300 mg PO once daily or 150 mg PO two times per day for age 16 yo or older. Epivir-HBV for chronic hepatitis B: 3 mg/kg (up to 100 mg) PO daily for age 2 yo or older. Coinfection with HIV and hepatitis B requires higher dose of lamivudine for HIV infection.

UNAPPROVED PEDS — Epivir for combination therapy for HIV infection. Infants, age younger than 30 days old: 2 mg/kg PO two times per day.

LAMIVUDINE (*cont.*)

FORMS — Generic/Trade: Tabs 150 (scored), 300 mg. Trade only (Epivir): Oral soln 10 mg/mL. Generic/Trade: Tabs 100 mg. Trade only (Epivir-HBV, Heptovir): Oral soln 5 mg/mL.

NOTES — Lamivudine-resistant hepatitis B reported. Epivir: Pancreatitis in children. Monitor for hepatic decompensation (potentially fatal), neutropenia, and anemia if also receiving interferon for hepatitis C. If hepatic decompensation occurs, consider discontinuing lamivudine, and reducing or discontinuing interferon, and/or ribavirin. Dosage reduction for CrCl less than 50 mL/min in prescribing information.

MOA — Nucleoside analog. Reduces HIV replication within infected cells by inhibiting HIV reverse transcriptase. Reduces hepatitis B replication by inhibiting HBV polymerase.

ADVERSE EFFECTS — Serious: Lactic acidosis/hepatic steatosis; exacerbation of hepatitis B after discontinuation of lamivudine; pancreatitis in children; hepatic decompensation in HCV/HIV coinfected patients. Frequent: Headache, fatigue, nausea, dizziness, nasal symptoms (well-tolerated compared with other NRTIs).

TENOFOVIR (*Viread, TDF*) ▶K ♀B ▶– $$$$$

WARNING — Stop tenofovir if hepatomegaly or steatosis occur, even if LFTs normal. Severe acute exacerbation of hepatitis B can occur after discontinuation of tenofovir in patients coinfected with HIV and hepatitis B. Monitor closely for at least 2 months after discontinuing tenofovir in such patients; consider treating hepatitis B.

ADULT — Combination therapy for HIV; chronic hepatitis B: 300 mg PO daily without regard to food. For adults who cannot swallow tabs, use 7.5 scoops of oral powder once daily. High rate of virologic failure with tenofovir + didanosine + lamivudine for HIV infection; avoid this regimen.

PEDS — Combination therapy of HIV. Oral powder, 2 yo and older: 8 mg/kg PO once daily (max 300 mg/day). Dosing scoop for oral powder delivers 40 mg tenofovir per scoop. Mix powder with 2 to 4 ounces of soft food that doesn't need chewing (applesauce, baby food, yogurt). Use immediately after mixing. Do not mix powder with liquid. Tabs, 2 yo and older and wt 17 kg or greater: Give PO once daily at dose of 150 mg for wt 17 kg to less than 22 kg; 200 mg for wt 22 kg to less than 28 kg; 250 mg for wt 28 kg to less than 35 kg; 300 mg for wt 35 kg or greater. Chronic hepatitis B, age 12 yo and older and wt 35 kg or greater: 300 mg PO daily without regard to meals. For patients who cannot swallow tabs, use 7.5 scoops of oral powder once daily.

FORMS — Trade only: Tabs 150, 200, 250, 300 mg. Oral powder 40 mg tenofovir/g.

NOTES — Decreased bone mineral density; consider bone mineral density monitoring if history of pathologic fracture or other risk factors for osteoporosis/bone loss. Consider calcium and vitamin D supplement. Tenofovir increases didanosine levels and possibly serious didanosine adverse effects (eg, pancreatitis, lactic acidosis, hyperlactatemia, neuropathy). If atazanavir is used with tenofovir, use 300 mg atazanavir + 100 mg ritonavir PO once daily. Atazanavir and lopinavir/ritonavir increase tenofovir levels; monitor and discontinue tenofovir if adverse effects. Tenofovir can cause renal impairment including acute renal failure and Fanconi syndrome. Evaluate renal function in patients who develop bone/extremity pain, fractures, muscle pain/weakness (signs of osteomalacia with proximal renal tubulopathy). Estimate CrCl before starting tenofovir. Avoid tenofovir if current/recent nephrotoxic drug use, including high-dose/multiple NSAIDs. Drugs that reduce renal function or undergo renal elimination (eg, acyclovir, adefovir, ganciclovir) may increase tenofovir levels; do not use with adefovir. Monitor CrCl, urine protein, urine glucose, serum phosphorus if mild renal impairment or at risk for renal impairment. Reduce dose for renal dysfunction: 300 mg once weekly (given after dialysis) for dialysis; 300 mg twice weekly if CrCl 10 to 29 mL/min; 300 mg q 48 h if CrCl 30 to 49 mL/min.

MOA — Nucleotide reverse transcriptase inhibitor. Similar mechanism of action as NRTIs, but does not require phosphorylation step required to activate NRTIs. Reduces HIV replication within infected cells by inhibiting HIV reverse transcriptase. Has activity against hepatitis B.

ADVERSE EFFECTS — Serious: Lactic acidosis/hepatic steatosis, renal impairment including acute renal failure and Fanconi syndrome, hypophosphatemia. Osteomalacia with proximal renal tubulopathy. Decreased bone mineral density in adults & children; fracture risk unknown. Immune reconstitution syndrome, including autoimmune disorders. Exacerbation of hepatitis B after discontinuation of tenofovir. Reports of syncope, usually with vagal syndrome. Frequent: GI complaints, dizziness.

ZIDOVUDINE (*Retrovir, AZT, ZDV*) ▶LK ♀C ▶– $$$$$

WARNING — Bone marrow suppression, myopathy.

ADULT — Combination therapy for HIV infection: 600 mg/day PO divided two or three times per day. IV dosing: 1 mg/kg IV administered over 1 h 5 to 6 times per day. Prevention of maternal-fetal HIV transmission, maternal dosing (after 14 weeks of pregnancy): 600 mg/day PO divided two or three times per day until start of labor. During labor, 2 mg/kg (total body wt) IV over 1 h, then 1 mg/kg/h until delivery.

PEDS — Combination therapy for HIV infection, age 4 weeks or older: Give 24 mg/kg/day divided two or three times per day for wt 4 to 8 kg; give 18 mg/kg/day divided two or three times per day for wt 9 kg to 29 kg; give 600 mg/day divided two or three times per day for wt 30 kg or greater. Alternative dose: 480 mg/m^2/day PO divided two or three times per day. Prevention of maternal-fetal HIV transmission, infant dosing: 2 mg/kg PO q 6 h from within 12 h of birth until 6 weeks old. Can also give infants 1.5 mg/kg IV over 30 min q 6 h.

(cont.)

ZIDOVUDINE (*cont.*)

FORMS — Generic/Trade: Caps 100 mg. Syrup 50 mg/5 mL (240 mL). Generic only: Tabs 300 mg.

NOTES — Not recommended as part of an initial HIV treatment regimen, primarily because of toxicity. Hematologic toxicity; monitor CBC. Increased bone marrow suppression with ganciclovir or valganciclovir. Granulocytopenia more common in children receiving zidovudine and nevirapine. Monitor for hepatic decompensation, neutropenia, and anemia if also receiving interferon regimen for hepatitis C. If hepatic decompensation occurs, consider discontinuing zidovudine, interferon, and/or ribavirin. See prescribing information for dosage adjustments for renal dysfunction or hematologic toxicity.

MOA — Decreases or inhibits HIV replication within infected cells by inhibiting HIV reverse transcriptase.

ADVERSE EFFECTS — Serious: Lactic acidosis/hepatic steatosis, lipoatrophy (possibly), hematologic toxicity, symptomatic myopathy, hepatic decompensation in HCV/HIV coinfected patients. Granulocytopenia more common in children receiving zidovudine and nevirapine. Frequent: GI intolerance, headache, insomnia, asthenia, anorexia.

ANTIMICROBIALS: Antiviral Agents—Anti-HIV—Protease Inhibitors

NOTE: Many serious drug interactions: Always check before prescribing. Protease inhibitors inhibit CYP3A4. Contraindicated with most antiarrhythmics, alfuzosin, ergot alkaloids, lovastatin, pimozide, rifampin, rifapentine, salmeterol, high-dose sildenafil for pulmonary hypertension, simvastatin, St. John's wort, triazolam. Midazolam contraindicated in labeling; but can use single dose IV cautiously with monitoring for procedural sedation. Monitor INR with warfarin. Avoid inhaled/nasal budesonide/fluticasone with ritonavir if possible; increased corticosteroid levels can cause Cushing's syndrome/adrenal suppression. Other protease inhibitors may increase budesonide/ fluticasone levels; find alternatives for long-term use. Reduce colchicine dose; do not coadminister colchicine and protease inhibitors in patients with renal or hepatic dysfunction. Adjust dose of bosentan or tadalafil for pulmonary hypertension. Erectile dysfunction: Single dose of sildenafil 25 mg q 48 h, tadalafil 5 mg (not more than 10 mg) q 72 h, or vardenafil initially 2.5 mg q 72 h. Adverse effects include spontaneous bleeding in hemophiliacs, hyperglycemia, hyperlipidemia, immune reconstitution syndrome, and fat redistribution. Coinfection with hepatitis C or other liver disease increases the risk of hepatotoxicity with protease inhibitors; monitor LFTs at least twice in 1st month of therapy, then q 3 months.

ATAZANAVIR (*Reyataz, ATV*) ▶L ♀B ▶– $$$$$

ADULT — Combination therapy for HIV infection. Therapy-naive patients: Atazanavir 300 mg + ritonavir 100 mg PO once daily OR atazanavir 400 mg PO once daily if ritonavir-intolerant. With tenofovir, therapy-naive: 300 mg + ritonavir 100 mg PO once daily. With efavirenz, therapy-naive: 400 mg + ritonavir 100 mg once daily. Therapy-experienced: 300 mg + ritonavir 100 mg once daily. Do not give atazanavir with efavirenz in therapy-experienced patients. Pregnancy or postpartum: Usual dose is 300 mg + 100 mg ritonavir PO once daily; do not use unboosted atazanavir. If given with tenofovir or an H2 blocker in treatment-experienced patients in 2nd or 3rd trimester, give atazanavir 400 mg + ritonavir 100 mg PO once daily. Atazanavir exposure can increase during the first 2 months postpartum; monitor for adverse effects. Give atazanavir with food; give 2 h before or 1 h after buffered didanosine.

PEDS — Combination therapy for HIV infection. Oral powder, age 3 mo and older and wt 10 kg to less than 25 kg: 200 mg atazanavir power (4 packets) with 80 mg ritonavir oral soln PO once daily for wt 10 kg to <15 kg; 250 mg atazanavir powder (5 packets) with 80 mg ritonavir oral soln PO once daily for wt 15 to <25 kg. Mix power with food or beverage and give ritonavir immediately after. Oral capsules, age 6 yo and older. Give atazanavir/ritonavir PO once daily 150/100 mg for wt 15 to less than 20 kg; 200/100 mg for wt 20 kg to less than 40 kg; 300/100 mg for wt 40 kg or greater. Therapy-naive, ritonavir-intolerant, age 13 yo or older and wt 40 kg or greater: 400 mg PO once daily with food. Do not give unboosted atazanavir to patients taking tenofovir, H2 blockers, or proton pump inhibitors. Give atazanavir with food. Max dose for atazanavir/ritonavir of 300/100 mg. Do not give to infants <3 mo due to risk of kernicterus.

FORMS — Trade only: Caps 150, 200, 300 mg. Powder packets (contain phenylalanine) 50 mg.

NOTES — Does not appear to increase cholesterol or triglycerides. Asymptomatic increases in indirect bilirubin due to inhibition of UDP-glucuronosyl transferase (UGT); may cause jaundice/scleral icterus. May cause nephrolithiasis/cholelithiasis. Do not use boceprevir with ritonavir-boosted atazanavir. Do not use with indinavir; both may increase bilirubin. Do not use with nevirapine. May inhibit irinotecan metabolism. Can prolong PR interval and rare cases of 2nd degree AV block reported; caution advised for patients with AV block or on drugs that prolong PR interval, especially if metabolized by CYP3A4. Monitor ECG with calcium channel blockers; consider reducing diltiazem dose by 50%. Reduce clarithromycin dose by 50%; consider alternative therapy for indications other than Mycobacterium avium complex. Acid required for absorption; acid-suppressing drugs can cause treatment failure. Proton pump inhibitors: In

ATAZANAVIR (cont.)

treatment-naive patients do not exceed dose equivalent of omeprazole 20 mg; give PPI 12 h before atazanavir 300 mg + ritonavir 100 mg. Do not use PPIs with unboosted atazanavir or in treatment-experienced patients. H2 blockers: Give atazanavir 300 mg + ritonavir 100 mg simultaneously with H2 blocker and/or at least 10 h after H2 blocker, with max dose equivalent of famotidine 40 mg two times per day for treatment-naive patients and 20 mg two times per day for treatment-experienced patients. For treatment-experienced patients receiving tenofovir and H2 blocker, give atazanavir 400 mg + ritonavir 100 mg once daily with food. If treatment-naive and ritonavir-intolerant, give atazanavir 400 mg PO once daily with food given at least 2 h before and at least 10 h after H2 blocker (max dose equivalent to famotidine 20 mg two times per day). For treatment-experienced pregnant women in 2nd or 3rd trimester receiving tenofovir or H2 blocker, give atazanavir 400 mg + ritonavir 100 mg once daily. Give atazanavir 2 h before or 1 h after antacids or buffered didanosine. Give atazanavir and delayed-release didanosine at different times. Inhibits CYP1A2, 2C9, and 3A4. Do not use unboosted atazanavir with buprenorphine; monitor for sedation if buprenorphine given with atazanavir/ritonavir. Use lowest possible dose of rosuvastatin (limit to 10 mg/day) or atorvastatin. Monitor levels of immunosuppressants, TCAs. Avoid carbamazepine/phenytoin/phenobarbital with unboosted atazanavir; may need dosage adjustment of carbamazepine/phenytoin/phenobarbital with ritonavir-boosted atazanavir. May need dosage adjustment of lamotrigine with ritonavir-boosted atazanavir; no dosage adjustment with unboosted atazanavir. Do not give voriconazole with ritonavir-boosted atazanavir unless necessary; monitor for voriconazole adverse effects and reduced response to voriconazole and ritonavir-boosted atazanavir. Use oral contraceptive with at least 35 mcg ethinyl estradiol with ritonavir-boosted atazanavir. Use oral contraceptive with 25 to 30 mcg ethinyl estradiol if atazanavir is not boosted by ritonavir. In mild to moderate hepatic impairment (Child-Pugh class B), consider dosage reduction to 300 mg PO daily with food. Do not use in Child-Pugh Class C. Dosage adjustment for hemodialysis: Atazanavir 300 mg + ritonavir 100 mg if treatment-naive; do not use atazanavir during hemodialysis if treatment-experienced.

MOA — Prevents cleavage of protein precursors required for HIV maturation, reproduction, and infection of new cells.

ADVERSE EFFECTS — Serious: Can prolong PR interval; second degree AV block reported rarely; serious skin reactions like Stevens-Johnson syndrome and DRESS; nephrolithiasis, cholelithiasis. Frequent: Increased indirect bilirubin, jaundice/scleral icterus, nausea, rash. Class effects: Hyperglycemia, fat redistribution, spontaneous bleeding in hemophiliacs.

DARUNAVIR (Prezista, DRV) ▶L ♀B ▶– $$$$$

ADULT — Combination therapy for HIV infection. Therapy-naive or experienced with no darunavir resistance substitutions: 800 mg + ritonavir 100 mg PO once daily. Therapy-experienced with at least 1 darunavir resistance substitution: 600 mg + ritonavir 100 mg PO two times per day. Take with food.

PEDS — Combination therapy for HIV infection, age 3 yo or older. Give darunavir PO with food. Treatment-naïve or treatment-experienced without resistance substitutions: Give darunavir + ritonavir both once daily according to wt: Darunavir 35 mg/kg + ritonavir 7 mg/kg for wt 10 to less than 15 kg; darunavir 600 mg + ritonavir 100 mg for wt 15 to less than 30 kg; darunavir 675 mg + ritonavir 100 mg for wt 30 to less than 40 kg; darunavir 800 mg + ritonavir 100 mg for wt 40 kg or greater. Treatment-experienced with at least 1 resistance substitution: Give darunavir + ritonavir both two times per day according to wt: Darunavir 20 mg/kg + ritonavir 7 mg/kg for wt 10 to less than 15 kg; darunavir 375 mg + ritonavir 48 mg for wt 15 to less than 30 kg; darunavir 450 mg + ritonavir 60 mg for wt 30 to less than 40 kg; darunavir 600 mg + ritonavir 100 mg for wt 40 kg or greater.

UNAPPROVED PEDS — Do not give darunavir-ritonavir to children younger than 3 yo; animal studies suggest toxicity in this age group.

FORMS — Trade only: Tabs 75, 150, 600, 800 mg. Susp 100 mg/mL (200 mL).

NOTES — Cross-sensitivity with sulfonamides possible; use caution in sulfonamide-allergic patients. Hepatotoxicity; monitor AST/ALT more frequently (especially during first few months of therapy) if patient already has liver dysfunction. Do not give with lopinavir/ritonavir or saquinavir. Reduce dose of clarithromycin if CrCl less than 60 mL/min (see clarithromycin entry for details). Do not use with more than 200 mg/day of ketoconazole or itraconazole. Ritonavir decreases voriconazole levels; do not use voriconazole with darunavir/ritonavir unless benefit exceeds risk. May decrease oral contraceptive efficacy; consider additional or alternative method. Give didanosine 1 h before or 2 h after darunavir/ritonavir. Use lowest possible dose of atorvastatin (not more than 20 mg/day), pravastatin, or rosuvastatin.

MOA — Prevents cleavage of protein precursors required for HIV maturation, reproduction, and infection of new cells.

ADVERSE EFFECTS — Severe: Stevens-Johnson syndrome and other severe skin reactions. Hepatotoxicity (esp if hepatitis B/C or baseline elevated transaminases). Frequent: Rash, diarrhea, nausea, headache, nasopharyngitis. Class effects: Hyperglycemia, fat redistribution, lipid abnormalities, spontaneous bleeding in hemophiliacs.

FOSAMPRENAVIR (Lexiva, FPV, ✱Telzir) ▶L ♀C ▶– $$$$$

ADULT — Combination therapy for HIV infection. Therapy-naive patients: Fosamprenavir 1400 mg PO two times per day (without ritonavir) OR fosamprenavir 1400 mg PO once daily + ritonavir 100 to

(cont.)

FOSAMPRENAVIR (*cont.*)

200 mg PO once daily OR fosamprenavir 700 mg PO + ritonavir 100 mg PO both two times per day. Protease inhibitor-experienced patients: 700 mg fosamprenavir + 100 mg ritonavir PO both two times per day. Do not use once-daily regimen. If once-daily ritonavir-boosted regimen given with efavirenz, increase ritonavir to 300 mg/day; no increase of ritonavir dose needed for two times per day regimen with efavirenz. Give nevirapine with fosamprenavir only if two times per day ritonavir-boosted regimen used. No meal restrictions for tabs; take susp with food. Re-dose if vomiting occurs within 30 min of giving oral susp.

PEDS — Combination therapy for HIV infection. Fosamprenavir/ritonavir for protease inhibitor-naïve patients 4 weeks or older, or protease inhibitor-experienced patients, 6 mo or older: Give PO two times per day according to wt: Fosamprenavir 45 mg/kg plus ritonavir 7 mg/kg for wt less than 11 kg; fosamprenavir 30 mg/kg plus ritonavir 3 mg/kg for wt 11 to less than 15 kg; fosamprenavir 23 mg/kg plus ritonavir 3 mg/kg for wt 15 to less than 20 kg; fosamprenavir 18 mg/kg plus ritonavir 3 mg/kg for wt 20 kg or greater. Do not exceed adult dose of fosamprenavir 700 mg plus ritonavir 100 mg both PO two times per day. For fosamprenavir/ritonavir, can use fosamprenavir tabs if wt 39 kg or greater and ritonavir caps if wt 33 kg or greater. Unboosted fosamprenavir for protease inhibitor-naïve patients, 2 yo and older: 30 mg/kg PO two times per day; can give 1400 mg as tabs PO two times per day if wt 47 kg or greater. Fosamprenavir is only for infants born at 38 wks gestation or more who have attained post-natal age of 28 days. Do not use once-daily dosing of fosamprenavir in children. Take tabs without regard to meals. Take susp with food. Re-dose if vomiting occurs within 30 min of giving oral susp.

FORMS — Trade only: Tabs 700 mg. Susp 50 mg/mL.

NOTES — Life-threatening skin reactions possible (reported with amprenavir). Cross-sensitivity with sulfonamides possible; use caution in sulfonamide-allergic patients. Increased cholesterol and triglycerides; monitor lipids. Do not give maraviroc with unboosted fosamprenavir. Do not give ritonavir-boosted fosamprenavir with boceprevir. Use lowest possible dose of atorvastatin (not more than 20 mg/day). Monitor CBC at least weekly if taking rifabutin. Monitor levels of immunosuppressants, TCAs. May need to increase dose of methadone. Do not use more than 200 mg/day ketoconazole/itraconazole with fosamprenavir + ritonavir; may need to reduce antifungal dose if patient is receiving more than 400 mg/day itraconazole or ketoconazole with unboosted fosamprenavir. Do not use more than 2.5 mg vardenafil q 24 h with unboosted fosamprenavir or q 72 h for fosamprenavir + ritonavir. Do not use hormonal contraceptives. More adverse reactions when fosamprenavir is given with Kaletra; appropriate dose for combination therapy unclear. Mild hepatic dysfunction (Child-Pugh score 5 to 6): 700 mg PO two times per day unboosted (for treatment-naive) or 700 mg PO two times per day plus ritonavir 100 mg PO once daily (for treatment-naive or -experienced). Moderate hepatic dysfunction (Child-Pugh score 7 to 9): 700 mg PO two times per day unboosted (for treatment-naive) or 450 mg PO two times per day plus ritonavir 100 mg PO once daily (for treatment-naive or -experienced). Severe hepatic dysfunction: fosamprenavir 350 mg PO two times per day unboosted (for treatment-naive) or 300 mg PO two times per day plus ritonavir 100 mg PO once daily (for treatment-naive or -experienced). No dosage adjustments available for peds patients with hepatic dysfunction. Refrigeration not required, but may improve taste of oral susp.

MOA — Prodrug of amprenavir. Prevents cleavage of protein precursors required for HIV maturation, reproduction, and infection of new cells.

ADVERSE EFFECTS — Severe: Life-threatening rash possible. Nephrolithiasis. Frequent: Diarrhea, N/V, headache, rash, pruritus, fatigue. GI intolerance more frequent with once-daily dosing. Class effects: Hyperglycemia, fat redistribution, lipid abnormalities, spontaneous bleeding in hemophiliacs.

INDINAVIR (*Crixivan, IDV*) ▶LK ♀C ▶– $$$$$

ADULT — Combination therapy for HIV infection: 800 mg PO q 8 h between meals with water (at least 48 oz/day).

PEDS — Not approved in children. Do not use in infants; may cause kernicterus.

UNAPPROVED ADULT — Combination therapy for HIV infection: Indinavir 800 mg PO with ritonavir 100 to 200 mg PO both two times per day; or indinavir 400 mg with ritonavir 400 mg both two times per day; or indinavir 600 mg PO with Kaletra 400/100 mg PO both two times per day. Can be given without regard to meals when given with ritonavir.

UNAPPROVED PEDS — Combination therapy for HIV infection: 350 to 500 mg/m^2/dose (max of 800 mg/dose) PO q 8 h for children; 800 mg PO q 8 h between meals with water (at least 48 oz/day) for adolescents.

FORMS — Trade only: Caps 200, 400 mg.

NOTES — Nephrolithiasis (especially in children), hemolytic anemia, indirect hyperbilirubinemia, possible hepatitis, interstitial nephritis with asymptomatic pyuria. Do not use with atazanavir; both may increase bilirubin. Do not give rivaroxaban with ritonavir-boosted indinavir. Avoid using with carbamazepine if possible. Give indinavir and buffered didanosine 1 h apart on empty stomach. Reduce indinavir dose to 600 mg PO q 8 h when given with ketoconazole or itraconazole 200 mg two times per day. Increase indinavir dose to 1000 mg PO q 8 h when given with efavirenz or nevirapine. Use lowest possible dose of atorvastatin or rosuvastatin. For mild to moderate hepatic cirrhosis, give 600 mg PO q 8 h. Indinavir not recommended in pregnancy because of dramatic reduction in blood levels.

INDINAVIR (cont.)

MOA — Prevents cleavage of protein precursors required for HIV maturation, reproduction, and infection of new cells.

ADVERSE EFFECTS — Serious: Nephrolithiasis, hematuria, and sterile leukocyturia (most frequent in children), interstitial nephritis with asymptomatic pyuria, hemolytic anemia. Frequent: GI complaints, headache, asthenia, blurred vision, dizziness, rash, metallic taste, indirect hyperbilirubinemia. Class effects: Hyperglycemia, fat redistribution, lipid abnormalities, spontaneous bleeding in hemophiliacs.

KALETRA PV/r (lopinavir-ritonavir) ▶L ♀C ▶– $$$$$

ADULT — Combination therapy for HIV infection: 400/100 mg PO two times per day (tabs or oral soln). Can use 800/200 mg PO once daily in patients with less than 3 lopinavir resistance-associated substitutions. Dosage adjustment for coadministration with efavirenz, nevirapine, fosamprenavir, or nelfinavir: 500/125 mg tabs (use two 200/50 mg + one 100/25 mg tab) or 533/133 mg oral soln (6.5 mL) PO two times per day. No once-daily dosing for pregnant patients; coadministration with carbamazepine, phenobarbital, phenytoin, efavirenz, nevirapine, fosamprenavir, or nelfinavir; or in patients with 3 or more lopinavir resistance-associated substitutions (L10F/I/R/V, K20M/N/R, L24I, L33F, M36I, I47V, G48V, I54L/T/V, V82A/C/F/S/T, and I84V). Give tabs without regard to meals; give oral soln with food.

PEDS — Combination therapy for HIV infection, age 14 days to 6 mo: Lopinavir 300 mg/m² or 16 mg/kg PO two times per day. Propylene glycol in oral soln can cause life-threatening toxicity in infants (especially preterm); do not give oral soln to neonates before postmenstrual age of 42 weeks and postnatal age of at least 14 days. Age 6 mo to 12 yo: Lopinavir 230 mg/m² or 12 mg/kg PO two times per day if wt less than 15 kg; 10 mg/kg PO two times per day if wt 15 to 40 kg. Dosage adjustment for coadministration with efavirenz, nevirapine, fosamprenavir, or nelfinavir: Lopinavir 300 mg/m² PO two times per day or 13 mg/kg PO two times per day for wt less than 15 kg; 11 mg/kg PO two times per day for wt 15 to 45 kg. Do not exceed adult dose. Give tabs without regard to meals; give oral soln with food. Beware of medication errors with oral soln; fatal overdose reported in infant given excessive volume of soln.

FORMS — Trade only (lopinavir/ritonavir): Tabs 200/50 mg, 100/25 mg. Oral soln 80/20 mg/mL (160 mL).

NOTES — Do not confuse Keppra (levetiracetam) with Kaletra. May cause pancreatitis. Ritonavir included in formulation to inhibit metabolism and boost levels of lopinavir. Do not give with boceprevir or rivaroxaban. Increases tenofovir levels; monitor for adverse reactions. Many other drug interactions including decreased efficacy of oral contraceptives. Limit rosuvastatin dose to 10 mg/day; use lowest possible dose of atorvastatin. Ritonavir decreases voriconazole levels; do not give with voriconazole unless benefit exceeds risk. Expected to increase fentanyl exposure. May require higher methadone dose. Reduce dose of clarithromycin if CrCl less than 60 mL/min (see clarithromycin entry for details). Give buffered didanosine 1 h before or 2 h after Kaletra oral soln. Kaletra tabs can be given at same time as didanosine without food. Do not give Kaletra with tipranavir 500 mg + ritonavir 200 mg both two times per day. Monitor lamotrigine and valproic acid levels. Do not give Kaletra once daily with phenytoin, phenobarbital, or carbamazepine; monitor for reduced phenytoin levels. Oral soln contains alcohol. Use oral soln within 2 months if stored at room temperature. Tabs do not require refrigeration. Do not crush, cut, or chew tabs.

MOA — Prevents cleavage of protein precursors required for HIV maturation, reproduction, and infection of new cells.

ADVERSE EFFECTS — Serious: Hepatitis, pancreatitis. Increased risk of MI possible with cumulative use of Kaletra. PR and QT interval prolongation reported; caution advised for patients at risk of cardiac conduction abnormalities or coadministration of other drugs that prolong PR or QT interval. Propylene glycol in oral soln can cause life-threatening toxicity in infants (especially preterm). Frequent: GI complaints (more common with once daily regimen), transaminase elevation. Class effects: Hyperglycemia, fat redistribution, lipid abnormalities, spontaneous bleeding in hemophiliacs.

NELFINAVIR (Viracept, NFV) ▶L ♀B ▶– $$$$$

ADULT — Combination therapy for HIV infection: 750 mg PO three times per day or 1250 mg PO two times per day with meals. Absorption improved when meal contains at least 500 calories with 11 to 28 g of fat.

PEDS — Combination therapy for HIV infection: 45 to 55 mg/kg PO two times per day or 25 to 35 mg/kg PO three times per day (up to 2500 mg/day) for age 2 yo or older. Take with meals. Absorption improved when meal contains at least 500 calories with 11 to 28 g of fat. Tabs can be dissolved in small amount of water.

FORMS — Trade only: Tabs 250, 625 mg.

NOTES — Diarrhea common. Use lowest possible dose of atorvastatin (not more than 40 mg/day) or rosuvastatin or consider pravastatin/fluvastatin. Decreases efficacy of oral contraceptives. May require higher methadone dose. Do not use with proton pump inhibitors. Give nelfinavir 2 h before or 1 h after buffered didanosine. No dosage adjustment for mild hepatic impairment (Child-Pugh Class A); not recommended for more severe hepatic failure (Child-Pugh B/C).

MOA — Prevents cleavage of protein precursors required for HIV maturation, reproduction, and infection of new cells.

ADVERSE EFFECTS — Frequent: Diarrhea, transaminase elevation. Class effects: Hyperglycemia, fat redistribution, lipid abnormalities, spontaneous bleeding in hemophiliacs.

RITONAVIR (*Norvir, RTV*) ▶L ♀B ▶– $$$$$
WARNING — Contraindicated with many drugs due to risk of drug interactions.
ADULT — See specific protease inhibitor entries for boosting doses of ritonavir. For initial antiretroviral regimens, HIV treatment guidelines recommend against ritonavir as the sole protease inhibitor, and prefer ritonavir boosting doses that do not exceed 100 mg/day. Adult doses of 100 to 400 mg/day PO are used to boost levels of other protease inhibitors. The full-dose regimen (600 mg PO two times per day) is poorly tolerated. Take ritonavir with food.
PEDS — See specific protease inhibitor entries for boosting doses of ritonavir. HIV treatment guidelines recommend against full-dose ritonavir or ritonavir as the sole protease inhibitor for initial therapy of HIV in children.Give ritonavir with meals. Oral soln contains 43.2% (v/v) alcohol and 26.6% (w/v) propylene glycol. It can cause propylene glycol toxicity in preterm infants; do not give oral soln to neonates before a postmenstrual age of 44 weeks. Medication errors or overdose of oral soln could lead to alcohol/propylene glycol toxicity in infants <6 mo.
FORMS — Trade only: Caps 100 mg, tabs 100 mg. Oral soln 80 mg/mL (240 mL).
NOTES — N/V, pancreatitis, alterations in AST, ALT, GGT, CPK, uric acid. Do not give with quinine or rivaroxaban. Ritonavir decreases voriconazole levels. Do not use ritonavir doses of 400 mg two times per day or greater with voriconazole; use ritonavir 100 mg two times per day with voriconazole only if benefit exceeds risk. Decreases efficacy of combined oral or patch contraceptives; consider alternative. May increases fentanyl levels; monitor for increase in fentanyl effects. Increases methadone dosage requirements. May cause serotonin syndrome with fluoxetine. Can prolong PR interval and rare cases of 2nd or 3rd degree AV block reported; caution advised for patients at risk for conduction problems or taking drugs that prolong PR interval, especially if metabolized by CYP3A4. Reduce clarithromycin dose if CrCl less than 60 mL/min (see clarithromycin entry for details). Give ritonavir 2.5 h before/after buffered didanosine. Monitor for increased digoxin levels. Caps and oral soln contain alcohol. Do not refrigerate oral soln. Try to refrigerate caps, but stable for 30 days at less than 77°F. Tabs do not require refrigeration, but must be taken with food.
MOA — Prevents cleavage of protein precursors required for HIV maturation, reproduction, and infection of new cells.
ADVERSE EFFECTS — Serious: Greater than 200% increase in triglycerides; hepatitis, pancreatitis. Can prolong PR interval; rare cases of second/third degree AV block reported. Frequent: GI complaints, paresthesias, asthenia, taste perversion, increased CPK & uric acid. Class effects: Hyperglycemia, fat redistribution, lipid abnormalities, spontaneous bleeding in hemophiliacs.

SAQUINAVIR (*Invirase, SQV*) ▶L ♀B ▶– $$$$$
ADULT — Combination therapy for HIV infection. Regimen must contain ritonavir. Saquinavir 1000 mg + ritonavir 100 mg PO both two times per day taken within 2 h after meals. Saquinavir 1000 mg + lopinavir-ritonavir (Kaletra) 400/100 mg PO both two times per day. If serious toxicity occurs, do not reduce Invirase dose; efficacy unclear for lower doses.
PEDS — Combination therapy for HIV, age 16 yo or older: Use adult dose. Pediatric dose that is effective without increasing risk of QT/PR interval prolongation has not been established.
FORMS — Trade only: Caps 200 mg. Tabs 500 mg.
NOTES — Can prolong QT (increase more than some other boosted protease inhibitors) and PR interval; rare cases of torsades and 2nd/3rd degree AV block. Get ECG at baseline, after 3 to 4 days of therapy, and periodically in at-risk patients. Do not use if baseline QT interval is longer than 450 msec. Discontinue if on-treatment QT interval is longer than 480 msec or interval increases by more than 20 msec over baseline. Do not use if refractory hypokalemia/hypomagnesemia, congenital long QT syndrome, complete AV block without pacemaker or at high risk for complete AV block, or severe hepatic impairment. Do not use with Class IA or III anti-arrhythmics, neuroleptics or antimicrobials that prolong QT interval, trazodone, drugs that both increase saquinavir levels and prolong the QT interval, or if QT interval increases by more than 20 msec after starting a drug that might increase the QT interval. Monitor if used with other drugs that prolong the PR interval (beta blockers, calcium channel blockers, digoxin, atazanavir). Do not use saquinavir with garlic supplements or tipranavir/ritonavir. Use lowest possible dose of atorvastatin (not more than 20 mg/day) or rosuvastatin. Proton pump inhibitors may increase saquinavir levels. Monitor for increased digoxin levels. May reduce methadone levels. Reduce dose of clarithromycin if CrCl less than 60 mL/min (see clarithromycin entry for details).
MOA — Prevents cleavage of protein precursors required for HIV maturation, reproduction, and infection of new cells.
ADVERSE EFFECTS — Frequent: GI complaints, headache, LFT elevation. Class effects: hyperglycemia, fat redistribution, lipid abnormalities, spontaneous bleeding in hemophiliacs.

TIPRANAVIR (*Aptivus, TPV*) ▶Feces ♀C ▶– $$$$$
WARNING — Potentially fatal hepatotoxicity. Monitor clinical status and LFTs frequently. Risk increased by coinfection with hepatitis B/C. Contraindicated in moderate to severe (Child-Pugh B/C) hepatic failure. Intracranial hemorrhage can occur with tipranavir + ritonavir; caution if at risk of bleeding from trauma, surgery, other medical conditions, or receiving antiplatelet agents or anticoagulants.
ADULT — Combination therapy for HIV infection, treatment-experienced patients with resistance to

TIPRANAVIR (*cont.*)

multiple protease inhibitors: 500 mg + ritonavir 200 mg PO both two times per day. Take tipranavir plus ritonavir capsules/soln without regard to meals; take tipranavir plus ritonavir tabs with meals.

PEDS — Combination therapy for HIV infection, treatment-experienced patients with resistance to multiple protease inhibitors, age 2 yo or older : 14 mg/kg with 6 mg/kg ritonavir (375 mg/m² with ritonavir 150 mg/m²) PO two times per day to max of 500 mg with ritonavir 200 mg two times per day. Dosage reduction for toxicity in patients infected with virus that is not resistant to multiple protease inhibitors: 12 mg/kg with 5 mg/kg ritonavir (290 mg/m² with 115 mg/m² ritonavir) PO two times per day. Take tipranavir plus ritonavir capsules/soln without regard to meals; take tipranavir plus ritonavir tabs with meals.

FORMS — Trade only: Caps 250 mg. Oral soln 100 mg/mL (95 mL in unit-of-use amber glass bottle).

NOTES — Contains sulfonamide moiety; potential for cross-sensitivity unknown. Al/Mg antacids may decrease absorption of tipranavir; separate doses. Contraindicated with CYP3A4 substrates that can cause life-threatening toxicity at high concentrations. Do not use with atorvastatin or etravirine. Monitor levels of immunosuppressants, TCAs. May need higher methadone dose. Ritonavir decreases voriconazole levels; do not give together unless benefit exceeds risk. Do not use tipranavir/ritonavir with Kaletra or saquinavir. Decreases ethinyl estradiol levels; consider nonhormonal contraception. Reduce clarithromycin dose if CrCl less than 60 mL/min (see clarithromycin entry for details). Caps contain alcohol. Refrigerate bottle of caps before opening. Use caps and oral soln within 60 days of opening container. Oral soln contains 116 international units/mL of vitamin E; advise patients not to take supplemental vitamin E other than a multivitamin.

MOA — Non-peptidic protease inhibitor. Prevents cleavage of protein precursors required for HIV maturation, reproduction, and infection of new cells.

ADVERSE EFFECTS — Serious: Life-threatening hepatotoxicity, intracranial hemorrhage. Frequent: Rash (high rate in women, especially those receiving ethinyl estradiol), diarrhea, N/V, fatigue, headache; increased LFTs, total cholesterol, and triglycerides. Class effects: Hyperglycemia, fat redistribution, lipid abnormalities, spontaneous bleeding in hemophiliacs.

ANTIMICROBIALS: Antiviral Agents—Anti-Herpetic

ACYCLOVIR (*Zovirax, Sitavig*) ▶K ♀B ▶+ $

ADULT — Genital herpes: 200 mg PO q 4 h (five times per day) for 10 days for first episode, for 5 days for recurrent episodes. Chronic suppression: 400 mg PO two times per day. Zoster: 800 mg PO q 4 h (five times per day) for 7 to 10 days. Chickenpox: 800 mg PO four times per day for 5 days. IV: 5 to 10 mg/kg IV q 8 h, each dose over 1 h. Zoster in immunocompromised patients: 10 mg/kg IV q 8 h for 7 days. Herpes simplex encephalitis: 10 mg/kg IV q 8 h for 10 days. Mucosal/cutaneous herpes simplex in immunocompromised patients: 5 mg/kg IV q 8 h for 7 days. Sitavig for recurrent herpes labialis in immunocompetent adults: Apply buccal tab once to upper gum above incisor within 1 h of prodromal symptom onset (before lesions appear). Apply to side of mouth with herpes symptoms. Hold in place with slight pressure to upper lip for 30 seconds to ensure adhesion.

PEDS — Safety and efficacy of PO acyclovir not established in children younger than 2 yo. Chickenpox: 20 mg/kg PO four times per day for 5 days. Use adult dose if wt greater than 40 kg. AAP does not recommend routine treatment of chickenpox with acyclovir, but it should be considered in patients older than 12 yo or with chronic cutaneous or pulmonary disease, chronic salicylate use, or short, intermittent, or inhaled courses of corticosteroid. Possibly also for secondary household cases. IV: 250 to 500 mg/m² q 8 h, each dose over 1 h. Zoster in immunocompromised patients younger than 12 yo: 20 mg/kg IV q 8 h for 7 days. Herpes simplex encephalitis: 20 mg/kg IV q 8 h for 10 days for age 3 mo to 12 yo; adult dose for age 13 yo or older. Neonatal herpes simplex (birth to 3 mo): 10 mg/kg IV q 8 h for 10 days; CDC regimen is 20 mg/kg IV q 8 h for 21 days for disseminated/CNS disease, for 14 days for skin/mucous membranes. Mucosal/cutaneous herpes simplex in immunocompromised patients: 10 mg/kg IV q 8 h for 7 days for age younger than 12 yo, adult dose for 13 yo or older. Treat ASAP after symptom onset. Sitavig buccal tabs are not approved in children, and not recommended for younger children due to potential risk of choking.

UNAPPROVED ADULT — Genital herpes: 400 mg PO three times per day for 7 to 10 days for first episode, for 5 days for recurrent episodes, for 5 to 10 days for recurrent episodes in HIV+ patients. Alternative regimens for recurrent episodes in HIV-negative patients: 800 mg PO two times per day for 5 days or 800 mg PO three times per day for 2 days. Chronic suppression of genital herpes in HIV+ patients: 400 to 800 mg PO two to three times per day. Orolabial herpes: 400 mg PO 5 times a day.

UNAPPROVED PEDS — Primary herpes gingivostomatitis: 15 mg/kg PO 5 times a day for 7 days. First episode genital herpes: 80 mg/kg/day PO divided three times per day (max 1.2 g/day) for 7 to 10 days. Use dose in unapproved adult for adolescents. Treat ASAP after symptom onset.

FORMS — Generic/Trade: Caps 200 mg. Tabs 400, 800 mg. Susp 200 mg/5 mL. Buccal tab (Sitavig-$$$$): Trade only: 50 mg.

NOTES — Maintain adequate hydration. Severe drowsiness with acyclovir plus zidovudine. Consider

(cont.)

ACYCLOVIR (*cont.*)

suppressive therapy for patients with at least 6 episodes of genital herpes per year. Reduce dose in renal dysfunction and in elderly. Base IV dose on ideal body wt in obese adults. Sitavig: Contraindicated if hypersensitivity to milk protein concentrate. Buccal tab is intended to remain in place until it dissolves. If it falls off within 6 h of application, reposition tab. If it does not stay in place, apply a new tab. If tab is swallowed within first 6 h, drink a glass of water and apply a new tab. No action is needed if tab falls off or is swallowed after it has been in place for at least 6 h. Do not chew gum while tab is in place.

MOA — Activated by viral thymidine kinase to become an inhibitor of viral DNA polymerase and block viral DNA synthesis.

ADVERSE EFFECTS — Serious: Encephalopathy, extravasation, crystalluria with IV. Frequent: GI distress & headache with PO. Sitavig buccal tabs: Application site irritation (rare).

FAMCICLOVIR (*Famvir*) ▶K ♀B ▶? $$

ADULT — Recurrent genital herpes: 1000 mg PO two times per day for 2 days. Chronic suppression of genital herpes: 250 mg PO two times per day. Recurrent herpes labialis: 1500 mg PO single dose. Recurrent orolabial/genital herpes in HIV patients: 500 mg PO two times per day for 7 days. Zoster: 500 mg PO three times per day for 7 days. Treat ASAP after symptom onset.

PEDS — Not approved in children.

UNAPPROVED ADULT — First episode genital herpes: 250 mg PO three times per day for 7 to 10 days. Chronic suppression of genital herpes in HIV+ patients: 500 mg PO two times per day. Chickenpox in young adults: 500 mg PO three times per day for 5 days. Bell's palsy: 750 mg PO three times per day plus prednisone 1 mg/kg PO daily for 7 days. Treat ASAP after symptom onset.

UNAPPROVED PEDS — Chickenpox in adolescents: 500 mg PO three times per day for 5 days. First episode genital herpes in adolescents: Use dose in unapproved adult.

FORMS — Generic/Trade: Tabs 125, 250, 500 mg.

NOTES — Consider suppressive therapy for patients with at least 6 episodes of genital herpes per year. Reduce dose for CrCl less than 60 mL/min.

MOA — Prodrug of penciclovir. Activated by viral thymidine kinase to become an inhibitor of viral DNA polymerase and block viral DNA synthesis.

ADVERSE EFFECTS — Similar to acyclovir. Frequent: Headache, nausea, diarrhea.

VALACYCLOVIR (*Valtrex*) ▶K ♀B ▶+ $$$$

ADULT — First episode genital herpes: 1 g PO two times per day for 10 days. Recurrent genital herpes: 500 mg PO two times per day for 3 days. Chronic suppression of genital herpes in immunocompetent patients: 1 g PO daily. Can use 500 mg PO daily if 9 or fewer recurrences per year; transmission of genital herpes reduced with use of this regimen by source partner, in conjunction with safer sex practices. Chronic suppression of genital herpes in HIV-infected patients: 500 mg PO two times per day. Herpes labialis: 2 g PO q 12 h for 2 doses. Zoster: 1 g PO three times per day for 7 days. Treat ASAP after symptom onset.

PEDS — Herpes labialis, age 12 yo or older: 2 g PO q 12 h for 2 doses. Chicken pox, age 2 to 17 yo: 20 mg/kg (max of 1 g) PO three times per day for 5 days. Treat ASAP after symptom onset.

UNAPPROVED ADULT — Recurrent genital herpes: 1 g PO daily for 5 days. First episode or recurrent genital herpes in HIV+ patients: 1 g PO two times per day for 5 to 14 days. Bell's palsy: 1 g PO two times per day plus prednisone 1 mg/kg PO daily for 7 days. Orolabial herpes in immunocompromised patients, including HIV infection: 1 g PO three times per day for 7 days. Chickenpox in young adults: 1 g PO three times per day for 5 days. Treat ASAP after symptom onset.

UNAPPROVED PEDS — First episode genital herpes in adolescents: Use adult dose. Treat ASAP after symptom onset.

FORMS — Generic/Trade: Tabs 500, 1000 mg.

NOTES — Consider suppressive therapy for patients with at least 6 episodes of genital herpes per year. Maintain adequate hydration. CNS and renal adverse effects more common if elderly or renal impairment; avoid inappropriately high doses in these patients. Reduce dose for CrCl less than 50 mL/min. Thrombotic thrombocytopenic purpura/hemolytic uremic syndrome at dose of 8 g/day.

MOA — Prodrug of acyclovir, which is activated by viral thymidine kinase to become an inhibitor of viral DNA polymerase and block viral DNA synthesis.

ADVERSE EFFECTS — Similar to acyclovir. CNS (e.g., agitation, hallucinations, confusion, encephalopathy): and renal adverse effects more common if elderly or renal impairment. Serious: Acute renal failure and anuria due to precipitation in renal tubules; may require hemodialysis to remove drug.

ANTIMICROBIALS: Antiviral Agents—Anti-Influenza

NOTE: Whenever possible, immunization is the preferred method of prophylaxis. Avoid anti-influenza antivirals from 48 hours before until 2 weeks after a dose of live influenza vaccine (FluMist) unless medically necessary. Patients with suspected influenza may have primary/concomitant bacterial pneumonia; antibiotics may be indicated.

AMANTADINE ▶K ♀C ▶? $$$$

ADULT — Influenza A: 100 mg PO two times per day; reduce dose to 100 mg PO daily for age 65 yo or

older. The CDC generally recommends against amantadine or rimantadine for treatment or prevention of influenza A in the United States due to

AMANTADINE (*cont.*)

high levels of resistance. Parkinsonism: 100 mg PO two times per day. Max 400 mg/day divided three to four times per day. Drug-induced extrapyramidal disorders: 100 mg PO two times per day. Max 300 mg/day divided three to four times per day.

PEDS — Safety and efficacy not established in infants age younger than 1 yo. Influenza A, treatment or prophylaxis: 5 mg/kg/day (up to 150 mg/day) PO divided two times per day for age 1 to 9 yo and any child wt less than 40 kg. 100 mg PO two times per day for age 10 yo or older. The CDC generally recommends against amantadine or rimantadine for treatment or prevention of influenza A in the United States due to high levels of resistance.

FORMS — Generic only: Caps 100 mg. Tabs 100 mg. Syrup 50 mg/5 mL (480 mL).

NOTES — CNS toxicity, suicide attempts, neuroleptic malignant syndrome with dosage reduction/withdrawal, anticholinergic effects, orthostatic hypotension. Do not stop abruptly in Parkinson's disease. Dosage reduction in adults with renal dysfunction: 200 mg PO once a week for CrCl less than 15 mL/min or hemodialysis. 200 mg PO 1st day, then 100 mg PO every other day for CrCl 15 to 29 mL/min. 200 mg PO 1st day, then 100 mg PO daily for CrCl 30 to 50 mL/min.

MOA — Appears to prevent viral replication by interfering with the function of the M2 protein in influenza virus. May facilitate dopamine release, and act as an NMDA receptor antagonist.

ADVERSE EFFECTS — Serious: Depression, suicidal ideation, seizures, orthostatic hypotension, neuroleptic malignant syndrome with dosage reduction/withdrawal (rare). Frequent: Anorexia, nausea, peripheral edema, CNS effects (esp. if elderly, renal dysfunction, seizure disorders, anticholinergics, or psychiatric disorder).

OSELTAMIVIR (*Tamiflu*) ▶LK ♀C, but + ▶? $$$$

ADULT — Influenza A/B, treatment: 75 mg PO two times per day for 5 days starting within 2 days of symptom onset. Prophylaxis: 75 mg PO daily. Start within 2 days of exposure and continue for 10 days. Take with food to improve tolerability.

PEDS — Influenza A/B treatment, age 2 weeks old and older: Give dose two times per day for 5 days starting within 2 days of symptom onset. Dose is: 3 mg/kg for age 2 weeks old to 11 mo; 30 mg for age at least 1 yo and wt 15 kg or less; 45 mg for wt 16 to 23 kg; 60 mg for wt 24 to 40 kg; 75 mg for wt >40 kg or age at least 13 yo. Influenza A/B prophylaxis, age 1 yo and older: Give once daily for 10 days starting within 2 days of exposure. Dose is 30 mg for age 1 yo or older and wt 15 kg or less, 45 mg for wt 16 to 23 kg, 60 mg for wt 24 to 40 kg, 75 mg for wt greater than 40 kg or age 13 yo and older. Prophylaxis can continue for up to 6 weeks during community outbreak. Can take with food to improve tolerability.

UNAPPROVED PEDS — Influenza treatment, age 9 to 11 mo (AAP recommended regimen): 3.5 mg/kg/dose PO two times per day for 5 days. Influenza prophylaxis, age 9 to 11 mo (AAP recommended regimen): 3.5 mg/kg/dose PO once daily for 10 days starting within 2 days of exposure. Influenza treatment, premature infants: 2 mg/kg/day PO divided two times per day. Influenza prophylaxis in infants 3 to 11 mo: 3 mg/kg/dose PO once daily for 10 days starting within 2 days of exposure. Due to limited data, prophylaxis is not recommended for infants younger than 3 mo unless the situation is critical. Can take with food to improve tolerability.

FORMS — Trade only: Caps 30, 45, 75 mg. Susp 6 mg/mL (60 mL) with 10 mL dosing device. Pharmacist can also compound susp (6 mg/mL).

NOTES — Previously not used in children younger than 1 yo; immature blood-brain barrier could lead to high oseltamivir levels in CNS. Increased INR with warfarin. Post-marketing reports (mostly from Japan) of self-injury and delirium, primarily among children and adolescents; monitor for abnormal behavior. Dosage adjustment for adults with CrCl 10 to 30 mL/min: 75 mg PO daily for 5 days for treatment, 75 mg PO every other day or 30 mg PO once daily for prophylaxis. Susp stable for 10 days at room temperature, 17 days refrigerated.

MOA — Oral neuraminidase inhibitor.

ADVERSE EFFECTS — Serious: Anaphylaxis, erythema multiforme, toxic epidermal necrolysis (these reactions rare). Frequent: N/V, stomach discomfort, headache. Post-marketing reports (mostly from Japan) of self-injury and delirium, primarily among children and adolescents.

RIMANTADINE (*Flumadine*) ▶LK ♀C ▶– $$

ADULT — Prophylaxis/treatment of influenza A: 100 mg PO two times per day. Start treatment within 2 days of symptom onset and continue for 7 days. Reduce dose to 100 mg PO once daily if severe hepatic dysfunction, CrCl less than 30 mL/min, or age older than 65 yo. The CDC generally recommends against amantadine/rimantadine for treatment/prevention of influenza A in the United States due to high levels of resistance.

PEDS — Influenza A prophylaxis: 5 mg/kg (up to 150 mg/day) PO once daily for age 1 to 9 yo; 100 mg PO two times per day for age 10 yo and older. The CDC generally recommends against amantadine/rimantadine for treatment/prevention of influenza A in the United States due to high levels of resistance.

UNAPPROVED PEDS — Influenza A treatment: 6.6 mg/kg (up to 150 mg/day) PO divided two times per day for age 1 to 9 yo; 100 mg PO two times per day for age 10 yo and older. Start treatment within 2 days of symptom onset and continue for 7 days. The CDC generally recommends against amantadine/rimantadine for treatment/prevention of influenza A in the United States due to high levels of resistance.

FORMS — Generic/Trade: Tabs 100 mg. Pharmacist can compound suspension.

MOA — Appears to prevent viral replication by interfering with the function of the M2 protein in influenza virus.

ADVERSE EFFECTS — GI effects similar to amantadine, but less CNS toxicity.

ZANAMIVIR (*Relenza*) ▶K ♀C ▶? $$$
ADULT — Influenza A/B treatment: 2 puffs two times per day for 5 days. Take 2 doses on day 1 at least 2 h apart. Start within 2 days of symptom onset. Influenza A/B prevention: 2 puffs once daily for 10 days, starting within 2 days of exposure.
PEDS — Influenza A/B treatment: 2 puffs two times per day for 5 days for age 7 yo or older. Take 2 doses on day 1 at least 2 h apart. Start within 2 days of symptom onset. Influenza A/B prevention: 2 puffs once daily for 10 days for age 5 yo or older, starting within 2 days of exposure.
FORMS — Trade only: Rotadisk inhaler 5 mg/puff (20 puffs).
NOTES — Contains lactose; contraindicated in patients with milk protein allergy. May cause bronchospasm and worsen pulmonary function in asthma or COPD; avoid if underlying airways disease. Stop if bronchospasm/decline in respiratory function. Show patient how to use inhaler.
MOA — Inhaled neuraminidase inhibitor.
ADVERSE EFFECTS — Serious: Bronchospasm in patients with reactive airway disease. Possible abnormal behavior and short-term delerium in children and adolescents; monitor for abnormal behavior. Frequent: Nasal and throat irritation.

ANTIMICROBIALS: Antiviral Agents—Other

ADEFOVIR (*Hepsera*) ▶K ♀C ▶− $$$$$
WARNING — Nephrotoxic; monitor renal function. May result in HIV resistance in untreated HIV infection; test for HIV before prescribing. Lactic acidosis with hepatic steatosis. Severe acute exacerbation of hepatitis B can occur after discontinuation of adefovir in patients with HIV and hepatitis B coinfection. Monitor closely for at least 2 months after discontinuing adefovir in such patients; consider retreating hepatitis B.
ADULT — Chronic hepatitis B: 10 mg PO daily.
PEDS — Chronic hepatitis B: 10 mg PO daily for age 12 yo or older.
FORMS — Generic/Trade: Tabs 10 mg.
NOTES — Monitor renal function. See prescribing information for dosage reduction if CrCl < 50 mL/min. Other nephrotoxic drugs may increase risk of nephrotoxicity; do not use with tenofovir. Use adefovir plus lamivudine instead of adefovir alone in patients with lamivudine-resistant hepatitis B. Adefovir resistance can cause viral load rebound. Consider change in therapy if persistent serum hepatitis B DNA > 1000 copies/mL.
MOA — Nucleotide reverse transcriptase inhibitor, similar mechanism of action as NRTIs. Negligible activity against HIV virus at 10 mg dose.
ADVERSE EFFECTS — Serious: Lactic acidosis/hepatic steatosis, nephrotoxicity, exacerbation of hepatitis B after discontinuation. Frequent: None.

BOCEPREVIR (*Victrelis*) ▶L ♀B ▶− $$$$$
ADULT — NOTE: Guidelines (www.hcvguidelines.org) do not recommend boceprevir-based regimens for the treatment of chronic hepatitis C. Chronic hepatitis C (genotype 1) including prior null/partial responders and relapsers: 800 mg PO three times per day (q 7 to 9 h) in combination with peginterferon and ribavirin. Take with food. Start boceprevir after 4 weeks of peginterferon plus ribavirin. Treatment duration is based on response at weeks 8, 12, and 24. Stop boceprevir if HCV-RNA is 1000 International units/mL or greater at week 8, 100 International units/mL or greater at week 12, or confirmed detectable at week 24.
PEDS — Safety and efficacy not established in children.
FORMS — Trade only: Caps 200 mg.
NOTES — Not for monotherapy. Strong inhibitor of CYP3A4. Many drug interactions. Contraindicated with alfuzosin, atorvastatin doses greater than 40 mg/day, carbamazepine, colchicine in patients with renal or hepatic impairment, doxazosin, drosperinone, ergot alkaloids, high-dose itraconazole or ketoconazole (>200 mg/day), lovastatin, oral midazolam, phenobarbital, phenytoin, pimozide, rifampin, salmeterol, high-dose sildenafil or tadalafil for pulmonary hypertension, silodosin, simvastatin, St. John's wort, tamsulosin, triazolam. Do not use with efavirenz, ritonavir-boosted atazanavir, ritonavir-darunavir, or lopinavir-ritonavir. Use lowest effective dose of atorvastatin (not more than 40 mg/day). Can substantially increase levels of cyclosporine and especially tacrolimus. Reduce doses of phosphodiesterase inhibitors for erectile dysfunction to not more than sildenafil 25 mg q 48 h, tadalafil 10 mg q 72 h, or vardenafil 2.5 mg q 24 h. Can increase digoxin levels; monitor levels and signs/sx of digoxin toxicity. Female patients or female partners of male patients must use 2 forms of contraception to avoid pregnancy because of ribavirin teratogenicity. A combined oral contraceptive containing at least 1 mg norethindrone can be used; avoid other hormonal contraceptives; contraceptives containing drospirenone are contraindicated. Can cause anemia,neutropenia, and pancytopenia; monitor CBC at baseline, weeks 2, 4, 8, 12, and prn. Can cause acute hypersensitivity reactions. Patients with compensated cirrhosis: 800 mg PO three times per day for 44 weeks in combination with peginterferon and ribavirin. Start boceprevir after 4 weeks of peginterferon plus ribavirin. Store in refrigerator before dispensing; patients can store at room temperature for 3 months.
MOA — Blocks viral replication by inhibiting hepatitis C virus non-structural protein 3 serine protease.
ADVERSE EFFECTS — Serious: Neutropenia, anemia (frequent), thrombocytopenia, pancytopenia, acute hypersensitivity reactions (including angioedema, urticaria). Frequent: Fatigue, nausea, headache, dysgeusia.

ENTECAVIR (*Baraclude*) ▶K ♀C ▶− $$$$$

WARNING — Nucleoside analogues can cause lactic acidosis with hepatic steatosis. Severe acute exacerbation of hepatitis B can occur after discontinuation. Monitor closely for at least 2 months after discontinuation. Patients coinfected with HIV and hepatitis B should not receive entecavir for hepatitis B unless they also receive HAART for HIV; failure to treat HIV in such patients could lead to HIV resistance to NRTIs.

ADULT — Chronic hepatitis B: 0.5 mg PO once daily if treatment-naive; 1 mg if lamivudine- or telbivudine-resistant, history of viremia despite lamivudine treatment, HIV coinfected, or decompensated liver disease. Give on empty stomach (2 h after last meal and 2 h before next meal).

PEDS — Chronic hepatitis B, age 2 yo and older. Treatment-naïve: Give oral soln PO once daily at a dose of 3 mL for 10 to 11 kg; 4 mL for >11 to 14 kg; 5 mL for >14 to 17 kg; 6 mL for >17 to 20 kg; 7 mL for >20 to 23 kg; 8 mL for >23 to 26 kg; 9 mL for >26 to 30 kg; 10 mL or 0.5 mg tab for >30 kg. Lamivudine-experienced: Give oral soln PO once daily at a dose of 6 mL for 10 to 11 kg; 8 mL for >11 to 14 kg; 10 mL for >14 to 17 kg; 12 mL for >17 to 20 kg; 14 mL for >20 to 23 kg; 16 mL for >23 to 26 kg; 18 mL for >26 to 30 kg; 20 mL or 1 mg tab for >30 kg. Age 16 yo or older: 0.5 mg PO once daily if treatment-naive; 1 mg if lamivudine- or telbivudine-resistant, history of viremia despite lamivudine treatment, HIV coinfected, or decompensated liver disease. Give on empty stomach (2 h after last meal and 2 h before next meal).

FORMS — Trade only: Tabs 0.5, 1 mg. Oral soln 0.05 mg/mL (210 mL).

NOTES — Entecavir treatment of coinfected patients not receiving HIV treatment may increase the risk of resistance to lamivudine or emtricitabine. Do not mix oral soln with water or other liquid. See product labeling for dosage adjustments for CrCl less than 50 mL/min or dialysis. Give dose after dialysis sessions.

MOA — Guanosine nucleoside analogue that inhibits hepatitis B polymerase. Partial inhibitor of HIV replication may select for lamivudine-resistant mutation.

ADVERSE EFFECTS — Serious: Nucleoside analogues can cause lactic acidosis/hepatic steatosis. Frequent: Headache, fatigue, dizziness, nausea.

INTERFERON ALFA-2B (*Intron A*) ▶K ♀C ▶?+ $$$$$

WARNING — May cause or worsen serious neuropsychiatric, autoimmune, ischemic, and infectious diseases. Frequent clinical and lab monitoring required. Stop interferon if signs/symptoms of these conditions are persistently severe or worsen.

ADULT — Chronic hepatitis B: 5 million units/day or 10 million units three times per week SC/IM for 16 weeks if HBeAg positive. Chronic hepatitis C: 3 million units SC/IM three times per week. Currently recommended hepatitis C treatment regimens (see www.hcvguidelines.org) include peginterferon rather than interferon. Other indications: Condylomata acuminata, AIDS-related Kaposi's sarcoma, hairy-cell leukemia, melanoma, and follicular lymphoma—see prescribing information for specific dose.

PEDS — Chronic hepatitis B: 3 million units/m² three times per week for 1st week, then 6 million units/m² (max 10 million units/dose) SC three times per week for age 1 yo or older. Chronic hepatitis C: Interferon alfa-2b 3 million units/m² SC three times per week for age 3 yo or older with PO ribavirin according to wt. Ribavirin: 200 mg two times per day for wt 25 to 36 kg; 200 mg q am and 400 mg q pm for wt 37 to 49 kg; 400 mg two times per day for wt 50 to 61 kg. Use adult dose for wt greater than 61 kg. If ribavirin contraindicated use interferon 3 to 5 million units/m² (max 3 million units/dose) SC/IM three times per week.

UNAPPROVED ADULT — Other indications: superficial bladder tumors, chronic myelogenous leukemia, cutaneous T-cell lymphoma, essential thrombocythemia, non-Hodgkin's lymphoma, and chronic granulocytic leukemia.

FORMS — Trade only: Powder/soln for injection 10, 18, 50 million units/vial. Soln for injection 18, 25 million units/multidose vial. Multidose injection pens 3, 5, 10 million units/0.2 mL (1.5 mL), 6 doses/pen.

NOTES — Monitor for depression, suicidal behavior (especially in adolescents), other severe neuropsychiatric effects. Thyroid abnormalities, hepatotoxicity, flu-like symptoms, pulmonary and cardiovascular reactions, retinal damage, neutropenia, thrombocytopenia, hypertriglyceridemia (consider monitoring). Monitor CBC, TSH, LFTs, electrolytes. Dosage adjustments for hematologic toxicity in prescribing information. Increases theophylline levels.

MOA — Interferons enhance phagocytic activity of macrophages and cytotoxicity of lymphocytes, and inhibit viral replication.

ADVERSE EFFECTS — Serious: May cause or worsen serious neuropsychiatric, autoimmune, ischemic, & infectious diseases (including thyroid abnormalities, hepatotoxicity, pulmonary & cardiovascular reactions, retinal damage, neutropenia, thrombocytopenia, hypertriglyceridemia, myelosuppression, psychiatric syndromes). May cause growth impairment in children that may rebound after discontinuation; possible reduction in adult height. Frequent: Flu-like syndrome, anorexia, dizziness, rash, depression.

INTERFERON ALFA-N3 (*Alferon N*) ▶K ♀C ▶− $$$$$

WARNING — Flu-like syndrome, myalgias, alopecia. Contraindicated in egg protein allergy.

ADULT — Intralesional injection for Condylomata acuminata.

PEDS — Not approved in children.

MOA — Interferons enhance phagocytic activity of macrophages and cytotoxicity of lymphocytes, and inhibit viral replication.

ADVERSE EFFECTS — Serious: Hypersensitivity. Frequent: Flu-like syndrome, myalgias.

PALIVIZUMAB (*Synagis*) ▶L ♀C ▶? $$$$$

PEDS — Prevention of respiratory syncytial virus pulmonary disease in high-risk infants: 15 mg/kg IM monthly for max of 5 doses per RSV season; give first injection before season starts (November to April in Northern hemisphere). See pediatrics. aappublications.org for eligibility criteria. Give a dose ASAP after cardiopulmonary bypass (due to decreased palivizumab levels) even if less than 1 month after last dose.

NOTES — AAP recommends stopping monthly prophylaxis after hospitalization for breakthrough RSV; also recommends against prophylaxis in second year of life (with rare exceptions). Preservative-free; use within 6 h of reconstitution. Not more than 1 mL per injection site. Can interfere with immunologic based diagnostic tests and viral culture assays for RSV, leading to false-negative diagnostic tests.

MOA — Monoclonal antibody against F glycoprotein on surface of respiratory syncytial virus provides passive immunity against the virus.

ADVERSE EFFECTS — Serious: Acute hypersensitivity reactions (rare); anaphylaxis after re-exposure (rare). Frequent: Increases aminotransferase activity, otherwise well-tolerated.

PEGINTERFERON ALFA-2A (*Pegasys*) ▶LK ♀C ▶– $$$$$

WARNING — May cause or worsen serious neuropsychiatric, autoimmune, ischemic, and infectious diseases. Frequent clinical and lab monitoring recommended. Discontinue if signs/symptoms of these conditions are persistently severe or worsen.

ADULT — Direct-acting agents with much greater efficacy are rapidly changing the treatment of chronic hepatitis C infection. A number of FDA-approved regimens are no longer recommended, including boceprevir regimens, ribavirin-interferon, and ribavirin-peginterferon (except as an alternative regimen for treatment-naïve patients with genotype 5 or 6). Some regimens of new direct-acting agents include weight-based ribavirin +/- peginterferon. See www.hcvguidelines.org for current treatment recommendations. Combination therapy of chronic hepatitis C, initial treatment: 180 mcg SC in abdomen or thigh once a week. Hepatitis B: 180 mcg SC in abdomen or thigh once a week for 48 weeks.

PEDS — Chronic hepatitis C, initial treatment, age 5 yo or older: 180 mcg/1.73 m² (max dose of 180 mcg) SC in abdomen or thigh once weekly. Give with PO ribavirin (see ribavirin-oral entry for dose based on wt). Treat genotype 2 or 3 for 24 weeks; treat genotypes 1 or 4 for 48 weeks.

FORMS — Trade only: 180 mcg/1 mL soln in single-use vial; 180 mcg/0.5 mL prefilled syringe; 180 mcg/0.5 mL, 135 mcg/0.5 mL auto-injector.

NOTES — In combination with ribavirin for chronic hepatitis C, peginterferon is preferred over interferon alfa because of substantially higher response rate. Contraindicated in autoimmune hepatitis; hepatic decompensation in cirrhotic patients (Child-Pugh score greater than 6 if HCV only; score 6 or greater if HIV coinfected). Growth delay possible in children. Monitor for depression, suicidal behavior, relapse of drug addiction, or other severe neuropsychiatric effects. Interferons can cause thrombocytopenia, neutropenia, thyroid dysfunction, hyperglycemia, hypoglycemia, cardiovascular events, colitis, pancreatitis, hypersensitivity, flu-like symptoms, pulmonary and ophthalmologic disorders. Risk of severe neutropenia/thrombocytopenia greater in HIV-infected patients. Monitor CBC, blood chemistry. Interferons increase risk of hepatic decompensation in hepatitis C/HIV coinfected patients receiving HAART with NRTI. Monitor LFTs and clinical status; discontinue peginterferon if Child-Pugh score 6 or greater. Exacerbation of hepatitis during treatment of hepatitis B; monitor LFTs more often and consider dosage reduction if ALT flares. Discontinue treatment if ALT increase is progressive despite dosage reduction or if flares accompanied by hepatic decompensation or bilirubin increase. May increase methadone levels. Use cautiously if CrCl less than 50 mL/min. Reduce adult dose to 135 mcg SC once weekly for CrCl <30 mL/min, ESRD, or hemodialysis. Dosage adjustments for adverse effects or hepatic dysfunction in prescribing information. Store in refrigerator.

MOA — Interferon alfa-2a that is conjugated to polyethylene glycol to increase duration of action. Interferons enhance phagocytic activity of macrophages and cytotoxicity of lymphocytes, and inhibit viral replication.

ADVERSE EFFECTS — Serious: Alpha interferons may cause or worsen serious neuropsychiatric, autoimmune, ischemic, & infectious diseases (including thyroid dysfunction, hyperglycemia, hypoglycemia, hepatotoxicity, colitis, pulmonary & cardiovascular reactions, neutropenia, thrombocytopenia, hypertriglyceridemia, myelosuppression, psychiatric syndromes, ophthalmologic disorders). Interferons increase risk of hepatic decompensation in hep C/HIV coinfected patients receiving HAART with NRTI. Exacerbation of hepatitis during treatment of hepatitis B. Acute hypersensitivity. Frequent: Psychiatric reactions, flu-like syndrome, hematologic toxicity, fatigue, injection site reactions, dizziness, pruritus, dermatitis, headache, alopecia, anorexia.

PEGINTERFERON ALFA-2B (*PEG-Intron*) ▶K? ♀C ▶– $$$$$

WARNING — May cause or worsen serious neuropsychiatric, autoimmune, ischemic, and infectious diseases. Frequent clinical and lab monitoring recommended. Discontinue if signs/symptoms of these conditions are persistently severe or worsen.

ADULT — Direct-acting agents with much greater efficacy are rapidly changing the treatment of chronic hepatitis C infection. A number of

PEGINTERFERON ALFA-2B (*cont.*)

FDA-approved regimens are no longer recommended, including boceprevir regimens, ribavirin-interferon, and ribavirin-peginterferon (except as an alternative regimen for treatment-naïve patients with genotype 5 or 6). Some regimens of new direct-acting agents include weight-based ribavirin and peginterferon. See www.hcvguidelines.org for current treatment recommendations. In combination with ribavirin for chronic hepatitis C, peginterferon is preferred over interferon alfa because of substantially higher response rate. Combination therapy with oral ribavirin (see ribavirin-oral entry for ribavirin dose): 1.5 mcg/kg/week given on the same day each week. To control amount injected, use vial strength based on wt: give 50 mcg (0.5 mL, 50 mcg/0.5 mL vial) for wt less than 40 kg, give 64 mcg (0.4 mL, 80 mcg/0.5 mL vial) for 40 to 50 kg, give 80 mcg (0.5 mL, 80 mcg/0.5 mL vial) for 51 to 60 kg, give 96 mcg (0.4 mL, 120 mcg/0.5 mL vial) for 61 to 75 kg, give 120 mcg (0.5 mL, 120 mcg/0.5 mL vial) for 76 to 85 kg, give 150 mcg (0.5 mL, 150 mcg/0.5 mL vial) for 86 kg or greater. Give at bedtime or with antipyretic to minimize flu-like symptoms.

PEDS — Chronic hepatitis C not previously treated with alfa-interferon, age 3 yo or older: 60 mcg/m^2 SC once a week with ribavirin 15 mg/kg/day PO divided two times per day (see ribavirin-oral entry for dosing of caps). Treat genotype 1 for 48 weeks. Treat genotype 2 or 3 for 24 weeks.

FORMS — Trade only: 50, 80, 120, 150 mcg/ 0.5 mL single-use vials with diluent, 2 syringes, and alcohol swabs. Disposable single-dose Redipen and Selectdose prefilled pens 50, 80, 120, 150 mcg.

NOTES — Contraindicated in autoimmune hepatitis; hepatic decompensation in cirrhotic patients (Child-Pugh score greater than 6). Coadministration with ribavirin contraindicated if CrCl less than 50 mL/min. Monitor for depression, suicidal behavior, exacerbation of substance use disorders, other severe neuropsychiatric effects. Thrombocytopenia, neutropenia, thyroid dysfunction, hyperglycemia, cardiovascular events, colitis, pancreatitis, hypersensitivity, flu-like symptoms, pulmonary damage. Monitor CBC, blood chemistry. May increase methadone levels. Dosage adjustments for adverse effects in prescribing information. Adult dosage reduction for renal dysfunction: 25% reduction for CrCl 30 to 50 mL/min; 50% reduction for CrCl <30 mL/min including hemodialysis. Peginterferon should be used immediately after reconstitution, but can be refrigerated for up to 24 h.

MOA — Interferon alfa-2b that is conjugated to polyethylene glycol. Binding of alpha interferon to cell surface receptors initiates intracellular events that enhances the phagocytic activity of macrophages and cytotoxicity of lymphocytes, and inhibits viral replication.

ADVERSE EFFECTS — Serious: May cause or worsen serious neuropsychiatric, autoimmune, ischemic, & infectious diseases (including thyroid abnormalities, hepatotoxicity, pulmonary & cardiovascular reactions, stroke, retinal damage, neutropenia, thrombocytopenia, hypertriglyceridemia, myelosuppression, psychiatric syndromes). Impaired growth in children during treatment with peginterferon plus ribavirin, with rebound after discontinuation. Frequent: Flu-like syndrome, anorexia, dizziness, rash, depression.

RIBAVIRIN—INHALED (*Virazole*) ▶Lung ♀X ▶– $$$$$

WARNING — Beware of sudden pulmonary deterioration with ribavirin. Drug precipitation may cause ventilator dysfunction.

PEDS — Severe respiratory syncytial virus infection: Aerosol 12 to 18 h/day for 3 to 7 days.

NOTES — Minimize exposure to healthcare workers, especially pregnant women.

MOA — Inhaled synthetic nucleoside that interferes with viral nucleic acid synthesis.

ADVERSE EFFECTS — Serious: Sudden pulmonary deterioration, ventilator dysfunction due to drug precipitation.

RIBAVIRIN—ORAL (*Rebetol, Copegus, Ribasphere*) ▶Cellular, K ♀X ▶– $$$$$

WARNING — Teratogen with extremely long half-life; contraindicated if pregnancy possible in patient/partner. Female patients and female partners of male patients must avoid pregnancy by using 2 forms of birth control during and for 6 months after stopping ribavirin. Obtain pregnancy test at baseline and monthly. Hemolytic anemia that may worsen cardiac disease. Assess for underlying heart disease before treatment with ribavirin. Do not use in significant/unstable heart disease. Baseline ECG if preexisting cardiac dysfunction.

ADULT — Direct-acting agents with much greater efficacy are rapidly changing the treatment of chronic hepatitis C infection. A number of FDA-approved regimens are no longer recommended, including boceprevir regimens, ribavirin-interferon, and ribavirin-peginterferon (except as an alternative regimen for initial treatment of patients with genotype 5 or 6). Some regimens of new direct-acting agents include weight-based ribavirin +/- peginterferon. See www.hcvguidelines.org for current treatment recommendations. Chronic hepatitis C, treatment-naive. Wt-based dosing of ribavirin for chronic hepatitis C in adults: Daily dose of 1000 mg/day PO for wt less than 75 kg, 1200 mg/day PO for wt 75 kg or greater. Divide daily dose of ribavirin two times per day and give with food. Copegus in combination with peginterferon alfa-2a (Pegasys): 1000 mg/day PO for wt less than 75 kg, 1200 mg/day PO for wt 75 kg or greater. Divide daily dose of ribavirin two times per day and give with food. Sofosbuvir-based regimens for genotypes 2 or 3 and HIV-coinfected patients give ribavirin at a dose of 1000 mg/day

(cont.)

RIBAVIRIN—ORAL (cont.)

PO for wt less than 75 kg, 1200 mg/day PO for wt 75 kg or greater.

PEDS — Chronic hepatitis C, initial treatment: Patients who start peginterferon plus ribavirin before their 18th birthday should continue with peds doses throughout treatment. Rebetol in combination with peginterferon alfa-2b (PegIntron), age 3 yo and older: For wt less than 47 kg or patients who cannot swallow caps: 15 mg/kg/day of soln PO divided two times per day. Caps: 400 mg two times per day for wt 47 to 59 kg, 400 mg q am and 600 mg q pm for wt 60 to 73 kg, 600 mg two times per day for wt greater than 73 kg. Take PO with food. Treat genotype 1 for 48 weeks, genotypes 2 and 3 for 24 weeks. Copegus tabs in combo with peginterferon alfa-2a (Pegasys), age 5 yo or older: 200 mg twice daily for 23 to 33 kg; 200 mg q am and 400 mg q pm for 34 to 46 kg; 400 mg twice daily for 47 to 59 kg; 400 mg q am and 600 mg q pm for 60 to 74 kg; 600 mg twice daily for 75 kg or more. Treat genotypes 2 and 3 for 24 weeks, other genotypes for 48 weeks. Take PO with food.

UNAPPROVED ADULT — Direct-acting agents with much greater efficacy are rapidly changing the treatment of chronic hepatitis C infection. A number of FDA-approved regimens are no longer recommended, including boceprevir regimens, ribavirin-interferon, and ribavirin-peginterferon (except as an alternative regimen for initial treatment of patients with genotype 5 or 6). Some regimens of new direct-acting agents include weight-based ribavirin +/- peginterferon. See www.hcvguidelines.org for current treatment recommendations. Chronic hepatitis C, genotype 2 or 3, initial treatment: sofosbuvir 400 mg PO once daily plus wt-based ribavirin (1000 mg/day PO for wt less than 75 kg, 1200 mg/day PO for wt 75 kg or greater). Divide daily dose of ribavirin two times per day and give with food. Treat genotype 2 for 12 weeks. Treat genotype 3 for 24 weeks. Chronic hepatitis C, genotypes 5 or 6, initial treatment: peginterferon alfa 2a 180 mcg SC once weekly + wt-based ribavirin (1000 mg/day PO for wt less than 75 kg, 1200 mg/day PO for wt 75 kg or greater) for 48 weeks. Divide daily dose of ribavirin two times per day and give with food.

UNAPPROVED PEDS — Chronic hepatitis C, age 2 yo and older: Treat for 48 weeks with peginterferon alfa-2b (PegIntron) in combination with ribavirin 15 mg/kg/day PO divided two times per day. The regimen provided here is from guideline for the management of chronic hepatitis C; it may vary from regimens in product labeling.

FORMS — Generic/Trade: Caps 200 mg, Tabs 200 mg. Generic only: Tabs 400, 500, 600 mg. Trade only (Rebetol): Oral soln 40 mg/mL (100 mL).

NOTES — Contraindicated in hemoglobinopathies; autoimmune hepatitis; hepatic decompensation in cirrhotic patients (Child-Pugh score greater than 6 if HCV only; score greater than 5 if HIV coinfected). Get CBC at baseline, weeks 2 and 4, and periodically. Risk of anemia increased if age older than 50 yo or renal dysfunction. Decreased INR with warfarin; monitor INR weekly for 4 weeks after ribavirin started/stopped. May increase risk of lactic acidosis with nucleoside reverse transcriptase inhibitors. Avoid didanosine or zidovudine. Coadministration with azathioprine can cause neutropenia; monitor CBC weekly for 1st month, every other week for next 2 months, then monthly or more frequently if doses are adjusted. Dosage adjustment for renal dysfunction in adults: Give 200 mg alternating with 400 mg every other day for CrCl 30 to 50 mL/min; 200 mg once daily for CrCl <30 mL/min, ESRD, or hemodialysis.

MOA — Oral synthetic nucleoside that interferes with viral nucleic acid synthesis.

ADVERSE EFFECTS — Serious and frequent: Hemolytic anemia (especially if older than 50 yo or if renal dysfunction). Frequent: Therapy with interferon plus ribavirin causes more cough, pruritus, and rash than interferon alone. Serious and rare: Severe acute hypersensitivity during co-therapy with interferon. Impaired growth of children during treatment with peginterferon plus ribavirin, with rebound after discontinuation.

SIMEPREVIR (Olysio, SMV✱Galexos) ▶L bile ♀C for simeprevir without ribavirin, X for simeprevir with ribavirin ▶- $$$$$

ADULT — Combination therapy of chronic hepatitis C, genotype 1: 150 mg PO once daily with food for 12 weeks with wt-based ribavirin (1000 mg/day PO for wt less than 75 kg; 1200 mg/day PO for wt 75 kg or greater, divided two times per day and taken with food) and peginterferon alfa 2a 180 mcg SC once weekly. Ribavirin and peginterferon continued for 12 additional weeks if initial treatment or prior relapse (total treatment duration of 24 weeks), 36 weeks if prior non-response (total treatment duration of 48 weeks). Stop regimen if HCV-RNA is 25 International units or greater at week 4, 12, or 24. Screen genotype 1a for Q80K polymorphism (reduced efficacy); consider alternative if present.

PEDS — Safety and efficacy not established in children.

UNAPPROVED ADULT — Combination therapy of chronic hepatitis C. Genotype 1, initial treatment and ineligible for interferon: Treat for 12 weeks with sofosbuvir 400 mg + simeprevir 150 mg both PO once daily +/- wt-based ribavirin (1000 mg/day PO for body wt less than 75 kg; 1200 mg/day PO for body wt 75 kg or greater). Genotype 4, initial treatment (alternative regimen): simeprevir 150 mg PO once daily for 12 weeks + wt-based ribavirin (1000 mg/day PO for body wt less than 75 kg; 1200 mg/day PO for body wt more than 75 kg) and peginterferon alfa 2a 180 mcg SC weekly for 24 to 48 weeks.

SIMEPREVIR (*cont.*)

FORMS — Trade only: Caps 150 mg.

NOTES — Cost is $22,120 per month. Not for monotherapy. Higher exposure in East Asians (dosage adjustment not established), leading to more frequent adverse events including rash and photosensitivity. Can cause severe photosensitivity (most common in first month); tell patients to use sun protection and limit exposure. Rash (most common in first month); discontinue if severe. Contains sulfonamide moiety; risk in sulfa allergy is unclear. For regimens containing ribavirin, avoid pregnancy in female patients or female partners of male patients because of ribavirin teratogenicity. Use 2 forms of contraception. Avoid moderate or strong inhibitors or inducers of CYP 3A4 (see P450 isozymes table), including IV/PO dexamethasone, nevirapine, HIV protease inhibitors. Simeprevir can increase exposure to digoxin, calcium channel blockers, some antiarrhythmics, and oral midazolam/ triazolam. Reduce initial rosuvastatin dose to 5 mg/day and max dose to 10 mg/day. Use lowest possible dose of atorvastatin, with max dose of 40 mg/day. Use lowest possible dose of simvastatin. Hepatitis C treatment guideline recommends against simeprevir-based regimens in decompensated cirrhosis (Child-Pugh class B/C) due to inadequate data. Guideline available at www.hcvguidelines.org.

MOA — Blocks viral replication by inhibiting hepatitis C virus non-structural protein 3 serine protease.

ADVERSE EFFECTS — Serious: Photosensitivity (most common in first month); rash (most common in first month). East Asians have higher simeprevir exposure (dosage adjustment not established), leading to more frequent adverse effects including rash and photosensitivity. Frequent: Rash, photosensitivity, pruritus, nausea, mild to moderate hyperbilirubinemia.

SOFOSBUVIR (*Sovaldi, SOF*) ▶LK ♀B for sofosbuvir, X for regimens that contain ribavirin ▶? $$$$$

ADULT — Combination therapy of chronic hepatitis C, genotypes 1, 2, 3, and 4: 400 mg PO once daily without regard to food. Genotype 1 or 4: Give with wt-based ribavirin (1000 mg/day PO for wt less than 75 kg; 1200 mg/day PO for wt 75 kg or greater, divided two times per day and taken with food) and peginterferon alfa 2a 180 mcg SC once weekly for 12 weeks. Genotype 1 ineligable for interferon (alternative regimen), genotype 3: Give with wt-based ribavirin for 24 weeks. Genotype 2: Give with wt-based ribavirin for 12 weeks. Hepatocellular cancer awaiting liver transplant: Give with ribavirin for up to 48 weeks or until transplant. Hepatitis C treatment recommendations available at www.hcvguidelines.org.

PEDS — Not approved in children.

UNAPPROVED ADULT — Combination therapy of chronic hepatitis C. Genotype I, initial treatment, interferon-ineligible: sofosbuvir 400 mg + simeprevir 150 mg both PO once daily +/- wt-based ribavirin (1000 mg/day PO for <75 kg; 1200 mg/day PO for 75 kg or greater) for 12 weeks. Give simeprevir and ribavirin with food. Genotype 3, initial treatment (alternative regimen): sofosbuvir 400 mg PO once daily + wt-based ribavirin for 12 weeks. Genotype 4, interferon-ineligible (alternative regimen): sofosbuvir 400 mg PO once daily and wt-based ribavirin for 24 weeks. Genotype 5 or 6: sofosbuvir 400 mg PO once daily with wt-based ribavirin and peginterferon (peginterferon alfa 2a 180 mcg SC once weekly) for 12 weeks.

FORMS — Trade only: Tabs 400 mg.

NOTES — Cost is $28,000/month. Not for monotherapy. For regimens that contain ribavirin, avoid pregnancy in female patients or female partners of male patients because of ribavirin teratogenicity. Use 2 nonhormonal contraceptives. Do not coadminister carbamazepine, oxcarbazepine, phenobarbital, phenytoin, rifabutin, rifampin, rifapentine, St. John's wort, or tipranvir-ritonavir. Dosage adjustment for CrCl <30 mL/min not established. No dosage adjustment needed for Child-Pugh Class A, B, or C. Hepatitis C treatment recommendations available at www.hcvguidelines.org.

MOA — Hepatitis C nucleotide analog NS5B RNA polymerase inhibitor. Prodrug is metabolized intracellularly to active form which is incorporated into viral RNA and acts as chain terminator.

ADVERSE EFFECTS — Frequent: Sofosbuvir plus ribavirin: fatigue, headache. Sofosbuvir plus peginterferon and ribavirin: fatigue, headache, nausea, insomnia, anemia, neutropenia.

TELAPREVIR (*Incivek*) ▶L ♀B ▶– $$$$$

WARNING — Telaprevir can cause serious skin reactions including Stevens-Johnson Syndrome, DRESS, and toxic epidermal necrolysis. Fatalities have occurred when telaprevir was continued in patients with progressive rash and systemic symptoms. Discontinue telaprevir, peginterferon and ribavirin immediately in patients with progressive severe rash or rash with systemic symptoms and refer patient to urgent medical care. Never restart telaprevir that was discontinued because of a serious skin reaction.

ADULT — NOTE: Guidelines (www.hcvguidelines.org) no longer recommend boceprevir- or telaprevir-based regimens for the treatment of chronic hepatitis C. Chronic hepatitis C (genotype 1) including prior null/partial responders or relapsers: 1125 mg PO two times per day taken 10-14 hours apart with food (not low fat). Give with peginterferon and ribavirin for 12 weeks. Give peginterferon and ribavirin for additional 12 to 36 weeks based on HCV RNA levels at weeks 4 and 12, and whether patient was partial/null responder to

(cont.)

TELAPREVIR (*cont.*)

prior therapy. Stop telaprevir if HCV RNA is greater than 1000 International units/mL at weeks 4 or 12, or detectable at week 24. Dosage adjustment for coadministration with efavirenz: 1125 mg PO q 8 h.

PEDS — Safety and efficacy not established in children.

FORMS — Trade only: 375 mg tabs in 28-day blister pack

NOTES — Not for monotherapy. Previous null responders have higher risk of resistance emerging and lower rate of sustained virologic response with telaprevir. Rash is common with telaprevir; monitor mild to moderate rash closely and discontinue therapy if it progresses or systemic symptoms develop. Strong inhibitor of CYP3A4. Many drug interactions. Contraindicated with alfuzosin, atorvastatin, carbamazepine, colchicine in patients with renal/hepatic impairment, most systemic corticosteroids, darunavir-ritonavir, ergot alkaloids, fosamprenavir-ritonavir, high-dose itraconazole or ketoconazole (>200 mg/day), lopinavir-ritonavir, lovastatin, oral midazolam, phenobarbital, phenytoin, pimozide, rifabutin, rifampin, salmeterol, high-dose sildenafil or tadalafil for pulmonary hypertension, simvastatin, St. John's wort, triazolam. Reduce doses of phosphodiesterase inhibitors for erectile dysfunction to not more than sildenafil 25 mg q 48 h, tadalafil 10 mg q 72 h, or vardenafil 2.5 mg q 72 h. May increase risk of QT-interval prolongation or torsades with CYP3A4 inhibitors that can prolong the QT interval (i.e., clarithromycin, erythromycin, voriconazole). Inhibits p-glycoprotein. Use lowest initial dose of digoxin and monitor digoxin levels. Avoid pregnancy in female patients or female partners of male patients because of ribavirin teratogenicity. May impair efficacy of hormonal contraceptives; use 2 nonhormonal contraceptives. Can cause anemia. Monitor Hb, CBC, TSH, chemistry panel, and LFTs at weeks 2, 4, 8, and 12, and prn. Do not use in moderate to severe hepatic impairment (Child-Pugh Class B/C, score of 7 or greater). Once bottle is opened, use within 28 days.

MOA — Blocks viral replication by inhibiting hepatitis C virus non-structural protein 3 serine protease.

ADVERSE EFFECTS — Serious: Stevens-Johnson syndrome, DRESS (rare), toxic epidermal necrolysis, anemia (frequent). Frequent: Rash, fatigue, pruritus, diarrhea, vomiting, hemorrhoids; anorectal discomfort, pruritus, or burning; dysgeusia, low platelet counts, increased bilirubin, increased uric acid.

TELBIVUDINE (*Tyzeka, ✚Sebivo*) ▶K ♀B ▶– $$$$$

WARNING — Nucleoside analogues can cause lactic acidosis with hepatic steatosis. Severe acute exacerbation of hepatitis B can occur after discontinuation. Monitor closely for at least 2 months after discontinuation.

ADULT — Chronic hepatitis B: 600 mg PO once daily. Refer to product labeling for baseline HBV DNA and ALT treatment criteria for HBeAg-positive and -negative patients. Choose alternate therapy if HBV DNA is detectable after 24 weeks of treatment.

PEDS — Chronic hepatitis B, age 16 yo or older: 600 mg PO once daily. Refer to product labeling for baseline HBV DNA and ALT treatment criteria for HBeAg-positive and -negative patients. Choose alternate therapy if HBV is detectable after 24 weeks of treatment.

FORMS — Trade only: Tabs 600 mg.

NOTES — Risk of peripheral neuropathy increased by peginterferon alfa 2a; do not coadminister. No dosage adjustment needed for hepatic dysfunction. Dosage adjustment for renal dysfunction: 600 mg PO q 96 h for ESRD, q 72 h for CrCl less than 30 mL/min but not hemodialysis, q 48 h for CrCl 30 to 49 mL/min. Give dose after hemodialysis session. Contains 47 mg sodium/30 mL of oral soln.

MOA — Thymidine nucleoside analogue that inhibits hepatitis B polymerase. It has no activity against HIV-1.

ADVERSE EFFECTS — Serious: Myopathy. Peripheral neuropathy (incidence and severity increased by peginterferon alfa 2a; do not coadminister). Nucleoside analogues can cause lactic acidosis/hepatic steatosis. Frequent: Headache, dizziness, fatigue, URI/nasopharyngitis/influenza/flu-like symptoms, cough, abdominal pain, increased CK levels, N/V, dyspepsia, diarrhea.

ANTIMICROBIALS: Carbapenems

NOTE: Carbapenems can dramatically reduce valproic acid levels; use another antibiotic (preferred) or add a supplemental anticonvulsant. Possible cross-sensitivity with other beta-lactams; –associated diarrhea; superinfection.

DORIPENEM (*Doribax*) ▶K ♀B ▶? $$$$$

ADULT — Complicated intra-abdominal infection: 500 mg IV q 8 h for 5 to 14 days. Complicated UTI or pyelonephritis: 500 mg IV q 8 h for 10 to 14 days.

PEDS — Not approved in children.

NOTES — Do not use for ventilator-associated bacterial pneumonia; doripenem had higher mortality and lower response rate than imipenem in clinical trial. May cause seizures, especially if pre-existing CNS disorder, renal impairment, or doses >1500 mg/day. Dose

(cont.)

DORIPENEM (*cont.*)

reduction in renal dysfunction: 250 mg q 12 h for CrCl 10 to 30 mL/min, 250 mg q 8 h for CrCl 30 to 50 mL/min.

MOA — Beta-lactam resistant to hydrolysis by most beta-lactamases, including extended-spectrum beta-lactamases.

ADVERSE EFFECTS — Serious: Cross-sensitivity with other beta-lactams; C. difficile associated diarrhea; superinfection; seizures (esp. if pre-existing CNS disorder, renal impairment, or doses >1500 mg/day). Frequent: Headache, nausea, diarrhea, rash, phlebitis.

ERTAPENEM (*Invanz*) ▶K ♀B ▶? $$$$$

ADULT — Community-acquired pneumonia, diabetic foot, complicated intra-abdominal, skin, urinary tract, acute pelvic infections: 1 g IM/IV over 30 min q 24 h for up to 14 days for IV, up to 7 days for IM. Prophylaxis, elective colorectal surgery: 1 g IV 1 h before incision.

PEDS — Community-acquired pneumonia, complicated intra-abdominal, skin, urinary tract, acute pelvic infections, 3 mo to 12 yo: 15 mg/kg IV/IM q 12 h (up to 1 g/day). Use adult dose for age 13 yo or older. Infuse IV over 30 min. Can give IV for up to 14 days, IM for up to 7 days.

NOTES — Seizures (especially if renal dysfunction or CNS disorder). Not active against Pseudomonas and Acinetobacter species. IM diluted with lidocaine; contraindicated if allergic to amide-type local anesthetics. For adults with renal dysfunction: 500 mg q 24 h for CrCl 30 mL/min or less or hemodialysis. Give 150 mg supplemental dose if daily dose given within 6 h before hemodialysis session. Do not dilute in dextrose.

MOA — Beta-lactam resistant to hydrolysis by most beta-lactamases, including extended-spectrum beta-lactamases.

ADVERSE EFFECTS — Serious: Cross-sensitivity with other beta-lactams, C. difficile-associated diarrhea, superinfection, seizures (0.5% of patients). Frequent: Diarrhea, N/V, infusion site reactions. Lidocaine diluent can cause allergy.

IMIPENEM-CILASTATIN (**Primaxin**) ▶K ♀C ▶? $$$$$

ADULT — Pneumonia, sepsis, endocarditis, polymicrobic, intra-abdominal, gynecologic, bone and joint, skin infections. Normal renal function, 70 kg or greater: mild infection: 250 to 500 mg IV q 6 h; moderate infection: 500 mg IV q 6 to 8 h or 1 g IV q 8 h; severe infection: 500 mg IV q 6 h to 1 g IV q 6 to 8 h. Complicated UTI: 500 mg IV q 6 h. See product labeling for doses in adults wt less than 70 kg. Can give up to 1.5 g/day IM for mild/moderate infections.

PEDS — Pneumonia, sepsis, endocarditis, polymicrobic, intra-abdominal, bone and joint, skin infections. 25 mg/kg IV q 12 h for age younger than 1 week old; 25 mg/kg IV q 8 h for age 1 to 4 weeks old; 25 mg/kg IV q 6 h for age 1 to 3 mo; 15 to 25 mg/kg IV q 6 h for

older than 3 mo. Not for children with CNS infections, or wt less than 30 kg with renal dysfunction.

UNAPPROVED ADULT — Malignant otitis externa, empiric therapy for neutropenic fever: 500 mg IV q 6 h.

NOTES — Seizures (especially if given with ganciclovir, elderly with renal dysfunction, or cerebrovascular or seizure disorder). See product labeling for dose if CrCl less than 70 mL/min. Not for CrCl less than 5 mL/min unless dialysis started within 48 h.

MOA — Beta-lactam resistant to hydrolysis by most beta-lactamases, including extended-spectrum beta-lactamases. Cilastatin inhibits renal tubular metabolism of imipenem.

ADVERSE EFFECTS — Serious: Cross-sensitivity with other beta-lactams (50% in patients with anaphylaxis to penicillin), C. difficile-associated diarrhea, superinfection. Frequent: Seizures in patients with risk factors (ganciclovir, elderly with renal dysfunction, cerebrovascular or seizure disorder).

MEROPENEM (*Merrem IV*) ▶K ♀B ▶? $$$$$

ADULT — Intra-abdominal infections: 1 g IV q 8 h. Complicated skin infections: 500 mg IV q 8 h; use 1 g IV q 8 h if P. aeruginosa skin infection.

PEDS — Meningitis: 40 mg/kg IV q 8 h for age 3 mo or older; 2 g IV q 8 h for wt greater than 50 kg. Intra-abdominal infection: 20 mg/kg IV q 8 h for age 3 mo or older; 1 g IV q 8 h for wt greater than 50 kg. Complicated skin infections: 10 mg/kg IV q 8 h for age 3 mo or older; 500 mg IV q 8 h for wt greater than 50 kg. Complicated skin infection caused by P. aeruginosa: 20 mg/kg IV q 8 h up to 1 g IV q 8 h; use 1 g IV q 8 h for wt >50 kg.

UNAPPROVED ADULT — Meningitis: 40 mg/kg (max 2 g) IV q 8 h. Hospital-acquired pneumonia, complicated UTI, malignant otitis externa: 1 g IV q 8 h.

UNAPPROVED PEDS — Infant wt greater than 2 kg: 20 mg/kg IV q 12 h for age younger than 1 week old, q 8 h for 1 to 4 weeks old.

NOTES — Seizures; thrombocytopenia in renal dysfunction. May cause motor impairment; tell patients to avoid driving or operating machinery. For adults with renal dysfunction: Give 50% of normal dose q 24 h for CrCl less than 10 mL/min, 50% of normal dose q 12 h for CrCl 10 to 25 mL/min, normal dose q 12 h for CrCl 26 to 50 mL/min.

MOA — Beta-lactam resistant to hydrolysis by most beta-lactamases, including extended-spectrum beta-lactamases.

ADVERSE EFFECTS — Serious: Cross-sensitivity with other beta-lactams, C. difficile-associated diarrhea, superinfection, seizures, thrombocytopenia in renal dysfunction. Frequent: Diarrhea, headache.

ANTIMICROBIALS: Cephalosporins—1st Generation

CEPHALOSPORINS: GENERAL ANTIMICROBIAL SPECTRUM

1st generation	gram-positive (including *S. aureus*); basic Gram-negative coverage
2nd generation	diminished *S. aureus*, improved gram-negative coverage compared to 1st generation; some with anaerobic coverage
3rd generation	further diminished *S. aureus*, further improved Gram-negative coverage compared to 1st and 2nd generation; some with Pseudomonal coverage & diminished Gram-positive coverage
4th generation	same as 3rd generation plus coverage against *Pseudomonas*
5th generation	Gram-negative coverage similar to 3rd generation; also active against *S. aureus* (including MRSA) and *S. pneumoniae*

NOTE: Cephalosporins are second-line to penicillins for group A strep pharyngitis, can rarely be cross-sensitive with penicillins, and can cause C. difficile associated diarrhea.

CEFADROXIL ▶K ♀B ▶+ $$$
ADULT — Simple UTI: 1 to 2 g/day PO divided one to two times per day. Other UTIs: 1 g PO two times per day. Skin infections: 1 g/day PO divided one to two times per day. Group A strep pharyngitis: 1 g/day PO divided one to two times per day for 10 days.
PEDS — UTIs, skin infections: 30 mg/kg/day PO divided two times per day. Group A streptococcal pharyngitis/tonsillitis, impetigo: 30 mg/kg/day PO divided one to two times per day. Treat pharyngitis for 10 days.
FORMS — Generic only: Tabs 1 g. Caps 500 mg. Susp 250, 500 mg/5 mL.
NOTES — Dosage adjustment for renal dysfunction in adults: 500 mg PO q 36 h for CrCl less than 10 mL/min; 500 mg PO q 24 h for CrCl 11 to 25 mL/min; 1 g load then 500 mg PO q 12 h for CrCl 26 to 50 mL/min.
MOA — Beta-lactam antibiotic that inhibits the biosynthesis of cell wall mucopeptide. (Beta-lactam fused to different ring structure from penicillins.)
ADVERSE EFFECTS — Serious: Cross-sensitivity with penicillins, C. difficile-associated diarrhea. Frequent: diarrhea.

CEFAZOLIN ▶K ♀B ▶+ $$
ADULT — Pneumonia, sepsis, endocarditis, skin, bone and joint, genital infections. Mild infections due to Gram-positive cocci: 250 to 500 mg IM/IV q 8 h. Moderate/severe infections: 0.5 to 1 g IM/IV q 6 to 8 h. Life-threatening infections: 1 to 1.5 g IV q 6 h. Simple UTI: 1 g IM/IV q 12 h. Pneumococcal pneumonia: 500 mg IM/IV q 12 h. Surgical prophylaxis: 1 g IM/IV 30 to 60 min preop, additional 0.5 to 1 g during surgery longer than 2 h, and 0.5 to 1 g q 6 to 8 h for 24 h postop. Prevention of perinatal group B streptococcal disease: Give to mother 2 g IV at onset of labor/after membrane rupture, then 1 g IV q 8 h until delivery. See table for prophylaxis of bacterial endocarditis.
PEDS — Pneumonia, sepsis, endocarditis, skin, bone and joint infections. Mild to moderate infections: 25 to 50 mg/kg/day IM/IV divided q 6 to 8 h for age 1 mo or older. Severe infections: 100 mg/kg/day IV divided q 6 to 8 h for age 1 mo or older. See table for prophylaxis of bacterial endocarditis.
NOTES — Dose reduction for renal dysfunction in adults: Usual first dose, then 50% of usual dose q 18 to 24 h for CrCl less than 10 mL/min; 50% of usual dose q 12 h for CrCl 11 to 34 mL/min; usual dose q 8 h for CrCl 35 to 54 mL/min. Dose reduction for renal dysfunction in children: Usual first dose, then 10% of usual dose q 24 h for CrCl 5 to 20 mL/min; 25% of usual dose q 12 h for CrCl 20 to 40 mL/min; 60% of usual dose q 12 h for CrCl 40 to 70 mL/min.
MOA — Beta-lactam antibiotic that inhibits the biosynthesis of cell wall mucopeptide. (Beta-lactam fused to different ring structure from penicillins.)
ADVERSE EFFECTS — Serious: Cross-sensitivity with penicillins, C. difficile-associated diarrhea. Frequent: Hypersensitivity.

CEPHALEXIN (*Keflex*) ▶K ♀B ▶? $$
ADULT — Pneumonia, bone, GU infections. Usual dose: 250 to 500 mg PO four times per day. Max: 4 g/day. Group A strep pharyngitis, skin infections, simple UTI: 500 mg PO two times per day. Treat pharyngitis for 10 days. See table for prophylaxis of bacterial endocarditis.
PEDS — Pneumonia, GU, bone, skin infections, group A strep pharyngitis. Usual dose: 25 to 50 mg/kg/day PO in divided doses. Max dose: 100 mg/kg/day. Can give two times per day for strep pharyngitis in children older than 1 yo, skin infections. Group A strep pharyngitis, skin infections, simple UTI in

CEPHALEXIN (cont.)

patients older than 15 yo: 500 mg PO two times per day. Treat pharyngitis for 10 days. Not for otitis media, sinusitis.

FORMS — Generic/Trade: Caps 250, 500, 750 mg. Generic only: Tabs 250, 500 mg. Susp 125, 250 mg/5 mL.

MOA — Beta-lactam antibiotic that inhibits the biosynthesis of cell wall mucopeptide. (Beta-lactam fused to different ring structure from penicillins.)

ADVERSE EFFECTS — Serious: Cross-sensitivity with penicillins, C. difficile-associated diarrhea. Frequent: Eosinophilia.

ANTIMICROBIALS: Cephalosporins—2nd Generation

NOTE: Cephalosporins are second-line to penicillins for group A strep pharyngitis, can rarely be cross-sensitive with penicillins, and can cause C. difficile–associated diarrhea.

CEFACLOR (★Ceclor) ▶K ♀B ▶? $$$$

ADULT — Pneumonia, group A strep pharyngitis, UTI, skin infections: 250 to 500 mg PO three times per day. Treat pharyngitis for 10 days.

PEDS — Pneumonia, group A streptococcal pharyngitis, UTI, skin infections: 20 to 40 mg/kg/day (up to 1 g/day) PO divided two times per day for pharyngitis, three times per day for other infections. Treat pharyngitis for 10 days.

FORMS — Generic only: Caps 250, 500 mg. Susp 125, 187, 250, 375 mg per 5 mL. Extended-release tab: 500 mg.

MOA — Serious: Cross-sensitivity with penicillins, C. difficile-associated diarrhea; serum sickness-like reactions with repeated use. Frequent: Headache.

ADVERSE EFFECTS — TAB006,TAB007

CEFOTETAN ▶K/Bile ♀B ▶? $$$$$

ADULT — Usual dose: 1 to 2 g IM/IV q 12 h. UTI: 0.5 to 2 g IM/IV q 12 h or 1 to 2 g IM/IV q 24 h. Pneumonia, gynecologic, intra-abdominal, bone and joint infections: 1 to 3 g IM/IV q 12 h. Skin infections: 1 to 2 g IM/IV q 12 h or 2 g IV q 24 h. Surgical prophylaxis: 1 to 2 g IV 30 to 60 min preop. Give after cord clamp for C-section.

PEDS — Not approved in children.

UNAPPROVED PEDS — Usual dose: 40 to 80 mg/kg/day IV divided q 12 h.

NOTES — Hemolytic anemia (higher risk than other cephalosporins), clotting impairment rarely. Disulfiram-like reaction with alcohol. Dosing reduction in adults with renal dysfunction: Usual dose q 48 h for CrCl less than 10 mL/min; usual dose q 24 h for CrCl 10 to 30 mL/min.

MOA — Beta-lactam antibiotic that inhibits the biosynthesis of cell wall mucopeptide. (Beta-lactam fused to different ring structure from penicillins.) Cefotetan has MTT side-chain.

ADVERSE EFFECTS — Serious: Cross-sensitivity with penicillins, C. difficile-associated diarrhea, hemolytic anemia, clotting impairment rarely, disulfiram-like reaction with alcohol.

CEFOXITIN ▶K ♀B ▶+ $

ADULT — Pneumonia, UTI, sepsis, intra-abdominal, gynecologic, skin, bone and joint infections. Uncomplicated: 1 g IV q 6 to 8 h. Moderate to severe: 1 g IV q 4 h or 2 g IV q 6 to 8 h. Infections requiring high doses: 2 g IV q 4 h or 3 g IV q 6 h. Uncontaminated GI surgery, vaginal/abdominal hysterectomy: 2 g IV 30 to 60 min preop, then 2 g IV q 6 h for 24 h. C-section: 2 g IV after cord clamped or 2 g IV q 4 h for 3 doses with 1st dose given after cord clamped.

PEDS — Pneumonia, UTI, sepsis, intra-abdominal, skin, bone and joint infections: 80 to 160 mg/kg/day (up to 12 g/day) IV divided into 4 to 6 doses for age 3 mo or older. Mild to moderate infections: 80 to 100 mg/kg/day IV divided into 3 to 4 doses. Surgical prophylaxis: 30 to 40 mg/kg IV 30 to 60 min preop; additional doses can be given q 6 h up to 24 h postop.

NOTES — Eosinophilia and increased AST with high doses in children. Dosing reduction in adults with renal dysfunction: Load with 1 to 2 g IV then 0.5 g IV q 24 to 48 h for CrCl less than 5 mL/min; 0.5 to 1 g IV q 12 to 24 h for CrCl 5 to 9 mL/min; 1 to 2 g IV q 12 to 24 h for CrCl 10 to 29 mL/min; 1 to 2 g IV q 8 to 12 h for CrCl 30 to 50 mL/min. Give 1 to 2 g supplemental dose after each hemodialysis.

MOA — Beta-lactam antibiotic that inhibits the biosynthesis of cell wall mucopeptide. (Beta-lactam fused to different ring structure from penicillins.)

ADVERSE EFFECTS — Serious: Cross-sensitivity with penicillins, C. difficile-associated diarrhea, eosinophilia & increased AST with high doses in children.

CEFPROZIL ▶K ♀B ▶+ $$$$

ADULT — Group A strep pharyngitis: 500 mg PO once daily for 10 days. Sinusitis: 250 to 500 mg PO two times per day. Acute exacerbation of chronic/secondary infection of acute bronchitis: 500 mg PO two times per day. Skin infections: 250 to 500 mg PO two times per day or 500 mg PO once daily.

PEDS — Otitis media: 15 mg/kg/dose PO two times per day. Group A strep pharyngitis: 7.5 mg/kg/dose PO two times per day for 10 days. Sinusitis: 7.5 to 15 mg/kg/dose PO two times per day. Skin infections: 20 mg/kg PO once daily. Use adult dose for age 13 yo or older.

FORMS — Generic only: Tabs 250, 500 mg. Susp 125, 250 mg/5 mL.

NOTES — Give 50% of usual dose at usual interval for CrCl less than 30 mL/min.

MOA — Beta-lactam antibiotic that inhibits the biosynthesis of cell wall mucopeptide. (Beta-lactam fused to different ring structure from penicillins.)

ADVERSE EFFECTS — Serious: Cross-sensitivity with penicillins, C. difficile-associated diarrhea, may cause serum sickness reaction. Frequent: None.

CEFUROXIME (*Zinacef, Ceftin*) ▶K ♀B ▶? $$$$
ADULT — Uncomplicated pneumonia, simple UTI, skin infections, disseminated gonorrhea: 750 mg IM/IV q 8 h. Bone and joint or severe/complicated infections: 1.5 g IV q 8 h. Sepsis: 1.5 g IV q 6 h to 3 g IV q 8 h. Gonorrhea: 1.5 g IM single dose split into 2 injections, given with probenecid 1 g PO. Surgical prophylaxis: 1.5 g IV 30 to 60 min preop, then 750 mg IM/IV q 8 h for prolonged procedures. Open heart surgery: 1.5 g IV q 12 h for 4 doses with 1st dose at induction of anesthesia. Cefuroxime axetil tabs: Group A strep pharyngitis, acute sinusitis: 250 mg PO two times per day for 10 days. Acute exacerbation of chronic/secondary infection of acute bronchitis, skin infections: 250 to 500 mg PO two times per day. Lyme disease: 500 mg PO two times per day for 14 days for early disease, for 28 days for Lyme arthritis. Simple UTI: 125 to 250 mg PO two times per day. Gonorrhea: 1 g PO single dose.
PEDS — Most infections: 50 to 100 mg/kg/day IM/IV divided q 6 to 8 h. Bone and joint infections: 150 mg/kg/day IM/IV divided q 8 h (up to adult dose). Cefuroxime axetil tabs: Group A strep pharyngitis: 125 mg PO two times per day for 10 days. Otitis media, sinusitis: 250 mg PO two times per day for 10 days. Cefuroxime axetil oral susp. Group A strep pharyngitis: 20 mg/kg/day (up to 500 mg/day) PO divided two times per day for 10 days. Otitis media, sinusitis, impetigo: 30 mg/kg/day (up to 1 g/day) PO divided two times per day for 10 days. Use adult dose for age 13 yo or older. For otitis media, AAP recommends 5 to 7 days of therapy for age 6 yo and older with mild to moderate symptoms, 7 days for age 2 to 5 yo with mild to moderate symptoms, and 10 days for age younger than 2 yo and childern with severe symptoms.
UNAPPROVED PEDS — Lyme disease: 30 mg/kg/day PO divided two times per day (max 500 mg/dose) for 14 days for early disease, for 28 days for Lyme arthritis. Community-acquired pneumonia: 150 mg/kg/day IV divided q 8 h.
FORMS — Generic/Trade: Tabs 250, 500 mg. Susp 125, 250 mg/5 mL.
NOTES — Dosage reduction for renal dysfunction in adults: 750 mg IM/IV q 24 h for CrCl < 10 mL/min, 750 mg IM/IV q 12 h for CrCl 10 to 20 mL/min. Give supplemental dose after hemodialysis. Tabs and susp not bioequivalent on mg/mg basis. Do not crush tabs.
MOA — Beta-lactam antibiotic that inhibits the biosynthesis of cell wall mucopeptide. (Beta-lactam fused to different ring structure from penicillins.)
ADVERSE EFFECTS — Serious: Cross-sensitivity with penicillins, C. difficile-associated diarrhea. Frequent: Anemia, eosinophilia.

ANTIMICROBIALS: Cephalosporins—3rd Generation

NOTE: Cephalosporins are 2nd-line to penicillins for group A strep pharyngitis, can rarely be cross-sensitive with penicillins, and can cause C. difficile–associated diarrhea.

CEFDINIR ▶K ♀B ▶? $$$$
ADULT — Community-acquired pneumonia, skin infections: 300 mg PO two times per day for 10 days. Sinusitis: 600 mg PO once daily or 300 mg PO two times per day for 10 days. Group A strep pharyngitis, acute exacerbation of chronic bronchitis: 600 mg PO once daily for 10 days or 300 mg PO two times per day for 5 to 10 days.
PEDS — Group A strep pharyngitis, otitis media: 14 mg/kg/day PO divided two times per day for 5 to 10 days or once daily for 10 days. See tables for management of otitis media and acute sinusitis. Sinusitis: 14 mg/kg/day PO divided once daily or two times per day for 10 days. Skin infections: 14 mg/kg/day PO divided two times per day for 10 days. Use adult dose for age 13 yo or older.
FORMS — Generic only: Caps 300 mg. Susp 125, 250 mg/5 mL.
NOTES — Give iron, multivitamins with iron, or antacids at least 2 h before or after cefdinir. Complexation of cefdinir with iron may turn stools red. Reduce dose for renal dysfunction: 300 mg PO daily for adults with CrCl less than 30 mL/min; 7 mg/kg/day PO once daily up to 300 mg/day for children with CrCl less than 30 mL/min. Hemodialysis: 300 mg or 7 mg/kg PO after hemodialysis, then 300 mg or 7 mg/kg PO q 48 h.
MOA — Beta-lactam antibiotic that inhibits the biosynthesis of cell wall mucopeptide. (Beta-lactam fused to different ring structure from penicillins.)
ADVERSE EFFECTS — Serious: Cross-sensitivity with penicillins, C. difficile-associated diarrhea. Frequent: Diarrhea.

CEFDITOREN (*Spectracef*) ▶K ♀B ▶? $$$$$
ADULT — Skin infections, group A strep pharyngitis: 200 mg PO two times per day for 10 days. Give 400 mg two times per day for 10 days for acute exacerbation of chronic bronchitis, for 14 days for community-acquired pneumonia. Take with food.
PEDS — Not approved for children younger than 12 yo. Skin infections, group A strep pharyngitis, adolescents age 12 yo or older: 200 mg PO two times per day with food for 10 days.
FORMS — Generic/Trade: Tabs 200, 400 mg.
NOTES — Contraindicated if milk protein allergy or carnitine deficiency. Not for long-term use due to potential risk of carnitine deficiency. Do not take with drugs that reduce gastric acid (antacids, H2 blockers, etc.). Dosage adjustment for renal dysfunction: Max 200 mg two times per day if CrCl 30 to 49 mL/min; max 200 mg once daily if CrCl less than 30 mL/min.
MOA — Beta-lactam antibiotic that inhibits the biosynthesis of cell wall mucopeptide. (Beta-lactam fused to different ring structure from penicillins.)
ADVERSE EFFECTS — Serious: Cross-sensitivity with penicillins, C. difficile-associated diarrhea. Frequent: N/V, diarrhea.

CEFIXIME (*Suprax*) ▶K/Bile ♀B ▶? $$$$
ADULT — Simple UTI, pharyngitis, acute bacterial bronchitis, acute exacerbation of chronic bronchitis: 400 mg PO once daily. Gonorrhea: 400 mg PO single dose. CDC now considers cefixime second-line for treatment of gonorrhea and requires test-of-cure. See STD table.
PEDS — Otitis media: 8 mg/kg/day susp/chew tab PO divided one to two times per day. Use only susp/chew tabs for otitis media (better blood levels). Pharyngitis: 8 mg/kg/day PO divided one to two times per day for 10 days. Use adult dose for wt >50 kg (>45 kg for 500 mg/5 mL susp) or age 13 yo or older.
UNAPPROVED PEDS — Febrile UTI (3 to 24 mo): 16 mg/kg PO on 1st day, then 8 mg/kg PO daily to complete 14 days. Gonorrhea: 8 mg/kg (max 400 mg) PO single dose for wt less than 45 kg, 400 mg PO single dose for 45 kg or greater. See table for management of acute sinusitis.
FORMS — Trade only: Susp 100, 200, 500 mg/5 mL. Chewable tabs 100, 150, 200 mg. Tabs 400 mg. Caps 400 mg.
NOTES — Poor activity against S. aureus. Increased INR with warfarin. May increase carbamazepine levels. Susp stable at room temp or refrigerated for 14 days. Reduce dose in renal dysfunction: 75% of usual dose at usual interval for CrCl 21 to 60 mL/min or hemodialysis; 50% of usual dose at usual interval for CrCl less than 20 mL/min or continuous peritoneal dialysis. Can cause false (+) on urine glucose test using Benedict's or Fehling's solution (Clinitest, etc); use glucose oxidase test (Clinistix, TesTape, etc) instead.
MOA — Beta-lactam antibiotic that inhibits the biosynthesis of cell wall mucopeptide. (Beta-lactam fused to different ring structure from penicillins.)
ADVERSE EFFECTS — Serious: Cross-sensitivity with penicillins, C. difficile-associated diarrhea. Frequent: N/V, diarrhea.

CEFOTAXIME (*Claforan*) ▶KL ♀B ▶+ $$$$
ADULT — Pneumonia, sepsis, GU and gynecologic, skin, intra-abdominal, bone and joint infections. Uncomplicated: 1 g IM/IV q 12 h. Moderate/severe: 1 to 2 g IM/IV q 8 h. Infections usually requiring high doses: 2 g IV q 6 to 8 h. Life-threatening: 2 g IV q 4 h. Meningitis: 2 g IV q 4 to 6 h. Gonorrhea: 0.5 to 1 g IM single dose.
PEDS — Pneumonia, sepsis, GU, skin, intra-abdominal, bone/joint, CNS infections. Labeled dose: 50 mg/kg/dose IV q 12 h for age younger than 1 week old; 50 mg/kg/dose IV q 8 h for age 1 to 4 weeks, 50 to 180 mg/kg/day IM/IV divided q 4 to 6 h for age 1 mo to 12 yo. AAP recommends 225 to 300 mg/kg/day IV divided q 6 to 8 h for S. pneumoniae meningitis. Mild to moderate infections: 75 to 100 mg/kg/day IV/IM divided q 6 to 8 h. Severe infections: 150 to 200 mg/kg/day IV/IM divided q 6 to 8 h.
UNAPPROVED ADULT — Disseminated gonorrhea, CDC regimen: 1 g IV q 8 h.
NOTES — Bolus injection through central venous catheter can cause arrhythmias. Decrease dose by 50% for CrCl less than 20 mL/min.

MOA — Beta-lactam antibiotic that inhibits the biosynthesis of cell wall mucopeptide. (Beta-lactam fused to different ring structure from penicillins.)
ADVERSE EFFECTS — Serious: Cross-sensitivity with penicillins, C. difficile-associated diarrhea. Frequent: Coombs + anemia, phlebitis.

CEFPODOXIME ▶K ♀B ▶? $$$$
ADULT — Acute exacerbation of chronic bronchitis, acute sinusitis: 200 mg PO two times per day for 10 days. Community-acquired pneumonia: 200 mg PO two times per day for 14 days. Group A strep pharyngitis: 100 mg PO two times per day for 5 to 10 days. Skin infections: 400 mg PO two times per day for 7 to 14 days. Simple UTI: 100 mg PO two times per day for 7 days. Approved for treatment of gonorrhea, but CDC does not recommend. Give tabs with food.
PEDS — 5 mg/kg PO two times per day for 5 days for otitis media, for 5 to 10 days for group A strep pharyngitis, for 10 days for sinusitis. Use adult dose for age 12 yo or older. For otitis media, AAP recommends 5 to 7 days of therapy for age 6 yo and older with mild to moderate symptoms, 7 days for age 2 to 5 yo with mild to moderate symptoms, and 10 days for age younger than 2 yo and children with severe symptoms. See tables for management of acute sinusitis and otitis media.
FORMS — Generic: Tabs 100, 200 mg. Susp 50, 100 mg/5 mL.
NOTES — Do not give antacids within 2 h before/after cefpodoxime. Reduce dose in renal dysfunction: Increase dosing interval to q 24 h for CrCl less than 30 mL/min. Give 3 times per week after dialysis session for hemodialysis patients. Susp stable for 14 days refrigerated.
MOA — Beta-lactam antibiotic that inhibits the biosynthesis of cell wall mucopeptide. (Beta-lactam fused to different ring structure from penicillins.)
ADVERSE EFFECTS — Serious: Cross-sensitivity with penicillins; C. difficile-associated diarrhea; acute hepatitis, bloody diarrhea, and pulmonary infiltrates (rare). Frequent: Diarrhea.

CEFTAZIDIME (*Fortaz, Tazicef*) ▶K ♀B ▶+ $$$$
ADULT — Simple UTI: 250 mg IM/IV q 12 h. Complicated UTI: 500 mg IM/IV q 8 to 12 h. Uncomplicated pneumonia, mild skin infections: 500 mg to 1 g IM/IV q 8 h. Serious gynecologic, intra-abdominal, bone and joint, life-threatening infections, meningitis, empiric therapy of neutropenic fever: 2 g IV q 8 h. Pseudomonas lung infections in cystic fibrosis: 30 to 50 mg/kg IV q 8 h (up to 6 g/day).
PEDS — Use sodium formulations in children (Fortaz, Tazicef). UTIs, pneumonia, skin, intra-abdominal, bone and joint infections: 100 to 150 mg/kg/day (up to 6 g/day) IV divided q 8 h for age 1 mo to 12 yo. Meningitis: 150 mg/kg/day (up to 6 g/day) IV divided q 8 h for age 1 mo to 12 yo; 30 mg/kg IV q 12 h for age younger than 4 weeks old. Use adult dose and formulations for age 12 yo or older.
UNAPPROVED ADULT — P. aeruginosa osteomyelitis of the foot from nail puncture: 2 g IV q 8 h.

(cont.)

CEFTAZIDIME (*cont.*)

UNAPPROVED PEDS — AAP recommends 50 mg/kg IV q 8 to 12 h for age younger than 1 week and wt greater than 2 kg, q 8 h for age 1 week old or older.

NOTES — High levels in renal dysfunction can cause CNS toxicity. Reduce dose in adults with renal dysfunction: load with 1 g then 500 mg q 48 h for CrCl less than 5 mL/min; load with 1 g then 500 mg q 24 h for CrCl 6 to 15 mL/min; 1 g IV q 24 h for CrCl 16 to 30 mL/min; 1 g IV q 12 h for CrCl 31 to 50 mL/min. 1 g IV load in hemodialysis patients, then 1 g IV after hemodialysis sessions.

MOA — Beta-lactam antibiotic that inhibits the biosynthesis of cell wall mucopeptide. (Beta-lactam fused to different ring structure from penicillins.)

ADVERSE EFFECTS — Serious: Cross-sensitivity with penicillins, C. difficile-associated diarrhea, CNS toxicity with high levels in patients with renal dysfunction. Frequent: Coombs + anemia, eosinophilia, increased LFTs.

CEFTIBUTEN (*Cedax*) ▶K ♀B ▶? $$$$$

ADULT — Group A streptococcal pharyngitis, acute exacerbation of chronic bronchitis, otitis media not due to S. pneumoniae: 400 mg PO once daily for 10 days.

PEDS — Group A streptococcal pharyngitis, otitis media not due to S. pneumoniae, age 6 mo or older: 9 mg/kg (up to 400 mg) PO once daily. Give susp on empty stomach.

FORMS — Trade only: Caps 400 mg. Susp 90 mg/5 mL.

NOTES — Poor activity against S. aureus and S. pneumoniae. Reduce dose in adults with renal dysfunction: 100 mg PO daily for CrCl 5 to 29 mL/min; 200 mg PO once daily for CrCl 30 to 49 mL/min. Reduce dose in children with renal dysfunction: 2.25 mg/kg PO once daily for CrCl 5 to 29 mL/min; 4.5 mg/kg PO once daily for CrCl 30 to 49 mL/min. Hemodialysis: Adults 400 mg PO and children 9 mg/kg PO after each dialysis session. Susp stable for 14 days refrigerated.

MOA — Beta-lactam antibiotic that inhibits the biosynthesis of cell wall mucopeptide. (Beta-lactam fused to different ring structure from penicillins.)

ADVERSE EFFECTS — Serious: Cross-sensitivity with penicillins, C. difficile-associated diarrhea. Frequent: Eosinophilia, nausea.

CEFTRIAXONE (*Rocephin*) ▶K/Bile ♀B ▶+ $

WARNING — Contraindicated in neonates who require (or are expected to require) IV calcium (including calcium in TPN); fatal lung/kidney precipitation of calcium ceftriaxone has been reported in neonates. In other patients, do not give ceftriaxone and calcium-containing solns simultaneously, but sequential administration is acceptable if lines are flushed with a compatible fluid between infusions. Do not dilute with Ringer's/Hartmann's soln or TPN containing calcium.

ADULT — Pneumonia, UTI, pelvic inflammatory disease (hospitalized), sepsis, meningitis, skin, bone and joint, intra-abdominal infections: Usual dose 1 to 2 g IM/IV q 24 h (max 4 g/day divided q 12 h). Gonorrhea: Single dose 250 mg IM. See STD table.

PEDS — Meningitis: 100 mg/kg/day (up to 4 g/day) IV divided q 12 to 24 h. Skin, pneumonia, other serious infections: 50 to 75 mg/kg/day (up to 2 g/day) IM/IV divided q 12 to 24 h. Otitis media: 50 mg/kg (up to 1 g) IM single dose. See table for treatment of acute otitis media in children.

UNAPPROVED ADULT — Lyme disease carditis, meningitis: 2 g IV once daily for 14 days. Chancroid: 250 mg IM single dose. Disseminated gonorrhea: 1 g IM/IV q 24 h. Prophylaxis, invasive meningococcal disease: 250 mg IM single dose.

UNAPPROVED PEDS — Otitis media, if initial antibiotic fails (at 48 to 72 hours): 50 mg/kg IM q day for 3 days. Otitis media, initial treatment if penicillin allergy: 50 mg/kg IM q day for 1 or 3 days. See tables for management of acute sinusitis and otitis media. Lyme disease carditis, meningitis: 50 to 75 mg/kg IM/IV once daily (up to 2 g/day) for 14 days. Prophylaxis, invasive meningococcal disease: Single IM dose of 125 mg for age younger than 16 yo, 250 mg for age 16 yo or older. Gonorrhea: 125 mg IM single dose; use adult regimens in STD table if wt 45 kg or greater. Gonococcal bacteremia/arthritis: 50 mg/kg (max 1 g for wt 45 kg or less) IM/IV once daily for 7 days. Gonococcal ophthalmia neonatorum/gonorrhea prophylaxis in newborn: 25 to 50 mg/kg up to 125 mg IM/IV single dose at birth. Disseminated gonorrhea, infants: 25 to 50 mg/kg/day IM/IV once daily for 7 days. Typhoid fever: 50 to 75 mg/kg IM/IV once daily for 14 days.

NOTES — Can cause prolonged prothrombin time (due to vitamin K deficiency), biliary sludging/symptoms of gallbladder disease. Do not give to neonates with hyperbilirubinemia. Dilute in 1% lidocaine for IM use. Do not exceed 2 g/day in patients with both hepatic and renal dysfunction.

MOA — Beta-lactam antibiotic that inhibits the biosynthesis of cell wall mucopeptide. (Beta-lactam fused to different ring structure from penicillins.)

ADVERSE EFFECTS — Serious: Cross-sensitivity with penicillins, C. difficile-associated diarrhea, prolonged prothrombin time due to vitamin K deficiency, biliary sludging/symptoms of gallbladder disease, hemolytic anemia. Fatal precipitation with calcium in lungs/kidneys of neonates. Frequent: Eosinophilia.

ANTIMICROBIALS: Cephalosporins—4th Generation

NOTE: Cross-sensitivity with penicillins possible. May cause C. difficile–associated diarrhea.

CEFEPIME (*Maxipime*) ▶K ♀B ▶? $$$$

ADULT — Mild, moderate UTI: 0.5 to 1 g IM/IV q 12 h. Severe UTI, skin, complicated intra-abdominal infections: 2 g IV q 12 h. Pneumonia: 1 to 2 g IV q 12 h. Empiric therapy of febrile neutropenia: 2 g IV q 8 h.

CEFEPIME (*cont.*)

PEDS — UTI, skin infections, pneumonia: 50 mg/kg IV q 12 h for wt 40 kg or less. Empiric therapy for febrile neutropenia: 50 mg/kg IV q 8 h for wt 40 kg or less. Do not exceed adult dose.

UNAPPROVED ADULT — P. aeruginosa osteomyelitis of the foot from nail puncture: 2 g IV q 12 h. Meningitis: 2 g IV q 8 h.

UNAPPROVED PEDS — Meningitis, cystic fibrosis, other serious infections: 50 mg/kg IV q 8 h (max of 6 g/day).

NOTES — An FDA safety review did not find higher mortality with cefepime than with other beta-lactams. High levels in renal dysfunction can cause CNS toxicity; dosing for CrCl less than 60 mL/min in package insert.

MOA — Beta-lactam antibiotic that inhibits the biosynthesis of cell wall mucopeptide. (Beta-lactam fused to different ring structure from penicillins.)

ADVERSE EFFECTS — Serious: Cross-sensitivity with penicillins, C. difficile-associated diarrhea, CNS toxicity (encephalopathy, myoclonus, seizures) due to high levels of cefepime, especially in patients with renal dysfunction. An FDA safety review did not find higher mortality with cefepime than with other beta lactams. Frequent: Coombs + anemia.

ANTIMICROBIALS: Cephalosporins—5th Generation

NOTE: Cephalosporins can be cross-sensitive with penicillins and can cause C. difficile associated diarrhea.

CEFTAROLINE (*Teflaro*) ▶K ♀B ▶? $$$$$

ADULT — Community-acquired bacterial pneumonia, acute bacterial skin and skin structure infections: 600 mg IV q12 h infused over 1 h.

PEDS — Not approved in children.

NOTES — Direct Coombs' test seroconversion reported; hemolytic anemia is possible. Dosage reduction for renal dysfunction: 400 mg IV q 12 h for CrCl 31 to 50 mL/min; 300 mg IV q 12 h for CrCl 15 to 30 mL/min; 200 mg IV q 12 h for ESRD including hemodialysis.

MOA — Beta-lactam antibiotic that inhibits the biosynthesis of cell wall mucopeptide. (Beta-lactam fused to different ring structure from penicillins).

ADVERSE EFFECTS — Serious: Serious: Cross-sensitivity with penicillins, C. difficile associated diarrhea. Coombs + anemia possible. Frequent: Diarrhea, nausea, rash.

ANTIMICROBIALS: Glycopeptides

DALBAVANCIN (*Dalvance*) ▶K ♀C ▶? $$$$$

ADULT — Gram-positive skin infections, including MRSA: 1000 mg followed 1 week later by 500 mg. Infuse IV over 30 minutes.

PEDS — Safety and efficacy not established in children.

NOTES — "Red Neck" (or "Red Man") syndrome with rapid IV administration. Dosage adjustment for renal impairment: 750 mg IV followed 1 week later by 375 mg for CrCl <30 mL/min and not receiving regular hemodialysis. Not removed by hemodialysis; dosage adjustment not required for hemodialysis and can be given without regard to timing of hemodialysis session.

MOA — Bacteriocidal lipoglycopeptide derived from teicoplanin that inhibits synthesis of cell wall peptidoglycan polymers.

SIDE EFFECTS — Serious: Anaphylaxis, skin reactions, increased ALT, C. difficile-associated diarrhea. "Red Neck" (or "Red Man") syndrome with rapid IV administration. Frequent: Nausea, headache, diarrhea.

ORITAVANCIN (*Orbactiv*) ▶K feces ♀C ▶? $$$$$

ADULT — Gram-positive skin infections, including MRSA: 1200 mg IV single dose infused over 3 h.

PEDS — Not approved for use in children.

NOTES — Can artificially prolong aPTT for up to 48 h; do not give IV unfractionated heparin for 48 h after a dose of oritavancin. Can artificially prolong PT and INR for up to 24 h, making INR monitoring of warfarin unreliable during that time. May increase INR and risk of bleeding with warfarin; coadministration is risk vs benefit decison. Can cause infusion reactions; slow or hold infusion if reaction develops. Hypersensitivity reactions. Cross-sensitivity with other glycopeptide antibiotics possible; monitor for hypersensitivity symptoms during infusion in patients with a history of glycopeptide allergy. Half-life of oritavancin is approximately 10 days. Risk of osteomyelitis higher with ortivancin than vancomycin in premarketing study; monitor for signs/symptoms of osteomyelitis. Incompatible with NS; flush IV line with D5W only. No dosage adjustment for mild to moderate hepatic or renal impairment.

MOA — Bacteriocidal lipoglycopeptide that is a vancomycin analog; inhibits 3 steps in synthesis of cell wall peptidoglycan polymers.

ADVERSE EFFECTS — Hypersensitivity reactions (median onset of 1.2 days and duration of 2.4 days in clinical trials). Infusion reactions (pruritus, urticaria, flushing). C. difficile-associated diarrhea. Frequent: Headache, N/V, diarrhea, limb and SC abcesses.

TELAVANCIN (*Vibativ*) ▶K ♀C ▶? $$$$$

WARNING — In patients with CrCl ≤50 mL/min treated for hospital-acquired/ventilator-associated pneumonia, there was higher mortality with telavancin than vancomycin. Do not use telavancin in patients with CrCl ≤50 mL/min unless potential benefit outweighs risk. Nephrotoxic; monitor renal function in all patients. Teratogenic in animal studies. Get serum pregnancy test before use in women

(cont.)

TELAVANCIN (*cont.*)

of child-bearing potential. Do not use in pregnancy unless potential benefit outweighs risk.

ADULT — Complicated skin infections including MRSA: 10 mg/kg IV once daily for 7 to 14 days. Hospital-acquired/ventilator-associated S. aureus pneumonia (not first-line): 10 mg/kg IV once daily for 7 to 21 days. Infuse over 1 h.

PEDS — Safety and efficacy not established in children.

NOTES — QT interval prolongation; do not use in congenital long QT syndrome, uncompensated heart failure, or severe left ventricular hypertrophy. Caution advised for coadministration with other drugs that prolong QT interval. Does not interfere with coagulation, but may affect some coagulation tests. To minimize interference, draw blood for INR, aPTT, clotting time, and factor Xa right before next dose of telavancin. Use IV solution within 4 h when stored at room temp. Nephrotoxicity; monitor renal function at least q 2 to 3 days. Efficacy may be decreased in patients with baseline CrCl ≤50 mL/min. Cyclodextrin vehicle may accumulate in renal dysfunction. Dosage adjustment for renal dysfunction in adults: 7.5 mg/kg IV q 24 h for CrCl 30 to 50 mL/min; 10 mg/kg q 48 h for CrCl 10 to 29 mL/min.

MOA — Bactericidal glycopeptide derivative of vancomycin that inhibits synthesis of cell wall peptidoglycan polymers. May also have other mechanisms of action.

ADVERSE EFFECTS — Serious: Nephrotoxicity (may be increased by NSAIDs, ACE inhibitors, loop diuretics); QT interval prolongation. Frequent: N/V, rash, foamy urine, metallic/soapy taste disturbance. May cause "Red Neck" (or "Red Man") syndrome with rapid IV administration.

VANCOMYCIN (*Vancocin*) ►K ♀C ▶? $$$$$

ADULT — Severe staph infections (including MRSA), endocarditis: 1 g IV q 12 h, each dose over 1 h or 30 mg/kg/day IV divided q 12 h. Empiric therapy, native valve endocarditis: 15 mg/kg (up to 2 g/day unless levels monitored) IV q 12 h with gentamicin. C. difficile–associated diarrhea: 125 mg PO four times per day for 10 days. IV administration ineffective for this indication. See table for management of C. difficile infection in adults, including higher dose of vancomycin plus metronidazole for severe complicated disease. Staphylococcal enterocolitis: 500 to 2000 mg/day PO divided three to four times per day for 7 to 10 days. See table for prophylaxis of bacterial endocarditis.

PEDS — Severe staph infections (including MRSA), endocarditis: 15 mg/kg IV load, then 10 mg/kg q 12 h for age younger than 1 week; 15 mg/kg IV load, then 10 mg/kg q 8 h for age 1 week to 1 mo; 10 mg/kg IV q 6 h for age older than 1 mo. C. difficile–associated diarrhea: 40 mg/kg/day (up to 2 g/day) PO divided four times per day for 10 days. IV administration ineffective for this indication.

UNAPPROVED ADULT — Usual dose: 15 to 20 mg/kg IV q 8 to 12 h. Consider loading dose of 25 to 30 mg/kg for severe infections. Infuse over 1 h; infuse over 1.5 to 2 h if dose greater than 1 g. Base IV dose on absolute body wt. In obese patients, base initial dose on absolute body wt, then adjust dose based on trough levels. C. difficile–associated diarrhea: 125 mg PO four times per day for 10 to 14 days. See table for management of C. difficile infection in adults, including higher dose of vancomycin plus metronidazole for severe complicated disease. Prevention of perinatal group B streptococcal disease: Give to mother 1 g IV q 12 h from onset of labor/after membrane rupture until delivery.

UNAPPROVED PEDS — Newborns: 10 to 15 mg/kg IV q 8 to 12 h for age younger than 1 week; 10 to 15 mg/kg IV q 6 to 8 h for age 1 week and older. Bacterial meningitis: 60 mg/kg/day IV divided q 6 h. Nonmeningeal pneumococcal infections: 40 to 45 mg/kg/day IV divided q 6 h.

FORMS — Generic/Trade: Caps 125, 250 mg.

NOTES — Maintain trough higher than 10 mg/L in all patients to avoid development of resistance; optimal trough for complicated infections is 15 to 20 mg/L. Draw trough just before the next dose after steady-state is reached (usually after 4th dose). Monitoring of peak levels no longer recommended. "Red Neck" (or "Red Man") syndrome with rapid IV administration, vein irritation with IV extravasation, reversible neutropenia, ototoxicity, or nephrotoxicity rarely. Enhanced effects of neuromuscular blockers. Use caution with other ototoxic/nephrotoxic drugs. Individualize dose if renal dysfunction. Oral vancomycin poorly absorbed; do not use for extraluminal infections.

MOA — Bactericidal glycopeptide that inhibits synthesis of cell wall peptidoglycan polymers. May also have other mechanisms of action.

ADVERSE EFFECTS — Serious: Reversible neutropenia, ototoxicity (rare and reversible with monotherapy) or nephrotoxicity (rare; risk may be increased by high doses, poor renal function, old age, or nephrotoxic drug), superinfection. Can cause C. difficile-associated diarrhea. Frequent: "Red Neck" (or "Red Man") syndrome with rapid IV administration, vein irritation with IV extravasation.

ANTIMICROBIALS: Macrolides

AZITHROMYCIN (*Zithromax, Zmax*) ►L ♀B ▶? $$

ADULT — Community-acquired pneumonia including Legionella, inpatient: 500 mg IV over 1 h daily for at least 2 days, then 500 mg PO daily for 7 to 10 days total. Pelvic inflammatory disease: 500 mg IV daily for 1 to 2 days, then 250 mg PO daily to complete 7 days. Oral for acute exacerbation of chronic bronchitis, community-acquired pneumonia, group A streptococcal pharyngitis (2nd line to penicillin), skin infections: 500 mg PO on 1st day, then 250 mg PO daily for 4 days. Acute sinusitis, alternative for acute exacerbation of chronic bronchitis: 500 mg PO daily for 3 days. Zmax for community-acquired pneumonia, acute sinusitis: 2 g PO single dose (contents

AZITHROMYCIN (cont.)

of full bottle) on empty stomach. Azithromycin is a poor option for acute sinusitis due to pneumococcal and H. influenzae resistance; see acute sinusitis treatment table for alternatives. Chlamydia, chancroid: 1 g PO single dose. Gonorrhea: 2 g PO single dose (CDC does not recommend azithromycin alone for routine treatment). Get culture (preferred) or NAAT 1 week after dose. Observe patient for at least 30 min for poor GI tolerability. See STD table. Prevention of disseminated Mycobacterium avium complex disease: 1200 mg PO once per week.

PEDS — Azithromycin is a poor option for otitis media and acute sinusitis due to pneumococcal and H. influenzae resistance; see otitis media and acute sinusitis treatment tables for alternatives. Oral for otitis media, community-acquired pneumonia: 10 mg/kg up to 500 mg PO on 1st day, then 5 mg/kg up to 250 mg PO daily for 4 days. Acute sinusitis: 10 mg/kg PO daily for 3 days. Zmax for community-acquired pneumonia, acute sinusitis: 60 mg/kg (max 2 g) PO single dose on empty stomach for age 6 mo or older; give adult dose of 2 g for wt 34 kg or greater. Otitis media: 30 mg/kg PO single dose or 10 mg/kg PO daily for 3 days. Group A streptococcal pharyngitis (2nd line to penicillin): 12 mg/kg up to 500 mg PO daily for 5 days. Take susp on empty stomach.

UNAPPROVED ADULT — See table for prophylaxis of bacterial endocarditis. Nongonococcal urethritis: 1 g PO single dose. See STD table for recurrent/persistent urethritis. Chlamydia in pregnancy: 1 g PO single dose. Campylobacter gastroenteritis: 500 mg PO daily for 3 days. For HIV-infected patients, treat mild/moderate disease for 7 to 10 days (not for bacteremia in HIV-infected patients). Traveler's diarrhea: 500 mg PO on 1st day, then 250 mg PO daily for 4 days; or 1 g PO single dose. Mycobacterium avium complex disease in AIDS, treatment: 500 mg PO daily (use at least 2 drugs for active infection). Pertussis treatment/postexposure prophylaxis: 500 mg PO on 1st day, then 250 mg PO daily for 4 days. Cholera: 1 g PO single dose (use this regimen in pregnancy).

UNAPPROVED PEDS — Prevention of disseminated Mycobacterium avium complex disease: 20 mg/kg PO once per week not to exceed adult dose. Mycobacterium avium complex disease treatment: 5 mg/kg PO daily (use at least 2 drugs for active infection). Cystic fibrosis patients colonized with P. aeruginosa, age 6 yo and older: 250 mg three days per week for 24 weeks for wt less than 40 kg, 500 mg PO three days per week for 24 weeks for wt 40 kg or greater. Chlamydia trachomatis: 1 g PO single dose for age younger than 8 yo and wt greater than 44 kg, and for age 8 yo or older for any wt. Pertussis treatment/postexposure prophylaxis: 10 mg/kg PO once daily for 5 days for infants younger than 6 mo; 10 mg/kg (max 500 mg) PO single dose on day 1, then 5 mg/kg (up to 250 mg) PO once daily for 4 days for age 6 mo or older. See table for bacterial endocarditis prophylaxis. Traveler's diarrhea: 5 to 10 mg/kg PO single dose. Cholera: 20 mg/kg up to 1 g PO single dose.

FORMS — Generic/Trade: Tabs 250, 500, 600 mg. Susp 100, 200 mg/5 mL. Packet 1000 mg. Z-Pak: #6, 250 mg tab. Tri-Pak: #3, 500 mg tab. Trade only: Extended-release oral susp (Zmax): 2 g in 60 mL single-dose bottle.

NOTES — Severe allergic/skin reactions rarely, IV site reactions, hearing loss with prolonged use, hepatotoxicity, exacerbation of myasthenia gravis. Can prolong QT interval and cause torsades. Consider risk vs benefit in at-risk patients: those with history of QT interval prolongation or torsades, uncompensated heart failure, ongoing proarrhythmic conditions such as uncorrected hypokalemia or hypomagnesemia, clinically significant bradycardia, or coadministration of Class IA or III antiarrhythmic drug. Azithromycin had additive dose-dependent QT interval prolongation with chloroquine. Does not inhibit CYP enzymes. Do not take at the same time as Al/Mg antacids (except Zmax which can be taken with antacids). Monitor INR with warfarin. Zmax: Store at room temperature and use within 12 h of reconstitution. Additional treatment required if vomiting occurs within 5 min of dose; consider for vomiting within 1 h of dose; unnecessary for vomiting more than 1 h after dose.

MOA — Inhibits protein synthesis in susceptible organisms by interfering with function of ribosomal 50s subunit. Mechanism of action in cystic fibrosis is unknown; macrolides may inhibit P. aeruginosa virulence factors or reduce inflammation.

ADVERSE EFFECTS — Serious: Allergic/skin reactions (rare), IV site reactions, hearing loss with prolonged use, hepatotoxicity, exacerbation of myasthenia gravis. Frequent: GI complaints, diarrhea, N/V most common with single-dose and 3-day regimens.

CLARITHROMYCIN (Biaxin, Biaxin XL) ▶KL ♀C ▶? $$$

ADULT — Group A streptococcal pharyngitis (2nd line to penicillin): 250 mg PO two times per day for 10 days. Acute exacerbation of chronic bronchitis (S. pneumoniae/M. catarrhalis), community-acquired pneumonia, skin infections: 250 mg PO two times per day for 7 to 14 days. Acute exacerbation of chronic bronchitis (H. influenzae): 500 mg PO two times per day for 7 to 14 days. H. pylori: See table in GI section. Mycobacterium avium complex disease prevention/treatment: 500 mg PO two times per day. Treat active mycobacterial infections with at least 2 drugs. Acute sinusitis: 500 mg PO two times per day for 14 days. Clarithromycin is a poor option for acute sinusitis due to pneumococcal and H. influenzae resistance; see acute sinusitis treatment table for alternatives. Biaxin XL: Acute sinusitis: 1000 mg PO daily for 14 days. Acute exacerbation of chronic bronchitis, community-acquired pneumonia: 1000 mg PO daily for 7 days. Take Biaxin XL with food.

PEDS — Group A streptococcal pharyngitis (2nd line to penicillin), community-acquired pneumonia, sinusitis, otitis media, skin infections: 7.5 mg/kg PO two times per day for 10 days. Clarithromycin is a poor option for acute sinusitis and otitis media due to pneumococcal and H. influenzae resistance;

(cont.)

CLARITHROMYCIN (*cont.*)

see acute sinusitis and otitis media treatment tables for alternatives. Mycobacterium avium complex prevention/treatment: 7.5 mg/kg up to 500 mg PO two times per day. Two or more drugs are needed for the treatment of active mycobacterial infections. UNAPPROVED ADULT — Pertussis treatment/postexposure prophylaxis: 500 mg PO two times per day for 7 days. Community-acquired pneumonia: 500 mg PO two times per day. See table for prophylaxis of bacterial endocarditis. UNAPPROVED PEDS — Pertussis treatment/postexposure prophylaxis (age 1 mo or older): 7.5 mg/kg (up to 500 mg) PO two times per day for 7 days. See table for prophylaxis of bacterial endocarditis. FORMS — Generic/Trade: Tabs 250, 500 mg. Extended-release tab 500 mg. Susp 125, 250 mg/5 mL. Trade only: Biaxin XL-Pak: #14, 500 mg tabs. NOTES — Can cause or exacerbate myasthenia gravis. Can prolong QT interval and cause torsades. Avoid in patients with history of QT prolongation or ventricular arrhythmia, ongoing proarrhythmic conditions such as uncorrected hypokalemia or hypomagnesemia, clinically significant bradycardia, or coadministration of Class IA or Class III antiarrhythmic drugs. Strong CYP3A4 inhibitor. Many drug interactions including increased levels of carbamazepine, cyclosporine, digoxin, disopyramide (monitor ECG), lovastatin (avoid), quinidine (monitor ECG), rifabutin, simvastatin (avoid), tacrolimus, theophylline. Toxicity with ergotamine, dihydroergotamine, or colchicine (reduce colchicine dose; contraindicated if renal/hepatic impairment). Reduce dose of sildenafil, tadalafil, tolterodine, vardenafil. Monitor INR with warfarin. Clarithromycin levels decreased by efavirenz (avoid concomitant use) and nevirapine enough to impair efficacy in Mycobacterium avium complex disease. Reduce clarithromycin dose by 50% if given with atazanavir; consider alternative for indications other than Mycobacterium avium complex. Dosage reduction for renal insufficiency in patients taking ritonavir, lopinavir/ritonavir (Kaletra), or ritonavir-boosted darunavir, fosamprenavir, saquinavir, or tipranavir: decrease dose by 75% for CrCl < 30 mL/min, decrease dose by 50% for CrCl 30 to 60 mL/min. Do not refrigerate susp. MOA — Inhibits protein synthesis in susceptible organisms by interfering with function of ribosomal 50s subunit. ADVERSE EFFECTS — Serious: Myasthenia gravis. Rare arrhythmias in patients with prolonged QT. Increased mortality reported 1 year after 2-week course of clarithromycin for prevention of cardiovascular mortality in patients with stable CHD. Frequent: Diarrhea, metallic taste.

ERYTHROMYCIN BASE (*Ery-Tab, P.C.E., ✝Eryc*) ▶L ♀B ▶+ $$$$

ADULT — Respiratory, skin infections: 250 to 500 mg PO four times per day or 333 mg PO three times per day. Pertussis, treatment/postexposure prophylaxis: 500 mg PO q 6 h for 14 days. S. aureus skin infections: 250 mg PO q 6 h or 500 mg PO q 12 h. Secondary prevention of rheumatic fever: 250 mg PO two times per day. Chlamydia in pregnancy, nongonococcal urethritis: 500 mg PO four times per day for 7 days. Alternative for chlamydia in pregnancy if high dose not tolerated: 250 mg PO four times per day for 14 days. Erythrasma: 250 mg PO three times per day for 21 days. Legionnaires' disease: 2 g/day PO in divided doses for 14 to 21 days. PEDS — Usual dose: 30 to 50 mg/kg/day PO divided four times per day for 10 days. Can double dose for severe infections. Pertussis: 40 to 50 mg/kg/day PO divided four times per day for 14 days (azithromycin preferred for age younger than 1 mo due to risk of hypertrophic pyloric stenosis with erythromycin). Chlamydia: 50 mg/kg/day PO divided four times per day for 14 days for wt less than 45 kg. UNAPPROVED ADULT — Chancroid: 500 mg PO three times per day for 7 days. Campylobacter gastroenteritis: 500 mg PO two times per day for 5 days. FORMS — Generic only: Tabs 250, 500 mg. Delayed-release cap 250 mg. Trade only: Delayed-release tab (Ery-Tab, PCE) 250, 333, 500 mg. NOTES — Can prolong QT interval and cause torsades. Avoid if QT interval prolonged, uncorrected hypokalemia or hypomagnesemia, clinically significant bradycardia, or coadministration of Class IA or III antiarrhythmic drug. Incidence of sudden death may be increased when erythromycin is combined with potent CYP3A4 inhibitors. Exacerbation of myasthenia gravis. Hypertrophic pyloric stenosis in infants primarily younger than 1 mo. CYP3A4 and 1A2 inhibitor. Many drug interactions including increased levels of carbamazepine, cyclosporine, digoxin, tacrolimus, theophylline, some benzodiazepines and statins (avoid simvastatin and lovastatin). Monitor INR with warfarin. MOA — Inhibits protein synthesis in susceptible organisms by interfering with function of ribosomal 50s subunit. ADVERSE EFFECTS — Serious: Arrhythmias in patients with prolonged QT (rare), aggravation of myasthenia gravis, hypertrophic pyloric stenosis in infants primarily younger than 1 month old. Incidence of sudden death may be increased when erythromycin is combined with potent CYP 3A4 inhibitors. Frequent: N/V, diarrhea.

ERYTHROMYCIN ETHYL SUCCINATE (*EES, EryPed*) ▶L ♀B ▶+ $

ADULT — Usual dose: 400 mg PO four times per day. Nongonococcal urethritis: 800 mg PO four times per day for 7 days. Chlamydia in pregnancy: 800 mg PO four times per day for 7 days or 400 mg PO four times per day for 14 days if high dose not tolerated. Secondary prevention of rheumatic fever: 400 mg PO two times per day. Legionnaires' disease: 3.2 g/day PO in divided doses for 14 to 21 days. PEDS — Usual dose: 30 to 50 mg/kg/day PO divided four times per day. Maximum dose: 100 mg/kg/day. Group A streptococcal pharyngitis: 40 mg/kg/day (up to 1 g/day) PO divided two to four times per

ERYTHROMYCIN ETHYL SUCCINATE (*cont.*)
day for 10 days. Secondary prevention of rheumatic fever: 400 mg PO two times per day. Pertussis: 40 to 50 mg/kg/day (up to 2 g/day) PO divided four times per day for 14 days.
FORMS — Generic/Trade: Tabs 400. Trade Only: Susp 200, 400 mg/5 mL.
NOTES — Can prolong QT interval and cause torsades. Avoid if QT interval prolonged, uncorrected hypokalemia or hypomagnesemia, clinically significant bradycardia, or coadministration of Class IA or III antiarrhythmic drug. Incidence of sudden death may be increased when erythromycin is combined with potent CYP3A4 inhibitors. May aggravate myasthenia gravis. Hypertrophic pyloric stenosis primarily in infants younger than 1 mo. CYP3A4 and 1A2 inhibitor. Many drug interactions including increased levels of carbamazepine, cyclosporine, digoxin, tacrolimus, theophylline, some benzodiazepines and statins (avoid simvastatin and lovastatin). Monitor INR with warfarin.
MOA — Inhibits protein synthesis in susceptible organisms by interfering with function of ribosomal 50s subunit.
ADVERSE EFFECTS — Serious: Arrhythmias in patients with prolonged QT (rare), aggravation of myasthenia gravis, hypertrophic pyloric stenosis primarily in infants younger than 1 month old. Coadministration of strong CYP 3A4 inhibitor with erythromycin may increase risk of sudden death. Frequent: N/V, diarrhea.

ERYTHROMYCIN LACTOBIONATE (*Erythrocin IV*) ▶L ♀B ▶+ $$$$$
ADULT — For severe infections/PO not possible: 15 to 20 mg/kg/day (up to 4 g/day) IV divided q 6 h. Legionnaires' disease: 4 g/day IV divided q 6 h.
PEDS — For severe infections/PO not possible: 15 to 20 mg/kg/day (up to 4 g/day) IV divided q 6 h.
UNAPPROVED PEDS — 20 to 50 mg/kg/day IV divided q 6 h.
NOTES — Dilute and give slowly to minimize venous irritation. Reversible hearing loss (increased risk in elderly given 4 g or more per day), allergic reactions, exacerbation of myasthenia gravis. Can prolong QT interval and cause torsades. Avoid if QT interval prolonged, uncorrected hypokalemia or hypomagnesemia, clinically significant bradycardia, or coadministration of Class IA or III antiarrhythmic drug. Incidence of sudden death may be increased when erythromycin is combined with potent CYP3A4 inhibitors. Hypertrophic pyloric stenosis primarily in infants younger than 1 mo. CYP3A4 and 1A2 inhibitor. Many drug interactions including increased levels of carbamazepine, cyclosporine, digoxin, disopyramide, tacrolimus, theophylline, some benzodiazepines and statins (avoid simvastatin and lovastatin). Monitor INR with warfarin.
MOA — Inhibits protein synthesis in susceptible organisms by interfering with function of ribosomal 50s subunit.
ADVERSE EFFECTS — Serious: Arrhythmias in patients with prolonged QT (rare), aggravation of myasthenia gravis, hypertrophic pyloric stenosis primarily in infants younger than 1 month old, reversible hearing loss with high doses (increased risk in elderly given 4 g/day or more), allergic reactions, venous irritation. Incidence of sudden death may be increased when erythromycin is combined with potent CYP3A4 inhibitors. Frequent: N/V, diarrhea.

FIDAXOMICIN (*Dificid*) ▶minimal absorption ♀B ▶? $$$$$
ADULT — C. difficile–associated diarrhea: 200 mg PO two times per day for 10 days.
PEDS — Safety and efficacy not established in children.
FORMS — Trade only: 200 mg tabs.
NOTES — Not for systemic infections. Only treats C. difficile–associated diarrhea.
MOA — Poorly absorbed macrolide that inhibits RNA synthesis by RNA polymerases. Bacteriocidal against C difficile.
ADVERSE EFFECTS — Serious: GI bleeding; acute hypersensitivity reactions (possible cross-reactivity with other macrolides). Frequent: N/V, abdominal pain.

ANTIMICROBIALS: Penicillins—1st Generation—Natural

PENICILLINS: GENERAL ANTIMICROBIAL SPECTRUM

1st generation	Most streptococci; oral anaerobic coverage
2nd generation	Most streptococci; *S. aureus* (but not MRSA)
3rd generation	Most streptococci; basic Gram-negative coverage
4th generation	*Pseudomonas*

NOTE: Anaphylaxis occurs rarely with penicillins; cross-sensitivity with cephalosporins is possible.

BENZATHINE PENICILLIN (*Bicillin L-A*) ▶K ♀B ▶? $$$
WARNING — Not for IV administration, which can cause cardiorespiratory arrest and death.
ADULT — Group A streptococcal pharyngitis: 1.2 million units IM single dose. Secondary prevention of rheumatic fever: 1.2 million units IM q month (q

(cont.)

BENZATHINE PENICILLIN (*cont.*)

3 weeks for high-risk patients) or 600,000 units IM q 2 weeks. Primary, secondary, early latent syphilis: 2.4 million units IM single dose. Tertiary, late latent syphilis: 2.4 million units IM q week for 3 doses.

PEDS — Group A streptococcal pharyngitis (AHA regimen): 600,000 units IM for wt 27 kg or less; 1.2 million units IM for wt greater than 27 kg. Secondary prevention of rheumatic fever: 600,000 units IM for wt 27 kg or less; 1.2 million units IM for wt greater than 27 kg; give q month (q 3 weeks for high-risk patients). Primary, secondary, early latent syphilis: 50,000 units/kg (up to 2.4 million units) IM single dose. Late latent syphilis: 50,000 units/kg (up to 2.4 million units) IM for 3 weekly doses.

UNAPPROVED ADULT — Prophylaxis of diphtheria/ treatment of carriers: 1.2 million units IM single dose.

UNAPPROVED PEDS — Prophylaxis of diphtheria/ treatment of carriers: 1.2 million units IM single dose for wt 30 kg or greater; 600,000 units IM single dose for wt less than 30 kg.

FORMS — Trade only: For IM use, 600,000 units/mL; 1, 2, 4 mL syringes.

NOTES — Do not give IV. Doses last 2 to 4 weeks. Not for neurosyphilis. IM injection less painful if warmed to room temp before giving.

MOA — Beta-lactam antibiotic that inhibits the biosynthesis of cell wall mucopeptide.

ADVERSE EFFECTS — Serious: Anaphylaxis (rare), cross-sensitivity with cephalosporins, transient CNS reactions (Hoigne's syndrome), Coombs + hemolytic anemia. Frequent: Allergy.

BICILLIN C-R (procaine penicillin + benzathine penicillin) ▶K ♀B ▐? $$$$

WARNING — Not for IV administration, which can cause cardiorespiratory arrest and death.

ADULT — Scarlet fever, erysipelas, upper-respiratory, skin, and soft-tissue infections due to group A strep: 2.4 million units IM single dose. Pneumococcal infections other than meningitis: 1.2 million units IM q 2 to 3 days until temperature normal for 48 h. Not for treatment of syphilis.

PEDS — Scarlet fever, erysipelas, upper-respiratory, skin, and soft-tissue infections due to group A strep: 600,000 units IM for wt less than 13.6 kg; 900,000 to 1.2 million units IM for wt 13.6 to 27 kg; 2.4 million units IM for wt greater than 27 kg. Pneumococcal infections other than meningitis: 600,000 units IM q 2 to 3 days until temperature normal for 48 h. Not for treatment of syphilis.

FORMS — Trade only: For IM use 300/300 and 450/150 (Peds) thousand units/mL procaine/ benzathine penicillin (600,000 units/mL); 2 mL syringe.

NOTES — Contraindicated if allergic to procaine. Do not give IV. Do not substitute Bicillin CR for Bicillin LA in treatment of syphilis.

MOA — Beta-lactam antibiotic that inhibits the biosynthesis of cell wall mucopeptide.

ADVERSE EFFECTS — Serious: Anaphylaxis (rare), cross-sensitivity with cephalosporins, Coombs + hemolytic anemia. Frequent: Allergy.

PENICILLIN G ▶K ♀B ▐? $$$$

ADULT — Penicillin-sensitive pneumococcal pneumonia: 8 to 12 million units/day IV divided q 4 to 6 h. Penicillin-sensitive pneumococcal meningitis: 24 million units/day IV divided q 2 to 4 h. Empiric therapy, native valve endocarditis: 20 million units/day IV continuous infusion or divided q 4 h plus nafcillin/oxacillin and gentamicin. Neurosyphilis: 18 to 24 million units/day continuous IV infusion or 3 to 4 million units IV q 4 h for 10 to 14 days. Bioterrorism anthrax: See www.bt.cdc.gov/bioterrorism/.

PEDS — Mild to moderate infections: 25,000 to 50,000 units/kg/day IV divided q 6 h. Severe infections including pneumococcal and meningococcal meningitis: 250,000 to 400,000 units/kg/day IV divided q 4 to 6 h. Neonates age younger than 1 week and wt greater than 2 kg: 25,000 to 50,000 units/kg IV q 8 h. Neonates age 1 week or older and wt greater than 2 kg: 25,000 to 50,000 units/kg IV q 6 h. Group B streptococcal meningitis: 250,000 to 450,000 units/kg/day IV divided q 8 h for age 1 week or younger; 450,000 to 500,000 units/kg/ day IV divided q 4 to 6 h for age older than 1 week. Congenital syphilis: 50,000 units/kg/dose IV q 12 h during first 7 days of life, then q 8 h thereafter to complete 10 days. Congenital syphilis or neurosyphilis: 50,000 units/kg IV q 4 to 6 h for 10 days for age older than 1 mo.

UNAPPROVED ADULT — Prevention of perinatal group B streptococcal disease: Give to mother 5 million units IV at onset of labor/after membrane rupture, then 2.5 to 3 million units IV q 4 h until delivery. Diphtheria: 100,000 to 150,000 units/kg/day IV divided q 6 h for 14 days.

UNAPPROVED PEDS — Diphtheria: 100,000 to 150,000 units/kg/day IV divided q 6 h for 14 days.

NOTES — Reduce dose in renal dysfunction.

MOA — Beta-lactam antibiotic that inhibits the biosynthesis of cell wall mucopeptide.

ADVERSE EFFECTS — Serious: Anaphylaxis (rare); cross-sensitivity with cephalosporins; hematologic and renal toxicity, and seizures with doses greater than 20 million units/day; Coombs + hemolytic anemia. Frequent: Allergy.

PENICILLIN V ▶K ♀B ▐? $

ADULT — Usual dose: 250 to 500 mg PO four times per day. AHA dosing for group A streptococcal pharyngitis: 500 mg PO two to three times per day for 10 days. Secondary prevention of rheumatic fever: 250 mg PO two times per day. Vincent's infection: 250 mg PO q 6 to 8 h.

PEDS — Usual dose: 25 to 50 mg/kg/day PO divided three to four times per day. Use adult dose for age 12 yo or older. AHA dosing for group

PENICILLIN V (cont.)

A streptococcal pharyngitis: 250 mg (for wt 27 kg or less) or 500 mg (wt greater than 27 kg) PO two or three times per day for 10 days. Secondary prevention of rheumatic fever: 250 mg PO two times per day.

UNAPPROVED PEDS — Prevention of pneumococcal infections in functional/anatomic asplenia: 125 mg PO two times per day for age younger than 3 yo; 250 mg PO two times per day for age 3 yo or older.

FORMS — Generic only: Tabs 250, 500 mg. Oral soln 125, 250 mg/5 mL.

NOTES — Oral soln stable in refrigerator for 14 days.

MOA — Beta-lactam antibiotic that inhibits the biosynthesis of cell wall mucopeptide.

ADVERSE EFFECTS — Serious: Anaphylaxis (rare), cross-sensitivity with cephalosporins, Coombs + hemolytic anemia. Frequent: Allergy.

PROCAINE PENICILLIN ►K ♀B ▶? $$$$$

ADULT — Pneumococcal and streptococcal infections, Vincent's infection, erysipeloid: 0.6 to 1 million units IM daily. Neurosyphilis: 2.4 million units IM daily plus probenecid 500 mg PO q 6 h, both for 10 to 14 days.

PEDS — Pneumococcal and streptococcal infections, Vincent's infection, erysipeloid, for wt less than 27 kg: 300,000 units IM daily. AAP dose for mild to moderate infections, age older than 1 mo: 25,000 to 50,000 units/kg/day IM divided one to two times per day. Congenital syphilis: 50,000 units/kg IM once daily for 10 days.

FORMS — Generic: For IM use, 600,000 units/mL; 1, 2 mL syringes.

NOTES — Peak 4 h, lasts 24 h. Contraindicated if procaine allergy; skin test if allergy suspected. Transient CNS reactions with high doses.

MOA — Beta-lactam antibiotic that inhibits the biosynthesis of cell wall mucopeptide.

ADVERSE EFFECTS — Serious: Anaphylaxis (rare), cross-sensitivity with cephalosporins, transient CNS reactions (Hoigne's syndrome), Coombs + hemolytic anemia. Frequent: Allergy.

ANTIMICROBIALS: Penicillins—2nd Generation—Penicillinase-Resistant

NOTE: Anaphylaxis occurs rarely with penicillins; cross-sensitivity with cephalosporins is possible.

DICLOXACILLIN ►KL ♀B ▶? $$

ADULT — Usual dose: 250 to 500 mg PO four times per day. Take on empty stomach.

PEDS — Mild to moderate upper respiratory, skin and soft-tissue infections: 12.5 mg/kg/day PO divided four times per day for age older than 1 mo. Pneumonia, disseminated infections: 25 mg/kg/day PO divided four times per day for age older than 1 mo. Follow-up therapy after IV antibiotics for staph osteomyelitis: 50 to 100 mg/kg/day PO divided four times per day. Use adult dose for wt 40 kg or greater. Give on empty stomach.

FORMS — Generic only: Caps 250, 500 mg.

MOA — Beta-lactam antibiotic that inhibits the biosynthesis of cell wall mucopeptide. Penicillinase-resistant penicillins are resistant to hydrolysis by the beta-lactamase, penicillinase.

ADVERSE EFFECTS — Serious: Anaphylaxis (rare), cross-sensitivity with cephalosporins.

NAFCILLIN ►L ♀B ▶? $$$$$

ADULT — Staph infections, usual dose: 500 mg IM q 4 to 6 h or 500 to 2000 mg IV q 4 h. Osteomyelitis: 1 to 2 g IV q 4 h. Empiric therapy, native valve endocarditis: 2 g IV q 4 h plus penicillin/ampicillin and gentamicin.

PEDS — Staph infections, usual dose: 25 mg/kg IM two times per day for pediatric patients who weigh less than 40 kg; give 10 mg/kg for neonates.

UNAPPROVED PEDS — Mild to moderate infections: 50 to 100 mg/kg/day IM/IV divided q 6 h. Severe infections: 100 to 200 mg/kg/day IM/IV divided q 4 to 6 h. Neonates, wt greater than 2 kg: 25 mg/kg IM/ IV q 8 h for age younger than 1 week old; 25 to 35 mg/kg IM/IV q 6 h for age 1 week or older.

NOTES — Reversible neutropenia with prolonged use. Decreased INR with warfarin. Decreased cyclosporine levels.

MOA — Beta-lactam antibiotic that inhibits the biosynthesis of cell wall mucopeptide. Penicillinase-resistant penicillins are resistant to hydrolysis by the beta-lactamase, penicillinase.

ADVERSE EFFECTS — Serious: Anaphylaxis (rare), cross-sensitivity with cephalosporins, extravasation, hypokalemia with dose of 200 mg/kg/ day or greater. Frequent: Reversible neutropenia with duration of therapy longer than 21 days, eosinophilia.

OXACILLIN ►KL ♀B ▶? $$$$$

ADULT — Staph infections: 250 mg to 2 g IM/IV q 4 to 6 h. Osteomyelitis: 1.5 to 2 g IV q 4 h. Empiric therapy, native valve endocarditis: 2 g IV q 4 h with penicillin/ampicillin and gentamicin.

PEDS — Mild to moderate infections: 100 to 150 mg/ kg/day IM/IV divided q 6 h. Severe infections: 150 to 200 mg/kg/day IM/IV divided q 4 to 6 h. Use adult dose for wt 40 kg or greater. Newborns, wt greater than 2 kg: 25 to 50 mg/kg IV q 8 h for age younger than 1 week old, increasing to q 6 h for age 1 week or older.

NOTES — Hepatic dysfunction possible with doses greater than 12 g/day; monitor LFTs.

MOA — Beta-lactam antibiotic that inhibits the biosynthesis of cell wall mucopeptide. Penicillinase-resistant penicillins are resistant to hydrolysis by the beta-lactamase, penicillinase.

ADVERSE EFFECTS — Serious: Anaphylaxis (rare), cross-sensitivity with cephalosporins, hepatic dysfunction possible with doses greater then 12 g/day. Frequent: Eosinophilia.

ANTIMICROBIALS: Penicillins—3rd Generation—Aminopenicillins

NOTE: Anaphylaxis occurs rarely with penicillins; cross-sensitivity with cephalosporins is possible. –associated diarrhea. High risk of rash in patients with mononucleosis or taking allopurinol.

AMOXICILLIN (*Moxatag*) ▶K ♀B ▶+ $
ADULT — ENT, skin, genitourinary infections: 250 to 500 mg PO three times per day or 500 to 875 mg PO two times per day. See table for management of acute sinusitis. Pneumonia: 500 mg PO three times per day or 875 mg PO two times per day. AHA dosing for group A streptococcal pharyngitis: 50 mg/kg (max 1 g) PO once daily for 10 days. Group A streptococcal pharyngitis/tonsillitis, for age 12 yo or older: 775 mg ER tab (Moxatag) PO once daily for 10 days. Do not chew/crush Moxatag tabs. H. pylori: See table in GI section. See table for prophylaxis of bacterial endocarditis.
PEDS — ENT, skin, GU infections: 20 to 40 mg/kg/day PO divided three times per day or 25 to 45 mg/kg/day PO divided two times per day. See tables for management of acute sinusitis and otitis media. Pneumonia: 40 mg/kg/day PO divided three times per day or 45 mg/kg/day PO divided two times per day. Infants, age younger than 3 mo: 30 mg/kg/day PO divided q 12 h. AHA dosing for group A streptococcal pharyngitis: 50 mg/kg (max 1 g) PO once daily for 10 days. Group A streptococcal pharyngitis/tonsillitis, for age 12 yo or older: 775 mg ER tab (Moxatag) PO once daily for 10 days. Do not chew/crush Moxatag tabs. See table for prophylaxis of bacterial endocarditis.
UNAPPROVED ADULT — High-dose for community-acquired pneumonia: 1 g PO three times per day. Lyme disease: 500 mg PO three times per day for 14 days for early disease, for 28 days for Lyme arthritis. Chlamydia in pregnancy: 500 mg PO three times per day for 7 days. Bioterrorism anthrax: See www.bt.cdc.gov/bioterrorism/.
UNAPPROVED PEDS — AAP otitis media: 80-90 mg/kg/day PO divided two times per day. Give 5 to 7 days of therapy for age 6 yo and older with mild to moderate symptoms, 7 days for age 2 to 5 yo with mild to moderate symptoms, and 10 days for age younger than 2 yo and children with severe symptoms. See table for treatment of otitis media in children. Community-acquired pneumonia: 80 to 100 mg/kg/day PO divided three to four times per day for age 4 mo to 4 yo. Lyme disease: 50 mg/kg/day (up to 1500 mg/day) PO divided three times per day for 14 days for early disease, for 28 days for Lyme arthritis. Bioterrorism anthrax: See www.bt.cdc.gov/bioterrorism/.
FORMS — Generic only: Caps 250, 500 mg. Tabs 500, 875 mg. Chewable tabs 125, 200, 250, 400 mg. Susp 125, 250 mg/5 mL. Susp 200, 400 mg/5 mL. Trade only: Extended-release tab (Moxatag) 775 mg.
NOTES — Reduce dose in adults with renal dysfunction: Give 250 to 500 mg PO daily for CrCl less than 10 mL/min or hemodialysis; 250 to 500 mg PO two times per day for CrCl 10 to 30 mL/min. Do not use 875 mg tab for CrCl less than 30 mL/min.

Give additional dose during and at end of dialysis. Oral susp and infant gtts stable for 14 days at room temperature or in the refrigerator.
MOA — Beta-lactam antibiotic that inhibits the biosynthesis of cell wall mucopeptide. Aminopenicillins are more active than natural penicillins against gram-negative cocci and Enterobacteriaceae.
ADVERSE EFFECTS — Serious: Anaphylaxis (rare), cross-sensitivity with cephalosporins. Frequent: Rash (nonallergic in patients with mononucleosis, chronic myelogenous leukemia, or allopurinol therapy), diarrhea.

AMPICILLIN ▶K ♀B ▶? $ PO $$$$$ IV
ADULT — Usual dose: 1 to 2 g IV q 4 to 6 h or 250 to 500 mg PO four times per day. Sepsis, meningitis: 150 to 200 mg/kg/day IV divided q 3 to 4 h. Empiric therapy, native valve endocarditis: 12 g/day IV continuous infusion or divided q 4 h plus nafcillin/oxacillin and gentamicin. See table for prophylaxis of bacterial endocarditis. Take oral ampicillin on an empty stomach.
PEDS — AAP recommendations: Mild to moderate infections: 100 to 150 mg/kg/day IM/IV divided q 6 h or 50 to 100 mg/kg/day PO divided four times per day. Severe infections: 200 to 400 mg/kg/day IM/IV divided q 6 h. Newborns, wt greater than 2 kg: 25 to 50 mg/kg IV given q 8 h for age younger than 1 week old, increase to q 6 h for age 1 week or older. Use adult doses for wt 40 kg or greater. Give oral ampicillin on an empty stomach. Group B streptococcal meningitis: 200 to 300 mg/kg/day IV divided q 8 h for age 7 days or younger; 300 mg/kg/day divided q 6 h for age older than 7 days. Give with gentamicin initially. See table for prophylaxis of bacterial endocarditis.
UNAPPROVED ADULT — Prevention of neonatal group B streptococcal disease: Give to mother 2 g IV at onset of labor/after membrane rupture, then 1 g IV q 4 h until delivery.
FORMS — Generic only: Caps 250, 500 mg. Susp 125, 250 mg/5 mL.
NOTES — Susp stable for 7 days at room temperature, 14 days in the refrigerator. Reduce dosing interval to q 12 to 24 h for CrCl less than 10 mL/min. Give dose after hemodialysis.
MOA — Beta-lactam antibiotic that inhibits the biosynthesis of cell wall mucopeptide. Aminopenicillins are more active than natural penicillins against gram-negative cocci and Enterobacteriaceae.
ADVERSE EFFECTS — Serious: Anaphylaxis (rare), cross-sensitivity with cephalosporins, C. difficile-associated diarrhea. Frequent: Nonallergic rash in patients with mononucleosis, chronic myelogenous leukemia, or allopurinol therapy; eosinophilia; diarrhea (especially with PO).

AMPICILLIN-SULBACTAM ►K ♀B ▶? $$$

ADULT — Skin, intra-abdominal, gynecologic infections: 1.5 to 3 g IM/IV q 6 h.

PEDS — Skin infections, for age 1 yo or older: 300 mg/kg/day IV divided q 6 h. Use adult dose for wt greater than 40 kg.

UNAPPROVED ADULT — Community-acquired pneumonia: 1.5 to 3 g IM/IV q 6 h with a macrolide or doxycycline.

UNAPPROVED PEDS — AAP regimens. Mild to moderate infections: 100 to 150 mg/kg/day of ampicillin IM/IV divided q 6 h. Severe infections: 200 to 400 mg/kg/day of ampicillin IM/IV divided q 6 h.

NOTES — Dosing for adults with renal impairment: Give usual dose q 24 h for CrCl 5 to 14 mL/min, q 12 h for CrCl 15 to 29 mL/min, q 6 to 8 h for adults with CrCl 30 mL/min or greater.

MOA — Beta-lactam antibiotic that inhibits the biosynthesis of cell wall mucopeptide. Aminopenicillins are more active than natural penicillins against gram-negative cocci and Enterobacteriaceae. Sulbactam is beta-lactamase inhibitor.

ADVERSE EFFECTS — Serious: Anaphylaxis (rare), cross-sensitivity with cephalosporins, C. difficile-associated diarrhea. Frequent: Rash (nonallergic in patients with mononucleosis, chronic myelogenous leukemia, or allopurinol therapy), eosinophilia, increased LFTs.

AUGMENTIN, AUGMENTIN ES-600, AUGMENTIN XR (amoxicillin-clavulanate, ★Clavulin) ►K ♀B ▶? $$$

ADULT — Pneumonia, otitis media, sinusitis, skin infections, UTIs: Usual dose 500 mg PO two times per day or 250 mg PO three times per day. More severe infections: 875 mg PO two times per day or 500 mg PO three times per day. Augmentin XR: 2 tabs PO q 12 h with meals for 10 days for acute sinusitis, give 7 to 10 days for community-acquired pneumonia. See table for management of acute sinusitis.

PEDS — 200, 400 mg chewables and 200, 400 mg/5 mL susp for two times per day administration. Pneumonia, otitis media, sinusitis: 45 mg/kg/day PO divided two times per day. Less severe infections such as skin, UTIs: 25 mg/kg/day PO divided two times per day. 125, 250 mg chewables and 125, 250 mg/ 5 mL susp for three times per day administration. Pneumonia, otitis media, sinusitis: 40 mg/kg/day PO divided three times per day. Less severe infections such as skin, UTIs: 20 mg/kg/day PO divided three times per day. Use 125 mg/5 mL susp and give 30 mg/kg PO q 12 hr for age younger than 3 mo. Give adult dose for wt 40 kg or greater. Augmentin ES-600 susp for age

3 mo or older and wt less than 40 kg. Recurrent/persistent otitis media with risk factors (antibiotics for otitis media in past 3 months and either in daycare or age 2 yo or younger): give 90 mg/kg/day PO divided two times per day with food for 10 days. See tables for management of acute sinusitis and otitis media.

UNAPPROVED ADULT — Treatment of infected dog/cat bite: 875 mg PO two times per day or 500 mg PO three times per day, duration of treatment based on response. See table for management of acute sinusitis.

UNAPPROVED PEDS — See tables for management of acute sinusitis and otitis media. IDSA recommends for community-acquired pneumonia, age older than 3 mo: 90 mg/kg/day PO divided two times per day (max dose of 2 g PO two times per day for age 5 yo and older). Treat for up to 10 days. AAP recommends for acute otitis media: 90 mg/kg/day PO divided two times per day. Give 5 to 7 days of therapy for children 6 yo and older with mild to moderate symptoms, 7 days for children 2 to 5 yo with mild to moderate symptoms, and 10 days for children younger than 2 yo and those with severe symptoms.

FORMS — Generic/Trade: (amoxicillin/clavulanate) Tabs 250/125, 500/125, 875/125 mg. Chewables, Susp 200/28.5, 400/57 mg per tab or 5 mL, 250/62.5 mg per 5 mL. (ES) Susp 600/42.9 mg per 5 mL. Extended-release tabs 1000/62.5 mg. Trade only: Susp 125/31.25 per 5 mL, 250/62.5 mg per 5 mL.

NOTES — Diarrhea common (less with twice daily dosing). Do not interchange Augmentin products with different clavulanate content. Do not use 250 mg amoxicillin + 125 mg clavulanate tab in children with wt less than 40 kg. Suspensions stable in refrigerator for 10 days. See prescribing information for dosage reduction of Augmentin tabs if CrCl < 30 mL/min. Augmentin XR contraindicated if CrCl < 30 mL/min.

MOA — Beta-lactam antibiotic that inhibits the biosynthesis of cell wall mucopeptide. Aminopenicillins are more active than natural penicillins against gram-negative cocci and Enterobacteriaceae. Clavulanate is beta-lactamase inhibitor.

ADVERSE EFFECTS — Serious: Anaphylaxis (rare), cross-sensitivity with cephalosporins, clavulanate-induced cholestatic hepatitis (esp. in elderly men treated for more than 2 weeks). Frequent: Diarrhea (less with bid dosing, incidence related to clavulanate dose), rash (nonallergic in patients with mononucleosis, chronic myelogenous leukemia, or allopurinol therapy).

ANTIMICROBIALS: Penicillins—4th Generation—Extended Spectrum

NOTE: Anaphylaxis occurs rarely with penicillins; cross-sensitivity with cephalosporins is possible. Hypokalemia; bleeding and coagulation abnormalities possible especially with renal impairment.

PIPERACILLIN-TAZOBACTAM (Zosyn, ★Tazocin) ►K ♀B ▶? $$$$$

ADULT — Appendicitis, peritonitis, skin infections, postpartum endometritis, pelvic inflammatory

disease, moderate community-acquired pneumonia: 3.375 g IV q 6 h. Nosocomial pneumonia: 4.5 g IV q 6 h (with aminoglycoside initially and if P aeruginosa is cultured).

(cont.)

PIPERACILLIN-TAZOBACTAM (*cont.*)

PEDS — Appendicitis/peritonitis: 80 mg/kg of piper-acillin IV q 8 h for age 2 to 9 mo; 100 mg/kg of piperacillin IV q 8 h for age older than 9 mo; use adult dose for wt greater than 40 kg.

UNAPPROVED ADULT — Serious infections: 4.5 g IV q 6 h.

UNAPPROVED PEDS — 150 to 300 mg/kg/day of piperacillin IV divided q 6 to 8 h for age younger than 6 mo, 300 to 400 mg/kg/day piperacillin IV divided q 6 to 8 h for age 6 mo or older.

NOTES — May prolong neuromuscular blockade with nondepolarizing muscle relaxants. False-positive result possible with Bio-Rad Laboratories Platelia Aspergillus EIA test. May reduce renal excretion of methotrexate; monitor methotrexate levels and toxicity. Reduce dosing in adults with renal impairment: 2.25 g IV q 8 h for CrCl less than 20 mL/min; 2.25 g IV q 6 h for CrCl 20 to 40 mL/min. Hemodialysis: Maximum dose of 2.25 g IV q 8 h plus 0.75 g after each dialysis.

MOA — Beta-lactam antibiotic that inhibits the bio-synthesis of cell wall mucopeptide. Tazobactam is beta-lactamase inhibitor.

ADVERSE EFFECTS — Serious: Anaphylaxis (rare); cross-sensitivity with cephalosporins; serious skin reactions like Stevens Johnson syndrome and toxic epidermal necrolysis (stop drug if progressive rash); hypokalemia; bleeding and coagulation abnormalities (especially with renal impairment). Frequent: N/V, diarrhea, headache.

TICARCILLIN-CLAVULANATE (Timentin) ▶K ♀B ▶? $$$$$

ADULT — Systemic infections or UTIs: 3.1 g IV q 4 to 6 h. Gynecologic infections. Moderate: 200 mg/kg/day IV divided q 6 h. Severe: 300 mg/kg/day IV divided q 4 h. Adults with wt less than 60 kg: 200 to 300 mg/kg/day (based on ticarcillin content) IV divided q 4 to 6 h. Use q 4 h dosing interval for Pseudomonas infections.

PEDS — Age 3 mo or older and wt less than 60 kg: 200 mg/kg/day (based on ticarcillin content) IV divided q 6 h for mild to moderate infections; 300 mg/kg/day IV divided q 4 h for severe infections. For wt 60 kg or greater: 3.1 g IV q 6 h for mild to moderate infections; 3.1 g IV q 4 h for severe infections.

NOTES — Timentin 3.1 g = 3 g ticarcillin and 0.1 g clavulanate. 4.75 mEq sodium per g of Timentin. Reduce dose in adults with renal dysfunction: Load with 3.1 g, then give 2 g daily for CrCl less than 10 mL/min and liver dysfunction; 2 g q 12 h for CrCl less than 10 mL/min; 2 g q 8 h for CrCl 10 to 30 mL/min; 2 g q 4 h for CrCl 30 to 60 mL/min. Peritoneal dialysis: 3.1 g q 12 h. Hemodialysis: 3.1 g load, then 2 g q 12 h and 3.1 g after each dialysis.

MOA — Beta-lactam antibiotic that inhibits the bio-synthesis of cell wall mucopeptide. Clavulanate is beta-lactamase inhibitor.

ADVERSE EFFECTS — Serious: Anaphylaxis (rare), cross-sensitivity with cephalosporins, hypokalemia, bleeding and coagulation abnormalities (especially with renal impairment), cholestatic hepatitis (due to clavulanate). Frequent: Eosinophilia, diarrhea.

ANTIMICROBIALS: Quinolones—2nd Generation

QUINOLONES: GENERAL ANTIMICROBIAL SPECTRUM

1st generation	1st generation quinolones are no longer available
2nd generation	Gram-negative (including *Pseudomonas*); *S. aureus* (but not MRSA or *pneumococcus*); some atypicals
3rd generation	Gram-negative (including *Pseudomonas*); Gram-positive, including *pneumococcus* and *S. aureus* (but not MRSA); expanded atypical coverage
4th generation	same as 3rd generation plus enhanced coverage of *pneumococcus*, decreased *Pseudomonas* activity

NOTE: As of April 2007, the CDC no longer recommends fluoroquinolones for gonorrhea because of high resistance rates. Fluoroquinolones can cause tendon rupture (rare; risk increased by corticosteroids, age older than 60 yo, or organ transplant), phototoxicity (risk varies among agents), C difficile-associated diarrhea (risk may vary among agents), QT interval prolongation (risk varies among agents; see QT drugs table), exacerbation of myasthenia gravis, CNS toxicity including seizures and increased intracranial pressure, peripheral neuropathy (rare), and hypersensitivity. Important quinolone drug interactions with antacids, iron, zinc, magnesium, sucralfate, buffered didanosine, cimetidine, caffeine, cyclosporine, phenytoin, anticoagulants, theophylline, etc.

CIPROFLOXACIN (*Cipro, Cipro XR*) ▶LK ♀C but terato-genicity unlikely ▶?+ $

WARNING — Tendon rupture (rare; risk increased by corticosteroids, age older than 60 yo, or organ transplant). Advise patients to stop fluoroquinolone, rest affected area, and seek medical advice for tendon swelling, pain, or inflammation. Avoid in patients with a history of myasthenia gravis; can exacerbate muscle weakness. Do not chew microcapsules in oral susp.

ADULT — UTI: 250 to 500 mg PO two times per day or 200 to 400 mg IV q 12 h. Simple UTI: 250 mg

CIPROFLOXACIN (*cont.*)

PO two times per day for 3 days or Cipro XR 500 mg PO once daily for 3 days. Cipro XR for complicated UTI, uncomplicated pyelonephritis: 1000 mg PO once daily for 7 to 14 days. Pneumonia, skin, bone/joint infections: 400 mg IV q 8 to 12 h or 500 to 750 mg PO two times per day. Treat bone/joint infections for 4 to 6 weeks. Acute sinusitis: 500 mg PO two times per day for 10 days. Chronic bacterial prostatitis: 500 mg PO two times per day for 28 days. Infectious diarrhea: 500 mg PO two times per day for 5 to 7 days. Typhoid fever: 500 mg PO two times per day for 10 days. Nosocomial pneumonia: 400 mg IV q 8 h. Complicated intra-abdominal infection (with metronidazole): 400 mg IV q 12 h, then 500 mg PO two times per day. Empiric therapy of febrile neutropenia: 400 mg IV q 8 h with piperacillin. Bioterrorism anthrax. Inhalation or severe cutaneous anthrax treatment: 400 mg IV q 12 h with at least 1 other drug initially, then monotherapy with 500 mg PO two times per day to complete 60 days. Monotherapy for postexposure prophylaxis or treatment of less severe cutaneous anthrax: 500 mg PO two times per day for 60 days. See www.bt.cdc.gov/bioterrorism/ for more info.

PEDS — Safety and efficacy not established for most indications in children; arthropathy in juvenile animals. Still limited data, but clinical trials in children show no evidence of arthropathy other than transient large-joint arthralgias. Musculoskeletal adverse events reported with ciprofloxacin treatment of complicated UTI in peds patients were mild to moderate in severity and resolved within 1 month after treatment. Complicated UTI, pyelonephritis, 1 to 17 yo: 6 to 10 mg/kg IV q 8 h, then 10 to 20 mg/kg PO q 12 h. Max of 400 mg IV or 750 mg PO per dose even for peds patients wt greater than 51 kg. Bioterrorism anthrax. Treatment of inhalation anthrax, severe cutaneous anthrax, or cutaneous anthrax in age younger than 2 yo: 10 to 15 mg/kg IV q 12 h with at least 1 other drug initially, then monotherapy with 10 to 15 mg/kg up to 500 mg PO two times per day to complete 60 days. Monotherapy for postexposure prophylaxis or less severe cutaneous anthrax treatment: 10 to 15 mg/kg up to 500 mg PO two times per day for 60 days. See www.bt.cdc.gov/bioterrorism/ for more info.

UNAPPROVED ADULT — Acute uncomplicated pyelonephritis: 500 mg PO two times per day for 7 days. Chancroid: 500 mg PO two times per day for 3 days. Prophylaxis, high-risk GU surgery: 500 mg PO or 400 mg IV. Prophylaxis, invasive meningococcal disease: 500 mg PO single dose. Traveler's diarrhea (treatment preferred over prophylaxis). Treatment: 500 mg PO two times per day for 1 to 3 days or 750 mg PO single dose. Prophylaxis: 500 mg PO daily for no more than 3 weeks. Infectious diarrhea: 500 mg PO two times per day for 1 to 3 days for Shigella, for 5 to 7 days for non-typhi Salmonella (usually not treated). Malignant otitis externa: 400 mg IV or 750 mg PO q 12 h. TB (2nd-line treatment): 750 to 1500 mg/day IV/PO. Salmonella gastroenteritis in HIV infection: 500 to 750 mg PO two times per day (400 mg IV q 12 h) for 7 to 14 days if CD4 count 200 or greater, for 2 to 6 weeks if CD4 count less than 200. Campylobacter in HIV infection: 500 to 750 mg PO (or 400 mg IV) two times per day for 7 to 10 days for mild/moderate disease, at least 14 days with aminoglycoside for bacteremia.

UNAPPROVED PEDS — Usual dose: 20 to 30 mg/kg/day IV/PO divided q 12 h (max 1.5 g/day PO; max 800 mg/day IV). Acute pulmonary exacerbation of cystic fibrosis: 10 mg/kg/dose IV q 8 h for 7 days, then 20 mg/kg/dose PO q 12 h to complete 10 to 21 days of treatment. TB (second-line treatment): 10 to 15 mg/kg PO two times per day (max: 1.5 g/day). Cholera: 20 mg/kg up to 750 mg PO single dose for age 2 to 15 yo.

FORMS — Generic/Trade: Tabs 100, 250, 500, 750 mg. Extended-release tabs 500, 1000 mg. Oral susp 250, 500 mg/5 mL.

NOTES — Crystalluria if alkaline urine. Ciprofloxacin inhibits CYP1A2, an enzyme that metabolizes caffeine, clozapine, tacrine, theophylline, and warfarin. Give ciprofloxacin immediate-release or Cipro XR 2 h before or 6 h after antacids, iron, sucralfate, calcium, zinc, buffered didanosine, or other highly buffered drugs. Can give with meals containing dairy products, but not with yogurt, milk, or calcium-fortified fruit juice alone. Do not give Cipro XR within 2 h of calcium doses greater than 800 mg. Watch for hypoglycemia with glyburide. Do not give oral susp in feeding or nasogastric tube. Cipro XR and immediate-release tabs are not inter-changeable. Do not split, crush, or chew Cipro XR. In patients with complicated UTI or acute pyelonephritis and CrCl less than 30 mL/min, reduce dose of Cipro XR to 500 mg daily. Reduce dose of immediate-release ciprofloxacin in adults with renal dysfunction: 250 to 500 mg PO q 24 h given after dialysis session for hemodialysis/peritoneal dialysis; 250 to 500 mg PO q 18 h or 200 to 400 mg IV q 18 to 24 h for CrCl 5 to 29 mL/min; 250 to 500 mg PO q 12 h for CrCl 30 to 50 mL/min.

MOA — Inhibits bacterial DNA synthesis by binding with DNA gyrase and topoisomerase IV.

ADVERSE EFFECTS — Serious: Tendon rupture (rare), phototoxicity, CNS toxicity, crystalluria if alkaline urine, peripheral neuropathy (rare), hypersensitivity. Theoretical risk of cartilage toxicity in children, but no clinical evidence of harm other than transient large-joint arthralgias. Musculoskeletal adverse events reported with ciprofloxacin treatment of complicated UTI in peds patients were mild to moderate in severity and resolved within 1 month after treatment. Frequent: N/V. More GI, neurologic, and musculoskeletal adverse reactions reported during postexposure prophylaxis of bioterrorism anthrax.

NORFLOXACIN (*Noroxin*) ▶LK ♀C ▶? $$

WARNING — Tendon rupture (rare; risk increased by corticosteroids, age older than 60 yo, or organ transplant). Advise patients to stop fluoroquinolone, rest

(cont.)

NORFLOXACIN *(cont.)*

affected area, and seek medical advice for tendon swelling, pain, or inflammation. Avoid in patients with a history of myasthenia gravis; can exacerbate muscle weakness.

ADULT — Simple UTI due to E. coli, K. pneumoniae, P. mirabilis: 400 mg PO two times per day for 3 days. UTI due to other organisms: 400 mg PO two times per day for 7 to 10 days. Complicated UTI: 400 mg PO two times per day for 10 to 21 days. Acute/chronic prostatitis: 400 mg PO two times per day for 28 days. Take on an empty stomach.

PEDS — Safety and efficacy of norfloxacin not established in children; arthropathy in juvenile animals.

UNAPPROVED ADULT — Traveler's diarrhea (treatment preferred over prophylaxis). Treatment: 400 mg PO two times per day for 1 to 3 days. Prophylaxis: 400 mg PO daily for up to 3 weeks. Infectious diarrhea: 400 mg PO two times per day for 5 to 7 days for non-typhi Salmonella (usually not treated), for 1 to 3 days for Shigella. Prevention of spontaneous bacterial peritonitis: 400 mg PO once daily. Take on an empty stomach.

FORMS — Trade only: Tabs 400 mg. Norfloxacin tabs discontinued from US market in April 2014.

NOTES — Crystalluria with high doses. Maintain adequate hydration. Norfloxacin inhibits CYP1A2, an enzyme that metabolizes caffeine, clozapine, ropinirole, tacrine, theophylline, tizanidine, and warfarin. Increased INR with warfarin. Do not take with dairy products. Give antacids, zinc, iron, sucralfate, multivitamins, or buffered didanosine 2 h before/after norfloxacin. Reduce dose in renal dysfunction: 400 mg PO daily for CrCl less than 30 mL/min.

MOA — Inhibits bacterial DNA synthesis by binding with DNA gyrase and topoisomerase IV.

ADVERSE EFFECTS — Serious: Tendon rupture (rare), phototoxicity, crystalluria (high doses), CNS toxicity, peripheral neuropathy (rare), and hypersensitivity. Frequent: None.

OFLOXACIN ▶LK ♀C ▶?+ $$$

WARNING — Tendon rupture (rare; risk increased by corticosteroids, age older than 60 yo, or organ transplant). Advise patients to stop fluoroquinolone, rest affected area, and seek medical advice for tendon swelling, pain, or inflammation. Avoid in patients with a history of myasthenia gravis; can exacerbate muscle weakness.

ADULT — Acute exacerbation of chronic bronchitis, community-acquired pneumonia, skin infections: 400 mg PO two times per day for 10 days. Simple UTI due to E. coli, K. pneumoniae: 200 mg PO two times per day for 3 days. Simple UTI due to other organisms: 200 mg PO two times per day for 7 days. Complicated UTI: 200 mg PO two times per day for 10 days. Chronic bacterial prostatitis: 300 mg PO two times per day for 6 weeks.

PEDS — Safety and efficacy of ofloxacin not established in children; arthropathy in juvenile animals.

UNAPPROVED ADULT — Epididymitis: 300 mg PO two times per day for 10 days. Traveler's diarrhea, treatment: 300 mg PO two times per day for 1 to 3 days. Infectious diarrhea: 300 mg PO two times per day for 1 to 3 days for Shigella, 5 to 7 days for non-typhi Salmonella (usually not treated). TB (2nd-line treatment): 600 to 800 mg PO daily.

FORMS — Generic only: Tabs 200, 300, 400 mg.

NOTES — May prolong QT interval; avoid using in proarrhythmic conditions or with drugs that prolong QT interval, including Class 1A and Class III antiarrhythmics. Give antacids, iron, sucralfate, multivitamins containing zinc, buffered didanosine 2 h before or after ofloxacin. May decrease metabolism of theophylline, increase INR with warfarin. Monitor glucose with antidiabetic agents. Can cause false positive on opiate urine screening immunoassay; may need confirmation test. Reduce dose in renal dysfunction: 50% of usual dose q 24 h for CrCl less than 20 mL/min; usual dose given q 24 h for CrCl 20 to 50 mL/min.

MOA — Inhibits bacterial DNA synthesis by binding with DNA gyrase and topoisomerase IV.

ADVERSE EFFECTS — Serious: Tendon rupture (rare), phototoxicity (risk varies among agents), QT interval prolongation, peripheral neuropathy (rare), CNS toxicity, and hypersensitivity. Frequent: N/V.

ANTIMICROBIALS: Quinolones—3rd Generation

NOTE: As of April 2007, the CDC no longer recommends fluoroquinolones for gonorrhea because of high resistance rates. Can cause tendon rupture (rare; risk increased by corticosteroids, age older than 60 yo, or organ transplant), C. difficile–associated diarrhea (risk may vary among agents), phototoxicity (risk varies among agents), CNS toxicity including seizures and increased intracranial pressure, peripheral neuropathy (rare), hypersensitivity, and QT interval prolongation (risk varies among agents; see QT drugs table). Avoid using in proarrhythmic conditions or with drugs that prolong QT including Class 1A and Class III antiarrhythmics. Important quinolone drug interactions with antacids, iron, zinc, magnesium, sucralfate, caffeine, cyclosporine, phenytoin, anticoagulants, theophylline, etc.

LEVOFLOXACIN *(Levaquin)* ▶KL ♀C ▶? $$$

WARNING — Tendon rupture (rare; risk increased by corticosteroids, age older than 60 yo, or organ transplant). Advise patients to stop fluoroquinolone, rest affected area, and seek medical advice for tendon swelling, pain, or inflammation. Avoid in patients with a history of myasthenia gravis; can exacerbate muscle weakness.

ADULT — IV and PO doses are the same. Community-acquired pneumonia: 750 mg once daily for 5 days or 500 mg once daily for 7 to 14 days. Nosocomial pneumonia: 750 mg once daily for 7 to 14 days. Acute sinusitis: 750 mg once daily for 5 days or 500 mg once daily for 10 to 14 days. See table for management of acute sinusitis. Acute exacerbation of chronic bronchitis: 500 mg once daily for

LEVOFLOXACIN (*cont.*)

7 days. Skin infections: 500 to 750 mg once daily for 7 to 14 days. Complicated UTI or pyelonephritis: 250 mg once daily for 10 days or 750 mg once daily for 5 days. Simple UTI: 250 mg once daily for 3 days. Chronic bacterial prostatitis: 500 mg once daily for 28 days. Postexposure prophylaxis for inhalation anthrax: 500 mg PO once daily for 60 days. See www.bt.cdc.gov/bioterrorism/ for more info. Plague: 500 mg once daily for 10 to 14 days. See www.bt.cdc.gov/bioterrorism/ for more info. Infuse IV doses over 60 min (250 to 500 mg) to 90 min (750 mg). Take oral soln on empty stomach.

PEDS — IV and PO doses are the same. Postexposure prophylaxis for inhalation anthrax, age 6 mo and older: Treat for 60 days with 8 mg/kg (max 250 mg/dose) two times per day if wt less than 50 kg; 500 mg once daily if wt greater than 50 kg. See www.bt.cdc.gov/bioterrorism/ for more info. Plague, age 6 mo and older: Treat for 10 to 14 days with 8 mg/kg (max 250 mg/dose) two times per day if wt less than 50 kg; 500 mg once daily if wt greater than 50 kg. See www.bt.cdc.gov/bioterrorism/ for more info. Clinical trials in children show no evidence of arthropathy other than transient large joint arthralgias. Infuse IV doses over 60 min (250 to 500 mg). Take oral soln on empty stomach.

UNAPPROVED ADULT — Legionnaires' disease: 1 g IV/PO on 1st day, then 500 mg IV/PO once daily. Chlamydia, epididymitis: See STD table. TB (2nd-line treatment): 500 to 1000 mg/day IV/PO. Traveler's diarrhea, treatment: 500 mg PO once daily for 1 to 3 days. Infectious diarrhea: 500 mg PO once daily for 1 to 3 days for Shigella, for 5 to 7 days for Salmonella.

UNAPPROVED PEDS — IV and PO doses are the same. Community-acquired pneumonia: 8 to 10 mg/kg two times per day for age 6 mo to 5 yo; 8 to 10 mg/kg/day once daily (max 750 mg once daily) for age 5 to 16 yo. Atypical pneumonia in adolescents with skeletal maturity: 500 mg PO once daily. Infuse IV doses over 60 min (250 to 500 mg). See table for management of acute sinusitis.

FORMS — Generic only: Tabs 250, 500, 750 mg. Oral soln 25 mg/mL

NOTES — Can prolong QT interval and cause torsades. Give Mg/Al antacids, iron, sucralfate, multivitamins containing zinc, buffered didanosine 2 h before/after PO levofloxacin. Increased INR with warfarin. Monitor glucose with antidiabetic agents. Can cause false positive on opiate urine screening immunoassay; may need confirmation test. Dosage adjustment in renal dysfunction is based on dose used in normal renal function. For dose of 750 mg in normal renal function: Give 750 mg q 48 h for CrCl 20 to 49 mL/min; give 750 mg load, then 500 mg q 48 h for CrCl 10 to 19 mL/min, hemodialysis or CAPD. For dose of 500 mg in normal renal function: Give 500 mg load, then 250 mg q 24 h for CrCl 20 to 49 mL/min; give 500 mg load, then 250 mg q 48 h for CrCl 10 to 19 mL/min, hemodialysis or CAPD. For dose of 250 mg in normal renal function: Give 250 mg q 48 h for CrCl 10 to 19 mL/min. Dosage adjustment not necessary for uncomplicated UTI if CrCl is 10 to 19 mL/min.

MOA — Inhibits bacterial DNA synthesis by binding with DNA gyrase and topoisomerase IV.

ADVERSE EFFECTS — Serious: QT interval prolongation and torsades (rare), tendon rupture (rare), phototoxicity (rare), peripheral neuropathy (rare), CNS toxicity, hepatotoxicity, and hypersensitivity. Frequent: Headache. Musculoskeletal disorders (arthralgia, arthritis, tendinopathy, gait abnormality) reported in children; safety for treatment duration more than 14 days not established.

ANTIMICROBIALS: Quinolones—4th Generation

NOTE: As of April 2007, the CDC no longer recommends fluoroquinolones for gonorrhea because of high resistance rates. Can cause tendon rupture (rare; risk increased by corticosteroids, age older than 60 yo, or organ transplant), C difficile-associated diarrhea (risk may vary among agents), phototoxicity (risk varies among agents), CNS toxicity including seizures and increased intracranial pressure, peripheral neuropathy (rare), hypersensitivity, and QT interval prolongation (risk varies among agents; see QT drugs table). Avoid using in proarrhythmic conditions or with drugs that prolong QT interval, including Class 1A and Class III antiarrhythmics. Important quinolone drug interactions with antacids, iron, zinc, magnesium, sucralfate, cimetidine, caffeine, cyclosporine, phenytoin, anticoagulants, theophylline, etc. Monitor INR with warfarin.

GEMIFLOXACIN (*Factive*) ▶Feces, K ♀C ▶– $$$$$

WARNING — Tendon rupture (rare; risk increased by corticosteroids, age older than 60 yo, or organ transplant). Advise patients to stop fluoroquinolone, rest affected area, and seek medical advice for tendon swelling, pain, or inflammation. Avoid in patients with a history of myasthenia gravis; can exacerbate muscle weakness.

ADULT — Acute exacerbation of chronic bronchitis: 320 mg PO daily for 5 days. Community-acquired pneumonia: 320 mg PO daily for 5 to 7 days (for 7 days for multidrug-resistant S. pneumoniae).

PEDS — Safety and efficacy of gemifloxacin not established in children; arthropathy in juvenile animals.

FORMS — Trade only: Tabs 320 mg.

NOTES — Maintain fluid intake to prevent crystalluria. Give 2 h before or 3 h after Al/Mg antacids, iron, multivitamins with zinc, buffered didanosine. Give at least 2 h before sucralfate. May increase INR with warfarin. Discontinue if rash develops. Reduce dose for CrCl 40 mL/min or less, hemodialysis, or CAPD: 160 mg PO daily.

MOA — Inhibits bacterial DNA synthesis by binding with DNA gyrase and topoisomerase IV.

(cont.)

GEMIFLOXACIN *(cont.)*

ADVERSE EFFECTS — Serious: QT interval prolongation, tendon rupture (rare), phototoxicity (rare), CNS toxicity, and hypersensitivity. Frequent: Rash (esp. in women younger than 40 yo or treatment duration more than 7 days).

MOXIFLOXACIN *(Avelox)* ▶LK ♀C ▶– $$$$

WARNING — Tendon rupture (rare; risk increased by corticosteroids, age older than 60 yo, or organ transplant). Advise patients to stop fluoroquinolone, rest affected area, and seek medical advice for tendon swelling, pain, or inflammation. Avoid in patients with a history of myasthenia gravis; can exacerbate muscle weakness.

ADULT — Chronic bronchitis exacerbation: 400 mg PO/IV daily for 5 days. Complicated intra-abdominal infection: (given IV initially) 400 mg PO/IV daily for 5 to 14 days. Community-acquired pneumonia, including penicillin-resistant S. pneumoniae: 400 mg PO/IV daily for 7 to 14 days. Acute sinusitis: 400 mg PO/IV daily for 10 days. See table for management of acute sinusitis. Uncomplicated skin infections: 400 mg PO/IV daily for 7 days. Complicated skin infections: 400 mg PO/IV daily for 7 to 21 days.

PEDS — Safety and efficacy of moxifloxacin not established in children; arthropathy in juvenile animals.

UNAPPROVED ADULT — TB (2nd-line treatment): 400 mg IV/PO daily.

UNAPPROVED PEDS — Atypical pneumonia in adolescents with skeletal maturity: 400 mg PO once daily.

FORMS — Generic/Trade: Tabs 400 mg.

NOTES — Can prolong the QT interval and cause torsades. Avoid if QT interval prolonged, uncorrected hypokalemia or hypomagnesemia, coadministration of class IA or III antiarrhythmic drugs. Do not exceed recommended IV dose or infusion rate due to QT prolongation risk. Contraindicated with ziprasidone. Give tabs at least 4 h before or 8 h after Mg/Al antacids, iron, multivitamins with zinc, sucralfate, buffered didanosine. Dosage adjustment not required for hepatic insufficiency.

MOA — Inhibits bacterial DNA synthesis by binding with DNA gyrase and topoisomerase IV.

ADVERSE EFFECTS — Serious: QT interval prolongation and torsades, tendon rupture (rare), phototoxicity, peripheral neuropathy (rare), CNS toxicity including seizures and increased intracranial pressure, and hypersensitivity. Frequent: Nausea, diarrhea.

ANTIMICROBIALS: Sulfonamides

NOTE: Sulfonamides can cause Stevens-Johnson syndrome; toxic epidermal necrolysis; hepatotoxicity; blood dyscrasias; hemolysis in glucose-6-phosphate dehydrogenase (G6PD) deficiency. Avoid maternal sulfonamides when the breastfed infant is ill, stressed, premature, has hyperbilirubinemia, or has G6PD deficiency. Not effective for streptococcal pharyngitis.

TRIMETHOPRIM-SULFAMETHOXAZOLE *(Bactrim, Septra, Sulfatrim Pediatric, cotrimoxazole, TMP-SMX)* ▶K ♀C ▶+ $

ADULT — UTI, shigellosis, acute exacerbation of chronic bronchitis: 1 tab PO two times per day, double strength (DS, 160 mg TMP/800 mg SMX). Travelers' diarrhea: 1 DS tab PO two times per day for 5 days. Pneumocystis treatment: 15 to 20 mg/kg/day (based on TMP) IV divided q 6 to 8 h or PO divided three times per day for 21 days total; can use 2 DS tabs PO three times per day for mild to moderate infection. Pneumocystis prophylaxis: 1 DS tab PO daily.

PEDS — UTI, shigellosis, otitis media: 1 mL/kg/day susp PO divided two times per day (up to 20 mL PO two times per day). Use adult dose for wt greater than 40 kg. TMP-SMX is a poor option for otitis media and sinusitis due to high pneumococcus and H. influenzae resistance rates; see otitis media and sinusitis treatment tables for alternatives. Pneumocystis treatment: 15 to 20 mg/kg/day (based on TMP) IV divided q 6 to 8 h or 5 mL susp/8 kg/dose PO q 6 h. Pneumocystis prophylaxis: 150 mg/m²/day (based on TMP) PO divided two times per day on 3 consecutive days each week. Do not use in infants younger than 2 mo; may cause kernicterus.

UNAPPROVED ADULT — Uncomplicated cystitis in women: 1 DS tab PO two times per day for 3 days. Do not use if resistance prevalence >20% or if used for

UTI in previous 3 months. Bacterial prostatitis: 1 DS tab PO two times per day for 10 to 14 days for acute, for 1 to 3 months for chronic. Burkholderia cepacia pulmonary infection in cystic fibrosis: 5 mg/kg (based on TMP) IV q 6 h. Pneumocystis prophylaxis: 1 SS tab PO daily. Primary prevention of toxoplasmosis in AIDS: 1 DS tab PO daily. Pertussis (2nd line to macrolides): 1 DS tab PO two times per day for 14 days. Community-acquired MRSA skin infections: 1 to 2 DS tabs PO two times per day for 5 to 10 days; 2 DS tabs PO bid for wt 100 kg or greater or BMI of 40 or greater. MRSA osteomyelitis: 4 mg/kg/dose (based on TMP) PO two times per day with rifampin 600 mg PO once daily. Prevention of spontaneous bacterial peritonitis: 1 DS tab PO once daily for 5 days per week.

UNAPPROVED PEDS — Community-acquired MRSA skin infections: 1 to 1.5 mL/kg/day PO divided two times per day for 5 to 10 days. Pertussis (2nd line to macrolides): 1 mL/kg/day PO divided two times per day for 14 days.

FORMS — Generic/Trade: Tabs 80 mg TMP/400 mg SMX (SS), 160 mg TMP/800 mg SMX (DS). Susp 40 mg TMP/200 mg SMX per 5 mL. 20 mL susp = 2 SS tabs = 1 DS tab.

NOTES — Not effective for streptococcal pharyngitis. AAP recommends against cotrimoxazole for acute otitis media in children because of high resistance rates. No activity against penicillin-nonsusceptible

TRIMETHOPRIM-SULFAMETHOXAZOLE (cont.)

pneumococci. Bone marrow depression with high IV doses. Significantly increased INR with warfarin; avoid concomitant use if possible. Increases levels of methotrexate, phenytoin. Rifampin reduces TMP-SMX levels. Do not give leucovorin during treatment of pneumocystis pneumonia; may increase treatment failure and mortality. Can cause hyperkalemia (risk increased by high doses of trimethoprim, renal impairment, other drugs that cause hyperkalemia). Dosing in renal dysfunction: Use 50% of usual dose for CrCl 15 to 30 mL/min. Do not use for CrCl less than 15 mL/min.

MOA — Sulfonamides (bacteriostatic) are structural analogs of PABA that bind with dihydropteroate synthetase and prevent bacterial folic acid synthesis. Trimethoprim inhibits dihydrofolate reductase, the enzyme after step in folic acid synthesis inhibited by sulfonamides. Trimethoprim acts like a potassium-sparing diuretic, reducing urinary potassium excretion.

ADVERSE EFFECTS — Serious: Stevens-Johnson syndrome, toxic epidermal necrolysis, hepatotoxicity, blood dyscrasias (thrombocytopenia risk possibly increased by thiazide diuretics), hemolysis in G6PD deficiency, hyperkalemia (risk increased by high doses of trimethoprim, renal impairment, or other drugs that cause hyperkalemia); hyponatremia with high doses; hypoglycemia in non-diabetic patients (esp. if renal/hepatic dysfunction, malnutrition, high doses). Bone marrow depression with high IV doses. Frequent: N/V, anorexia, allergic skin reactions, photosensitivity.

SULFADIAZINE ▶K ♀C ▶+ $$$$$

ADULT — Usual dose: 2 to 4 g PO initially, then 2 to 4 g/day divided into 3 to 6 doses. Secondary prevention of rheumatic fever: 1 g PO daily. Toxoplasmosis treatment: 1 to 1.5 g PO four times per day with pyrimethamine and leucovorin.

PEDS — Not for infants younger than 2 mo, except as adjunct to pyrimethamine for congenital toxoplasmosis. Usual dose: Give 75 mg/kg PO initially, then 150 mg/kg/day up to 6 g/day divided into 4 to 6 doses. Secondary prevention of rheumatic fever, for wt 27 kg or less: 500 mg PO daily. Use adult dose for wt greater than 27 kg.

UNAPPROVED ADULT — CNS toxoplasmosis in AIDS. Acute therapy: For wt less than 60 kg give pyrimethamine 200 mg PO for first dose, then 50 mg PO once daily with sulfadiazine 1000 mg PO q 6 h and leucovorin 10 to 25 mg PO once daily (up to 50 mg once daily or two times per day) . For wt 60 kg or greater give pyrimethamine 200 mg PO for first dose, then 75 mg PO once daily with sulfadiazine 1500 mg PO q 6 h and leucovorin 10 to 25 mg PO once daily (up to 50 mg once daily or two times per day). Secondary prevention: Pyrimethamine 25 to 50 mg PO once daily with sulfadiazine 2000 to 4000 mg/day PO divided two to four times per day and leucovorin 10 to 25 mg PO once daily.

UNAPPROVED PEDS — Not for age younger than 2 mo, except as adjunct to pyrimethamine for congenital toxoplasmosis. AAP regimen for toxoplasmosis: 100 to 200 mg/kg/day PO with pyrimethamine and leucovorin (duration varies). Secondary prevention after CNS toxoplasmosis in HIV infection: 85 to 120 mg/kg/day PO divided in 2 to 4 doses with pyrimethamine and leucovorin.

FORMS — Generic only: Tabs 500 mg.

NOTES — Maintain fluid intake to prevent crystalluria and stone formation. Reduce dose in renal insufficiency. May increase INR with warfarin. May increase levels of methotrexate, phenytoin.

MOA — Structural analog of PABA that binds with dihydropteroate synthetase and prevents nucleic acid synthesis. Bacteriostatic.

ADVERSE EFFECTS — Serious: Stevens-Johnson syndrome, toxic epidermal necrolysis, hepatotoxicity, blood dyscrasias, hemolysis in G6PD deficiency, crystalluria and stone formation. Frequent: Rash, N/V, diarrhea, fever.

ANTIMICROBIALS: Tetracyclines

NOTE: Tetracyclines can cause photosensitivity and pseudotumor cerebri (avoid with isotretinoin which is also linked to pseudotumor cerebri). May decrease efficacy of oral contraceptives. Increased INR with warfarin. May increase risk of ergotism with ergot alkaloids. Use tetracyclines with caution in renal dysfunction; doxycycline preferred.

DEMECLOCYCLINE ▶K, feces ♀D ▶?+ $$$$

ADULT — Usual dose: 150 mg PO four times per day or 300 mg PO two times per day on empty stomach.

PEDS — Avoid in age younger than 8 yo due to teeth staining. Usual dose: 6.6 to 13.2 mg/kg/day PO given in 2 to 4 divided doses on empty stomach.

UNAPPROVED ADULT — SIADH: 600 to 1200 mg/day PO given in 3 to 4 divided doses.

FORMS — Generic/Trade: Tabs 150, 300 mg.

NOTES — Can cause diabetes insipidus, high risk of photosensitivity. Absorption impaired by iron, calcium, Al/Mg antacids. Take with fluids (not milk) to decrease esophageal irritation. SIADH onset of action occurs within 5 to 14 days; do not increase dose more frequently than q 3 to 4 days.

MOA — Inhibits bacterial protein synthesis by binding with ribosomal 30S subunit and blocking addition of amino acids to peptide chain. Active against intracellular bacteria. Bacteriostatic. Blocks action of ADH at level of collecting duct and distal tubule.

ADVERSE EFFECTS — Serious: Pseudotumor cerebri, nephrotoxicity, photosensitivity (high risk), teeth staining in children younger than 8 yo, diabetes insipidus. Frequent: N/V, heartburn, epigastric distress, diarrhea.

DOXYCYCLINE (*Doryx, Monodox, Oracea, Periostat, Vibramycin, Acticlate, Adoxa, ✱Doxycin*) ▶LK ♀D ▶?+ $

ADULT — Usual dose: 100 mg PO two times per day on 1st day, then 100 mg/day PO daily or divided two times per day. Severe infections: 100 mg PO two times per day. Chlamydia, nongonococcal urethritis: 100 mg PO two times per day for 7 days. Doryx for chlamydia urethritis/cervicitis: 200 mg PO once daily for 7 days. Acne vulgaris: Up to 100 mg PO two times per day. Oracea for inflammatory rosacea (papules and pustules): 40 mg PO once q am on empty stomach. Community-acquired MRSA skin infections: 100 mg PO two times per day for 5 to 10 days. Periostat for periodontitis: 20 mg PO two times per day 1 h before breakfast and dinner. Cholera: 300 mg PO single dose. Primary, secondary, early latent syphilis if penicillin-allergic: 100 mg PO two times per day for 14 days. Late latent or tertiary syphilis if penicillin-allergic: 100 mg PO two times per day for 4 weeks. Not for neurosyphilis. Malaria prophylaxis: 100 mg PO daily starting 1 to 2 days before exposure until 4 weeks after. IV: 200 mg on 1st day in 1 to 2 infusions, then 100 to 200 mg/day in 1 to 2 infusions. Bioterrorism anthrax: 100 mg two times per day for 60 days. Use IV with at least 1 other drug for initial treatment of inhalation or severe cutaneous anthrax. PO monotherapy for less severe cutaneous anthrax or postexposure prophylaxis. See http://www.bt.cdc.gov/bioterrorism/ for more info.

PEDS — Avoid in age younger than 8 yo due to teeth staining. Usual dose: 4.4 mg/kg/day PO divided two times per day on 1st day, then 2.2 to 4.4 mg/kg/day PO divided daily or two times per day for wt 45 kg or less. Use adult dose for wt greater than 45 kg. Malaria prophylaxis: 2 mg/kg/day up to 100 mg PO daily starting 1 to 2 days before exposure until 4 weeks after. Most PO and IV doses are equivalent. Bioterrorism anthrax: 100 mg two times per day for age older than 8 yo and wt greater than 45 kg; 2.2 mg/kg two times per day for age older than 8 yo and wt 45 kg or less, or age 8 yo or younger. Treat for 60 days. Use IV with at least 1 other drug for initial treatment of inhalation anthrax, severe cutaneous anthrax, or cutaneous anthrax in age younger than 2 yo. PO monotherapy for less severe cutaneous anthrax and postexposure prophylaxis. See http://www.bt.cdc.gov/bioterrorism/ for more info.

UNAPPROVED ADULT — See table for management of acute sinusitis. See STD table for granuloma inguinale, lymphogranuloma venereum, pelvic inflammatory disease treatment. Lyme disease: 100 mg PO two times per day for 14 days for early disease, for 28 days for Lyme arthritis. Prevention of Lyme disease in highly endemic area, with deer tick attachment at least 48 h: 200 mg PO single dose with food within 72 h of tick bite. Ehrlichiosis: 100 mg IV/PO two times per day for 7 to 14 days. Malaria, co-therapy with quinine/quinidine: 100 mg IV/PO two times per day for 7 days. Lymphatic filariasis: 100 mg PO two times per day for 8 weeks.

UNAPPROVED PEDS — Community-acquired MRSA skin infections: 2 mg/kg/dose PO q 12 h for wt 45 kg or less; 100 mg PO two times per day for wt greater than 45 kg. Treat for 5 to 10 days. Avoid in age younger than 8 yo due to teeth staining. Cholera: 2 to 4 mg/kg PO single dose for all ages.

FORMS — Monohydrate salt. Generic/Trade: Caps 50, 75, 100, 150 mg. Tabs 50, 75, 100, 150 mg. Trade only: Delayed-release caps 40 mg (Oracea $$$$$). Susp (Vibramycin) 25 mg/5 mL. Hyclate salt. Tabs: Trade only: 75, 150 mg. Generic/Trade: 20 mg. Generic only: 100 mg. Caps: Generic only: 50 mg. Generic/Trade: 100 mg. Delayed-release Tabs: Generic Only: 75, 100 mg. Generic/Trade: 150 mg. Trade only: 200 mg (Doryx $$$$$). Delayed-release caps: Generic only: 75, 100 mg. Calcium salt. Trade only: Susp (Vibramycin) 50 mg/5 mL. Monohydrate formulations may have better GI tolerability than hyclate formulations.

NOTES — Photosensitivity, pseudotumor cerebri, increased BUN, painful IV infusion. Do not use Oracea for treatment of infections. Do not give antacids or calcium supplements within 2 h of doxycycline. Barbiturates, carbamazepine, rifampin, and phenytoin may decrease doxycycline levels. Take with fluids to decrease esophageal irritation; can take with food/milk. Can break Doryx tabs and give immediately in a spoonful of applesauce. Do not crush or chew delayed-release pellets in tab. Maternal antimalarial prophylaxis does not harm breastfed infant or protect infant from malaria.

MOA — Inhibits bacterial protein synthesis by binding with ribosomal 30S subunit and blocking addition of amino acids to peptide chain. Active against intracellular bacteria. Bacteriostatic. Subantimicrobial doses have anti-inflammatory effects.

ADVERSE EFFECTS — Serious: Pseudotumor cerebri, Steven-Johnson syndrome, toxic epidermal necrolysis, DRESS, increased BUN, erosive esophagitis if taken lying down, teeth staining in children younger than 8 yo. Frequent: Photosensitivity, vaginitis, painful IV infusion.

MINOCYCLINE (*Minocin, Dynacin, Solodyn*) ▶LK ♀D ▶?+ $

ADULT — Usual dose: 200 mg IV/PO 1st dose, then 100 mg q 12 h. IV and PO doses are the same. Not more than 400 mg/day IV. Community-acquired MRSA skin infections: 200 mg PO first dose, then 100 mg PO two times per day for 5 to 10 days. Solodyn ($$$$$) for inflammatory nonnodular moderate to severe acne: 1 mg/kg PO once daily. Dose is 45 mg for wt 45 to 54 kg, 65 mg for wt 55 to 77 kg, 90 mg for 78 to 102 kg, 115 mg for wt 103 to 125 kg, 135 mg for 126 to 136 kg.

PEDS — Avoid in age younger than 8 yo due to teeth staining. Usual dose: 4 mg/kg PO 1st dose, then

MINOCYCLINE (cont.)

2 mg/kg two times per day. Community-acquired MRSA skin infection: 4 mg/kg PO first dose, then 2 mg/kg/dose PO two times per day for 5 to 10 days. Do not exceed adult dose. IV and PO doses are the same. Solodyn ($$$$$) for inflammatory nonnodular moderate to severe acne, age 12 yo or older: Give PO once daily at dose of 45 mg for wt 45 to 54 kg, 65 mg for wt 55 to 77 kg, 90 mg for 78 to 102 kg, 115 mg for wt 103 to 125 kg, 135 mg for 126 to 136 kg.

UNAPPROVED ADULT — Acne vulgaris (traditional dosing, not for Solodyn): 50 mg PO two times per day. RA: 100 mg PO two times per day.

FORMS — Generic/Trade: Caps, Tabs ($) 50, 75, 100 mg. Extended-release tabs ($$$$$) 45, 90, 135 mg. Trade only: Extended-release tabs (Solodyn-$$$$$) 55, 65, 80, 105, 115 mg.

NOTES — Dizziness, hepatotoxicity, lupus. Do not use Solodyn for treatment of infections. Do not give antacids or calcium supplements within 2 h of minocycline. Take with fluids (not milk) to decrease esophageal irritation. Do not chew, crush, or split Solodyn or Ximino.

MOA — Inhibits bacterial protein synthesis by binding with ribosomal 30S subunit and blocking addition of amino acids to peptide chain. Active against intracellular bacteria. Bacteriostatic. Subantimicrobial doses have anti-inflammatory effects.

ADVERSE EFFECTS — Serious: Pseudotumor cerebri, serum sickness, Stevens-Johnson syndrome, drug rash with eosinophilia and systemic symptoms (DRESS), increased BUN, photosensitivity, hepatotoxicity, lupus, hypersensitivity pneumonitis, hyperpigmentation, teeth staining in children younger than 8 yo. Frequent: Dizziness/vestibular toxicity.

TETRACYCLINE ▶LK ♀D ▶?+ $

ADULT — Usual dose: 250 to 500 mg PO four times per day on empty stomach. H. pylori: See table in GI section. Primary, secondary, early latent syphilis if penicillin-allergic: 500 mg PO four times per day for 14 days. Late latent syphilis if penicillin-allergic: 500 mg PO four times per day for 28 days.

PEDS — Avoid in children younger than 8 yo due to teeth staining. Usual dose: 25 to 50 mg/kg/day PO divided in 2 to 4 doses on empty stomach.

UNAPPROVED ADULT — Malaria, co-therapy with quinine: 250 mg PO four times per day for 7 days.

UNAPPROVED PEDS — Avoid in children younger than 8 yo due to teeth staining. Malaria, co-therapy with quinine: 25 mg/kg/day PO divided four times per day for 7 days.

FORMS — Generic only: Caps 250, 500 mg.

NOTES — Increased BUN/hepatotoxicity in patients with renal dysfunction. Do not give antacids or calcium supplements within 2 h of tetracycline. Take with fluids (not milk) to decrease esophageal irritation.

MOA — Inhibits bacterial protein synthesis by binding with ribosomal 30S subunit and blocking addition of amino acids to peptide chain. Active against intracellular bacteria. Bacteriostatic.

ADVERSE EFFECTS — Serious: Pseudotumor cerebri, increased BUN/hepatotoxicity in patients with renal dysfunction, photosensitivity, teeth staining in children younger than 8 yo.

ANTIMICROBIALS: Other Antimicrobials

AZTREONAM (Azactam, Cayston) ▶K ♀B ▶+ $$$$$

ADULT — UTI: 500 mg to 1 g IM/IV q 8 to 12 h. Pneumonia, sepsis, skin, intra-abdominal, gynecologic: Moderate infections, 1 to 2 g IM/IV q 8 to 12 h. P. aeruginosa or severe infections, 2 g IV q 6 to 8 h. Use IV route for doses greater than 1 g. Cystic fibrosis respiratory symptoms: 1 vial Cayston nebulized three times per day for 28 days, followed by cycle of 28 days off treatment.

PEDS — Serious Gram-negative infections, usual dose: 30 mg/kg/dose IV q 6 to 8 h. Cystic fibrosis respiratory symptoms, age 7 yo and older: 1 vial Cayston nebulized three times per day for 28 days, followed by cycle of 28 days off treatment.

UNAPPROVED ADULT — Meningitis: 2 g IV q 6 to 8 h.

UNAPPROVED PEDS — P. aeruginosa pulmonary infection in cystic fibrosis: 50 mg/kg/dose IV q 6 to 8 h.

FORMS — Trade only (Cayston): 75 mg/vial with diluent for inhalation.

NOTES — Dosing in adults with renal dysfunction: 1 to 2 g IV load, then 50% of usual dose for CrCl 10 to 30 mL/min; 0.5 to 2 g IV load, then 25% of usual dose for CrCl less than 10 mL/min. For life-threatening infections, also give 12.5% of initial dose after each hemodialysis. Cayston: Use bronchodilator before each dose (short acting bronchodilator 15 min to 4 h before or long-acting bronchodilator 30 min to 12 h before). Give immediately after reconstitution only with Altera nebulizer. Order of administration is bronchodilator, mucolytic, then Cayston. Stable at room temperature for 28 days.

MOA — Monobactam (monocyclic beta-lactam) that binds only to penicillin-binding proteins in gram-negative organisms.

ADVERSE EFFECTS — Serious: Cross-sensitivity with ceftazidime possible, but unlikely, C. difficile–associated diarrhea. Frequent: Eosinophilia. Cayston for inhalation: Bronchospasm, cough, wheezing, fever.

CHLORAMPHENICOL ▶LK ♀C ▶– $$$$$

WARNING — Serious and fatal blood dyscrasias. Dose-dependent bone marrow suppression common.

ADULT — Typhoid fever, rickettsial infections: 50 mg/kg/day IV divided q 6 h. Up to 75 to 100 mg/kg/day IV for serious infections untreatable with other agents.

(cont.)

CHLORAMPHENICOL (*cont.*)

PEDS — Severe infections including meningitis: 50 to 100 mg/kg/day IV divided q 6 h. AAP recommends 75 to 100 mg/kg/day for invasive pneumococcal infections only in patients with life-threatening beta-lactam allergy.

NOTES — Monitor CBC q 2 days. Monitor serum levels. Therapeutic peak: 10 to 20 mcg/mL. Trough: 5 to 10 mcg/mL. Use cautiously in acute intermittent porphyria/G6PD deficiency. Gray baby syndrome in preemies and newborns. Barbiturates, rifampin decrease chloramphenicol levels. Chloramphenicol increases barbiturate, phenytoin levels and may increase INR with warfarin. Dosing in adults with hepatic dysfunction: 1 g IV load, then 500 mg q 6 h.

MOA — Inhibits bacterial protein synthesis by interfering with ribosomal 50S subunit. Bacteriostatic/cidal depending on pathogen.

ADVERSE EFFECTS — Serious: Fatal blood dyscrasias, dose-dependent bone marrow suppression common. Gray baby syndrome in preemies and newborns.

CLINDAMYCIN (*Cleocin, ✦Dalacin C*) ▶L ♀B ▶?+ $

WARNING — Can cause C. difficile–associated diarrhea.

ADULT — Serious anaerobic, streptococcal, staph infections: 600 to 900 mg IV q 8 h or 150 to 450 mg PO four times per day. Community-acquired MRSA skin infections: 300 to 450 mg PO three times per day for 5 to 10 days. Complicated MRSA skin infection: 600 mg IV/PO q 8 h for 7 to 14 days. MRSA pneumonia: 600 mg IV/PO q 8 h for 7 to 21 days. MRSA osteomyelitis: 600 mg IV/PO q 8 h. See tables for prophylaxis of bacterial endocardits and treatment of STDs (pelvic inflammatory disease).

PEDS — Serious anaerobic, streptococcal, staph infections: 20 to 40 mg/kg/day IV divided q 6 to 8 h or 8 to 20 mg/kg/day (as caps) PO divided three to four times per day or 8 to 25 mg/kg/day (as palmitate oral soln) PO divided three to four times per day. MRSA pneumonia, osteomyelitis, complicated skin infection: 40 mg/kg/day IV divided q 6 to 8 h. Do not use doses which are less than 37.5 mg of oral soln PO three times per day for children with wt less than 11 kg. Infants age younger than 1 mo: 15 to 20 mg/kg/day IV divided three to four times per day. See table for prophylaxis of bacterial endocarditis.

UNAPPROVED ADULT — Bacterial vaginosis: 300 mg PO two times per day for 7 days. Oral/dental infection: 300 mg PO four times per day. Prevention of perinatal group B streptococcal disease: 900 mg IV to mother q 8 h until delivery. CNS toxoplasmosis, AIDS (with leucovorin, pyrimethamine): Acute treatment 600 mg PO/IV q 6 h; secondary prevention 300 to 450 mg PO q 6 to 8 h. AHA dose for group A streptococcal pharyngitis in penicillin-allergic patients: 20 mg/kg/day (max 1.8 g/day) PO divided three times per day for 10 days. Group A streptococcal pharyngitis, repeated culture-positive episodes: 20 mg/kg/day (max 1.8 g/day) PO divided three times per day for 10 days. Malaria, co-therapy with quinine/quinidine: 10 mg/kg base IV loading dose followed by 5 mg/kg IV q 8 h or 20 mg/kg/day base PO divided three times per day to complete 7 days.

UNAPPROVED PEDS — Community-acquired MRSA skin infections: 10 to 13 mg/kg/dose PO q 6 to 8 h for 5 to 10 days (max 40 mg/kg/day). AHA dose for group A streptococcal pharyngitis in penicillin-allergic patients: 20 mg/kg/day (max 1.8 g/day) PO divided three times per day for 10 days. Group A streptococcal pharyngitis, repeated culture-positive episodes: 20 to 30 mg/kg/day PO divided q 8 h for 10 days. Otitis media, after failure of initial antibiotic treatment: 30 to 40 mg/kg/day PO divided three times per day plus third-generation cephalosporin. For oral therapy of acute otitis media, AAP recommends 5 to 7 days of therapy for children 6 yo and older with mild to moderate symptoms, 7 days for children 2 to 5 yo with mild to moderate symptoms, and 10 days for children younger than 2 yo and children with severe symptoms. See tables for management of otitis media and acute sinusitis in children. Toxoplasmosis, substitute for sulfadiazine in sulfonamide-intolerant children: 5 to 7.5 mg/kg (up to 600 mg/dose) PO/IV q 6 h + pyrimethamine + leucovorin. Malaria, co-therapy with quinine/quinidine: 10 mg/kg base IV loading dose followed by 5 mg/kg IV q 8 h or 20 mg/kg/day base PO divided three times per day to complete 7 days.

FORMS — Generic/Trade: Caps 75, 150, 300 mg. Oral soln 75 mg/5 mL (100 mL).

NOTES — Not for meningitis. Not more than 600 mg/IM injection site. Avoid if lincomycin hypersensitivity. Consider D-test for MRSA inducible resistance.

MOA — Semisynthetic derivative of lincomycin that inhibits RNA-dependent protein synthesis in susceptible organisms by interfering with function of ribosomal 50S subunit. Bacteriostatic.

ADVERSE EFFECTS — Serious: C. difficile-associated diarrhea. Frequent: Diarrhea, allergic reactions.

COLISTIMETHATE (*Coly-Mycin M Parenteral*) ▶K ♀C ▶? $$$$

ADULT — Gram-negative infections, esp. P. aeruginosa: 2.5 to 5 mg/kg/day IM/IV divided q 6 to 12 h or IV continuous infusion. Max dose is 5 mg/kg/day (colistin base activity) in patients with normal renal function. Inject IV slowly over 3 to 5 minutes q 12 h. For continuous infusion, inject half of daily dose over 3 to 5 minutes; give remainder as continuous infusion over 22 to 23 h, starting 1 to 2 h after first injection. Base dose on ideal body wt in obesity.

PEDS — Gram-negative infections, esp. P. aeruginosa: 2.5 to 5 mg/kg/day IM/IV divided q 6 to 12 h or IV continuous infusion. Max dose is 5 mg/kg/day (colistin base activity) in patients with normal renal function. Inject IV slowly over 3 to 5 minutes q 12 h. For continuous infusion, inject half of daily dose over 3 to 5 minutes; give remainder as continuous infusion over 22 to 23 h, starting 1 to 2 h after first injection. Base dose on ideal body wt in obesity.

UNAPPROVED ADULT — Cystic fibrosis: Use nebulizer soln promptly after it is made. Storage for longer

COLISTIMETHATE *(cont.)*

than 24 h increases the formation of polymyxin E1 which may cause pulmonary toxicity.

FORMS — Generic/Trade: Each vial contains colistimethate sodium equivalent to 150 mg colistin base activity.

NOTES — Each vial contains 150 mg colistin base activity. May enhance neuromuscular junction blockade by aminoglycosides, neuromuscular blockers; extreme caution advised for coadministration. Can cause transient neurologic symptoms that can be relieved by dosage reduction. Dose-dependent, reversible nephrotoxicity. Dosage adjustment in adults with renal dysfunction: 2.5 to 3.8 mg/kg divided into 2 doses per day for CrCl 50 to 79 mL/min; 2.5 mg/kg once daily or divided into 2 doses per day for CrCl 30 to 49 mL/min; 1.5 mg/kg q 36 h for CrCl 10 to 29 mL/min.

MOA — Polypeptide antibiotic that penetrates and disrupts bacterial cell membrane.

ADVERSE EFFECTS — Dose-dependent, reversible nephrotoxicity. Reports of respiratory arrest after IM administration. Transient neurologic symptoms including perioral paresthesia, numbness, vertigo, dizziness, slurred speech, generalized pruritus.

DAPTOMYCIN (*Cubicin*) ▶K ♀B ▶? $$$$$

ADULT — Complicated skin infections (including MRSA): 4 mg/kg IV once daily for 7 to 14 days. S. aureus bacteremia (including MRSA), including endocarditis: 6 mg/kg IV once daily for at least 2 to 6 weeks. Infuse over 30 min or inject over 2 min.

PEDS — Not approved in children.

UNAPPROVED ADULT — MRSA bacteremia/endocarditis, high-dose regimen: 8 to 10 mg/kg IV once daily. Vancomycin-resistant MRSA bacteremia: 10 mg/kg IV once daily in combo with another antibiotic. MRSA osteomyelitis: 6 mg/kg IV once daily.

UNAPPROVED PEDS — MRSA bacteremia/endocarditis: 6 to 10 mg/kg IV once daily. MRSA osteomyelitis: 6 mg/kg IV once daily.

NOTES — May cause myopathy (with doses of 6 mg/kg/day or greater), neuropathy, eosinophilic pneumonia (rare), C. difficile–associated diarrhea. Monitor CK levels weekly. Stop if myopathy symptoms and CK more than 5 times upper limit of normal, or no symptoms and CK at least 10 times upper limit of normal. Consider withholding statins during daptomycin treatment. Can falsely elevate PT with certain thromboplastin reagents; minimize effect by drawing PT/INR sample just before daptomycin dose or use another reagent. Not effective for pneumonia (inactivated by surfactant). Reduce dose in adults with CrCl less than 30 mL/min: 4 mg/kg IV q 48 h for complicated skin infections; 6 mg/kg IV q 48 h for S. aureus bacteremia. Give dose after hemodialysis sessions. Efficacy may be reduced in patients with CrCl less than 50 mL/min. Reconstituted soln stable for up to 12 h at room temp or 48 h in refrigerator (combined time in vial and IV bag). Do not use in Readymed

elastomeric infusion pump due to leaching of MBT impurity.

MOA — Cyclic lipopeptide that depolarizes bacterial membrane potential. Inhibition of DNA, RNA, and protein synthesis kills bacteria.

ADVERSE EFFECTS — Serious: Myopathy (with doses of 6 mg/kg/day or greater), neuropathy, eosinophilic pneumonia (rare), C difficile-associated diarrhea. Frequent: Increased CK levels, constipation, nausea, headache, abnormal LFTs, dyspnea.

FOSFOMYCIN (*Monurol*) ▶K ♀B ▶? $$$

ADULT — Simple UTI in women: One 3 g packet PO single dose. Dissolve granules in ½ cup of water.

PEDS — Not approved for age younger than 12 yo.

FORMS — Trade only: 3 g packet of granules.

NOTES — Metoclopramide decreases urinary excretion of fosfomycin. No additional benefit with multiple dosing. Single dose less effective than ciprofloxacin or TMP-SMX; equivalent to nitrofurantoin.

MOA — Inactivates enolpyruvyl transferase, irreversibly blocking an early step in bacterial cell wall synthesis. Also reduces bacterial adherence to uroepithelial cells. Bactericidal in urine.

ADVERSE EFFECTS — Serious: None. Frequent: Diarrhea.

LINCOMYCIN (*Lincocin*) ▶LK ♀C ▶– $$$$

WARNING — C. difficile–associated diarrhea.

ADULT — Serious Gram-positive infections: 600 mg IM q 12 to 24 h. 600 to 1000 mg IV q 8 to 12 h. Max IV daily dose is 8 g. Dilute to 1 g/100 mL or less, and infuse over at least 1 h. Reserve for patients who are allergic to or do not respond to penicillins.

PEDS — Serious Gram-positive infections, age older than 1 mo: 10 to 20 mg/kg/day IV divided q 8 to 12 h. Dilute to 1 g/100 mL or less, and infuse over at least 1 h. Reserve for patients who are allergic to or do not respond to penicillins.

NOTES — Do not use in patients with clindamycin hypersensitivity. Monitor hepatic and renal function and CBC during prolonged therapy. Do not coadminister with erythromycin due to potential antagonism. May enhance effects of neuromuscular blockers. Reduce dose by 25% to 30% in patients with severe renal dysfunction and consider monitoring levels.

MOA — Inhibits RNA-dependent protein synthesis in susceptible organisms by interfering with function of ribosomal 50S subunit.

ADVERSE EFFECTS — Serious: C. difficile-associated diarrhea; severe hypersensitivity reactions; Stevens-Johnson syndrome; neutropenia; thrombocytopenia; renal dysfunction. Hypotension/cardiopulmonary arrest possible if IV infusion too rapid. Frequent: No data.

LINEZOLID (*Zyvox,* ✦*Zyvoxam*) ▶Oxidation/K ♀C ▶? $$$$$

ADULT — IV and PO doses are the same. Vancomycin-resistant E. faecium infections: 600 mg IV/PO q 12 h for 14 to 28 days. Pneumonia, complicated skin infections (including MRSA and diabetic foot): 600

(cont.)

LINEZOLID (*cont.*)

mg IV/PO q 12 h for 10 to 14 days. IV infused over 30 to 120 min.

PEDS — Pneumonia, complicated skin infections (including MRSA): 10 mg/kg (up to 600 mg) IV/PO q 8 h for age younger than 12 yo; 600 mg IV/PO q 12 h for age 12 yo or older. Treat for for 10 to 14 days. Vancomycin-resistant E. faecium infections: 10 mg/kg IV/PO q 8 h (up to 600 mg) for age younger than 12 yo; 600 mg IV/PO q 12 h for age 12 yo or older. Treat for 14 to 28 days. Uncomplicated skin infections: 10 mg/kg PO q 8 h for age younger than 5 yo; 10 mg/kg PO q 12 h for age 5 to 11 yo; 600 mg PO q 12 h for age 12 yo or older. Treat for 10 to 14 days. Preterm infants (less than 34 weeks gestational age): 10 mg/kg q 12 h, increase to 10 mg/kg q 8 h by 7 days of life. IV infused over 30 to 120 min.

UNAPPROVED ADULT — Community-acquired MRSA skin infection: 600 mg PO two times per day for 5 to 10 days.

UNAPPROVED PEDS — Community-acquired MRSA skin infection: 10 mg/kg (up to 600 mg) PO q 8 h for age younger than 12 yo; 600 mg PO q 12 h for age 12 yo or older. Treat for 5 to 10 days.

FORMS — Trade only: Tabs 600 mg. Susp 100 mg/5 mL.

NOTES — Myelosuppression. Monitor CBC weekly, especially if more than 2 weeks of therapy, pre-existing myelosuppression, other myelosuppressive drugs, or chronic infection treated with other antibiotics. Consider stopping if myelosuppression occurs or worsens. Peripheral and optic neuropathy, primarily in those treated for more than 1 month. Ophthalmic exam recommended for visual changes at any time; monitor visual function in all patients treated for 3 months or longer. In a study comparing linezolid with vancomycin, oxacillin, or dicloxacillin for catheter-related bloodstream infections, mortality was increased in linezolid-treated patients infected only with Gram-negative bacteria. Inhibits MAO; may interact with adrenergic and serotonergic drugs, high-tyramine foods. Limit tyramine to less than 100 mg/meal. Reduce initial dose of dopamine/epinephrine. Serotonin syndrome reported with concomitant administration of serotonergic drugs (SSRIs). Rifampin can reduce linezolid exposure; clinical significance unclear. Hypoglycemia reported in diabetics treated with insulin or oral hypoglycemics. Store susp at room temperature; stable for 21 days. Gently turn bottle over 3 to 5 times before giving a dose; do not shake.

MOA — Oxazolidinone that inhibits bacterial protein synthesis by binding with 50S ribosome (may compete for binding with chloramphenicol). Bacteriostatic.

ADVERSE EFFECTS — Serious: Myelosuppression, reports of serotonin syndrome, peripheral and optic neuropathy (with long-term use; optic neuropathy sometimes progressing to vision loss), lactic acidosis (immediate evaluation if recurrent

N/V, unexplained acidosis, low bicarbonate). Hypoglycemia reported in diabetics treated with insulin or oral hypoglycemics. In a study comparing linezolid with vancomycin, oxacillin, dicloxacillin for catheter-related bloodstream infections, mortality was increased in linezolid-treated patients infected only with gram-negative bacteria. Frequent: Thrombocytopenia, N/V, diarrhea. Tooth discoloration (removable with cleaning).

METHENAMINE HIPPURATE (*Hiprex, Urex*) ▶KL ♀C ▶? $$$$

ADULT — Long-term suppression of UTI: 1 g PO two times per day.

PEDS — Long-term suppression of UTI: 0.5 to 1 g PO two times per day for 6 to 12 yo; 1 g PO two times per day for older than 12 yo.

FORMS — Generic/Trade: Tab 1 g.

NOTES — Not for UTI treatment. Contraindicated if renal or severe hepatic impairment, severe dehydration. Acidify urine if Proteus, Pseudomonas infections. Give 1 to 2 g vitamin C PO q 4 h if urine pH > 5. Avoid sulfonamides, alkalinizing foods and medications.

MOA — Releases formaldehyde (bactericidal) in acidic urine.

ADVERSE EFFECTS — Frequent: N/V, rash, dysuria.

METRONIDAZOLE (*Flagyl, Flagyl ER, ✲Nidazol*) ▶KL ♀B ▶?- $

WARNING — Carcinogenic in animal studies; avoid unnecessary use.

ADULT — Trichomoniasis: Treat patient and sex partners with 2 g PO single dose (may be used in pregnancy per CDC), 250 mg PO three times per day for 7 days, or 375 mg PO two times per day for 7 days. Flagyl ER for bacterial vaginosis: 750 mg PO daily for 7 days on empty stomach. H. pylori: See table in GI section. Anaerobic bacterial infections: Load 1 g or 15 mg/kg IV, then 500 mg or 7.5 mg/kg IV/PO q 6 to 8 h (up to 4 g/day), each IV dose over 1 h. Prophylaxis, colorectal surgery: 15 mg/kg IV completed 1 h preop, then 7.5 mg/kg IV q 6 h for 2 doses. Acute amebic dysentery: 750 mg PO three times per day for 5 to 10 days. Amebic liver abscess: 500 to 750 mg IV/PO three times per day for 10 days.

PEDS — Amebiasis: 35 to 50 mg/kg/day PO (up to 750 mg/dose) divided three times per day for 10 days.

UNAPPROVED ADULT — Bacterial vaginosis: 500 mg PO two times per day for 7 days. Bacterial vaginosis in pregnancy: 500 mg PO two times per day or 250 mg PO three times per day for 7 days. Trichomoniasis (CDC alternative to single dose): 500 mg PO two times per day for 7 days. Pelvic inflammatory disease, recurrent/persistent urethritis: See STD table. C. difficile–associated diarrhea, mild/moderate: 500 mg PO three times per day for 10 to 14 days. C. difficile–associated diarrhea, severe complicated: 500 mg IV q 8 h with PO/PR vancomycin. See table for management of C. difficile infection in adults.

(cont.)

METRONIDAZOLE *(cont.)*

Giardia: 250 mg PO three times per day for 5 to 7 days.
UNAPPROVED PEDS — C. difficile–associated diarrhea: 30 mg/kg/day PO divided four times per day for 10 to 14 days (not to exceed adult dose). Trichomoniasis: 5 mg/kg PO three times per day (max 2 g/day) for 7 days. Giardia: 15 mg/kg/day PO divided three times per day for 5 to 7 days. Anaerobic bacterial infections: 30 mg/kg/day IV/PO divided q 6 h, each IV dose over 1 h (up to 4 g/day).
FORMS — Generic/Trade: Tabs 250, 500 mg. Trade only: Caps 375 mg. Extended-release tab: 750 mg.
NOTES — Peripheral neuropathy (chronic use), seizures, encephalopathy, aseptic meningitis, optic neuropathy. Avoid long-term use. Disulfiram reaction; avoid alcohol until at least 1 day after treatment with tabs, at least 3 days with caps/Flagyl ER. Do not give within 2 weeks of disulfiram. Interacts with barbiturates, lithium, phenytoin. Increased INR with warfarin. Darkens urine. Give iodoquinol or paromomycin after treatment for amebic dysentery or liver abscess. Can minimize infant exposure by withholding breastfeeding for 12 to 24 h after maternal single dose. Decrease dose in liver dysfunction.
MOA — Bactericidal agent that is reduced intracellularly to toxic intermediates/free radicals that damage DNA or other macromolecules.
ADVERSE EFFECTS — Serious: Peripheral neuropathy (chronic use), seizures, encephalopathy, aseptic meningitis, optic neuropathy. Frequent: Darkens urine, N/V, diarrhea, metallic aftertaste, disulfiram-like reaction.

NITROFURANTOIN *(Furadantin, Macrodantin, Macrobid)* ▶KL ♀B ▶+? $$
ADULT — Uncomplicated UTI: 50 to 100 mg PO four times per day for 7 days or until 3 days after sterile urine. Long-term suppressive therapy: 50 to 100 mg PO at bedtime. Macrobid for uncomplicated UTI: 100 mg PO two times per day for 7 days. Take nitrofurantoin with food.
PEDS — Uncomplicated UTI: 5 to 7 mg/kg/day PO divided four times per day for 7 days or until 3 days after sterile urine. Long-term suppressive therapy: Doses as low as 1 mg/kg/day PO divided one to two times per day. Macrobid for uncomplicated UTI, age older than 12 yo: 100 mg PO two times per day for 7 days. Take nitrofurantoin with food.
UNAPPROVED ADULT — Uncomplicated cystitis in women: IDSA recommends 100 mg Macrobid PO two times per day for 5 days (avoid if early pyelonephritis suspected).
FORMS — Generic/Trade: Caps (Macrodantin) 25, 50, 100 mg. Caps (Macrobid) 100 mg. Susp (Furadantin) 25 mg/5 mL.
NOTES — Contraindicated if CrCl less than 60 mL/min, pregnancy 38 weeks or longer, infant age younger than 1 mo. Hemolytic anemia in G6PD deficiency (including susceptible infants exposed through breastmilk), hepatotoxicity (monitor LFTs periodically), peripheral

neuropathy. May turn urine brown. Do not use for complicated UTI or pyelonephritis.
MOA — Appears to interact with ribosomal proteins and damage bacterial DNA.
ADVERSE EFFECTS — Serious: Pulmonary fibrosis with prolonged use, hepatotoxicity, peripheral neuropathy, hemolytic anemia in G6PD deficiency. Frequent: N/V, allergy, brown discoloration of urine.

RAXIBACUMAB ▶? ♀B ▶?
ADULT — Inhalation anthrax, treatment in combo with antibiotics or for prevention when other options are not available or inappropriate: 40 mg/kg single dose IV over 135 minutes. Premedicate with diphenhydramine 25 to 50 mg IV/PO within 1 h before infusion. See www.bt.cdc.gov/bioterrorism/ for more info.
PEDS — Inhalation anthrax, treatment in combo with antibiotics or for prevention when other options are not available or inappropriate: Infuse IV over 135 minutes a single dose of 80 mg/kg for wt 15 kg or less, 60 mg/kg for wt 15 to 50 kg, 40 mg/kg for wt greater than 50 kg. Premedicate with diphenhydramine 25 to 50 mg IV/PO within 1 h before infusion. See www.bt.cdc.gov/bioterrorism/ for more info.
FORMS — Not available commercially. Distribution of raxibacumab managed by CDC.
NOTES — Does not cross blood-brain barrier; does not treat or prevent meningitis. Efficacy is based on animal studies. Reduce infusion rate or interrupt infusion if infusion reaction (rash, pruritus, urticaria) occurs.
MOA — Anthrax antitoxin. Raxibacumab is a monoclonal antibody that neutralizes anthrax toxin (no direct antibacterial activity).
ADVERSE EFFECTS — Infusion-related rash (reduced by diphenhydramine pretreatment), extremity pain, pruritus, somnolence, mild clonus, moderate dyspnea.

RIFAXIMIN *(Xifaxan)* ▶feces ♀C ▶? $$$$
ADULT — Traveler's diarrhea: 200 mg PO three times per day for 3 days. Prevention of recurrent hepatic encephalopathy ($$$$$): 550 mg PO two times per day.
PEDS — Not approved for age younger than 12 yo.
UNAPPROVED ADULT — Irritable bowel syndrome, non-constipation with bloating: 550 mg PO two to three times per day for 14 days.
FORMS — Trade only: Tabs 200, 550 mg.
NOTES — Not effective for diarrhea complicated by fever/blood in stool or caused by pathogens other than E. coli. Consider switching to another agent if diarrhea persists for 24 to 48 h or worsens. P-glycoprotein inhibitors (e.g., cyclosporine; see p-glycoprotein table) can substantially increase rifaximin exposure, esp. if hepatic impairment. Rifaximin exposure may increase in severe hepatic impairment.
MOA — Rifamycin structurally related to rifampin. Inhibits bacterial RNA synthesis by binding with beta-subunit of bacterial DNA-dependent RNA

(cont.)

RIFAXIMIN (*cont.*)

polymerase. Active against entero-toxigenic or -aggregative E Coli.
ADVERSE EFFECTS — Serious: None found. Frequent: None found.

SYNERCID (**quinupristin + dalfopristin**) ▶Bile ♀B ▶? $$$$$
ADULT — Complicated staphylococcal/streptococcal skin infections: 7.5 mg/kg IV q 12 h. Infuse over 1 h.
PEDS — Safety and efficacy not established in children.
UNAPPROVED ADULT — MRSA bacteremia (2nd line): 7.5 mg/kg IV q 8 h.
UNAPPROVED PEDS — Complicated staphylococcal/ streptococcal skin infections: 7.5 mg/kg IV q 12 h. Infuse over 1 h.
NOTES — Indication for vancomycin-resistant E. faecium infections was removed from labeling because efficacy was not demonstrated in clinical trials. Venous irritation (flush with D5W after peripheral infusion; do not use normal saline/heparin), arthralgias/myalgias, hyperbilirubinemia. Infuse by central venous catheter to avoid dose-related vein irritation. CYP3A4 inhibitor. Increases levels of cyclosporine, midazolam, nifedipine, and others.
MOA — Streptogramin fixed-dose combination that inhibits bacterial protein synthesis by binding to different sites of the 50S ribosomal subunit and forming a stable tertiary complex with each other and the ribosome.
ADVERSE EFFECTS — Serious: None. Frequent: Venous irritation after peripheral infusion, arthralgia/myalgia, hyperbilirubinemia.

TEDIZOLID (*Sivextro*) ▶L ♀C ▶? $$$$$
ADULT — Skin infections, including MRSA: 200 mg IV/PO once daily for 6 days. Infuse IV over 1 hour.
PEDS — Safety and efficacy not established in children.
FORMS — Trade only: Tabs 200 mg.
NOTES — Consider alternatives in neutropenic patients; tedizolid was not evaluated in neutropenic patients and antibacterial activity was reduced in the absence of granulocytes in an animal model. Tedizolid is a weak, reversible MAO inhibitor in vitro. The FDA briefing document for tedizolid concluded that no restrictions are necessary for coadministration with adrenergic or serotonergic drugs and tyramine-rich foods. Phase 3 clinical trials excluded MOA inhibitors,serotonergic drugs, and a high-tyramine diet.
MOA — Oxazolidinone that inhibits bacterial protein synthesis by binding with 50S ribosome. Bacteriostatic.
ADVERSE EFFECTS — Serious: C. difficile-associated diarrhea. Frequent: N/V, diarrhea, headache, dizziness.

TELITHROMYCIN (*Ketek*) ▶LK ♀C ▶? $$$$
WARNING — Contraindicated in myasthenia gravis due to reports of exacerbation, including fatal acute respiratory depression. Warn patients about exacerbation of myasthenia gravis, hepatotoxicity, visual disturbances, and loss of consciousness.
ADULT — Community-acquired pneumonia: 800 mg PO daily for 7 to 10 days. Indications for acute sinusitis and acute exacerbation of chronic bronchitis removed from labeling because potential benefit no longer justifies risk of adverse effects.
PEDS — Safety and efficacy not established in children.
FORMS — Trade only: Tabs 300, 400 mg.
NOTES — May prolong QT interval. Avoid in proarrhythmic conditions or with drugs that prolong QT interval. Life-threatening hepatotoxicity. Monitor for signs/symptoms of hepatitis. Contraindicated if history of hepatitis due to any macrolide or telithromycin. Contraindicated in myasthenia gravis. CYP3A4 substrate and inhibitor. Contraindicated with pimozide, rifampin, ergot alkaloids. Withhold simvastatin, lovastatin, or atorvastatin during course of telithromycin. Consider monitoring INR with warfarin. Give telithromycin and theophylline at least 1 h apart. Monitor for increased toxicity of digoxin, midazolam, metoprolol. CYP3A4 inducers (i.e., phenytoin, carbamazepine) could reduce telithromycin levels. Dosage adjustment for CrCl less than 30 mL/min (including hemodialysis) is 600 mg once daily. On dialysis days, give after hemodialysis session. Dosage adjustment for CrCl less than 30 mL/min with hepatic dysfunction is 400 mg once daily.
MOA — Ketolide; structure and mechanism of action similar to macrolides. Inhibits protein synthesis in susceptible organisms by interfering with function of ribosomal 50S subunit. Methoxy and ketone groups enhance acid stability and ribosomal binding, and reduce susceptibility to drug efflux pumps.
ADVERSE EFFECTS — Serious: Exacerbation of myasthenia gravis; hepatotoxicity. Frequent: Diarrhea, nausea, dizziness, elevated LFTs. Other: Visual disturbances, esp. difficulty in accommodation (rare; most cases occur after 1st or 2nd dose in women less than 40 yo), transient loss of consciousness.

TIGECYCLINE (*Tygacil*) ▶Bile, K ♀D ▶?+ $$$$$
WARNING — Tigacycline had 0.6% higher mortality rate than comparators in meta-analysis of phase 3 and 4 clinical trials. Use it only when alternatives are not appropriate.
ADULT — Complicated skin infections, complicated intra-abdominal infections, community-acquired pneumonia: 100 mg IV 1st dose, then 50 mg IV q 12 h. Infuse over 30 to 60 min. Not approved for hospital-acquired or ventilator-associated pneumonia (decreased efficacy and higher mortality) or diabetic foot infection (decreased efficacy).
PEDS — Not approved in children. Avoid in children age younger than 8 yo due to permanent teeth staining.
NOTES — Caution advised for tigecycline monotherapy of complicated intra-abdominal infection due to intestinal perforation. Discard reconstituted tigacycline if it does not have yellow-orange

(cont.)

TIGECYCLINE (*cont.*)

color. May decrease efficacy of oral contraceptives. Monitor INR with warfarin. Dosage adjustment for severe liver dysfunction (Child-Pugh C): 100 mg IV 1st dose, then 25 mg IV q 12 h.

MOA — Inhibits bacterial protein synthesis by binding with ribosomal 30S subunit and blocking addition of amino acids to peptide chain. Bacteriostatic.

ADVERSE EFFECTS — Serious: Higher mortality than other antibiotics, especially in ventilator-associated pneumonia. Anaphylaxis/anaphylactoid rxns, acute pancreatitis, hepatic dysfunction. Other adverse effects may be similar to tetracyclines (Serious: Pseudotumor cerebri, anti-anabolic effects, photoxxsxxxxensitivity, permanent teeth staining in children younger than 8 yo.) Frequent: N/V.

TRIMETHOPRIM (*Primsol, ✦Proloprim*) ▶K ♀C ▶– $

ADULT — Uncomplicated UTI: 100 mg PO two times per day or 200 mg PO daily.

PEDS — Safety not established in age younger than 2 mo. Otitis media (not for M. catarrhalis): 10 mg/kg/day PO divided two times per day for 10 days for age 6 mo or older. Trimethoprim is not a good option for otitis media; see otitis media treatment table for alternatives.

UNAPPROVED ADULT — Prophylaxis of recurrent UTI: 100 mg PO at bedtime. Pneumocystis treatment: 5 mg/kg PO three times per day with dapsone 100 mg PO daily for 21 days.

FORMS — Generic only: Tabs 100 mg. Trade only (Primsol): Oral soln 50 mg/5 mL.

NOTES — Contraindicated in megaloblastic anemia due to folate deficiency. Blood dyscrasias. Inhibits metabolism of phenytoin. Can cause hyperkalemia (risk increased by high doses of trimethoprim, renal impairment, or other drugs that cause hyperkalemia). Dosing in adults with renal dysfunction: 50 mg PO q 12 h for CrCl 15 to 30 mL/min. Do not use if CrCl < 15 mL/min.

MOA — Folate antagonist; inhibits bacterial dihydrofolate reductase, the enzyme after step in folate synthesis inhibited by sulfonamides.

ADVERSE EFFECTS — Serious: Blood dyscrasias. Frequent: Rash, pruritus.

CARDIOVASCULAR

ACE INHIBITOR DOSING

ACE INHIBITOR DOSING	HTN		Heart Failure	
	Initial	*Max/day*	*Initial*	*Max/day*
benazepril (*Lotensin*)	10 mg daily*	80 mg	-	-
captopril (*Capoten*)	25 mg bid/tid	450 mg	6.25 mg tid	450 mg
enalapril (*Vasotec*)	5 mg daily*	40 mg	2.5 mg bid	40 mg
fosinopril (*Monopril*)	10 mg daily*	80 mg	5-10 mg daily	40 mg
lisinopril (*Zestril/ Prinivil*)	10 mg daily	80 mg	2.5-5 mg daily	40 mg
moexipril (*Univasc*)	7.5 mg daily*	30 mg	-	-
perindopril (*Aceon*)	4 mg daily*	16 mg	2 mg daily	16 mg
quinapril (*Accupril*)	10-20 mg daily*	80 mg	5 mg bid	40 mg
ramipril (*Altace*)	2.5 mg daily*	20 mg	1.25-2.5 mg bid	10 mg
trandolapril (*Mavik*)	1-2 mg daily*	8 mg	1 mg daily	4 mg

bid=two times per day; tid=three times per day.

Data taken from prescribing information and *Circulation* 2013;128:e240-e327.

* May require bid dosing for 24-h BP control.

LIPID CHANGE BY CLASS/AGENT[1]

Drug class/agent	LDL-C	HDL-C	TG
Atorvastatin+ezetimibe[2]	↓ 53–61%	↑ 5–9%	↓ 30–40%
Bile acid sequestrants[3]	↓ 15–30%	↑ 3–5%	No change or ↑
Cholesterol absorption inhibitor[4]	↓ 18%	↑ 1%	↓ 8%
Fibrates[5]	↓ 5–20%	↑ 10–20%	↓ 20–50%
Lovastatin+ext'd release niacin[6]*	↓ 30–42%	↑ 20–30%	↓ 32–44%
Niacin[7]*	↓ 5–25%	↑ 15–35%	↓ 20–50%
Omega3 fatty acids[8]	↓ 5% or ↑ 44%	↓ 4% or ↑ 9%	↓ 27–45%
Statins[9]	↓ 18–63%	↑ 5–15%	↓ 7–35%
Simvastatin+ezetimibe[10]	↓ 45–59%	↑ 6–10%	↓ 23–31%

LDL-C= low density lipoprotein cholesterol. HDL-C = high density lipoprotein cholesterol. TG = triglycerides.
[1]Adapted from prescribing information.
[2]Liptruzet® (10/10–10/80 mg).
[3]Cholestyramine (4–16 g), colestipol (5–20 g), colesevelam (2.6–3.8 g).
[4]Ezetimibe (10 mg). When added to statin therapy, will ↓ LDL-C 25%, ↑ HDL-C 3%, ↓ TG 14% in addition
 to statin effects.
[5]Fenofibrate (145–200 mg), gemfibrozil (600 mg two times per day).
[6]Advicor® (20/1000–40/2000 mg).
[7]Extended release nicotinic acid (Niaspan® 1–2 g), immediate release (crystalline) nicotinic acid (1.5–3 g),
 sustained release nicotinic acid (Slo-Niacin® 1–2 g).
[8]Epanova® (4 g), Lovaza® (4 g), Vascepa® (4 g)
[9]Atorvastatin (10–80 mg), fluvastatin (20–80 mg), lovastatin (20–80 mg), pravastatin (20–80 mg),
 rosuvastatin (5–40 mg), simvastatin (20–40 mg).
[10]Vytorin® (10/10–10/40 mg).
*Lowers lipoprotein a.

CARDIAC PARAMETERS AND FORMULAS

Cardiac output (CO) = heart rate × CVA volume [normal 4 to 8 L/min]
Cardiac index (CI) = CO/BSA [normal 2.8 to 4.2 L/min/m^2]
MAP (mean arterial pressure) = [(SBP − DBP)/3] + DBP [normal 80 to 100 mmHg]
SVR (systemic vascular resistance) = (MAP − CVP) × (80)/CO [normal 800 to 1200 dyne x sec/cm^5]
PVR (pulmonary vasc resisistance) = (PAM − PCWP) × (80)/CO [normal 45 to 120 dyne x sec/cm^5]
QTc = QT/square root of RR [normal 0.38 to 0.42]
Right atrial pressure (central venous pressure) [normal 0 to 8 mmHg]
Pulmonary artery systolic pressure (PAS) [normal 20 to 30 mmHg]
Pulmonary artery diastolic pressure (PAD) [normal 10 to 15 mmHg]
Pulmonary capillary wedge pressure (PCWP) [normal 8 to 12 mmHg (post-MI ~16 mmHg)]

ANTIHYPERTENSIVE COMBINATION PRODUCTS

ACEI + Diuretic	Accuretic, Capozide, ♣ Inhibace Plus, Lotensin HCT, Monopril HCT, Prinzide, Uniretic, Vaseretic, Zestoretic
ACEI + CCB	Lotrel, Tarka
ARB + Diuretic	Atacand HCT, ♣ Atacand Plus, Avalide, Benicar HCT, Diovan HCT, Edarbyclor, Hyzaar, ♣ Micardis Plus, Micardis HCT, Teveten HCT
ARB + CCB	Azor, Exforge, Twynsta
ARB + CCB + Diuretic	Exforge HCT, Tribenzor
Beta-blocker + Diuretic	Corzide, Dutoprol, Inderide, Lopressor HCT, Tenoretic, Ziac
CCB + Statin	Caduet
Direct Renin Inhibitor + CCB	Tekamlo
Direct Renin Inhibitor + CCB + Diuretic	Amturnide
Direct Renin Inhibitor + Diuretic	♣ Rasilez HCT, Tekturna HCT
Diuretic combinations	Aldactazide, Dyazide, Maxzide, ♣ Moduret, Moduretic, ♣ Triazide
Diuretic + Miscellaneous Antihypertensive	Aldoril, Apresazide, Clorpres, Minizide

ACEI = ACE inhibitor; ARB = angiotensin receptor blocker; CCB = calcium channel blocker.

CHOLESTEROL TREATMENT RECOMMENDATIONS (AGES ≥ 21 YEARS)

Consider benefits, risks, drug–drug interactions, adverse effects, and patient preferences before initiating statin therapy.

[1]Rule out secondary causes. If non-fasting triglycerides ≥ 500 mg/dL, then a fasting lipid panel is needed.

[2]High-intensity statin = atorvastatin 40, 80 mg; rosuvastatin 20, 40 mg. Moderate-intensity statin is acceptable if patient is not a candidate for high-intensity statin therapy. Moderate-intensity statin = atorvastatin 10, 20 mg; fluvastatin 40 mg twice daily, fluvastatin XL 80 mg; lovastatin 40 mg; pitavastatin 2, 4 mg; pravastatin 40, 80 mg; rosuvastatin 5, 10 mg; simvastatin 20, 40 mg.

[3]Calculator available: http://tools.cardiosource.org/ASCVD-Risk-Estimator/

ASCVD = atherosclerotic cardiovascular disease (includes coronary heart disease, stroke, and peripheral artery disease. DM = Diabetes mellitus. LCL-C = low-density lipoprotein cholesterol. Rx = prescription strength.

Adapted from: *J Am Coll Cardiol.* 2014; 63(25_PA), *Circulation.* 2011; 123: 2292–2333.

HIGH- AND MODERATE-INTENSITY STATIN DOSES

Statin	High-Intensity Dose (Lowers LDL-C at least 50%)	Moderate-Intensity Dose (Lowers LDL-C 30% to <50%)
atorvastatin	40, 80 mg	10, 20 mg
fluvastatin XL	n/a	80 mg
fluvastatin	n/a	40 mg twice daily
lovastatin	n/a	40 mg
pitavastatin	n/a	2, 4 mg
pravastatin	n/a	40, 80 mg
rosuvastatin	20, 40 mg	5, 10 mg
simvastatin	n/a	20, 40 mg

LDL-C = low density lipoprotein cholesterol. Will get ~6% decrease in LDL-C with every doubling of dose.

Adapted from *J Am Coll Cardiol.* 2014; 63(25_PA).

HTN THERAPY FOR ADULTS ≥ 18 YEARS OLD

Patient Information		BP Target (mm Hg)	Preferred therapy	Comments
All patients with CKD (with or without DM)	Any age	< 140/90	Start ACEI or ARB; alone or in combination with drug from another class[1]	Implement lifestyle interventions; reinforce adherence during patient encounters. Drug treatment strategy based on response and tolerance: Either, titrate first drug to max dose before adding second; add second drug before reaching max dose of first drug; or start with 2 drug classes separately or as fixed dose combinations.[2,3]
Nonblack (no CKD)	Any age + DM	< 140/90	Start ACEI, ARB, CCB, or thiazide; alone or combination[1]	
	Age < 60 yo (no DM or CKD)	< 140/90		
	Age ≥ 60 yo (no DM or CKD)	< 150/90		
Black (no CKD)	Any age + DM	< 140/90	Start CCB or thiazide; alone or combination[1]	
	Age < 60 yo (no DM or CKD)	< 140/90		
	Age ≥ 60 yo (no DM or CKD)	< 150/90		

[1]Do not combine ACEI and ARB therapy.

[2]Consider starting with 2 drugs when SBP is > 160 mmHg and/or DBP is > 100 mm Hg, or if SBP is > 20 mm Hg above goal and/or DBP is > 10 mm Hg above goal. If goal BP is not achieved with 2 drugs, select a third drug from the list. Titrate prn.

[3] If needed, may add another drug (eg, beta-blocker, aldosterone antagonist, others) and/or refer to physician with HTN management expertise. ACEI = angiotensin converting enzyme inhibitor; ARB = angiotensin-receptor blocker; CCB = calcium-channel blocker; CKD = chronic kidney disease.

SELECTED DRUGS THAT MAY PROLONG THE QT INTERVAL

alfuzosin	dronedarone*	isradipine	promethazine
amantadine	droperidol*	lapatinib	quetiapine
amiodarone*	eribulin	levofloxacin*	quinidine*
anagrelide*	erythromycin*	lithium	ranolazine
arsenic trioxide*	escitalopram*	methadone*	risperidone
atazanavir	famotidine	mirabegron	saquinavir
azithromycin*	felbamate	mirtazapine	sevoflurane*
bedaquiline	fingolimod	moexipril/HCTZ	sotalol*
chloroquine*	flecainide*	moxifloxacin*	sunitinib
chlorpromazine*	foscarnet	nicardipine	tacrolimus
cisapride*	fosphenytoin	nilotinib	tamoxifen
citalopram*	gatifloxacin	ofloxacin	telithromycin
clarithromycin*	gemifloxacin	olanzapine	thioridazine*
clozapine	granisetron	ondansetron*	tizanidine
cocaine*	halofantrine*	oxytocin	tolterodine
dexmedetomidine	haloperidol*	paliperidone	vandetanib*
disopyramide*	ibutilide*	pentamidine*	vardenafil
dofetilide*	iloperidone	perflutren lipid	venlafaxine
dolasetron	indapamide	microspheres	voriconazole
		pimozide*	ziprasidone
		procainamide*	

NOTE: This table may not include all drugs that prolong the QT interval or cause torsades. Risk of drug-induced QT prolongation may be increased in women, elderly, hypokalemia, hypomagnesemia, bradycardia, starvation, CHF, and CNS injuries. Hepatorenal dysfunction and drug interactions can increase the concentration of QT interval-prolonging drugs. Coadministration of QT interval prolonging drugs can have additive effects. Avoid these (and other) drugs in congenital prolonged QT syndrome (www.crediblemeds.org).

*Torsades reported in product labeling/case reports.

THROMBOLYTIC THERAPY FOR ST-SEGMENT ELEVATION MI (STEMI)

Indications (if high-volume cath lab unavailable)	Clinical history and presentation strongly suggestive of MI within 12 h plus at least 1 of the following: 1 mm ST elevation in at least 2 contiguous leads; new left BBB; or 2 mm ST depression in V1-4 suggestive of true posterior MI.
Absolute contraindications	Previous intracranial hemorrhage; known cerebral vascular lesion (arteriovenous malformation); known malignant intracranial neoplasm; recent (<3 months) ischemic CVA (except acute ischemic CVA <4.5 h); aortic dissection; active bleeding or bleeding diathesis (excluding menses); significant closed head or facial trauma (<3 months); intracranial or intraspinal surgery (<2 months); severe uncontrolled HTN (unresponsive to emergency therapy); for streptokinase: prior exposure (<6 months).
Relative contraindications	Severe uncontrolled HTN (>180/110 mm Hg) on presentation or chronic severe HTN; prior ischemic CVA (>3 months), dementia, other intracranial pathology; traumatic/prolonged (>10 min) cardiopulmonary resuscitation; major surgery (<3 weeks); recent (within 2–4 weeks) internal bleeding; puncture of noncompressible vessel; pregnancy; active peptic ulcer disease; current use of anticoagulants.

Reference: *Circulation* 2013;127:e362-425

CARDIOVASCULAR: ACE Inhibitors

NOTE: See also Antihypertensive Combinations. Contraindicated in pregnancy or with history of angioedema. Women of child bearing age should use reliable form of contraception; discontinue ACE inhibitor as soon as pregnancy is detected. Do not use with aliskiren in patients with DM or CrCl < 60 mL/min. Dual inhibition of renin-angiotensin system increases risk of renal impairment, hypotension, and hyperkalemia. Hyperkalemia possible, especially if used concomitantly with other drugs that increase K+ (including K+ containing salt substitutes) and in patients with heart failure, DM, or renal impairment. An increase in serum creatinine up to 35% above baseline is acceptable and is not reason to withhold therapy unless hyperkalemia occurs. Concomitant NSAID, including selective COX-2 inhibitors, may further deteriorate renal function and decrease antihypertensive effects. Consider intestinal angioedema if abdominal pain (with or without N/V). African Americans and smokers may be at higher risk for angioedema. Concomitant mTOR inhibitor (eg, temsirolimus) may increase angioedema risk. Swelling of tongue, glottis, or larynx may result in airway obstruction, especially with history of airway surgery. Increases risk of hypotension with volume depleted or hyponatremic patients. African Americans may need higher dose to achieve adequate response. Renoprotection and decreased cardiovascular morbidity/mortality seen with some ACE inhibitors are most likely a class effect. Anaphylactoid reactions have been reported when ACE inhibitor patients are dialyzed with high-flux membranes (eg, AN69) or undergoing low-density lipoprotein apheresis with dextran sulfate absorption. Nitroid reactions (facial flushing, N/V, hypotension) have been reported with concomitant gold injections. Cholestatic hepatitis or acute liver failure have been reported with ACE inhibitor use; if patient develops jaundice or marked elevations of hepatic enzymes, discontinue ACE inhibitor.

BENAZEPRIL (*Lotensin*) ▶LK ♀D ▶? $$

WARNING — Do not use in pregnancy.

ADULT — HTN: Start 10 mg PO daily, usual maintenance dose 20 to 40 mg PO daily or divided two times per day, max 80 mg/day, but added effect not apparent above 40 mg/day. Elderly, renal impairment, or concomitant diuretic therapy: Start 5 mg PO daily.

PEDS — HTN: Start 0.2 mg/kg/day (max 10 mg/day) as monotherapy; doses greater than 0.6 mg/kg/day or 40 mg/day have not been studied. Do not use if age younger than 6 yo or if glomerular filtration rate less than 30 mL/min.

UNAPPROVED ADULT — Renoprotective dosing: 10 mg PO daily. Heart failure: Start 5 mg PO daily, usual 5 to 20 mg/day, max 40 mg/day (in 1 to 2 doses).

FORMS — Generic/Trade: Tabs, unscored 5, 10, 20, 40 mg.

NOTES — Twice daily dosing may be required for 24 h BP control.

MOA — Inhibits angiotensin-converting enzyme which converts angiotensin I to angiotensin II.

ADVERSE EFFECTS — Serious: Angioedema, hyperkalemia, renal impairment. Frequent: Cough.

CAPTOPRIL (*Capoten*) ▶LK ♀D ▶+ $$$

WARNING — Do not use in pregnancy.

ADULT — HTN: Start 25 mg PO two to three times per day, usual maintenance dose 25 to 150 mg PO two to three times per day, max 450 mg/day. Elderly, renal impairment, or concomitant diuretic therapy: Start 6.25 to 12.5 mg PO two to three times per day. Heart failure: Start 6.25 to 12.5 mg PO three times per day, usual 50 to 100 mg PO three times per day, max 450 mg/day. Diabetic nephropathy: 25 mg PO three times per day.

PEDS — Not approved in children.

UNAPPROVED ADULT — Hypertensive urgency: 12.5 to 25 mg PO, repeated once or twice if necessary at intervals of 30 to 60 min.

UNAPPROVED PEDS — Neonates: 0.1 to 0.4 mg/kg/day PO divided q 6 to 8 h. Infants: Initial dose 0.15 to 0.3 mg/kg/dose, titrate to effective dose, max dose 6 mg/kg/day divided one to four times per day. Children: Initial dose 0.3 to 0.5 mg/kg/dose PO q 8 h, titrate to effective dose, maximum dose 6 mg/kg/day (not to exceed 450 mg/day) divided two to four times per day.

FORMS — Generic only: Tabs, scored 12.5, 25, 50, 100 mg.

NOTES — A captopril soln or susp (1 mg/mL) can be made by dissolving tabs in distilled water or flavored syrup. The soln is stable for 7 days at room temperature.

MOA — Inhibits angiotensin-converting enzyme which converts angiotensin I to angiotensin II.

ADVERSE EFFECTS — Serious: Angioedema, hyperkalemia, renal impairment. Frequent: Cough, rash.

CILAZAPRIL (✱*Inhibace*) ▶LK ♀D ▶? $

WARNING — Do not use in pregnancy.

ADULT — Canada only. HTN: Initial dose 2.5 mg PO daily, usual maintenance dose 2.5 to 5 mg daily, max 10 mg daily. Elderly or concomitant diuretic therapy: Initiate 1.25 mg PO daily. Heart failure adjunct: Initially 0.5 mg PO daily, increase to usual maintenance of 1 to 2.5 mg daily. Renal impairment with CrCl 10 to 40 mL/min, initiate 0.5 mg daily, max 2.5 mg/day. CrCl less than 10 mL/min, 0.25 to 0.5 mg once or twice per week, adjust dose according to BP response.

PEDS — Not approved in children.

FORMS — Generic/Trade: Not available in US. Tabs, scored 1, 2.5, 5 mg.

NOTES — Reduce dose in hepatic/renal impairment.

MOA — Inhibits angiotensin-converting enzyme which converts angiotensin I to angiotensin II.

ADVERSE EFFECTS — Serious: Angioedema, hyperkalemia, renal impairment. Frequent: Cough.

ENALAPRIL (*enalaprilat, Vasotec, Epaned*) ▶LK ♀D ▶+ $$

WARNING — Do not use in pregnancy.

ADULT — HTN: Start 5 mg PO daily, usual maintenance dose 10 to 40 mg PO daily or divided two times per day, max 40 mg/day. If oral therapy not possible, can use enalaprilat 1.25 mg IV q 6 h over 5 min, and increase up to 5 mg IV q 6 h if needed. Renal impairment or concomitant diuretic therapy: Start 2.5 mg PO daily. Heart failure: Start 2.5 mg PO two times per day, usual dose 10 to 20 mg PO two times per day, max 40 mg/day.

PEDS — HTN, age 1 mo or older: Start 0.08 mg/kg/day (max 5 mg/day; doses greater than 0.58 mg/kg/day or 40 mg/day have not been studied.

UNAPPROVED ADULT — Hypertensive crisis: Enalaprilat 1.25 to 5 mg IV q 6 h. Renoprotective dosing: 10 to 20 mg PO daily.

UNAPPROVED PEDS — HTN: Start 0.1 mg/kg/day PO daily or divided two times per day, titrate to effective dose, maximum dose 0.5 mg/kg/day; 0.005 to 0.01 mg/kg/dose IV q 8 to 24 h.

FORMS — Generic/Trade: Tabs, scored 2.5, 5 mg, unscored 10, 20 mg. Trade only: Oral Soln 1 mg/mL (Epaned-$$$$$)

NOTES — Twice daily dosing may be required for 24 h BP control. An enalapril oral susp (0.2 mg/mL) can be made by dissolving one 2.5 mg tab in 12.5 mL sterile water, use immediately. Enalaprilat is the active metabolite of enalapril.

MOA — Inhibits angiotensin-converting enzyme which converts angiotensin I to angiotensin II.

ADVERSE EFFECTS — Serious: Angioedema, hyperkalemia, renal impairment. Frequent: Cough.

FOSINOPRIL ▶LK ♀D ▶? $$

WARNING — Do not use in pregnancy.

ADULT — HTN: Start 10 mg PO daily, usual maintenance dose 20 to 40 mg PO daily or divided two times per day, max 80 mg/day, but added effect not apparent above 40 mg/day. Elderly, renal impairment, or concomitant diuretic therapy: Start 5 mg PO daily. Heart failure: Start 5 to 10 mg PO daily, usual 20 to 40 mg PO daily, max 40 mg/day.

PEDS — HTN age 6 to 16 yo and wt greater than 50 kg: 5 to 10 mg PO daily.

UNAPPROVED ADULT — Renoprotective dosing: 10 to 20 mg PO daily.

FORMS — Generic only: Tabs, scored 10, unscored 20, 40 mg.

NOTES — Twice daily dosing may be required for 24 h BP control. Elimination 50% renal, 50% hepatic. Accumulation of drug negligible with impaired renal function. The brand name product (Monopril) is no longer available.

MOA — Inhibits angiotensin-converting enzyme which converts angiotensin I to angiotensin II.

ADVERSE EFFECTS — Serious: Angioedema, hyperkalemia, renal impairment. Frequent: Cough.

LISINOPRIL (*Prinivil, Zestril*) ▶K ♀D ▶? $

WARNING — Do not use in pregnancy.

ADULT — HTN: Start 10 mg PO daily, usual maintenance dose 20 to 40 mg PO daily, max 80 mg/day, but added effect not apparent above 40 mg/day. Renal impairment or concomitant diuretic therapy: Start 2.5 to 5 mg PO daily. Heart failure, acute MI: Start 2.5 to 5 mg PO daily, usual 5 to 20 mg PO daily, max 40 mg/day.

PEDS — HTN age older than 6 yo: 0.07 mg/kg PO daily; 5 mg/day max. Not recommended for age younger than 6 yo or with glomerular filtration rate less than 30 mL/min/1.73 m².

UNAPPROVED ADULT — Renoprotective dosing: 10 to 20 mg PO daily.

FORMS — Generic/Trade: Tabs, unscored (Zestril) 2.5, 5, 10, 20, 30, 40 mg. Tabs, scored (Prinivil) 10, 20, 40 mg.

MOA — Inhibits angiotensin-converting enzyme which converts angiotensin I to angiotensin II.

ADVERSE EFFECTS — Serious: Angioedema, hyperkalemia, renal impairment. Frequent: Cough.

MOEXIPRIL (*Univasc*) ▶LK ♀D ▶? $$

WARNING — Do not use in pregnancy.

ADULT — HTN: Start 7.5 mg PO daily, usual maintenance dose 7.5 to 30 mg PO daily or divided two times per day, max 30 mg/day. Renal impairment or concomitant diuretic therapy: Start 3.75 mg PO daily; max 15 mg/day with renal impairment.

PEDS — Not approved in children.

FORMS — Generic/Trade: Tabs scored 7.5, 15 mg.

NOTES — Twice daily dosing may be required for 24 h BP control.

MOA — Inhibits angiotensin-converting enzyme which converts angiotensin I to angiotensin II.

ADVERSE EFFECTS — Serious: Angioedema, hyperkalemia, renal impairment. Frequent: Cough.

PERINDOPRIL (*Aceon, ✦Coversyl*) ▶K ♀D ▶? $$$

WARNING — Do not use in pregnancy.

ADULT — HTN: Start 4 mg PO daily, usual maintenance dose 4 to 8 mg PO daily or divided two times per day, max 16 mg/day. Renal impairment or concomitant diuretic therapy: Start 2 mg PO daily or divided two times per day, max 8 mg/day. Reduction of cardiovascular events in stable CAD: Start 4 mg PO daily for 2 weeks, max 8 mg/day. Elderly (age older than 65 yo): 4 mg PO daily, max 8 mg/day.

PEDS — Not approved in children.

UNAPPROVED ADULT — Heart failure: Start 2 mg PO daily, max dose 16 mg daily. Recurrent CVA prevention: 4 mg PO daily with indapamide.

FORMS — Generic/Trade: Tabs scored 2, 4, 8 mg.

NOTES — Twice daily dosing may be required for 24 h BP control.

MOA — Inhibits angiotensin-converting enzyme which converts angiotensin I to angiotensin II.

ADVERSE EFFECTS — Serious: Angioedema, hyperkalemia, renal impairment. Frequent: Cough.

QUINAPRIL (*Accupril*) ▶LK ♀D ▶? $$

WARNING — Do not use in pregnancy.

ADULT — HTN: Start 10 to 20 mg PO daily (start 10 mg/day if elderly), usual maintenance dose 20 to 80 mg PO daily or divided two times per day, max

QUINAPRIL (cont.)

80 mg/day, but added effect not apparent above 40 mg/day. Renal impairment or concomitant diuretic therapy: Start 2.5 to 5 mg PO daily. Heart failure: Start 5 mg PO two times per day, usual maintenance dose 20 to 40 mg/day divided two times per day.
PEDS — Not approved in children.
FORMS — Generic/Trade: Tabs scored 5, unscored 10, 20, 40 mg.
NOTES — Twice daily dosing may be required for 24 h BP control.
MOA — Inhibits angiotensin-converting enzyme which converts angiotensin I to angiotensin II.
ADVERSE EFFECTS — Serious: Angioedema, hyperkalemia, renal impairment. Frequent: Cough.

RAMIPRIL (*Altace*) ▶LK ♀D ▶? $
WARNING — Do not use in pregnancy.
ADULT — HTN: Start 2.5 mg PO daily, usual maintenance dose 2.5 to 20 mg PO daily or divided two times per day, max 20 mg/day. Renal impairment or concomitant diuretic therapy: Start 1.25 mg PO daily. Heart failure/post-MI: Start 2.5 mg PO two times per day, usual maintenance dose 5 mg PO two times per day. Reduce risk of MI, CVA, death from cardiovascular causes: Start 2.5 mg PO daily for 1 week, then 5 mg daily for 3 weeks, increase as tolerated to maintenance dose 10 mg daily.
PEDS — Not approved in children.

UNAPPROVED ADULT — Renoprotective dosing: Titrate to 10 mg PO daily.
FORMS — Generic/Trade: Caps 1.25, 2.5, 5, 10 mg.
NOTES — Twice daily dosing may be required for 24 h BP control. Cap contents can be sprinkled on applesauce and eaten or mixed with 120 mL of water or apple juice and swallowed. Mixtures are stable for 24 h at room temperature or 48 h refrigerated. Concomitant insulin or hypoglycemic agents may increase hypoglycemia risk.
MOA — Inhibits angiotensin-converting enzyme which converts angiotensin I to angiotensin II.
ADVERSE EFFECTS — Serious: Angioedema, hepatotoxicity, hyperkalemia, pancreatitis, renal impairment. Frequent: Cough.

TRANDOLAPRIL (*Mavik*) ▶LK ♀D ▶? $
WARNING — Do not use in pregnancy.
ADULT — HTN: Start 1 mg PO daily, usual maintenance dose 2 to 4 mg PO daily or divided two times per day, max 8 mg/day, but added effect not apparent above 4 mg/day. Heart failure/post-MI: Start 1 mg PO daily, titrate to target dose 4 mg PO daily. Renal impairment or concomitant diuretic therapy: Start 0.5 mg PO daily.
PEDS — Not approved in children.
FORMS — Generic/Trade: Tabs, scored 1, unscored 2, 4 mg.
NOTES — Twice daily dosing may be required for 24 h BP control.
MOA — Serious: Angioedema, hyperkalemia, renal impairment. Frequent: Cough.
ADVERSE EFFECTS — TAB013

CARDIOVASCULAR: Aldosterone Antagonists

NOTE: Hyperkalemia possible, especially if used concomitantly with other drugs that increase K+ (including K+ containing salt substitutes) and in patients with heart failure, DM, or renal impairment. Adding an aldosterone antagonist is recommended in select patients with heart failure and reduced LVEF with careful monitoring for preserved renal function and normal K+ concentration. Serum creatinine should be less than 2.5 mg/dL in men or less than 2.0 mg/dL in women; and K+ should be less than 5.0 mEq/L.

EPLERENONE (*Inspra*) ▶L ♀B ▶? $$$$
ADULT — HTN: Start 50 mg PO daily, increase after 4 weeks if needed to max dose 50 mg two times per day. Start 25 mg daily with concomitant moderate CYP3A4 inhibitor (eg, erythromycin, verapamil, fluconazole, saquinavir). Improve survival of stable patients with LV systolic dysfunction (LVEF 40% or less) and heart failure/post-MI: Start 25 mg PO daily; titrate to target dose 50 mg PO daily within 4 weeks, if tolerated.
PEDS — Not approved in children.
FORMS — Generic/trade: Tabs, unscored 25, 50 mg.
NOTES — Contraindicated with potassium > 5.5 mEq/L; CrCl < 30 mL/min; strong CYP3A4 inhibitors (ketoconazole, itraconazole, nefazodone, troleandomycin, clarithromycin, ritonavir, nelfinavir). For treatment of HTN, contraindications include Type 2 DM with microalbuminuria; serum creatinine > 2 mg/dL in males or > 1.8 mg/dL in females; CrCl < 50 mL/min; concomitant therapy with K+ supplements, K+-sparing diuretics. Hyperkalemia more common with concomitant ACE inhibitors/ARBs.

Measure serum K+ before initiating, within first week, at 1 month after starting treatment or dose adjustment, then prn. With concomitant moderate CYP3A4 inhibitor (e.g., erythromycin, fluconazole, saquinavir, verapamil) check K+ and serum creatinine within 3 to 7 days of initiating eplerenone. Monitor lithium levels with concomitant lithium therapy.
MOA — Blocks the binding of aldosterone to mineralocorticoid receptors.
ADVERSE EFFECTS — Serious: Hyperkalemia, hyponatremia (rare). Frequent: Headache, dizziness.

SPIRONOLACTONE (*Aldactone*) ▶LK ♀D ▶+ $
WARNING — Use only for approved indications. Tumorigen in rats.
ADULT — HTN: 50 to 100 mg PO daily or divided two times per day, increase dose prn after 2 weeks based on serum potassium and BP. Edema (heart failure, hepatic disease, nephrotic syndrome): Start 100 mg PO daily or divided two times per day, maintain for 5 days, increase prn to achieve diuretic response, usual dose range 25 to 200 mg/day. Other diuretics

(cont.)

SPIRONOLACTONE (*cont.*)

may be needed. Diuretic-induced hypokalemia: 25 to 100 mg PO daily when potassium supplements/ sparing regimens inappropriate. Severe heart failure (NYHA III or IV): Start 25 mg PO daily, max 50 mg daily. Primary hyperaldosteronism, maintenance therapy: 100 to 400 mg/day PO until surgery or indefinitely if surgery not an option.

PEDS — Edema: 3.3 mg/kg PO daily or divided two times per day.

UNAPPROVED ADULT — Hirsutism: 50 to 200 mg PO daily, maximal regression of hirsutism in 6 months. Acne: 50 to 200 mg PO daily.

UNAPPROVED PEDS — Edema/HTN: 1 to 3.3 mg/kg/ day, PO daily or divided two times per day, max 200 mg/day.

FORMS — Generic/Trade: Tabs, unscored 25 mg, scored 50, 100 mg.

NOTES — May be helpful in patients with resistant hypertension. Contraindicated with anuria, renal insufficiency, hyperkalemia, Addison's disease, or other conditions associated with hyperkalemia. Dosing more frequently than bid not necessary. Hyperkalemia more likely with doses 50 mg/day or more and with concomitant ACEIs or K+ supplements. Measure serum K+ and SrCr before initiating, after 1 week, monthly for the first 3 months, quarterly for 1 year, then every 6 months after starting treatment or dose adjustment.

MOA — Blocks the binding of aldosterone to mineralocorticoid receptors.

ADVERSE EFFECTS — Serious: Agranulocytosis, hyperkalemia (rare), hypersensitivity, Stevens-Johnson Syndrome. Frequent: Gynecomastia, headache, impotence, irregular menses.

CARDIOVASCULAR: Angiotensin Receptor Blockers (ARBs)

NOTE: See also antihypertensive combinations. Avoid concomitant ACE inhibitor use. Contraindicated in pregnancy. Women of child bearing age should use reliable form of contraception; discontinue ARB as soon as pregnancy is detected. Do not use with aliskiren in patients with DM or CrCl < 60 mL/min. Dual inhibition of renin-angiotensin system increases risk of renal impairment, hypotension, and hyperkalemia. Hyperkalemia possible, especially if used concomitantly with other drugs that increase K+ (including K+ containing salt substitutes) and in patients with heart failure, DM, or renal impairment. An increase in serum creatinine up to 35% above baseline is acceptable and is not reason to withhold therapy unless hyperkalemia occurs. Concomitant NSAID, including selective COX-2 inhibitors, may further deteriorate renal function and decrease antihypertensive effects. May increase lithium levels. Rare cases of angioedema and rhabdomyolysis have been reported with ARBs.

AZILSARTAN (*Edarbi*) ▶L - ♀D ♀? $$$$

WARNING — Do not use in pregnancy.

ADULT — HTN: Start 80 mg daily, max 80 mg daily. Start 40 mg daily with concomitant high-dose diuretic therapy.

FORMS — Trade only: Tabs, unscored 40, 80 mg.

MOA — Blocks binding of angiotensin II to the angiotensin subtype I receptor.

ADVERSE EFFECTS — Serious: angioedema, hyperkalemia, renal impairment.

CANDESARTAN (*Atacand*) ▶K ♀D ♀? $$$

WARNING — Do not use in pregnancy.

ADULT — HTN: Start 16 mg PO daily, max 32 mg/ day. Reduce cardiovascular death and hospitalizations from heart failure (NYHA II–IV and LVEF 40% or less): Start 4 mg PO daily, may double dose q 2 weeks; maximum 32 mg/day.

PEDS — HTN: For age 1 to 5 yo: Start 0.20 mg/kg (oral suspension), dose range 0.05 to 0.4 mg/kg/day. For age 6 to 16 yo and wt less than 50 kg: Start 4 to 8 mg/day, range 4 to 16 mg/day. For age 6 to 16 yo, wt greater than 50 kg: Start 8 to 16 mg/day, range 4 to 32 mg/day. Doses higher than 0.4 mg/kg/day (in ages 1 to 5 yo) or 32 mg (ages 6 to 16 yo) have not been studied.

FORMS — Generic/Trade: Tabs 4, 8, 16, 32 mg.

MOA — Blocks binding of angiotensin II to the angiotensin subtype 1 receptor.

ADVERSE EFFECTS — Serious: Hyperkalemia, renal impairment.

EPROSARTAN (*Teveten*) ▶Fecal excretion ♀D ♀? $$$$

WARNING — Do not use in pregnancy.

ADULT — HTN: Start 600 mg PO daily, maximum 800 mg/day given daily or divided two times per day.

PEDS — Not approved in children.

FORMS — Generic/Trade: Tabs, unscored 600 mg. Trade only: Tabs, unscored 400 mg.

MOA — Serious: Hyperkalemia, renal impairment.

IRBESARTAN (*Avapro*) ▶L ♀D ♀? $

WARNING — Do not use in pregnancy.

ADULT — HTN: Start 150 mg PO daily, max 300 mg/ day. Volume-depleted patients: Start 75 mg PO daily. Type 2 diabetic nephropathy: Start 150 mg PO daily, target dose 300 mg daily.

PEDS — Not approved in children.

FORMS — Generic/Trade: Tabs unscored 75, 150, 300 mg.

MOA — Serious: Hyperkalemia, renal impairment.

LOSARTAN (*Cozaar*) ▶L ♀D ♀? $

WARNING — Do not use in pregnancy.

ADULT — HTN: Start 50 mg PO daily, max 100 mg/day given daily or divided two times per day. Volume-depleted patients or history of hepatic impairment: Start 25 mg PO daily. CVA risk reduction in patients with HTN and LV hypertrophy (may not be effective in black patients): Start 50 mg PO daily. If need more BP reduction add HCTZ 12.5 mg PO daily; then increase losartan to 100 mg/day, then increase HCTZ to 25 mg/day. Type 2 diabetic nephropathy: Start 50 mg PO daily, target dose 100 mg daily.

LOSARTAN (*cont.*)

PEDS — HTN: Start 0.7 mg/kg/day (up to 50 mg), doses greater than 1.4 mg/kg/day or above 100 mg have not been studied. Do not use for age younger than 6 yo or if glomerular filtration rate less than 30 mL/min.

UNAPPROVED ADULT — Heart failure: Start 12.5 mg PO daily, target dose 50 mg daily. Renoprotective dosing: Start 50 mg PO daily, increase to 100 mg daily prn for BP control.

FORMS — Generic/Trade: Tabs, unscored 25, 50, 100 mg.

NOTES — Monitor BP control when adding or discontinuing rifampin, fluconazole, or erythromycin.

MOA — Blocks binding of angiotensin II to the angiotensin subtype 1 receptor.

ADVERSE EFFECTS — Serious: Hyperkalemia, renal impairment, thrombocytopenia (rare).

OLMESARTAN (*Benicar, ✦Olmetec*) ▶K ♀D ▶? $$$$

WARNING — Do not use in pregnancy.

ADULT — HTN: Start 20 mg PO daily, maximum 40 mg/day.

PEDS — HTN, 6 to 16 yo: Weight 20 to less than 35 kg: Start 10 mg PO daily, max 20 mg/day. Weight 35 kg or more: Start 20 mg PO daily, max 40 mg/day. Contraindicated in children < 1 yo.

FORMS — Trade only: Tabs, unscored 5, 20, 40 mg.

NOTES — Take at least 4 h prior to colesevelam. Some patients may develop sprue enteropathy with significant weight loss months to years after starting olmesartan; teach patients to report severe, chronic diarrhea with substantial weight loss; discontinue olmesartan if these symptoms occur.

MOA — Blocks binding of angiotensin II to the angiotensin subtype 1 receptor.

ADVERSE EFFECTS — Serious: Hyperkalemia, renal impairment, sprue enteropathy.

TELMISARTAN (*Micardis*) ▶L ♀D ▶? $$$$

WARNING — Do not use in pregnancy.

ADULT — HTN: Start 40 mg PO daily, maximum 80 mg/day. Cardiovascular risk reduction in patients older than 55 yo unable to take ACE inhibitors: Start 80 mg PO daily, max 80 mg/day.

PEDS — Not approved in children.

FORMS — Generic/Trade: Tabs, unscored 20, 40, 80 mg.

NOTES — Swallow tabs whole, do not break or crush. May increase digoxin level.

MOA — Blocks binding of angiotensin II to the angiotensin subtype 1 receptor.

ADVERSE EFFECTS — Serious: Hyperkalemia, renal impairment.

VALSARTAN (*Diovan*) ▶L ♀D ▶? $$$$

WARNING — Do not use in pregnancy.

ADULT — HTN: Start 80 to 160 mg PO daily, max 320 mg/day. Heart failure: Start 40 mg PO two times per day, target dose 160 mg two times per day; there is no evidence of added benefit when used with adequate dose of ACE inhibitor. Reduce mortality/morbidity post-MI with LV systolic dysfunction/failure: Start 20 mg PO two times per day, increase to 40 mg PO two times per day within 7 days, target dose 160 mg two times per day.

PEDS — HTN: Start 1.3 mg/kg/day (up to 40 mg), max 2.7 mg/kg/day (or 160 mg). Do not use if younger than 6 yo.

UNAPPROVED ADULT — Renoprotective dosing: 80 to 160 mg PO daily.

FORMS — Generic/Trade: Tabs, scored 40 mg, unscored 80, 160, 320 mg.

MOA — Serious: Hyperkalemia, renal impairment.

CARDIOVASCULAR: Anti-Dysrhythmics/Cardiac Arrest

ADENOSINE (*Adenocard*) ▶Plasma ♀C ▶? $

ADULT — PSVT conversion (not A-fib): 6 mg rapid IV and flush, preferably through a central line. If no response after 1 to 2 min then 12 mg. A 3rd dose of 12 mg may be given prn.

PEDS — PSVT conversion wt less than 50 kg: Initial dose 50 to 100 mcg/kg IV, give subsequent doses q 1 to 2 min prn and increase the dose 50 to 100 mcg/kg each time, up to a max single dose of 300 mcg/kg or 12 mg (whichever is less). PST coversion wt 50 kg or greater: Use adult dosage.

NOTES — Half-life is less than 10 sec. Give doses by rapid IV push followed by NS flush. Need higher dose if on theophylline or caffeine, lower dose if on dipyridamole or carbamazepine. May cause respiratory collapse in patients with asthma, COPD. Use in setting with cardiac resuscitation readily available. Do not use with acute myocardial ischemia, unstable angina, or cardiovascular instability. Do not confuse with adenosine phosphate used for the symptomatic relief of varicose vein complications.

MOA — Blocks cardiac conduction through the AV node.

ADVERSE EFFECTS — Serious: Arrhythmias, heart block, bronchoconstriction, seizures. Frequent: Flushing, chest tightness.

AMIODARONE (*Pacerone, Cordarone*) ▶L ♀D ▶– $$$$

WARNING — May cause potentially fatal toxicities, including pulmonary toxicity, hepatic injury, and worsened arrhythmia. Only use for adults with life-threatening ventricular arrhythmias when other treatments ineffective or not tolerated.

ADULT — Life-threatening ventricular arrhythmia without cardiac arrest: Load 150 mg IV over 10 min, then 1 mg/min for 6 h, then 0.5 mg/min for 18 h. Mix in D5W. Oral loading dose 800 to 1600 mg PO daily for 1 to 3 weeks, reduce dose to 400 to 800 mg daily for 1 month when arrhythmia is controlled or adverse effects are prominent, then reduce to lowest effective dose, usually 200 to 400 mg daily.

PEDS — Not approved in children.

UNAPPROVED ADULT — Atrial fibrillation (refractory or with accessory pathway): Loading dose 600 to

(cont.)

AMIODARONE (cont.)

800 mg PO daily for 7 to 14 days, then 200 to 400 mg daily. Maintain sinus rhythm with A-fib: 100 to 400 mg PO daily. Shock-refractory VF/pulseless VT: 300 mg or 5 mg/kg IV bolus followed by unsynchronized shock, additional 150 mg bolus may be given if serious arrhythmias recur. Stable monomorphic ventricular tachycardia: 150 mg IV over 10 min, repeat q 10 to 15 min prn.

UNAPPROVED PEDS — May cause death or other serious side effects in children (see NOTES); do not use in infants younger than 30 days of age and use only if medically warranted if 30 days of age or older. Ventricular arrhythmia: IV therapy limited data; 5 mg/kg IV over 30 min; followed by 5 mcg/kg/min infusion; increase infusion prn up to max 10 mcg/kg/min or 20 mg/kg/day. Give loading dose in 1 mg/kg aliquots with each aliquot given over 5 to 10 min; do not exceed 30 mg/min.

FORMS — Trade only (Pacerone): Tabs, unscored 100 mg. Generic/Trade: Tabs, scored 200, 400 mg.

NOTES — Proarrhythmic. Contraindicated in cardiogenic shock and in profound/symptomatic bradycardia (whether from AV block or sinus-node dysfunction) in the absence of a functioning pacemaker. Consider inpatient rhythm monitoring during initiation of therapy, especially when treating life-threatening arrhythmias. Consult cardiologist before using with other antiarrhythmic agents. Do not use with iodine allergy. Photosensitivity and skin discoloration (blue/gray color) with oral therapy. Hypo- or hyperthyroidism possible. Monitor LFTs, TFTs, and PFTs. Baseline and regular eye exams. Prompt ophthalmic examination needed with changes in visual acuity or decreased peripheral vision. Most manufacturers of laser refractive devices contraindicate eye laser surgery when taking amiodarone. Long elimination half-life, approximately 26 to 107 days. Drug interactions may persist after discontinuance due to long half-life. May increase levels of substrates of p-glycoprotein and drugs metabolized by CYP 450 enzymes (CYP1A2, CYP2C9, CYP2D6, CYP3A4). Coadministration of fluoroquinolones, macrolides, loratadine, trazodone, azoles, or Class IA and III antiarrhythmic drugs may prolong QTc. May double or triple phenytoin level. May increase cyclosporine level. May increase digoxin level; discontinue digoxin or reduce dose by 50%. May increase INR with warfarin therapy; reduce warfarin dose by 33 to 50%. Do not use with simvastatin doses greater than 20 mg/day, lovastatin doses greater than 40 mg/day; may increase atorvastatin level (use lower dose); increases risk of myopathy and rhabdomyolysis. Coadministration with clopidogrel may result in ineffective platelet inhibition. Do not use with grapefruit juice. Use cautiously with beta-blockers and calcium channel blockers. Protease inhibitors, cimetidine may increase levels. Give two times per day if intolerable GI effects occur with once daily dosing. IV therapy may cause hypotension and bradycardia in adults. Administer IV infusion using a nonevacuated glass bottle and in-line IV filter. Use central line when concentration exceeds 2 mg/mL. May cause congenital hypothyroidism and hyperthyroidism if given during pregnancy. Avoid use in children younger than 1 mo: IV form contains benzyl alcohol, which may cause gasping syndrome (gasping respirations, hypotension, bradycardia, and cardiovascular collapse). In children 1 mo to 15 yo may cause life-threatening hypotension, bradycardia, and AV block. May adversely affect male reproductive tract development in infants and toddlers from plasticizer exposure from IV tubing; use syringes instead of IV tubing to administer doses to infants and toddlers.

MOA — Prolongs cardiac repolarization (Class III antiarrhythmic properties). Also has sodium channel blockade, beta adrenergic blockade, and calcium channel blockade effects (Class I, II, IV effects).

ADVERSE EFFECTS — Serious: Pulmonary toxicity, thyroid toxicity, bradycardia/heart block, arrhythmias, rhabdomyolysis, blindness, visual impairment, SIADH, hepatotoxicity, acute renal failure, agranulocytosis. Frequent: Hypotension, elevated LFTs, photosensitivity, GI intolerance, corneal microdeposits.

ATROPINE (AtroPen) ▶K ♀C ▶– $

ADULT — Bradyarrhythmia/CPR: 0.5 to 1 mg IV q 3 to 5 min, max 0.04 mg/kg (3 mg). Treatment of muscarinic symptoms of insecticide or nerve agent poisonings: Mild symptoms: 1 injection of 2 mg auto-injector pen, 2 additional injections after 10 min may be given in rapid succession if severe symptoms develop. Severe symptoms: 3 injections of 2 mg pen in rapid succession. Administer in mid-lateral thigh. Max 3 injections.

PEDS — CPR: 0.02 mg/kg/dose IV q 5 min for 2 to 3 doses prn (max single dose 0.5 mg); minimum single dose, 0.1 mg; max cumulative dose 1 mg. Treatment of muscarinic symptoms of insecticide or nerve agent poisonings: Follow adult dosing instructions, but if wt less than 7 kg use 0.25 mg pen, if wt 7 to 18 kg use 0.5 mg pen, if wt 18 to 41 kg use 1 mg pen, if wt greater than 41 kg use 2 mg pen.

UNAPPROVED ADULT — ET administration prior to IV access: 2 to 2.5 times the recommended IV dose in 10 mL of NS or distilled water.

FORMS — Trade only: Prefilled auto-injector pen: 0.25 mg (yellow), 0.5 mg (blue), 1 mg (dark red), 2 mg (green).

NOTES — Injector should be used by someone who has adequate training in recognizing and treating nerve agent or insecticide intoxication. Seek immediate medical attention after injection(s).

MOA — Blocks acetylcholine activity leading to increased cardiac chronotropic effect.

ADVERSE EFFECTS — Serious: Arrhythmias, tachycardia, paradoxical bradycardia (rare), paralysis (large doses). Frequent: Dry mouth, blurred vision, mydriasis, confusion, palpitations, urinary hesitancy, anhidrosis, constipation, injection site pain.

DIGOXIN (*Lanoxin, Digitek,* ✢*Toloxin*) ▶KL ♀C ▶+ $
ADULT — Systolic heart failure/rate control of chronic A-fib: age younger than 70 yo: 0.25 mg PO daily; age 70 yo or older: 0.125 mg PO daily; impaired renal function: 0.0625 to 0.125 mg PO daily; titrate based on response. Rapid A-fib: Total loading dose (TLD), 10 to 15 mcg/kg IV/PO, give in 3 divided doses every 6 to 8 h; give ~50% TLD for 1 dose, then ~25% TLD for 2 doses (e.g., 70 kg with normal renal function: 0.5 mg, then 0.25 mg q 6 to 8 h for 2 doses). Impaired renal function, 6 to 10 mcg/kg IV/PO TLD, given in 3 divided doses every 6 to 8 h. Titrate to minimum effective dose. Other agents (i.e., beta blockers, diltiazem, verapamil) more effective in controlling ventricular rate in A-fib.
PEDS — Heart failure with normal sinus rhythm: IV loading based on age: premature neonate: 15 to 25 mcg/kg; full-term neonate: 20 to 30 mcg/kg; age 1 to 24 mo: 30 to 50 mcg/kg; age 2 to 5 yo: 25 to 35 mcg/kg; age 5 to 10 yo: 15 to 30 mcg/kg; age older than 10 yo: 8 to 12 mcg/kg. Start by administering half of the total loading dose and then reassess in 4 to 8 h to determine need for second half of loading dose. Daily IV maintenance: Use 20 to 30% of actual IV loading dose for premature neonate; use 25 to 35% of actual IV loading dose for ages full-term to older than 10 yo; use divided two times per day for age younger than 10 yo. Daily PO maintenance: age 2 to 5 yo: 10 to 15 mcg/kg; age 6 to 10 yo: 7 to 10 mcg/kg; age older than 10 yo: 3 to 5 mcg/kg. Caution: Pediatric doses are in mcg, elixir product is labeled in mg/mL. Atrial fibrillation: Titrate to minimum dose needed to achieve desired ventricular rate without undesirable side effects.
UNAPPROVED ADULT — Reentrant PSVT (after carotid massage, IV adenosine, IV beta-blocker, IV diltiazem): 8 to 15 mcg/kg (based on ideal body wt) IV, give 50% of total dose initially, 25% 4 to 6 h later, and then the final 25% 4 to 6 h later.
FORMS — Generic/Trade: Tabs, scored (Lanoxin, Digitek) 0.125, 0.25 mg. Generic Only; elixir 0.05 mg/mL.
NOTES — Proarrhythmic. Consider patient-specific characteristics (lean/ideal wt, CrCl, age, concomitant disease states, concomitant medications, and factors likely to alter pharmacokinetic/dynamic profile of digoxin) when dosing; see prescribing information for alterations based on wt and renal function. Assess electrolytes, renal function, levels periodically. Elimination prolonged with renal impairment. Maintain normal potassium, magnesium, and calcium levels. Adjust dose based on response and therapeutic serum levels (range from 0.8 to 2 ng/mL); the risk of adverse events increases when the level is more than 1.2 ng/mL. Lower serum trough levels (0.5 to 1 ng/mL) may be appropriate for heart failure; A-fib may need higher levels. Nausea, vomiting, visual disturbances, and cardiac arrhythmias may indicate toxicity. Avoid administering IM due to severe local irritation.

Many interactions with other drugs and nutritional supplements. See prescribing information for full information before using in patients with sinus node disease, AV block, accessory AV pathway, certain heart failure disorders with preserved LV function, hypermetabolic states, thyroid disease, beri beri heart disease, or planned cardioversion. Do not use with acute MI or myocarditis. Therapeutic doses may cause ECG changes (PR-interval prolongation, ST-segment depression) and false positive ST-T changes during exercise testing; these are expected and do not indicate toxicity.
MOA — Slows cardiac conduction through the AV node, increases force of myocardial contraction.
ADVERSE EFFECTS — Serious: Arrhythmias, heart block. Frequent: Dizziness, headache, mental disturbances, N/V, diarrhea.

DIGOXIN IMMUNE FAB (*Digibind, DigiFab*) ▶K ♀C ▶? $$$$$
ADULT — Digoxin toxicity: Acute ingestion of known amount: 1 vial binds approximately 0.5 mg digoxin. Acute ingestion of unknown amount: 10 vials IV, may repeat once. Toxicity during chronic therapy: 6 vials usually adequate; one formula is: Number vials = (serum dig level in ng/mL) × (kg)/100.
PEDS — Digoxin toxicity: Dose varies. Acute ingestion of known amount: One vial binds approximately 0.5 mg digoxin. Acute ingestion of unknown amount: 10 vials IV, may repeat once; monitor for volume overload. Toxicity during chronic therapy: 1 vial usually adequate for infants and small children (less than 20 kg); one formula is: Number vials = (serum dig level in ng/mL) × (kg)/100.
NOTES — After digoxin immune fab infusion, use free digoxin level to guide therapy. Total serum digoxin concentration will be falsely elevated for several days.
MOA — Binds digoxin preventing interaction with sodium pump receptor.
ADVERSE EFFECTS — Serious: Hypersensitivity (rare), hypokalemia.

DISOPYRAMIDE (*Norpace, Norpace CR*) ▶KL ♀C ▶+ $$$
WARNING — Proarrhythmic. Contraindicated in preexisting/congenital QT prolongation, history of torsade de pointes, cardiogenic shock; 2nd/3rd degree heart block without pacemaker Only use for adults with life-threatening ventricular arrhythmias; increased mortality in patients with non-life-threatening ventricular arrhythmias and structural heart disease (ie, MI, LV dysfunction).
ADULT — Rarely indicated, consult cardiologist. Ventricular arrhythmia: 400 to 800 mg PO daily in divided doses (immediate-release is divided q 6 h: Extended-release is divided q 12 h). With cardiomyopathy or possible cardiac decompensation, limit initial dose to 100 mg of immediate-release q 6 to 8 h; do not give a loading dose. With liver disease or moderate renal impairment (CrCl > 40 mg/dL): 400 mg/day PO in divided doses. Use immediate-release form when CrCl is less than 40 mg/dL: Give 100 mg

(cont.)

DISOPYRAMIDE (*cont.*)

q 8 h for CrCl 30 to 40 mg/dL, give 100 mg q 12 h for CrCl 15 to 30 mg/dL, give 100 mg q 24 h for CrCl < 15 mg/dL.

PEDS — Ventricular arrhythmia: Divide all doses q 6 h. Younger than 1 yo: 10 to 30 mg/kg/day; age 1 to 4 yo: 10 to 20 mg/kg/day; age 4 to 12 yo:10 to 15 mg/kg/day; age 12 to 18 yo: 6 to 15 mg/kg/day .

UNAPPROVED ADULT — Maintain sinus rhythm with A-fib: 400 to 750 mg/day in divided doses.

FORMS — Generic/Trade: Caps, immediate-release 100, 150 mg. Trade only: Caps, extended-release 100, 150 mg.

NOTES — Proarrhythmic. Consider inpatient rhythm monitoring during initiation of therapy, especially when treating life-threatening arrhythmias. Anticholinergic side effects (dry mouth, constipation, blurred vision, urinary hesitancy) commonly occur. Reduce dose in patients with CrCl < 40 mL/min. Initiate as an outpatient with extreme caution. May start 6 to 12 h after last dose of quinidine, or 3 to 6 h after last dose of procainamide. May start extended-release form 6 h after last dose of immediate-release form.

MOA — Depresses phase 0 depolarization, prolongs cardiac action potential duration (Class 1A).

ADVERSE EFFECTS — Serious: Arrhythmias. Frequent: Dizziness, headache, hypotension, dry mouth, blurred vision, urinary retention, constipation.

DOFETILIDE (*Tikosyn*) ▶KL ♀C ▶– $$$$$

WARNING — Available only to hospitals and prescribers who have received appropriate dosing and treatment initiation education. Must be initiated or reinitiated in a facility that can provide CrCl calculation, ECG monitoring, and cardiac resuscitation. Monitor on telemetry for a minimum of 3 days.

ADULT — Conversion of A-fib/flutter: Specialized dosing based on CrCl and QTc interval.

PEDS — Not approved in children.

FORMS — Trade only: Caps, 0.125, 0.25, 0.5 mg.

NOTES — Proarrhythmic. Rarely indicated. Contraindicated in acquired/congenital QT prolongation; CrCl less than 20 mL/min; baseline QTc interval more than 440 msec or more than 500 msec in patients with ventricular conduction abnormalities; or with concomitant HCTZ, verapamil, cimetidine, dolutegravir, ketoconazole, megestrol, prochlorperazine, or trimethoprim. Use with heart rate below 50 bpm has not been studied. Serum K^+, Mg^{++} should be within normal range prior to initiating and during therapy. Monitor K^+ and Mg^{++} (low levels increase risk of arrhythmias). Assess CrCl and QTc prior to first dose. Continuously monitor ECG during hospital initiation and adjust dose based on QTc interval. Do not discharge within 12 h after conversion to normal sinus rhythm. Effects may be increased by known CYP3A4 inhibitors and drugs that inhibit renal elimination. Using with phenothiazines, cisapride, TCAs, macrolides, fluoroquinolones may increase QTc.

MOA — Prolongs cardiac repolarization (Class III antiarrhythmic properties).

ADVERSE EFFECTS — Serious: Arrhythmias. Common: Chest pain, headache.

DRONEDARONE (*Multaq*) ▶L ♀X ▶– $$$$$

WARNING — Contraindicated with NYHA Class IV heart failure, symptomatic heart failure with recent decompensation requiring hospitalization, or atrial fibrillation who will not or cannot be cardioverted into normal sinus rhythm. Increases risk of death, stroke, and heart failure in patients with decompensated heart failure or permanent atrial fibrillation.

ADULT — Reduce hospitalization risk for patients with atrial fib who are in sinus rhythm and have a history of paroxysmal or persistent atrial fib: 400 mg PO two times per day with morning and evening meals.

PEDS — Not approved in children.

FORMS — Trade only: Tabs, unscored 400 mg.

NOTES — Proarrhythmic. Do not use with 2nd or 3rd degree AV block or sick sinus syndrome without functioning pacemaker; bradycardia < 50 bpm; QTc Bazett interval > 500 ms; liver or lung toxicity related to previous amiodarone use; severe hepatic impairment; pregnancy; lactation; grapefruit juice; drugs or herbals that increase QT interval; Class I or III antiarrhythmic agents; potent inhibitors of CYP3A4 enzyme system (clarithromycin, itraconazole, ketoconazole, nefazodone, ritonavir, voriconazole); or inducers of CYP3A4 enzyme system (carbamazepine, phenytoin, phenobarbital, rifampin, St. John's wort). Correct hypo/hyperkalemia and hypomagnesium before giving. Monitor ECG every 3 months; if in atrial fib, then either stop dronedarone or cardiovert. May initiate or exacerbate heart failure symptoms; teach patients to report symptoms of new or worsening heart failure (e.g., wt gain, edema, dyspnea). May be associated with hepatic injury; teach patients to report symptoms of hepatic injury (e.g., anorexia, nausea, vomiting, fatigue, malaise, right upper quadrant discomfort, jaundice, dark urine); discontinue if hepatic injury is suspected. Serum creatinine may increase (~0.1 mg/dL) during first weeks, but does not reflect change in renal function; reversible when discontinued. Monitor renal function periodically. Give with appropriate antithrombotic therapy. May increase INR when used with warfarin. May increase dabigatran or other p-glycoprotein substrates level. May increase digoxin level; discontinue digoxin or reduce dose by 50%; monitor for digoxin toxicity. Use cautiously with beta-blockers (BB) and calcium channel blockers (CCB); initiate lower doses of BB or CCB; initiate at low dose and monitor ECG. Do not use with more than 10 mg of simvastatin. May increase level of sirolimus, tacrolimus, or CYP3A4 substrates with narrow therapeutic index.

MOA — Has sodium channel blockade, beta-adrenergic blockade, cardiac repolarization, and calcium channel blockade effects (Class I, II, III, IV effects).

DRONEDARONE (*cont.*)

ADVERSE EFFECTS — Serious: New/worsening heart failure, bradycardia/heart block, arrhythmias, hepatotoxicity, pulmonary toxicity. Frequent: Abdominal pain, asthenia, diarrhea, nausea.

FLECAINIDE (*Tambocor*) ▶K ♀C ▶– $$$$

WARNING — Proarrhythmic. Increased mortality in patients with non-life-threatening ventricular arrhythmias with history of MI; not recommended for use with chronic atrial fibrillation.

ADULT — Prevention of paroxysmal atrial fib/ flutter or PSVT, with symptoms and no structural heart disease: Start 50 mg PO q 12 h, may increase by 50 mg two times per day q 4 days, max 300 mg/day. Life-threatening ventricular arrhythmias without structural heart disease: Start 100 mg PO q 12 h, may increase by 50 mg two times per day q 4 days, max 400 mg/day. With CrCl less than 35 mL/min: Start 50 mg PO two times per day.

PEDS — Consult pediatric cardiologist.

UNAPPROVED ADULT — Cardioversion of recent onset atrial fib: 200 to 300 mg PO single dose. Maintain sinus rhythm with A-fib: 200 to 300 mg/day in divided doses.

FORMS — Generic/Trade: Tabs, unscored 50, scored 100, 150 mg.

NOTES — Contraindicated in cardiogenic shock; sick sinus syndrome or significant conduction delay; 2nd/3rd degree heart block or bundle brand block without pacemaker; acquired/congenital QT prolongation; or patients with history of torsades de pointes. Consider inpatient rhythm monitoring during initiation of therapy, especially when treating life-threatening arrhythmias. Use with AV nodal slowing agent (beta-blocker, verapamil, diltiazem) to minimize risk of 1:1 atrial flutter. Reduce dose if QRS widening more than 20% from baseline or if 2nd/3rd degree AV block. Correct hypo/hyperkalemia before giving. Increases digoxin level 13 to 19%. Consult cardiologist before using with other antiarrhythmic agents. Reduce dose of flecainide 50% when used with amiodarone. Quinidine, cimetidine may increase levels. Use cautiously with disopyramide, verapamil, or impaired hepatic function. Use cautiously with impaired renal function; will take more than 4 days to reach new steady state level. Target trough level 0.2 to 1 mcg/mL.

MOA — Depresses phase 0 depolarization significantly, slows cardiac conduction significantly (Class 1C).

ADVERSE EFFECTS — Serious: Arrhythmias, depressed conduction/widened QRS at higher heart rates. Frequent: Dizziness, headache, nausea, dyspnea, fatigue, visual disturbances.

IBUTILIDE (*Corvert*) ▶K ♀C ▶? $$$$$

WARNING — Proarrhythmic; only administer by trained personnel with continuous ECG monitoring, capable of identifying and treating acute ventricular arrhythmias. Potentially fatal ventricular arrhythmias may occur with/without QT prolongation and can lead to torsade de pointes.

ADULT — Recent onset A-fib/flutter: Give 0.01 mg/kg over 10 min for wt less than 60 kg, may repeat if no response after 10 min. Give 1 mg (10 mL) IV over 10 min for wt 60 kg or greater, may repeat once if no response after 10 min. Useful in combination with DC cardioversion if DC cardioversion alone is unsuccessful.

PEDS — Not approved in children.

NOTES — Proarrhythmic. Serum K+, Mg++ should be within normal range prior to initiating and during therapy. Monitor K+ and Mg++ (low levels increase risk of arrhythmias). Keep on cardiac monitor at least 4 h. Use with caution, if at all, when QT interval is > 500 msec, severe LV dysfunction, or in patients already using class Ia or III antiarrhythmics. Stop infusion when arrhythmia is terminated.

MOA — Prolongs cardiac repolarization (Class III antiarrhythmic properties).

ADVERSE EFFECTS — Serious: Arrhythmias.

ISOPROTERENOL (*Isuprel*) ▶LK ♀C ▶? $$$$$

ADULT — Refractory bradycardia or 3rd degree AV block: Bolus method: 0.02 to 0.06 mg IV: infusion method, dilute 2 mg in 250 mL D5W (8 mcg/mL), a rate of 37.5 mL/h delivers 5 mcg/min. General dose range 2 to 20 mcg/min.

PEDS — Refractory bradycardia or 3rd degree AV block: Dilute 2 mg in 250 mL D5W (8 mcg/mL). Start IV infusion 0.05 mcg/kg/min, increase every 5 to 10 min by 0.1 mcg/kg/min until desired effect or onset of toxicity, max 2 mcg/kg/min. For a 10 kg child, a rate of 8 mL/h delivers 0.1 mcg/kg/min.

MOA — Serious: Arrhythmias, tachycardia. Frequent: Hypertension, palpitations, flushing, sweating, dizziness.

ADVERSE EFFECTS — TAB015,TAB016

LIDOCAINE (*Xylocaine, Xylocard*) ▶LK ♀B ▶? $

ADULT — Ventricular arrhythmia: Load 1 mg/kg IV, then 0.5 mg/kg IV q 8 to 10 min prn to max 3 mg/kg. IV infusion: 4 g in 500 mL D5W (8 mg/mL) at 1 to 4 mg/min.

PEDS — Ventricular arrhythmia: Loading dose 1 mg/kg IV/intraosseous slowly; may repeat for 2 doses 10 to 15 min apart; max 3 to 5 mg/kg in 1 h. ET tube: Use 2 to 2.5 times IV dose. IV infusion: 4 g in 500 mL D5W (8 mg/mL) at 20 to 50 mcg/kg/min. For a 10 kg child a rate of 3 mL/h delivers 40 mcg/kg/min.

UNAPPROVED ADULT — ET administration prior to IV access: 2 to 2.5 times the recommended IV dose in 10 mL of NS or distilled water. Shock refractory VF/pulseless VT: 1 to 1.5 mg/kg IV push once, then 0.5 to 0.75 mg/kg IV push q 5 to 10 min prn to max 3 mg/kg.

NOTES — Reduce infusion in heart failure, liver disease, elderly. Not for routine use after acute MI. Monitor for CNS side effects with prolonged infusions.

MOA — Depresses phase 0 depolarization slightly, shortens cardiac action potential duration (Class 1B).

ADVERSE EFFECTS — Serious: Arrhythmias, hypersensitivity (rare), seizures (rare). Frequent: Hypotension, dizziness, drowsiness.

MEXILETINE (*Mexitil*) ▶L ♀C ▶– $$$$
  WARNING — Proarrhythmic. Increased mortality in patients with non-life-threatening ventricular arrhythmias and structural heart disease (i.e., MI, LV dysfunction).
  ADULT — Rarely indicated, consult cardiologist. Ventricular arrhythmia: Start 200 mg PO q 8 h with food or antacid, max dose 1200 mg/day. Patients responding to q 8 h dosing may be converted to q 12 h dosing with careful monitoring, max 450 mg/dose q 12 h.
  PEDS — Not approved in children.
  FORMS — Generic only: Caps 150, 200, 250 mg.
  NOTES — Patients may require decreased dose with severe liver disease. CNS side effects may limit dose titration. Monitor level when given with phenytoin, rifampin, phenobarbital, cimetidine, fluvoxamine. May increase theophylline level.
  MOA — Depresses phase 0 depolarization slightly, shortens cardiac action potential duration (Class 1B).
  ADVERSE EFFECTS — Serious: Arrhythmias, blood dyscrasias, pulmonary infiltrates/fibrosis. Frequent: N/V, diarrhea, dizziness, nervousness, headache, blurred vision, tremor, ataxia.

PROCAINAMIDE ▶LK ♀C ▶? $$
  WARNING — Proarrhythmic. Increased mortality in patients with non-life-threatening ventricular arrhythmias and structural heart disease (i.e., MI, LV dysfunction). Contraindicated with systemic lupus erythematosus. Has been associated with blood dyscrasias.
  ADULT — Ventricular Arrhythmia: Loading dose: 100 mg IV q 10 min or 20 mg/min (150 mL/h) until QRS widens more than 50%, dysrhythmia suppressed, hypotension, or total of 17 mg/kg or 1000 mg delivered. Infusion: Dilute 2 g in 250 mL D5W (8 mg/mL) run at rate of 15 to 45 mL/h to deliver 2 to 6 mg/min. If rhythm unresponsive, guide therapy by serum procainamide/NAPA levels.
  PEDS — Not approved in children.
  UNAPPROVED ADULT — Restoration of sinus rhythm in atrial fibrillation with accessory pathway (preexcitation): 100 mg IV q 10 min or 20 mg/min. until: QRS widens more than 50%, dysrhythmia suppressed, hypotension, or total of 17 mg/kg or 1000 mg delivered.
  UNAPPROVED PEDS — Arrhythmia: 2 to 6 mg/kg IV over 5 min, max loading dose 100 mg, repeat loading dose q 5 to 10 min prn up to max 15 mg/kg; 20 to 80 mcg/kg/min IV infusion, max dose 2 g/day. Consult pedi cardiologist or intensivist.
  NOTES — Proarrhythmic. Use lower dose or longer dosing interval with liver disease. Use cautiously with renal impairment or failure. Avoid with preexisting peripheral neuropathy. If positive antinuclear antibody (ANA) test develops, weigh risk/benefit of continued therapy. Evaluate complete blood count, including white cell, differential, and platelet counts, weekly for first 12 weeks of therapy and periodically afterward, and if patient develops unusual bleeding/bruising or signs of infection.

If hematologic disorders are identified, discontinue therapy. The brand-name products (Procan, Pronestyl) are no longer available.
  MOA — Depresses phase 0 depolarization, prolongs cardiac action potential duration (Class 1A).
  ADVERSE EFFECTS — Serious: Arrhythmias, blood dyscrasias (rare), SLE. Frequent: Hypotension, fever, headache.

PROPAFENONE (*Rythmol, Rythmol SR*) ▶L ♀C ▶? $$
  WARNING — Proarrhythmic. Increased mortality in patients with non-life-threatening ventricular arrhythmias and structural heart disease (i.e., MI, LV dysfunction).
  ADULT — Prevention of paroxysmal atrial fib/flutter or PSVT, with symptoms and no structural heart disease; or life-threatening ventricular arrhythmias: Start (immediate-release) 150 mg PO q 8 h; may increase after 3 to 4 days to 225 mg PO q 8 h; max 900 mg/day. Prolong time to recurrence of symptomatic atrial fib without structural heart disease: 225 mg SR PO q 12 h, may increase after 5 days to 325 mg PO q 12 h, max 425 mg q 12 h.
  PEDS — Not approved in children.
  UNAPPROVED ADULT — Cardioversion of recent onset atrial fib: 600 mg PO single dose. Outpatient prn therapy for recurrent atrial fib in highly select patients ("pill-in-the-pocket"): Single dose PO of 450 mg for wt less than 70 kg, 600 mg for wt 70 kg or greater.
  FORMS — Generic/Trade: Tabs, immediate-release scored 150, 225 mg. Caps, sustained-release, (SR-$$$$$) 225, 325, 425 mg. Generic only: Tabs, immediate-release, scored 300 mg.
  NOTES — Contraindicated with heart failure; cardiogenic shock; SA, AV or intraventricular disorders of impulse generation or conduction (e.g., sick sinus node syndrome, AV block) without pacemaker; hypotension; bradycardia; known Brugada Syndrome; bronchospastic disorders and severe COPD; electrolyte imbalance. Use inpatient rhythm monitoring prior to and during therapy; discontinue propafenone if changes are suggestive of Brugada Syndrome. Consider using with AV nodal blocking agent (beta-blocker, verapamil, diltiazem) to minimize risk of 1:1 atrial flutter. Reduce dose if QRS widening more than 20% from baseline or if 2nd/3rd degree AV block. Correct hypo/hyperkalemia and hypomagnesium before giving. Reduce dose 70 to 80% with impaired hepatic function. Use cautiously with impaired renal function. Poorly metabolized by 10% population; reduce dose and monitor for toxicity. Consult cardiologist before using with other antiarrhythmic agents. Do not use with amiodarone; quinidine; or the combination of CYP3A4 and CYP2D6 inhibitors (or CYP2D6 deficiency). CYP2D6 inhibitors (e.g., desipramine, paroxetine, ritonavir, sertraline); CYP3A4 inhibitors (e.g., ketoconazole, ritonavir, saquinavir, erythromycin, grapefruit juice); CYP1A2 inhibitors (e.g., amiodarone, cigarette smoke); cimetidine; fluoxetime may increase levels. Rifampin reduces level.

PROPAFENONE (cont.)

Orlistat reduces level; taper orlistat withdrawal in patients stabilized on propafenone. May increase digoxin level 35 to 85%. May increase beta-blocker levels. May increase INR when used with warfarin. Concomitant lidocaine increases risk of CNS side effects. Instruct patient to report any changes in OTC, prescription, supplement use and symptoms that may be associated with altered electrolytes (prolonged/excessive diarrhea, sweating, vomiting, thirst, appetite loss). May affect artificial pacemakers; monitor pacemaker function. May exacerbate myasthenia gravis. Bioavailability of 325 mg SR two times per day is equivalent to 150 mg immediate-release three times per day.

MOA — Depresses phase 0 depolarization significantly, slows cardiac conduction significantly (Class 1C).

ADVERSE EFFECTS — Serious: Agranulocytosis, arrhythmias, heart block. Frequent: Dizziness, headache, nausea, dyspnea, fatigue, blurred vision, metallic taste.

QUINIDINE ▸LK ♀C ▶+ $

WARNING — Proarrhythmic. Associated with QT prolongation and torsades de pointes. Contraindicated with complete AV block or left bundle branch block. Increased mortality in patients with non-life-threatening arrhythmias and structural heart disease (i.e., MI, LV dysfunction).

ADULT — Arrhythmia: Gluconate, extended-release: 324 to 648 mg PO q 8 to 12 h; sulfate, immediate-release: 200 to 400 mg PO q 6 to 8 h; sulfate, extended-release: 300 to 600 mg PO q 8 to 12 h. Consider inpatient rhythm and QT monitoring during initiation of therapy. Life-threatening malaria: Load with 10 mg/kg (max 600 mg) IV over 1 to 2 h, then 0.02 mg/kg/min for at least 24 h. Dose given as quinidine gluconate. When parasitemia less than 1% and PO meds tolerated, convert to PO quinine to complete 3 days (Africa/South America) or 7 days (Southeast Asia). Also give doxycycline, tetracycline, or clindamycin.

PEDS — Not approved in children.

UNAPPROVED PEDS — Arrhythmia: Test dose (oral sulfate or IM/IV gluconate) 2 mg/kg (max 200 mg). Sulfate: 15 to 60 mg/kg/day PO divided q 6 h. Life-threatening malaria: Load with 10 mg/kg IV over 1 to 2 h, then 0.02 mg/kg/min for at least 24 h. Dose given as quinidine gluconate. When parasitemia < 1% and PO meds tolerated, convert to PO quinine to complete 3 days (Africa/South America) or 7 days (Southeast Asia). Also give doxycycline, tetracycline, or clindamycin.

FORMS — Generic only: Gluconate, Tabs ($$$$), extended-release, unscored 324 mg. Sulfate, Tabs ($), scored immediate-release 200, 300 mg, Tabs, extended-release, ($$$$) 300 mg.

NOTES — Proarrhythmic. QRS widening, QT interval prolongation (risk increased by hypokalemia, hypomagnesemia, or bradycardia), hypotension, hypoglycemia. Use cautiously with renal impairment/failure or hepatic disease. Use extreme caution with history of QT prolongation or torsades de pointes.

Contraindicated with ziprasidone. Monitor ECG and BP. Drug interactions with some antiarrhythmics, digoxin, phenytoin, phenobarbital, rifampin, verapamil. Do not chew, break, or crush extended-release tabs. Do not use with digitalis toxicity, hypotension, AV/bundle branch block, or myasthenia gravis. Quinidine gluconate 267 mg = quinidine sulfate 200 mg.

MOA — Depresses phase 0 depolarization, prolongs cardiac action potential duration (Class 1A). Unknown antimalarial mechanism.

ADVERSE EFFECTS — Serious: Arrhythmias, syncope (rare), hypersensitivity (rare). Frequent: Diarrhea, hypotension, N/V, cinchonism (disturbed hearing, headaches, visual changes, confusion).

SODIUM BICARBONATE ▸K ♀C ▶? $

ADULT — Cardiac arrest: 1 mEq/kg/dose IV initially, followed by repeat doses up to 0.5 mEq/kg at 10 min intervals during continued arrest. Severe acidosis: 2 to 5 mEq/kg dose IV administered as a 4 to 8 h infusion. Repeat dosing based on lab values.

PEDS — Cardiac arrest: Neonates or infants age younger than 2 yo, 1 mEq/kg dose IV slow injection initially, followed by repeat doses up to 1 mEq/kg at 10 min intervals during continued arrest. To avoid intracranial hemorrhage due to hypertonicity, use a 1:1 dilution of 8.4% (1 mEq/mL) sodium bicarbonate and dextrose 5% or use the 4.2% (0.5 mEq/mL) product.

UNAPPROVED ADULT — Prevention of contrast-induced nephropathy: Administer 154 mEq/L soln at 3 mL/kg/h IV for 1 h before contrast, followed by infusion of 1 mL/kg/h for 6 h post procedure. If wt greater than 110 kg then dose based on 110 kg wt.

NOTES — Full correction of bicarbonate deficit should not be attempted during the first 24 h. May exacerbate intracellular acidosis.

MOA — Replacement therapy, urinary alkalinization.

ADVERSE EFFECTS — Serious: Hypernatremia (rapid infusion), edema (rapid infusion). Frequent: None.

SOTALOL (**Betapace, Betapace AF, ✦Rylosol**) ▸K ♀B ▶– $$$$

WARNING — Initiate or re-initiate this product in a facility with cardiac resuscitation capacity, continuous ECG and CrCl monitoring. Do not substitute Betapace for Betapace AF.

ADULT — Ventricular arrhythmia (Betapace), symptomatic A-fib/A-flutter (Betapace AF): Start 80 mg PO two times per day, usual maintenance dose 160 to 320 mg/day divided two times per day, max 640 mg/day. Adjust dose if CrCl < 60 mL/min.

PEDS — Not approved in children.

FORMS — Generic/Trade: Tabs, scored 80, 120, 160, 240 mg. Tabs, scored (Betapace AF) 80, 120, 160 mg.

NOTES — Proarrhythmic. Caution, higher incidence of torsades de pointes with doses higher than 320 mg/day, in women, or heart failure.

MOA — Prolongs cardiac repolarization (Class III antiarrhythmic properties).

ADVERSE EFFECTS — Serious: Arrhythmias, bradycardia, exacerbation of heart failure.

CARDIOVASCULAR: Anti-Hyperlipidemic Agents—Bile Acid Sequestrants

CHOLESTYRAMINE (*Questran, Questran Light, Prevalite, ★Olestyr*) ▶Not absorbed ♀C ▶+ $$$$
ADULT — Elevated LDL-C: Start 4 g PO daily to two times per day before meals, usual maintenance 12 to 24 g/day in divided doses two to four times per day before meals, max 24 g/day.
PEDS — Not approved in children.
UNAPPROVED ADULT — Cholestasis-associated pruritus: 4 to 8 g two to three times per day. Diarrhea: 4 to 16 g/day.
UNAPPROVED PEDS — Elevated LDL-C: Start 240 mg/kg/day PO divided three times per day before meals, usual maintenance 8 to 16 g/day divided three times per day.
FORMS — Generic/Trade: Powder for oral susp, 4 g cholestyramine resin/9 g powder (Questran), 4 g cholestyramine resin/5 g powder (Questran Light), 4 g cholestyramine resin/5.5 g powder (Prevalite). Each available in bulk powder and single-dose packets.
NOTES — Administer other drugs at least 2 h before or 4 to 6 h after cholestyramine to avoid decreased absorption of the other agent. May divide up to 6 times per day. Mix powder with 60 to 180 mL of water, milk, fruit juice, or drink. Avoid carbonated liquids for mixing. GI problems common, mainly constipation. May cause elevated triglycerides; do not use when triglycerides exceed 400 mg/dL.
MOA — Binds bile acid in the intestine, preventing their reabsorption.
ADVERSE EFFECTS — Serious: Fecal impaction (rare). Frequent: Constipation.

COLESEVELAM (*Welchol, ★Lodalis*) ▶Not absorbed ♀B ▶+ $$$$$
ADULT — LDL-C reduction or glycemic control of type 2 DM: 3.75 g once daily or 1.875 g PO two times per day, max 3.75 g/day. Give with meal and 4 to 8 ounces of water, fruit juice, or diet soft drink. 3.75 g is equivalent to 6 tabs; 1.875 g is equivalent to 3 tabs.
PEDS — Hyperlipidemia, 10 yo or older: 3.75 g once daily or 1.875 g PO two times per day, max 3.75 g/

day. Give with meal and 4 to 8 ounces of water, fruit juice, or diet soft drink. 3.75 g is equivalent to 6 tabs; 1.875 g is equivalent to 3 tabs.
FORMS — Trade only: Tabs, unscored 625 mg. Powder single-dose packets 3.75 g.
NOTES — Powder packets contain phenylalanine 13.5 mg per colesevelam 1.875 g. GI problems common, mainly constipation. May cause elevation of triglycerides. Do not use with triglycerides >500 mg/dL, or history of bowel obstruction or hypertriglyceridemia-induced pancreatitis. May decrease levels of cyclosporine, glyburide, levothyroxine, oral contraceptives containing ethinyl estradiol and norethindrone, phenytoin, warfarin.
MOA — Binds bile acid in the intestine, preventing their reabsorption.
ADVERSE EFFECTS — Serious: Fecal impaction (rare). Frequent: Constipation, dyspepsia, nausea.

COLESEVELAM (*Colestid, Colestid Flavored*) ▶Not absorbed ♀B ▶+ $$$
ADULT — Elevated LDL-C: Tabs: Start 2 g PO daily to two times per day with full glass of liquid, max 16 g/day. Granules: Start 5 g PO one to two times per day, increase by 5 g increments as tolerated at 1- to 2-month intervals, max 30 g/day. Mix granules in at least 90 mL of non-carbonated liquid.
PEDS — Not approved in children.
UNAPPROVED PEDS — 125 to 250 mg/kg/day PO in divided doses two to four times per day, dosing range 10 to 20 g/day.
FORMS — Generic/Trade: Tabs 1 g. Granules for oral susp, 5 g/7.5 g powder. Available in bulk powder and individual packets
NOTES — Administer other drugs at least 1 h before or 4 to 6 h after colestipol to avoid decreased absorption of the other agent. Swallow tabs whole. GI problems common, mainly constipation. May increase triglycerides; do not use when triglycerides above 400 mg/dL.
MOA — Binds bile acid in the intestine, preventing their reabsorption.
ADVERSE EFFECTS — Serious: Fecal impaction (rare). Frequent: Constipation.

CARDIOVASCULAR: Anti-Hyperlipidemic Agents—Fibrates

NOTE: Contraindicated with active liver disease, gall bladder disease, and/or CrCl less than 30 mL/min. Evaluate renal function (SrCr and estimated glomerular filtration rate [eGFR] based on creatinine) at baseline, within 3 months after initiation, q 6 months thereafter. Monitor LFTs (baseline, periodically as indicated). Increased risk of myopathy and rhabdomyolysis when used with a statin or colchicine. May cause paradoxical decrease in HDL; if severely depressed HDL is detected, discontinue fibrate, monitor HDL until it returns to baseline, and do not restart fibrate. May increase cholesterol excretion into bile, leading to cholelithiasis; if suspected, do gall bladder studies. May increase the effect of warfarin; reduce dose of warfarin; monitor INR. Take either at least 2 h before or 4 h after bile acid sequestrants.

BEZAFIBRATE (*★Bezalip SR*) ▶K ♀D ▶– $$$
ADULT — Canada only. Hyperlipidemia/hypertriglyceridemia: 200 mg of immediate-release PO two to three times per day, or 400 mg of sustained-release PO q am or q pm with or after

food. Reduce dose in renal insufficiency or dialysis. The 400 mg SR tab should not be used if CrCl less than 60 mL/min or creatinine greater than 1.5 mg/dL.
PEDS — Not approved in children.

BEZAFIBRATE (cont.)

FORMS — Canada Trade only: Sustained-release tab 400 mg.

MOA — Triglyceride reduction — Inhibits lipolysis, decreases FFA uptake, inhibits hepatic VLDL secretion HDL increase – unknown mechanism.

ADVERSE EFFECTS — Serious: Myopathy/rhabdomyolysis (rare), hepatotoxicity (rare), cholelithiasis (rare). Frequent: Epigastric distress, nausea, diarrhea, flatulence.

FENOFIBRATE (*TriCor, Antara, Fenoglide, Lipofen, Triglide, ✦Lipidil Micro, Lipidil Supra, Lipidil EZ*) ▶LK ♀C ▶– $$$

ADULT — Hypertriglyceridemia: Tricor tabs: Start 48 to 145 mg PO daily, max 145 mg/day. Antara: 43 to 130 mg PO daily; max 130 mg daily. Fenoglide: 40 to 120 mg PO daily; max 120 mg daily. Lipofen: 50 to 150 mg PO daily, max 150 mg daily. Triglide: 50 to 160 mg PO daily, max 160 mg daily. Generic tabs: 54 to 160 mg, max 160 mg daily. Generic caps: 67 to 200 mg PO daily, max 200 mg daily. Hypercholesterolemia/mixed dyslipidemia: Tricor tabs: 145 mg PO daily. Antara: 130 mg PO daily. Fenoglide: 120 mg daily. Lipofen: 150 mg daily. Triglide: 160 mg daily. Generic tabs: 160 mg daily. Generic caps: 200 mg PO daily. Renal impairment, elderly: Tricor tabs: Start 48 mg PO daily; Antara: Start 43 mg PO daily; Fenoglide: 40 mg daily/Lipofen: Start 50 mg daily; Triglide: Start 50 mg PO daily; generic tabs: Start 40 to 54 mg PO daily; generic caps 43 mg PO daily.

PEDS — Not approved in children.

FORMS — Generic only: Tabs, unscored 54, 160 mg. Generic caps 67, 134, 200 mg. Generic/Trade: Tabs (TriCor), unscored 48, 145 mg. Caps, (Antara) 43, 130 mg. Trade only: (Fenoglide) unscored 40, 120 mg. Tabs (Lipofen), unscored 50, 150 mg. Tabs (Triglide), unscored 50, 160 mg.

NOTES — May consider concomitant therapy with a low- or moderate-intensity statin if the benefits from CVD risk reduction or triglyceride lowering (when 500 mg/dL or more) outweigh the risk of adverse effects. May increase serum creatinine level without changing eGFR. All formulations, except Antara, Tricor, and Triglide, should be taken with food to increase plasma concentrations. Conversion between forms: Generic 200 mg cap with food is equivalent to 145 mg Tricor; Tricor 48 mg and 145 mg replaced micronized Tricor 54 mg and 160 mg.

MOA — Activates lipoprotein lipase and reduces apoprotein C-III leading to elimination of triglycerides.

ADVERSE EFFECTS — Serious: Tumor (rare), hepatotoxicity (rare), myopathy/rhabdomyolysis (rare), cholelithiasis (rare).

FENOFIBRIC ACID (*Fibricor, TriLipix*) ▶LK ♀C ▶– $$$

ADULT — Mixed dyslipidemia and CHD or CHD risk equivalent in combination with optimal statin therapy: TriLipix: 135 mg PO daily. Hypertriglyceridemia: Fibricor: 35 to 105 mg PO daily, max 105 mg daily. TriLipix: 45 to 135 mg PO daily, max 135 mg daily. Hypercholesterolemia/mixed dyslipidemia: Fibricor: 105 mg PO daily. TriLipix: 135 mg PO daily. Renal impairment: Fibricor: 35 mg PO daily. TriLipix: 45 mg PO daily.

PEDS — Not approved in children.

FORMS — Trade only: Caps (Trilipix) delayed-release 45, 135 mg. Tabs (Fibricor) 35, 105 mg. Generic only: Tabs 35, 105 mg.

NOTES — May consider concomitant therapy with a low- or moderate-intensity statin if the benefits from CVD risk reduction or triglyceride lowering (when 500 mg/dL or more) outweigh the risk of adverse effects. May increase serum creatinine level without changing eGFR. Co-administration of immunosuppressant or other potentially nephrotoxic medications may increase the risk of nephrotoxicity.

MOA — Activates lipoprotein lipase and reduces apoprotein C-III leading to elimination of triglycerides.

ADVERSE EFFECTS — Serious: Tumor (rare), hepatotoxicity (rare), myopathy/rhabdomyolysis (rare), cholelithiasis (rare).

GEMFIBROZIL (*Lopid*) ▶LK ♀C ▶? $

ADULT — Hypertriglyceridemia/primary prevention of artery heart disease: 600 mg PO two times per day 30 min before meals.

PEDS — Not approved in children.

FORMS — Generic/Trade: Tabs, scored 600 mg.

NOTES — Do not use with statin; increases risk of myopathy and rhabdomyolysis. Do not use with repaglinide; increases risk of hypoglycemia. Consider alternative therapy when baseline serum creatinine is greater than 2 mg/dL.

MOA — Activates lipoprotein lipase and reduces apoprotein C-III leading to elimination of triglycerides.

ADVERSE EFFECTS — Serious: Hepatotoxicity (rare), myopathy/rhabdomyolysis (rare), cholelithiasis (rare), angioedema. Frequent: Dyspepsia, abdominal pain, nausea, diarrhea, headache.

CARDIOVASCULAR: Anti-Hyperlipidemic Agents—HMG-CoA Reductase Inhibitors ("Statins") and combinations

NOTE: Each statin has restricted maximum doses that are lower than typical maximum doses when used with certain interacting medications; see prescribing information for complete information. Consider patient characteristics that may modify the decision to use higher intensity statin therapy, including history of hemorrhagic stroke or Asian descent. Evaluate muscle symptoms before initiating statin therapy and at each follow-up visit. Measure creatinine kinase before starting statin, if patient at risk for adverse muscle events. Risk of muscle issues increase with advanced age (65 yo or more), female gender, uncontrolled hypothyroidism, low vitamin D level, renal impairment, higher statin doses, history of muscle disorders, and concomitant use of certain medicines (ex. fibrates, niacin 1 gram or more, colchicine, or ranolazine). Teach patients to report promptly unexplained muscle pain, tenderness, or weakness; rule out common causes;

discontinue if myopathy diagnosed or suspected. Obtain creatine kinase, TSH, vitamin D level when patient complains of muscle soreness, tenderness, weakness, or pain. With tolerable muscle complaints or asymptomatic creatine kinase increase < 10 times upper limit of normal, continue statin at same or reduced dose; use symptoms to guide continuing/discontinuing statin. With intolerable muscle symptoms with/without creatine kinase elevation, discontinue statin; when asymptomatic, may restart same/different statin at same/lower dose. With rhabdomyolysis, discontinue statin, provide IV hydration; weigh risk/benefit of statin therapy when recovered. Rare reports of immune-mediated necrotizing myopathy. : Rare. Monitor ALT before initiating statin therapy and as clinically indicated thereafter. May initiate, continue, or increase dose of statin with modest LFT elevation (less than 3 times upper limit of normal). Repeat LFTs and rule out other causes with isolated, asymptomatic LFT elevation less than 3 times upper limit of normal. Consider continuing vs. discontinuing statin or reducing statin dose. Discontinue statin with persistent ALT elevations more than 3 times the upper limit of normal or objective evidence of liver injury; seek cause; consider referral to gastroenterologist or hepatologist. : Measure A1c before starting statin, if diabetes status unknown. Statins may increase the risk of hyperglycemia and type 2 diabetes in patients with risk factors for diabetes. In 100 individuals treated with statin therapy for 1 year, the risk of diabetes is ~0.1 and ~0.3 excess cases with a moderate-intensity and high-intensity statin respectively. Benefits outweighs risks. : The 2013 ACC/AHA cholesterol guidelines expert panel did not find evidence that statins adversely affect cognition. If patient complains of confusion or memory impairment while on statin therapy, consider all possible causes, including other drugs (eg, sleep aides, analgesics, OTC antihistamines) and medical conditions (eg, depression, anxiety, sleep apnea) that affect memory.

ADVICOR (lovastatin + niacin) ▶LK ♀X ▶– $$$$
ADULT — Hyperlipidemia: 1 tab PO at bedtime with a low-fat snack, max 40/2000 mg/day. Establish dose using extended-release niacin first. If already on lovastatin, substitute combo product with lowest niacin dose. If therapy is discontinued more than 7 days, reinstitute therapy with lowest dose. See component drugs for other dosing restrictions.
PEDS — Not approved in children.
FORMS — Trade only: Tabs, unscored extended-release lovastatin/niacin 20/500, 20/750, 20/1000, 40/1000 mg.See component drug for other dose restrictions.
NOTES — Swallow whole; do not break, chew, or crush. Immediate-release aspirin or NSAID 30 min prior may decrease niacin flushing reaction. Niacin may worsen glucose control, peptic ulcer disease, gout, headaches, and menopausal flushing.
MOA — See component drugs.
ADVERSE EFFECTS — See component drugs.

ATORVASTATIN (Lipitor) ▶L ♀X ▶– $
ADULT — Hyperlipidemia/prevention of cardiovascular events: Start 10 mg PO daily, 40 mg daily for LDL-C reduction > 45%, increase at intervals of 4 weeks or more to a max of 80 mg/day. Do not give with cyclosporine; tipranavir + ritonavir; or telaprevir. Use with caution and lowest dose necessary with lopinavir + ritonavir. Do not exceed 20 mg/day when given with clarithromycin, itraconazole, other protease inhibitors (saquinavir + ritonavir, darunavir + ritonavir, fosamprenavir, or fosamprenavir + ritonavir). Do not exceed 40 mg/day when given with boceprevir or nelfinavir.
PEDS — Hyperlipidemia, 10 yo or older: Start 10 mg daily, max 20 mg/day. See prescribing information for more information.
FORMS — Generic/Trade: Tabs, unscored 10, 20, 40, 80 mg.
NOTES — Metabolized by CYP3A4 enzyme system. May give any time of day. May increase digoxin level. Take concomitant rifampin at the same time with atorvastatin to avoid reduction of atorvastatin level. May increase levels or norethindrone and

ethinyl estradiol. Patients with recent CVA/TIA and no CHD who received atorvastatin 80 mg/day had a higher incidence of hemorrhagic stroke and non-fatal hemorrhagic stroke than placebo group in the posthoc analysis of the SPARCL trial.
MOA — Inhibits 3-hydroxy-3-methyl-glutaryl-coenzyme A (HMG-CoA) reductase which converts HMG-CoA to mevalonate in cholesterol biosynthesis.
ADVERSE EFFECTS — Serious: Hepatotoxicity (rare), myopathy/rhabdomyolysis (rare). Frequent: Headache, dyspepsia.

CADUET (amlodipine + atorvastatin) ▶L ♀X ▶– $$$$$
ADULT — Simultaneous treatment of HTN and hypercholesterolemia: Establish dose using component drugs first. See component drug for other dose restrictions. Dosing interval: Daily.
PEDS — Not approved in children.
FORMS — Generic/Trade: Tabs, 2.5/10, 2.5/20, 2.5/40, 5/10, 5/20, 5/40, 5/80, 10/10, 10/20, 10/40, 10/80 mg.
MOA — See component drugs.
ADVERSE EFFECTS — TAB017

FLUVASTATIN (Lescol, Lescol XL) ▶L ♀X ▶– $$$$
ADULT — Hyperlipidemia: Start 20 mg PO at bedtime for LDL-C reduction of less than 25%, 40 to 80 mg at bedtime for LDL-C reduction of 25% or more, max 80 mg/day, give 80 mg daily (Lescol XL) or 40 mg two times per day. Prevention of cardiac events post-percutaneous coronary intervention: 80 mg of extended-release PO daily, max 80 mg daily. Do not exceed 20 mg/day when given with cylosporine or fluconazole.
PEDS — Hyperlipidemia: Start 20 mg PO at bedtime, max 80 mg daily (XL) or divided two times per day. See prescribing information for more information.
FORMS — Generic/Trade: Caps 20, 40 mg. Trade only: Tab, extended-release, unscored 80 mg.
NOTES — Mainly metabolized by the CYP2C9, so less potential for drug interactions. Monitor blood sugar levels when given with glyburide and the dose of fluvastatin is changed. Monitor phenytoin levels when given with phenytoin and fluvastatin is initiated or

FLUVASTATIN (cont.)

the dose is changed. Monitor INR when given with warfarin and fluvastatin is initiated, discontinued or the dose is changed.

MOA — Inhibits 3-hydroxy-3-methyl-glutaryl-coenzyme A (HMG-CoA) reductase which converts HMG-CoA to mevalonate in cholesterol biosynthesis.

ADVERSE EFFECTS — Serious: Hepatotoxicity (rare), myopathy/rhabdomyolysis (rare). Frequent: Headache, dyspepsia.

LIPTRUZET (ezetimibe + atorvastatin) ▶L - ♀X ▶- $$$$

ADULT — Hyperlipidemia: Start 10/10 or 10/20 mg PO daily, max 10/80 mg/day. See component drug for other dose restrictions.

PEDS — Not approved in children.

FORMS — Trade only: Tabs, unscored ezetimibe/atorvastatin 10/10, 10/20, 10/40, 10/80 mg.

NOTES — Take either at least 2 h before or 4 h after bile acid sequestrants.

MOA — See compenent drugs.

ADVERSE EFFECTS — See component drugs.

LOVASTATIN (Mevacor, Altoprev) ▶L ♀X ▶- $$$

ADULT — Hyperlipidemia/prevention of cardiovascular events: Start 20 mg PO daily with the evening meal, increase at intervals of 4 weeks or more to max 80 mg/day (daily or divided two times per day). Altoprev dosed daily with max dose 60 mg/day. Do not use with boceprevir, clarithromycin, cobicistat-containing products, cyclosporine, erythromycin, gemfibrozil, grapefruit juice, HIV protease inhibitors, itraconazole, ketoconazole, nefazodone, posaconazole, telaprevir, telithromycin, or voriconazole; increases risk of myopathy. Do not exceed 20 mg/day when used with danazol, diltiazem, dronedarone, verapamil, or CrCl less than 30 mL/min. Do not exceed 40 mg/day when used with amiodarone.

PEDS — Hyperlipidemia, 10 yo or older: Start 10 mg PO q PM, max 40 mg/day. See prescribing information for more information.

FORMS — Generic/Trade: Tabs, unscored 20, 40 mg. Generic Only: Tabs unscored, 10 mg. Trade Only: Tabs extended-release (Altoprev) 20, 40, 60 mg.

NOTES — Metabolized by CYP3A4 enzyme system.

MOA — Inhibits 3-hydroxy-3-methyl-glutaryl-coenzyme A (HMG-CoA) reductase which converts HMG-CoA to mevalonate in cholesterol biosynthesis.

ADVERSE EFFECTS — Serious: Hepatotoxicity (rare), myopathy/rhabdomyolysis (rare). Frequent: Headache, dyspepsia.

PITAVASTATIN (Livalo) ▶L - ♀X ▶- $$$$

ADULT — Hyperlipidemia: Start 2 mg PO at bedtime, max 4 mg daily. CrCl 15 to 59 mL/min or end-stage renal disease receiving hemodialysis: Max start 1 mg PO daily, max 2 mg daily. Do not use with cyclosporine. Do not exceed 1 mg/day when given with erythromycin. Do not exceed 2 mg/day when given with rifampin.

PEDS — Not approved in children.

FORMS — Trade only: Tabs 1, 2, 4 mg.

NOTES — Mainly metabolized by CYP2C9.

MOA — Inhibits 3-hydroxy-3-methyl-glutaryl-coenzyme A (HMG-CoA) reductase which converts HMG-CoA to mevalonate in cholesterol biosynthesis.

ADVERSE EFFECTS — Serious: Hepatotoxicity (rare), myopathy/rhabdomyolysis (rare). Frequent: Constipation, diarrhea, myalgia.

PRAVASTATIN (Pravachol) ▶L ♀X ▶- $$$

ADULT — Hyperlipidemia/prevention of cardiovascular events: Start 40 mg PO daily, increase at intervals of 4 weeks or more to max 80 mg/day. Renal or hepatic impairment: Start 10 mg PO daily. Do not exceed 20 mg/day when given with cyclosporine. Do not exceed 40 mg/day when given with clarithromycin.

PEDS — Hyperlipidemia, 8 to 13 yo: 20 mg PO daily; 14 to 18 yo: 40 mg PO daily. See prescribing information for more information.

FORMS — Generic/Trade: Tabs, unscored 10, 20, 40, 80 mg.

NOTES — Not metabolized substantially by the CYP isoenzyme system, less potential for drug interactions.

MOA — Inhibits 3-hydroxy-3-methyl-glutaryl-coenzyme A (HMG-CoA) reductase, which converts HMG-CoA to mevalonate in cholesterol biosynthesis.

ADVERSE EFFECTS — Serious: Hepatotoxicity (rare), myopathy/rhabdomyolysis (rare). Frequent: Headache, dyspepsia.

ROSUVASTATIN (Crestor) ▶L ♀X ▶- $$$$$

ADULT — Hyperlipidemia/slow progression of atherosclerosis/primary prevention of cardiovascular disease: Start 10 to 20 mg daily, may adjust dose after 2 to 4 weeks, max 40 mg/day. Do not start with 40 mg; use 40 mg only when treatment goal not achieved with 20 mg/day. Renal impairment (CrCl less than 30 mL/min and not on hemodialysis): Start 5 mg PO daily, max 10 mg/day. Asians: Start 5 mg PO daily. When given with atazanavir with or without ritonavir or lopinavir with ritonavir, do not exceed 10 mg/day. When given with cyclosporine, do not exceed 5 mg/day. Avoid using with gemfibrozil; if used concomitantly, do not exceed 10 mg/day. When given with colchicine, do not exceed 5 mg/day.

PEDS — Hyperlipidemia, 10 yo or older: Start 5 to 20 mg PO daily, max 20 mg/day. See prescribing information for more information. Canada only: May use with age older than 8 yo with homozygous familial hypercholesterolemia.

UNAPPROVED ADULT — Primary prevention of major cardiovascular events in patients with LDL-C less than 130 mg/dL and high-sensitivity CRP 2 mg/dL or greater: 20 mg PO daily.

FORMS — Trade only: Tabs, unscored 5, 10, 20, 40 mg.

NOTES — Partially metabolized by CYP2C9 enzyme system. Potentiates effects of warfarin; monitor INR. Give aluminum- and magnesium-containing antacids more than 2 h after rosuvastatin. Proteinuria, with unknown clinical significance, reported with 40 mg/day; consider dose reduction when using 40 mg/day with unexplained persistent proteinuria.

(cont.)

ROSUVASTATIN (cont.)

MOA — Inhibits 3-hydroxy-3-methyl-glutaryl-coenzyme A (HMG-CoA) reductase which converts HMG-CoA to mevalonate in cholesterol biosynthesis.

ADVERSE EFFECTS — Serious: Hepatotoxicity (rare), myopathy/rhabdomyolysis (rare). Frequent: Myalgia, constipation, nausea, asthenia, abdominal pain, proteinuria (transient), hematuria (transient).

SIMCOR (simvastatin + niacin) ▶LK ♀X ▶– $$$$

ADULT — Hyperlipidemia: 1 tab PO at bedtime with a low-fat snack, max 40/2000 mg/day. If niacin-naive or switching from immediate-release niacin, start: 20/500 mg PO q pm. If receiving extended-release niacin, do not start with more than 40/2000 mg PO q pm. Do not use with boceprevir, clarithromycin, cyclosporine, danazol, diltiazem, erythromycin, fenofibrate, gemfibrozil, grapefruit juice, HIV protease inhibitors, itraconazole, ketoconazole, nefazodone, posaconazole, strong CYP3A4 inhibitors, telaprevir, telithromycin, verapamil; increases risk of myopathy. Do not exceed 20/1000 mg/day when used in Chinese patients or with amiodarone, amlodipine or ranolazine; increases risk of myopathy.

PEDS — Not approved in children.

FORMS — Trade only: Tabs, unscored extended-release simvastatin/niacin 20/500, 20/750, 20/1000, 40/500, 40/1000 mg.

NOTES — Swallow whole; do not break, chew, or crush. Immediate-release aspirin or NSAID 30 min prior may decrease niacin flushing reaction. Niacin may worsen glucose control, peptic ulcer disease, gout, headaches, and menopausal flushing. May increase INR when given with warfarin.

MOA — See component drugs.

ADVERSE EFFECTS — See component drugs.

SIMVASTATIN (Zocor) ▶L ♀X ▶– $

ADULT — Do not initiate therapy with or titrate to 80 mg/day; only use 80 mg/day in patients who have taken this dose for more than 12 months without evidence of muscle toxicity. Hyperlipidemia: Start 10 to 20 mg PO q pm, max 40 mg/day. Reduce cardiovascular mortality/events in high risk for coronary heart disease event: Start 40 mg PO q pm, max 40 mg/day. Severe renal impairment: Start 5

mg/day, closely monitor. Chinese patients: Do not exceed 20 mg/day with niacin 1 g or more daily. Do not use with boceprevir, clarithromycin, cobicistat-containing products, cyclosporine, danazol, erythromycin, gemfibrozil, grapefruit juice, HIV protease inhibitors, itraconazole, ketoconazole, nefazodone, posaconazole, strong CYP3A4 inhibitors, telaprevir, telithromycin, voriconazole; increases risk of myopathy. Do not exceed 10 mg/day when used with diltiazem, dronedarone, or verapamil. Do not exceed 20 mg/day when used with amiodarone, amlodipine or ranolazine. Do not exceed 20 mg/day when used with lomitapide; if patient has been on simvastatin 80 mg/day for at least 1 year without muscle toxicity, then do not exceed 40 mg/day when used with lomitapide.

PEDS — Hyperlipidemia, 10 yo or older: Start 10 mg PO q pm, max 40 mg/day. See prescribing information for more information.

FORMS — Generic/Trade: Tabs, unscored 5, 10, 20, 40, 80 mg.

NOTES — May increase INR when given with warfarin.

MOA — Inhibits 3-hydroxy-3-methyl-glutaryl-coenzyme A (HMG-CoA) reductase which converts HMG-CoA to mevalonate in cholesterol biosynthesis.

ADVERSE EFFECTS — Serious: Hepatotoxicity, myopathy/rhabdomyolysis (rare). Frequent: Headache, dyspepsia.

VYTORIN (ezetimibe + simvastatin) ▶L ♀X ▶– $$$$

ADULT — Hyperlipidemia: Start 10/10 or 10/20 mg PO q pm, max 10/40 mg/day. Restrict the use of the 10/80 mg dose to patients who have taken it at least 12 months without muscle toxicity. See simvastatin monograph for other dose restrictions.

PEDS — Not approved in children.

UNAPPROVED ADULT — Reduce risk of CV events in patients with CKD, not on dialysis: 10/20 mg/day.

FORMS — Trade only: Tabs, unscored ezetimibe/simvastatin 10/10, 10/20, 10/40, 10/80 mg.

NOTES — Give at least 2 h before or 4 h after bile acid sequestrant. May increase INR when given with warfarin.

MOA — See component drugs.

ADVERSE EFFECTS — See component drugs.

CARDIOVASCULAR: Anti-Hyperlipidemic Agents—Omega Fatty Acids

NOTE: FDA-approved fish oil. Swallow whole; do not crush, break, or chew. Prolongs bleeding time, may potentiate warfarin. Monitor AST/ALT if hepatic impairment. Use caution in patients with known hypersensitivity to fish and/or shellfish.

ICOSAPENT ETHYL (Vascepa) ▶L ♀C ▶? $$$$$

ADULT — Adjunct to diet to reduce high triglycerides (500 mg/dL or above): 4 caps PO daily or divided two times per day. Contains EPA+DHA.

PEDS — Not approved in children.

FORMS — Trade only: Caps 1 g.

MOA — May reduce hepatic VLDL-TG synthesis and/or secretion; enhances TG clearance from circulating VLDL particles.

ADVERSE EFFECTS — Serious: Hypersensitivity. Frequent: Arthralgia.

OMEGA-3-ACID ETHYL ESTERS (Lovaza) ▶L ♀C ▶? $$$$$

ADULT — Adjunct to diet to reduce high triglycerides (500 mg/dL or above): 4 caps PO daily or divided two times per day. Contains EPA+DHA.

PEDS — Not approved in children.

FORMS — Generic/Trade: 1 g cap.

MOA — May reduce hepatic VLDL-TG synthesis and/or secretion; enhances TG clearance from circulating VLDL particles.

OMEGA-3-ACID ETHYL ESTERS (*cont.*)

ADVERSE EFFECTS — Serious: Hypersensitivity. Frequent: Belching, dyspepsia, taste changes.

OMEGA-3-CARBOXYLIC ACIDS (*Epanova*) ▶L ♀C ▶? $$$$$

ADULT — Adjunct to diet to reduce high triglycerides (500 mg/dL or above): 2 or 4 caps PO daily. Contains EPA.

PEDS — Not approved in children.

FORMS — Trade only: Caps 1 g.

MOA — May reduce hepatic VLDL-TG synthesis and/or secretion; enhances TG clearance from circulating VLDL particles.

ADVERSE EFFECTS — Serious: Hypersensitivity. Frequent: abdominal pain, belching, diarrhea, nausea.

CARDIOVASCULAR: Anti-Hyperlipidemic Agents—Other

EZETIMIBE (*Zetia, ✦Ezetrol*) ▶L ♀C ▶? $$$$

WARNING — May increase cyclosporine levels.

ADULT — Hyperlipidemia: 10 mg PO daily alone or in combination with statin or fenofibrate.

PEDS — Not approved in children.

UNAPPROVED PEDS — Hyperlipidemia, 10 yo or older: 10 mg PO daily coadministered with simvastatin.

FORMS — Trade only: Tabs, unscored 10 mg.

NOTES — Take either at least 2 h before or 4 h after bile acid sequestrants. Monitor cyclosporine levels (may increase). When used with statin, monitor LFTs before initiating and as clinically indicated thereafter. Do not use with fibrate other than fenofibrate. Concomitant fenofibrate increases ezetimibe level and may increase risk of cholelithiasis.

MOA — Selectively inhibits small intestine cholesterol absorption.

ADVERSE EFFECTS — Serious: Anaphylaxis, angioedema, cholelithiasis, cholecystitis, myopathy/rhabdomyolysis (rare), pancreatitis, thrombocytopenia. Frequent: Arthralgia, back pain, diarrhea, rash.

LOMITAPIDE (*Juxtapid*) ▶L ♀X ▶– $$$$$

WARNING — May elevate liver transaminases. Measure ALT, AST, alkaline phosphatase, total bilirubin before starting therapy; measure ALT and AST regularly as recommended. Adjust dose if ALT or AST 3 or more times the upper limit of normal. Discontinue with clinically significant liver toxicity. Increases hepatic steatosis, which may be a risk factor for progressive liver disease, including steatohepatitis and cirrhosis. Only available through restricted Juxtapid REMS program.

ADULT — Only approved in patients with homozygous familial hypercholesterolemia: Start 5 mg PO once daily. May increase as tolerated to 10 mg daily after at least 2 weeks; then to 20 mg daily after at least 4 weeks; then to 40 mg daily after at least 4 weeks; max 60 mg/day. End-stage renal disease on dialysis or with baseline mild hepatic impairment: Do not exceed 40 mg daily. Before initiating therapy: measure ALT, AST, alkaline phosphatase, and total bilirubin; obtain a negative pregnancy test in women of childbearing age; initiate low-fat diet with <20% of energy from fat. Swallow whole; take with water, without food at least 2 hours after evening meal. Depletes absorption of fat-soluble vitamins/fatty acids; patient should take daily vitamin E 400 international units and at least linoleic acid 200 mg, alpha-linolenic acid (ALA) 210 mg, eicosapentaenoic acid (EPA) 110 mg, and docosahexaenoic acid (DHA) 80 mg. Do not use with strong or moderate CYP3A4 inhibitors, moderate or severe hepatic impairment, active liver disease, or unexplained persistent abnormal liver function tests. Do not exceed 30 mg daily with concomitant weak CYP3A4 inhibitors, including atorvastatin and oral contraceptives. May increase warfarin levels; monitor INR. May increase levels of simvastatin, lovastatin, p-glycoprotein substrates; limit doses of these when used concomitantly with lomitapide. Give bile acid sequestrants at least 4 hours before or after lomitapide.

PEDS — Not approved in children.

FORMS — Trade only: Caps 5, 10, 20 mg.

MOA — Decreases the synthesis of chylomicrons and VLDL by inhibiting microsomal triglyceride transfer protein.

ADVERSE EFFECTS — Serious: Hepatotoxicity. Frequent: Abdominal pain, diarrhea, dyspepsia, nausea, vomiting.

MIPOMERSEN (*Kynamro*) ▶tissues - ♀B ▶? $$$$$

WARNING — May elevate liver transaminases. Measure ALT, AST, alkaline phosphatase, total bilirubin before starting therapy; measure ALT and AST regularly as recommended. Hold dose if ALT or AST 3 or more times the upper limit of normal. Discontinue with clinically significant liver toxicity. Increases hepatic steatosis, which may be a risk factor for progressive liver disease, including steatohepatitis and cirrhosis. Only available through restricted Kynamro REMS program.

ADULT — Only approved in patients with homozygous familial hypercholesterolemia: 200 mg subcutaneously once weekly. Before initiating therapy: measure ALT, AST, alkaline phosphatase, and total bilirubin. Do not use as adjunct to LDL apheresis. Do not use with moderate or severe hepatic impairment, active liver disease, or unexplained persistent abnormal liver function tests.

PEDS — Not approved in children.

FORMS — Trade only: Single-use vial or prefilled syringe containing 1 mL of a 200 mg/mL solution.

MOA — Inhibits apolipoprotein B-100 synthesis.

ADVERSE EFFECTS — Serious: Hepatotoxicity. Frequent: flu-like symptoms, headache, injection site reactions, nausea.

CARDIOVASCULAR: Antiadrenergic Agents

CLONIDINE (*Catapres, Catapres-TTS, Kapvay, ✱Dixarit*)
▶LK ♀C ▶? $
ADULT — HTN, immediate-release: Start 0.1 mg PO two times per day, may increase by 0.1 mg/day each week, usual maintenance dose 0.2 to 0.6 mg/day in 2 to 3 divided doses, max 2.4 mg/day. HTN, transdermal (Catapres-TTS): Start 0.1 mg/24 h patch q week, titrate to desired effect, max effective dose 0.6 mg/24 h (two 0.3 mg/24 h patches).
PEDS — HTN: Start 5 to 7 mcg/kg/day PO divided q 6 to 12 h, titrate at 5 to 7 days intervals to 5 to 25 mcg/kg/day divided q 6 h; max 0.9 mg/day. Transdermal therapy not recommended in children. ADHD (6 to 17 yo), extended-release (KapVay): Start 0.1 mg PO at bedtime; may increase by 0.1 mg/day each week; give twice daily with equal or higher dose at bedtime, max 0.4 mg daily.
UNAPPROVED ADULT — HTN urgency: Initially 0.1 to 0.2 mg PO, followed by 0.1 mg q 1 h prn up to a total dose of 0.5 to 0.7 mg. Menopausal flushing: 0.1 to 0.4 mg/day PO divided two to three times per day; transdermal applied weekly 0.1 mg/day. Tourette syndrome: 3 to 5 mcg/kg/day PO divided two to four times per day. Opioid withdrawal, adjunct: 0.1 to 0.3 mg PO three to four times per day or 0.1 to 0.2 mg PO q 4 h tapering off over days 4 to 10. Alcohol withdrawal, adjunct: 0.1 to 0.2 mg PO q 4 h prn. Smoking cessation: Start 0.1 mg PO two times per day, increase 0.1 mg/day at weekly intervals to 0.75 mg/day as tolerated; transdermal (Catapres-TTS): 0.1 to 0.2 mg/24 h patch q week for 2 to 3 weeks after cessation. ADHD: 5 mcg/kg/day PO for 8 weeks. Posttraumatic stress disorder: Start 0.1 mg PO bedtime, max 0.6 mg/day in divided doses.
UNAPPROVED PEDS — ADHD: Start 0.05 mg PO at bedtime, titrate based on response over 8 weeks to max 0.2 mg/day (for wt less 45 kg) or to max 0.4 mg/day (wt 45 kg or greater) in 2 to 4 divided doses. Tourette syndrome: 3 to 5 mcg/kg/day PO divided two to four times per day.
FORMS — Generic/Trade: Tabs, immediate-release, unscored (Catapres) 0.1, 0.2, 0.3 mg. Transdermal weekly patch ($$$$$) 0.1 mg/day (TTS-1), 0.2 mg/day (TTS-2), 0.3 mg/day (TTS-3). Tabs, extended-release, unscored ($$$$$) 0.1 mg. Trade only: Tabs, extended-release, unscored (Kapvay-$$$$$) 0.2 mg.
NOTES — The sympatholytic action of clonidine may worsen sinus node dysfunction and atrioventricular block, especially in patients taking other sympatholytic drugs. Monitor for bradycardia when taking concomitant digoxin, nondihydropyridine calcium channel blockers, or beta blockers. Use lower initial dose with renal impairment. Rebound HTN with abrupt discontinuation of tabs, especially at doses that exceed 0.7 mg/day. Taper therapy slowly q 3 to 7 days to avoid rebound HTN. Dispose of used patches carefully, keep away from children. Remove patch before defibrillation, cardioversion, or MRI to avoid skin burns. Transdermal therapy should not be interrupted during the surgical period. Oral therapy should be continued within 4 h of surgery and restarted as soon as possible afterward. May potentiate the CNS depressive effects of alcohol, barbiturates, or other sedating drugs. Concomitant TCAs may reduce the BP lowering effects. Concomitant neuroleptics may induce or exacerbate, orthostatic regulation disturbances (eg, orthostatic hypotension, dizziness, fatigue). With alcoholic delirium, high intravenous doses of clonidine may increase the arrhythmogenic potential (QT-prolongation, ventricular fibrillation) of high IV doses of haloperidol. Do not crush, chew, or break extended-release tablets. Monitor response and side effects when interchanging between clonidine products; many are not equivalent on mg:mg basis.
MOA — Centrally acting alpha-2 agonist.
ADVERSE EFFECTS — Serious: Rebound hypertension, orthostatic hypotension, depression, bradycardia, syncope. Frequent: Dry mouth, constipation, drowsiness, dizziness, sedation, sexual dysfunction, rash.

DOXAZOSIN (*Cardura, Cardura XL*) ▶L ♀C ▶? $$
WARNING — Not first-line agent for HTN. Increased risk of heart failure in patients who used doxazosin compared to diuretic in treating HTN.
ADULT — BPH, immediate-release: Start 1 mg PO at bedtime, titrate by doubling the dose over at least 1- to 2-week intervals up to a maximum of 8 mg PO at bedtime. BPH, extended-release (not approved for HTN): Start 4 mg PO q am with breakfast, titrate dose in 3 to 4 weeks to max dose 8 mg PO q am. HTN, immediate-release: Start 1 mg PO at bedtime, max 16 mg/day. Avoid use of doxazosin alone to treat combined HTN and BPH.
PEDS — Not approved in children.
UNAPPROVED ADULT — Promote spontaneous passage of ureteral calculi: 4 mg (XL formulation only) PO daily usually combined with an NSAID, antiemetic, and opioid of choice.
FORMS — Generic/Trade: Tabs, scored 1, 2, 4, 8 mg. Trade only (Cardura XL): Tabs, extended-release, 4, 8 mg.
NOTES — Orthostatic hypotension is common. Bedtime dosing may minimize side effects. Initial 1 mg dose is used to decrease postural hypotension that may occur after the 1st few doses. If therapy is interrupted for several days, restart at the 1 mg dose. Increased risk of hypotension when used with erectile dysfunction medication (e.g., sildenafil, tadalafil, vardenafil); use lowest dose of erectile dysfunction medication. Use caution with concomitant strong CYP3A4 inhibitor (e.g., clarithromycin, itraconazole, ketoconazole, nefazodone, protease inhibitor, telithromycin, or voriconazole). Intraoperative floppy iris syndrome may occur during cataract surgery, if patient is on or previously taken alpha-1 blocker.

DOXAZOSIN (*cont.*)

MOA — Blocks binding of catecholamines to post-synaptic alpha-1 receptors; decreases urethral resistance.

ADVERSE EFFECTS — Serious: Postural hypotension, heart failure. Frequent: Headache, dizziness, fatigue, nausea, constipation.

GUANFACINE (*Tenex,* ✽*Intuniv XR*) ▶K ♀B ▶? $

ADULT — HTN: Start 1 mg PO at bedtime, increase to 2 to 3 mg at bedtime if needed after 3 to 4 weeks, max 3 mg/day.

PEDS — HTN age 12 yo and older: Use adult dosage.

UNAPPROVED PEDS — ADHD: Start 0.5 mg PO daily, titrate by 0.5 mg q 3 to 4 days as tolerated to 0.5 mg PO three times per day.

FORMS — Generic/Trade: Tabs unscored 1, 2 mg.

NOTES — Most of antihypertensive effect is seen at 1 mg/day. Rebound HTN with abrupt discontinuation.

MOA — Centrally acting alpha-2 agonist.

ADVERSE EFFECTS — Serious: Syncope, rebound hypertension, hallucinations. Frequent: Sedation, dizziness, dry mouth, constipation, impotence.

METHYLDOPA ▶LK ♀B ▶+ $

ADULT — HTN: Start 250 mg PO two to three times per day usual maintenance dose 500 to 3000 mg/day divided two to four times per day, max 3000 mg/day. Hypertensive crisis: 250 to 500 mg IV q 6 h, maximum 1 g IV q 6 h, maximum 4000 mg/day.

PEDS — HTN: 10 mg/kg/day PO divided two to four times per day, titrate dose to a max dose 65 mg/kg/day or 3000 mg/day, whichever is less.

FORMS — Generic only: Tabs, unscored 250, 500 mg.

NOTES — May be used to manage BP during pregnancy. IV form has a slow onset of effect and other agents preferred for rapid reduction of BP. Hemolytic anemia possible. The brand name product (Aldomet) is no longer available.

MOA — Stimulates central alpha-adrenergic receptors reducing sympathetic outflow.

ADVERSE EFFECTS — Serious: Hemolytic anemia (rare), LFT abnormalities. Frequent: Sedation, dizziness, dry mouth, constipation, impotence.

PRAZOSIN (*Minipress*) ▶L ♀C ▶? $$

WARNING — Not first line agent for HTN. Increased risk of heart failure in patients who used related drug doxazosin compared to diuretic in treating HTN.

ADULT — HTN: Start 1 mg PO two to three times per day, usual maintenance dose 20 mg/day divided two to three times per day, max 40 mg/day, but doses higher than 20 mg/day usually do not increase efficacy.

PEDS — Not approved in children.

UNAPPROVED ADULT — Posttraumatic stress disorder nightmares: Start 1 mg PO bedtime, increase weekly by 1 to 2 mg/day to max dose of 20 mg/day. Doses greater than 10 mg/day are divided early evening and at bedtime.

UNAPPROVED PEDS — HTN: Start 0.005 mg/kg PO single dose; increase slowly prn up to maintenance dose 0.025 to 0.150 mg/kg/day divided q 6 h; max dose 0.4 mg/kg/day.

FORMS — Generic/Trade: Caps 1, 2, 5 mg.

NOTES — Othostatic hypotension common; to avoid, start with 1 mg at bedtime, and increase dose gradually. Increased risk of hypotension when used with erectile dysfunction medication (e.g., sildenafil, tadalafil, verdenafil); use lowest dose of erectile dysfunction medication. Intraoperative floppy iris syndrome may occur during cataract surgery, if patient is on or previously taken alpha-1 blocker.

MOA — Blocks binding of catecholamines to post-synaptic alpha-1 receptors.

ADVERSE EFFECTS — Serious: Postural hypotension, heart failure. Frequent: Headache, dizziness

RESERPINE ▶LK ♀C ▶– $$

ADULT — HTN: Start 0.05 to 0.1 mg PO daily or 0.1 mg PO every other day, max dose 0.25 mg/day.

PEDS — Not approved in children.

FORMS — Generic only: Tabs, scored 0.1, 0.25 mg.

NOTES — Should be used in combination with a diuretic to counteract fluid retention and augment BP control. May cause depression at higher doses, avoid use in patients with uncontrolled depression or active peptic ulcer disease.

MOA — Blocks transport of norepinephrine into storage granules.

ADVERSE EFFECTS — Serious: None. Frequent: Nasal stuffiness.

TERAZOSIN ▶LK ♀C ▶? $$

WARNING — Not first-line for HTN. Increased risk of heart failure in patients who used related drug doxazosin compared to diuretic in treating HTN.

ADULT — HTN: Start 1 mg PO at bedtime usual effective dose 1 to 5 mg PO daily or divided two times per day, max 20 mg/day. BPH: Start 1 mg PO at bedtime titrate dose in a stepwise fashion to 2, 5, or 10 mg PO at bedtime to desired effect. Treatment with 10 mg PO at bedtime for 4 to 6 weeks may be needed to assess benefit. Maximum 20 mg/day.

PEDS — Not approved in children.

FORMS — Generic only: Caps 1, 2, 5, 10 mg.

NOTES — Orthostatic hypotension is common. Bedtime dosing may minimize side effects. Initial 1 mg dose is used to decrease postural hypotension that may occur after the first few doses. If therapy is interrupted for several days, restart at the 1 mg dose. Increased risk of hypotension when used with erectile dysfunction medication (e.g., sildenafil, tadalafil, verdenafil); use lowest dose of erectile dysfunction medication. Intraoperative floppy iris syndrome may occur during cataract surgery, if patient is on or previously taken alpha-1 blocker. The brand name product (Hytrin) is no longer available.

MOA — Blocks binding of catecholamines to post-synaptic alpha-1 receptors, increases urinary flow rate.

ADVERSE EFFECTS — Serious: Postural hypotension, heart failure. Frequent: Headache, dizziness.

CARDIOVASCULAR: Antihypertensive Combinations

NOTE: In general, establish dose using component drugs first. See component drugs for metabolism, pregnancy, and lactation.

***ACCURETIC* (quinapril + hydrochlorothiazide)** ▶See component drugs ♀See component drugs ▶See component drugs $$
WARNING — Do not use in pregnancy.
ADULT — HTN: Dosing interval: Daily.
PEDS — Not approved in children.
FORMS — Generic/Trade: Tabs, scored 10/12.5, 20/12.5, unscored 20/25 mg.
MOA — See component drugs.

***ALDACTAZIDE* (spironolactone + hydrochlorothiazide)** ▶See component drugs ♀See component drugs ▶See component drugs $$
WARNING — Spironolactone is a tumorigen in rats. Use only for approved indications and only if necessary. Should not be used for initial therapy of edema or HTN; these conditions require individualized dosing. Treatment of HTN and edema should be reevaluated as patient's condition warrants.
ADULT — HTN: Dosing interval: Daily to two times per day.
PEDS — Not approved in children.
FORMS — Generic/Trade: Tabs, unscored 25/25 mg. Trade only: Tabs, scored 50/50 mg.
MOA — See component drugs.

***ALDORIL* (methyldopa + hydrochlorothiazide)** ▶See component drugs ♀See component drugs ▶See component drugs $$
WARNING — Titrate component drugs first to avoid hypotension.
ADULT — HTN: Dosing interval: two times per day.
PEDS — Not approved in children.
FORMS — Generic only: Tabs, unscored, 250/15, 250/25 mg.
MOA — See component drugs.

***AMTURNIDE* (aliskiren + amlodipine + hydrochlorothiazide)** ▶See component drugs - ♀D ▶- $$$$
WARNING — Do not use in pregnancy.
ADULT — HTN: Dosing interval: daily.
PEDS — Not approved in children.
FORMS — Trade only: Tabs, unscored 150/5/12.5, 300/5/12.5, 300/5/25, 300/10/12.5, 300/10/25 mg.

***ATACAND HCT* (candesartan + hydrochlorothiazide, ✶*Atacand Plus*)** ▶See component drugs ♀See component drugs ▶See component drugs $$$$
WARNING — Do not use in pregnancy.
ADULT — HTN: Dosing interval: Daily.
PEDS — Not approved in children.
FORMS — Generic/Trade: Tabs, unscored 16/12.5, 32/12.5, 32/25 mg.
MOA — See component drugs.

***AVALIDE* (irbesartan + hydrochlorothiazide)** ▶See component drugs ♀See component drugs ▶See component drugs $
WARNING — Do not use in pregnancy.
ADULT — HTN, initial therapy for patients needing multiple medications: Start 150/12.5 PO daily, may increase after 1 to 2 weeks, max 300/25 daily.
PEDS — Not approved in children.
FORMS — Generic/Trade: Tabs, unscored 150/12.5, 300/12.5.
MOA — See component drugs.

***AZOR* (amlodipine + olmesartan)** ▶See component drugs ♀See component drugs ▶See component drugs $$$
WARNING — Do not use in pregnancy.
ADULT — HTN, initial therapy for patients needing multiple medications: Start 5/20 mg PO daily, may increase after 1 to 2 weeks, max 10/40 daily.
PEDS — Not approved in children.
FORMS — Trade only: Tabs, unscored 5/20, 5/40, 10/20, 10/40 mg.
MOA — See component drugs.

***CAPOZIDE* (captopril + hydrochlorothiazide)** ▶See component drugs ♀See component drugs ▶See component drugs $$
WARNING — Do not use in pregnancy.
ADULT — HTN: Dosing interval: two to three times per day.
PEDS — Not approved in children.
FORMS — Generic only: Tabs, scored 25/15, 25/25, 50/15, 50/25 mg.
MOA — See component drugs.

***CLORPRES* (clonidine + chlorthalidone)** ▶See component drugs ♀See component drugs ▶See component drugs $$$$$
ADULT — HNT: Dosing interval: two to three times per day.
PEDS — Not approved in children.
FORMS — Trade only: Tabs, scored 0.1/15, 0.2/15, 0.3/15 mg.
MOA — See component drugs.

***CORZIDE* (nadolol + bendroflumethiazide)** ▶See component drugs ♀See component drugs ▶See component drugs $$$
WARNING — Avoid abrupt cessation in coronary heart disease or HTN.
ADULT — HTN: Dosing interval: Daily.
PEDS — Not approved in children.
FORMS — Generic/Trade: Tabs 40/5, 80/5 mg.
MOA — See component drugs.

***DIOVAN HCT* (valsartan + hydrochlorothiazide)** ▶See component drugs ♀See component drugs ▶See component drugs $$$$
WARNING — Do not use in pregnancy.
ADULT — HTN, initial therapy for patients needing multiple medications: Start 160/12.5 PO daily, may increase after 1 to 2 weeks, max 300/25 daily.
PEDS — Not approved in children.
FORMS — Generic/Trade: Tabs, unscored 80/12.5, 160/12.5, 320/12.5, 160/25, 320/25 mg.
MOA — See component drugs.

DUTOPROL (metoprolol succinate + hydrochloro-thiazide) ▶See component drugs - ♀See component drugs. ▶ $
WARNING — Avoid abrupt cessation in coronary heart disease or HTN.
ADULT — HTN: Dosing interval: Daily.
FORMS — Trade only: Tabs, unscored 25/12.5, 50/12.5, 100/12.5.
MOA — See component drugs.
ADVERSE EFFECTS — See component drugs.

DYAZIDE (triamterene + hydrochlorothiazide) ▶See component drugs ♀See component drugs ▶See component drugs $
ADULT — HTN: Dosing interval: Daily.
PEDS — Not approved in children.
FORMS — Generic/Trade: Caps, (Dyazide) 37.5/25 mg. Generic only: Caps, 50/25 mg.
NOTES — Dyazide 37.5/25 cap same combination as Maxzide-25 tab.
MOA — See component drugs.
ADVERSE EFFECTS — See component drugs.

EDARBYCLOR (azilsartan + chlorthalidone) ▶See component drugs - See component drugs ♀D ▶? $$$$
WARNING — Do not use in pregnancy.
ADULT — HTN, intial therapy for patients needing multiple medications: Start 40/12.5 PO daily, may increase after 2 to 4 weeks, max 40/25 daily.
FORMS — Trade only: Tabs, unscored 40/12.5, 40/25 mg.
MOA — See component drugs.
ADVERSE EFFECTS — See component drugs.

EXFORGE (amlodipine + valsartan) ▶See component drugs ♀See component drugs ▶See component drugs $$$$
WARNING — Do not use in pregnancy.
ADULT — HTN, initial therapy for patients needing multiple medications: Start 5/160 PO daily, may increase after 1 to 2 weeks, max 10/320 daily.
PEDS — Not approved in children.
FORMS — Trade only: Tabs, unscored 5/160, 5/320, 10/160, 10/320 mg.
MOA — See component drugs.

EXFORGE HCT (amlodipine + valsartan + hydrochlo-rothiazide) ▶See component drugs ♀See component drugs ▶See component drugs $$$$
WARNING — Do not use in pregnancy.
ADULT — HTN, add-on/switch therapy when HTN not adequately controlled on any two of the following classes: calcium channel blockers, angiotensin receptor blockers, and diuretics: Dosing interval: Daily.
PEDS — Not approved in children.
FORMS — Trade only: Tabs, unscored 5/160/12.5, 5/160/25, 10/160/12.5, 10/160/25, 10/320/25 mg.
MOA — See component drugs.

HYZAAR (losartan + hydrochlorothiazide) ▶See component drugs ♀See component drugs ▶See component drugs $$$
WARNING — Do not use in pregnancy.
ADULT — HTN, initial therapy for patients needing multiple medications: Start 50/12.5 mg PO daily,

may increase after 2 to 4 weeks, max 100/25 mg daily. CVA risk reduction in HTN and LV hypertro-phy (CVA risk reduction may not occur in patients of African descent): Establish dose using component drugs first. Dosing interval: Daily.
PEDS — Not approved in children.
FORMS — Generic/Trade: Tabs, unscored 50/12.5, 100/12.5, 100/25 mg.
MOA — See component drugs.

INDERIDE (propranolol + hydrochlorothiazide) ▶See component drugs ♀See component drugs ▶See component drugs $$$
WARNING — Avoid abrupt cessation in coronary heart disease or HTN.
ADULT — HTN: Dosing interval: Daily to two times per day.
PEDS — Not approved in children.
FORMS — Generic only: Tabs, scored 40/25, 80/25 mg.
NOTES — Do not crush or chew cap contents. Swallow whole.
MOA — See component drugs.
ADVERSE EFFECTS — See component drugs.

INHIBACE PLUS (cilazapril + hydrochlorothiazide) ▶See component drugs ♀See component drugs ▶See component drugs $$
WARNING — Do not use in pregnancy.
ADULT — Canada only, HTN: Dosing interval daily.
PEDS — Not approved in children.
FORMS — Trade: Tabs, scored 5/12.5 mg.
MOA — See component drugs.

LOPRESSOR HCT (metoprolol + hydrochlorothiazide) ▶See component drugs ♀See component drugs ▶See component drugs $$$
WARNING — Abrupt cessation in coronary heart dis-ease or HTN.
ADULT — HTN: Dosing interval: Daily to two times per day.
PEDS — Not approved in children.
FORMS — Generic/Trade: Tabs, scored 50/25, 100/25 mg. Generic only: Tabs, scored 100/50 mg.
MOA — See component drugs.

LOTENSIN HCT (benazepril + hydrochlorothiazide) ▶See component drugs ♀See component drugs ▶See component drugs $$$
WARNING — Do not use in pregnancy.
ADULT — HTN: Dosing interval: Daily.
PEDS — Not approved in children.
FORMS — Generic/Trade: Tabs, scored 5/6.25, 10/12.5, 20/12.5, 20/25 mg.
MOA — See component drugs.

LOTREL (amlodipine + benazepril) ▶See component drugs ♀See component drugs ▶See component drugs $$$
WARNING — Do not use in pregnancy.
ADULT — HTN: Dosing interval: Daily.
PEDS — Not approved in children.
FORMS — Generic/Trade: Caps, 2.5/10, 5/10, 5/20, 10/20, 5/40, 10/40 mg.
MOA — See component drugs.

MAXZIDE (triamterene + hydrochlorothiazide, ✸*Triazide*) ▶See component drugs ♀See component drugs ▶See component drugs $
ADULT — HTN: Dosing interval: Daily.

(cont.)

MAXZIDE (cont.)
PEDS — Not approved in children.
FORMS — Generic/Trade: Tabs, scored 75/50 mg.
MOA — See component drugs.
MAXZIDE-25 (triamterene + hydrochlorothiazide) ▶See component drugs ♀See component drugs ▶See component drugs $
ADULT — HTN: Dosing interval: Daily.
PEDS — Not approved in children.
FORMS — Generic/Trade: Tabs, scored 37.5/25 mg
MOA — See component drugs.
MICARDIS HCT (telmisartan + hydrochlorothiazide, ✽*Micardis Plus*) ▶See component drugs ♀See component drugs ▶See component drugs $$$$
WARNING — Do not use in pregnancy.
ADULT — HTN: Dosing interval: Daily.
PEDS — Not approved in children.
FORMS — Generic/Trade: Tabs, unscored 40/12.5, 80/12.5, 80/25 mg.
NOTES — Swallow tabs whole, do not break or crush. Caution in hepatic insufficiency.
MOA — See component drugs.
ADVERSE EFFECTS — See component drugs.
MINIZIDE (prazosin + polythiazide) ▶See component drugs ♀See component drugs ▶See component drugs $$$
ADULT — HTN: Dosing interval: two to three times per day.
PEDS — Not approved in children.
FORMS — Trade only: Caps, 1/0.5, 2/0.5, 5/0.5 mg.
MOA — See component drugs.
MODURETIC (amiloride + hydrochlorothiazide, ✽*Moduret*) ▶See component drugs ♀See component drugs ▶See component drugs $
ADULT — HTN: Dosing interval: Daily. The brand name product (Moduretic) is no longer available.
PEDS — Not approved in children.
FORMS — Generic only: Tabs, scored 5/50 mg.
MOA — See component drugs.
MONOPRIL HCT (fosinopril + hydrochlorothiazide) ▶See component drugs ♀See component drugs ▶See component drugs $$
WARNING — Do not use in pregnancy.
ADULT — HTN: Dosing interval: Daily.
PEDS — Not approved in children.
FORMS — Generic only: Tabs, unscored 10/12.5, scored 20/12.5 mg.
MOA — See component drugs.
BENICAR HCT (olmesartan + hydrochlorothiazide, ✽*Olmetec Plus*) ▶See component drugs ♀See component drugs ▶See component drugs $$$$
WARNING — Do not use in pregnancy.
ADULT — HTN: Dosing interval: Daily.
PEDS — Not approved in children.
FORMS — Trade only: Tabs, unscored 20/12.5, 40/12.5, 40/25 mg.
MOA — See component drugs.
PRINZIDE (lisinopril + hydrochlorothiazide) ▶See component drugs ♀See component drugs ▶See component drugs $
WARNING — Do not use in pregnancy.

ADULT — HTN: Dosing interval: Daily.
PEDS — Not approved in children.
FORMS — Generic/Trade: Tabs, unscored 10/12.5, 20/12.5, 20/25 mg.
MOA — See component drugs.
TARKA (trandolapril + verapamil) ▶See component drugs ♀See component drugs ▶See component drugs $$$$
WARNING — Do not use in pregnancy.
ADULT — HTN: Dosing interval: Daily.
PEDS — Not approved in children.
FORMS — Trade only: Tabs, unscored 2/180, 1/240, 2/240, 4/240 mg.
NOTES — Contains extended-release form of verapamil. Do not chew or crush, swallow whole. Hypotension, bradyarrhythmias, and lactic acidosis have occurred in patients receiving concurrent erythromycin or clarithromycin.
MOA — See component drugs.
ADVERSE EFFECTS — See component drugs.
TEKAMLO (aliskiren + amlodipine) ▶See component drugs - ♀D ▶– $$$$
WARNING — Do not use in pregnancy.
ADULT — HTN, initial or add-on therapy for patients needing multiple medications: Start 150/5 mg daily, may increase after 1 to 2 weeks, max 300/10 mg daily.
FORMS — Trade only: Tabs unscored 150/5, 150/10, 300/5, 300/10 mg.
TEKTURNA HCT (aliskiren + hydrochlorothiazide, ✽*Rasilez HCT*) ▶See component drugs ♀See component drugs ▶See component drugs $$$
WARNING — Avoid in pregnancy.
ADULT — HTN, initial therapy for patients needing multiple medications: Start 150/12.5 PO daily, may increase after 2 weeks, max 300/25 daily.
PEDS — Not approved in children.
FORMS — Trade only: Tabs, unscored 150/12.5, 150/25, 300/12.5, 300/25 mg.
MOA — See component drugs.
TENORETIC (atenolol + chlorthalidone) ▶See component drugs ♀See component drugs ▶See component drugs $
WARNING — Avoid abrupt cessation in coronary heart disease or HTN.
ADULT — HTN: Dosing interval: Daily.
PEDS — Not approved in children.
FORMS — Generic/Trade: Tabs, scored 50/25, unscored 100/25 mg.
MOA — See component drugs.
TEVETEN HCT (eprosartan + hydrochlorothiazide, ✽*Teveten Plus*) ▶See component drugs ♀See component drugs ▶See component drugs $$$$
WARNING — Do not use in pregnancy.
ADULT — HTN: interval: Daily.
PEDS — Not approved in children.
FORMS — Trade only: Tabs, unscored 600/12.5, 600/25 mg.
MOA — See component drugs.
TRIBENZOR (amlodipine + olmesartan + hydrochlorothiazide) ▶See component drugs - ♀D ▶– $$$$$
WARNING — Do not use in pregnancy.
ADULT — HTN, add-on/switch therapy when HTN not adequately controlled on any two of the following

TRIBENZOR (cont.)
classes: calcium channel blockers, angiotensin receptor blockers, and diuretics: Dosing interval: Daily.
PEDS — Not approved in children.
FORMS — Trade only: Tabs, unscored 5/20/12.5, 5/40/12.5, 5/40/25, 10/40/12.5, 10/40/25 mg.
MOA — See component drugs.

TWYNSTA (amlodipine + telmisartan) ▶See component drugs ♀▶ $$$$
WARNING — Do not use in pregnancy.
ADULT — HTN, initial therapy for patients needing multiple medications: Start 5/40 to 5/80 mg PO daily, may increase after 2 weeks, max 10/80 mg daily. Do not use as initial therapy in patients 75 yo or older or with hepatic impairment.
PEDS — Not approved in children.
FORMS — Generic/Trade: Tabs, unscored 5/40, 5/80, 10/40, 10/80 mg.
MOA — See component drugs.

UNIRETIC (moexipril + hydrochlorothiazide) ▶See component drugs♀See component drugs ▶See component drugs $$
WARNING — Do not use in pregnancy.
ADULT — HTN: Dosing interval: Daily to two times per day.
PEDS — Not approved in children.
FORMS — Generic/Trade: Tabs, scored 7.5/12.5, 15/12.5, 15/25 mg.
MOA — See component drugs.

VASERETIC (enalapril + hydrochlorothiazide) ▶See component drugs ♀See component drugs ▶See component drugs $$
WARNING — Do not use in pregnancy.
ADULT — HTN: Dosing interval: Daily to two times per day.
PEDS — Not approved in children.
FORMS — Generic/Trade: Tabs, unscored 5/12.5, 10/25 mg.
MOA — See component drugs.

ZESTORETIC (lisinopril + hydrochlorothiazide) ▶See component drugs ♀See component drugs ▶See component drugs $$
WARNING — Do not use in pregnancy.
ADULT — HTN: Dosing interval: Daily.
PEDS — Not approved in children.
FORMS — Generic/Trade: Tabs, unscored 10/12.5, 20/12.5, 20/25 mg.
MOA — See component drugs.

ZIAC (bisoprolol + hydrochlorothiazide) ▶See component drugs ♀See component drugs ▶See component drugs $$
WARNING — Avoid abrupt cessation in coronary heart disease or HTN.
ADULT — HTN: Dosing interval: Daily.
PEDS — Not approved in children.
FORMS — Generic/Trade: Tabs, unscored 2.5/6.25, 5/6.25, 10/6.25 mg.
MOA — See component drugs.

CARDIOVASCULAR: Antihypertensives—Other

ALISKIREN (Tekturna, ✷Rasilez) ▶LK ♀D ▶–? $$$$
WARNING — Avoid in pregnancy.
ADULT — HTN: 150 mg PO daily, max 300 mg/day.
PEDS — Not approved in children.
FORMS — Trade only: Tabs, unscored 150, 300 mg.
NOTES — Women of child-bearing age should use reliable form of contraception; discontinue aliskiren as soon as pregnancy is detected. Do not use with ACE inhibitors or angiotensin receptor blockers in patients with DM or CrCl <60 mL/min. Dual inhibition of renin-angiotensin system increases risk of renal impairment, hypotension, and hyperkalemia. Do not use with cyclosporine or itraconazole. Concomitant NSAID, including selective COX-2 inhibitors, may further deteriorate renal function (usually reversible) and decrease antihypertensive effects. Hyperkalemia possible, especially if used concomitantly with other drugs that increase K+ (including K+-containing salt substitutes) and in patients with heart failure, DM, or renal impairment. Monitor potassium and renal function periodically. May increase creatine kinase, uric acid levels. Best absorbed on empty stomach; high-fat meals decrease absorption.
MOA — Direct renin inhibitor.
ADVERSE EFFECTS — Serious: Angioedema, hypotension, seizures. Frequent: Diarrhea, cough, dyspepsia, rash, GERD.

FENOLDOPAM (Corlopam) ▶LK ♀B ▶? $$$$
ADULT — Severe HTN: Dilute 10 mg in 250 mL D5W (40 mcg/mL), rate at 11 mL/h delivers 0.1 mcg/kg/min for 70 kg adult, titrate q 15 min, usual effective dose 0.1 to 1.6 mcg/kg/min. Lower initial doses (0.03 to 0.1 mcg/kg/min) associated with less reflex tachycardia.
PEDS — Reduce BP: Start 0.2 mcg/kg/min, increase by up to 0.3 to 0.5 mcg/kg/min q 20 to 30 min. Max infusion 0.8 mcg/kg/min. Administer in hospital by continuous infusion pump; use max 4 h; monitor BP and HR continuously. Refer to prescribing information for dilution instructions and infusion rates.
UNAPPROVED ADULT — Prevention of contrast nephropathy in those at risk (conflicting evidence of efficacy): Start 0.03 mcg/kg/min infusion 60 min prior to dye. Titrate infusion q 15 min up to 0.1 mcg/kg/min if BP tolerates. Maintain infusion (with concurrent saline) up to 4 to 6 h after procedure.
NOTES — Avoid concomitant beta-blocker use due to hypotension. Use cautiously with glaucoma or increased intraocular HTN.
MOA — Stimulates dopamine-1 receptors and alpha-2 receptors causing vasodilation.
ADVERSE EFFECTS — Serious: Hypotension, tachycardia, hypokalemia (rare). Frequent: Headache, flushing, nausea.

HYDRALAZINE (*Apresoline*) ▶LK ♀C ▶+ $$$
ADULT — HTN: Start 10 mg PO two to four times per day for 2 to 4 days, increase to 25 mg two to four times per day, then 50 mg two to four times per day if necessary, max 300 mg/day. Hypertensive emergency: 10 to 20 mg IV; if no IV access, 10 to 50 mg IM. Use lower doses initially and repeat prn to control BP. Preeclampsia/eclampsia: 5 to 10 mg IV initially, followed by 5 to 10 mg IV every 20 to 30 min prn to control BP.
PEDS — Not approved in children.
UNAPPROVED ADULT — Heart failure: Start 10 to 25 mg PO three times per day, target dose 75 mg three times per day, max 100 mg three times per day. Use in combination with isosorbide dinitrate for patients intolerant to ACE inhibitors.
UNAPPROVED PEDS — HTN: Start 0.75 to 1 mg/kg/day PO divided two to four times per day, increase slowly over 3 to 4 weeks up to 7.5 mg/kg/day; initial IV dose 1.7 to 3.5 mg/kg/day divided in 4 to 6 doses. HTN urgency: 0.1 to 0.2 mg/kg IM/IV q 4 to 6 h prn. Max single dose, 25 mg PO and 20 mg IV.
FORMS — Generic only: Tabs, unscored 10, 25, 50, 100 mg.
NOTES — Headache, nausea, dizziness, tachycardia, peripheral edema, systemic lupus erythematosus-like syndrome. Usually used in combination with diuretic and beta-blocker to counter side effects.
MOA — Relaxes peripheral arterial smooth muscle (vasodilation).
ADVERSE EFFECTS — Serious: SLE, angina exacerbation, rash. Frequent: Tachycardia, headache, edema.

MECAMYLAMINE (*Vecamyl*) ▶K - ♀C ▶– $$$$$
ADULT — Moderately severe or severe essential HTN or uncomplicated malignant HTN: Start 2.5 mg PO two times daily, increase as needed by 2.5 mg increments no sooner than every 2 days, usual maintenance dose 25 mg/day divided two to four times.
PEDS — Not approved in children.
FORMS — Trade only: Tabs unscored, 2.5 mg.
NOTES — Do not give with coronary insufficiency, recent AMI, glaucoma, organic pyloric stenosis, renal insufficiency, uremia, antibiotics, or sulfonamides. Orthostatic hypotension common, especially during dosage titration. If taken after eating, may give gradual absorption and smoother control of excessively high BP. Monitor BP standing and supine. Rebound, severe hypertension with sudden drug withdrawal. Discontinue slowly and use other antihypertensives.
MOA — Blocks nerve transmission in sympathetic and parasympathetic ganglia
ADVERSE EFFECTS — Serious: syncope, rebound hypertension, ileus, tremors (rare), choreiform movements (rare). Frequent: postural hypotension, dizziness, sedation, dry mouth, anorexia, N/V, diarrhea, constipation, urinary retention, impotence.

METYROSINE (*Demser*) ▶K ♀C ▶? $$$$$
ADULT — Pheochromocytoma: Start 250 mg PO four times per day, increase by 250 to 500 mg/day prn, max dose 4 g/day.

PEDS — Pheochromocytoma age older than 12 yo: Use adult dosage.
FORMS — Trade only: Caps, 250 mg.
MOA — Decreases excess production of catecholamines by blocking tyrosine hydroxylase, the rate-limiting enzyme of catecholamine synthesis.
ADVERSE EFFECTS — Serious: Crystalluria (rare). Frequent: Sedation, drooling, speech difficulty, tremor, disorientation, diarrhea.

MINOXIDIL ▶K ♀C ▶+ $$
WARNING — Potent vasodilator; may produce serious complications from hypotension and reflex tachycardia. Relatively contraindicated in patients with coronary disease (i.e., recent/acute MI, CAD, angina). May increase pulmonary artery pressure. Has been associated with development of pericardial effusion and tamponade; more likely to occur in patients with renal disease.
ADULT — Refractory HTN: Start 2.5 to 5 mg PO daily, increase at no less than 3-day intervals, usual dose 10 to 40 mg daily, max 100 mg/day.
PEDS — Not approved in children younger than 12 yo.
UNAPPROVED PEDS — HTN: Start 0.2 mg/kg PO daily, increase q 3 days prn up to 0.25 to 1 mg/kg/day daily or divided two times per day; max 50 mg/day.
FORMS — Generic only: Tabs, scored 2.5, 10 mg.
NOTES — Usually used in combination with a diuretic and a beta-blocker to counteract side effects. Relatively contraindicated with renal disease, pre-existing pulmonary hypertension, or chronic heart failure not secondary to HTN (drug may increase pulmonary artery pressure).
MOA — Relaxes peripheral arterial smooth muscle (vasodilation).
ADVERSE EFFECTS — Serious: Pericardial effusion (rare), angina exacerbation, heart failure exacerbation. Frequent: Tachycardia, headache, edema, hair growth.

NITROPRUSSIDE (*Nitropress*) ▶RBCs ♀C ▶– $
WARNING — May cause significant hypotension. Reconstituted soln must be further diluted before use. Cyanide toxicity may occur, especially with high infusion rates (10 mcg/kg/min), hepatic/renal impairment, and prolonged infusions (longer than 3 to 7 days). Protect from light.
ADULT — Hypertensive emergency: 50 mg in 250 mL D5W (200 mcg/mL), start at 0.3 mcg/kg/min (for 70 kg adult give 6 mL/h) via IV infusion, titrate slowly, usual range 0.3 to 10 mcg/kg/min, max 10 mcg/kg/min.
PEDS — Severe HTN: Use adult dosage.
NOTES — Discontinue if inadequate response to 10 mcg/kg/min after 10 min. Cyanide toxicity with high doses, hepatic/renal impairment, and prolonged infusions; check thiocyanate levels. Protect IV infusion minibag from light.
MOA — Relaxes peripheral arterial and venous smooth muscle.
ADVERSE EFFECTS — Serious: Cyanide toxicity (rare), thiocyanate toxicity (rare), methemoglobinemia (rare), severe hypotension. Frequent: N/V, sweating, flushing, weakness.

PHENOXYBENZAMINE (*Dibenzyline*) ▶KL ♀C ▶? $$$$$
ADULT — Pheochromocytoma: Start 10 mg PO two times per day, increase slowly every other day prn, usual dose 20 to 40 mg two to three times per day, max 120 mg/day.
PEDS — Not approved in children.
UNAPPROVED PEDS — Pheochromocytoma: 0.2 mg/kg/day PO daily in divided doses two to three times per day; initial dose no more than 10 mg, increase slowly every other day prn, usual dose 0.4 to 1.2 mg/kg/day.
FORMS — Trade only: Caps, 10 mg.
NOTES — Patients should be observed after each dosage increase for symptomatic hypotension and other adverse effects. Do not use for essential HTN.
MOA — Blocks binding of catecholamines to presynaptic and postsynaptic alpha receptors.
ADVERSE EFFECTS — Serious: Hypotension. Frequent: Dizziness, nasal congestion, tachycardia, miosis.

PHENTOLAMINE (*Regitine, Rogitine*) ▶Plasma ♀C ▶? $$$$
ADULT — Diagnosis of pheochromocytoma: 5 mg IV/IM. Rapid IV administration is preferred. An immediate, marked decrease in BP should occur, typically, 60 mmHg SBP and 25 mmHg DBP decrease in 2 min. HTN during pheochromocytoma surgery: 5 mg IV/IM 1 to 2 h preop, 5 mg IV during surgery prn.
PEDS — Diagnosis of pheochromocytoma: 0.05 to 0.1 mg/kg IV/IM, up to 5 mg/dose. Rapid IV administration is preferred. An immediate, marked decrease in BP should occur, typically, 60 mmHg SBP and 25 mmHg DBP decrease in 2 min. HTN during pheochromocytoma surgery: 0.05 to 0.1 mg/kg IV/IM 1 to 2 h preop, repeat q 2 to 4 h prn.
UNAPPROVED ADULT — IV extravasation of catecholamines: 5 to 10 mg in 10 mL NS, inject 1 to 5 mL SC (in divided doses) around extravasation site. Hypertensive crisis: 5 to 15 mg IV.
UNAPPROVED PEDS — IV extravasation of catecholamines: Neonates, 2.5 to 5 mg in 10 mL NS, inject 1 mL SC (in divided doses) around extravasation site; children, Use adult dosage.
NOTES — Weakness, flushing, hypotension; priapism with intracavernous injection. Use within 12 h of extravasation. Distributed to hospital pharmacies, at no charge, only for use in life-threatening situations. Call (888) 669-6682 for ordering.
MOA — Blocks binding of catecholamines to presynaptic and postsynaptic alpha receptors.
ADVERSE EFFECTS — Serious: Hypotension, tachycardia, arrhythmias. Frequent: Weakness, dizziness, flushing, nasal congestion.

CARDIOVASCULAR: Antiplatelet Drugs

ABCIXIMAB (*ReoPro*) ▶Plasma ♀C ▶? $$$$$
ADULT — Platelet aggregation inhibition, prevention of acute cardiac ischemic events associated with PTCA: 0.25 mg/kg IV bolus over 1 min via separate infusion line 10 to 60 min before procedure, then 0.125 mcg/kg/min up to 10 mcg/min infusion for 12 h. Unstable angina not responding to standard therapy when percutaneous coronary intervention (PCI) is planned within 24 h: 0.25 mg/kg IV bolus over 1 min via separate infusion line, followed by 10 mcg/min IV infusion for 18 to 24 h, concluding 1 h after PCI.
PEDS — Not approved in children.
NOTES — Thrombocytopenia possible. Discontinue abciximab, heparin, and aspirin if uncontrollable bleeding occurs.
MOA — Inhibits platelet aggregation by blocking the effects of fibrinogen and other substances at platelet glycoprotein IIb/IIIa receptors.
ADVERSE EFFECTS — Serious: Bleeding, hypersensitivity (rare), thrombocytopenia (rare). Frequent: Pain.

AGGRENOX (acetylsalicylic acid + dipyridamole) ▶LK ♀D ▶? $$$$$
ADULT — Prevention of CVA after TIA/CVA: 1 cap PO two times per day. Headache is a common adverse effect.
PEDS — Not approved in children.
FORMS — Trade only: Caps, 25 mg aspirin/200 mg extended-release dipyridamole.
NOTES — Do not crush or chew Caps. May need supplemental aspirin for prevention of MI. Concomitant anticoagulants, NSAIDs, or antiplatelet agents increase risk of bleeding.
MOA — See component drugs.
ADVERSE EFFECTS — See component drugs.

CLOPIDOGREL (*Plavix*) ▶LK ♀B ▶? $
WARNING — Requires activation to an active metabolite by the CYP system, mainly CYP2C19. When treated at recommended doses, poor metabolizers have higher cardiovascular event rates after acute coronary syndrome or percutaneous coronary intervention than patients with normal CYP2C19 function. Tests to determine a patient's CYP2C19 genotype may aid in determining therapeutic strategy. Consider alternative treatment or treatment strategies in patients identified as CYP2C19 poor metabolizers.
ADULT — Reduction of thrombotic events after recent acute MI, recent CVA, established peripheral arterial disease: 75 mg PO daily. Non-ST segment elevation acute coronary syndrome: 300 mg loading dose, then 75 mg PO daily in combination with aspirin PO daily. ST segment elevation MI: Start with/without 300 mg loading dose, then 75 mg PO daily in combination with aspirin, with/without thrombolytic.
PEDS — Not approved in children.
UNAPPROVED ADULT — Medical treatment, without stent, of unstable angina/non-ST segment elevation MI: 300 to 600 mg loading dose, then 75 mg daily in combination with aspirin for at least 1 month and up to 1 year. Medical treatment, without stent and with/without thrombolytics, of ST segment elevation MI: 300 mg loading dose, then 75 mg daily in

(cont.)

CLOPIDOGREL (*cont.*)

combination with aspirin for at least 14 days and up to 1 year. When early percutaneous coronary intervention is planned: 600 mg loading dose; consider using 300 mg if patient received thrombolytic within 12 to 24 h, then 150 mg once a day for 6 days, then 75 mg daily for at least 1 year. Post bare-metal stent placement or post drug-eluting stent placement: 75 mg daily in combination with aspirin for at least 1 year (in patients not at high risk for bleeding). Post-percutaneous coronary brachytherapy: 75 mg daily in combination with aspirin for at least one year. Acute coronary syndrome with aspirin allergy or reduction of thrombotic events in high-risk patient after TIA: 75 mg PO daily.

FORMS — Generic/Trade: Tabs, unscored 75, 300 mg.

NOTES — Allergic cross-reactivity may occur among thienopyridines. Effectiveness is reduced with impaired CYP2C19 function; avoid drugs that are strong or moderate CYP2C19 inhibitors (e.g., omeprazole, esomeprazole, cimetidine, etravirine, felbamate, fluconazole, fluoxetine, fluvoxamine, ketoconazole, voriconazole). Contraindicated with active pathologic bleeding (peptic ulcer or intracranial bleed). Prolongs bleeding time. Discontinue use 5 days before elective surgery, except in 1st year post coronary stent implantation; premature discontinuation increases risk of cardiovascular events. Concomitant aspirin, SSRI, or SNRI increases bleeding risk. Cardiovascular (but not CVA) patients may receive additional benefit when given with aspirin. Should not be used with aspirin for primary prevention of cardiovascular events.

MOA — Inhibits platelet aggregation by blocking the effects of adenosine diphosphate at its platelet receptor.

ADVERSE EFFECTS — Serious: Acute liver failure, anaphylaxis, angioedema, aplastic anemia, agranulocytosis, bleeding, pancreatitis, Stevens-Johnson syndrome, thrombotic thrombocytopenia purpura. Frequent: Pruritus, purpura, diarrhea, rash.

DIPYRIDAMOLE (*Persantine*) ▶L ♀B ▶? $$$

ADULT — Prevention of thromboembolic complications of cardiac valve replacement: 75 to 100 mg PO four times per day in combination with warfarin.

PEDS — Not approved in children younger than 12 yo.

UNAPPROVED ADULT — Platelet aggregation inhibition: 150 to 400 mg/day PO divided three to four times per day.

FORMS — Generic/Trade: Tabs, unscored 25, 50, 75 mg.

NOTES — May cause chest pain when used in CAD.

MOA — Inhibits platelet adhesion by inhibiting phosphodiesterase. Increases coronary blood flow by selective dilation of the coronary arteries.

ADVERSE EFFECTS — Serious: Angioedema, bronchospasm, thrombocytopenia. Frequent: Headache, dizziness, abdominal discomfort, perioperative bleeding (rare).

EPTIFIBATIDE (*Integrilin*) ▶K ♀B ▶? $$$$$

ADULT — Acute coronary syndrome (unstable angina/non-ST segment elevation MI): Load 180 mcg/kg IV bolus, then IV infusion 2 mcg/kg/min for up to 72 h. If percutaneous coronary intervention (PCI) occurs during the infusion, continue infusion for 18 to 24 h after procedure. PCI: Load 180 mcg/kg IV bolus just before procedure, followed by infusion 2 mcg/kg/min and a second 180 mcg/kg IV bolus 10 min after the first bolus. Continue infusion for up to 18 to 24 h (minimum 12 h) after the procedure. Renal impairment (CrCl < 50 mL/min): No change in bolus dose; decrease infusion to 1 mcg/kg/min. For obese patient (greater than 121 kg): max bolus dose 22.6 mg; max infusion rate 15 mg/h. Renal impairment and obese: max bolus dose 22.6 mg; max infusion rate 7.5 mg/h.

PEDS — Not approved in children.

NOTES — Discontinue infusion prior to CABG. Give with aspirin and heparin (unless contraindicated); discontinue heparin after percutaneous coronary intervention. Contraindicated in patients on dialysis, with a history of bleeding diathesis or active abnormal bleeding within past 30 days, severe hypertension (SBP > 200 mmHg or DBP > 110 mmHg) not controlled on antihypertensive therapy; major surgery within past 6 weeks; stroke within 30 days or any history of hemorrhagic stroke. Thrombocytopenia possible; monitor platelets. If profound thrombocytopenia occurs or platelets decrease to < 100,000 mm^3, discontinue eptifibatide and heparin and monitor serial platelet counts, assess for drug-dependent antibodies, and treat as appropriate.

MOA — Inhibits platelet aggregation by blocking the effects of fibrinogen and other substances at platelet glycoprotein IIb/IIIa receptors.

ADVERSE EFFECTS — Serious: Bleeding, thrombocytopenia (rare). Frequent: Pain.

PRASUGREL (*Effient*) ▶LK ♀B ▶? $$$$$

WARNING — May cause significant, fatal bleeding. Do not use with active bleeding or history of TIA or CVA. Generally not recommend for patients 75 yo and older. Do not start in patients likely to need urgent CABG. When possible, discontinue 7 days prior to any surgery. Risk factors for bleeding: Body wt less than 60 kg, propensity to bleed, concomitant medications that increase bleeding risk. Suspect bleeding with hypotension and recent coronary angiography, PCI, CABG, or other surgical procedure. Premature discontinuation increases risk of stent thrombosis, MI, and death.

ADULT — Reduction of thrombotic events, including stent thrombosis, after acute coronary syndrome managed with percutaneous coronary intervention (PCI): 60 mg loading dose, then 10 mg PO daily in combination with aspirin. Wt less than 60 kg: consider lower maintenance dose, 5 mg PO daily.

PEDS — Not approved in children.

FORMS — Trade only: Tabs, unscored 5, 10 mg.

NOTES — Concomitant warfarin or NSAID increases bleeding risk. Allergic cross-reactivity may occur among thienopyridines.

PRASUGREL *(cont.)*

MOA — Inhibits platelet activation and aggregation by blocking the effects of adenosine diphosphate at its platelet receptor.

ADVERSE EFFECTS — Serious: Angioedema, bleeding.

TICAGRELOR (*Brilinta*) ▶L - ♀C ▶? $$$$$

WARNING — May cause significant, fatal bleeding. Do not use with active bleeding or history of intracranial hemorrhage. Do not start in patients likely to need urgent CABG. When possible, discontinue 5 days prior to any surgery. Suspect bleeding with hypotension and recent coronary angiography, PCI, CABG, or other surgical procedure. If possible, manage bleeding without discontinuing ticagrelor; discontinuation increases risk of cardiovascular events. After the initial dose of aspirin, use with aspirin 75-100 mg daily; doses of aspirin greater than 100 mg daily reduce the effectiveness of ticagrelor.

ADULT — Reduction of thrombotic events in patients with acute coronary syndrome (MI or unstable angina): 180 mg loading dose, then 90 mg PO two times daily in combination with aspirin. After the initial dose of aspirin, do not use more than 100 mg of aspirin daily with ticagrelor.)

PEDS — Not approved in children.

FORMS — Trade only: Tabs, unscored 90 mg.

NOTES — Do not use with strong CYP3A inhibitors (e.g., clarithromycin, HIV protease inhibitors, itraconazole, ketoconazole, nefazodone, telithromycin, voriconazole), CYP3A inducers (e.g., carbamazepine, dexamethasone, phenobarbital, phenytoin, rifampin), or severe hepatic impairment. P-glycoprotein inhibitors (e.g., cyclosporine) increase ticagrelor levels. Monitor digoxin levels when initiating or changing ticagrelor therapy. Increases risk of statin-related side effects when used concomitantly with more than 40 mg daily of simvastatin or lovastatin.

MOA — Inhibits platelet activation by reversibly interacting with the adenosine diphosphate receptor.

ADVERSE EFFECTS — Serious: Angioedema, bleeding. Frequent: Dyspnea.

TICLOPIDINE ▶L ♀B ▶? $$$$

WARNING — May cause life-threatening neutropenia, agranulocytosis, and thrombotic thrombocytopenia purpura (TTP). During 1st 3 months of treatment, monitor patient clinically and hematologically for neutropenia or TTP; discontinue if evidence is seen.

ADULT — Due to adverse effects, other antiplatelet agents preferred. Platelet aggregation inhibition/reduction of thrombotic CVA: 250 mg PO twice daily with food. Prevention of cardiac stent occlusion: 250 mg PO twice daily in combo with aspirin 325 mg PO daily for up to 30 days post-stent implantation.

PEDS — Not approved in children.

UNAPPROVED ADULT — Prevention of graft occlusion with CABG: 250 mg PO two times per day.

FORMS — Generic/Trade: Tabs, unscored 250 mg.

NOTES — Allergic cross-reactivity may occur among thienopyridines. Check CBC q 2 weeks during the first 3 months of therapy. Neutrophil counts usually return to normal within 1 to 3 weeks following discontinuation. Loading dose 500 mg PO on day 1 may be used for prevention of cardiac stent occlusion. The brand name product (Ticlid) is no longer available.

MOA — Inhibits platelet aggregation by blocking the effects of adenosine diphosphate at its platelet receptor.

ADVERSE EFFECTS — Serious: Bleeding, thrombocytopenia (rare), neutropenia (rare). Frequent: Diarrhea, nausea, dyspepsia.

TIROFIBAN (*Aggrastat*) ▶K ♀B ▶? $$$$$

ADULT — Non-ST segment elevation acute coronary syndromes: Give 25 mcg/kg over 3 min, then 0.15 mcg/kg/min for up to 18 h. Renal impairment (CrCl 60 mL/min or less): Give 25 mcg/kg over 3 min, then 0.075 mcg/kg/min.

PEDS — Not approved in children.

NOTES — Thrombocytopenia possible. Concomitant aspirin and heparin/enoxaparin use recommended, unless contraindicated. Dose heparin to keep PTT 2 times normal.

MOA — Inhibits platelet aggregation by blocking the effects of fibrinogen and other substances at platelet glycoprotein IIb/IIIa receptors.

ADVERSE EFFECTS — Serious: Bleeding, thrombocytopenia (rare). Frequent: Pain.

CARDIOVASCULAR: Beta-Blockers

NOTE: See also Antihypertensive Combinations. Not first line for HTN (unless concurrent angina, post MI, or heart failure with reduced ejection fraction). Atenolol may be less effective for HTN than other beta-blockers. Non-selective beta-blockers, including carvedilol and labetalol, are contraindicated with asthma; use agents with beta-1 selectivity and monitor cautiously; beta-1 selectivity diminishes at high doses. Contraindicated with acute decompensated heart failure, sick sinus syndrome without pacer, cardiogenic shock, heart block greater than first degree, or severe bradycardia. Agents with intrinsic sympathomimetic activity (eg, pindolol) are contraindicated post acute MI. Abrupt cessation may precipitate angina, MI, arrhythmias, tachycardia, rebound HTN; or with thyrotoxicosis, thyroid storm; discontinue by tapering over 1 to 2 weeks. Do not routinely stop chronic beta blocker therapy prior to surgery. Discontinue beta-blocker several days before discontinuing concomitant clonidine to minimize the risk of rebound HTN. Some inhalation anesthetics may increase the cardiodepressant effect of beta-blockers. With pheochromocytoma, give beta-blocker only after initiating alpha-blocker; using beta-blocker alone may increase BP due to the attenuation of beta-mediated vasodilatation in skeletal muscle (unopposed alpha stimulation). Patients actively using cocaine should avoid beta-blockers with unopposed alpha-adrenergic vasoconstriction, because this will promote coronary artery vasoconstriction/spasm (carvedilol or labetalol have additional alpha-1-blocking effects and are safer). Concomitant amiodarone, disopyramide, clonidine, digoxin, or nondihydropyridine calcium channel blockers may increase risk of bradycardia. Monitor for heart failure exacerbation and hypotension (particularly orthostatic) when titrating dose. May increase blood sugar or mask tachycardia occurring with hypoglycemia. May aggravate psoriasis or symptoms of arterial insufficiency. Intraoperative floppy iris syndrome may occur during cataract surgery, if patient is on or has previously taken agents with alpha-1 blocking activity.

ACEBUTOLOL (*Sectral*, ✦*Rhotral*) ▶LK ♀B ▶– $$
WARNING — Avoid abrupt cessation in coronary heart disease or HTN.
ADULT — HTN: Start 400 mg PO daily or 200 mg PO two times per day, usual maintenance 400 to 800 mg/day, max 1200 mg/day. Twice daily dosing appears to be more effective than daily dosing.
PEDS — Not approved in children age younger than 12 yo.
UNAPPROVED ADULT — Angina: Start 200 mg PO two times per day, increase prn up to 800 mg/day.
FORMS — Generic/Trade: Caps 200, 400 mg.
NOTES — Beta-1 receptor selective; has mild intrinsic sympathomimetic activity.
MOA — Blocks binding of catecholamines to beta-1 receptors.
ADVERSE EFFECTS — Serious: Bronchoconstriction (high doses), masks hypoglycemic response and slow recovery, rebound hypertension/angina. Frequent: Bradycardia, fatigue, impotence.

ATENOLOL (*Tenormin*) ▶K ♀D ▶– $
WARNING — Avoid abrupt cessation in coronary heart disease or HTN.
ADULT — Acute MI: 50 to 100 mg PO daily or in divided doses. HTN: Start 25 to 50 mg PO daily or divided two times per day, maximum 100 mg/day. Renal impairment, elderly: Start 25 mg PO daily, increase prn. Angina: Start 50 mg PO daily or divided two times per day, increase prn to max of 200 mg/day.
PEDS — Not approved in children.
UNAPPROVED ADULT — Reduce perioperative cardiac events (death) in high-risk patients undergoing noncardiac surgery: Start 5 to 10 mg IV prior to anesthesia, then 50 to 100 mg PO daily during hospitalization (max 7 days). Maintain HR between 55 to 65 bpm. Hold dose for HR less than 55 bpm and SBP less than 100 mm Hg. Reentrant PSVT associated with ST-elevation MI (after carotid massage, IV adenosine): 2.5 to 5 mg over 2 min to 10 mg max over 10 to 15 min. Rate control of atrial fibrillation/flutter: Start 25 mg PO daily, titrate to desired heart rate.
UNAPPROVED PEDS — HTN: 1 to 1.2 mg/kg/dose PO daily, max 2 mg/kg/day.
FORMS — Generic/Trade: Tabs, unscored 25, 100 mg; scored, 50 mg.
NOTES — Beta-1 receptor selective. Doses greater than 100 mg/day usually do not provide further BP lowering. Risk of hypoglycemia to neonates born to mothers using atenolol at parturition or while breastfeeding. May be less effective for HTN and lowering CV event risk than other beta-blockers.

MOA — Blocks binding of catecholamines to beta-1 receptors.
ADVERSE EFFECTS — Serious: Bronchoconstriction (high doses), masks hypoglycemic response and slow recovery, rebound hypertension/angina. Frequent: Bradycardia, fatigue, impotence.

BETAXOLOL (*Kerlone*) ▶LK ♀C ▶? $
WARNING — Avoid abrupt cessation in coronary heart disease or HTN.
ADULT — HTN: Start 5 to 10 mg PO daily, max 20 mg/day. Renal impairment, elderly: Start 5 mg PO daily, increase prn.
PEDS — Not approved in children.
FORMS — Generic/Trade: Tabs scored 10 mg, unscored 20 mg.
NOTES — Beta-1 receptor selective.
MOA — Blocks binding of catecholamines to beta-1 receptors.
ADVERSE EFFECTS — Serious: Bronchoconstriction (high doses), masks hypoglycemic response and slow recovery, rebound hypertension/angina. Frequent: Bradycardia, fatigue, impotence.

BISOPROLOL (*Zebeta*, ✦*Monocor*) ▶LK ♀C ▶? $$
WARNING — Avoid abrupt cessation in coronary heart disease or HTN.
ADULT — HTN: Start 2.5 to 5 mg PO daily, max 20 mg/day. Renal impairment: Start 2.5 mg PO daily, increase prn.
PEDS — Not approved in children.
UNAPPROVED ADULT — Compensated heart failure: Start 1.25 mg PO daily, double dose q 2 weeks as tolerated to goal 10 mg/day. Reduce perioperative cardiac events (death, MI) in high-risk patients undergoing noncardiac surgery: Start 5 mg PO daily, at least 1 week prior to surgery, increase to 10 mg daily to maintain HR less than 60 bpm, continue for 30 days postop. Hold dose for HR less than 50 bpm or SBP less than 100 mm Hg.
FORMS — Generic/Trade: Tabs, scored 5 mg, unscored 10 mg.
NOTES — Monitor closely for heart failure exacerbation and hypotension when titrating dose. Avoid in decompensated heart failure (i.e., NYHA class IV heart failure or pulmonary edema). Stabilize dose of digoxin, diuretics, and ACE inhibitor before starting bisoprolol. Highly beta-1 receptor selective.
MOA — Blocks binding of catecholamines to beta-1 receptors.
ADVERSE EFFECTS — Serious: Bronchoconstriction (high doses), masks hypoglycemic response and slow recovery, rebound hypertension/angina. Frequent: Bradycardia, fatigue, impotence.

CARVEDILOL (*Coreg, Coreg CR*) ▶L ♀C ▶? $$$
WARNING — Avoid abrupt cessation in coronary heart disease or HTN.
ADULT — Heart failure: Immediate-release: Start 3.125 mg PO two times per day, double dose q 2 weeks as tolerated up to max of 25 mg two times per day (for wt 85 kg or less) or 50 mg two times per day (for wt 85 kg or greater). Heart failure, sustained-release: Start 10 mg PO daily, double dose q 2 weeks as tolerated up to max of 80 mg/day. Reduce cardiovascular risk in post MI with LV dysfunction, immediate-release: Start 3.125 to 6.25 mg PO two times per day, double dose q 3 to 10 days as tolerated to max of 25 mg two times per day. LV dysfunction post MI, sustained-release: Start 10 to 20 mg PO daily, double dose q 3 to 10 days as tolerated to max of 80 mg/day. HTN, immediate-release: Start 6.25 mg PO two times per day, double dose q 7 to 14 days as tolerated to max 50 mg/day. HTN, sustained-release: Start 20 mg PO daily, double dose q 7 to 14 days as tolerated to max 80 mg/day.
PEDS — Not approved in children.
FORMS — Generic/Trade: Tabs, immediate-release, unscored 3.125, 6.25, 12.5, 25 mg. Trade only: Caps, extended-release 10, 20, 40, 80 mg.
NOTES — Alpha-1, beta-1, and beta-2 receptor blocker. Avoid in hepatic impairment. May reversibly elevate LFTs. Amiodarone may increase carvedilol levels. May increase digoxin levels. Reduce the dose with bradycardia (< 55 bpm). Take with food to decrease orthostatic hypotension. Separate Coreg CR and alcohol (including medications containing alcohol) by at least 2 h. Give Coreg CR in the morning. The contents of Coreg CR may be sprinkled over applesauce and consumed immediately. Dosing conversion from immediate-release to sustained-release: 3.125 mg two times per day = 10 mg CR; 6.25 mg two times per day = 20 mg CR; 12.5 mg two times per day = 40 mg CR; 25 mg two times per day = 80 mg CR.
MOA — Blocks binding of catecholamines to postsynaptic alpha-1, beta-1, and beta-2 receptors.
ADVERSE EFFECTS — Serious: Anaphylaxis, angioedema, bronchoconstriction, masks hypoglycemic response and slow recovery, rebound hypertension/angina. Frequent: Bradycardia, fatigue, impotence, hypotension.

ESMOLOL (*Brevibloc*) ▶K ♀C ▶? $$$$$
ADULT — SVT/HTN emergency: Load 500 mcg/kg over 1 min (dilute 5 g in 500 mL (10 mg/mL) and give 3.5 mL to deliver 35 mg bolus for 70 kg patient) then start infusion 50 to 200 mcg/kg/min (42 mL/h delivers 100 mcg/kg/min for 70 kg patient). If optimal response is not attained, repeat IV load and increase IV infusion to 100 mcg/kg/min for 4 min. If necessary, additional boluses (500 mcg/kg/min over 1 min) may be given followed by IV infusion with increased dose by 50 mcg/kg/min for 4 min. Max IV infusion rate 200 mcg/kg/min.
PEDS — Not approved in children.
UNAPPROVED PEDS — Same schedule as adult except loading dose 100 to 500 mcg/kg IV over 1 min and IV infusion 25 to 100 mcg/kg/min. IV infusions may be increased by 25 to 50 mcg/kg/min q 5 to 10 min. Titrate dose based on response.

NOTES — Hypotension. Beta-1 receptor selective. Half-life is 9 min.
MOA — Blocks binding of catecholamines to beta-1 receptors.
ADVERSE EFFECTS — Serious: Bronchoconstriction (high doses), masks hypoglycemic response and slow recovery, rebound hypertension/angina. Frequent: Bradycardia, fatigue.

LABETALOL (*Trandate*) ▶LK ♀C ▶+ $$$
WARNING — Avoid abrupt cessation in coronary heart disease or HTN.
ADULT — HTN: Start 100 mg PO two times per day, usual maintenance dose 200 to 600 mg two times per day, max 2400 mg/day. HTN emergency: Start 20 mg slow IV injection, then 40 to 80 mg IV q 10 min prn up to 300 mg total cumulative dose or start 0.5 to 2 mg/min IV infusion, adjust rate prn up to total cumulative dose 300 mg.
PEDS — Not approved in children.
UNAPPROVED PEDS — HTN: 4 mg/kg/day PO divided two times per day, increase prn up to 40 mg/kg/day. IV: Start 0.3 to 1 mg/kg/dose (max 20 mg) slow IV injection q 10 min or 0.4 to 1 mg/kg/h IV infusion up to 3 mg/kg/h.
FORMS — Generic/Trade: Tabs, scored 100, 200, 300 mg.
NOTES — Alpha-1, beta-1, and beta-2 receptor blocker. May be used to manage BP during pregnancy. The brand name product (Normodyne) is no longer available.
MOA — Blocks binding of catecholamines to postsynaptic alpha-1, beta-1, and beta-2 receptors.
ADVERSE EFFECTS — Serious: Bronchoconstriction, hepatotoxicity, masks hypoglycemic response and slow recovery, rebound hypertension/angina. Frequent: Bradycardia, fatigue, impotence, hypotension.

METOPROLOL (*Lopressor, Toprol-XL, ✱Betaloc*) ▶L ♀C ▶? $$
WARNING — Avoid abrupt cessation in coronary heart disease or HTN.
ADULT — Acute MI: 50 to 100 mg PO q 12 h; or 5 mg IV q 5 to 15 min up to 15 mg, then start 50 mg PO q 6 h for 48 h, then 100 mg PO two times per day as tolerated. HTN (immediate-release): Start 100 mg PO daily or in divided doses, increase prn up to 450 mg/day; may require multiple daily doses to maintain 24 h BP control. HTN (extended-release): Start 25 to 100 mg PO daily, increase prn q 1 week up to 400 mg/day. Heart failure: Start 12.5 to 25 mg (extended-release) PO daily, double dose q 2 weeks as tolerated up to max 200 mg/day. Angina: Start 50 mg PO two times per day (immediate-release) or 100 mg PO daily (extended-release), increase prn up to 400 mg/day. Immediate-release form is metoprolol tartrate; extended-release form is metoprolol succinate. Take with food.
PEDS — HTN 6 yo or older: Start 1 mg/kg, max 50 mg/ daily. Not recommended for younger than 6 yo.
UNAPPROVED ADULT — Atrial tachyarrhythmia, except with Wolff-Parkinson-White syndrome: 2.5

(cont.)

METOPROLOL (*cont.*)

to 5 mg IV q 2 to 5 min prn to control rapid ventricular response, max 15 mg over 10 to 15 min. Reentrant PSVT (after carotid massage, IV adenosine): 2.5 to 5 mg q 2 to 5 min to 15 mg max over 10 to 15 min. Reduce perioperative cardiac events (death) in high-risk patients undergoing noncardiac surgery: Start 100 mg (extended-release) 2 h prior to anesthesia, then 50 to 100 mg (extended-release) PO daily or 2.5 to 5 mg IV q 6 h during hospitalization (max 7 days). Maintain HR between 55 to 65 bpm. Hold dose for HR < 55 bpm and SBP < 100 mmHg. Rate control of atrial fibrillation/flutter: Start 25 mg PO two times per day, titrate to desired heart rate.

FORMS — Generic/Trade: Tabs, immediate release, tartrate, scored 50, 100 mg, extended-release, succinate, 25, 50, 100, 200 mg. Generic only: Tabs, extended-release, tartrate, scored 25 mg.

NOTES — Beta-1 receptor selective. The immediate and extended-release products may not give same clinical response on mg:mg basis; monitor response and side effects when interchanging between metoprolol products. Do not start high-dose extended-release form in patients undergoing noncardiac surgery. Monitor closely for heart failure exacerbation and hypotension when titrating dose. Stabilize dose of diuretics and ACE inhibitor before starting metoprolol. May need lower doses in elderly and in patients with liver impairment. Extended-release tabs may be broken in half, but do not chew or crush.

MOA — Blocks binding of catecholamines to beta-1 receptors.

ADVERSE EFFECTS — Serious: Bronchoconstriction (high doses), masks hypoglycemic response and slow recovery, rebound hypertension/angina. Frequent: Bradycardia, fatigue, impotence.

NADOLOL (*Corgard*) ▶K ♀C ▶– $$$$

WARNING — Avoid abrupt cessation in coronary heart disease or HTN.

ADULT — HTN: Start 20 to 40 mg PO daily, usual maintenance dose 40 to 80 mg/day, max 320 mg/day. Renal impairment: Start 20 mg PO daily, adjust dosage interval based on severity of renal impairment: For CrCl < 10 mL/min give q 40 to 60 h; for CrCl 10 to 30 mL/min give q 24 to 48 h; for CrCl 31 to 50 mL/min give q 24 to 36 h. Angina: Start 40 mg PO daily, usual maintenance dose 40 to 80 mg/day, max 240 mg/day.

PEDS — Not approved in children.

UNAPPROVED ADULT — Prevent rebleeding esophageal varices: 40 to 160 mg/day PO. Titrate dose to reduce heart rate to 25% below baseline.

FORMS — Generic/Trade: Tabs scored 20, 40, 80 mg.

NOTES — Beta-1 and beta-2 receptor blocker.

MOA — Blocks binding of catecholamines to beta-1 and beta-2 receptors.

ADVERSE EFFECTS — Serious: Bronchoconstriction, masks hypoglycemic response and slow recovery, rebound hypertension/angina. Frequent: Bradycardia, fatigue, impotence.

NEBIVOLOL (*Bystolic*) ▶L ♀C ▶– $$$

WARNING — Avoid abrupt cessation in coronary heart disease or HTN.

ADULT — HTN: Start 5 mg PO daily, maximum 40 mg/day. Severe renal impairment (CrCl < 30 mL/min), moderate hepatic impairment: Start 2.5 mg PO daily, increase cautiously.

PEDS — Not approved in children.

FORMS — Trade only: Tabs unscored 2.5, 5, 10, 20 mg.

NOTES — Do not use with severe liver impairment.

MOA — At doses of 10 mg or less or for extensive metabolizers: beta-1 receptor selective. At doses greater than 10 mg or poor metazolizers: beta-1 and beta-2 receptor blocker.

ADVERSE EFFECTS — Serious: Bronchoconstriction. Frequent: Dizziness, fatigue, headache.

PENBUTOLOL (*Levatol*) ▶LK ♀C ▶? $$$$

WARNING — Avoid abrupt cessation in coronary heart disease or HTN.

ADULT — HTN: Start 20 mg PO daily, usual maintenance dose 20 to 40 mg, max 80 mg/day.

PEDS — Not approved in children.

FORMS — Trade only: Tabs, scored 20 mg.

NOTES — Beta-1 and beta-2 receptor blocker; has mild intrinsic sympathomimetic activity.

MOA — Blocks binding of catecholamines to beta-1 and beta-2 receptors.

ADVERSE EFFECTS — Serious: Bronchoconstriction, masks hypoglycemic response and slow recovery, rebound hypertension/angina. Frequent: Bradycardia, fatigue, dizziness, impotence.

PINDOLOL ▶K ♀B ▶? $$$

WARNING — Avoid abrupt cessation in coronary heart disease or HTN.

ADULT — HTN: Start 5 mg PO two times per day, usual maintenance dose 10 to 30 mg/day, max 60 mg/day.

PEDS — Not approved in children.

UNAPPROVED ADULT — Angina: 15 to 40 mg/day PO in divided doses three to four times per day.

FORMS — Generic only: Tabs, scored 5, 10 mg.

NOTES — Has intrinsic sympathomimetic activity (partial beta-agonist activity); beta-1 and beta-2 receptor blocker. The brand name product (Visken) is no longer available.

MOA — Blocks binding of catecholamines to beta-1 and beta-2 receptors.

ADVERSE EFFECTS — Serious: Bronchoconstriction, masks hypoglycemic response and slow recovery, rebound hypertension/angina. Frequent: Bradycardia, fatigue, impotence.

PROPRANOLOL (*Inderal, Inderal LA, InnoPran XL*) ▶L ♀C ▶+ $$

WARNING — Avoid abrupt cessation in coronary heart disease or HTN.

ADULT — HTN: Start 20 to 40 mg PO two times per day, usual maintenance dose 160 to 480 mg/day, max 640 mg/day; extended-release (Inderal LA): Start 60 to 80 mg PO daily, usual maintenance dose 120 to 160 mg/day, max 640 mg/day;

PROPRANOLOL (*cont.*)

extended-release (InnoPran XL): Start 80 mg at bedtime (10 pm), max 120 mg at bedtime. Angina: Start 10 to 20 mg PO three to four times per day, usual maintenance 160 to 240 mg/day, max 320 mg/day; extended-release (Inderal LA): Start 80 mg PO daily, same usual dosage range and max for HTN. Migraine prophylaxis: Start 40 mg PO two times per day or 80 mg PO daily (extended-release), max 240 mg/day. Supraventricular tachycardia or rapid atrial fibrillation/flutter: 10 to 30 mg PO three to four times per day. MI: 180 to 240 mg/day PO in divided doses two to four times per day. Pheochromocytoma surgery: 60 mg PO in divided doses two to three times per day beginning 3 days before surgery, use in combination with an alpha-blocking agent. IV: Reserved for life-threatening arrhythmia, 1 to 3 mg IV, repeat dose in 2 min if needed, additional doses only after 4 h. Not for use in hypertensive emergency. Essential tremor: Start 40 mg PO two times per day, titrate prn to 120 to 320 mg/day.

PEDS — HTN: Start 1 mg/kg/day PO divided two times per day, usual maintenance dose 2 to 4 mg/kg/day PO divided two times per day, max 16 mg/kg/day.

UNAPPROVED ADULT — Prevent rebleeding esophageal varices: 20 to 180 mg PO two times per day. Titrate dose to reduce heart rate to 25% below baseline. Control heart rate with A-fib: 80 to 240 mg/day daily or in divided doses. Thyrotoxicosis: 60 to 80 mg every 4 h; or IV 0.5 to 1 mg over 10 min every 3 h.

UNAPPROVED PEDS — Arrhythmia: 0.01 to 0.1 mg/kg/dose (max 1 mg/dose) by slow IV push. Manufacturer does not recommend IV propranolol in children.

FORMS — Generic/Trade: Tabs, scored 40, 60, 80 mg. Caps, extended-release 60, 80, 120, 160 mg. Generic only: Soln 20, 40 mg/5 mL. Tabs, 10, 20 mg. Trade only: (InnoPran XL at bedtime) 80, 120 mg.

NOTES — Beta-1 and beta-2 receptor blocker. The immediate and extended-release products may not give same clinical response on mg:mg basis; monitor response and side effects when interchanging between products. Extended-release caps (Inderal LA) may be opened, and the contents sprinkled on food for administration, cap contents should be swallowed whole without crushing or chewing. InnoPran XL is a chronotherapeutic product; give at bedtime to blunt early morning surge in BP. Acute alcohol use may increase propranolol level; chronic alcohol use may decrease propranolol level.

MOA — Blocks binding of catecholamines to beta-1 and beta-2 receptors.

ADVERSE EFFECTS — Serious: Anaphylaxis, agranulocytosis, bronchoconstriction, masks hypoglycemic response and slows recovery, rebound hypertension/angina, Stevens-Johnson syndrome. Frequent: Bradycardia, fatigue, dizziness, impotence.

TIMOLOL (*Blocadren*) ▶LK ♀C ▶+ $$$

WARNING — Avoid abrupt cessation in coronary heart disease or HTN.

ADULT — HTN: Start 10 mg PO two times per day, usual maintenance 20 to 40 mg/day, max 60 mg/day. MI: 10 mg PO two times per day, started 1 to 4 weeks post MI. Migraine headaches: Start 10 mg PO two times per day, use 20 mg/day daily or divided two times per day for prophylaxis, increase prn up to max 60 mg/day; stop therapy if satisfactory response not obtained after 6 to 8 weeks of max dose.

PEDS — Not approved in children.

UNAPPROVED ADULT — Angina: 15 to 45 mg/day PO divided three to four times per day.

FORMS — Generic only: Tabs, 5, 10, 20 mg.

NOTES — Beta-1 and beta-2 receptor blocker.

MOA — Blocks binding of catecholamines to beta-1 and beta-2 receptors.

ADVERSE EFFECTS — Serious: Bronchoconstriction, masks hypoglycemic response and slow recovery, rebound hypertension/angina. Frequent: Bradycardia, fatigue, impotence.

CARDIOVASCULAR: Calcium Channel Blockers (CCBs)—Dihydropyridines

NOTE: See also Antihypertensive Combinations. Avoid in decompensated heart failure. Peripheral edema, especially with higher doses. Extended/controlled/sustained-release tabs should be swallowed whole; do not chew or crush. Avoid grapefruit juice, which may enhance effect.

AMLODIPINE (*Norvasc*) ▶L ♀C ▶– $

ADULT — HTN, CAD: Start 5 mg PO daily, max 10 mg/day. Elderly, small, frail, or with hepatic insufficiency: Start 2.5 mg PO daily.

PEDS — HTN (6 to 17 yo): 2.5 to 5 mg PO daily.

UNAPPROVED PEDS — HTN: Start 0.1 to 0.2 mg/kg/day PO daily, max 0.3 mg/kg/day (max 10 mg daily).

FORMS — Generic/Trade: Tabs, unscored 2.5, 5, 10 mg.

NOTES — Do not use with more than 20 mg of simvastatin. Use cautiously with aortic valve stenosis or severe obstructive coronary artery disease. Strong or moderate CYP3A4 inhibitors may increase levels and effects of amlodipine.

MOA — Blocks calcium-dependent contractions in cardiac and peripheral smooth muscle leading to vasodilation.

ADVERSE EFFECTS — Serious: None. Frequent: Peripheral edema, headache, palpitations.

CLEVIDIPINE (*Cleviprex*) ▶KL ♀C ▶? $$$$$

ADULT — HTN: Start 1 to 2 mg/h IV, double dose q 1.5 min as approaches BP goal, then titrate at smaller increments q 5 to 10 min to desired BP, usual maintenance dose 4 to 6 mg/h, max 32 mg/h IV. An increase of 1 to 2 mg/h will decrease SBP approximately 2 to 4 mm Hg.

PEDS — Not approved in children.

(cont.)

CLEVIDIPINE (*cont.*)

NOTES — Contraindicated with egg or soy allergy, defective lipid metabolism, or severe aortic stenosis. May exacerbate heart failure.

MOA — Blocks calcium-dependent contractions in cardiac and peripheral smooth muscle leading to vasodilation.

ADVERSE EFFECTS — Serious: Acute renal failure, atrial fib. Frequent: Headache, nausea, vomiting.

FELODIPINE (*Plendil, ✦Renedil*) ▶L ♀C ▶? $$

ADULT — HTN: Start 2.5 to 5 mg PO daily, usual maintenance dose 5 to 10 mg/day, max 10 mg/day.

PEDS — Not approved in children.

FORMS — Generic/Trade: Tabs, extended-release, unscored 2.5, 5, 10 mg.

NOTES — Extended-release tab. May increase tacrolimus level. Concomitant CYP3A4 inhibitors (e.g., ketoconazole, itraconazole, erythromycin, grapefruit juice, cimetidine) may increase felodipine level.

MOA — Blocks calcium-dependent contractions in cardiac and peripheral smooth muscle leading to vasodilation.

ADVERSE EFFECTS — Serious: None. Frequent: Peripheral edema, headache, palpitations.

ISRADIPINE ▶L ♀C ▶? $$$$

ADULT — HTN: Start 2.5 mg PO two times per day, usual maintenance 5 to 10 mg/day, max 20 mg/day divided two times per day (max 10 mg/day in elderly).

PEDS — Not approved in children.

FORMS — Generic only: Immediate-release caps 2.5, 5 mg.

NOTES — The brand name product (DynaCirc) is no longer available.

MOA — Blocks calcium-dependent contractions in cardiac and peripheral smooth muscle leading to vasodilation.

ADVERSE EFFECTS — Serious: Angioedema. Frequent: Peripheral edema, headache, palpitations.

NICARDIPINE (*Cardene, Cardene SR*) ▶L ♀C ▶? $$$

ADULT — HTN: Sustained-release (Cardene SR): Start 30 mg PO two times per day, usual maintenance dose 30 to 60 mg PO two times per day, max 120 mg/day; immediate-release, start 20 mg PO three times per day, usual maintenance dose 20 to 40 mg PO three times per day, max 120 mg/day. Angina: Immediate-release, start 20 mg PO three times per day, usual maintenance dose 20 to 40 mg three times per day. Short-term management of HTN, patient not receiving PO nicardipine: Begin IV infusion at 5 mg/h, titrate infusion rate by 2.5 mg/h q 5 to 15 min prn, max 15 mg/h. Short-term management of HTN, patient receiving PO nicardipine: If using 20 mg PO q 8 h, give 0.5 mg/h IV; if using 30 mg PO q 8 h, give 1.2 mg/h IV; if using 40 mg PO q 8 h, give 2.2 mg/h. When discontinuing IV nicardipine and transitioning to an oral BP regimen: Administer first dose of nicardipine PO 1 h prior to discontinuing IV infusion; or initiate BP-lowering agent other than nicardipine upon discontinuation of IV infusion.

PEDS — Not approved in children.

UNAPPROVED PEDS — HTN: 0.5 to 3 mcg/kg/min IV infusion.

FORMS — Generic/Trade: Caps, immediate-release 20, 30 mg. Trade only: Caps, sustained-release 30, 45, 60 mg.

NOTES — Decrease dose if hepatically impaired. Titrate carefully if renally impaired. Use sustained-release caps for HTN only, not for angina. May increase cyclosporine level. Concomitant cimetidine may increase nicardipine level.

MOA — Blocks calcium-dependent contractions in cardiac and peripheral smooth muscle leading to vasodilation.

ADVERSE EFFECTS — Serious: Hypotension. Frequent: Peripheral edema, headache, palpitations.

NIFEDIPINE (*Procardia, Adalat, Procardia XL, Adalat CC, Afeditab CR, ✦Adalat XL*) ▶L ♀C ▶– $$

ADULT — HTN: Extended-release Start 30 to 60 mg PO daily, max 120 mg/day. Angina: Extended-release, Start 30 to 60 mg PO daily, max 120 mg/day; immediate-release, Start 10 mg PO three times per day, usual maintenance dose 10 to 20 mg tid, max 120 mg/day.

PEDS — Not approved in children.

UNAPPROVED ADULT — Preterm labor: Loading dose 10 mg PO q 20 to 30 min if contractions persist up to 40 mg within the first h. After contractions are controlled, maintenance dose: 10 to 20 mg PO q 4 to 6 h or 60 to 160 mg extended-release PO daily. Duration of treatment has not been established. Promotes spontaneous passage of ureteral calculi: Extended-release, 30 mg PO daily for 10 to 28 days.

UNAPPROVED PEDS — HTN: 0.25 to 0.5 mg/kg/dose PO q 4 to 6 h prn, max 10 mg/dose or 3 mg/kg/day. Doses less than 0.25 mg/kg may be effective.

FORMS — Generic/Trade: Caps 10, 20 mg. Tabs, extended-release (Adalat CC, Afeditab CR, Procardia XL) 30, 60 mg; (Adalat CC, Procardia XL) 90 mg.

NOTES — Do not use immediate-release caps for treating HTN, hypertensive emergencies, or ST-elevation MI. Immediate-release cap should not be chewed and swallowed or given sublingually; may cause excessive hypotension, CVA. Extended-release tabs can be substituted for immediate-release caps at the same dose in patients whose angina is controlled. Extended-release tab has been associated with gastrointestinal obstruction; use extended-release tab cautiously in patients with pre-existing severe gastrointestinal narrowing. Metabolized by the CYP3A4 enzyme system. Use alternative BP lowering medication when patient on carbamazepine, phenobarbital, phenytoin, rifampin, or St. John's wort; these reduce levels of nifidepine significantly. Concomitant clarithromycin, erythromycin, fluconazole, fluoxetine, grapefruit, HIV protease inhibitors, ketoconazole, itraconazole, or nefazodone increases nifedipine level. Increases tacrolimus level. Avoid grapefruit juice while taking nifedipine. Severe hypotension and/or increased fluid volume requirements may occur when used with beta-blocker for patient who had surgery using high dose fentanyl

NIFEDIPINE (cont.)

anesthesia; when appropriate, discontinue nifedipine at least 36 hours prior to surgery that may require high dose fentanyl anesthesia.
MOA — Blocks calcium-dependent contractions in cardiac and peripheral smooth muscle leading to vasodilation. Tocolytic.
ADVERSE EFFECTS — Serious: Hypotension, gastrointestinal obstruction (extended-release tab). Frequent: Peripheral edema, headache, palpitations, flushing.

NISOLDIPINE (Sular) ▶L ♀C ▶? $$$$$

ADULT — HTN: Start 17 mg PO daily, may increase by 8.5 mg weekly, max 34 mg/day. Impaired hepatic function, elderly: Start 8.5 mg PO daily, titrate prn.

PEDS — Not approved in children.
FORMS — Generic/Trade: Tabs, extended-release 8.5, 17, 25.5, 34 mg. These replace the former 10, 20, 30, 40 mg tabs. Generic only: Tabs, extended-release 20, 30, 40 mg.
NOTES — Take on an empty stomach. Sular 8.5, 17, 25.5, 34 mg replace 10, 20, 30, 40 mg respectively.
MOA — Blocks calcium-dependent contractions in cardiac and peripheral smooth muscle leading to vasodilation.
ADVERSE EFFECTS — Serious: None. Frequent: Peripheral edema, headache, palpitations.

CARDIOVASCULAR: Calcium Channel Blockers (CCBs)—Non-Dihydropyridines

NOTE: See also Antihypertensive Combinations. Avoid in decompensated heart failure, 2nd/3rd degree heart block without pacemaker, acute MI and pulmonary congestion, or systolic blood pressure less than 90 mm Hg systolic.

DILTIAZEM (Cardizem, Cardizem LA, Cardizem CD, Cartia XT, Dilacor XR, Diltiazem CD, Diltzac, Diltia XT, Matzim LA, Tiazac, Taztia XT) ▶L ♀C ▶+ $$

ADULT — Atrial fibrillation/flutter, PSVT: 20 mg (0.25 mg/kg) IV bolus over 2 min. If needed and patient tolerated IV bolus with no hypotension, rebolus 15 min later with 25 mg (0.35 mg/kg). IV infusion: Start 10 mg/h, increase by 5 mg/h (usual range 5 to 15 mg/h). HTN, once a day, extended-release (Cardizem CD, Cartia XT, Dilacor XR, Diltia XT, Taztia XT, Tiazac): Start 120 to 240 mg PO daily, usual maintenance range 240 to 360 mg/day, max 540 mg/day. HTN, once a day, graded extended-release (Cardizem LA): Start 180 to 240 mg, max 540 mg/day. HTN, twice a day, sustained-release (Cardizem SR): Start 60 to 120 mg PO two times per day, max 360 mg/day. Angina, immediate-release: Start 30 mg PO four times per day, max 360 mg/day divided three to four times per day. Angina, extended-release: 120 to 180 mg PO daily, max 540 mg/day. Angina, once a day, graded extended-release (Cardizem LA): Start 180 mg PO daily, doses greater than 360 mg may provide no additional benefit.
PEDS — Not approved in children. Diltiazem injection should be avoided in neonates due to potential toxicity from benzyl alcohol in the injectable product.
UNAPPROVED ADULT — Control heart rate with chronic A-fib: 120 to 360 mg/day daily or in divided doses.
UNAPPROVED PEDS — HTN: Start 1.5 to 2 mg/kg/day PO divided three to four times per day, max 3.5 mg/kg/day.
FORMS — Generic/Trade: Tabs, immediate-release, unscored (Cardizem) 30 mg, scored 60, 90, 120 mg. Caps, extended-release (Cardizem CD, Cartia XT daily) 120, 180, 240, 300, 360 mg, (Diltzac, Taztia XT, Tiazac daily) 120, 180, 240, 300, 360, 420 mg, (Dilacor XR, Diltia XT) 120, 180, 240 mg. Tabs, extended-release (Cardizem LA daily, Matzim LA) 180,

240, 300, 360, 420 mg. Generic only: Caps, extended release (twice daily) 60, 90, 120 mg. Trade only: Tabs, extended-release (Cardizem LA daily) 120 mg.
NOTES — Sinus bradycardia resulting in hospitalization and pacemaker insertion has been reported with concomitant clonidine; monitor heart rate. May increase levels of buspirone, lovastatin, quinidine, simvastatin. Do not use with more than 10 mg of simvastatin or 20 mg of lovastatin. Contents of extended-release caps may be sprinkled over food. Do not chew or crush cap contents. May accumulate with hepatic impairment. Monitor response and side effects when interchanging between diltiazem products; many are not equivalent on mg:mg basis. Cardizem LA is a chronotherapeutic product; give at bedtime to blunt early morning surge in BP.
MOA — Blocks calcium-dependent contractions in cardiac and peripheral smooth muscle leading to vasodilation; slows cardiac conduction through the AV node.
ADVERSE EFFECTS — Serious: Bradycardia, heart block (rare). Frequent: Peripheral edema, headache.

VERAPAMIL (Isoptin SR, Calan, Calan SR, Verelan, Verelan PM, ✱Veramil) ▶L ♀C ▶– $$

ADULT — SVT: 5 to 10 mg (0.075 to 0.15 mg/kg) IV over 2 min; a 2nd dose of 10 mg IV may be given 15 to 30 min later if needed. PSVT/rate control with atrial fibrillation: 240 to 480 mg/day PO divided three to four times per day. Angina: Start 40 to 80 mg PO three to four times per day, max 480 mg/day; sustained-release (Isoptin SR, Calan SR, Verelan), start 120 to 240 mg PO daily, max 480 mg/day (use twice daily dosing for doses greater than 240 mg/day with Isoptin SR and Calan SR). HTN: Same as angina, except (Verelan PM) start 100 to 200 mg PO at bedtime max 400 mg/day; immediate-release tabs should be avoided in treating HTN.
PEDS — SVT: age 1 to 15 yo: 2 to 5 mg (0.1 to 0.3 mg/kg) IV, max dose 5 mg. Repeat dose once in 30 min if

(cont.)

VERAPAMIL (cont.)

needed, max second dose 10 mg. Immediate-release and sustained-release tabs not approved in children.

FORMS — Generic/Trade: Tabs, immediate-release, scored (Calan) 40, 80, 120 mg. Tabs, sustained-release, unscored (Isoptin SR, Calan SR) 120, scored 180, 240 mg. Caps, sustained-release (Verelan) 120, 180, 240, 360 mg. Caps, extended-release (Verelan PM) 100, 200, 300 mg.

NOTES — Contraindicated in severe LV dysfunction, A-fib/flutter conducted via accessory pathway (i.e., Wolff-Parkinson-White). Grapefruit juice may increase level. Do not use with more than 10 mg of simvastatin or 20 mg of lovastatin. Hypotension, bradyarrhythmias, and lactic acidosis have been reported with concomitant telithromycin. Sinus bradycardia resulting in hospitalization and pacemaker insertion has been reported with concomitant clonidine; monitor heart rate. May increase digoxin level 50 to 75%. May increase doxorubicin level. May change the level of certain chemotherapeutic agents; may get reduced absorption of verapamil with some chemotherapeutic regimens; see prescribing information for complete list. Scored, sustained-release tabs (Calan SR, Isoptin SR) may be broken and each piece swallowed whole, do not chew or crush. Monitor response and side effects when interchanging between verapamil products; many are not equivalent on mg:mg basis. Contents of sustained-release caps may be sprinkled on food (e.g., apple sauce). Do not chew or crush cap contents. Use cautiously with impaired renal/hepatic function. Verelan PM is a chronotherapeutic product; give at bedtime to blunt early morning surge in BP.

MOA — Blocks calcium-dependent contractions in cardiac and peripheral smooth muscle leading to vasodilation; slows cardiac conduction through the SA node.

ADVERSE EFFECTS — Serious: Bradycardia, heart block (rare). Frequent: Constipation, headache.

CARDIOVASCULAR: Diuretics—Loop

NOTE: Thiazides are preferred diuretics for HTN. With decreased renal function (CrCl less than 30 mL/min), loop diuretics may be more effective than thiazides for HTN. Rare hypersensitivity in patients allergic to sulfa-containing drugs, except ethacrynic acid. For diuretics given twice daily, give second dose in mid-afternoon to avoid nocturia.

BUMETANIDE (Bumex, ✽Burinex) ▶K ♀C ▶? $

ADULT — Edema: 0.5 to 2 mg PO daily, repeat doses at 4 to 5 h intervals prn until desired response is attained, max 10 mg/day; 0.5 to 1 mg IV/IM, repeat doses at 2 to 3 h intervals prn until desired response is attained, max 10 mg/day. Dosing for 3 to 4 consecutive days followed by no drug for 1 to 2 days is acceptable. Twice daily dosing may enhance diuretic effect. IV injections should be over 1 to 2 min. An IV infusion may be used, change bag q 24 h.

PEDS — Not approved in children.

UNAPPROVED PEDS — Edema: 0.015 to 0.1 mg/kg/dose PO/IV/IM daily or every other day, max 0.1 mg/kg/day or 10 mg/day.

FORMS — Generic only: Tabs, scored 0.5, 1, 2 mg.

NOTES — Bumetanide 1 mg is roughly equivalent to furosemide 40 mg. IV administration is preferred when GI absorption is impaired.

MOA — Block chloride reabsorption by inhibiting the Na$^+$/K$^+$/Cl$^-$ cotransport system in the thick ascending limb of the loop of Henle.

ADVERSE EFFECTS — Serious: Electrolyte imbalances (hypokalemia, hyponatremia, hypochloremic alkalosis, hypomagnesemia, hypocalcemia, hyperuricemia), dehydration, ototoxicity (rare), skin reactions. Frequent: Dizziness, headache, fatigue, muscle cramps, impotence.

ETHACRYNIC ACID (Edecrin) ▶K ♀B ▶? $$$$$

ADULT — Edema: 0.5 to 1 mg/kg IV, max 100 mg/dose; 25 mg PO daily on day 1, followed by 50 mg PO two times per day on day 2, followed by 100 mg PO in the morning and 50 to 100 mg PO in the evening depending on the response to the morning dose, max 400 mg/day.

PEDS — Not approved in children.

UNAPPROVED ADULT — HTN: 25 mg PO daily, max 100 mg/day divided two to three times per day.

UNAPPROVED PEDS — Edema: 1 mg/kg IV; 25 mg PO daily, increase slowly by 25 mg increments prn. Ethacrynic acid should not be administered to infants.

FORMS — Trade only: Tabs, scored 25 mg.

NOTES — Ototoxicity possible. Does not contain a sulfonamide group; can be safely used in patients with true sulfa allery. Do not administer SC or IM due to local irritation. IV ethacrynic acid should be reconstituted to a concentration of 50 mg/mL and given slowly by IV infusion over 20 to 30 min. May increase lithium levels.

MOA — Block chloride reabsorption by inhibiting the Na$^+$/K$^+$/Cl$^-$ cotransport system in the thick ascending limb of the loop of Henle.

ADVERSE EFFECTS — Serious: Electrolyte imbalances (hypokalemia, hyponatremia, hypochloremic alkalosis, hypomagnesemia, hypocalcemia, hyperuricemia), dehydration, pancreatitis (rare), photosensitivity (rare), ototoxicity (rare). Frequent: Dizziness, headache, fatigue, muscle cramps, impotence.

FUROSEMIDE (Lasix) ▶K ♀C ▶? $

ADULT — HTN: Start 10 to 40 mg PO twice daily, max 600 mg daily. Edema: Start 20 to 80 mg IV/IM/PO, increase dose by 20 to 40 mg in 6 to 8 h until desired response is achieved, max 600 mg/day. Give maintenance dose daily or divided two times per day. IV infusion: 0.05 mg/kg/h, titrate rate to desired response.

PEDS — Edema: 0.5 to 2 mg/kg/dose IV/IM/PO q 6 to 12 h, max 6 mg/kg/dose. IV infusion: 0.05 mg/kg/h, titrate rate to achieve desired response.

UNAPPROVED ADULT — Ascites: 40 mg PO daily in combination with spironolactone; may increase dose after 2 to 3 days if no response.

FUROSEMIDE (*cont.*)

FORMS — Generic/Trade: Tabs, unscored 20, scored 40, 80 mg. Generic only: Oral soln 10 mg/mL, 40 mg/5 mL.

NOTES — Oral absorption may decrease in acute heart failure exacerbation. Bioequivalence of oral form is 50% of IV dose. Monitor renal function in elderly. Do not use with lithium. Increases risk of ototoxicity when used with other drugs associated with ototoxicity, especially with renal dysfunction. May potentiate renal dysfunction when used with other drugs associated with renal dysfunction. May antagonize the muscle-relaxing effects of tubocurarine. Ototoxicity is associated with rapid IV administration (more than 4 mg/min).

MOA — Block chloride reabsorption by inhibiting the $Na^+/K^+/Cl^-$ cotransport system in the thick ascending limb of the loop of Henle.

ADVERSE EFFECTS — Serious: Electrolyte imbalances (hypokalemia, hyponatremia, hypochloremic alkalosis, hypomagnesemia, hypocalcemia, hyperuricemia), dehydration, pancreatitis (rare), photosensitivity (rare), hypersensitivity (rare), ototoxicity (rare), dermatologic-hypersensitivity reactions. Frequent: Dizziness, headache, fatigue, muscle cramps, impotence.

TORSEMIDE (*Demadex*) ▶LK ♀B ▶? $

ADULT — HTN: Start 5 mg PO daily, increase prn q 4 to 6 weeks, max 10 mg daily. Edema: Start 10 to 20 mg IV/PO daily, double dose prn, max 200 mg IV/PO daily. Ascites: 5 to 10 mg IV/PO daily, double dose prn, max 40 mg daily.

PEDS — Not approved in children.

FORMS — Generic/Trade: Tabs, scored 5, 10, 20, 100 mg.

MOA — Block chloride reabsorption by inhibiting the $Na^+/K^+/Cl^-$ cotransport system in the thick ascending limb of the loop of Henle.

ADVERSE EFFECTS — Serious: Electrolyte imbalances (hypokalemia, hyponatremia, hypochloremic alkalosis, hypomagnesemia, hypocalcemia, hyperuricemia), dehydration, pancreatitis (rare), photosensitivity (rare), hypersensitivity (rare). Frequent: Dizziness, headache, fatigue, muscle cramps, impotence.

CARDIOVASCULAR: Diuretics—Potassium Sparing

NOTE: See also antihypertensive combinations and aldosterone antagonists. May cause hyperkalemia; greater incidence with renal impairment, diabetes, or elderly. Monitor potassium levels before initiating therapy, when adjusting diuretic doses, and with illness that may alter renal function. Use cautiously with other agents that may cause hyperkalemia (ie, ACE inhibitors, ARBs, aliskiren, potassium containing salt substitutes).

AMILORIDE (*Midamor*) ▶LK ♀B ▶? $$$

WARNING — May cause hyperkalemia.

ADULT — Diuretic-induced hypokalemia: Start 5 mg PO daily, increase prn, max 20 mg/day. Edema/HTN: Start 5 mg PO daily in combination with another diuretic, usually a thiazide for HTN, increase prn, max 20 mg/day. Other diuretics may need to be added when treating edema.

PEDS — Not approved in children.

UNAPPROVED ADULT — Hyperaldosteronism: 10 to 40 mg PO daily. Do not use combination product (Moduretic) for treatment of primary hyperaldosteronism.

UNAPPROVED PEDS — Edema: 0.625 mg/kg daily for children weighing 6 to 20 kg.

FORMS — Generic only: Tabs, unscored 5 mg.

NOTES — Spironolactone is generally preferred for treating primary hyperaldosteronism.

MOA — Block sodium reabsorption and potassium excretion in the distal tubule.

ADVERSE EFFECTS — Serious: Hyperkalemia (rare). Frequent: Headache.

TRIAMTERENE (*Dyrenium*) ▶LK ♀B ▶– $$$

WARNING — May cause hyperkalemia. Incidence is greater with renal impairment, diabetes, or elderly. Monitor potassium frequently, before initiation, when adjusting diuretic doses, and with illness that may alter renal function.

ADULT — Edema (cirrhosis, nephrotic syndrome, heart failure): Start 100 mg PO two times per day, max 300 mg/day. Most patients can be maintained on 100 mg PO daily or every other day after edema is controlled. Other diuretics may be needed.

PEDS — Not approved in children.

UNAPPROVED PEDS — Edema: 4 mg/kg/day divided two times per day after meals, increase to 6 mg/kg/day if needed, max 300 mg/day.

FORMS — Trade only: Caps 50, 100 mg.

NOTES — Combo product with HCTZ (e.g., Dyazide, Maxzide) available for HTN.

MOA — Block sodium reabsorption and potassium excretion in the distal tubule.

ADVERSE EFFECTS — Serious: Hyperkalemia (rare). Frequent: Headache.

CARDIOVASCULAR: Diuretics—Thiazide Type

NOTE: See also Antihypertensive Combinations. Possible hypersensitivity in sulfa allergy. Should be used for most patients with HTN, alone or combined with other antihypertensive agents. Thiazides are not recommended for gestational HTN. Coadministration with NSAIDs, including selective COX-2 inhibitors, may reduce the antihypertensive, diuretic, and natriuretic effects of thiazides. Thiazide-induced hypokalemia is associated with increased fasting blood glucose and new onset diabetes; keep potassium 4.0 mg/dL or greater to minimize risk; may use thiazide in combination with oral potassium supplementation, ACE inhibitor, ARB, or potassium-sparing diuretic to maintain K+ level.

CHLOROTHIAZIDE (*Diuril*) ▶L ♀C, D if used in pregnancy-induced HTN ▶+ $
ADULT — HTN: Start 125 to 250 mg PO daily or divided two times per day, max 1000 mg/day divided two times per day. Edema: 500 to 2000 mg PO/IV daily or divided two times per day. Dosing on alternate days or for 3 to 4 consecutive days followed by no drug for 1 to 2 days is acceptable.
PEDS — Edema: Infants: Start 10 to 20 mg/kg/day PO daily or divided two times per day, up to 30 mg/kg/day divided two times per day. Children 6 mo to 2 yo: 10 to 20 mg/kg/day PO daily or divided two times per day, max 375 mg/day. Children 2 to 12 yo: Start 10 to 20 mg/kg/day PO daily or divided two times per day, up to 1 g/day. IV formulation not recommended for infants or children.
FORMS — Trade only: Susp 250 mg/5 mL. Generic only: Tabs, scored 250, 500 mg.
NOTES — Do not administer SC or IM.
MOA — Blocks sodium and chloride reabsorption in the distal tubules.
ADVERSE EFFECTS — Serious: Electrolyte imbalances (hypokalemia, hyponatremia, hypomagnesemia, hypercalcemia, hyperuricemia), pancreatitis (rare), photosensitivity (rare), hypersensitivity (rare). Frequent: Dizziness, headache, fatigue, muscle cramps, impotence.

CHLORTHALIDONE ▶L ♀B, D if used in pregnancy-induced HTN ▶+ $
ADULT — HTN: For generic, start 12.5 to 25 mg PO daily, usual maintenance dose 12.5 to 50 mg/day, max 50 mg/day. Edema: For generic, start 50 to 100 mg PO daily or 100 mg every other day or 100 mg 3 times a week, usual maintenance dose 150 to 200 mg/day, max 200 mg/day.
PEDS — Not approved in children.
UNAPPROVED ADULT — Nephrolithiasis: 25 to 50 mg PO daily.
UNAPPROVED PEDS — Edema: 2 mg/kg PO 3 times a week.
FORMS — Generic only: Tabs, unscored 25, 50 mg.
NOTES — Doses greater than 50 mg/day for HTN have significantly more hypokalemia with no greater antihypertensive effects.
MOA — Blocks sodium and chloride reabsorption in the distal tubules and decreases urinary calcium excretion.
ADVERSE EFFECTS — Serious: Agranulocytosis, aplastic anemia, electrolyte imbalances (hypokalemia, hyponatremia, hypomagnesemia, hypercalcemia, hyperuricemia), pancreatitis (rare), photosensitivity (rare), hypersensitivity (rare), thrombocytopenia. Frequent: Dizziness, headache, fatigue, muscle cramps, impotence.

HYDROCHLOROTHIAZIDE (*HCTZ, Oretic, Microzide*) ▶L ♀B, D if used in pregnancy-induced HTN ▶+ $
ADULT — HTN: Start 12.5 to 25 mg PO daily, usual maintenance dose 25 mg/day, max 50 mg/day. Edema: 25 to 100 mg PO daily or in divided doses or 50 to 100 mg PO every other day or 3 to 5 days/week, max 200 mg/day.

PEDS — Edema: 1 to 2 mg/kg/day PO daily or divided two times per day, max 37.5 mg/day in infants up to 2 yo, max 100 mg/day in children 2 to 12 yo.
UNAPPROVED ADULT — Nephrolithiasis: 50 to 100 mg PO daily.
FORMS — Generic/Trade: Tabs, scored 25, 50 mg, Caps 12.5 mg.
NOTES — Doses 50 mg/day or greater may cause hypokalemia with little added BP control.
MOA — Blocks sodium and chloride reabsorption in the distal tubules and decreases urinary calcium excretion.
ADVERSE EFFECTS — Agranulocytosis, aplastic anemia, electrolyte imbalances (hypokalemia, hyponatremia, hypomagnesemia, hypercalcemia, hyperuricemia),acute myopia and secondary acute angle closure glaucoma, pancreatitis (rare), photosensitivity (rare), hypersensitivity (rare), thrombocytopenia. Frequent: Dizziness, headache, fatigue, muscle cramps, impotence.

INDAPAMIDE (*✴Lozide*) ▶L ♀B, D if used in pregnancy-induced HTN ▶? $
ADULT — HTN: Start 1.25 to 2.5 mg PO daily, max 5 mg/day. Edema/Heart failure: 2.5 to 5 mg PO q am.
PEDS — Not approved in children.
FORMS — Generic only: Tabs, unscored 1.25, 2.5 mg.
NOTES — The brand name product (Lozol) is no longer available.
MOA — Blocks sodium and chloride reabsorption in the distal tubules.
ADVERSE EFFECTS — Serious: Electrolyte imbalances (hypokalemia, hyponatremia, hypomagnesemia, hypercalcemia, hyperuricemia), pancreatitis (rare), photosensitivity (rare), hypersensitivity (rare). Frequent: Dizziness, headache, fatigue, muscle cramps, impotence.

METHYCLOTHIAZIDE (*Enduron*) ▶L ♀B, D if used in pregnancy-induced HTN ▶? $$$
ADULT — HTN: Start 2.5 mg PO daily, usual maintenance dose 2.5 to 5 mg/day. Edema: Start 2.5 mg PO daily, usual maintenance dose 2.5 to 10 mg/day.
PEDS — Not approved in children.
FORMS — Generic only: Tabs, scored, 5 mg.
MOA — Blocks sodium and chloride reabsorption in the distal tubules.
ADVERSE EFFECTS — Serious: Electrolyte imbalances (hypokalemia, hyponatremia, hypomagnesemia, hypercalcemia, hyperuricemia), pancreatitis (rare), photosensitivity (rare), hypersensitivity (rare). Frequent: Dizziness, headache, fatigue, muscle cramps, impotence.

METOLAZONE (*Zaroxolyn*) ▶L ♀B, D if used in pregnancy-induced HTN ▶? $$$
ADULT — Edema (heart failure, renal disease): 5 to 10 mg PO daily, max 10 mg/day in heart failure, 20 mg/day in renal disease. If used with loop diuretic, start with 2.5 mg PO daily. Reduce to lowest effective dose as edema resolves. May be given every other day as edema resolves.
PEDS — Not approved in children.

METOLAZONE (cont.)

UNAPPROVED PEDS — Edema: 0.2 to 0.4 mg/kg/day daily or divided two times per day.

FORMS — Generic/Trade: Tabs 2.5, 5, 10 mg.

NOTES — Generally used for diuretic resistance, not HTN. When used with furosemide or other loop diuretics, administer metolazone 30 min before IV loop diuretic. Correct electrolyte imbalances before initiating therapy. Combination diuretic therapy may increase the risk of electrolyte disturbances.

MOA — Blocks sodium and chloride reabsorption in the distal tubules.

ADVERSE EFFECTS — Serious: Electrolyte imbalances (hypokalemia, hyponatremia, hypomagnesemia, hypercalcemia, hyperuricemia), pancreatitis (rare), photosensitivity (rare), hypersensitivity (rare). Frequent: Dizziness, headache, fatigue, muscle cramps, impotence.

CARDIOVASCULAR: Nitrates

NOTE: Avoid if systolic BP below 90 mmHg or below baseline by more than 30 mmHg, severe bradycardia (less than 50 bpm), tachycardia (greater than 100 bpm), or right ventricular infarction. Avoid in those who have received erectile dysfunction therapy, with sildenafil or vardenafil, in the last 24 h. Only with close medical supervision and hemodynamic monitoring, may give nitrate 12 h after avanafil or 48 h after tadalafil.

ISOSORBIDE DINITRATE (Isordil, Dilatrate-SR) ▶L ♀C ▶? $

ADULT — Acute angina: 2.5 to 10 mg SL or chewed immediately, repeat prn q 5 to 10 min up to 3 doses in 30 min. SL and chew Tabs may be used prior to events likely to provoke angina. Angina prophylaxis: Start 5 to 20 mg PO three times per day (7 am, noon, and 5 pm), max 40 mg three times per day. Sustained-release (Dilatrate SR): Start 40 mg PO two times per day, max 80 mg PO two times per day (8 am and 2 pm).

PEDS — Not approved in children.

UNAPPROVED ADULT — Heart failure: 10 to 40 mg PO three times per day, max 80 mg three times per day. Use in combination with hydralazine.

FORMS — Generic/Trade: Tabs, scored 5, 10, 20, 30 mg. Trade only: Tabs, (Isordil) 40 mg. Caps, extended-release (Dilatrate-SR) 40 mg. Generic only: Tabs, sustained-release 40 mg. Tabs, sublingual 2.5, 5 mg.

NOTES — Use SL or chew Tabs for an acute angina attack. Extended-release tab may be broken, but do not chew or crush, swallow whole; do not use for acute angina. Allow for a nitrate-free period of 10 to 14 h each day to avoid nitrate tolerance.

MOA — Relaxes cardiac and peripheral smooth muscle (venous greater than arterial).

ADVERSE EFFECTS — Serious: Hypotension, methemoglobinemia (rare). Frequent: Headache, tachycardia, dizziness, flushing.

ISOSORBIDE MONONITRATE (ISMO, Monoket, Imdur) ▶L ♀C ▶? $$

ADULT — Angina: 20 mg PO two times per day (8 am and 3 pm). Extended-release (Imdur): Start 30 to 60 mg PO daily, max 240 mg/day.

PEDS — Not approved in children.

FORMS — Generic/Trade: Tabs, unscored (ISMO, two times per day dosing) 20 mg, scored (Monoket, two times per day dosing) 10, 20 mg extended-release, scored (Imdur, daily dosing) 30, 60, unscored 120 mg.

NOTES — Extended-release tab may be broken, but do not chew or crush, swallow whole. Do not use for acute angina.

MOA — Relaxes cardiac and peripheral smooth muscle (venous greater than arterial).

ADVERSE EFFECTS — Serious: Hypotension, methemoglobinemia (rare). Frequent: Headache, tachycardia, dizziness, flushing.

NITROGLYCERIN INTRAVENOUS INFUSION ▶L ♀C ▶? $

ADULT — Perioperative HTN, acute MI/heart failure, acute angina: Mix 50 mg in 250 mL D5W (200 mcg/mL), start at 10 to 20 mcg/min IV (3 to 6 mL/h), then titrate upward by 10 to 20 mcg/min q 3 to 5 min until desired effect is achieved.

PEDS — Not approved in children.

UNAPPROVED ADULT — Hypertensive emergency: Start 10 to 20 mcg/min IV infusion, titrate up to 100 mcg/min. Antihypertensive effect is usually evident in 2 to 5 min. Effect may persist for only 3 to 5 min after infusion is stopped.

UNAPPROVED PEDS — IV infusion: Start 0.25 to 0.5 mcg/kg/min, increase by 0.5 to 1 mcg/kg/min q 3 to 5 min prn, max 5 mcg/kg/min.

NOTES — Nitroglycerin migrates into polyvinyl chloride (PVC) tubing. Use lower initial doses (5 mcg/min) with non-PVC tubing. Use with caution in inferior/right ventricular MI.

MOA — Relaxes cardiac and peripheral smooth muscle (venous greater than arterial).

ADVERSE EFFECTS — Serious: Hypotension, methemoglobinemia (rare). Frequent: Headache, tachycardia, dizziness, flushing.

NITROGLYCERIN OINTMENT (Nitro-BID) ▶L ♀C ▶? $

ADULT — Angina prophylaxis: Start 0.5 inch q 8 h applied to nonhairy skin area, maintenance 1 to 2 inch q 8 h, maximum 4 inch q 4 to 6 h.

PEDS — Not approved in children.

FORMS — Trade only: Ointment, 2%, tubes 1, 30, 60 g (Nitro-BID).

NOTES — Do not use for acute angina attack. One inch ointment contains about 15 mg nitroglycerin. Allow for a nitrate-free period of 10 to 14 h each day to avoid nitrate tolerance. Generally change to oral tabs or transdermal patch for long-term therapy.

MOA — Relaxes cardiac and peripheral smooth muscle (venous greater than arterial).

(cont.)

NITROGLYCERIN OINTMENT (*cont.*)

ADVERSE EFFECTS — Serious: Hypotension, methemoglobinemia (rare). Frequent: Headache, tachycardia, dizziness, flushing.

NITROGLYCERIN SPRAY (*Nitrolingual, NitroMist*) ▶L ♀C ▶? $$$$

ADULT — Acute angina: 1 to 2 sprays under the tongue at the onset of attack, repeat prn, max 3 sprays in 15 min. A dose may be given 5 to 10 min before activities that might provoke angina.

PEDS — Not approved in children.

FORMS — Trade only: Nitrolingual soln, 4.9, 12 mL. 0.4 mg/spray (60 or 200 sprays/canister); NitroMist aerosol 0.4 mg/spray (230 sprays/canister).

NOTES — AHA guidelines recommend calling 911 if chest pain not relieved or gets worse after using 1 dose of nitroglycerin. May be preferred over SL tabs in patients with dry mouth. Patient can see how much medicine is left in the upright bottle. Nitrolingual: Replace bottle when fluid is below level of center tube; NitroMist: Replace bottle when fluid reaches the bottom of the hole in the side of the container. Before initial use, prime pump: Nitrolingual, spray 5 times into air (away from self and others); NitroMist, spray 10 times into air (away from self and others). Prime at least once q 6 weeks if not used: Nitrolingual spray 1 time into the air (away from self and others); NitroMist spray twice into the air (away from self and others). Do not shake NitroMist before using.

MOA — Relaxes cardiac and peripheral smooth muscle (venous greater than arterial).

ADVERSE EFFECTS — Serious: Hypotension. Frequent: Headache, tingling/mouth burning, tachycardia, dizziness, flushing.

NITROGLYCERIN SUBLINGUAL (*Nitrostat, NitroQuick*) ▶L ♀B ▶? $

ADULT — Acute angina: 0.4 mg under tongue or between the cheek and gum, repeat dose q 5 min prn up to 3 doses in 15 min. A dose may be given 5 to 10 min before activities that might provoke angina.

PEDS — Not approved in children.

FORMS — Generic/Trade: Sublingual tabs, unscored 0.3, 0.4, 0.6 mg; in bottles of 100 or package of 4 bottles with 25 tabs each.

NOTES — AHA guidelines recommend calling 911 if chest pain not relieved or gets worse after using 1 dose of nitroglycerin. May produce a burning/tingling sensation when administered, although this should not be used to assess potency. Store in original glass bottle to maintain potency/stability. Traditionally, unused tabs should be discarded 6 months after the original bottle is opened; however, the Nitrostat product is stable for 24 months after the bottle is opened or until the expiration date on the bottle, whichever is earlier. If used rarely, prescribe package with 4 bottles with 25 Tabs each.

MOA — Relaxes cardiac and peripheral smooth muscle (venous greater than arterial).

ADVERSE EFFECTS — Serious: Hypotension. Frequent: Headache, tingling/mouth burning, tachycardia, dizziness, flushing.

NITROGLYCERIN SUSTAINED RELEASE ▶L ♀C ▶? $

ADULT — Angina prophylaxis: Start 2.5 mg PO two to three times per day, then titrate upward prn.

PEDS — Not approved in children.

FORMS — Generic only: Caps, extended-release 2.5, 6.5, 9 mg.

NOTES — Do not use for acute angina attack. Swallow whole, do not chew or crush. Allow for a nitrate-free period of 10 to 14 h each day to avoid nitrate tolerance.

MOA — Relaxes cardiac and peripheral smooth muscle (venous greater than arterial).

ADVERSE EFFECTS — Serious: Hypotension, methemoglobinemia (rare). Frequent: Headache, tachycardia, dizziness, flushing.

NITROGLYCERIN TRANSDERMAL (*Minitran, Nitro-Dur, ✦Trinipatch, Transderm-Nitro*) ▶L ♀C ▶? $$

ADULT — Angina prophylaxis: Start with lowest dose and apply 1 patch for 12 to 14 h each day to non-hairy skin.

PEDS — Not approved in children.

FORMS — Generic/Trade: Transdermal system 0.1, 0.2, 0.4, 0.6 mg/h. Trade only: (Nitro-Dur) 0.3, 0.8 mg/h.

NOTES — Do not use for acute angina attack. Allow for a nitrate-free period of 10 to 14 h each day to avoid nitrate tolerance.

MOA — Relaxes cardiac and peripheral smooth muscle (venous greater than arterial).

ADVERSE EFFECTS — Serious: Hypotension, methemoglobinemia (rare). Frequent: Headache, rash, tachycardia, dizziness, drug tolerance, flushing.

CARDIOVASCULAR: Pressors/Inotropes

DOBUTAMINE ▶Plasma ♀D ▶– $

ADULT — Inotropic support in cardiac decompensation (heart failure, cardiogenic shock, surgical procedures): 2 to 20 mcg/kg/min. Mix 250 mg in 250 mL D5W (1 mg/mL); a rate of 21 mL/h delivers 5 mcg/kg/min for a 70 kg patient; alternatively mix 200 mg in 100 mL D5W (2 mg/mL) set at a rate of 10.5 mL/h delivers 5 mcg/kg/min for a 70 kg patient.

PEDS — Not approved in children.

UNAPPROVED ADULT — Refractory septic shock: 2 to 20 mcg/kg/min.

UNAPPROVED PEDS — Use adult dosage. Use lowest effective dose.

NOTES — For short-term use, up to 72 h.

MOA — Stimulates beta-1 receptors (primarily increases cardiac contractility) and stimulates beta-2 receptors (mild peripheral vasodilation).

ADVERSE EFFECTS — Serious: Arrhythmias, tachycardia. Frequent: Hypertension or hypotension.

DOPAMINE ▶Plasma ♀C ▶– $

WARNING — Avoid extravasation; peripheral ischemia, necrosis, gangrene may occur. If

DOPAMINE (*cont.*)

extravasation occurs, infiltrate the area as soon as possible with a phentolamine and normal saline solution.

ADULT — Pressor: Start 5 mcg/kg/min, increase prn by 5 to 10 mcg/kg/min increments at 10 min intervals, max 50 mcg/kg/min. Mix 400 mg in 250 mL D5W (1600 mcg/mL); a rate of 13 mL/h delivers 5 mcg/kg/min in a 70 kg patient. Alternatively, mix 320 mg in 100 mL D5W (3200 mcg/mL) set at a rate of 6.5 mL/h delivers 5 mcg/kg/min in a 70 kg patient.

PEDS — Not approved in children.

UNAPPROVED ADULT — Symptomatic bradycardia unresponsive to atropine: 5 to 20 mcg/kg/min IV infusion.

UNAPPROVED PEDS — Pressor: Use adult dosage.

NOTES — Doses in mcg/kg/min: 2 to 4 is the traditional renal dose; recent evidence suggests ineffective and active at dopaminergic receptors; 5 to 10 is the cardiac dose: Active at dopaminergic and beta-1 receptors; greater than 10 is active at the dopaminergic, beta-1, and alpha-1 receptors.

MOA — Stimulates beta-1 receptors (increases cardiac contractility and chronotropic effect), stimulates alpha receptors (peripheral vasoconstriction), and stimulates renal dopaminergic receptors (increases renal perfusion).

ADVERSE EFFECTS — Serious: Arrhythmias, tachycardia. Frequent: Hypotension, N/V, palpitations, headache, dyspnea.

EPHEDRINE ▶K ♀C ▶? $

ADULT — Pressor: 10 to 25 mg IV slow injection, with repeat doses q 5 to 10 min prn, max 150 mg/day. Orthostatic hypotension: 25 mg PO daily to four times per day. Bronchospasm: 25 to 50 mg PO q 3 to 4 h prn.

PEDS — Not approved in children.

UNAPPROVED PEDS — Pressor: 3 mg/kg/day SC or IV in 4 to 6 divided doses.

FORMS — Generic only: Caps, 50 mg.

MOA — Stimulates beta-1 receptors (increases cardiac contractility and chronotropic effect), stimulates alpha receptors (peripheral vasoconstriction), stimulates beta-2 receptors (mild peripheral vasodilation).

ADVERSE EFFECTS — Serious: Arrhythmias, tachycardia. Frequent: Hypertension, headache, palpitations, flushing, sweating, dizziness.

EPINEPHRINE (*EpiPen, EpiPen Jr, Auvi-Q, Adrenalin*) ▶Plasma ♀C ▶– $

ADULT — Cardiac arrest: 1 mg (1:10,000 soln) IV, repeat every 3 to 5 min if needed; infusion 1 mg in 250 mL D5W (4 mcg/mL) at rate of 15 to 60 mL/h delivers 1 to 4 mcg/min. Anaphylaxis: 0.1 to 0.5 mg SC/IM (1:1000 soln), may repeat SC dose every 10 to 15 min for anaphylactic shock. Acute asthma and Hypersensitivity reactions: 0.1 to 0.3 mg of 1:1000 soln SC or IM. Hypersensitivity reactions: 0.01 mg/kg SC autoinjector.

PEDS — Cardiac arrest: 0.01 mg/kg IV/intraosseous (IO) (max 1 mg/dose) or 0.1 mg/kg ET (max 10

mg/dose), repeat 0.1 to 0.2 mg/kg IV/IO/ET every 3 to 5 min if needed. Neonates: 0.01 to 0.03 mg/kg IV (preferred) or up to 0.1 mg/kg ET, repeat q 3 to 5 min if needed; IV infusion start 0.1 mcg/kg/min, increase in increments of 0.1 mcg/kg/min if needed, max 1 mcg/kg/min. Anaphylaxis: 0.01 mg/kg (0.01 mL/kg of 1:1000 injection) SC, may repeat SC dose at 20 min to 4 h intervals depending on severity of condition. Acute asthma: 0.01 mL/kg (up to 0.5 mL) of 1:1000 soln SC or IM; repeat q 15 min for 3 to 4 doses prn. Hypersensitivity reactions: 0.01 mg/kg SC autoinjector.

UNAPPROVED ADULT — Symptomatic bradycardia unresponsive to atropine: 2 to 10 mcg/min IV infusion. ET administration prior to IV access: 2 to 2.5 times the recommended IV dose in 10 mL of NS or distilled water.

FORMS — Soln for injection: 1:1000 (1 mg/mL in 1 mL amps or 10 mL vial). Trade only: EpiPen Autoinjector delivers one 0.3 mg (1:1000, 0.3 mL) IM/SQ dose. EpiPen Jr. Autoinjector delivers one 0.15 mg (1:2000, 0.3 mL) IM/SQ dose. Auvi-Q Auto-injector delivers one 0.15 mg (1:1000, 0.15 mL) or 0.3 mg (1:1000, 0.3 mL) IM/SQ dose. EpiPen and Auvi-Q only available in a 2-pack

NOTES — Cardiac arrest: Adult: Use the 1:10,000 injectable soln for IV use in cardiac arrest (10 mL = 1 mg); Peds: Use 1:10,000 for initial IV dose, then 1:1000 for subsequent dosing or ET doses. Anaphylaxis: Use the 1:1000 injectable soln for SC/IM (0.1 mL = 0.1 mg);. consider EpiPen Jr. in patients weighing less than 30 kg. Directions for Epi-Pen: Remove cap. Place black tip end on thigh and push down to inject. Hold in place for 10 sec. May be injected directly through clothing.

MOA — Stimulates beta-1 receptors (increases cardiac contractility and chronotropic effect), stimulates alpha receptors (peripheral vasoconstriction), stimulates beta-2 receptors (peripheral vasodilation).

ADVERSE EFFECTS — Serious: Arrhythmias, tachycardia. Frequent: Hypertension, headache, palpitations, flushing, sweating, dizziness.

MIDODRINE (*✷Amatine*) ▶LK ♀C ▶? $$$$$

WARNING — May cause significant supine HTN. Contraindicated with severe cardiac disease or persistent/excessive supine HTN.

ADULT — The last daily dose should be no later than 6 pm to avoid supine HTN during sleep. Orthostatic hypotension: Start 10 mg PO three times per day, increase dose prn to max 40 mg/day. Renal impairment: Start 2.5 mg three times per day.

PEDS — Not approved in children.

FORMS — Generic: Tabs, scored 2.5, 5, 10 mg.

NOTES — The last daily dose should be no later than 6 pm to avoid supine HTN during sleep.

MOA — Stimulates alpha receptors (peripheral vasoconstriction).

ADVERSE EFFECTS — Serious: Hypertension. Frequent: Paresthesia, piloerection, pruritus, dysuria, chills.

MILRINONE ▸K ♀C ▶? $$

ADULT — Systolic heart failure (NYHA class III, IV): Load 50 mcg/kg IV over 10 min, then begin IV infusion of 0.375 to 0.75 mcg/kg/min. Renal impairment: Infusion rate for CrCl 5 mL/min or less: 0.2 mcg/kg/min; CrCl 6 to 10 mL/min: 0.23 mcg/kg/min; CrCl 11 to 20 mL/min: 0.28 mcg/kg/min; CrCl 21 to 30 mL/min: 0.33 mcg/kg/min; CrCl 31 to 40 mL/min: 0.38 mcg/kg/min; CrCl 41 to 50 mL/min: 0.43 mcg/kg/min.

PEDS — Not approved in children.

UNAPPROVED PEDS — Inotropic support: Limited data, 50 mcg/kg IV bolus over 10 min, followed by 0.5 to 1 mcg/kg/min IV infusion, titrate to effect within dosing range.

NOTES — The brand name product (Primacor) is no longer available.

MOA — Inhibits phosphodiesterase enzyme leading to increased intracellular cAMP (positive inotropic effect).

ADVERSE EFFECTS — Serious: Arrhythmias. Frequent: None.

NOREPINEPHRINE (Levophed) ▸Plasma ♀C ▶? $

WARNING — Tissue ischemia, necrosis, gangrene may occur with extravasation. If extravasation occurs, infiltrate affected area with a soln of phentolamine in NS as soon as possible.

ADULT — Acute hypotension: Start 8 to 12 mcg/min, adjust to maintain BP, average maintenance rate 2 to 4 mcg/min, mix 4 mg in 500 mL D5W (8 mcg/mL); a rate of 22.5 mL/h delivers 3 mcg/min. Ideally through central line.

PEDS — Not approved in children.

UNAPPROVED PEDS — Acute hypotension: Start 0.05 to 0.1 mcg/kg/min IV infusion, titrate to desired effect, max dose 2 mcg/kg/min.

NOTES — Avoid extravasation, do not administer IV push or IM.

MOA — Stimulates beta-1 receptors (increases cardiac contractility and chronotropic effect) and stimulates alpha receptors (peripheral vasoconstriction).

ADVERSE EFFECTS — Serious: Arrhythmias, tissue hypoxia. Frequent: Hypertension, headache.

PHENYLEPHRINE – INTRAVENOUS ▸Plasma ♀C ▶– $

WARNING — Avoid with severe cardiac disease, including CAD and dilated cardiomyopathy. Tissue ischemia, necrosis, gangrene may occur with extravasation. If extravasation occurs, infiltrate affected area with a soln of phentolamine in NS as soon as possible.

ADULT — Mild to moderate hypotension: 0.1 to 0.2 mg slow IV injection, do not exceed 0.5 mg in initial dose, repeat dose prn no less than q 10 to 15 min; 1 to 10 mg SC/IM, initial dose should not exceed 5 mg. Infusion for severe hypotension: 20 mg in 250 mL D5W (80 mcg/mL), start 100 to 180 mcg/min (75 to 135 mL/h), usual dose once BP is stabilized 40 to 60 mcg/min.

PEDS — Not approved in children.

UNAPPROVED PEDS — Mild to moderate hypotension: 5 to 20 mcg/kg IV bolus every 10 to 15 min prn; 0.1 to 0.5 mcg/kg/min IV infusion, titrate to desired effect.

NOTES — Avoid SC or IM administration during shock, use IV route to ensure drug absorption.

MOA — Stimulates alpha receptors (peripheral vasoconstriction).

ADVERSE EFFECTS — Serious: Arrhythmias. Frequent: Hypertension, headache, N/V, sweating, dizziness.

CARDIOVASCULAR: Pulmonary Arterial Hypertension

AMBRISENTAN (Letairis, ✽Volibris) ▸L ♀X ▶– $$$$$

WARNING — Contraindicated with idiopathic pulmonary fibrosis or pregnancy. Women of childbearing age need pregnancy test prior to starting therapy, monthly during treatment, and 1 month after stopping treatment. Prevent pregnancy during treatment and for one month after stopping treatment with acceptable methods of contraception. Only available through restricted program; prescribers, pharmacies, female patients must enroll.

ADULT — Pulmonary arterial hypertension: Start 5 mg PO daily; if tolerated, may increase to 10 mg/day.

PEDS — Not approved in children.

FORMS — Trade only: Tabs, unscored 5, 10 mg.

NOTES — Monitor hemoglobin at initiation, after 1 month of therapy, then periodically. If pulmonary edema occurs, consider veno-occlusive disease; if confirmed, discontinue therapy. Not recommended with moderate or severe hepatic impairment. Do not exceed 5 mg when given with cyclosporine. May reduce sperm count. Do not split, crush, or chew tablets.

MOA — Endothelin receptor antagonist.

ADVERSE EFFECTS — Serious: Pulmonary veno-occlusive disease. Frequent: Fluid retention, flushing, nasal congestion, peripheral edema, sinusitis.

BOSENTAN (Tracleer) ▸L ♀X ▶–? $$$$$

WARNING — Hepatotoxicity; monitor LFTs prior to starting therapy and monthly thereafter. Discontinue bosentan with aminotransferase elevations accompanied by signs/symptoms of liver dysfunction/injury or increases in bilirubin 2 or more times the upper limit of normal. Contraindicated in pregnancy due to birth defects; women of childbearing age need pregnancy test prior to starting therapy & monthly thereafter. Prevent pregnancy during treatment and for one month after stopping treatment with two acceptable methods of contraception, unless the patient had tubal sterilization or uses Copper T 380A IUD or LNg 20 IUS.

ADULT — Pulmonary arterial hypertension: Start 62.5 mg PO two times per day for 4 weeks, increase to 125 mg two times per day maintenance dose. With low body wt (less than 40 kg) and older than 12 yo: 62.5 mg PO two times per day. Stop bosentan more than 36 hr prior to initiating ritonavir; when

BOSENTAN (*cont.*)

on ritonavir more than 10 days, give bosentan 62.5 mg PO daily or every other day.
PEDS — Not approved in children.
FORMS — Trade only: Tabs, unscored 62.5, 125 mg.
NOTES — Available only through access program by calling 866-228-3546. Avoid with moderate or severe liver impairment or aminotransferases more than 3 times upper limit of normal prior to initiation. Concomitant glyburide or cyclosporine is contraindicated. Induces metabolism of other drugs (e.g., contraceptives, simvastatin, lovastatin, atorvastatin). Do not use with both CYP2C9 inhibitor (e.g., amiodarone, fluconazole) and strong CYP3A4 inhibitor (e.g., ketoconazole, itraconazole, ritonavir) or moderate CYP3A4 inhibitor (e.g., amprenavir, erythromycin, fluconazole, diltiazem); will increase levels of bosentan. May decrease warfarin plasma concentration; monitor INR. Rifampin alters bosentan levels; monitor LFTs weekly for 4 weeks, followed by normal monitoring. If pulmonary edema occurs, consider veno-occlusive disease; if confirmed, discontinue therapy. Monitor hemoglobin after 1 and 3 months of therapy, then q 3 months. May reduce sperm count.
MOA — Endothelin receptor antagonist.
ADVERSE EFFECTS — Serious: Hepatotoxicity, pulmonary veno-occlusive disease. Frequent: Anemia, fluid retention, flushing, rash.

EPOPROSTENOL (*Flolan*) ▶Plasma ♀B ▶? $$$$$
ADULT — Pulmonary arterial hypertension (PAH): Acute dose ranging, 2 ng/kg/min increments via IV infusion until the patient develops symptomatic intolerance (mean maximal dose without symptoms 8.6 ng/kg/min), start continuous IV infusion at 4 ng/kg/min or less than the patient's maximum-tolerated infusion (MTI) rate for acute dose ranging. If the MTI rate is less than 5 ng/kg/min, start chronic IV infusion at ½ the MTI.
PEDS — Not approved in children.
NOTES — Avoid abrupt cessation or dose decreases. Administer by continuous IV infusion via a central venous catheter. Temporary peripheral IV infusions may be used until central access is established. May potentiate bleeding risk of anticoagulants. May potentiate hypotensive effects of other medications. If pulmonary edema occurs, consider veno-occlusive disease; if confirmed, discontinue therapy.
MOA — Naturally occuring prostaglandin. Dilates pulmonary and sytemic arteries. Inhibits platelet aggregation.
ADVERSE EFFECTS — Serious: Hypotension, may increase risk of bleeding, veno-occlusive disease, sepsis. Frequent: Dizziness, flushing, headache, myalgia, N/V.

ILOPROST (*Ventavis*) ▶L ♀C ▶? $$$$$
ADULT — Pulmonary arterial hypertension: Start 2.5 mcg/dose by inhalation (as delivered at mouthpiece); if well tolerated increase to 5 mcg/dose by inhalation (as delivered at mouthpiece). Use 6 to 9 times a day (minimum of 2 h between doses) during waking h.

PEDS — Not approved in children.
NOTES — Only administer with I-neb AAD Systems. Each single-use ampule delivers 20 mcg to medication chamber of nebulizer and 2.5 or 5 mcg to the mouthpiece; discard remaining soln after each inhalation. Do not mix with other medications. Avoid contact with skin/eyes or oral ingestion. Monitor vital signs when initiating therapy. Do not initiate therapy if SBP less than 85 mm Hg. With Child-Pugh Class B or C hepatic impairment, consider increasing the dosing interval (e.g., 3 to 4 h between doses) depending on patient's response at end of dosing interval. May potentiate bleeding risk of anticoagulants. May potentiate hypotensive effects of other medications. Discontinue therapy if pulmonary edema occurs; this may be sign of pulmonary venous hypertension. May induce bronchospasm; carefully monitor patients with COPD, severe asthma, or acute pulmonary infection.
MOA — Prostacyclin analogue. Dilates systemic and pulmonary arteries Inhibits platelet aggregation.
ADVERSE EFFECTS — Serious: Bronchospasm, hepatotoxicity, hypotension, syncope, pneumonia, thrombosis. Frequent: Cough, flushing, headache, hemoptysis, insomnia, myalgia, N/V, tongue pain, trismus.

MACITENTAN (*Opsumit*) ▶L ♀X ▶– $$$$$
WARNING — Contraindicated with pregnancy. Women of childbearing age need pregnancy test prior to starting therapy, monthly during treatment, and 1 month after stopping treatment. Prevent pregnancy during treatment and for one month after stopping treatment with acceptable methods of contraception. Only available through restricted program; prescribers, pharmacies, female patients must enroll.
ADULT — Pulmonary arterial hypertension: 10 mg PO daily.
PEDS — Not approved in children.
FORMS — Trade: Tabs 10 mg.
NOTES — Measure baseline hemoglobin and LFTs; monitor when clinically indicated. If pulmonary edema occurs, consider veno-occlusive disease; if confirmed, discontinue therapy. Avoid concomitant strong CYP3A4 inducers (e.g., rifampin) and strong CYP3A4 inhibitors (e.g., ketoconazole, ritonavir). May reduce sperm count.
MOA — Endothelin receptor antagonist.
ADVERSE EFFECTS — Serious: Anemia, pulmonary veno-occlusive disease. Frequent: bronchitis, headache, influenza, pharyngitis, UTI.

RIOCIGUAT (*Adempas*) ▶LK ♀X ▶– $$$$$
WARNING — Contraindicated with pregnancy. Women of childbearing age need pregnancy test prior to starting therapy, monthly during treatment, and 1 month after stopping treatment. Prevent pregnancy during treatment and for one month after stopping treatment with acceptable methods of contraception. Only available through restricted program; prescribers, pharmacies, female patients must enroll.
ADULT — Pulmonary arterial hypotension: Start 1 mg PO three times daily; may increase by 0.5 mg q 2

(cont.)

RIOCIGUAT (*cont.*)

weeks as tolerated, max 2.5 mg three times daily. If patient may not tolerate hypotensive effects, start 0.5 mg PO three times daily. Not recommended with CrCl less than 15 mL/min, dialysis, or severe (Child Pugh C) hepatic impairment.

PEDS — Not approved in children.

FORMS — Trade: Tabs 0.5, 1, 1.5, 2, 2.5 mg.

NOTES — Contraindicated with nitrates, nitric oxide donors, phosphodiesterase inhibitors. Separate from antacid administration by at least 1 h. Concomitant strong CYP and p-glycoprotein/breast cancer resistance protein inhibitors (e.g., ketoconazole, itraconazole, ritonavir) increase risk of hypotension; consider initiating 0.5 mg PO three times daily; monitor for hypotension. Smoking reduces plasma concentrations 50–60%; if patient smokes, may need more than 2.5 mg PO three times daily; decrease dose if patient stops smoking. If pulmonary edema occurs, consider veno-occlusive disease; if confirmed, discontinue therapy. May increase bleeding risk.

MOA — Guanylate cyclase stimulator.

ADVERSE EFFECTS — Serious: Anemia, hypotension, may increase risk of bleeding. Frequent: Constipation, diarrhea, dizziness, dyspnea, GERD, headache, N/V.

SILDENAFIL (*Revatio*) ▶LK ♀B ▶– $$$$

ADULT — Pulmonary arterial hypertension: 5 mg or 20 mg PO three times per day, with doses 4-6 h apart; or 2.5 mg or 10 mg IV three times per day.

PEDS — Not approved in children.

FORMS — Generic/Trade: Tabs 20 mg. Trade only: Suspension 10 mg/mL.

NOTES — Contraindicated with nitrates. Coadministration is not recommended with ritonavir, potent CYP3A inhibitors, or other phosphodiesterase-5 inhibitors. Concomitant alpha-blockers or amlodipine may potentiate hypotension. Use not recommended for patients with pulmonary veno-occlusive disease or pediatric patients (1-17 yo). Sudden vision loss due to nonarteritic ischemic optic neuropathy has been reported. Discontinue with sudden decrease/loss of hearing. Teach patients to seek medical attention for vision loss, hearing loss, or in men if erections last longer than 4 h. Safety and efficacy in treating patients with pulmonary hypertension secondary to sickle cell disease have not been established; may increase risk for vaso-occlusive crisis.

MOA — Selectively inhibits phosphodiesterase-5 resulting in relaxation of pulmonary vascular smooth muscle bed.

ADVERSE EFFECTS — Serious: MI, CVA, hypotension, syncope, cerebral thrombosis, retinal hemorrhage, vision loss (nonarteritic ischemic optic neuropathy). Frequent: Dyspepsia, dyspnea, erythema, epistaxis, flushing, headache, insomnia, rhinitis.

TADALAFIL (*Adcirca*) ▶L ♀B ▶– $$$$

ADULT — Pulmonary arterial hypertension: 40 mg PO daily, 20 mg if CrCl less than 80 mL/min or mild to moderate hepatic impairment. Avoid with CrCl less than 30 mL/min or severe hepatic impairment.

PEDS — Not approved in children.

FORMS — Trade only (Adcirca): Tabs 20 mg.

NOTES — Contraindicated with nitrates; If nitrates needed and had tadalafil in last 48 h, give nitrate under close medical supervision with hemodynamic monitoring. Coadministration is not recommended with potent CYP3A inhibitors (itraconazole, ketoconazole), potent CYP3A inducers (rifampin), or other phosphodiesterase-5 inhibitors. Caution with ritonavir, see prescribing info for specific dose adjustments. Alpha-blockers or alcohol may potentiate hypotension. Use not recommended for patients with pulmonary veno-occlusive disease. Sudden vision loss due to nonarteritic ischemic optic neuropathy has been reported. Retinal artery occlusion has been reported. Discontinue with sudden decrease/loss of hearing. Transient global amnesia. Teach patients to seek medical attention for vision loss, hearing loss, or in men if erections last longer than 4 h.

MOA — Selectively inhibits phosphodiesterase-5 resulting in relaxation of pulmonary vascular smooth muscle bed.

ADVERSE EFFECTS — Serious: Priapism, hypotension, myocardial infarction, vision loss (nonarteritic ischemic optic neuropathy), retinal artery occlusion. Frequent: Headache, flushing, dyspepsia, back pain.

TREPROSTINIL SODIUM—INJECTABLE (*Remodulin*) ▶KL ♀B ▶? $$$$$

ADULT — Pulmonary arterial hypertension: Continuous SC (preferred) or central IV infusion. Start 1.25 ng/kg/min based on ideal body wt. Reduce to 0.625 ng/kg/min if initial dose not tolerated. Dose based on clinical response and tolerance. Increase by no more than 1.25 ng/kg/min/week in first 4 weeks, then increase by no more than 2.5 ng/kg/min/week. Mild to moderate hepatic insufficiency: Start 0.625 ng/kg/min based on ideal body wt; increase cautiously. Not studied with severe hepatic insufficiency. Transitioning from epoprostenol: Must be done in hospital; initiate at 10% epoprostenol dose; gradually increase dose as epoprostenol dose is decreased (see chart in prescribing information).

PEDS — Not approved in children.

NOTES — Avoid abruptly lowering the dose or cessation. Use cautiously in the elderly and those with liver or renal dysfunction. Initiate in setting with personnel and equipment for physiological monitoring and emergency care. Administer by continuous infusion using infusion pump. Patient must have access to backup infusion pump and infusion sets. Must dilute prior to giving IV; use infusion set with in-line filter; see prescribing information for details. May potentiate bleeding risk for patients on anticoagulants. May potentiate hypotensive effects of other medications.

MOA — Prostacyclin analogue. Dilates systemic and pulmonary arteries. Inhibits platelet aggregation.

TREPROSTINIL SODIUM—INJECTABLE (cont.)

ADVERSE EFFECTS — Serious: Hypotension, may increase risk of bleeding, sepsis (from indwelling central venous catheter). Frequent: Pain at infusion site, local reaction at infusion site, dizziness, headache, diarrhea, nausea, pruritus, jaw pain, vasodilation.

TREPROSTINIL—INHALED SOLUTION (Tyvaso) ▶KL - ♀B ▶? $$$$$

ADULT — Pulmonary arterial hypertension: Start 3 breaths (18 mcg) per treatment session four times per day during waking hours; treatments should be at least 4 h apart; may reduce initial dose to 1 to 2 breaths per treatment session if 3 breaths not tolerated. May increase by 3 breaths q 1 to 2 weeks as tolerated, max 9 breaths (54 mcg) per treatment four times per day.

PEDS — Not approved in children.

FORMS — 1.74 mg in 2.9 mL inhalation solution

NOTES — Administer undiluted with the Tyvaso Inhalation System. A single breath delivers about 6 mcg treprostinil; discard remaining solution at the end of each day. Do not mix with other medications. Avoid contact with skin/eyes or oral ingestion. Safety and efficacy not established with existing lung disease (asthma, COPD). Carefully monitor patients with acute pulmonary infection. May need to adjust doses if CYP2C8 inducers (e.g., rifampin) or CYP2C8 inhibitors (e.g., gemfibrozil) are added or withdrawn. Use cautiously in the elderly and those with liver or renal dysfunction. May potentiate bleeding risk of anticoagulants. May potentiate hypotensive effects of other medications.

MOA — Prostacyclin analogue. Dilates systemic and pulmonary arteries. Inhibits platelet aggregation.

ADVERSE EFFECTS — Serious: Hypotension, may increase risk of bleeding. Frequent: Cough, diarrhea, dizziness, flushing, headache, nausea, pharyngollaryngeal pain.

TREPROSTINIL—ORAL (Orenitram) ▶L ♀C ▶? $$$$$

ADULT — Pulmonary artery hypertension: Start 0.25 mg PO two times daily; increase by 0.25 to 0.5 mg two times daily or 0.125 mg three times daily every 3 to 4 days as tolerated. Mild liver impairment (Child Pugh Class A) or with strong CYP2C8 inhibitor (ie, gemfibrozil): Start 0.125 mg PO two times daily; increase by 0.125 mg two times daily every 3 to 4 days as tolerated.

PEDS — Not approved in children.

FORMS — Trade: Extended-release tabs 0.125, 0.25, 1, 2.5 mg.

NOTES — Take with food. Swallow whole. Do not abruptly discontinue. Avoid use with moderate or severe hepatic impairment. Avoid alcohol; may increase rate of release of treprostinil. May increase bleeding risk. In patients with diverticulosis, may become lodged in diverticulum.

MOA — Prostacyclin analogue. Dilates systemic and pulmonary arteries. Inhibits platelet aggregation.

ADVERSE EFFECTS — Serious: Hypotension, may increase risk of bleeding. Frequent: Diarrhea, headache, nausea.

CARDIOVASCULAR: Thrombolytics

ALTEPLASE (tpa, t-PA, Activase, Cathflo, *Activase rt-PA) ▶L ♀C ▶? $$$$$

ADULT — Acute MI: wt 67 kg or less, give 15 mg IV bolus, then 0.75 mg/kg (max 50 mg) over 30 min, then 0.5 mg/kg (max 35 mg) over the next 60 min; wt greater than 67 kg, give 15 mg IV bolus, then 50 mg over 30 min, then 35 mg over the next 60 min. Acute ischemic CVA with symptoms 3 h or less: 0.9 mg/kg (max 90 mg); give 10% of total dose as an IV bolus, and the remainder IV over 60 min. Multiple exclusion criteria. Select patients may receive with symtoms 4.5 h or less (age < 80 yo; baseline NIHSS score 25 or less; no anticoagulant use; or no combination of prior stroke and diabetes). Acute pulmonary embolism: 100 mg IV over 2 h, then restart heparin when PTT twice normal or less. Occluded central venous access device: 2 mg/mL in catheter for 2 h. May use second dose if needed.

PEDS — Occluded central venous access device: Wt at least 10 kg but less than 30 kg: Dose equal to 110% of the internal lumen volume, not to exceed 2 mg/2 mL. Other uses not approved in children.

NOTES — Must be reconstituted. Soln must be used within 8 h after reconstitution.

MOA — Enhances conversion of plasminogen to plasmin to achieve fibrinolysis.

ADVERSE EFFECTS — Serious: Bleeding, intracranial hemorrhage, hypersensitivity. Frequent: N/V, bleeding, hypotension, fever.

RETEPLASE (Retavase) ▶L ♀C ▶? $$$$$

ADULT — Acute MI: 10 units IV over 2 min; repeat 1 dose in 30 min.

PEDS — Not approved in children.

NOTES — Must be reconstituted with sterile water for injection to 1 mg/mL concentration. Soln must be used within 4 h after reconstitution.

MOA — Enhances conversion of plasminogen to plasmin.

ADVERSE EFFECTS — Serious: Bleeding. Frequent: None.

STREPTOKINASE (Streptase, Kabikinase) ▶L ♀C ▶? $$$$$

ADULT — Acute MI: 1.5 million units IV over 60 min. Pulmonary embolism: 250,000 units IV loading dose over 30 min, followed by 100,000 units/h IV infusion for 24 h (maintain infusion for 72 h if concurrent DVT suspected). DVT: 250,000 units IV loading dose over 30 min, followed by 100,000 units/h IV infusion for 24 h. Occluded arteriovenous catheter: 250,000 units instilled into the catheter, remove soln containing 250,000 units of drug from catheter after 2 h using a 5 mL syringe.

PEDS — Not approved in children.

(cont.)

STREPTOKINASE (*cont.*)
NOTES — Must be reconstituted. Soln must be used within 8 h of reconstitution. Do not shake vial. Do not repeat use in less than 1 year. Do not use with history of severe allergic reaction.
MOA — Enhances conversion of plasminogen to plasmin.
ADVERSE EFFECTS — Serious: Bleeding, hypersensitivity (rare). Frequent: None.

TENECTEPLASE (*TNKase*) ▶L ♀C ▶? $$$$$
ADULT — Acute MI: Single IV bolus dose over 5 sec based on body wt: wt less than 60 kg: 30 mg; wt 60–69 kg: 35 mg; wt 70–79 kg: 40 mg; wt 80–89 kg: 45 mg; wt 90 kg or more: 50 mg.
PEDS — Not approved in children.
NOTES — Must be reconstituted. Soln must be used within 8 h after reconstitution.
MOA — Enhances conversion of plasminogen to plasmin.
ADVERSE EFFECTS — Serious: Bleeding. Frequent: None.

UROKINASE (*Kinlytic*) ▶L ♀B ▶? $$$$$
ADULT — Pulmonary embolism: 4400 units/kg IV loading dose over 10 min, followed by IV infusion 4400 units/kg/h for 12 h.
PEDS — Not approved in children.
UNAPPROVED ADULT — Occluded IV catheter: 5000 units in catheter for 1-4 h.
UNAPPROVED PEDS — Arterial or venous thrombosis: 4400 units/kg IV loading dose over 10 min, followed by 4400 units/kg/h for 12 to 72 h. Occluded IV catheter: 5000 units in the catheter for 1-4 h.
NOTES — Must be reconstituted. Do not shake vial.
MOA — Enhances conversion of plasminogen to plasmin.
ADVERSE EFFECTS — Serious: Bleeding, hypersensitivity (rare). Frequent: None.

CARDIOVASCULAR: Volume Expanders

ALBUMIN (*Albuminar, Buminate, Albumarc, ✸Plasbumin*) ▶L ♀C ▶? $$$$$
ADULT — Shock, burns: 500 mL of 5% soln (50 mg/mL) infused as rapidly as tolerated. Repeat infusion in 30 min if response is inadequate. 25% soln may be used with or without dilution. Undiluted 25% soln should be infused at 1 mL/min to avoid too rapid plasma volume expansion.
PEDS — Shock, burns: 10 to 20 mL/kg IV infusion at 5 to 10 mL/min using 50 mL of 5% soln.
UNAPPROVED PEDS — Shock/hypovolemia: 1 g/kg/dose IV rapid infusion. Hypoproteinemia: 1 g/kg/dose IV infusion over 30 to 120 min.
NOTES — Fever, chills. Monitor for plasma volume overload (dyspnea, fluid in lungs, abnormal increase in BP or CVP). Less likely to cause hypotension than plasma protein fraction, more purified. In treating burns, large volumes of crystalloid solns (0.9% sodium chloride) are used to maintain plasma volume with albumin. Use 5% soln in pediatric hypovolemic patients. Use 25% soln in pediatric patients with volume restrictions.
MOA — Expands plasma volume.
ADVERSE EFFECTS — Serious: Pulmonary edema (rapid infusion), hypersensitivity (rare), bleeding. Frequent: Hypotension (rapid infusion), fever, chills, itching.

DEXTRAN (*Rheomacrodex, Gentran, Macrodex*) ▶K ♀C ▶? $$
ADULT — Shock/hypovolemia: Dextran 40, Dextran 70 and 75, up to 20 mL/kg during the first 24 h, up to 10 mL/kg/day thereafter, do not continue for longer than 5 days. The first 500 mL may be infused rapidly with CVP monitoring. DVT/PE prophylaxis during surgery: Dextran 40, 50 to 100 g IV infusion the day of surgery, continue for 2 to 3 days postop with 50 g/day. 50 g/day may be given every 2nd or 3rd day thereafter up to 14 days.
PEDS — Total dose should not exceed 20 mL/kg.
UNAPPROVED ADULT — DVT/PE prophylaxis during surgery: Dextran 70 and 75 solns have been

used. Other uses: To improve circulation with sickle cell crisis, prevention of nephrotoxicity with radiographic contrast media, toxemia of late pregnancy.
NOTES — Monitor for plasma volume overload (dyspnea, fluid in lungs, abnormal increase in BP or CVP) and anaphylactoid reactions. May impair platelet function. Less effective that other agents for DVT/PE prevention.
MOA — Expands plasma volume.
ADVERSE EFFECTS — Serious: Pulmonary edema (rapid infusion), anaphylaxis (rare), bleeding. Frequent: Hypotension (rapid infusion), fever, chills, itching.

HETASTARCH (*Hespan, Hextend*) ▶K ♀C ▶? $$
WARNING — Do not use in critically ill adult patients, including those with sepsis or in ICU; associated with increased risk of death and renal injury.
ADULT — Shock/hypovolemia: 500 to 1000 mL IV infusion, total daily dose usually should not exceed 20 mL/kg (1500 mL). Renal impairment: CrCl less than 10 mL/min, usual initial dose followed by 20 to 25% of usual dose.
PEDS — Not approved in children.
UNAPPROVED PEDS — Shock/hypovolemia: 10 mL/kg/dose; do not exceed 20 mL/kg/day.
NOTES — Monitor for volume overload. Little or no antigenic properties compared to dextran.
MOA — Expands plasma volume.
ADVERSE EFFECTS — Serious: Pulmonary edema (rapid infusion), hypersensitivity (rare), bleeding. Frequent: Hypotension (rapid infusion), fever, chills, itching.

PLASMA PROTEIN FRACTION (*Plasmanate, Protenate, Plasmatein*) ▶L ♀C ▶? $$$
ADULT — Shock/hypovolemia: Adjust initial rate according to clinical response and BP, but rate should not exceed 10 mL/min. As plasma volume normalizes, infusion rate should not exceed 5 to 8 mL/min. Usual dose 250 to 500 mL. Hypoproteinemia: 1000 to 1500 mL/day IV infusion.
PEDS — Shock/hypovolemia: Initial dose 6.6 to 33 mL/kg infused at a rate of 5 to 10 mL/min.

PLASMA PROTEIN FRACTION (*cont.*)

NOTES — Fever, chills, hypotension with rapid infusion. Monitor for volume overload. Less pure than albumin products.

MOA — Expands plasma volume.
ADVERSE EFFECTS — Serious: Pulmonary edema (rapid infusion), hypersensitivity (rare), bleeding. Frequent: Hypotension (rapid infusion), fever, chills, itching.

CARDIOVASCULAR: Other

BIDIL **(hydralazine + isosorbide dinitrate)** ▶LK ♀C ▶? $$$$$
ADULT — Heart failure (adjunct to standard therapy in black patients): Start 1 tab PO three times per day, increase as tolerated to max 2 tabs three times per day. May decrease to ½ tab three times per day with intolerable side effects; try to increase dose when side effects subside.
PEDS — Not approved in children.
FORMS — Trade only: Tabs, scored 37.5/20 mg.
NOTES — See component drugs.
MOA — See component drugs.
ADVERSE EFFECTS — See component drugs

CILOSTAZOL (*Pletal*) ▶L ♀C ▶? $$$$
WARNING — Contraindicated in heart failure of any severity due to decreased survival.
ADULT — Intermittent claudication: 100 mg PO twice daily on empty stomach. 50 mg PO twice daily with CYP3A4 inhibitors (e.g., ketoconazole, itraconazole, erythromycin, diltiazem) or CYP2C19 inhibitors (e.g., omeprazole). Beneficial effect may take up to 12 weeks.
PEDS — Not approved in children.
FORMS — Generic/Trade: Tabs 50, 100 mg.
NOTES — Caution with moderate/severe liver impairment or CrCl less than 25 mL/min. Give with other antiplatelet therapy (aspirin or clopidogrel) when treating peripheral arterial disease to reduce cardiovascular risk. Grapefruit juice may increase levels and the risk of side effects.
MOA — Inhibits platelet aggregation and causes vasodilation by blocking the effects of phosphodiesterase III enzyme.
ADVERSE EFFECTS — Serious: Heart failure exacerbation, cerebral/pulmonary hemorrhage, Stevens-Johnson syndrome, thrombocytopenia. Frequent: Palpitations, dizziness, nausea, diarrhea, dyspepsia, headache.

NESIRITIDE (*Natrecor*) ▶K, plasma ♀C ▶? $$$$$
ADULT — Hospitalized patients with decompensated heart failure with dyspnea at rest: 2 mcg/kg IV bolus over 1 min, then 0.01 mcg/kg/min IV infusion for up to 48 h. Bolus dose may not be appropriate for patients with SBP less than 110 or with recent use of afterload reducer (eg, nitroglycerin). Do not initiate at higher doses. Limited experience with increased doses: 0.005 mcg/kg/min increments, preceded by 1 mcg/kg bolus, no more frequently than q 3 h up to max infusion dose 0.03 mcg/kg/min. Mix 1.5 mg vial in 250 mL D5W (6 mcg/mL). A bolus of 23.3 mL is 2 mcg/kg for a 70 kg patient, infusion set at rate 7 mL/h delivers a 0.01 mcg/kg/min for a 70 kg patient.
PEDS — Not approved in children.
NOTES — Contraindicated with cardiogenic shock or SBP less than 100 mm Hg. May increase mortality;

meta-analysis showed nonstatistically significant increased risk of death within 30 days post treatment compared with noninotropic control group. Not indicated for outpatient infusion, for scheduled repetitive use, to improve renal function, or to enhance diuresis. Discontinue if dose-related symptomatic hypotension occurs and support BP prn. May restart infusion with dose reduced by 30% (no bolus dose) once BP stabilized. May worsen renal impairment. Do not shake reconstituted vial, and dilute vial prior to administration. Incompatible with most injectable drugs; administer agents using separate IV lines. Do not measure BNP levels while infusing; may measure BNP at least 2 to 6 h after infusion completion.
MOA — Human B-type natriuretic peptide that relaxes cardiac smooth muscle (arterial and venous vasodilation).
ADVERSE EFFECTS — Serious: Arrhythmias, altered kidney function. Frequent: Hypotension, headache, insomnia, dizziness, nausea.

PENTOXIFYLLINE (*Trental*) ▶L ♀C ▶? $$$
ADULT — Intermittent claudication: 400 mg PO three times per day with meals. With CNS/GI adverse effects, may decrease to two times per day. CrCl less than 30 mL/min: 400 mg PO daily. Beneficial effect may take up to 8 weeks. May be less effective in relieving cramps, tiredness, tightness, and pain during exercise.
PEDS — Not approved in children.
FORMS — Generic/Trade: Tabs, extended-release 400 mg.
NOTES — Contraindicated with recent cerebral/retinal bleed. Increases theophylline levels. Increases INR with warfarin.
MOA — Decreases blood viscosity and improves erythrocyte flexibility.
ADVERSE EFFECTS — None.

RANOLAZINE (*Ranexa*) ▶LK ♀C ▶? $$$$$
ADULT — Chronic angina: 500 mg PO two times per day, increase to 1000 mg PO two times per day prn based on clinical symptoms, max 2000 mg daily. Max 500 mg two times per day, if used with diltiazem, verapamil, or moderate CYP3A inhibitors.
PEDS — Not approved in children.
FORMS — Trade only: Tabs, extended-release 500, 1000 mg.
NOTES — Baseline and follow-up ECGs; may prolong QT interval. If CrCl < 60 mL/min at baseline, monitor renal function after initiation and periodically; discontinue ranolazine if acute renal failure occurs. Contraindicated with hepatic cirrhosis, potent CYP3A4 inhibitors (eg, clarithromycin, protease inhibitors, itraconazole, ketoconazole, nefazodone),

(cont.)

RANOLAZINE (*cont.*)

CYP3A inducers (e.g., carbamazepine, phenobarbital, phenytoin, rifabutin, rifapentin, rifampin, St. John's wort). Limit dose of ranolazine to max 500 mg two times per day with moderate CYP3A inhibitors (e.g., diltiazem, erythromycin, fluconazole, grapefruit juice-containing products, verapamil). Limit simvastatin to 20 mg when used with ranolazine. Limit metformin to 1700 mg daily when used with ranolazine 1000 mg twice daily. P-glycoprotein inhibitors (e.g., cyclosporine) increase ranolazine levels; titrate ranolazine based on clinical response. Increases levels of CYP3A substrates (e.g., lovastatin, simvastatin), CYP2D6 substrates (e.g., antipsychotic agents, TCAs), OCT2 substrates (e.g., metformin), cyclosporine, tacrolimus, sirolimus, drugs transported by p-glycoprotein (e.g., digoxin); may need dose adjustments. Swallow whole; do not crush, break, or chew. May be less effective in women. Teach patients to report palpitations or fainting spells.

MOA — Unknown; inhibits late sodium current at therapeutic levels. Antianginal and anti-ischemic effects not dependent on HR or BP.

ADVERSE EFFECTS — Serious: Acute renal failure, QT prolongation. Frequent: Constipation, dizziness, headache, nausea.

CONTRAST MEDIA

CONTRAST MEDIA: MRI Contrast—Gadolinium-Based

NOTE: Avoid gadolinium-based contrast agents if severe renal insufficiency (GFR less than 30 mL/min/1.73 m2) due to risk of nephrogenic systemic fibrosis/nephrogenic fibrosing dermopathy. Similarly avoid in acute renal insufficiency of any severity due to hepatorenal syndrome or during the perioperative phase of liver transplant.

GADOBENATE (*MultiHance*) ▶K ♀C ▶? $$$$
ADULT — Noniodinated, nonionic IV contrast for MRI.
PEDS — Not approved in children.
MOA — Gadolinium-based noniodinated, nonionic IV contrast for MRI.
ADVERSE EFFECTS — Serious: Hypersensitivity, nephropathy. Frequent: None.

GADOBUTROL (*Gadavist, ✱Gadavist*) ▶K - ♀C ▶? ©V $$$$
ADULT — 0.1 mL/kg for age 2 yo or older up to a maximum of 14 mLs
PEDS — 0.1 mL/kg for age 2 yo or older
NOTES — Formulated at a higher concentration (1 mmol/mL) compared to certain other gadolinium based contrast agents, resulting in a lower volume of administration.
MOA — Gadolinium based IV contrast for MRI
ADVERSE EFFECTS — Serious: Hypersensitivity, nephrogenic systemic fibrosis, dermopathy. Frequent: None

GADODIAMIDE (*Omniscan*) ▶K ♀C ▶? $$$$
ADULT — Noniodinated, nonionic IV contrast for MRI.
PEDS — Noniodinated, nonionic IV contrast for MRI.
NOTES — Use caution if renal disease. May falsely lower serum calcium. Not for intrathecal use.
MOA — Gadolinium-based noniodinated, nonionic IV contrast for MRI.
ADVERSE EFFECTS — Serious: Hypersensitivity, nephropathy. Frequent: None.

GADOPENTETATE (*Magnevist*) ▶K ♀C ▶? $$$
ADULT — Noniodinated IV contrast for MRI.
PEDS — Age older than 2 yo: Noniodinated IV contrast for MRI.
NOTES — Use caution in sickle cell and renal disease.

MOA — Gadolinium-based noniodinated IV contrast for MRI.
ADVERSE EFFECTS — Serious: Black Box Warning for Nephrogenic Systemic Fibrosis in patients with reduced GFR. Serious: Hypersensitivity, nephropathy. Frequent: None.

GADOTERATE MEGLUMINE (*Dotarem*) ▶K - ♀C ▶? $$$$
ADULT — Gadolinium based macrocyclic and ionic IV contrast for MRI of the CNS and blood brain barrier and/or abnormal vascularity: dose is 0.2 mL/kg (0.1 mmol/kg) IV bolus infused at rate of 2 mL/second
PEDS — Age older than 2 yo: 0.2 mL/kg (0.1 mmol/kg) IV bolus infused at rate of 1 to 2 mL/second. Not approved age less than 2 yo
ADVERSE EFFECTS — Hypersensitivity, headache

GADOTERIDOL (*Prohance*) ▶K ♀C ▶? $$$$
ADULT — Noniodinated, nonionic IV contrast for MRI.
PEDS — Age older than 2 yo: Noniodinated, nonionic IV contrast for MRI.
NOTES — Use caution in sickle cell and renal disease.
MOA — Gadolinium-based noniodinated, nonionic IV contrast for MRI.
ADVERSE EFFECTS — Serious: Hypersensitivity, nephropathy. Frequent: None.

GADOVERSETAMIDE (*OptiMARK*) ▶K ♀C ▶– $$$$
ADULT — Noniodinated IV contrast for MRI.
PEDS — Not approved in children.
NOTES — Use caution in sickle cell and renal disease.
MOA — Gadolinium-based noniodinated IV contrast for MRI.
ADVERSE EFFECTS — Serious: Hypersensitivity, nephropathy. Frequent: None.

CONTRAST MEDIA: MRI Contrast—Other

FERUMOXIDES (*Feridex*) ▶L ♀C ▶? $$$$
ADULT — Noniodinated, nonionic, iron-based IV contrast for hepatic MRI.
PEDS — Not approved in children.
NOTES — Contains dextran.
MOA — Noniodinated, nonionic, iron-based IV contrast for hepatic MRI.
ADVERSE EFFECTS — Serious: Hypersensitivity. Frequent: None.

FERUMOXSIL (*GastroMARK*) ▶L ♀B ▶? $$$$
ADULT — Noniodinated, nonionic, iron-based, oral GI contrast for MRI.
PEDS — Not approved in children younger than 16 yo.

MOA — Noniodinated, nonionic, iron-based, oral GI contrast for MRI.
ADVERSE EFFECTS — Serious: Hypersensitivity. Frequent: Abdominal pain, N/V.

MANGAFODIPIR (*Teslascan*) ▶L ♀– ▶– $$$$
ADULT — Non-iodinated IV contrast for MRI.
PEDS — Not approved in children.
NOTES — Contains manganese.
MOA — Non-iodinated IV contrast for MRI.
ADVERSE EFFECTS — Serious: Hypersensitivity. Frequent: Headache.

CONTRAST MEDIA: Radiography Contrast

NOTE: Beware of allergic or anaphylactoid reactions. Avoid IV contrast in renal insufficiency or dehydration. Hold metformin (Glucophage) prior to or at the time of iodinated contrast dye use and for 48 h after procedure. Restart after procedure only if renal function is normal.

BARIUM SULFATE ▶Not absorbed ♀? ▶+ $
ADULT — Noniodinated GI (e.g., oral, rectal) contrast.
PEDS — Noniodinated GI (e.g., oral, rectal) contrast.
NOTES — Contraindicated if suspected esophageal, gastric, or intestinal perforation. Use with caution in GI obstruction. May cause abdominal distention, cramping, and constipation with oral use.
MOA — Noniodinated GI contrast.
ADVERSE EFFECTS — Serious: Hypersensitivity, worsening of bowel obstruction. Frequent: Constipation. None.

DIATRIZOATE (*Cystografin, Gastrografin, Hypaque, MD-Gastroview, RenoCal, Reno-DIP, Reno-60, Renografin*) ▶K ♀C ▶? $
WARNING — Not for intrathecal or epidural use.
ADULT — Iodinated, ionic, high osmolality IV, or GI contrast.
PEDS — Iodinated, ionic, high osmolality IV, or GI contrast.
NOTES — High osmolality contrast may cause tissue damage if infiltrated/extravasated. IV: Hypaque, Renografin, Reno-DIP, RenoCal. GI: Gastrografin, MD-Gastroview.
MOA — Iodinated, ionic, high-osmolality IV or GI contrast.
ADVERSE EFFECTS — Serious: Hypersensitivity. Frequent: None.

IODIXANOL (*Visipaque*) ▶K ♀B ▶? $$$
ADULT — Iodinated, nonionic, iso-osmolar IV contrast.
PEDS — Iodinated, nonionic, iso-osmolar IV contrast.
NOTES — Not for intrathecal use.
MOA — Iodinated, nonionic, low osmolality IV contrast.
ADVERSE EFFECTS — Serious: Hypersensitivity. Frequent: None.

IOHEXOL (*Omnipaque*) ▶K ♀B ▶? $$$
ADULT — Iodinated, nonionic, low osmolality IV, and oral/body cavity contrast.
PEDS — Iodinated, nonionic, low osmolality IV, and oral/body cavity contrast.
MOA — Iodinated, nonionic, low osmolality IV and oral/body cavity contrast.
ADVERSE EFFECTS — Serious: Hypersensitivity. Frequent: None.

IOPAMIDOL (*Isovue*) ▶K ♀? ▶? $$
ADULT — Iodinated, nonionic, low-osmolality IV contrast.

PEDS — Iodinated, nonionic, low-osmolality IV contrast.
MOA — Iodinated, nonionic, low osmolality IV contrast.
ADVERSE EFFECTS — Serious: Hypersensitivity. Frequent: None.

IOPROMIDE (*Ultravist*) ▶K ♀B ▶? $$$
ADULT — Iodinated, nonionic, low osmolality IV contrast.
PEDS — Iodinated, nonionic, low osmolality IV contrast.
MOA — Iodinated, nonionic, low osmolality IV contrast.
ADVERSE EFFECTS — Serious: Hypersensitivity. Frequent: None.

IOTHALAMATE (*Conray, ✶Vascoray*) ▶K ♀B ▶− $
ADULT — Iodinated, ionic, high osmolality IV contrast.
PEDS — Iodinated, ionic, high osmolality IV contrast.
NOTES — High osmolality contrast may cause tissue damage if infiltrated/extravasated.
MOA — Iodinated, ionic, high osmolality IV contrast.
ADVERSE EFFECTS — Serious: Hypersensitivity. Frequent: None.

IOVERSOL (*Optiray*) ▶K ♀B ▶? $$
ADULT — Iodinated, nonionic, low osmolality IV contrast.
PEDS — Iodinated, nonionic, low osmolality IV contrast.
MOA — Iodinated, nonionic, low osmolality IV contrast.
ADVERSE EFFECTS — Serious: Hypersensitivity. Frequent: None.

IOXAGLATE (*Hexabrix*) ▶K ♀B ▶− $$$
ADULT — Iodinated, ionic, low osmolality IV contrast.
PEDS — Iodinated, ionic, low osmolality IV contrast.
MOA — Iodinated, ionic, low osmolality IV contrast.
ADVERSE EFFECTS — Serious: Hypersensitivity. Frequent: None.

IOXILAN (*Oxilan*) ▶K ♀B ▶− $$$
ADULT — Iodinated, nonionic, low osmolality IV contrast.
PEDS — Iodinated, nonionic, low osmolality IV contrast.
MOA — Iodinated, nonionic, low osmolality IV contrast.
ADVERSE EFFECTS — Serious: Hypersensitivity. Frequent: None.

CONTRAST MEDIA: Other

INDIGOTINDISULFONATE (*Indigo Carmine*) ▶K ♀C ▶? $
ADULT — Identification of ureteral tears during surgery: 5 mL IV.
PEDS — Identification of ureteral tears during surgery: Use less than the adult dose.
FORMS — Trade only: 40 mg/5 mL vial.

MOA — Blue dye excreted in urine.
ADVERSE EFFECTS — Serious: Hypersensitivity. Frequent: None.
ISOSULFAN BLUE (*Lymphazurin*) ▶LK ♀? ▶? $$$$$
ADULT — Lymphography, identification of lymphatics during cancer surgery: 0.5 to 3 mL SC.

ISOSULFAN BLUE (*cont.*)

PEDS — Optimal dosing not defined.

FORMS — Trade only: 1% (10 mg/ mL) 5 mL vial.

MOA — Blue dye for delineation of lymphatic vessels.

ADVERSE EFFECTS — Serious: Hypersensitivity including anaphylaxis. Frequent: Swelling at injection site.

PENTETATE INDIUM (*Indium DTPA*) ▶K ♀C ▮? $$$$$

ADULT — Radionuclide cisternography.

PEDS — Not approved in children.

FORMS — 1 mci/mL, 1.5 mL vial.

MOA — Radiopharmaceutical

ADVERSE EFFECTS — Serious: Aseptic meningitis, pyogenic reactions. Frequent: skin reactions, vomiting.

DERMATOLOGY

CORTICOSTEROIDS: TOPICAL

Potency*	Generic	Trade Name	Forms	Frequency
Low	alclometasone dipropionate	Aclovate	0.05% C/O	bid-tid
Low	clocortolone pivalate	Cloderm	0.1% C	tid
Low	desonide	DesOwen, Tridesilon	0.05% C/L/O	bid-tid
Low	hydrocortisone	Hytone, others	0.5% C/L/O; 1% C/L/O; 2.5% C/L/O	bid-qid
Low	hydrocortisone acetate	Cortaid, Corticaine	0.5% C/O; 1% C/O/Sp	bid-qid
Medium	betamethasone valerate	Luxiq	0.1% C/L/O; 0.12% F (Luxiq)	qd-bid
Medium	desoximetasone‡	Topicort	0.05% C	bid
Medium	fluocinolone	Synalar	0.01% C/S; 0.025% C/O	bid-qid
Medium	flurandrenolide	Cordran	0.025% C/O; 0.05% C/L/O/T	bid-qid
Medium	fluticasone propionate	Cutivate	0.005% O; 0.05% C/L	daily-bid
Medium	hydrocortisone butyrate	Locoid	0.1% C/O/S	bid-tid
Medium	hydrocortisone valerate	Westcort	0.2% C/O	bid-tid
Medium	mometasone furoate	Elocon	0.1% C/L/O	qd
Medium	triamcinolone‡	Aristocort, Kenalog	0.025% C/L/O; 0.1% C/L/O/S	bid-tid
High	amcinonide	Cyclocort	0.1% C/L/O	bid-tid
High	betamethasone dipropionate‡	Maxivate, others	0.05% C/L/O (non-Diprolene)	qd-bid
High	desoximetasone‡	Topicort	0.05% G; 0.25% C/O	bid
High	diflorasone diacetate‡	Maxiflor	0.05% C/O	bid
High	fluocinonide	Lidex	0.05% C/G/O/S	bid-qid
High	halcinonide	Halog	0.1% C/O/S	bid-tid
High	triamcinolone‡	Aristocort, Kenalog	0.5% C/O	bid-tid
Very high	betamethasone dipropionate‡	Diprolene, Diprolene AF	0.05% C/G/L/O	qd-bid
Very high	clobetasol	Temovate, Cormax, Olux	0.05% C/G/O/L/S/Sp/F (Olux)	bid
Very high	diflorasone diacetate‡	Psorcon	0.05% C/O	qd-tid
Very high	halobetasol propionate	Ultravate	0.05% C/O	qd-bid

bid=two times per day; tid=three times per day; qid=four times per day.
*Potency based on vasoconstrictive assays, which may not correlate with efficacy. Not all available products are listed, including those lacking potency ratings.
‡These drugs have formulations in more than once potency category.
C, cream; O, ointment; L, lotion; T, tape; F, foam; S, solution; G, gel; Sp, spray

DERMATOLOGY: Acne Preparations

NOTE: For topical agents, wash area prior to application. Wash hands before and after application; avoid eye area.

ACANYA (clindamycin—topical + benzoyl peroxide) ▶K ♀C ▶+ $$$$
ADULT — Acne: Apply once daily.
PEDS — Not approved in children 12 yo or younger.
FORMS — Trade only: Gel (clindamycin 1.2% + benzoyl peroxide 2.5%) 50 g.
NOTES — Expires 2 months after mixing.
MOA — Antibacterial + drying and sebostatic effects.
ADVERSE EFFECTS — Frequent: Dryness, scaling, erythema, burning, pruritus. Severe: C. difficile-associated diarrhea, anaphylaxis.

ADAPALENE (*Differin*) ▶bile ♀C ▶? $$$$
ADULT — Acne: Apply at bedtime.
PEDS — Not approved in children.
UNAPPROVED PEDS — Acne: Apply at bedtime.
FORMS — Generic/Trade: Gel 0.1%. Cream 0.1% (45 g). Trade only: Gel 0.3% (45 g). Soln 0.1% (59 mL).
NOTES — During early weeks of therapy, acne exacerbation may occur. May cause erythema, scaling, dryness, pruritus, and burning in up to 40% of patients. Therapeutic results take 8 to 12 weeks.
MOA — Modulates cellular differentiation, inflammation, keratinization.
ADVERSE EFFECTS — Frequent: Dryness, scaling, erythema, burning, pruritus.

AZELAIC ACID (*Azelex, Finacea, Finevin*) ▶K ♀B ▶? $$$$
ADULT — Acne (Azelex, Finevin): Apply two times per day. Rosacea (Finacea): Apply two times per day.
PEDS — Not approved in children.
UNAPPROVED ADULT — Melasma: Apply two times per day.
UNAPPROVED PEDS — Acne: Apply at bedtime.
FORMS — Trade only: Cream 20%, 30, 50 g (Azelex). Gel 15% 50 g (Finacea).
NOTES — Improvement of acne occurs within 4 weeks. Monitor for hypopigmentation especially in patients with dark complexions. Avoid use of occlusive dressings.
MOA — May possess antibacterial activity.
ADVERSE EFFECTS — Frequent: Dryness, scaling, erythema, burning, stinging, tingling, pruritus.

BENZACLIN (clindamycin—topical + benzoyl peroxide) ▶K ♀C ▶+ $$$$
ADULT — Acne: Apply two times per day.
PEDS — Not approved in children.
UNAPPROVED PEDS — Acne: Apply at bedtime.
FORMS — Generic/Trade: Gel (clindamycin 1% + benzoyl peroxide 5%) 50 g (jar). Trade only: 25, 35 g (jar) and 50 g (pump).
NOTES — Expires 10 weeks after mixing.
MOA — Antibacterial + drying and sebostatic effects.
ADVERSE EFFECTS — Frequent: Dryness, scaling, erythema, burning, pruritus. Severe: C. difficile-associated diarrhea, allergic reactions/hypersensitivity.

BENZAMYCIN (erythromycin base—topical + benzoyl peroxide) ▶LK ♀C ▶? $$$
ADULT — Acne: Apply two times per day.
PEDS — Not approved in children.
UNAPPROVED PEDS — Acne: Apply at bedtime.
FORMS — Generic/Trade: Gel (erythromycin 3% + benzoyl peroxide 5%) 23.3, 46.6 g. Trade only: Benzamycin Pak, #60 gel pouches.
NOTES — Must be refrigerated, expires 3 months after pharmacy dispensing.
MOA — Antibacterial + drying and sebostatic effects.
ADVERSE EFFECTS — Frequent: Dryness, scaling, erythema, burning, pruritus.

BENZOYL PEROXIDE (*Benzac, Benzagel 10%, Desquam, Clearasil, ✱Solugel*) ▶LK ♀C ▶? $
ADULT — Acne: Cleansers: Wash one to two times per day. Creams/gels/lotion: Apply daily initially, gradually increase to two to three times per day if needed.
PEDS — Not approved in children.
UNAPPROVED PEDS — Acne: Cleansers: Wash one to two times per day. Creams/gels/lotion: Apply daily initially, gradually increase to two to three times per day if needed.
FORMS — OTC and Rx generic: Liquid 2.5, 5, 10%. Bar 5, 10%. Mask 5%. Lotion 4, 5, 8, 10%. Cream 5, 10%. Gel 2.5, 4, 5, 6, 10, 20%. Pad 3, 4, 6, 8, 9%. Other strengths available.
NOTES — If excessive drying or peeling occurs, reduce frequency of application. Use with PABA-containing sunscreens may cause transient skin discoloration. May bleach fabric.
MOA — Antibacterial + drying and sebostatic effects.
ADVERSE EFFECTS — Frequent: Dryness, scaling, erythema, burning, pruritus.

CLENIA (sulfacetamide—topical + sulfur) ▶K ♀C ▶? $$$
ADULT — Acne, rosacea, seborrheic dermatitis: Apply cream/lotion daily to three times per day, foaming wash daily to two times per day.
PEDS — Not approved in children.
FORMS — Generic only: Lotion (sodium sulfacetamide 10%/sulfur 5%) 25, 30, 45, 60 g. Trade only: Cream (sodium sulfacetamide 10%/sulfur 5%) 28 g. Generic/Trade: Foaming Wash 170, 340 g.
NOTES — Avoid with sulfa allergy, renal failure.
MOA — Antibacterial.
ADVERSE EFFECTS — Frequent: Local irritation, stinging, burning.

CLINDAMYCIN—TOPICAL (*Cleocin T, Clindagel, ClindaMax, Evoclin, ✱Dalacin T*) ▶L ♀B ▶– $
ADULT — Acne: Apply daily (Evoclin, Clindagel) or two times per day (Cleocin T).
PEDS — Not approved in children.
UNAPPROVED ADULT — Rosacea: Apply lotion two times per day.
UNAPPROVED PEDS — Acne: Apply two times per day.

(cont.)

CLINDAMYCIN—TOPICAL (*cont.*)

FORMS — Generic/Trade: Gel 1% 30, 60 g. Lotion 1% 60 mL. Soln 1% 30, 60 mL. Trade only: Foam 1% 50, 100 g (Evoclin). Gel 1% 40, 75 mL (Clindagel).

NOTES — Concomitant use with erythromycin may decrease effectiveness. Most common adverse effects dryness, erythema, burning, peeling, oiliness, and itching. C. difficile–associated diarrhea has been reported with topical use.

MOA — Antibacterial.

ADVERSE EFFECTS — Frequent: Dryness, burning, pruritus. Severe: C. difficile-associated diarrhea.

***DIANE-35* (cyproterone + ethinyl estradiol)** ▶L ♀X ▶– $$

WARNING — Not recommended in women who smoke. Increased risk of thromboembolism, CVA, MI, hepatic neoplasia, and gallbladder disease. Nausea, breast tenderness, and breakthrough bleeding are common, transient side effects. Nighttime dosing may minimize nausea. Effectiveness is reduced by hepatic enzyme-inducing drugs such as certain anticonvulsants and barbiturates, rifampin, rifabutin, griseofulvin, and protease inhibitors. Antibiotics or products that contain St. John's wort may reduce efficacy.

ADULT — Canada only. In women, severe acne unresponsive to oral antibiotics and other treatments, with associated symptoms of androgenization, including seborrhea and mild hirsutism: 1 tab PO daily for 21 consecutive days, stop for 7 days, repeat cycle.

PEDS — Not approved in children.

FORMS — Canada Generic/Trade: Blister pack of 21 tabs 2 mg cyproterone acetate/0.035 mg ethinyl estradiol.

NOTES — Higher thromboembolic risk than other oral contraceptives, therefore only indicated for acne, and not solely for contraception (although effective for the latter). Same warnings, precautions, and contraindications as other oral contraceptives.

MOA — Cyproterone: Potent antiandrogenic, progestogenic and antigonadotrophic activity; blocks androgen receptors and reduces androgen synthesis. Ethinyl estradiol increases levels of sex hormone binding globulin, and decreases circulating plasma levels of androgens. The combination also prevents ovulation and possible conception.

ADVERSE EFFECTS—Serious: DVT/PE, stroke, MI, hepatic neoplasia, gallbladder disease. Frequent: Nausea, breast tenderness, and breakthrough bleeding.

***DUAC* (clindamycin—topical + benzoyl peroxide,** ✱*Clindoxyl*) ▶K ♀C ▶+ $$$$

ADULT — Acne: Apply at bedtime.

PEDS — Not approved in children.

UNAPPROVED PEDS — Acne: Apply at bedtime.

FORMS — Trade only: Gel (clindamycin 1% + benzoyl peroxide 5%) 45 g.

NOTES — Expires 2 months after pharmacy dispensing.

MOA — Antibacterial + drying and sebostatic effects.

ADVERSE EFFECTS — Frequent: Dryness, scaling, erythema, burning, pruritus. Severe: C. difficile-associated diarrhea, anaphylaxis.

***EPIDUO* (adapalene + benzoyl peroxide,** ✱*Tactuo*) ▶Bile, K ♀C ▶? $$$$$

ADULT — Acne: Apply daily.

PEDS — Not approved in children younger than 9 years. Acne: Children 9 years and older: apply daily.

FORMS — Trade only: Gel (0.1% adapalene + benzoyl peroxide 2.5%) 45 g.

NOTES — During early weeks of therapy, acne exacerbation may occur. May cause erythema, scaling, dryness, pruritus, and burning.

MOA — Modulates cellular differentiation, inflammation, keratinization + drying and sebostatic effects.

ADVERSE EFFECTS — Frequent: Erythema, scaling, dryness, stinging, burning.

ERYTHROMYCIN—TOPICAL (*Eryderm, Erycette, Erygel, A/T/S,* ✱*Sans-Acne, Erysol*) ▶L ♀B ▶? $

ADULT — Acne: Apply two times per day.

PEDS — Not approved in children.

UNAPPROVED PEDS — Acne: Apply two times per day.

FORMS — Generic/Trade: Soln 2% 60 mL. Pads 2%. Gel 2% 30, 60 g. Ointment 2% 25 g. Generic only: Soln 1.5% 60 mL.

NOTES — May be more irritating when used with other acne products. Concomitant use with clindamycin may decrease effectiveness.

MOA — Antibacterial.

ADVERSE EFFECTS — Frequent: Dryness, pruritus, erythema, scaling.

ISOTRETINOIN (*Amnesteem, Claravis, Sotret, Absorica, Myorisan, Zenatane,* ✱*Accutane Roche, Clarus*) ▶LK ♀X ▶– $$$$$

WARNING — Contraindicated in pregnant women or in women who may become pregnant. If used in a woman of childbearing age, patient must have severe, disfiguring acne, be reliable, comply with mandatory contraceptive measures, receive written and oral instructions about hazards of taking during pregnancy, have 2 negative pregnancy tests prior to beginning therapy. Must use 2 forms of effective contraception from 1 month prior until 1 month after discontinuation of therapy, unless absolute abstinence is chosen or patient has undergone a hysterectomy. Men should not father children. May cause depression, suicidal thought, and aggressive or violent behavior; monitor for symptoms. Obtain written informed consent. Write prescription for no more than a 1-month supply. Informed consent documents available from the manufacturer.

ADULT — Severe, recalcitrant cystic acne: 0.5 to 2 mg/kg/day PO divided two times per day for 15 to 20 weeks. Typical target dose is 1 mg/kg/day. May repeat 2nd course of therapy after at least 2 months off therapy.

PEDS — Not approved in children.

UNAPPROVED ADULT — Prevention of 2nd primary tumors in patients treated for squamous cell carcinoma of the head and neck: 50 to 100 mg/m^2/day PO. Also been used in keratinization disorders.

ISOTRETINOIN (cont.)

UNAPPROVED PEDS — Severe, recalcitrant cystic acne: 0.5 to 2 mg/kg/day PO divided two times per day for 15 to 20 weeks. Typical target dose is 1 mg/kg/day. Maintenance therapy for neuroblastoma: 100 to 250 mg/m²/day PO in 2 divided doses.

FORMS — Generic: Caps 10, 20, 40 mg. Generic only (Sotret, Absorica, and Claravis): Caps 30 mg.

NOTES — Prescription can be for a maximum of a 1-month supply. May cause headache, cheilitis, drying of mucous membranes including eyes, nose, mouth, hair loss, abdominal pain, pyuria, joint and muscle pain/stiffness, conjunctivitis, elevated ESR, and changes in serum lipids and LFTs. Effect on bone loss unknown; use caution in patients predisposed to osteoporosis. In children in whom skeletal growth is not complete, do not exceed the recommended dose for the recommended duration of treatment. Pseudotumor cerebri has occurred during therapy often when used with a tetracycline; avoid concomitant vitamin A, tetracycline, minocycline. May cause corneal opacities, decreased night vision, and inflammatory bowel disease. May decrease carbamazepine concentrations. Avoid excessive exposure to sunlight.

MOA — Decreases sebaceous gland size and sebum production.

ADVERSE EFFECTS — Frequent: Dryness, burning, pruritus, inflammation, photosensitivity, xerostomia, increased triglycerides, bone pain, arthralgias, myalgias, epistaxis. Severe: Teratogenic, possible depression, aggressive or violent behavior, premature epiphyseal closure, osteoporosis, osteopenia, delayed bone healing, pseudotumor cerebri, corneal opacities, hepatitis, back pain, severe skin reactions including Stevens-Johnson syndrome.

ROSULA (sulfacetamide—topical + sulfur) ▶K ♀C ▶? $$$$

ADULT — Acne, rosacea, seborrheic dermatitis: Apply cream/gel/aqueous cleanser one to three times per day, foaming wash one to two times per day.

PEDS — Not approved in children.

FORMS — Trade only: Gel (sodium sulfacetamide 10%/sulfur 5%) 45 g. Aqueous cleanser (sodium sulfacetamide 10%/sulfur 5%) 355 mL. Soap (sodium sulfacetamide 10%/sulfur 4%) 473 mL.

NOTES — Avoid with sulfa allergy or renal failure.

MOA — Antibacterial.

ADVERSE EFFECTS — Frequent: Local irritation, stinging, burning.

SALICYLIC ACID (Akurza, Clearasil Cleanser, Stridex Pads) ▶not absorbed ♀? ▶? $

ADULT — Acne (OTC): Apply/wash area up to 3 times a day. Removal of excessive keratin in hyperkeratotic disorders (Rx): Apply to affected area at bedtime and cover. Hydrate skin before application.

PEDS — Acne: Apply/wash area up to 3 times a day.

FORMS — OTC Generic/Trade: Pads, Gel, Lotion, Liquid, Mask scrub, 0.5%, 1%, 2%. Rx Trade only (Akurza): Cream 6% 340 g. Lotion 6%, 355 mL.

MOA — Keratolytic.

ADVERSE EFFECTS — Frequent: Irritation, stinging, burning.

SULFACET-R (sulfacetamide—topical + sulfur) ▶K ♀C ▶? $$$

ADULT — Acne, rosacea, seborrheic dermatitis: Apply one to three times per day.

PEDS — Not approved in children.

FORMS — Generic/Trade: Lotion (sodium sulfacetamide 10%/sulfur 5%) 25 g.

NOTES — Avoid with sulfa allergy or renal failure.

MOA — Antibacterial.

ADVERSE EFFECTS — Frequent: Local irritation, stinging, burning.

SULFACETAMIDE—TOPICAL (Klaron) ▶K ♀C ▶? $$$$

ADULT — Acne: Apply two times per day.

PEDS — Not approved in children.

FORMS — Generic/Trade: Lotion 10% 118 mL.

NOTES — Cross-sensitivity with sulfa or sulfite allergy.

MOA — Antibacterial.

ADVERSE EFFECTS — Frequent: Irritation, stinging, burning. Severe: Stevens-Johnson syndrome, systemic lupus erythematosus.

TAZAROTENE (Tazorac, Avage) ▶L ♀X ▶? $$$$

ADULT — Acne (Tazorac): Apply 0.1% cream at bedtime. Palliation of fine facial wrinkles, mottled hyper- and hypopigmentation, benign facial lentigines (Avage): Apply at bedtime. Psoriasis: Apply 0.05% cream at bedtime, increase to 0.1% prn.

PEDS — Not approved in children.

UNAPPROVED PEDS — Acne: Apply 0.1% cream at bedtime. Psoriasis: Apply 0.05% cream at bedtime.

FORMS — Trade only (Tazorac): Cream 0.05% and 0.1% 30, 60 g. Gel 0.05% and 0.1% 30, 100 g. Trade only (Avage): Cream 0.1% 15, 30 g.

NOTES — Avoid using gel formulation with other medications or cosmetics that are considered drying. In psoriasis, may reduce irritation and improve efficacy by using topical corticosteroid in morning and tazarotene at bedtime. Desquamation, burning, dry skin, erythema, pruritus may occur in up to 30% of patients. May cause photosensitivity.

MOA — Modulates cellular differentiation, keratinization; anti-inflammatory, immunologic activity.

ADVERSE EFFECTS — Frequent: Pruritus, burning, erythema, rash changes in pigmentation. Severe: blister.

TRETINOIN—TOPICAL (Retin-A, Retin-A Micro, Renova, Retisol-A, ✱Stieva-A, Rejuva-A, Vitamin A Acid Cream) ▶LK ♀C ▶? $$$

ADULT — Acne (Retin A, Retin-A Micro): Apply at bedtime. Wrinkles, hyperpigmentation, tactile roughness (Renova): Apply at bedtime.

PEDS — Not approved in children.

UNAPPROVED ADULT — Used in skin cancer and lamellar ichthyosis, mollusca contagiosa, verrucae plantaris, verrucae planae juvenilis, hyperpigmented lesions in black individuals, ichthyosis vulgaris, and pityriasis rubra pilaris.

FORMS — Generic/Trade: Cream 0.025% 20, 45 g; 0.05% 20, 45 g; 0.1% 20, 45 g. Gel 0.025% 15, 45 g;

(cont.)

TRETINOIN—TOPICAL (cont.)

0.01% 15, 45 g. Micro gel 0.04%, 0.1% 20, 45g, and 50 g pump. Trade only: Renova cream 0.02% 40, 60 g.

NOTES — May induce erythema, peeling. Minimize sun exposure. Concomitant use with sulfur, resorcinol, benzoyl peroxide, or salicylic acid may result in skin irritation. Gel preps are flammable.

MOA — Induces loosening of keratinocytes, inhibits microcomedone formation.

ADVERSE EFFECTS — Frequent: Dryness, erythema, scaling. Severe: Contraindicated in pregnancy.

VELTIN (clindamycin⊠topical + tretinoin) ▶LK ♀C ▶? $$$$

WARNING — Clindamycin has been reproted to cause severe colitis.

ADULT — Acne: Apply at bedtime.

PEDS — Has not been studied in children younger than 12 yo.

FORMS — Trade: Gel clindamycin 1.2% + tretinoin 0.025%, 30 g.

MOA — antibiotic + retinoid

ADVERSE EFFECTS — Frequent: dryness, irritation, exfoliation, erythema, pruritis.

ZIANA (clindamycin—topical + tretinoin) ▶LK ♀C ▶? $$$$

ADULT — Acne: Apply at bedtime.

PEDS — Use adult dose for age 12 yo or older.

FORMS — Trade only: Gel clindamycin 1.2% + tretinoin 0.025% 30, 60 g.

NOTES — May induce erythema, peeling. Minimize sun exposure.

MOA — Induces loosening of keratinocytes, inhibits microcomedone formation, antibacterial.

ADVERSE EFFECTS — Frequent: Dryness, erythema, scaling.

DERMATOLOGY: Actinic Keratosis Preparations

AMINOLEVULINIC ACID (Levulan Kerastick) ▶Not absorbed ♀C ▶? $$$$

ADULT — Non-hyperkeratotic actinic keratoses: Apply soln to lesions on scalp or face; expose to special light source 14 to 18 h later.

PEDS — Not approved in children.

FORMS — Trade only: 20% soln, single-use applicator stick.

NOTES — Soln should be applied by healthcare personnel. Advise patients to avoid sunlight during 14 to 18 h period before blue light illumination.

MOA—Photosensitizer as precursor to protoporphyrin.

ADVERSE EFFECTS — Frequent: Scaling, pruritus, hypo- or hyperpigmentation, erosions, stinging, burning.

DICLOFENAC—TOPICAL (Solaraze, Voltaren, Pennsaid) ▶L ♀B ▶? $$$

ADULT — Actinic/solar keratoses: Apply two times per day to lesions for 60 to 90 days (Solaraze). Osteoarthritis of areas amenable to topical therapy: 2 g (upper extremities) to 4 g (lower extremities) four times per day (Voltaren). 40 gtts to knee(s) four times daily (Pennsaid).

PEDS — Not approved in children.

FORMS — Generic/Trade: Gel 3% (Solaraze) 100 g. Soln 1.5% (Pennsaid) 150 mL. Trade only: Gel 1% (Voltaren) 100 g. Soln 2.0% Pump (Pennsaid) 112 gm.

NOTES — Avoid exposure to sun and sunlamps. Use caution in aspirin-sensitive patients. When using for OA (Voltaren), maximum daily dose 16 g to any single lower extremity joint, 8 g to any single upper extremity joint.

MOA — Inhibits prostaglandins at level of cyclooxygenase.

ADVERSE EFFECTS — Frequent: Rash, abdominal cramps, nausea, indigestion.

FLUOROURACIL—TOPICAL (5-FU, Carac, Efudex, Fluoroplex) ▶L ♀X ▶– $$$

WARNING — Contraindicated in pregnant women or women who plan to get pregnant during therapy. Avoid application to mucous membranes.

ADULT — Actinic or solar keratoses: Apply two times per day to lesions for 2 to 6 weeks. Superficial basal cell carcinomas: Apply 5% cream/soln two times per day.

PEDS — Not approved in children.

UNAPPROVED ADULT — Condylomata acuminata: 1% soln in 70% ethanol and the 5% cream has been used.

FORMS — Trade only: Cream 0.5% 30 g (Carac), 5% 25 g (Efudex), 1% 30 g (Fluoroplex). Generic/Trade: Soln 2%, 5% 10 mL (Efudex). Cream 5% 40 g.

NOTES — May cause severe irritation and photosensitivity. Contraindicated in women who are or who may become pregnant during therapy. Avoid application to mucous membranes.

MOA — Pyrimidine anti-metabolite that interferes with DNA synthesis.

ADVERSE EFFECTS — Frequent: Dermatitis, pruritic maculopapular rash, alopecia, heartburn, nausea, inflammation along segments of the GI tract, diarrhea. Severe: Myelosuppression, mucositis.

INGENOL (Picato) ▶not absorbed ♀C ▶? $$$

ADULT — Actinic keratosis on face and scalp: Apply 0.015% gel to affected areas once daily for 3 days. Actinic keratosis on trunk and extremities: Apply 0.05% gel to affected areas once daily for 2 days.

PEDS — Not approved in children.

FORMS — Trade: Gel 0.015% 0.25 g, 0.05% 0.25 g.

NOTES — Avoid contact with the periocular area.

MOA — Induces cell death by unknown mechanism.

ADVERSE EFFECTS — Frequent: local skin reactions, application site pain, application site pruritus, application site irritation, application site infection, periorbital edema.

METHYLAMINOLEVULINATE (Metvix, Metvixia) ▶not absorbed ♀C ▶?

ADULT — Non-hyperkeratotic actinic keratoses of face/scalp: Apply cream 1 mm thick (max 1 gram) to lesion and 5 mm surrounding area; cover with dressing for 3 h; remove dressing and

METHYLAMINOLEVULINATE (cont.)

cream and perform illumination therapy. Repeat in 7 days.

PEDS — Not approved in children.

FORMS — Trade only: Cream 16.8%, 2 g tube.

NOTES — Use in immunocompetent individuals. Lesion debridement should be performed prior to application of cream. Formulated in peanut and almond oil; has not been tested in patients allergic to peanuts.

MOA — Photosensitizer as precursor to photoactive porphyrin.

ADVERSE EFFECTS — Frequent: Peeling, pruritus, edema, ulceration, bleeding, blisters, stinging, burning, pain, crusting, contact sensitization. Severe: angioedema.

DERMATOLOGY: Antibacterials (Topical)

BACITRACIN—TOPICAL ▶not absorbed ♀C ▶? $

ADULT — Minor cuts, wounds, burns, or skin abrasions: Apply one to three times per day.

PEDS — Not approved in children.

UNAPPROVED PEDS — Minor cuts, wounds, burns, or skin abrasions: Apply one to three times per day.

FORMS — OTC Generic/Trade: Ointment 500 units/g 1, 15, 30 g.

NOTES — May cause contact dermatitis or anaphylaxis.

MOA — Antibacterial, inhibit bacterial wall synthesis.

ADVERSE EFFECTS — Frequent: None.

FUSIDIC ACID—TOPICAL (Fucidin) ▶L ♀? ▶? $

ADULT — Canada only. Skin infections: Apply three to four times per day.

PEDS — Canada only. Skin infections: Apply three to four times per day.

FORMS — Canada trade only: Cream 2% fusidic acid 5, 15, 30 g. Ointment 2% sodium fusidate 5, 15, 30 g.

NOTES — Contains lanolin; possible hypersensitivity.

MOA — Antibacterial, interferes with bacterial protein synthesis.

ADVERSE EFFECTS — Serious: Hypersensitivity. Frequent: Mild irritation, pain.

GENTAMICIN—TOPICAL ▶K ♀D ▶? $

ADULT — Skin infections: Apply three to four times per day.

PEDS — Skin infections in children older than 1 yo: Apply three to four times per day.

FORMS — Generic only: Ointment 0.1% 15, 30 g. Cream 0.1% 15, 30 g.

MOA — Antibacterial, interferes with bacterial protein synthesis.

ADVERSE EFFECTS — Frequent: Neurotoxicity (when applied to large areas), gait instability, ototoxicity, nephrotoxicity.

MAFENIDE (Sulfamylon) ▶LK ♀C ▶? $$$

ADULT — Adjunctive treatment of burns: Apply one to two times per day.

PEDS — Adjunctive treatment of burns: Apply one to two times per day.

FORMS — Generic/Trade: Topical Soln 50 g packets. Trade only: Cream 5% 57, 114, 454 g.

NOTES — Can cause metabolic acidosis. Contains sulfonamides.

MOA — Antibacterial, interferes with bacterial folic acid synthesis.

ADVERSE EFFECTS — Frequent: Burning, pain, excoriation.

METRONIDAZOLE—TOPICAL (Noritate, MetroCream, MetroGel, MetroLotion, ✱Rosasol) ▶KL ♀B(- in 1st trimester) ▶- $$$

ADULT — Rosacea: Apply daily (1%) or two times per day (0.75%).

PEDS — Not approved in children.

UNAPPROVED ADULT — A 1% soln prepared from the oral tabs has been used in the treatment of infected decubitus ulcers.

FORMS — Trade only: Gel (MetroGel) 1% 45, 60 g. Cream (Noritate) 1% 60 g. Generic/Trade: Gel 0.75% 45 g. Cream 0.75% 45 g. Lotion (MetroLotion) 0.75% 59 mL.

NOTES — Results usually noted within 3 weeks, with continuing improvement through 9 weeks. Avoid using vaginal prep on face due to irritation because of formulation differences.

MOA — Antibacterial, breakage of bacterial DNA, antiinflammatory.

ADVERSE EFFECTS — Frequent: Dizziness, headache, nausea, diarrhea, anorexia, vomiting.

MUPIROCIN (Bactroban, Centany) ▶not absorbed ♀B ▶? $$

ADULT — Impetigo: Apply three times per day for 3 to 5 days. Infected wounds: Apply three times per day for 10 days. Nasal MRSA eradication: 0.5 g in each nostril two times per day for 5 days.

PEDS — Impetigo (mupirocin cream/ointment): Apply three times per day. Infected wounds: Apply three times per day for 10 days. Nasal form not approved in children younger than 12 yo.

FORMS — Generic/Trade: Ointment 2% 22 g. Nasal ointment 2% 1 g single-use tubes (for MRSA eradication). Trade only: Cream 2% 15, 30 g.

MOA — Antibacterial; inhibits bacterial protein and RNA synthesis.

ADVERSE EFFECTS — Frequent: Dryness, burning, erythema, stinging, tenderness.

NEOSPORIN CREAM (neomycin—topical + polymyxin—topical + bacitracin—topical) ▶K ♀C ▶? $

ADULT — Minor cuts, wounds, burns, or skin abrasions: Apply one to three times per day.

PEDS — Not approved in children.

UNAPPROVED PEDS — Minor cuts, wounds, burns, or skin abrasions: Apply one to three times per day.

FORMS — OTC Trade only: neomycin 3.5 mg/g + polymyxin 10,000 units/g; 15 g and unit dose 0.94 g.

NOTES — Neomycin component can cause contact dermatitis.

MOA — Antibacterial.

ADVERSE EFFECTS — Frequent: None.

NEOSPORIN OINTMENT (bacitracin—topical + neo-mycin—topical + polymyxin—topical) ▶K ♀C ▶? $
ADULT — Minor cuts, wounds, burns, or skin abrasions: Apply one to three times per day.
PEDS — Not approved in children.
UNAPPROVED PEDS — Minor cuts, wounds, burns, or skin abrasions: Apply one to three times per day.
FORMS — OTC Generic/Trade: bacitracin 400 units/g + neomycin 3.5 mg/g + polymyxin 5000 units/g 15, 30 g and "to go" 0.9 g packets.
NOTES — Also known as triple antibiotic ointment. Neomycin component can cause contact dermatitis.
MOA — Antibacterial.
ADVERSE EFFECTS — Frequent: None.
POLYSPORIN (bacitracin—topical + polymyxin—topical, *Polytopic*) ▶K ♀C ▶? $
ADULT — Minor cuts, wounds, burns, or skin abrasions: Apply one to three times per day.
PEDS — Not approved in children.
UNAPPROVED PEDS — Minor cuts, wounds, burns, or skin abrasions: Apply one to three times per day.
FORMS — OTC Trade only: Ointment 15, 30 g and unit dose 0.9 g. Powder 10 g.
NOTES — May cause allergic contact dermatitis and rarely contact anaphylaxis.
MOA — Antibacterial.
ADVERSE EFFECTS — May cause allergic contact dermatitis and rarely contact anaphylaxis.
RETAPAMULIN (*Altabax*) ▶not absorbed ♀B ▶? $$$
ADULT — Impetigo: Apply thin layer (up to 100 cm2 in total area) two times per day for 5 days.
PEDS — Impetigo (9 mo or older): Apply thin layer (up to 2% total body surface area in pediatric patients) two times per day for 5 days.
FORMS — Trade only: Ointment 1% 5, 10, 15 g.

NOTES — Do not apply to nasal mucosa.
MOA — Antibacterial; inhibits bacterial protein and RNA synthesis.
ADVERSE EFFECTS — Frequent: Skin irritation.
SILVER SULFADIAZINE (*Silvadene, *Flamazine*) ▶LK ♀B ▶– $$
ADULT — Burns: Apply one to two times per day.
PEDS — Not approved in children.
UNAPPROVED ADULT — Has been used for pressure ulcers.
UNAPPROVED PEDS — Burns: Apply one to two times per day.
FORMS — Generic/Trade: Cream 1% 20, 50, 85, 400, 1000 g.
NOTES — Avoid in sulfa allergy. Leukopenia, primarily decreased neutrophil count in up to 20% of patients. Significant absorption may occur and serum sulfa concentrations approach therapeutic levels. Avoid in G6PD deficiency. Has been associated with blood dyscrasias including agranulocytosis, aplastic anemia, thrombocytopenia, and hemolytic anemia; dermatologic and allergic reactions, including life-threatening cutaneous reactions such as Stevens-Johnson syndrome, toxic epidermal necrolysis and exfoliative dermatitis; gastrointestinal reactions; hepatitis and hepatocellular necrosis; CNS reactions; and toxic nephrosis. Use caution in pregnancy nearing term, premature infants, infants 2 mo or younger and in patients with renal or hepatic dysfunction.
MOA — Antibacterial; acts on bacterial cell wall.
ADVERSE EFFECTS — Frequent: Pruritus, rash. Severe: Erythema multiforme, hemolytic anemia, leukopenia, agranulocytosis, aplastic anemia, interstitial nephritis, hepatitis.

DERMATOLOGY: Antifungals (Topical)

BUTENAFINE (*Lotrimin Ultra, Mentax*) ▶L ♀B ▶? $
ADULT — Treatment of tinea pedis: Apply daily for 4 weeks or two times per day for 7 days. Tinea corporis, tinea versicolor, or tinea cruris: Apply daily for 2 weeks.
PEDS — Not approved in children.
FORMS — Rx Trade only: Cream 1% 15, 30 g (Mentax). OTC Trade only: Cream 1% 12, 24 g (Lotrimin Ultra).
NOTES — Most common adverse effects include contact dermatitis, burning, and worsening of condition. If no improvement in 4 weeks, reevaluate diagnosis.
MOA — Antifungal; binds to fungal cell membrane.
ADVERSE EFFECTS — Frequent: Burning, stinging, erythema, irritation.
CICLOPIROX (*Loprox, Loprox TS, Penlac, *Stieprox shampoo*) ▶K ♀B ▶? $$$$
ADULT — Tinea pedis, cruris, corporis, and versicolor, candidiasis (cream, lotion): Apply two times per day. Onychomycosis of fingernails/toenails (Penlac): Apply daily to affected nails; apply over previous coat; remove with alcohol q 7 days.

Seborrheic dermatitis (Loprox shampoo): Shampoo twice weekly for 4 weeks.
PEDS — Onychomycosis of fingernails/toenails in children age 12 yo or older (Penlac): Apply daily to affected nails; apply over previous coat; remove with alcohol q 7 days. Not approved in children younger than 12 yo.
FORMS — Trade only: Shampoo (Loprox) 1% 120 mL. Generic/Trade: Gel 0.77% 30, 45, 100 g. Nail soln (Penlac) 8% 6.6 mL. Cream (Loprox) 0.77% 15, 30, 90 g. Lotion (Loprox TS) 0.77% 30, 60 mL.
NOTES — Clinical improvement of tinea usually occurs within 1st week. Patients with tinea versicolor usually exhibit clinical and mycological clearing after 2 weeks. If no improvement in 4 weeks, reevaluate diagnosis. Do not get shampoo in eyes. No safety information available in diabetes or immunocompromise. Shampoo may affect hair color in those with light-colored hair. For nail soln, infected portion of each nail should be removed by healthcare professional as frequently as monthly. Oral antifungal therapy is more effective for onychomycosis than Penlac.

CICLOPIROX (*cont.*)
MOA — Antifungal; inhibits fungal DNA, RNA, protein synthesis.
ADVERSE EFFECTS — Frequent: Pruritus, erythema, burning.

CLOTRIMAZOLE—TOPICAL (*Lotrimin AF, Mycelex, ✦Canesten, Clotrimaderm*) ▶L ♀B ▶? $
ADULT — Treatment of tinea pedis, cruris, corporis, and versicolor, and cutaneous candidiasis: Apply two times per day.
PEDS — Treatment of tinea pedis, cruris, corporis, versicolor, cutaneous candidiasis: Apply two times per day.
FORMS — Note that Lotrimin brand cream, lotion, soln are clotrimazole, while Lotrimin powders and liquid spray are miconazole. Rx Generic only: Cream 1% 15, 30, 45 g. Soln 1% 10, 30 mL. OTC Trade only (Lotrimin AF): Cream 1% 12, 24 g. Soln 1% 10 mL.
NOTES — If no improvement in 4 weeks, reevaluate diagnosis.
MOA — Antifungal; alters fungal cell wall permeability.
ADVERSE EFFECTS — Frequent: Burning, irritation, stinging.

ECONAZOLE (*Ecoza*) ▶not absorbed ♀C ▶? $$
ADULT — Treatment of tinea pedis, cruris, corporis, and versicolor: Apply daily. Cutaneous candidiasis: Apply two times per day.
PEDS — Not approved in children.
FORMS — Generic only: Cream 1% 15, 30, 85 g. Trade only: Foam 1% 70 g (Ecoza-$$$$$)
NOTES — Treat candidal infections, tinea cruris and tinea corporis for 2 weeks and tinea pedis for 1 month to reduce risk of recurrence.
MOA — Antifungal; alters fungal cell wall permeability.
ADVERSE EFFECTS — Frequent: Burning, stinging, pruritus, erythema.

EFINACONAZOLE (*Jublia*) ▶minimal absorption ♀C ▶? $$$$$
ADULT — Onchomycosis of toenail: apply once daily to affected toenail.
PEDS — Not approved for use in children.
FORMS — Trade: soln 1%, 4 mL, 8 mL.
MOA — Inhibits ergosterol.
ADVERSE EFFECTS — Common: ingrown toenail, application site vesicles and pain.

KETOCONAZOLE—TOPICAL (*Extina, Nizoral, Nizoral AD, Xolegel, ✦Ketoderm*) ▶L ♀C ▶? $$
ADULT — Shampoo (2%): Tinea versicolor: Apply to affected area, leave on for 5 min, rinse. Cream: Cutaneous candidiasis, tinea corporis, tinea cruris, and tinea versicolor: Apply daily. Seborrheic dermatitis: Apply cream (2%) two times per day for 4 weeks or gel daily for 2 weeks or foam two times per day for 4 weeks. Dandruff: Apply shampoo (Nizoral AD 1%) twice a week.
PEDS — Not approved in children younger than 12 yo.
UNAPPROVED ADULT — Seborrheic dermatitis: Apply cream (2%) daily.

UNAPPROVED PEDS — Shampoo (2%): Tinea versicolor: Apply to affected area, leave on for 5 min, rinse. Cream: Cutaneous candidiasis, tinea corporis, tinea cruris, and tinea versicolor: Apply daily. Seborrheic dermatitis: Apply cream (2%) two times per day. Dandruff: Apply shampoo (1%) twice a week.
FORMS — Generic/Trade: Cream 2% 15, 30, 60 g. Shampoo 2% 120 mL. Trade only: Shampoo 1% 120, 210 mL (OTC Nizoral AD). Gel 2% 15 g (Xolegel). Foam 2% 50, 100 g (Extina).
NOTES — Treat candidal infections, tinea cruris, tinea corporis, and tinea versicolor for 2 weeks. Treat seborrheic dermatitis for 4 weeks. Treat tinea pedis for 6 weeks.
MOA — Antifungal; alters fungal cell wall permeability.
ADVERSE EFFECTS — Frequent: Burning, stinging, irritation, erythema. Severe: angioedema.

LULICONAZOLE (*Luzu*) ▶minimal absorption ♀C ▶? $$$$$
ADULT — Tinea pedis: apply one daily for 2 weeks. Tinea cruris, tinea coproris: apply once daily for 1 week.
PEDS — Not approved for use in children.
FORMS — Trade: 1% cream, 30g, 60g.
MOA — Inhibits ergosterol synthesis
ADVERSE EFFECTS — Common: application site reactions.

MICONAZOLE—TOPICAL (*Micatin, Lotrimin AF, ZeaSorb AF*) ▶L ♀+ ▶? $
ADULT — Tinea pedis, cruris, corporis, and versicolor, cutaneous candidiasis: Apply two times per day.
PEDS — Not approved in children.
UNAPPROVED PEDS — Tinea pedis, cruris, corporis, and versicolor, cutaneous candidiasis: Apply two times per day.
FORMS — Note that Lotrimin brand cream, lotion, soln are clotrimazole, while Lotrimin powders and liquid spray are miconazole. OTC Trade only: Powder 2% 70, 160 g. Spray powder 2% 90, 100, 140 g. Spray liquid 2% 90, 105 mL. Gel 2% 24 g.
NOTES — Symptomatic relief generally occurs in 2 to 3 days. Treat candida, tinea cruris, tinea corporis for 2 weeks, tinea pedis for 1 month to reduce risk of recurrence.
MOA — Antifungal; alters fungal cell wall permeability.
ADVERSE EFFECTS — Frequent: Rash, pruritus.

NAFTIFINE (*Naftin*) ▶LK ♀B ▶? $$$$$
ADULT — Tinea pedis, cruris, and corporis: Apply daily (cream) or two times per day (gel).
PEDS — Not approved in children.
FORMS — Trade only: Cream 1% 60, 90 g, cream 1% Pump 90 g. Gel 1% 40, 60, 90 g. Cream 2% 45g.
NOTES — If no improvement in 4 weeks, reevaluate diagnosis.
MOA — Antifungal; alters fungal cell wall synthesis.
ADVERSE EFFECTS — Frequent: Burning, stinging, erythema, irritation, pruritus.

NYSTATIN—TOPICAL (*Mycostatin, ♣Nyaderm*) ▶not absorbed ♀C ▶? $
ADULT — Cutaneous or mucocutaneous Candida infections: Apply two to three times per day.
PEDS — Cutaneous or mucocutaneous Candida infections: Apply two to three times per day.
FORMS — Generic/Trade: Cream, Ointment 100,000 units/g 15, 30 g. Powder 100,000 units/g 15, 30, 60 g.
NOTES — Ineffective for dermatophytes/tinea. For fungal infections of the feet, dust feet and footwear with powder.
MOA — Antifungal; alters fungal cell wall permeability.
ADVERSE EFFECTS — Frequent: Contact dermatitis, N/V, diarrhea, stomach pain. Severe: Stevens-Johnson syndrome, hypersensitivity.

OXICONAZOLE (*Oxistat, Oxizole*) ▶minimal absorption ♀B ▶? $$$
ADULT — Tinea pedis, cruris, and corporis: Apply one to two times per day. Tinea versicolor (cream only): Apply daily.
PEDS — Cream: Tinea pedis, cruris, and corporis: Apply one to two times per day. Tinea versicolor: Apply daily.
FORMS — Trade only: Cream 1% 15, 30, 60 g. Lotion 1% 30 mL.
MOA — Antifungal; alters fungal cell wall integrity.
ADVERSE EFFECTS — Frequent: Burning, stinging, erythema, irritation, pruritus, xeroderma.

SERTACONAZOLE (*Ertaczo*) ▶minimal absorption ♀C ▶? $$$
ADULT — Tinea pedis: Apply two times per day.
PEDS — Not approved for children younger than 12 yo.
FORMS — Trade only: Cream 2% 30, 60 g.
MOA — Antifungal; alters fungal cell wall integrity.

ADVERSE EFFECTS — Frequent: Burning, dermatitis, dry skin.

TERBINAFINE—TOPICAL (*Lamisil, Lamisil AT*) ▶L ♀B ▶? $
ADULT — Tinea pedis: Apply two times per day. Tinea cruris and corporis: Apply one to two times per day. Tinea versicolor (soln): Apply two times per day.
PEDS — Not approved in children.
UNAPPROVED ADULT — Cutaneous candidiasis.
UNAPPROVED PEDS — Tinea pedis: Apply two times per day. Tinea cruris and corporis: Apply one to two times per day. Tinea versicolor (soln): Apply two times per day.
FORMS — OTC Trade only (Lamisil AT): Cream 1% 12, 24 g. Spray pump soln 1% 30 mL. Gel 1% 6, 12 g.
NOTES — In many patients, improvement noted within 3 to 4 days, but therapy should continue for a minimum of 1 week, maximum of 4 weeks. Topical therapy not effective for nail fungus.
MOA — Antifungal; alters fungal cell wall synthesis.
ADVERSE EFFECTS — Frequent: Contact dermatitis, burning, irritation, pruritus.

TOLNAFTATE (*Tinactin*) ▶? ♀? ▶? $
ADULT — Tinea pedis, tinea cruris, tinea corporis, and tinea versicolor: Apply two times per day. Prevention of tinea pedis (powder and aerosol): Apply prn.
PEDS — Tinea pedis, tinea cruris, tinea corporis, and tinea versicolor: Apply two times per day for older than 2 yo. Prevention of tinea pedis (powder and aerosol): Apply prn.
FORMS — OTC Generic/Trade: Cream 1% 15, 30 g. Soln 1% 10 mL. Powder 1% 45 g. OTC Trade only: Gel 1% 15 g. Powder 1% 90 g. Spray powder 1% 100, 133, 150 g. Spray liquid 1% 100, 113 mL.
MOA — Antifungal; inhibits fungal cell growth.
ADVERSE EFFECTS — Frequent: Contact dermatitis, stinging, irritation, pruritus.

DERMATOLOGY: Antiparasitics (Topical)

A-200 (pyrethrins + piperonyl butoxide, *♣R&C*) ▶L ♀C ▶? $
ADULT — Lice: Apply shampoo, wash after 10 min. Reapply in 5 to 7 days.
PEDS — Lice: Apply shampoo, wash after 10 min. Reapply in 5 to 7 days.
FORMS — OTC Generic/Trade: Shampoo (0.33% pyrethrins, 4% piperonyl butoxide) 60, 120 mL.
NOTES — Use caution if allergic to ragweed. Avoid contact with mucous membranes. A-200 brand name no longer available.
MOA — Neuronal toxin to lice; inhibits pyrethrin metabolism.
ADVERSE EFFECTS — Frequent: Burning, stinging, pruritus.

BENZYL ALCOHOL (*Ulesfia*) ▶not absorbed - ♀B ▶? $$$$
WARNING — Flammable.
ADULT — Lice: Apply to dry hair to saturate scalp and hair. Amount depends on hair length. Rinse after 10 minutes. Reapply in 7 days, if necessary.

PEDS — Lice, 6 mo or older: Apply to dry hair to saturate scalp and hair. Rinse after 10 minutes. Reapply in 7 days, if necessary.
FORMS — Lotion 5% 60 mL and in 2-pack with nit comb.
MOA — Asphyxiation.
ADVERSE EFFECTS — Frequent: eye irritation, scalp irritation and anesthesia.

CROTAMITON (*Eurax*) ▶? ♀C ▶? $$
ADULT — Scabies: Massage cream/lotion into entire body from chin down, repeat 24 h later, bathe 48 h later. Pruritus: Massage into affected areas prn.
PEDS — Not approved in children.
UNAPPROVED PEDS — Scabies: Massage cream/lotion into entire body from chin down, repeat 24 h later, bathe 48 h later. Pruritus: Massage into affected areas prn.
FORMS — Trade only: Cream 10% 60 g. Lotion 10% 60, 480 mL.
NOTES — Advise patients to ensure application under nails. Patients with scabies should change

CROTAMITON (*cont.*)

bed linen and clothing in am after 2nd application and bathe 48 h after last application. Consider treating entire family if treating scabies.
MOA — Scabicidal; mechanism of action unknown.
ADVERSE EFFECTS — Frequent: None.

LINDANE ▶L ♀B ▶? $

WARNING — For use only in patients who have failed other agents. Seizures and deaths have been reported with repeat or prolonged use. Use caution with infants, children, elderly, those who weigh less than 50 kg. Contraindicated in premature infants and patients with uncontrolled seizures.
ADULT — Head/crab lice: Lotion: Apply 30 to 60 mL to affected area, wash off after 12 h. Shampoo: Apply 30 to 60 mL, wash off after 4 min. Scabies (lotion): Apply 30 to 60 mL to total body from neck down, wash off after 8 to 12 h.
PEDS — Lindane penetrates human skin and has potential for CNS toxicity. Studies indicate potential toxic effects of topical lindane are greater in young. Maximum dose for age younger than 6 yo is 30 mL.
FORMS — Generic only: Lotion 1% 60, 480 mL. Shampoo 1% 60, 480 mL.
NOTES — For lice, reapply if living lice noted after 7 days. After shampooing, comb with fine tooth comb to remove nits. Consider treating entire family if treating scabies.
MOA — Nervous system stimulant lethal to ova and parasites.
ADVERSE EFFECTS — Frequent: None. Severe: CNS side effects—headache, restlessness, seizures, aplastic anemia, arrhythmias, hepatitis, pulmonary edema, hematuria.

MALATHION (*Ovide*) ▶? ♀B ▶? $$$$

ADULT — Lice: Apply to dry hair, let dry naturally, wash off in 8 to 12 h.
PEDS — Lice in children: Apply to dry hair, let dry naturally, wash off in 8 to 12 h for 6 yo or older.
FORMS — Generic/Trade only: Lotion 0.5% 59 mL.
NOTES — Do not use hair dryer; flammable. Avoid contact with eyes. Use a fine tooth comb to remove nits and dead lice. Application may be repeated in 7 to 9 days.
MOA — Kills lice and their ova.
ADVERSE EFFECTS — Frequent: None.

PERMETHRIN (*Elimite, Acticin, Nix, ✦Kwellada-P*) ▶L ♀B ▶? $$

ADULT — Scabies (cream): Massage cream into entire body (avoid mouth, eyes, nose), wash off after 8 to 14 h. 30 g is typical adult dose. Repeat in 7 days. Lice (liquid): Apply to clean, towel-dried hair, saturate hair and scalp, wash off after 10 min.
PEDS — Scabies (cream) age older than 2 mo: Massage cream into entire body (avoid mouth, eyes, nose), wash off after 8 to 14 h. Lice (liquid) in age older than 2 yo: Saturate hair and scalp, wash off after 10 min.
FORMS — Generic/Trade: Cream (Elimite, Acticin) 5% 60 g. OTC Generic/Trade: Liquid creme rinse (Nix) 1% 60 mL.
NOTES — If necessary, may repeat application in 7 days. Consider treating entire family if treating scabies.
MOA — Neuronal toxin which paralyzes lice.
ADVERSE EFFECTS — Frequent: Burning, stinging, erythema, numbness, pruritus.

RID (**pyrethrins + piperonyl butoxide**) ▶L ♀C ▶? $

ADULT — Lice: Apply shampoo/mousse, wash after 10 min. Reapply in 5 to 10 days prn.
PEDS — Lice: Apply shampoo/mousse, wash after 10 min. Reapply in 5 to 10 days prn.
FORMS — OTC Generic/Trade: Shampoo 60, 120, 240 mL. OTC Trade only: Mousse 5.5 oz.
NOTES — Use caution if allergic to ragweed. Avoid contact with mucous membranes. Available alone or as part of a RID 1-2-3 kit containing shampoo, egg, and nit comb-out gel and home lice control spray for nonwashable items.
MOA — Neuronal toxin to lice; inhibits pyrethrin metabolism.
ADVERSE EFFECTS — Frequent: Burning, stinging, pruritus.

SPINOSAD (*Natroba*) ▶not absorbed - ♀B ▶? $$$$$

ADULT — Lice: Apply to dry hair/scalp to cover. Leave on 10 minutes then rinse. Retreat if live lice seen after 7 days.
PEDS — 4 yo and older: Lice: Apply to dry hair/scalp to cover. Leave on 10 minutes then rinse. Retreat if live lice seen after 7 days.
FORMS — Topical susp, 0.9%, 120 mL.
MOA — Neuronal excitation of lice.
ADVERSE EFFECTS — Frequent: erythema, irritation.

DERMATOLOGY: Antipsoriatics

ACITRETIN (*Soriatane*) ▶L ♀X ▶– $$$$$

WARNING — Contraindicated in pregnancy and avoid pregnancy for 3 years following medication discontinuation. Major human fetal abnormalities have been reported. Females of child bearing age must avoid alcohol while on medication and for 2 months following therapy since alcohol prolongs elimination of a teratogenic metabolite. Use in reliable females of reproductive potential only if they have severe, unresponsive psoriasis, have received written and oral warnings of the teratogenic potential, are using 2 reliable forms of contraception, and have 2 negative pregnancy tests within 1 week prior to starting therapy. Contraception should start at least 1 month prior to therapy and continue for 3 years following discontinuation. Must have negative monthly pregnancy test during treatment. Therefore, prescribe limited amount and do not allow refill until documented negative pregnancy test. Following discontinuation, repeat pregnancy test q 3 months. It is unknown whether residual acitretin in seminal fluid poses a risk to the fetus while a male patient is taking the drug or after it is discontinued.

(cont.)

ACITRETIN *(cont.)*

ADULT — Severe psoriasis: Initiate at 25 to 50 mg PO daily.

PEDS — Not approved in children.

UNAPPROVED ADULT — Lichen planus: 30 mg/day PO for 4 weeks, then titrate to 10 to 50 mg/day for 12 weeks total. Sjögren-Larsson syndrome: 0.47 mg/kg/day PO. Also used in Darier's disease, palmoplantar pustulosis, nonbullous and bullous ichthyosiform erythroderma, lichen sclerosus et atrophicus of the vulva, palmoplantar lichen nitidus and chemoprevention for high-risk immunosuppressed patients with history of squamous cell carcinomas of the skin. Pityriasis rubra pilaris: 25 mg to 50 mg PO once daily.

UNAPPROVED PEDS — Has been used in children with lamellar ichthyosis. Pediatric use is not recommended. Adverse effects on bone growth are suspected.

FORMS — Generic/Trade only: Caps 10, 17.5, 25 mg.

NOTES — Transient worsening of psoriasis may occur, and full benefit may take 2 to 3 months. Elevated LFTs may occur in one-third of patients; monitor LFTs at 1 to 2 weeks intervals until stable and then periodically thereafter. Monitor serum lipid concentrations q 1 to 2 weeks until response to drug is established. May decrease tolerance to contact lenses due to dry eyes. Avoid prolonged exposure to sunlight. May cause hair loss. May cause depression. May cause bone changes, especially with use more than 6 months. Many adverse drug reactions.

MOA — Unknown.

ADVERSE EFFECTS — Frequent: Cheilitis, xerostomia, rhinitis, epistaxis, alopecia, skin peeling, pruritus, erythematous rash, rigors, arthralgias, xerophthalmus. Severe: Hepatitis, pancreatitis, pseudotumor cerebri.

ANTHRALIN (*Drithocreme*) ▶? ♀C �D– $$$

ADULT — Chronic psoriasis: Apply daily.

PEDS — Not approved in children.

UNAPPROVED ADULT — Alopecia areata.

UNAPPROVED PEDS — Chronic psoriasis: Apply daily.

FORMS — Trade only: Cream 0.5, 1% 50 g.

NOTES — Short contact periods (i.e., 15 to 20 min) followed by removal with an appropriate solvent (soap or petrolatum) may be preferred. May stain fabric, skin, or hair.

MOA — Inhibits proliferation of epidermal cells in psoriasis.

ADVERSE EFFECTS — Frequent: Irritation, discoloration of skin and clothing.

CALCIPOTRIENE (*Dovonex, Sorilux*) ▶L ♀C �D? $$$$

ADULT — Moderate plaque psoriasis: Apply two times per day.

PEDS — Not approved in children.

UNAPPROVED ADULT — Has been used for vitiligo and morphea.

UNAPPROVED PEDS — Moderate plaque psoriasis: Apply two times per day. Has been used for vitiligo.

FORMS — Trade only: Ointment 0.005% 30, 60, 100 g (Dovonex). Cream 0.005% 30, 60, 100 g (Dovonex). Foam for scalp 0.005% 60, 120 g (Sorilux). Generic/Trade: Scalp soln 0.005% 60 mL.

NOTES — Avoid contact with face. Do not exceed 100 g/week to minimize risk of hypercalcemia, hypercalciuria. Burning, itching, and skin irritation may occur in 10 to 15% of patients.

MOA — Regulates skin cell production and proliferation.

ADVERSE EFFECTS — Frequent: Burning, irritation, drying, rash, worsening of psoriasis, pruritus.

METHOXSALEN (*8-MOP, Oxsoralen-Ultra, Uvadex*) ▶skin ♀C �D? $$$$$

WARNING — Should only be perscribed by physicians who have special training. For the treatment of patients with psoriasis, restrict to severe cases. Possibility of ocular damage, aging of the skin, and skin cancer (including melanoma).Women of childbearing potential should avoid becoming pregnant

ADULT — Psoriasis: Dose based on wt (0.4 mg/kg/dose), 1½ to 2 h before ultraviolet light exposure. Specialized dosing of sterile solution for photopheresis (Uvadex).

PEDS — Not approved in children.

FORMS — Generic/Trade: Soft gelcap 10 mg (Oxsoralen-Ultra). Trade only: Hard gelcap 10 mg (8-MOP). Sterile solution for use in photopheresis 20 mcg/mL (Uvadex)

NOTES — Oxsoralen-Ultra (soft gelcap) cannot be interchanged with 8-MOP (hard gelcap) due to significant bioavailability differences and photosensitization onset times. Take with food or milk. Wear ultraviolet light-blocking glasses and avoid sun exposure after ingestion and for remainder of day.

MOA — DNA photodamage and decreased cell proliferation.

ADVERSE EFFECTS — Frequent: Nausea, pruritus, erythema, nervousness, insomnia. Severe: Depression, skin cancer with prolonged use, cataracts.

TACLONEX (calcipotriene + betamethasone—topical) ▶L ♀C �D? $$$$$

ADULT — Psoriasis: Apply daily for up to 4 weeks.

PEDS — Not approved in children.

FORMS — Calcipotriene 0.005% + betamethasone dipropionate 0.064%. Generic/Trade: Ointment 60, 100 g. Trade only: Topical susp (Taclonex) 60, 120 g.

NOTES — Do not exceed 100 g/week due to risk of hypercalcemia. Do not use on more than 30% of body surface area. Do not apply to face, groin, or axillae to avoid irritant dermatitis.

MOA — Vitamin D3 analog that inhibits cell proliferation, regulates skin cell production, anti-inflammatory.

ADVERSE EFFECTS — See calcipotriene and betamethasone.

USTEKINUMAB (*Stelara*) ▶L ♀B �D? $$$$$

WARNING — Can cause serious infections. Discontinue if serious infection. Caution if high risk of malignancy or a history of malignancy. Theoretical risk of infection from Mycobacterium, Salmonella, and BCG vaccine. Evaluate patients for TB prior to therapy. Risk of reversible posterior leukoencephalopathy syndrome.

USTEKINUMAB (cont.)

ADULT — Severe plaque psoriasis, active psoriatic arthritis, wt less than 100 kg: 45 mg SC initially and again 4 weeks later, followed by 45 mg SC q 12 weeks. For wt greater than 100 kg and psoriatic arthritis with moderate to severe plaque psoriasis: 90 mg SC initially and again 4 weeks later, followed by 90 mg SC q 12 weeks.

PEDS — Not approved in children.
FORMS — Trade only: 45 and 90 mg prefilled syringe and vial.
NOTES — After proper training, may be self-administered at home, if appropriate.
MOA — Interleukin antagonist.
ADVERSE EFFECTS — Frequent: Headache, fatigue. Severe: Serious infection, malignancy, disseminated TB-reversible posterior leukoencephalopathy syndrome.

DERMATOLOGY: Antivirals (Topical)

ACYCLOVIR—TOPICAL (Zovirax) ▶K ♀C ▶? $$$$$
ADULT — Initial episodes of herpes genitalis: Apply ointment q 3 h (6 times per day) for 7 days. Non-life-threatening mucocutaneous herpes simplex in immunocompromised patients: Apply ointment q 3 h (6 times per day) for 7 days. Recurrent herpes labialis: Apply cream 5 times per day for 4 days.
PEDS — Recurrent herpes labialis: Apply cream 5 times per day for 4 days for age 12 yo or older.
UNAPPROVED PEDS — Initial episodes of herpes genitalis: Apply ointment q 3 h (6 times per day) for 7 days. Non-life-threatening mucocutaneous herpes simplex in immunocompromised patients: Apply ointment q 3 h (6 times per day) for 7 days.
FORMS — Generic/Trade: Ointment 5% 15, 30 g. Trade only: Cream 5% 5 g.
NOTES — Use finger cot or rubber glove to apply ointment to avoid dissemination. Burning/stinging may occur in up to 28% of patients. Oral form more effective than topical for herpes genitalis.
MOA — Antiviral; inhibits DNA synthesis and viral replication.
ADVERSE EFFECTS — Frequent: Rash (oint). Skin irritation (cream). Severe: Cutaneous sensitization.

DOCOSANOL (Abreva) ▶not absorbed ♀B ▶? $
ADULT — Oral-facial herpes (cold sores): Apply 5 times per day until healed.
PEDS — Oral-facial herpes (cold sores): Use adult dose for age 12 years or older.
FORMS — OTC Trade only: Cream 10% 2 g.
MOA — Inhibits entry of lipid-enveloped viruses.
ADVERSE EFFECTS — Frequent: Headache, site reaction, rash, pruritus, dry skin, ache.

IMIQUIMOD (Aldara, Zyclara, ✦Vyloma) ▶not absorbed ♀C ▶? $$$$$
ADULT — External genital and perianal warts, 3.75% cream: Apply 3 times a week at bedtime for up to 16 weeks. Wash off after 8 h. Non-hyperkeratotic, non-hypertrophic actinic keratoses on face/scalp in immunocompetent adults, 2.5% or 3.75% cream: Apply to face or scalp (but not both) twice a week for up to 16 weeks (Aldara) or once daily for two 2-week periods separated by a 2 week break (Zyclara). Wash off after 8 h. Primary superficial basal cell carcinoma: Apply 5 times per week for 6 weeks (Aldara). Wash off after 8 h.
PEDS — External genital and perianal warts: Apply 3 times per week at bedtime and wash off after 6 to 10 h for age 12 yo or older (Aldara) or once daily for two 2-week periods separated by a 2 week break (Zyclara).
UNAPPROVED ADULT — Molluscum contagiosum. Apply 3 times per week, wash off after 6 to 10 h.
UNAPPROVED PEDS — Molluscum contagiosum.
FORMS — Generic/Trade: Cream 5% (Aldara) single-use packets. Trade only: Cream 3.75% (Zyclara) single-use packets, box of 28. Cream 2.5% single-use packets and 7.5 g pump .
NOTES — May weaken condoms and diaphragms. Avoid sexual contact while cream is on when used for genital/perianal warts. Most common adverse effects include erythema, itching, erosion, burning, excoriation, edema, and pain. Discard partially used packets.
MOA — Mechanism unknown but may increase cytokine concentrations.
ADVERSE EFFECTS — Frequent: Pruritus, erythema, burning, erosion, edema, flu-like symptoms. Severe: Erythema, erosion, edema, severe local inflammation of the external female genitalia leading to urinary retention.

PENCICLOVIR (Denavir) ▶not absorbed ♀B ▶? $$
ADULT — Recurrent herpes labialis (cold sores): Apply q 2 h while awake for 4 days.
PEDS — Not approved in children.
UNAPPROVED PEDS — Recurrent herpes labialis: Apply q 2 h while awake for 4 days.
FORMS — Trade only: Cream 1% tube 1.5 g.
NOTES — Start therapy as soon as possible during prodrome. For moderate to severe cases of herpes labialis, systemic treatment with famciclovir or acyclovir may be preferred.
MOA — Antiviral: Inhibits viral DNA synthesis and replication.
ADVERSE EFFECTS — Frequent: Headache, erythema.

PODOFILOX (Condylox, ✦Condyline, Wartec) ▶? ♀C ▶? $$$$
ADULT — External genital warts (gel and soln) and perianal warts (gel only): Apply two times per day for 3 consecutive days of a weeks and repeat for up to 4 weeks.
PEDS — Not approved in children.
FORMS — Generic/Trade: Soln 0.5% 3.5 mL. Trade only: Gel 0.5% 3.5 g.
MOA — Unknown.
ADVERSE EFFECTS — Frequent: Inflammation, burning, erosion, pain, pruritus, bleeding.

PODOPHYLLIN (*Podocon-25, Podofin, Podofilm*) ▶?
♀– ▶– $$$
ADULT — Genital wart removal: Initial application: Apply to wart and leave on for 30 to 40 min to determine patient's sensitivity. Thereafter, use minimum contact time necessary (1 to 4 h depending on result). Remove dried podophyllin with alcohol or soap and water.
PEDS — Not approved in children.
FORMS — Not to be dispensed to patients. For hospital/clinic use; not intended for outpatient prescribing. Trade only: Liquid 25% 15 mL.
NOTES — Do not treat large areas or numerous warts all at once. Contraindicated in diabetics, pregnancy, patients using steroids or with poor circulation, and on bleeding warts.
MOA — Arrests mitosis by binding to microtubule spindle.
ADVERSE EFFECTS — Frequent: Pruritus, N/V, abdominal pain, diarrhea. Severe: Hallucination,

hepatotoxicity, leukopenia, thrombocytopenia, renal failure.

SINECATECHINS (*Veregen*) ▶minimal absorption ♀C ▶? $$$$$
ADULT — Apply three times per day to external genital warts for up to 16 weeks.
PEDS — Not approved in children.
FORMS — Trade only: Ointment 15% 15, 30 g.
NOTES — Botanical drug product. Contains a partially purified fraction of the water extract of green tea leaves. Do not use on open wounds. Do not use in immunocompromised patients. Generic name used to be kunecatechins.
MOA — Unknown, but thought to be immunomodulatory.
ADVERSE EFFECTS — Frequent: Burning, pain, erythema at application site, erosion, edema, induration, rash.

DERMATOLOGY: Atopic Dermatitis Preparations

NOTE: Long-term safety has not been established. Avoid use in immunocompromised patients and in children younger than 2 yo. Use minimum amount to control symptoms.

PIMECROLIMUS (*Elidel*) ▶L ♀C ▶? $$$$
WARNING — Use minimum amount, only on involved areas and avoid occlusion.
ADULT — Atopic dermatitis: Apply two times per day.
PEDS — Atopic dermatitis: Apply two times per day for age 2 yo or older.
UNAPPROVED ADULT — Perioral dermatitis, oral lichen planus, intertriginous/facial psoriasis.
FORMS — Trade only: Cream 1% 30, 60, 100 g.
NOTES — Long-term safety unclear.
MOA — Calcineurin inhibitor modulator.
ADVERSE EFFECTS — Frequent: Burning headache, nasopharyngitis, cough, influenza, pyrexia, viral infection.

TACROLIMUS—TOPICAL (*Protopic*) ▶minimal absorption ♀C ▶? $$$$$
WARNING — May be associated with skin cancer or lymphoma. Avoid continuous long-term use. Avoid in children less than 2 yo.

ADULT — Atopic dermatitis: Apply two times per day.
PEDS — Atopic dermatitis: Apply 0.03% ointment two times per day for age 2 to 15 yo.
UNAPPROVED ADULT — Vitiligo: Apply 0.1% two times per day. Chronic allergic contact dermatitis (e.g., nickel-induced): Apply 0.1% ointment two times per day.
FORMS — Trade only: Ointment 0.03%, 0.1% 30, 60, 100 g.
NOTES — Do not use with an occlusive dressing. Continue treatment for 1 week after clearing of symptoms.
MOA — Topical immunomodulator that suppresses T-cell activation and cytokine release.
ADVERSE EFFECTS — Frequent: Skin burning/tingling, pruritus, flu-like symptoms, erythema, headache, urticaria, acne. Severe: LFT increase, anaphylactoid reaction, angina, angioedema.

DERMATOLOGY: Corticosteroid/Antimicrobial Combinations

Cortisporin (neomycin—topical + polymyxin—topical + hydrocortisone—topical) ▶LK ♀C ▶? $$$
ADULT — Corticosteroid-responsive dermatoses with secondary infection: Apply two to four times per day.
PEDS — Not approved in children.
UNAPPROVED PEDS — Corticosteroid-responsive dermatoses with secondary infection: Apply two to four times per day.
FORMS — Trade only: Cream 7.5 g. Ointment (also contains bacitracin) 15 g.
NOTES — Due to concerns about nephrotoxicity and ototoxicity associated with neomycin, do not use over wide areas or for prolonged periods of time.
MOA — Antibacterial + anti-inflammatory.

ADVERSE EFFECTS — Ocular: Frequent: Blurred vision, itching, elevation of intraocular pressure, glaucoma. Severe: Hypersensitivity, anaphylaxis.

FUCIDIN H (fusidic acid—topical + hydrocortisone—topical) ▶L ♀? ▶? $$
ADULT — Canada only. Atopic dermatitis: Apply three times per day.
PEDS — Canada only. Atopic dermatitis: Apply three times per day for age 3 yo or older.
FORMS — Canada Trade only: Cream (2% fusidic acid, 1% hydrocortisone acetate) 30 g.
NOTES — Not to be used longer than 2 weeks; notify prescriber if improvement not seen after 1 week.

FUCIDIN H (cont.)

MOA — Antibacterial, interferes with bacterial protein synthesis + anti-inflammatory.

ADVERSE EFFECTS — Serious: Hypersensitivity. Frequent: Mild irritation, flare of dermatitis.

LOTRISONE (clotrimazole—topical + betamethasone—topical, ✷**Lotriderm**) ▶L ♀C ▶? $$$

ADULT — Tinea pedis, cruris, and corporis: Apply two times per day.

PEDS — Not approved in children younger than 17 years.

FORMS — Generic/Trade: Cream (clotrimazole 1% + betamethasone 0.05%) 15, 45 g. Lotion (clotrimazole 1% + betamethasone 0.05%) 30 mL.

NOTES — Treat tinea cruris and corporis for 1 week (no longer than) 2 weeks and tinea pedis for 2 weeks (no longer than 4 weeks). Do not use for diaper dermatitis.

MOA — Antifungal + anti-inflammatory.

ADVERSE EFFECTS — Frequent: Erythema, stinging, blistering, peeling, edema, pruritus, urticaria, irritation, telangiectasia.

MYCOLOG II (nystatin—topical + triamcinolone—topical) ▶L ♀C ▶? $

ADULT — Cutaneous candidiasis: Apply two times per day.

PEDS — Not approved in children.

UNAPPROVED PEDS — Sometimes used for diaper dermatitis, but not recommended due to risk of adrenal suppression.

FORMS — Generic only: Cream, Ointment 15, 30, 60, 120, 454 g.

NOTES — Avoid occlusive dressings.

MOA — Antifungal + anti-inflammatory.

ADVERSE EFFECTS — Frequent: None. Severe: Stevens-Johnson syndrome.

DERMATOLOGY: Corticosteroids (Topical)

NOTE: After long-term use, do not discontinue abruptly; switch to a less potent agent or alternate use of corticosteroids and emollient products. Monitor for hyperglycemia/adrenal suppression if used for long period of time or over a large area of the body, especially in children. Chronic administration may cause skin atrophy and interfere with pediatric growth and development.

ALCLOMETASONE DIPROPIONATE (Aclovate) ▶L ♀C ▶? $$

ADULT — Inflammatory and pruritic manifestations of corticosteroid-responsive dermatoses: Apply sparingly two to three times per day.

PEDS — Inflammatory and pruritic manifestations of corticosteroid-responsive dermatoses: Apply sparingly two to three times per day for age 1 yo or older. Safety and efficacy for more than 3 weeks have not been established.

FORMS — Generic/Trade: Ointment, Cream 0.05% 15, 45, 60 g.

MOA — Anti-inflammatory; suppresses DNA synthesis, decreases WBC influx.

ADVERSE EFFECTS — Frequent: Burning, pruritus, dryness, irritation, erythema.

AMCINONIDE (Cyclocort) ▶L ♀C ▶? $$

ADULT — Inflammatory and pruritic manifestations of corticosteroid-responsive dermatoses: Apply sparingly two to three times per day.

PEDS — Inflammatory and pruritic manifestations of corticosteroid-responsive dermatoses: Apply sparingly two to three times per day.

FORMS — Generic only: Cream, Ointment 0.1% 15, 30, 60 g. Lotion 0.1% 60 mL.

MOA — Anti-inflammatory; suppresses DNA synthesis, decreases WBC influx.

ADVERSE EFFECTS — Frequent: Burning, pruritus, dryness, irritation, erythema. Severe: Steroid atrophy, hypothalamic axis suppression with higher potency preparations.

AUGMENTED BETAMETHASONE DIPROPIONATE (Diprolene, Diprolene AF, ✷Topilene Glycol) ▶L ♀C ▶? $$$

ADULT — Inflammatory and pruritic manifestations of corticosteroid-responsive dermatoses: Apply sparingly one to two times per day.

PEDS — Not approved younger than 12 yo.

FORMS — Generic/Trade: Diprolene: Ointment 0.05% 15, 50 g. Lotion 0.05% 30, 60 mL. Diprolene AF: Cream 0.05% 15, 50 g. Generic only: Gel 0.05% 15, 50 g.

NOTES — Do not use occlusive dressings. Do not use for longer than 2 consecutive week and do not exceed a total dose of 45 to 50 g per weeks or 50 mL per weeks of the lotion.

MOA — Anti-inflammatory; suppresses DNA synthesis, decreases WBC influx.

ADVERSE EFFECTS — Frequent: Burning, pruritus, dryness, irritation, erythema. Severe: Steroid atrophy, hypothalamic axis suppression with higher potency preparations.

BETAMETHASONE DIPROPIONATE (Diprosone, Maxivate, ✷Propaderm, TARO-sone) ▶L ♀C ▶? $

ADULT — Inflammatory and pruritic manifestations of corticosteroid-responsive dermatoses: Apply sparingly one to two times per day.

PEDS — Inflammatory and pruritic manifestations of corticosteroid-responsive dermatoses: Apply sparingly one to two times per day.

FORMS — Generic only: Ointment, Cream 0.05% 15, 45 g. Lotion 0.05% 30, 60 mL.

NOTES — Do not use occlusive dressings.

MOA — Anti-inflammatory; suppresses DNA synthesis, decreases WBC influx.

ADVERSE EFFECTS — Frequent: Burning, pruritus, dryness, irritation, erythema. Severe: Steroid atrophy, hypothalamic axis suppression with higher potency preparations.

BETAMETHASONE VALERATE (Luxiq foam, Beta-Val, ✷Betaderm) ▶L ♀C ▶? $$

ADULT — Inflammatory and pruritic manifestations of corticosteroid-responsive dermatoses: Apply sparingly one to two times per day. Dermatoses of

(cont.)

BETAMETHASONE VALERATE (*cont.*)

scalp: Apply small amount of foam to scalp two times per day.

PEDS — Inflammatory and pruritic manifestations of corticosteroid-responsive dermatoses: Apply sparingly one to two times per day.

FORMS — Generic only: Ointment, Cream 0.1% 15, 45 g. Lotion 0.1% 60 mL. Generic/Trade: Foam (Luxiq) 0.12% 50, 100g.

MOA — Anti-inflammatory; suppresses DNA synthesis, decreases WBC influx.

ADVERSE EFFECTS — Frequent: Burning, pruritus, dryness, irritation, erythema. Severe: Steroid atrophy, hypothalamic axis suppression with higher potency preparations.

CLOBETASOL (*Temovate, Olux, Clobex, Cormax, ✷Dermasone*) ▶L ♀C ▶? $$

ADULT — Inflammatory and pruritic manifestations of corticosteroid-responsive dermatoses: Apply sparingly two times per day. For scalp apply foam two times per day.

PEDS — Not approved in children.

FORMS — Generic/Trade: Cream, Ointment 0.05% 15, 30, 45, 60 g. Scalp application 0.05% 25, 50 mL. Gel 0.05% 15, 30, 60 g. Foam (Olux) 0.05% 50, 100 g. Lotion (Clobex) 0.05% 30, 60, 120 mL. Shampoo 0.05% 118 mL. Trade only (Clobex): Spray 0.05% 60, 125 mL.

NOTES — Adrenal suppression at doses as low as 2 g per day. Do not use occlusive dressings. Do not use for longer than 2 consecutive weeks and do not exceed a total dose of 50 g per weeks.

MOA — Anti-inflammatory; suppresses DNA synthesis, decreases WBC influx.

ADVERSE EFFECTS — Frequent: Burning, pruritus, dryness, irritation, erythema, alopecia. Severe: Steroid atrophy, hypothalamic axis suppression with higher potency preparations.

CLOCORTOLONE PIVALATE (*Cloderm*) ▶L ♀C ▶? $$$

ADULT — Inflammatory and pruritic manifestations of corticosteroid-responsive dermatoses: Apply sparingly three times per day.

PEDS — Inflammatory and pruritic manifestations of corticosteroid-responsive dermatoses: Apply sparingly three times per day.

FORMS — Trade only: Cream 0.1% 30, 45, 75, 90 g.

MOA — Anti-inflammatory; suppresses DNA synthesis, decreases WBC influx.

ADVERSE EFFECTS — Frequent: Burning, pruritus, dryness, irritation, erythema. Severe: Hypothalamic axis suppression with higher potency preparations.

DESONIDE (*DesOwen, Desonate, Tridesilon, Verdeso*) ▶L ♀C ▶? $$

ADULT — Inflammatory and pruritic manifestations of corticosteroid-responsive dermatoses: Apply sparingly two to three times per day.

PEDS — Inflammatory and pruritic manifestations of corticosteroid-responsive dermatoses: Apply sparingly two to three times per day.

FORMS — Generic/Trade: Cream, Ointment 0.05%, 15, 60 g. Lotion 0.05%, 60, 120 mL. Trade only: Gel (Desonate) 0.05% 60 g, Foam (Verdeso) 0.05%, 50, 100 g.

NOTES — Do not use with occlusive dressings.

MOA — Anti-inflammatory; suppresses DNA synthesis, decreases WBC influx.

ADVERSE EFFECTS — Frequent: Burning, pruritus, dryness, irritation, erythema.

DESOXIMETASONE (*Topicort, Topicort LP, ✷Desoxi*) ▶L ♀C ▶? $$$$

ADULT — Inflammatory and pruritic manifestations of corticosteroid-responsive dermatoses: Apply sparingly two times per day.

PEDS — Safety and efficacy have not been established for Topicort 0.25% ointment. For inflammatory and pruritic manifestations of corticosteroid-responsive dermatoses (cream and gel): Apply sparingly two times per day.

FORMS — Generic/Trade: Cream, Gel 0.05% 15, 60 g. Cream, Ointment 0.25% 15, 60, 100 g. Trade only: Spray 0.25% 100 mL.

MOA — Anti-inflammatory; suppresses DNA synthesis, decreases WBC influx.

ADVERSE EFFECTS — Frequent: Burning, pruritus, dryness, irritation, erythema. Severe: Steroid atrophy, hypothalamic axis suppression with higher potency preparations.

DIFLORASONE (*Psorcon E, Maxiflor*) ▶L ♀C ▶? $$$

ADULT — Inflammatory and pruritic manifestations of corticosteroid-responsive dermatoses: Apply sparingly one to three times per day.

PEDS — Not approved in children.

FORMS — Generic/Trade: Cream, Ointment 0.05% 15, 30, 60 g.

NOTES — Doses of 30 g/day of diflorasone 0.05% cream for 1 week resulted in adrenal suppression in some psoriasis patients.

MOA — Anti-inflammatory; suppresses DNA synthesis, decreases WBC influx.

ADVERSE EFFECTS — Frequent: Burning, pruritus, dryness, irritation, erythema. Severe: Steroid atrophy, hypothalamic axis suppression with higher potency preparations.

FLUOCINOLONE—TOPICAL (*Synalar, Capex, Derma-Smoothe/FS*) ▶L ♀C ▶? $

ADULT — Inflammatory and pruritic manifestations of corticosteroid-responsive dermatoses: Apply sparingly two to three times per day. Psoriasis of the scalp (Derma-Smoothe/FS): Massage into scalp, cover with shower cap and leave on 4 or more hours or overnight and then wash off.

PEDS — Inflammatory and pruritic manifestations of corticosteroid-responsive dermatoses: Apply sparingly two to four times per day. Atopic dermatitis: Moisten skin and apply to affected areas two times per day for up to 4 weeks (Derma-Smoothe/FS).

FORMS — Generic/Trade: Cream, Ointment 0.025% 15, 60, 120 g. Soln 0.01% 60 mL, 90 mL. (Derma-Smoothe/FS): Topical oil 0.01% 120 mL. Generic

FLUOCINOLONE—TOPICAL (cont.)

only: Cream 0.01% 15, 60 g. Trade only (Capex) Shampoo 0.01% 120 mL.

MOA — Anti-inflammatory; suppresses DNA synthesis, decreases WBC influx.

ADVERSE EFFECTS — Frequent: Burning, pruritus, dryness, irritation, erythema. Severe: Hypothalamic axis suppression with higher potency preparations.

FLUOCINONIDE (Lidex, Lidex-E, Vanos, ✷Lidemol, Topsyn, Tiamol) ▶L ♀C ▶? $$

ADULT — Inflammatory and pruritic manifestations of corticosteroid-responsive dermatoses: Apply sparingly two to four times per day. Plaque-type psoriasis: Apply 0.1% cream (Vanos) one to two times per day for 2 consecutive weeks only; no more than 60 g per week. Atopic dermatitis: Apply 0.1% cream (Vanos) once a day.

PEDS — Inflammatory and pruritic manifestations of corticosteroid-responsive dermatoses: Apply sparingly two to four times per day.

FORMS — Generic/Trade: Cream, Ointment, Gel 0.05% 15, 30, 60 g. Soln 0.05% 20, 60 mL. Cream (Vanos) 0.1% 30, 60, 120 g .

MOA — Anti-inflammatory by inhibiting production of prostaglandins and leukotrienes; suppresses DNA synthesis, decreases WBC influx.

ADVERSE EFFECTS — Frequent: Burning, pruritus, dryness, irritation, erythema. Severe: Immunosuppression (with more than 2 weeks use), steroid atrophy, hypothalamic axis suppression with higher potency preparations.

FLURANDRENOLIDE (Cordran, Cordran SP) ▶L ♀C ▶? $$$

ADULT — Inflammatory and pruritic manifestations of corticosteroid-responsive dermatoses: Apply sparingly two to three times per day.

PEDS — Inflammatory and pruritic manifestations of corticosteroid-responsive dermatoses: Apply sparingly two to three times per day.

FORMS — Trade only: Ointment, Cream 0.05% 15, 30, 60 g. Lotion 0.05% 15, 60 mL. Tape 4 mcg/cm².

MOA — Anti-inflammatory; suppresses DNA synthesis, decreases WBC influx.

ADVERSE EFFECTS — Frequent: Burning, pruritus, dryness, irritation, erythema. Severe: Hypothalamic axis suppression with higher potency preparations.

FLUTICASONE—TOPICAL (Cutivate) ▶L ♀C ▶? $$

ADULT — Eczema: Apply sparingly one to two times per day. Other inflammatory and pruritic manifestations of corticosteroid-responsive dermatoses: Apply sparingly two times per day.

PEDS — Children older than 3 mo: Eczema: Apply sparingly one to two times per day. Other inflammatory and pruritic manifestations of corticosteroid-responsive dermatoses: Apply sparingly two times per day.

FORMS — Generic/Trade: Cream 0.05% 15, 30, 60 g. Ointment 0.005% 15, 30, 60 g. Lotion 0.05% 60, 120 mL.

NOTES — Do not use with an occlusive dressing.

MOA — Anti-inflammatory; suppresses DNA synthesis, decreases WBC influx.

ADVERSE EFFECTS — Frequent: Burning, pruritus, dryness, irritation, erythema. Severe: Hypothalamic axis suppression with higher potency preparations.

HALCINONIDE (Halog) ▶L ♀C ▶? $$

ADULT — Inflammatory and pruritic manifestations of corticosteroid-responsive dermatoses: Apply sparingly two to three times per day.

PEDS — Inflammatory and pruritic manifestations of corticosteroid-responsive dermatoses: Apply sparingly two to three times per day.

FORMS — Trade only: Cream, Ointment 0.1% 15, 30, 60 g. Soln 0.1% 20, 60 mL.

MOA — Anti-inflammatory; suppresses DNA synthesis, decreases WBC influx.

ADVERSE EFFECTS — Frequent: Burning, pruritus, dryness, irritation, erythema. Severe: Steroid atrophy, hypothalamic axis suppression with higher potency preparations.

HALOBETASOL PROPIONATE (Ultravate) ▶L ♀C ▶? $$

ADULT — Inflammatory and pruritic manifestations of corticosteroid-responsive dermatoses: Apply sparingly one to two times per day.

PEDS — Not approved in children.

FORMS — Generic/Trade: Cream, Ointment 0.05% 15, 50 g.

NOTES — Do not use occlusive dressings. Do not use for more than 2 consecutive weeks and do not exceed a total dose of 50 g/week.

MOA — Anti-inflammatory; suppresses DNA synthesis, decreases WBC influx.

ADVERSE EFFECTS — Frequent: Burning, pruritus, dryness, irritation, erythema. Severe: Steroid atrophy, hypothalamic axis suppression with higher potency preparations.

HYDROCORTISONE ACETATE (Cortaid, Corticaine, Cortifoam, Micort-HC Lipocream, ✷Hyderm, Cortamed) ▶L ♀C ▶? $

ADULT — Inflammatory and pruritic manifestations of corticosteroid-responsive dermatoses: Apply sparingly two to four times per day.

PEDS — Inflammatory and pruritic manifestations of corticosteroid-responsive dermatoses: Apply sparingly two to four times per day.

FORMS — OTC Generic/Trade: Ointment 0.5% 15 g. Ointment 1% 15, 30 g. Cream 0.5% 15 g. Cream 1% 15, 30, 60 g. Topical spray 1% 60 mL. Rx Trade only: Cream 2.5% 30 g (Micort-HC Lipocream). Rectal foam 15 g (Cortifoam).

MOA — Anti-inflammatory; suppresses DNA synthesis, decreases WBC influx.

ADVERSE EFFECTS — Frequent: Burning, pruritus, dryness, irritation, erythema.

HYDROCORTISONE BUTYRATE (Locoid, Locoid Lipocream) ▶L ♀C ▶? $$

ADULT — Inflammatory and pruritic manifestations of corticosteroid-responsive dermatoses: Apply sparingly two to three times per day. Seborrheic dermatitis (soln only): Apply two to three times per day.

(cont.)

HYDROCORTISONE BUTYRATE (cont.)

PEDS — Inflammatory and pruritic manifestations of corticosteroid-responsive dermatoses: Apply sparingly two to three times per day. Seborrheic dermatitis (soln only): Apply two to three times per day.

FORMS — Generic/Trade: Cream, Ointment 0.1% 15, 45 g. Soln 0.1% 20, 60 mL. Trade only: Cream 0.1% (Lipocream) 15, 45, 60 g.

MOA — Anti-inflammatory; suppresses DNA synthesis, decreases WBC influx.

ADVERSE EFFECTS — Frequent: Burning, pruritus, dryness, irritation, erythema. Severe: Hypothalamic axis suppression with higher potency preparations.

HYDROCORTISONE PROBUTATE (Pandel) ▶L ♀C ▶? $$

ADULT — Inflammatory and pruritic manifestations of corticosteroid-responsive dermatoses: Apply sparingly one to two times per day.

PEDS — Not approved in children.

FORMS — Trade only: Cream 0.1% 15, 45, 80 g.

MOA — Anti-inflammatory; suppresses DNA synthesis, decreases WBC influx.

ADVERSE EFFECTS — Frequent: Burning, pruritus, dryness, irritation, erythema. Severe: Hypothalamic axis suppression with higher potency preparations.

HYDROCORTISONE VALERATE (Westcort, ＊Hydroval) ▶L ♀C ▶? $$

ADULT — Inflammatory and pruritic manifestations of corticosteroid-responsive dermatoses: Apply sparingly two to three times per day.

PEDS — Safety and efficacy of Westcort ointment have not been established in children. Inflammatory and pruritic manifestations of corticosteroid-responsive dermatoses (cream only): Apply sparingly two to three times per day.

FORMS — Generic/Trade: Cream, Ointment 0.2% 15, 45, 60 g.

MOA — Anti-inflammatory; suppresses DNA synthesis, decreases WBC influx.

ADVERSE EFFECTS — Frequent: Burning, pruritus, dryness, irritation, erythema. Severe: Hypothalamic axis suppression with higher potency preparations.

HYDROCORTISONE—TOPICAL (Cortizone, Hycort, Hytone, Tegrin-HC, Dermolate, Synacort, Anusol-HC, Proctocream HC, ＊Cortoderm, Prevex-HC, Cortate, Emo-Cort) ▶L ♀C ▶? $

ADULT — Inflammatory and pruritic manifestations of corticosteroid-responsive dermatoses: Apply sparingly two to four times per day. External anal itching: Apply cream three to four times per day prn or suppository two times per day or rectal foam one to two times per day.

PEDS — Inflammatory and pruritic manifestations of corticosteroid-responsive dermatoses: Apply sparingly two to four times per day.

FORMS — Products available OTC and Rx depending on labeling. 2.5% preparation available Rx only. Generic/Trade: Ointment 0.5% 30 g. Ointment 1% 15, 20, 30, 60, 454 g. Ointment 2.5% 5, 20, 30, 454 g. Cream 0.5% 30 g. Cream 1% 5, 15, 20, 30,

120 g. Cream 2.5% 5, 20, 30, 454 g. Lotion 1% 120 mL. Lotion 2.5% 60 mL. Anal preparations: Generic/Trade: Cream 2.5% 30 g (Anusol HC, Proctocream HC). Suppositories 25 mg (Anusol HC).

MOA — Anti-inflammatory; suppresses DNA synthesis, decreases WBC influx.

ADVERSE EFFECTS — Frequent: Burning, pruritus, dryness, irritation, erythema.

MOMETASONE—TOPICAL (Elocon, ＊Elocom) ▶L ♀C ▶? $

ADULT — Inflammatory and pruritic manifestations of corticosteroid-responsive dermatoses: Apply sparingly once a day.

PEDS — Inflammatory and pruritic manifestations of corticosteroid-responsive dermatoses: Apply sparingly once a day for age 2 yo or older. Safety and efficacy for more than 3 weeks have not been established.

FORMS — Generic/Trade: Cream, Ointment 0.1% 15, 45 g. Lotion 0.1% 30, 60 mL.

NOTES — Do not use an occlusive dressing. Not for ophthalmic use.

MOA — Anti-inflammatory; suppresses DNA synthesis, decreases WBC influx.

ADVERSE EFFECTS — Frequent: Burning, pruritus, dryness, irritation, erythema. Severe: Hypothalamic axis suppression with higher potency preparations, skin atrophy.

PREDNICARBATE (Dermatop) ▶L ♀C ▶? $$

ADULT — Inflammatory and pruritic manifestations of corticosteroid-responsive dermatoses: Apply sparingly two times per day.

PEDS — Inflammatory and pruritic manifestations of corticosteroid-responsive dermatoses: Apply sparingly two times per day for age 1 yo or older. Safety and efficacy for more than 3 weeks have not been established.

FORMS — Generic/Trade: Cream, Ointment 0.1% 15, 60 g.

NOTES — Can damage latex (condoms, diaphragms, etc.). Avoid contact with latex.

MOA — Anti-inflammatory; suppresses DNA synthesis, decreases WBC influx.

ADVERSE EFFECTS — Frequent: Burning, pruritus, dryness, irritation, erythema. Severe: Hypothalamic axis suppression with higher potency preparations.

TRIAMCINOLONE—TOPICAL (Kenalog, Kenalog in Orabase, Trianex, ＊Oracort, Triaderm) ▶L ♀C ▶? $

ADULT — Inflammatory and pruritic manifestations of corticosteroid-responsive dermatoses: Apply sparingly three to four times per day. Oral paste: Aphthous ulcers: Using finger, apply about 1 cm of paste to oral lesion and a thin film will develop. Apply paste two to three times per day, ideally after meals and at bedtime.

PEDS — Inflammatory and pruritic manifestations of corticosteroid-responsive dermatoses: Apply sparingly three to four times per day.

FORMS — Generic Only: Cream, 0.1% 15, 30, 80, 454 g. Cream 0.5% 15 g. Cream 0.025% 15, 80, 454 g. Ointment, 0.1% 15, 80, 454g. Ointment,

TRIAMCINOLONE—TOPICAL (*cont.*)

0.5% 15 g, Ointment, 0.025% 15, 80, 454 g. Lotion 0.025% and 0.1% 60 mL. Generic/Trade: Oral paste (in Orabase) 0.1% 5 g. Trade only: Ointment (Trianex), 0.05% 17, 85g. Aerosol topical spray 0.147 mg/g, 63, 100 g.

MOA — Anti-inflammatory; suppresses DNA synthesis, decreases WBC influx.
ADVERSE EFFECTS — Frequent: Burning, pruritus, dryness, irritation, erythema. Severe: Steroid atrophy, hypothalamic axis suppression with higher potency preparations.

DERMATOLOGY: Hemorrhoid Care

ANALPRAM-HC, EPIFOAM, PROCTOFOAM HC (hydrocortisone—topical + pramoxine—topical) ▶L ♀C ▶? $$$
ADULT — Inflammatory and pruritic manifestations of corticosteroid-responsive dermatoses of the anal region: Apply two to four times per day.
PEDS — Use with caution. Inflammatory and pruritic manifestations of corticosteroid-responsive dermatoses of the anal region: Apply two to four times per day.
FORMS — Trade only: Topical aerosol foam (Proctofoam HC, Epifoam 1% hydrocortisone + 1% pramoxine) 10 g. Cream (Analpram-HC 1% hydrocortisone + 1% pramoxine, 2.5% hydrocortisone + 1% pramoxine) 4 g, 30 g. Lotion (Analpram-HC 2.5% hydrocortisone + 1% pramoxine) 60 mL.
MOA — Combination of local anesthetic and anti-inflammatory; suppresses DNA synthesis, decreases WBC influx.
ADVERSE EFFECTS — Frequent: Redness, irritation, pain.

DIBUCAINE (*Nupercainal*) ▶L ♀? ▶? $
ADULT — Hemorrhoids or other anorectal disorders: Apply three to four times per day prn.
PEDS — Not approved in children.
UNAPPROVED PEDS — Hemorrhoids or other anorectal disorders: Apply three to four times per day prn for age older than 2 yo or wt greater than 35 lbs or 15.9 kg.
FORMS — OTC Trade only: Ointment 1% 30, 60 g.
NOTES — Do not use if younger than 2 yo or wt less than 35 pounds.

MOA — Anesthetic, anti-inflammatory.
ADVERSE EFFECTS — Frequent: None.
PRAMOXINE (*Tucks Hemorrhoidal Ointment, Fleet Pain Relief, ProctoFoam NS*) ▶not absorbed ♀+ ▶+ $
ADULT — Hemorrhoids: Apply ointment, pads, or foam up to 5 times per day prn.
PEDS — Not approved in children.
FORMS — OTC Trade only: Ointment (Tucks Hemorrhoidal Ointment) 30 g. Pads (Fleet Pain Relief) 100 each. Aerosol foam (ProctoFoam NS) 15 g.
MOA — Anesthetic.
ADVERSE EFFECTS — Frequent: Redness, irritation, swelling, pain.
STARCH (*Tucks Suppositories*) ▶not absorbed ♀+ ▶+ $
ADULT — Hemorrhoids: 1 suppository PR up to 6 times per day prn or after each bowel movement.
PEDS — Not approved in children.
FORMS — OTC Trade only: Suppository (51% topical starch; vegetable oil, tocopheryl acetate) 12, 24 each.
MOA — Lubricant.
ADVERSE EFFECTS — Frequent: None.
WITCH HAZEL (*Tucks*) ▶? ♀+ ▶+ $
ADULT — Hemorrhoids: Apply to anus/perineum up to 6 times per day prn.
PEDS — Not approved in children.
FORMS — OTC Generic/Trade: Pads 50% 12, 40, 100 ea, generically available in various quantities.
MOA — Astringent.
ADVERSE EFFECTS — Frequent: None.

DERMATOLOGY: Other Dermatologic Agents

ALITRETINOIN (*Panretin, ✣Toctino*) ▶not absorbed ♀D ▶– $$$$$
WARNING — May cause fetal harm if significant absorption were to occur. Women of child-bearing age should be advised to avoid becoming pregnant during treatment.
ADULT — Cutaneous lesions of AIDS-related Kaposi's sarcoma: Apply two to four times per day.
PEDS — Not approved in children.
FORMS — Trade only: Gel 0.1% 60 g.
MOA — Binds retinoid receptors to inhibit Kaposi's sarcoma.
ADVERSE EFFECTS — Frequent: Pain, rash, pruritus, paresthesia, edema, dermatitis.
ALUMINUM CHLORIDE (*Drysol, Certain Dri*) ▶K ♀? ▶? $
ADULT — Hyperhidrosis: Apply at bedtime. For maximum effect, cover area with plastic wrap held in place with tight shirt and wash area following

morning. Once excessive sweating stopped, use once a week or twice a week.
PEDS — Not approved in children.
FORMS — Rx Trade only: Soln 20% 37.5 mL bottle, 35, 60 mL bottle with applicator. OTC Trade only (Certain Dri): Soln 12.5% 36 mL bottle.
NOTES — To prevent irritation, apply to dry area.
MOA — Astringent.
ADVERSE EFFECTS — Frequent: Irritation, burning, prickling.
BECAPLERMIN (*Regranex*) ▶minimal absorption ♀C ▶? $$$$$
WARNING — Increased rate of mortality due to malignancy in patients who used 3 or more tubes. Use with caution in patients with known malignancy.
ADULT — Diabetic neuropathic ulcers: Apply daily and cover with saline-moistened gauze for 12 h. Rinse after 12 h and cover with saline gauze without medication.

(cont.)

BECAPLERMIN (*cont.*)

PEDS — Not approved in children.

FORMS — Trade only: Gel 0.01%, 2, 15 g.

NOTES — Length of gel to be applied calculated by size of wound (length × width × 0.6 = amount of gel in inches). If ulcer does not decrease by 30% in size by 10 weeks or complete healing has not occurred by 20 weeks, continued therapy should be reassessed. Ineffective for stasis ulcers and pressure ulcers. Increased cancer mortality in patients who use 3 or more tubes of the product.

MOA — Recombinant human platelet-derived growth factor, which promotes cellular proliferation and angiogenesis, enhances new granulation tissue, and induces fibroblast proliferation and differentiation.

ADVERSE EFFECTS — Frequent: None Severe: Increased cancer mortality.

BRIMONIDINE (*Mirvaso*) ▶L ♀B ▶- $$$$$

ADULT — Persistent erythema associated with rosacea: Apply once daily to chin, forehead, nose, and each cheek.

PEDS — Not approved in children younger than 18 years.

FORMS — 0.33% gel, 30 g.

NOTES — Use caution in patients with severe or uncontrolled CV disease. May potentiate vascular insufficiency.

MOA — alpha adrenergic agonist.

ADVERSE EFFECTS — Common: erythema, flushing, burning, contact dermatitis.

CALAMINE ▶? ♀? ▶? $

ADULT — Itching due to poison ivy/oak/sumac, insect bites, or minor irritation: Apply up to three to four times per day prn.

PEDS — Itching due to poison ivy/oak/sumac, insect bites, or minor irritation: Apply up to three to four times per day prn for age older than 2 yo.

FORMS — OTC Generic only: Lotion 120, 240, 480 mL.

MOA — Astringent.

ADVERSE EFFECTS — Frequent: Dryness.

CAPSAICIN (*Zostrix, Zostrix-HP, Qutenza*) ▶? ♀? ▶? $

ADULT — Pain due to RA, OA, and neuralgias such as zoster or diabetic neuropathies: Apply to affected area up to three to four times per day. Post herpetic neuralgia: 1 patch (Qutenza) applied for one h in medical office, may repeat q 3 months.

PEDS — Children older than 2 yo: Pain due to RA, OA, and neuralgias such as zoster or diabetic neuropathies: Apply to affected area up to three to four times per day.

UNAPPROVED ADULT — Psoriasis and intractable pruritus, postmastectomy/postamputation neuromas (phantom limb pain), vulvar vestibulitis, apocrine chromhidrosis, and reflex sympathetic dystrophy.

FORMS — Rx: Patch 8% (Qutenza). OTC Generic/Trade: Cream 0.025% 60 g, 0.075% (HP) 60 g. OTC Generic only: Lotion 0.025% 59 mL, 0.075% 59 mL.

NOTES — Burning occurs in 30% or more of patients but diminishes with continued use. Pain more commonly occurs when applied less than three to four times per day. Wash hands immediately after application.

MOA — Counter-irritant, releases Substance P.

ADVERSE EFFECTS — Frequent: Burning, redness, sensation of warmth.

COAL TAR (*Polytar, Tegrin, Cutar, Tarsum*) ▶? ♀? ▶? $

ADULT — Dandruff, seborrheic dermatitis: Apply shampoo at least twice a week. Psoriasis: Apply to affected areas one to four times per day or use shampoo on affected areas.

PEDS — Children older than 2 yo: Dandruff, seborrheic dermatitis: Apply shampoo at least twice a week. Psoriasis: Apply to affected areas one to four times per day or use shampoo on affected areas.

FORMS — OTC Generic/Trade: Shampoo, cream, ointment, gel, lotion, liquid, oil, soap.

NOTES — May cause photosensitivity for up to 24 h after application.

MOA — Unknown.

ADVERSE EFFECTS — Frequent: folliculitis, skin and hair staining, photosensitivity, contact dermatitis.

DEET (*Off, Cutter, Repel, Ultrathon, n-n-diethyl-m-toluamide*) ▶L ♀+ ▶+ $

ADULT — Mosquito repellant: 10% to 50% every 2 to 6 h. Higher concentration products do not work better, but have a longer duration of action.

PEDS — Up to 30% spray/lotion every 2 to 6 h for age 2 mo or older.

FORMS — OTC Generic/Trade: Spray, lotion, towelette 4.75% to 100%.

NOTES — Duration of action varies by concentration. For example, 23.8% DEET provides approximately 5 h of protection from mosquito bites, 20% DEET provides approximately 4 h of protection, 6.65% DEET provides approximately 2 h of protection and products with 4.75% DEET provides approximately 1.5 h of protection. Apply sunscreen prior to application of DEET-containing products.

MOA — Repels female mosquitos; does not kill them.

ADVERSE EFFECTS — Frequent: Dermatitis.

DOXEPIN—TOPICAL (*Zonalon*) ▶L ♀B ▶- $$$$

ADULT — Pruritus associated with atopic dermatitis, lichen simplex chronicus, eczematous dermatitis: Apply four times per day for up to 8 days.

PEDS — Not approved in children.

FORMS — Trade only: Cream 5% 30, 45 g.

NOTES — Risk of systemic toxicity increased if applied to more than 10% of body. Can cause contact dermatitis.

MOA — Inhibits pre-synaptic uptake of serotonin +/- norepinephrine.

ADVERSE EFFECTS — Frequent: None.

EFLORNITHINE (*Vaniqa*) ▶K ♀C ▶? $$$

ADULT — Reduction of facial hair: Apply to face two times per day at least 8 h apart.

PEDS — Not approved in children.

FORMS — Trade only: Cream 13.9% 30 g.

NOTES — Takes 4 to 8 weeks or more to see an effect.

EFLORNITHINE (*cont.*)

MOA — Specific, irreversible inhibition of ornithine decarboxylase, reduces length of growing cycle so hair becomes progressively shorter.

ADVERSE EFFECTS — Frequent: Stinging, burning, tingling, erythema, rash.

EMLA (**prilocaine—topical + lidocaine—topical**) ▶LK ♀B ▶? $$

ADULT — Topical anesthesia for minor dermal procedures (e.g., IV cannulation, venipuncture): apply 2.5 g over 20 to 25 cm² area or 1 disc at least 1 h prior to procedure, for major dermal procedures (i.e., skin grafting harvesting) apply 2 g/10 cm² area at least 2 h prior to procedure.

PEDS — Prior to circumcision in infants older than 37 weeks gestation: Apply a max dose 1 g over max of 10 cm². Topical anesthesia: Children age 1 to 3 mo or less than 5 kg: Apply a max 1 g dose over max of 10 cm²; age 4 to 12 mo and more than 5 kg: Apply max 2 g dose over a max of 20 cm²; age 1 to 6 yo and more than 10 kg: Apply max dose 10 g over max of 100 cm²; age 7 to 12 yo and more than 20 kg: Apply max dose 20 g over max of 200 cm².

FORMS — Generic/Trade: Cream (2.5% lidocaine + 2.5% prilocaine) 5, 30 g.

NOTES — Cover cream with an occlusive dressing. Do not use in children younger than 12 mo if child is receiving treatment with methemoglobin-inducing agents. Do not use on open wounds. Patients with glucose-6-phosphate deficiencies are more susceptible to methemoglobinemia. Use caution with amiodarone, bretylium, sotalol, dofetilide; possible additive cardiac effects. Dermal analgesia increases for up to 3 h under occlusive dressings and persists for 1 to 2 h after removal.

MOA — Anesthetic.

ADVERSE EFFECTS — Frequent: None. Severe: CNS effects, tachycardia, bronchospasm, hypotension.

HYALURONIC ACID (**Bionect, Restylane, Perlane**) ▶? ♀? ▶? $$$

ADULT — Moderate to severe facial wrinkles: Inject into wrinkle/fold (Restylane, Perlane). Protection of dermal ulcers: Apply gel/cream/spray to wound two or three times per day (Bionect).

PEDS — Not approved in children.

FORMS — OTC Trade only: Cream 2% 15, 30 g. Rx Generic/Trade: Soln 3% 30 mL. Gel 4% 30 g. Cream 4% 15, 30, 60 g. Injectable gel 2%.

NOTES — Do not use more than 1.5 mL of injectable form per treatment area. Injectable product contains trace amounts of Gram-positive bacterial proteins; contraindicated if history of anaphylaxis or severe allergy.

MOA — Increases volume under skin to smooth out wrinkle.

ADVERSE EFFECTS — Frequent (injectable product): Bruising, redness, swelling, pain, tenderness, itching. Severe (injectable product): Bacterial infections, anaphylaxis, severe allergic reactions.

IVERMECTIN—TOPICAL (**Sklice**) ▶minimal absorption - ♀C ▶? $$$$

ADULT — Head lice: Apply to dry hair and scalp. Rinse after 10 minutes. Second application not necessary.

PEDS — Not approved in children younger than 6 mo. In children 6 mo and older, use adult dosing.

FORMS — Trade: Lotion 0.5%, 120 mL.

MOA — Selectively binds glutamate-gated chloride channels, resulting in louse paralysis and death.

ADVERSE EFFECTS — Frequent: conjunctivitis, ocular hyperemia, eye irritation, dandruff, dry skin, and skin burning sensation.

LACTIC ACID (**Lac-Hydrin, AmLactin, ✤Dermalac**) ▶? ♀? ▶? $$

ADULT — Ichthyosis vulgaris and xerosis (dry, scaly skin): Apply two times per day to affected area.

PEDS — Ichthyosis vulgaris and xerosis (dry, scaly skin) in children older than 2 yo: Apply two times per day to affected area.

FORMS — Trade only: Lotion 12% 150, 360 mL. OTC: Cream 12% 140, 385 g. AmLactin AP is lactic acid (12%) with pramoxine (1%).

NOTES — Frequently causes irritation in non-intact skin. Minimize exposure to sun, artificial sunlight.

MOA — Humectant, reduce corneocyte cohesion.

ADVERSE EFFECTS — Frequent: Stinging, burning.

LIDOCAINE—TOPICAL (**Xylocaine, Lidoderm, Numby Stuff, LMX, Zingo, ✤Maxilene**) ▶LK ♀B ▶+ $ - varies by therapy

WARNING — Contraindicated in allergy to amide-type anesthetics.

ADULT — Topical anesthesia: Apply to affected area prn. Dose varies with anesthetic procedure, degree of anesthesia required and individual patient response. Postherpetic neuralgia (patch): Apply up to 3 patches to affected area at once for up to 12 h within a 24 h period.

PEDS — Topical anesthesia: Apply to affected area prn. Dose varies with anesthetic procedure, degree of anesthesia required and individual patient response. Max 3 mg/kg/dose, do not repeat dose within 2 h. Intradermal powder injection for venipuncture/IV cannulation, for age 3 to 18 yo (Zingo): 0.5 mg to site 1 to 10 min prior.

UNAPPROVED PEDS — Topical anesthesia prior to venipuncture: Apply 30 min prior to procedure (ELA-Max 4%).

FORMS — For membranes of mouth and pharynx: Spray 10%, Ointment 5%, Liquid 5%, Soln 2%, 4%, Dental patch. For urethral use: Jelly 2%. Patch (Lidoderm $$$$$) 5%. Intradermal powder injection system: 0.5 mg (Zingo). OTC Trade only: Liposomal lidocaine 4% (ELA-Max).

NOTES — Apply patches only to intact skin to cover the most painful area. Patches may be cut into smaller sizes with scissors prior to removal of the release liner. Store and dispose out of the reach of children and pets to avoid possible toxicity from ingestion.

MOA — Anesthetic.

(cont.)

LIDOCAINE—TOPICAL (*cont.*)

ADVERSE EFFECTS — Frequent: Skin irritation. Severe: CNS effects, bradycardia, bronchospasm, hypotension, allergic reactions.

MINOXIDIL—TOPICAL (*Rogaine, Women's Rogaine, Rogaine Extra Strength, Minoxidil for Men*) ▶K ♀C ▶– $

ADULT — Androgenetic alopecia in men or women: 1 mL to dry scalp two times per day.

PEDS — Not approved in children.

UNAPPROVED ADULT — Alopecia areata.

UNAPPROVED PEDS — Alopecia: Apply to dry scalp two times per day.

FORMS — OTC Generic/Trade: Soln 2% 60 mL (Rogaine, Women's Rogaine). Soln 5% 60 mL (Rogaine Extra Strength, Theroxidil Extra Strength—for men only). Foam 5% 60 g (Rogaine Extra Strength).

NOTES — 5% strength for men only. Alcohol content may cause burning and stinging. Evidence of hair growth usually takes at least 4 months. If treatment is stopped, new hair will be shed in a few months.

MOA — Promotes hair growth.

ADVERSE EFFECTS — None.

MONOBENZONE (*Benoquin*) ▶minimal absorption ♀C ▶? $$$

ADULT — Extensive vitiligo: Apply two to three times per day.

PEDS — Not approved age in children younger than 12 yo.

FORMS — Trade only: Cream 20% 35.4 g.

NOTES — Avoid prolonged exposure to sunlight. May take 1 to 4 months for depigmentation to occur. Depigmentation is permanent and can cause lifelong increase in photosensitivity.

MOA — Increases excretion of melanin from melanocytes.

ADVERSE EFFECTS — Frequent: Minor skin irritation.

OATMEAL (*Aveeno*) ▶not absorbed ♀? ▶? $

ADULT — Pruritus from poison ivy/oak, varicella: Apply lotion four times per day prn. Also available in packets to be added to bath.

PEDS — Pruritus from poison ivy/oak, varicella: Apply lotion four times per day prn. Also available in bath packets for tub.

FORMS — OTC Generic/Trade: Lotion. Bath packets.

MOA — Anti-pruritic, lubricating.

ADVERSE EFFECTS — Frequent: None.

PANAFIL (papain + urea + chlorophyllin copper complex) ▶? ♀? ▶? $$$

ADULT — Debridement of acute or chronic lesions: Apply to clean wound and cover one to two times per day.

PEDS — Not approved in children.

FORMS — Trade only: Ointment 6, 30 g. Spray 33 mL.

NOTES — Longer redressings (2 to 3 days) are acceptable. May be applied under pressure dressings. Hydrogen peroxide inactivates papain; avoid concomitant use.

MOA — Enzymatic debridement.

ADVERSE EFFECTS — Frequent: Burning, profuse exudates.

PLIAGLIS (tetracaine—topical + lidocaine—topical) ▶minimal absorption ♀B ▶? $$

WARNING — Contraindicated in allergy to amide-type anesthetics.

ADULT — Prior to venipuncture, intravenous cannulation, superficial dermatological procedure: Apply 20 to 30 min prior to procedure. Tattoo removal: Apply 60 min prior to procedure.

PEDS — Not approved in children.

FORMS — Trade only: Cream lidocaine 7% + tetracaine 7%.

MOA — Topical anesthetic.

ADVERSE EFFECTS — Frequent: Skin irritation, erythema, blanching, rash. Severe: CNS effects, bradycardia, bronchospasm, hypotension.

POLIDOCANOL (*Asclera*) ▶minimal absorption ♀C ▶? $$$$$

ADULT — Varicose veins: Variable dose injected into varicose vein, depending on size and extent of varicose vein.

PEDS — Not approved for use in children.

FORMS — Trade: Inj soln 0.5% and 1%.

MOA — Sclerosing agent.

ADVERSE EFFECTS — Common: mild, local reactions at site of injection. Severe: anaphylaxis

POLY-L-LACTIC ACID (*Sculptra*) ▶not absorbed ♀? ▶? $$$$$

ADULT — Restoration of facial fat loss due to HIV lipoatrophy: Dose based on degree of correction needed.

PEDS — Not approved in children younger than 18 years.

MOA — Biocompatible, biodegradable, synthetic polymer.

ADVERSE EFFECTS — Frequent: Bruising, edema, discomfort, hematoma, inflammation, erythema, injection site papule.

PRAMOSONE (pramoxine—topical + hydrocortisone—topical, ✱*Pramox HC*) ▶not absorbed ♀C ▶? $$$

ADULT — Apply three to four times per day.

PEDS — Apply two to three times per day.

FORMS — Trade only: 1% pramoxine/1% hydrocortisone: Cream 30, 60 g. Ointment 30 g. Lotion 60, 120, 240 mL. 1% pramoxine/2.5% hydrocortisone acetate: Cream 30, 60 g. Ointment 30 g. Lotion 60, 120 mL.

NOTES — Monitor for hyperglycemia/adrenal suppression if used for long period of time or over a large area of the body, especially in children. Chronic administration may interfere with pediatric growth and development.

MOA — Anti-inflammatory; suppresses DNA synthesis, decreases WBC influx.

ADVERSE EFFECTS — Frequent: Burning, pruritus, dryness, irritation, erythema.

SELENIUM SULFIDE (*Selsun, Exsel, Versel*) ▶? ♀C ▶? $

ADULT — Dandruff, seborrheic dermatitis: Massage 5 to 10 mL of shampoo into wet scalp, allow to remain 2 to 3 min, rinse. Apply twice a week for 2 weeks. For maintenance, less frequent administration needed.

SELENIUM SULFIDE (*cont.*)

Tinea versicolor: Apply 2.5% shampoo/lotion to affected area, allow to remain on skin 10 min, rinse. Repeat daily for 7 days.

PEDS — Dandruff, seborrheic dermatitis: Massage 5 to 10 mL of shampoo into wet scalp, allow to remain 2 to 3 min, rinse. Apply twice a week for 2 weeks. For maintenance, less frequent administration needed. Tinea versicolor: Apply 2.5% lotion/shampoo to affected area, allow to remain on skin 10 min, rinse. Repeat daily for 7 days.

FORMS — OTC Generic/Trade: Lotion/Shampoo 1% 120, 210, 240, 325 mL, 2.5% 120 mL. Rx Generic/Trade: Lotion/Shampoo 2.5% 120 mL.

MOA — May inhibit epidermal growth enzymes.

ADVERSE EFFECTS — Frequent: Unusual dryness, oiliness of skin.

***SOLAGE* (mequinol + tretinoin)** ▶not absorbed ♀X ▶? $$$$
ADULT — Canada only. Solar lentigines: Apply two times per day separated by at least 8 h.

PEDS — Not approved in children.

FORMS — Trade only: Soln 30 mL (mequinol 2% + tretinoin 0.01%).

NOTES — Use in non-Caucasians has not been evaluated. Avoid in patients taking photosensitizers. Minimize exposure to sunlight.

MOA — Competitively inhibits melantin precursors.

ADVERSE EFFECTS — Frequent: Erythema, burning, stinging, pruritus, desquamation.

SUNSCREEN ▶minimal absorption ♀? ▶+ $
ADULT — Apply at least 2 tablespoons for full body coverage 30 minutes before going outdoors. If in the sun between 10 am and 4 pm, reapply sunscreen q 2 h (more often if swimming or sweating).

PEDS — Avoid sun exposure if younger than 6 mo. For age 6 mo or older: Apply at least 2 tablespoons for full body coverage 30 minutes before going outdoors. If in the sun between 10 am and 4 pm, reapply sunscreen q 2 h (more often if swimming or sweating). Apply prior to sun exposure.

FORMS — Many formulations available.

NOTES — Sun protection factor (SPF) numbers equal the ratio of doses of ultraviolet radiation (predominantly UVB radiation) that result in sunburn with protection to the doses that result in erythema without protection. SPF 2 equals a 50% block, SPF 15 equals a 93% block, and SPF 45 equals a 98% block.

MOA — Physical block from sun (eg, zinc, titanium oxide); or absorption of high-energy ultraviolet rays and release as lower-energy rays, thereby preventing the skin-damaging ultraviolet rays from reaching the skin (eg, avobenzone).

ADVERSE EFFECTS — Frequent: irritation.

***SYNERA* (tetracaine—topical + lidocaine—topical)** ▶minimal absorption ♀B ▶? $$
WARNING — Contraindicated in allergy to amide-type anesthetics.

ADULT — Prior to venipuncture, intravenous cannulation, superficial dermatological procedure: Apply 20 to 30 min prior to procedure.

PEDS — Children 3 yo or older: Prior to venipuncture, IV cannulation, superficial dermatological procedure: Apply 20 to 30 min prior to procedure.

FORMS — Trade only: Topical patch (lidocaine 70 mg + tetracaine 70 mg.

NOTES — Do not cut patch or remove top cover.

MOA — Topical anesthetic.

ADVERSE EFFECTS — Frequent: Skin irritation, erythema, blanching, rash. Severe: CNS effects, bradycardia, bronchospasm, hypotension.

***TRI-LUMA* (fluocinolone—topical + hydroquinone + tretinoin)** ▶minimal absorption ♀C ▶? $$$$
ADULT — Melasma of the face: Apply at bedtime for 4 to 8 weeks.

PEDS — Not approved in children.

FORMS — Trade only: Cream 30 g (fluocinolone 0.01% + hydroquinone 4% + tretinoin 0.05%).

NOTES — Minimize exposure to sunlight. Not intended for melasma maintenance therapy.

MOA — Competitively inhibits melantin precursors, anti-inflammatory.

ADVERSE EFFECTS — Frequent: Erythema, desquamation, burning, dryness, pruritus, acne.

***VUSION* (miconazole—topical + zinc oxide + white petrolatum)** ▶minimal absorption ♀C ▶? $$$$$
ADULT — Not approved in adults.

PEDS — Apply to affected diaper area with each change for 7 days.

FORMS — Trade only: Ointment 50 g.

NOTES — Use only in documented cases of candidiasis.

MOA — Antifungal; alters fungal cell wall permeability; barrier.

ADVERSE EFFECTS — Frequent: None.

***XERESE* (acyclovir + hydrocortisone)** ▶minimal absorption ♀B ▶? $$$$$
ADULT — Recurrent herpes labialis: Apply 5 times a day, starting at the first signs and symptoms.

PEDS — Recurrent herpes labialis (6 years or older): Apply 5 times a day, starting at the first signs and symptoms.

MOA — Herpes simplex virus analog DNA polymerase inhibitor

ADVERSE EFFECTS — Frequent: dryness, flaking of skin, burning, tingling. erythema, pigmentation changes, inflammation.

ENDOCRINE AND METABOLIC

A1C REDUCTION IN TYPE 2 DIABETES

Intervention	Expected A1C Reduction with Monotherapy
Alpha-glucosidase inhibitors	0.5–0.8%
DPP-4 Inhibitors (gliptins)	0.5–0.8%
GLP-1 agonists	0.5–1%
Insulin	1.5–3.5%
Lifestyle modifications	1–2%
Meglitinides	0.5–1.5%
Metformin	1–2%
Pramlintide	0.5–1%
SGLT2 inhibitors	0.7–1%
Sulfonylureas	1–2%
Thiazolidinediones	0.5–1.4%

References: *Diabetes Care* 2009; 32:195. *Diabetes Obes Metab* 2013;15:372–82. Farxiga product information, 1/2014.

CORTICOSTEROIDS

CORTICOSTEROIDS	Approximate Equivalent Dose (mg)	Relative Anti-inflammatory Potency	Relative Mineralocorti-coid Potency	Biological Half-life (h)
betamethasone	0.6–0.75	20–30	0	36–54
cortisone	25	0.8	2	8–12
dexamethasone	0.75	20–30	0	36–54
fludrocortisone	n.a	10	125	18–36
hydrocortisone	20	1	2	8–12
methylprednisolone	4	5	0	18–36
prednisolone	5	4	1	18–36
prednisone	5	4	1	18–36
triamcinolone	4	5	0	12–36

n.a., not available.

DIABETES NUMBERS*

Criteria for diagnosis	Self-monitoring glucose goals
Pre- diabetes: Fasting glucose 100–125 mg/dL or A1C 5.7–6.4% or 140–199 mg/dL 2 h after 75 g oral glucose load	Preprandial: 70–130 mg/dL Postprandial: < 180 mg/dL
Diabetes:[†] A1C ≥ 6.5% Fasting glucose ≥ 126 mg/dL Random glucose with symptoms: ≥ 200 mg/dL, or ≥ 200 mg/dL 2 h after 75 g oral glucose load	**A1C goal:** < 7% for most non-pregnant adults, individualize based on age, comorbid conditions, microvascular complications, known cardiovascular disease hypoglycemia, and other patient specific factors. A1C goal < 7.5% for pediatric Type 1 Diabetes.

Hospitalized patients: may consider more stringent goal if safely achievable without hypoglycemia
Critically ill glucose goal: 140–180 mg/d

Non-critically ill glucose goal (hospitalized patients): premeal blood glucose < 140 mg/dL, random < 180 mg/dL

Estimated average glucose (eAG): eAG (mg/dL) = (28.7 x A1C) − 46.7

Complications prevention & management: ASA[‡] (75–162 mg/day) in Type 1 & 2 adults for primary prevention if 10-year cardiovascular risk > 10% (includes most men older than 50 yo or women older than 60 yo with at least one other major risk factor) and secondary prevention (those with vascular disease); statin therapy to achieve goal LDL regardless of baseline LDL (for those with vascular disease, those older than 40 yo and additional risk factor, or those younger than 40 yo but LDL > 100 mg/dL); ACE inhibitor or ARB if hypertensive or albuminuria; pneumococcal vaccine (revaccinate one time if age 65 yo or older and previously received vaccine at age younger than 65 and more than 5 years ago); hepatitis B vaccine if previously unvaccinated and 19 to 59 yo, consider if age 60 yo or older.

Every visit: Measure wt & BP (goal < 140/80 mm Hg[§]); visual foot exam; review self-monitoring glucose record; review/adjust meds; review self-mgmt skills, dietary needs, and physical activity; smoking cessation counseling.

Twice a year: A1C in those meeting treatment goals with stable glycemia (quarterly if not); dental exam.
Annually: Fasting lipid profile** [goal LDL < 100 mg/dL, cardiovascular disease consider LDL < 70 mg/dL; HDL > 40 mg/dL (> 50 mg/dL in women), TG < 150 mg/dL], q 2 years with low-risk lipid values; creatinine; albumin to creatinine ratio spot collection; dilated eye exam (q2 years if no evidence of retinopathy); flu vaccine.

*See recommendations at: care.diabetesjournals.org. References: Diabetes Care 2014;37(Suppl 1): S14–80. Diabetes Care. 2014;37:2034–2054.
Glucose values are plasma.
[†]In the absence of symptoms, confirm diagnosis with glucose testing on subsequent day.
[‡]Avoid ASA if younger than 21 yo due to Reye's Syndrome risk; use if younger than 30 yo has not beenstudied.
[§]Lower systolic targets (i.e. < 130 mm Hg) may be considered on a patient-specific basis if treatment goals can be met without excessive treatment burden.
**LDL is primary target of therapy, consider 30 to 40% LDL reduction from baseline as alternate goal if unable to reach targets on maximal tolerated statin.

IV SOLUTIONS

Solution	Dextrose	Calories/ Liter	Na*	Ca*	Lactate*	Osm*
0.9 NS	0 g/L	0	154	0	0	310
LR	0 g/L	9	130	3	28	273
D5 W	50 g/L	170	0	0	0	253
D5 0.2 NS	50 g/L	170	34	0	0	320
D5 0.45 NS	50 g/L	170	77	0	0	405
D5 0.9 NS	50 g/L	170	154	0	0	560
D5 LR	50 g/L	170	130	2.7	28	527

* All given in mEq/L

ENDOCRINE AND METABOLIC: Androgens / Anabolic Steroids

NOTE: See OB/GYN section for other hormones.

FLUOXYMESTERONE (*Halotestin, Androxy*) ▶L ♀X ▶? ©III $$$$
ADULT — Palliative treatment of androgen-responsive recurrent breast cancer in women who are 1 to 5 years postmenopausal: 5 to 10 mg PO two to four times per day for 1 to 3 months.
PEDS — Delayed puberty in males: 2.5 to 10 mg PO daily for 4 to 6 months.
FORMS — Generic only: Tabs 10 mg.
NOTES — Transdermal or injectable therapy preferred for hypogonadism. Pediatric use by specialists who monitor bone maturation q 6 months. Prolonged high-dose use may cause hepatic adenomas, hepatocellular carcinoma, and peliosis hepatitis. Monitor LFTs. Monitor Hb for polycythemia.
MOA — Steroid with anabolic and androgenic actions.
ADVERSE EFFECTS — Serious: Peliosis hepatitis, liver tumors, cholestatic hepatitis, habituation, heart failure exacerbation, polycythemia. Frequent: Virilization, testicular atrophy, oligospermia, excitation, insomnia, anxiety, depression, paresthesia, altered libido, bladder irritability, menstrual irregularity, gynecomastia, acne, edema, lipid abnormalities.

METHYLTESTOSTERONE (*Android, Methitest, Testred, Virilon*) ▶L ♀X ▶? ©III $$$
ADULT — Advancing inoperable breast cancer in women who are 1 to 5 years postmenopausal: 50 to 200 mg/day PO in divided doses.
PEDS — Delayed puberty in males: 10 mg PO daily for 4 to 6 months.
FORMS — Trade/Generic: Caps 10 mg, Tabs 10, 25 mg.
NOTES — Transdermal or injectable therapy preferred to oral for hypogonadism. Pediatric use by specialists who monitor bone maturation q 6 months. Prolonged high-dose use may cause hepatic adenomas, hepatocellular carcinoma, and peliosis hepatitis. Monitor LFTs. Monitor Hb for polycythemia.
MOA — Steroid with anabolic and androgenic actions.
ADVERSE EFFECTS — Serious: Peliosis hepatitis, liver tumors, cholestatic hepatitis, habituation, heart failure exacerbation, polycythemia. Frequent: Virilization, testicular atrophy, oligospermia, excitation, insomnia, anxiety, depression, paresthesia, altered libido, bladder irritability, menstrual irregularity, gynecomastia, acne, edema, lipid abnormalities.

OXANDROLONE (*Oxandrin*) ▶L ♀X ▶? ©III $$$$$
WARNING — Peliosis hepatitis, liver cell tumors, and lipid changes have occurred secondary to anabolic steroid use.
ADULT — Weight gain promotion following extensive surgery, chronic infection, or severe trauma; in some patients who fail to gain or maintain wt without a physiologic cause; to offset protein catabolism associated with long-term corticosteroid therapy: 2.5 mg/day to 20 mg/day PO divided two to four times per day for 2 to 4 weeks. May repeat therapy intermittently as indicated.
PEDS — Weight gain: Up to 0.1 mg/kg or up to 0.045 mg/pound PO divided two to four times per day for 2 to 4 weeks. May repeat therapy intermittently as indicated.
FORMS — Generic/Trade: Tabs 2.5, 10 mg.
NOTES — Contraindicated in known or suspected prostate/breast cancer. Not shown to enhance athletic ability. Associated with dyslipidemia; monitor lipids. Pediatric use by specialists who monitor bone maturation q 6 months. Long-term use may cause hepatic adenomas, hepatocellular carcinoma, and peliosis hepatitis; monitor LFTs. May increase anticoagulant effects of warfarin. Monitor Hb for polycythemia.
MOA — Steroid with anabolic and androgenic actions.
ADVERSE EFFECTS — Serious: Peliosis hepatitis, liver tumors, cholestatic hepatitis, habituation, heart failure exacerbation, polycythemia. Frequent: Virilization, testicular atrophy, oligospermia, excitation, insomnia, anxiety, depression, paresthesia, altered libido, bladder irritability, menstrual irregularity, gynecomastia, acne, edema, lipid abnormalities.

TESTOSTERONE (*Androderm, AndroGel, Axiron, Aveed, Delatestryl, Depo-Testosterone, Striant, Testim, Testopel, Testro AQ, ✦Andriol*) ▶L ♀X ▶? ©III $ - varies by therapy
WARNING — Risk of transfer and secondary exposure with topical products. Virilization has been reported in children after secondary exposure to gel. Women and children should avoid contact with skin areas to which gel has been applied. Advise patient to wash hands with soap and water following application and cover area with clothing once gel has dried. Aveed: serious pulmonary oil microembolism reactions and anaphylaxis reported; observe for 30 min following dose. Aveed only available via restricted program.
ADULT — Hypogonadism in men: Injectable enanthate or cypionate, 50 to 400 mg IM q 2 to 4 weeks. Injectable undecanoate (Aveed): 750 mg IM, repeat in 4 weeks then every 10 weeks thereafter. Testopel: 2 to 6 pellets (150 to 450 mg testosterone) SC q 3 to 6 months. 2 pellets for each 25 mg testosterone propionate required weekly. Transdermal: Androderm: Start 4 mg patch at bedtime to clean, dry area of skin on back, abdomen, upper arms, or thighs. Nonvirilized patients start with 2 mg patch at bedtime. Adjust based on serum testosterone concentrations; see product information. AndroGel 1%: Apply 5 g from gel pack

TESTOSTERONE (cont.)

or 4 pumps (5 g gel; 50 mg testosterone) from dispenser daily to clean, dry, intact skin of the shoulders, upper arms, or abdomen. May increase dose to 7.5 to 10 g (100 mg testosterone) after 2 weeks. Androgel 1.62%: Apply 2 pumps (40.5 mg testosterone) from dispenser daily to shoulders or upper arms. Adjust based on serum testosterone concentration q14 to 28 days. Dose range 1 to 4 pumps daily. Axiron: 60 mg (1 pump of 30 mg to each axilla) once daily. Testim: 1 tube (5 g) daily to the clean, dry intact skin of the shoulders or upper arms. May increase dose to 2 tubes (10 g) after 2 weeks. Buccal (Striant): 30 mg q 12 h on upper gum above the incisor tooth; alternate sides for each application.

PEDS — Not approved in children.

FORMS — Trade only: Patch 2, 4 mg/24 h (Androderm). Gel 1% 2.5, 5 g packet, 75 g multidose pump (AndroGel 1% 1.25 g gel containing 12.5 mg testosterone per actuation). Gel 1.62%, 20.25 mg testosterone/actuation (AndroGel 1.62%). Gel 1.62% (Androgel 1.62%) 1.25, 2.5gm (package of 30) Gel 1%, 5 g tube (Testim). Solution 90 mL multidose pump (Axiron, 30 mg/actuation). Gel (Fortesta) 10mg/actuation. Pellet 75 mg (Testopel). Buccal: Blister packs: 30 mg (Striant). IM injection (Aveed): 750 mg/3 mL through restricted access program. Generic/Trade: Injection 100, 200 mg/mL (cypionate), 200 mg/mL (ethanate).

NOTES — Do not apply Androderm or AndroGel to scrotum. Apply Axiron only to axilla. Do not apply Testim to the scrotum or abdomen. Wash hands after topical product administration. Do not shower or swim for 5 hours after applying AndroGel. Pellet implantation is less flexible for dosage adjustment, therefore, take great care when estimating the amount of testosterone. For testosterone gel form, obtain serum testosterone level 2 weeks after initiation, then increase dose if necessary. Inject IM formulations slowly into gluteal muscle; rare reports of cough or respiratory distress following injection. Prolonged high-dose use of oral forms of testosterone have caused hepatic adenomas, hepatocellular carcinoma, and peliosis hepatitis. The overall risk of testosterone use on heart disease and the prostate (including prostate cancer) remain uncertain. Monitor prostate exam, PSA, and hemoglobin to detect polycythemia. Advise patient to regularly inspect the gum region where Striant is applied and report any abnormality; refer for dental consultation as appropriate. Injectable forms less expensive than gel or patch. Reports of venous thromboembolism; evaluate for DVT/PE if lower extremity swelling or shortness of breath.

MOA — Steroid with anabolic and androgenic actions.

ADVERSE EFFECTS — Serious: Peliosis hepatitis, liver tumors, cholestatic hepatitis, habituation, heart failure exacerbation, polycythemia, venous thromboembolism, serious pulmonary oil microembolism reactions, anaphylaxis. Frequent: Virilization, testicular atrophy, oligospermia, excitation, insomnia, anxiety, depression, paresthesia, altered libido, bladder irritability, menstrual irregularity, gynecomastia, acne, edema, gum or mouth irritation (buccal), transient cough (IM).

ENDOCRINE AND METABOLIC: Bisphosphonates

NOTE: Supplemental Vitamin D and calcium are recommended for osteoporosis prevention and treatment. Osteonecrosis of the jaw has been reported with bisphosphonates; generally associated with tooth extraction and/or local infection with delayed healing. Prior to treatment, consider dental exam and appropriate preventative dentistry, particularly with risk factors (eg, cancer, chemotherapy, corticosteroids, poor oral hygiene). While on bisphosphonate therapy, avoid invasive dental procedures when possible. Severe musculoskeletal pain has been reported; may occur at any time during therapy. Atypical, low trauma femoral shaft fractures have been reported; evaluate new thigh/groin pain for possible fracture. AACE guidelines recommend considering a drug holiday for 1-2 years in patients with stable bone mineral density after 4 to 5 years of treatment in patients with mild osteoporosis and after 10 years of treatment in patients with high fracture risk. Monitor bone density and resume treatment if it declines, if bone turnover markers increase or if fracture.

ALENDRONATE (Fosamax, Fosamax Plus D, Binosto, ✦Fosavance) ▶K ♀C ▶– $

ADULT — Prevention of postmenopausal osteoporosis (Fosamax): 5 mg PO daily or 35 mg PO weekly. Treatment of postmenopausal osteoporosis (Fosamax, Fosamax Plus D, Binosto): 10 mg daily, 70 mg PO weekly, 70 mg/vitamin D3 2800 international units PO weekly, or 70 mg/vitamin D3 5600 international units PO weekly. Treatment of glucocorticoid-induced osteoporosis (Fosamax): 5 mg PO daily in men and women or 10 mg PO daily in postmenopausal women not taking estrogen. Treatment of osteoporosis in men (Fosamax, Fosamax Plus D, Binosto): 10 mg PO daily, 70 mg PO weekly, or 70 mg/vitamin D3 2800 international units PO weekly, or 70 mg/vit D3 5600 international units PO weekly. Paget's disease (Fosamax): 40 mg PO daily for 6 months.

PEDS — Not approved in children.

UNAPPROVED ADULT — Prevention of glucocorticoid-induced osteoporosis men and women: 5 mg PO daily or 35 mg PO weekly; 10 mg PO daily or 70 mg PO weekly (postmenopausal women not taking estrogen). Treatment of glucocorticoid-induced

(cont.)

ALENDRONATE (cont.)

osteoporosis in men and women: 35 mg weekly or 70 mg weekly (postmenopausal women not taking estrogen).

FORMS — Generic/Trade (Fosamax): Tabs 5, 10, 35, 40, 70 mg. Trade only: Fosamax Plus D: 70 mg + either 2800 or 5600 units of vitamin D3. Binosto: 70 mg effervescent tab.

NOTES — May cause esophagitis, esophageal ulcers and esophageal erosions, occasionally with bleeding and rarely followed by esophageal stricture or perforation. Monitor frequently for dysphagia, odynophagia, and retrosternal pain. Not recommended if CrCl less than 35 mL/min. For patients requiring invasive dental procedures, discontinuation may reduce the risk for osteonecrosis of the jaw. All products: Take 30 min before first food, beverage, and medication of the day. Remain in upright position for at least 30 min following dose. Fosamax/Fosamax Plus D: Take with a full glass of water only. Binosto: dissolve in 4 oz plain water, wait 5 min after effervescence stops, stir then drink.

MOA — Inhibits osteoclast-mediated bone resorption, increases bone mineral density.

ADVERSE EFFECTS — Serious: Esophageal disease (ulcers, erosion, esophagitis, stricture, perforation), gastric/duodenal ulcer, osteonecrosis of the jaw, severe skin reactions. Low-energy femoral shaft and subtrochanteric fractures, asthma exacerbation. Frequent: Headache, musculoskeletal pain, abdominal pain, diarrhea, dizziness, joint swelling, rash, photosensitivity.

CLODRONATE (✱Clasteon, Bonefos) ▶K ♀D ▶– $$$$$

ADULT — Canada only. Hypercalcemia of malignancy; management of osteolysis resulting from bone metastases of malignant tumors: IV single dose, 1500 mg slow infusion over at least 4 h. IV multiple dose, 300 mg slow infusion daily over 2 to 6 h up to 10 days. Oral, following IV therapy, maintenance 1600 to 2400 mg/day in single or divided doses. Max PO dose 3200 mg/day; duration of therapy is usually 6 months.

PEDS — Not approved in children.

FORMS — Generic/Trade: Caps 400 mg.

NOTES — Contraindicated if creatinine more than 5 mg/dL or if severe GI tract inflammation. Avoid rapid bolus which may cause severe local reactions, thrombophlebitis, or renal failure. Do not mix with calcium-containing infusions. Ensure adequate hydration prior to infusion. Normocalcemia usually occurs within 2 to 5 days after initiation of therapy with multiple dose infusion. Monitor serum calcium, renal function in those with renal insufficiency, LFTs and hematological parameters.

MOA — Inhibits osteoclast-mediated bone resorption without an inhibitory effect on mineralization, decreases serum calcium.

ADVERSE EFFECTS — Serious: Hypersensitivity, decreased renal function, hypocalcemia. Frequent: N/V, anorexia, abdominal pain, diarrhea (with oral form), infusion site reaction.

ETIDRONATE (Didronel) ▶K ♀C ▶? $$$$$

ADULT — Paget's disease: 5 to 10 mg/kg PO daily for 6 months or 11 to 20 mg/kg daily for 3 months. Heterotopic ossification with hip replacement: 20 mg/kg/day PO for 1 month before and 3 months after surgery. Heterotopic ossification with spinal cord injury: 20 mg/kg/day PO for 2 weeks, then 10 mg/kg/day PO for 10 weeks.

PEDS — Not approved in children.

FORMS — Generic/Trade: Tabs 400 mg. Generic only: Tabs 200 mg.

NOTES — Divide dose if GI discomfort occurs. Avoid in abnormalities of the esophagus that may delay esophageal emptying (e.g., stricture). Avoid food, vitamins with minerals, or antacids within 2 h of dose.

MOA — Inhibits osteoclast-mediated bone resorption, blocks growth and mineralization of hydroxyapatite crystals.

ADVERSE EFFECTS — Serious: Esophageal disease (ulcers, esophagitis, perforation), peptic ulcer disease, agranulocytosis, pancytopenia, leukopenia, fractures, osteonecrosis of the jaw, asthma exacerbation. Frequent: Headache, gastritis, leg cramps, arthralgia, bone pain.

IBANDRONATE (Boniva) ▶K ♀C ▶? $$$$

ADULT — Prevention and treatment of postmenopausal osteoporosis. Oral: 150 mg PO q month. IV: 3 mg IV q 3 months.

PEDS — Not approved in children.

FORMS — Generic/Trade: Tab 150 mg. IV: 3 mg.

NOTES — May cause esophagitis. Avoid in abnormalities of the esophagus that may delay esophageal emptying (e.g., stricture). Avoid if CrCl less than 30 mL/min. Oral: Take 1 h before first food/beverage with a full glass of plain water; remain in upright position 1 h after taking. IV: Administer over 15 to 30 sec. Anaphylaxis reported with injection.

MOA — Inhibits osteoclast-mediated bone resorption, increases bone mineral density.

ADVERSE EFFECTS — Serious: Esophageal disease (ulcer, esophagitis), osteonecrosis of the jaw, asthma exacerbation, anaphylaxis (IV). Frequent: Back pain, dyspepsia, diarrhea, myalgia, headache, injection site reaction.

PAMIDRONATE (Aredia) ▶K ♀D ▶? $$$$$

WARNING — Single dose should not exceed 90 mg due to risk of renal impairment/failure.

ADULT — Hypercalcemia of malignancy, moderate (corrected Ca in the range of 12 to 13.5 mg/dL): 60 to 90 mg IV single dose infused over 2 to 24 h. Hypercalcemia of malignancy, severe (Ca more than 13.5 mg/dL): 90 mg IV single dose infused over 2 to 24 h. Wait at least 7 days before considering retreatment. Paget's disease: 30 mg IV over 4 h daily for 3 days. Osteolytic bone lesions: 90 mg IV over 4 h once a month. Osteolytic bone metastases: 90 mg IV over 2 h q 3 to 4 weeks.

PEDS — Not approved in children.

UNAPPROVED ADULT — Mild hypercalcemia: 30 mg IV single dose over 4 h. Treatment of osteoporosis:

PAMIDRONATE (*cont.*)

30 mg IV q 3 months. Prevention of bone loss during androgen deprivation treatment for prostate cancer: 60 mg IV q 12 weeks.

NOTES — Fever occurs in more than 20% of patients. Monitor creatinine (prior to each dose), lytes, calcium, phosphate, magnesium, and CBC (regularly). Avoid in severe renal impairment and hold dosing if worsening renal function. Longer infusions (more than 2 h) may reduce renal toxicity. Not studied in patients with SCr above 3 mg/dL. Maintain adequate hydration.

MOA — Inhibits osteoclast-mediated bone resorption, decreases serum calcium.

ADVERSE EFFECTS — Serious: Atrial fibrillation, syncope, hypertension, tachycardia, osteonecrosis of the jaw, severe musculoskeletal pain, orbital inflammation, atypical femoral shaft fracture, renal tubular disorders, glomerulonephropathy, adult respiratory distress syndrome, interstitial lung disease. Frequent: Electrolyte depletion (potassium, magnesium, calcium, phosphate), fever, infusion site reaction, bone pain, dyspepsia, anorexia, nausea, diarrhea.

RISEDRONATE (*Actonel, Atelvia*) ▶K ♀C ▶? $$$$$

ADULT — Prevention and treatment of postmenopausal osteoporosis: 5 mg PO daily, 35 mg PO weekly or 150 mg once a month. Treatment of osteoporosis in men: 35 mg PO weekly. Prevention and treatment of glucocorticoid-induced osteoporosis: 5 mg PO daily. Paget's disease: 30 mg PO daily for 2 months.

PEDS — Not approved in children.

UNAPPROVED ADULT — Prevention and treatment of glucocorticoid-induced osteoporosis: 35 mg PO weekly.

FORMS — Generic/Trade: Tabs 150 mg. Trade only: Tabs 5, 30, 35 mg. Delayed-release tab (Atelvia): 35 mg.

NOTES — May cause esophagitis, monitor frequently for dysphagia, odynophagia, and retrosternal pain. Remain in upright position for at least 30 min following dose. Take Actonel 30 min before first food, beverage, or medication of the day with a full glass of water only. Take delayed-release (Atelvia) in the morning immediately following breakfast with 4 oz. or more of water only. Avoid in abnormalities of the esophagus that may delay esophageal emptying (eg, stricture).

MOA — Inhibits osteoclast-mediated bone resorption, increases bone mineral density.

ADVERSE EFFECTS — Serious: Esophageal disease (ulcers, erosion, esophagitis, stricture, perforation), gastric/duodenal ulcer, hypersensitivity, asthma exacerbation. Frequent: Headache, musculoskeletal pain, abdominal pain, diarrhea.

TILUDRONATE (*Skelid*) ▶K ♀C ▶? $$$$$

ADULT — Paget's disease: 400 mg PO daily for 3 months.

PEDS — Not approved in children.

FORMS — Trade only: Tabs 200 mg.

NOTES — May cause esophagitis, esophageal ulcers and esophageal erosions, occasionally with bleeding and rarely followed by esophageal stricture or perforation. Monitor frequently for dysphagia, odynophagia, and retrosternal pain. Take 30 min before first food, beverage, or medication of the day with a full glass of water only. Remain in upright position for at least 30 min following dose.

MOA — Inhibits osteoclast-mediated bone resorption, increases bone mineral density.

ADVERSE EFFECTS — Serious: Esophageal disease (ulcers, erosion, esophagitis, stricture, perforation), gastric/duodenal ulcer, hyperparathyroidism, cataract, glaucoma. Frequent: Edema, diarrhea, nausea.

ZOLEDRONIC ACID (*Reclast, Zometa, ✦Aclasta*) ▶K ♀D ▶? $$$$$

ADULT — Treatment of osteoporosis (Reclast): 5 mg once yearly IV infusion over 15 min or longer. Prevention of postmenopausal osteoporosis: (Reclast) 5 mg IV infusion every 2 years. Prevention and treatment of glucocorticoid-induced osteoporosis in patients expected to receive glucocorticoids for at least 12 months (Reclast): 5 mg once yearly IV infusion over 15 min or longer. Hypercalcemia of malignancy (corrected Ca at least 12 mg/dL, Zometa): 4 mg single-dose IV infusion over 15 min or longer. Wait at least 7 days before considering retreatment. Paget's disease (Reclast): 5 mg IV single dose. Multiple myeloma and metastatic bone lesions from solid tumors (Zometa): 4 mg (CrCl more than 60 mL/min), 3.5 mg (CrCl 50 to 60 mL/min), 3.3 mg (CrCl 40 to 49 mL/min) or 3 mg (CrCl 30 to 39 mL/min) IV infusion over 15 min or longer q 3 to4 weeks.

PEDS — Not approved in children.

UNAPPROVED ADULT — Osteoporosis (Zometa): 4 mg once yearly IV infusion over 15 min or longer. Paget's disease (Zometa; approved in Canada): 5 mg IV single dose. Treatment of hormone-refractory prostate cancer metastatic to bone (Zometa): 4 mg IV q 3 to 4 weeks. Prevention of bone loss during androgen-deprivation treatment for non-metastatic prostate cancer (Zometa): 4 mg IV q 3 months for 1 year or 4 mg q 12 months. Prevention of bone loss during aromatase inhibitor use in breast cancer (Zometa): 4 mg IV q 6 months. Suppression of breast cancer in combination with adjuvant endocrine therapy (tamoxifen): 4 mg IV q 6 months for 3 years.

FORMS — Generic/Trade: 4 mg/5 mL IV (Zometa), 5 mg/100 mL IV (Reclast)

NOTES — Contraindicated in severe renal impairment (CrCl less than 35 mL/min) and hold dosing with worsening renal function. Monitor creatinine (before each dose), electrolytes, calcium, phosphate, magnesium, and Hb/HCT (regularly). Avoid single doses higher than 4 mg (Zometa) or higher than 5 mg (Reclast), infusions less than 15 min. Fever occurs in more than 15%. Correct preexisting hypocalcemia before therapy; life-threatening hypocalcemia reported (cardiac arrthymias, seizures). Maintain adequate hydration for those with

(cont.)

ZOLEDRONIC ACID *(cont.)*

hypercalcemia of malignancy, and give 500 mg calcium supplement and vitamin D 400 international units PO daily to those with multiple myeloma or metastatic bone lesions. Acute phase reactions reported (fever, fatigue, bone pain/arthralgias, myalgias, flu-like illness); typically onset is within 3 days and usually resolves within 7 to 14 days.

MOA — A bisphosphonate that inhibits osteoclast-mediated bone resorption, increases bone mineral density, decreases serum calcium.

ADVERSE EFFECTS — Serious: Hypotension, renal impairment, granulocytopenia, thrombocytopenia, pancytopenia, osteonecrosis of the jaw, severe musculoskeletal pain, ocular inflammation, atypical femoral shaft fracture, acute phase reaction, bronchospasm, interstitial lung disease, asthma exacerbation, acute phase reaction, hypocalcemia, cardiac arrhythmias, seizures. Frequent: Electrolyte depletion (potassium, magnesium, calcium, phosphate), flu-like symptoms, fever, infusion site reaction, N/V, skeletal pain, constipation, diarrhea, conjunctivitis.

ENDOCRINE AND METABOLIC: Corticosteroids

NOTE: See also Dermatology, Ophthalmology.

BETAMETHASONE (*Celestone, Celestone Soluspan, ♣Betaject*) ▶L ♀C ▶– $$$$$

ADULT — Anti-inflammatory/Immunosuppressive: 0.6 to 7.2 mg/day PO divided two to four times per day or up to 9 mg/day IM. 0.25 to 2 mL intra-articular depending on location and size of joint.

PEDS — Dosing guidelines not established.

UNAPPROVED ADULT — Fetal lung maturation, maternal antepartum between 24 and 34 weeks gestation: 12 mg IM q 24 h for 2 doses.

UNAPPROVED PEDS — Anti-inflammatory/Immunosuppressive: 0.0175 to 0.25 mg/kg/day PO divided three to four times per day. Fetal lung maturation, maternal antepartum: 12 mg IM q 24 h for 2 doses.

FORMS — Trade only: Syrup 0.6 mg/5 mL.

NOTES — Avoid prolonged use in children due to possible bone growth retardation. If such therapy necessary monitor growth and development.

MOA — Long-acting glucocorticoid.

ADVERSE EFFECTS — Serious: Hypertension, diabetes, osteoporosis, immunosuppression, impaired wound healing, adrenal suppression, peptic ulcer disease, cataracts. Frequent: Cushingoid state, N/V, weight gain, myopathy, leukocytosis, skin atrophy, edema.

CORTISONE (*Cortone*) ▶L ♀D ▶– $

ADULT — Adrenocortical insufficiency: 25 to 300 mg PO daily.

PEDS — Dosing guidelines not established.

UNAPPROVED PEDS — Adrenocortical insufficiency: 0.5 to 0.75 mg/kg/day PO divided q 8 h.

FORMS — Generic only: Tabs 25 mg.

MOA — Short-acting glucocorticoid with mineralocorticoid activity at higher doses.

ADVERSE EFFECTS — Serious: Hypertension, diabetes, osteoporosis, immunosuppression, impaired wound healing, adrenal suppression, peptic ulcer disease, cataracts. Frequent: Cushingoid state, N/V, weight gain, myopathy, leukocytosis, skin atrophy, edema.

DEXAMETHASONE (*Decadron, Dexpak, ♣Dexasone*) ▶L ♀C ▶– $

ADULT — Anti-inflammatory/immunosuppressive: 0.5 to 9 mg/day PO/IV/IM divided two to four times per day. Cerebral edema: 10 to 20 mg IV load, then 4 mg IM q 6 h (off-label IV use common) or 1 to 3 mg PO three times per day.

PEDS — Dosing varies by indication; start 0.02 to 0.3 mg/kg/day divided three to four times per day.

UNAPPROVED ADULT — Initial treatment of immune thrombocytopenic purpura: 40 mg PO daily for 4 days. Fetal lung maturation, maternal antepartum between 24 and 34 weeks gestation: 6 mg IM q 12 h for 4 doses. Bacterial meningitis (controversial): 0.15 mg/kg IV q 6 h for 2 to 4 days; start 10 to 15 min before the 1st dose of antibiotic. Antiemetic, prophylaxis: 8 mg IV or 12 mg PO prior to chemotherapy; 8 mg PO daily for 2 to 4 days. Antiemetic, treatment: 10 to 20 mg PO/IV q 4 to 6 h.

UNAPPROVED PEDS — Anti-inflammatory/immunosuppressive: 0.08 to 0.3 mg/kg/day PO/IV/IM divided q 6 to 12 h. Croup: 0.6 mg/kg PO/IV/IM for one dose. Bacterial meningitis (controversial): 0.15 mg/kg IV q 6 h for 2 to 4 days; start 10 to 15 min before the 1st dose of antibiotic. Bronchopulmonary dysplasia in preterm infants: 0.5 mg/kg PO/IV divided q 12 h for 3 days, then taper. Acute asthma: Older than 2 yo: 0.6 mg/kg to max 16 mg PO daily for 2 days.

FORMS — Generic/Trade: Tabs 0.5, 0.75. Generic only: Tabs 0.25, 1.0, 1.5, 2, 4, 6 mg; elixir 0.5 mg/5 mL; Soln 0.5 mg/5 mL, 1 mg/1 mL (concentrate). Trade only: DexPak 13 day (51 total 1.5 mg tabs for a 13-day taper), DexPak 10 day (35 total 1.5 mg tabs for 10-day taper), DexPak 6 days (21 total 1.5 mg tabs for 6-day taper).

NOTES — Avoid prolonged use in children due to possible bone growth retardation. If such therapy necessary monitor growth and development.

MOA — Long-acting glucocorticoid.

ADVERSE EFFECTS — Serious: Hypertension, diabetes, osteoporosis, immunosuppression, impaired wound healing, adrenal suppression, peptic ulcer disease, cataracts. Frequent: Cushingoid state, N/V, weight gain, myopathy, leukocytosis, skin atrophy, edema.

FLUDROCORTISONE (*Florinef*) ▶L ♀C ▶? $

ADULT — Adrenocortical insufficiency/Addison's disease: 0.1 mg PO 3 times a week to 0.2 mg PO daily. Salt-losing adrenogenital syndrome: 0.1 to 0.2 mg PO daily.

FLUDROCORTISONE (*cont.*)

PEDS — Not approved in children.

UNAPPROVED ADULT — Postural hypotension: 0.05 to 0.4 mg PO daily.

UNAPPROVED PEDS — Adrenocortical insufficiency: 0.05 to 0.2 mg PO daily.

FORMS — Generic only: Tabs 0.1 mg.

NOTES — For primary adrenocortical insufficiency usually given in conjunction with cortisone or hydrocortisone .

MOA — Potent mineralocorticoid with high glucocorticoid activity; primarily used for its mineralocorticoid effects.

ADVERSE EFFECTS — Serious: Hypokalemic alkalosis, hypertension, diabetes, osteoporosis, immunosuppression, impaired wound healing, adrenal suppression, peptic ulcer disease, cataracts. Frequent: Edema, cushingoid state, N/V, weight gain, myopathy, leukocytosis, skin atrophy.

HYDROCORTISONE (*Cortef, Cortenema, Solu-Cortef*) ▶L ♀C ▶– $

ADULT — Adrenocortical insufficiency: 20 to 240 mg/day PO divided three to four times per day or 100 to 500 mg IV/IM q 2 to 10 h prn (sodium succinate). Ulcerative colitis: 100 mg retention enema at bedtime (laying on side for 1 h or longer) for 21 days. May use for 2 to 3 months for severe cases; when course extends more than 3 weeks then discontinue gradually by decreasing frequency to every other night for 2 to 3 weeks. Multiple sclerosis acute exacerbation: 800 mg daily then 320 mg every other day for 1 month.

PEDS — Dosing guidelines not established. Prescribing information suggests tailoring doses to the specific disease being treated with a range of initial doses of 0.56 to 8 mg/kg/day IV/PO divided three to four times per day.

UNAPPROVED ADULT — Adrenocortical insufficiency: 15-25 mg/day PO divided two to three times per day with one-half to two-thirds of dose given in AM.

UNAPPROVED PEDS — Chronic adrenocortical insufficiency: 0.5 to 0.75 mg/kg/day PO divided q 8 h or 0.25 to 0.35 mg/kg/day IM daily. Acute adrenocortical insufficiency: Infants and young children 1 to 2 mg/kg IV bolus, then 25 to 150 mg/day divided q 6 to 8 h. Older children 1 to 2 mg/kg IV bolus, then 150 to 250 mg/day IV q 6 to 8 h.

FORMS — Generic/Trade: Tabs 5, 10, 20 mg; Enema 100 mg/60 mL.

NOTES — Agent of choice for adrenocortical insufficiency because of mixed glucocorticoid and mineralocorticoid properties at doses more than 100 mg/day.

MOA — Short-acting glucocorticoid with mineralocorticoid activity at higher doses.

ADVERSE EFFECTS — Serious: Hypertension, diabetes, osteoporosis, immunosuppression, impaired wound healing, adrenal suppression, peptic ulcer disease, cataracts. Frequent: Cushingoid state, N/V, weight gain, myopathy, leukocytosis, skin atrophy, edema.

METHYLPREDNISOLONE (*Solu-Medrol, Medrol, Depo-Medrol*) ▶L ♀C ▶– $

ADULT — Anti-inflammatory/Immunosuppressive: Parenteral (Solu-Medrol) 10 to 250 mg IV/IM q 4 h prn. Oral (Medrol) 4 to 48 mg PO daily. Medrol Dosepak tapers 24 to 0 mg PO over 7 days. IM/joints (Depo-Medrol) 4 to 120 mg IM q 1 to 2 weeks. Multiple sclerosis flare: 200 mg PO/IV daily for 1 week followed by 80 mg PO daily for 1 month.

PEDS — Dosing guidelines not established.

UNAPPROVED ADULT — Acute asthma exacerbation ("burst" therapy): 40 to 60 mg PO daily or divided two times per day for 3 to 10 days. Acute asthma exacerbation (vomiting or nonadherent): 240 mg IM once. Optic neuritis: 1 g IV daily (or in divided doses) for 3 days, then PO prednisone 1 mg/kg/day for 11 days (followed by a 3-day taper). Multiple sclerosis flare: 1 g IV daily (or in divided doses) for 3 to 5 days. May follow with PO prednisone 1 mg/kg/day for 14 days, then taper off. Spinal cord injury: 30 mg/kg IV over 15 min, followed in 45 min by 5.4 mg/kg/h IV infusion for 23 h (if initiated within 3 h of injury) or for 47 h (if initiated 3 to 8 h after injury). Due to insufficient evidence, routine use in spinal cord injury not recommended.

UNAPPROVED PEDS — Anti-inflammatory/Immunosuppressive: 0.5 to 1.7 mg/kg/day PO/IV/IM divided q 6 to 12 h. Spinal cord injury: 30 mg/kg IV over 15 min, followed in 45 min by 5.4 mg/kg/h IV infusion for 23 h. Due to insufficient evidence, routine use in spinal cord injury not recommended. Acute asthma exacerbation ("burst" therapy): 1 to 2 mg/kg/day PO; max 60 mg daily for 3 to 10 days. Acute asthma exacerbation (vomiting or nonadherent): Age younger than 5 yo: 7.5 mg/kg IM once; age 5 to 11 yo: 240 mg IM once; age at least 12: 240 mg IM once.

FORMS — Trade only: Tabs 2, 16, 32 mg. Generic/Trade: Tabs 4, 8 mg. Medrol Dosepak (4 mg, 21 tabs).

NOTES — Other dosing regimens have been used for MS and optic neuritis. Avoid initial treatment of optic neuritis with oral steroids, as it may increase the risk of new episodes. Contains benzyl alcohol, contraindicated in premature infants and for intrathecal administration. Do not use for traumatic brain injury.

MOA — Intermediate-acting glucocorticoid.

ADVERSE EFFECTS — Serious: Cardiac arrest or arrhythmia (with IV), hypertension, osteoporosis, immunosuppression, impaired wound healing, adrenal suppression, peptic ulcers, cataracts, postinjection flare, HPA axis suppression. Frequent: Cushingoid state, N/V, weight gain, edema, hyperglycemia, hypokalemia, injection site hypo/hyperpigmentation, myopathy, dermal or subdermal changes, deltoid muscle atrophy with IM injection.

PREDNISOLONE (*Flo-Pred, Prelone, Pediapred, Orapred, Orapred ODT*) ▶L ♀C ▶+ $$

ADULT — Anti-inflammatory/Immunosuppressive: 5 to 60 mg/day PO; individualize to severity of disease and response. Multiple sclerosis: 200 mg PO daily for 1 week, then 80 mg every other day for 1 month.

(cont.)

PREDNISOLONE (*cont.*)

PEDS — Anti-inflammatory/Immunosuppressive: 0.14 to 2 mg/kg/day PO divided three to four times per day (4 to 60 mg/m²/day); individualize to severity of disease and response. Acute asthma: 1 to 2 mg/kg/day daily or divided two times per day for 3 to 10 days. Nephrotic syndrome: 60 mg/m²/day divided three times per day for 4 weeks; then 40 mg/m²/day every other day for 4 weeks.

UNAPPROVED ADULT — Acute asthma exacerbation ("burst" therapy): 40 to 60 mg PO daily or divided two times per day for 3 to 10 days.

UNAPPROVED PEDS — Acute asthma exacerbation ("burst" therapy): 1 to 2 mg/kg/day PO; max 60 mg daily for 3 to 10 days. Early active RA: 10 mg/day PO.

FORMS — Generic/Trade: Syrup 15 mg/5 mL (Prelone; wild cherry flavor). Soln 5 mg/5 mL (Pediapred, raspberry flavor), 15 mg/5 mL (Orapred; grape flavor). Trade only: Orally disintegrating tabs 10, 15, 30 mg (Orapred ODT); Susp 5 mg/5 mL, 15 mg/5 mL (Flo-Pred; cherry flavor). Generic only: Tabs 5 mg. Syrup 5 mg/5 mL.

MOA — Intermediate-acting glucocorticoid with mineralocorticoid activity; primarily used for its glucocorticoid effects.

ADVERSE EFFECTS — Serious: Hypertension, diabetes, osteoporosis, immunosuppression, impaired wound healing, adrenal suppression, peptic ulcer disease, cataracts. Frequent: Cushingoid state, N/V, weight gain, myopathy, leukocytosis, skin atrophy, edema.

PREDNISONE (*Rayos, Prednisone Intensol, ✦Winpred*) ▶L ♀C ▶+ $

ADULT — Anti-inflammatory/immunosuppressive: 5 to 60 mg/day PO daily or divided two to four times per day. If using delayed-release tabs (Rayos), start 5 mg PO daily if steroid-naive.

PEDS — Dosing guidelines not established.

UNAPPROVED ADULT — Acute asthma exacerbation ("burst" therapy): 40 to 60 mg PO daily or divided two times per day for 3 to 10 days.

UNAPPROVED PEDS — Anti-inflammatory/immunosuppressive: 0.05 to 2 mg/kg/day divided one to four times per day. Acute asthma exacerbation ("burst" therapy): 1 to 2 mg/kg/day PO; max 60 mg daily for 3 to 10 days.

FORMS — Generic only: Tabs 1, 2.5, 5, 10, 20, 50 mg. Soln 5 mg/5 mL, 5 mg/mL (Prednisone Intensol). Dosepacks (5 mg tabs: Tapers 30 to 5 mg PO over 6 days or 30 to 10 mg over 12 days), Dosepacks Double Strength (10 mg tabs: Tapers 60 to 10 mg over 6 days, or 60 to 20 mg PO over 12 days) taper packs. Trade only: Delayed-release tabs 1, 2, 5 mg.

NOTES — Conversion to prednisolone may be impaired in liver disease.

MOA — Intermediate-acting glucocorticoid with mineralocorticoid activity; primarily used for its glucocorticoid effects.

ADVERSE EFFECTS — Serious: Hypertension, diabetes, osteoporosis, immunosuppression, impaired wound healing, adrenal suppression, peptic ulcer disease, cataracts, psychosis, depression. Frequent: Cushingoid state, N/V, weight gain, myopathy, leukocytosis, skin atrophy, edema.

TRIAMCINOLONE (*Aristospan, Kenalog, Trivaris*) ▶L ♀C ▶– $

ADULT — Anti-inflammatory/Immunosuppressive: 4 to 48 mg/day PO divided one to four times per day. 2.5 to 60 mg IM daily (Kenalog, Trivaris). Intra-articular: Small joints 2.5 to 5 mg (Kenalog, Trivaris), 2 to 6 mg (Aristospan); large joints 5 to 15 mg (Kenalog, Trivaris); 10 to 20 mg (Aristospan). Intravitreal: 4 mg (Trivaris).

PEDS — Dosing guidelines not established.

UNAPPROVED PEDS — Anti-inflammatory/Immunosuppressive: 0.117 to 1.66 mg/kg/day PO divided four times per day.

FORMS — Trade only: Injection 10 mg/mL, 40 mg/mL (Kenalog), 5 mg/mL, 20 mg/mL (Aristospan), 8 mg (80 mg/mL) syringe (Trivaris).

NOTES — Parenteral form not for IV use. Kenalog and Aristospan contain benzyl alcohol; do not use in neonates. Due to Trivaris availability in a syringe, multiple injections may be required for dose.

MOA — Intermediate-acting glucocorticoid.

ADVERSE EFFECTS — Serious: Hypertension, diabetes, osteoporosis, immunosuppression, impaired wound healing, adrenal suppression, peptic ulcer disease, cataracts, postinjection flare, anaphylaxis, angioedema. Frequent: Cushingoid state, N/V, wt gain, myopathy, leukocytosis, skin atrophy, injection site hyper/hypopigmentation, edema.

ENDOCRINE AND METABOLIC: Diabetes-Related—Alpha-Glucosidase Inhibitors

NOTE: No clinical studies have established conclusive evidence of decreased macrovascular outcomes with antidiabetic drugs. Alpha-glucosidase inhibitor administered alone should not cause hypoglycemia. If hypoglycemia occurs, treat with oral glucose rather than sucrose (table sugar). Adverse GI effects (ie, flatulence, diarrhea, abdominal pain) may occur with initial therapy.

ACARBOSE (*Precose, ✦Glucobay*) ▶Gut/K ♀B ▶– $$$

ADULT — DM, Type 2: Initiate therapy with 25 mg PO three times per day with the first bite of each meal. May start with 25 mg PO daily to minimize GI adverse effects. May increase to 50 mg PO three times per day after 4 to 8 weeks. Usual range is 50 to 100 mg PO three times per day. Maximum dose for patients wt 60 kg or less is 50 mg three times per day, wt greater than 60 kg max is 100 mg three times per day.

PEDS — Not approved in children.

UNAPPROVED ADULT — DM prevention, Type 2: 100 mg PO three times per day or to maximum tolerated dose.

ACARBOSE (cont.)

FORMS — Generic/Trade: Tabs 25, 50, 100 mg.

MOA — Inhibits intestinal alpha-glucoside hydrolase and pancreatic alpha-amylase and delays glucose absorption.

ADVERSE EFFECTS — Serious: Elevated serum transaminases, hypersensitivity, ileus, thrombocytopenia, pneumatosis cystoidis intestinalis, fulminant hepatitis. Frequent: Flatulence, diarrhea, abdominal pain.

MIGLITOL (*Glyset*) ▶K ♀B ▶– $$$

ADULT — DM, Type 2: Initiate therapy with 25 mg PO three times per day with the first bite of each meal.

Use 25 mg PO daily to start if GI adverse effects. May increase dose to 50 mg PO three times per day after 4 to 8 weeks, max 300 mg/day.

PEDS — Not approved in children.

FORMS — Trade only: Tabs 25, 50, 100 mg.

NOTES — Consider reducing dose of insulin or sulfonylurea if used in combination.

MOA — Inhibits intestinal alpha-glucoside hydrolase and delays glucose absorption.

ADVERSE EFFECTS — Serious: ileus, pneumatosis cystoides intestinalis. Frequent: Flatulence, diarrhea, abdominal pain, rash, transient decrease in serum iron.

ENDOCRINE AND METABOLIC: Diabetes-Related—Combinations

NOTE: No clinical studies have established conclusive evidence of decreased macrovascular outcomes with antidiabetic drugs. may cause life-threatening lactic acidosis, usually in setting of decreased tissue perfusion, hypoxia, hepatic dysfunction, or impaired renal clearance. Hold prior to IV contrast agents and for 48 h after. Avoid if ethanol abuse, heart failure (requiring treatment), hepatic or renal impairment (creatinine 1.4 mg/dL or greater in women, 1.5 mg/dL or greater in men), or hypoxic states (cardiogenic shock, septicemia, acute MI). Initial GI upset may be minimized by starting with lower dose of metformin component. may cause edema, wt gain, new heart failure, or exacerbate existing heart failure (avoid in NYHA Class III or IV). Monitor for signs of heart failure (rapid wt gain, dyspnea, edema) following initiation or dose increase. If occurs, manage fluid retention and consider discontinuation or dosage decrease. Rosiglitazone (Avandia) is not recommended with nitrates or insulin, and its labeling includes boxed warning regarding increased risk of myocardial ischemic events and notes that studies are currently inconclusive. Avoid if liver disease or ALT > 2.5 times normal. Monitor LFTs before therapy and periodically thereafter. Discontinue if ALT > 3 times upper normal limit. Full effect may not be apparent for up to 12 weeks. May cause resumption of ovulation in premenopausal anovulatory women; recommend contraception use. can lead to hemolytic anemia in patients with G6PD deficiency; use caution or consider alternate agents. : Report pancreatitis and discontinue drug if occurs.

ACTOPLUS METACTOPLUS MET XR (pioglitazone + metformin) ▶KL ♀C ▶? $$$$$

ADULT — DM, Type 2: 1 tab PO daily to two times per day. If inadequate control with metformin monotherapy, start 15/500 or 15/850 mg PO one to two times per day. If inadequate control with pioglitazone monotherapy, start 15/500 mg two times per day or 15/850 mg daily. Max 45/2550 mg/day. Extended release, start 1 tab (15/100 mg or 30/1000 mg) daily with evening meal. Max: 45/2000 mg/day.

PEDS — Not approved nor recommended in children.

FORMS — Generic/Trade: Tabs 15/500, 15/850 mg Trade only: Extended-release (Actoplus Met XR), tabs: 15/1000 mg, 30/1000 mg.

NOTES — Urinary bladder tumors reported; advise patients to report macroscopic hematuria or dysuria.

MOA — Combination product that increases insulin sensitivity, decreases hepatic gluconeogenesis.

ADVERSE EFFECTS — Serious: Potential hepatotoxicity, heart failure exacerbation, resumption of ovulation, macular edema, lactic acidosis, decreased vitamin B12, fracture, bladder tumor. Frequent: Asthenia, anemia, edema, wt gain, headache, dyslipidemia, diarrhea, increased LFTs, N/V, flatulence, abdominal discomfort, diarrhea, headache, taste disturbance.

AVANDAMET (rosiglitazone + metformin) ▶KL ♀C ▶? $$$$$

ADULT — DM, Type 2, initial therapy (drug-naive): Start 2/500 mg PO one or two times per day. If

inadequate control with metformin alone, select tab strength based on adding 4 mg/day rosiglitazone to existing metformin dose. If inadequate control with rosiglitazone alone, select tab strength based on adding 1000 mg/day metformin to existing rosiglitazone dose. Max 8/2000 mg/day.

PEDS — Not approved in children.

FORMS — Trade only: Tabs 2/500, 4/500, 2/1000, 4/1000 mg.

NOTES — Due to potential for elevated cardiovascular risks, rosiglitazone products restricted by FDA to use in patients where other medications cannot control Type 2 diabetes. May be given concomitantly with sulfonylureas.

MOA — Combination product that increases insulin sensitivity, decreases hepatic gluconeogenesis.

ADVERSE EFFECTS — Serious: Potential hepatotoxicity, heart failure, resumption of ovulation, lactic acidosis, decreased vitamin B12, macular edema, fracture in women, myocardial infarction. Frequent: Asthenia, anemia, edema, weight gain or loss, headache, dyslipidemia, diarrhea, increased LFTs, N/V, flatulence, abdominal discomfort, headache, taste disturbance.

AVANDARYL (rosiglitazone + glimepiride) ▶LK ♀C ▶? $$$$

ADULT — DM, Type 2, initial therapy (drug-naive): Start 4/1 mg PO daily. If switching from monotherapy with a sulfonylurea or glitazone, consider 4/2

(cont.)

AVANDARYL (cont.)

mg PO daily. Max 8/4 mg/day. Give with breakfast or the first main meal of the day. Use low starting dose of 4/1 mg and titrate more slowly in elderly, malnourished and in renal and hepatic impairment.

PEDS — Not approved in children.

FORMS — Trade only (restricted access): Tabs 4/1, 4/2, 4/4, 8/2, 8/4 mg rosiglitazone/glimepiride.

NOTES — Due to potential for elevated cardiovascular risks, rosiglitazone products restricted by FDA to use in patients where other medications cannot control Type 2 diabetes.

MOA — Combination product that stimulates pancreatic beta-cell insulin release and increases insulin sensitivity in adipose tissue, skeletal muscle, and liver.

ADVERSE EFFECTS — Serious: Potential hepatotoxicity, heart failure, resumption of ovulation, macular edema, hypoglycemia, hypersensitivity, SIADH, disulfiram-like reaction, cholestatic jaundice, marrow suppression, hemolytic anemia, eosinophilia, hepatic porphyria, increased LFTs, fracture, myocardial infarction. Frequent: Edema, weight gain, upper respiratory tract infection, headache, fatigue, N/V/D, dyspepsia, rash, pruritus, blurred vision.

DUETACT (pioglitazone + glimepiride) ▶LK ♀C ▶– $$$$$

ADULT — DM, Type 2: Start 30/2 mg PO daily. Start up to 30/4 mg PO daily if prior glimepiride therapy, or 30/2 mg PO daily if prior pioglitazone therapy; max 30/4 mg/day. Give with breakfast or the first main meal of the day. In the elderly, the malnourished, or those with renal/hepatic impairment, precede therapy with trial of glimepiride 1 mg/day and then titrate Duetact more slowly.

PEDS — Not approved nor recommended in children.

FORMS — Generic/Trade: Tabs 30/2, 30/4 mg pioglitazone/glimepiride.

NOTES — Urinary bladder tumors reported; advise patients to report macroscopic hematuria or dysuria.

MOA — Combination product that stimulates pancreatic beta-cell insulin release and increases insulin sensitivity in adipose tissue, skeletal muscle, and liver.

ADVERSE EFFECTS — Serious: Potential hepatotoxicity, heart failure exacerbation, resumption of ovulation, hypoglycemia, hypersensitivity, SIADH, disulfiram-like reaction, cholestatic jaundice, marrow suppression, hemolytic anemia, eosinophilia, hepatic porphyria, increased LFTs, macular edema, fracture, bladder tumor. Frequent: Edema, wt gain, upper respiratory tract infection, headache, fatigue, N/V/D, dyspepsia, rash, pruritus, blurred vision. Fracture risk in PI for women; in men citation is: Arch Intern Med. 2008;168(8):820-825.

GLUCOVANCE (glyburide + metformin) ▶KL ♀B ▶? $$$

WARNING — Contraindicated with bosentan.

ADULT — DM, Type 2, initial therapy (drug-naive): Start 1.25/250 mg PO daily or two times per day with meals; maximum 10/2000 mg daily. Inadequate control with a sulfonylurea or metformin alone: Start 2.5/500 or 5/500 mg PO two times per day with meals; maximum 20/2000 mg daily.

PEDS — Not approved in children.

FORMS — Generic/Trade: Tabs 1.25/250, 2.5/500, 5/500 mg.

MOA — Combination product that stimulates pancreatic beta-cell insulin release, decreases hepatic gluconeogenesis, and increases insulin sensitivity.

ADVERSE EFFECTS — Serious: Hypoglycemia, hypersensitivity, SIADH, disulfiram-like reaction, cholestatic jaundice, aplastic anemia, hemolytic anemia, leukopenia, thrombocytopenia, agranulocytosis, pancytopenia, eosinophilia, hepatic porphyria, increased LFTs, hepatitis, liver failure, lactic acidosis, decreased serum vitamin B12. Frequent: Diarrhea, N/V, flatulence, abdominal discomfort, headache, fatigue, rash, weight gain or loss, taste disturbance.

JANUMET, JANUMET XR (sitagliptin + metformin) ▶K ♀B ▶? $$$$

ADULT — DM, Type 2: Individualize based on patient's current therapy. Immediate-release: Start 1 tab PO two times per day. Extended-release: 1 tab PO daily. If inadequate control with metformin monotherapy, start 50/500 or 50/1000 two times per day based on current metformin dose. Extended-release: start 100 mg sitagliptin daily plus current daily metformin. If inadequate control on sitagliptin monotherapy: Immediate-release: start 50/500 two times per day. Extended-release: Start 100/1000 mg daily. Max 100/2000 mg daily. Give with meals.

PEDS — Not approved in children.

FORMS — Trade only: Immediate-release tabs 50/500, 50/1000 mg, extended-release tabs 100/1000, 50/500, 50/1000 mg sitagliptin/metformin.

NOTES — Not for use in Type 1 DM or DKA. Assess renal function and hematologic parameters prior to initiating and at least annually thereafter. Assess renal function more often if risk factors for dysfunction and discontinue if renal dysfunction. Do not split, crush or chew extended-release formulation. Discontinue if signs of hypersensitivity, including anaphylaxis, angioedema and severe dermatologic reactions.

MOA — Combination product that decreases hepatic gluconeogenesis, increases insulin sensitivity and slows inactivation of incretin hormones.

ADVERSE EFFECTS — Serious: Lactic acidosis, hypersensitivity, decreased serum vitamin B12, pancreatitis. Frequent: Diarrhea, N/V, flatulence, abdominal discomfort, headache, wt loss, taste disturbance, URI, nasopharyngitis, athralgia, myalgia, pain in extremity and back pain.

JENTADUETO (linagliptin + metformin) ▶KL - ♀B ▶? $$$$$

ADULT — DM, Type 2: If prior metformin, start 2.5 mg linagliptin and current metformin dose two times per day. If no prior metformin, start 2.5/5 mg PO two times per day. If current linagliptin/metformin, start at current doses. Max 2.5/1000 mg.

JENTADUETO (cont.)

PEDS — Not approved in peds.

FORMS — Trade only: 2.5/500, 2.5/850, 2.5/1000 mg.

NOTES — Not for use in Type 1 DM or DKA. May cause hypoglycemia when added to sulfonylurea or insulin therapy; consider reducing dose of sulfonylurea or insulin to decrease risk of hypoglycemia. Metformin may lower B12 levels, monitor hematologic parameters annually. Monitor for pancreatitis at initiation of therapy and dosage increases; discontinue drug if occurs. Monitor for and discontinue if hypersensitivity reaction; reaction can occur early or late in therapy.

MOA — Combination product that decreases hepatic gluconeogenesis, increases insulin sensitivity and slows inactivation of incretin hormones.

ADVERSE EFFECTS — Serious: Hypoglycemia, pancreatitis, hypersensitivity, lactic acidosis, B12 deficiency. Frequent: nasophayngitis, diarrhea, N/V, flatulence, myalgia.

JUVISYNC (sitagliptin + simvastatin) ►KL - ♀X ▶? $$$$$

ADULT — DM, Type 2 with hyperlipidemia: 100/40 (sitagliptin/simvastatin) mg PO once daily in evening. Or, may start on current dose of sitagliptin/simvastatin.

PEDS — Not approved in pediatrics.

FORMS — Trade only: Tabs 100/10, 100/20, 100/40 mg sitagliptin/simvastatin.

NOTES — Not for use in Type 1 DM or DKA. Assess renal function periodically; as sitagliptin should be dose adjusted with CrCl < 50 mL/min combination product may no longer be feasible. Not studied in combination with insulin. When adding to sulfonylurea therapy, consider reducing dose of sulfonylurea to decrease risk of hypoglycemia. Discontinue if signs of hypersensitivity, including anaphylaxis, angioedema and severe dermatologic reactions. Monitor for myopathy. Check LFTs at baseline and when clinically indicated; discontinue of persistent elevations. Chinese patients: Do not exceed 20 mg/day with niacin 1 g or more daily. Do not use with strong CYP3A4 inhibitors, gemfibrozil, cyclosporine, or danazol. See simvastatin notes/warnings for additional considerations and dosing with drug interactions.

MOA — Dipeptidyl peptidase IV (DPP-IV) inhibitor that slows inactivation of incretin hormones, resulting in increased glucose-stimulated insulin secretion and decreased glucagon secretion with HMG-CoA reducase inhibitor which inhibits HMG-CoA to mevalonate in cholesterol biosynthesis.

ADVERSE EFFECTS — Serious: Hypersensitivity, anaphylaxis, angioedema, pancreatitis, hepatotoxicity, myopathy, rhabdomyolysis. Frequent: URI, nasopharyngitis, headache, abdominal pain, constipation, nausea, arthralgia, back pain, pain in extremity.

KAZANO (alogliptin + metformin) ►K - ♀B ▶? $$$$$

ADULT — DM, Type 2: Individualize based on patient's current therapy. 1 tab PO two times per day. Max 25/2000 mg/day. Give with meals.

PEDS — Not approved in children.

FORMS — Trade only: 12.5/500, 12.5/1000 mg alogliptin/metformin.

NOTES — Not for use in Type 1 DM or DKA. Assess renal function and hematologic parameters prior to initiating and at least annually thereafter. Assess renal function more often if risk factors for dysfunction and discontinue if renal dysfunction. Discontinue if signs of hypersensitivity, including anaphylaxis, angioedema and severe dermatologic reactions.

MOA — Combination product that decreases hepatic gluconeogenesis, increases insulin sensitivity and slows inactivation of incretin hormones.

ADVERSE EFFECTS — Serious: Lactic acidosis, hypersensitivity, decreased serum vitamin B12, hepatic failure, pancreatitis. Frequent: Diarrhea, N/V, flatulence, abdominal discomfort, headache, taste disturbance, URI, nasopharyngitis, UTI, back pain, HTN.

KOMBIGLYZE XR (saxagliptin + metformin, ✱Komboglyze) ▶ ♀B ▶? $$$$$

ADULT — DM, Type 2: If inadequately controlled on metformin alone, start 2.5 to 5 mg of saxagliptin plus current dose of metformin; give once daily with evening meal. If inadequately controlled on saxagliptin, start 5/500 mg once daily with evening meal. Max: 5/2000 mg/day.

PEDS — Not approved in children.

FORMS — Trade only: Tabs 5/500, 2.5/1000, 5/1000 mg.

NOTES — Reduce saxagliptin dose to 2.5 mg when administered with strong CYP3A4/5 inhibitors such as ketoconazole; use individual products instead of combination product if needed to achieve appropriate dose. Not for use in Type 1 DM or DKA. Assess renal function periodically. To minimize risk of hypoglycemia if used with insulin or a sulfonylurea, consider lower dose of insulin or sulfonylurea. Do not split, crush or chew. Hypersensitivity, including angioedema, reported; caution if history of angioedema to other DPP4 inhibitors.

MOA — Combination product with dipeptidyl peptidase IV (DPP-IV) inhibitor that slows inactivation of incretin hormones, resulting in increased glucose-stimulated insulin secretion and decreased glucagon secretion and a biguanide that decreases hepatic gluconeogenesis and increases insulin sensitivity.

ADVERSE EFFECTS — Serious: Lactic acidosis, decreased serum vitamin B12, hypersensitivity, angioedema, hypoglycemia, lymphopenia, pancreatitis. Frequent: Diarrhea, N/V, flatulence, abdominal discomfort, headache, wt loss, taste disturbance, URI, UTI, nasopharyngitis, peripheral edema.

METAGLIP (glipizide + metformin) ►KL ♀C ▶? $$$

ADULT — DM, Type 2, initial therapy (drug-naive): Start 2.5/250 mg PO daily to 2.5/500 mg PO twice per day with meals; max 10/2000 mg daily. Inadequate control with a sulfonylurea or metformin alone: Start 2.5/500 or 5/500 mg

(cont.)

METAGLIP (cont.)

PO twice per day with meals; max 20/2000 mg daily.

PEDS — Not approved in children.

FORMS — Generic/Trade: Tabs 2.5/250, 2.5/500, 5/500 mg.

NOTES — May add thiazolidinedione if glycemic control is not obtained.

MOA — Combination product that stimulates pancreatic beta-cell insulin release, decreases hepatic gluconeogenesis, and increases insulin sensitivity.

ADVERSE EFFECTS — Serious: Hypoglycemia, hypersensitivity, SIADH, disulfiram-like reaction, cholestatic jaundice, hepatocellular jaundice, aplastic anemia, hemolytic anemia, leukopenia, thrombocytopenia, agranulocytosis, pancytopenia, eosinophilia, hepatic porphyria, increased LFTs, lactic acidosis, decreased serum vitamin B12. Frequent: Weight gain or loss, fatigue, diarrhea, nausea, dyspepsia, rash, vomiting, flatulence, asthenia, abdominal discomfort, headache, taste disturbance.

OSENI (alogliptin + pioglitazone) ▶KL - ♀C ▶? $$$$$

ADULT — DM, Type 2: Individualize based on patient's current therapy. 1 tab PO daily. Max 25/45 mg/day. If CrCl 30 to 59 mL/min reduce dose of alogliptin to 12.5 mg daily.

PEDS — Not approved in children

FORMS — Trade only: Tabs 12.5/15, 12.5/30, 12.5/45, 25/15, 25/30, 25/45 mg alogliptin/pioglitazone.

NOTES — Do not use in Type 1 DM or DKA. Discontinue if signs of hypersensitivity, including anaphylaxis, angioedema and severe dermatologic reactions. Urinary bladder tumors reported with pioglitazone; advise patients to report macroscopic hematuria or dysuria. Reports of fracture risk with pioglitazone.

MOA — Combination of dipeptidyl peptidase IV (DPP-IV) inhibitor that slows inactivation of incretin hormones, resulting in increased glucose-stimulated insulin secretion and decreased glucagon secretion and thiazolidinedione that increases insulin sensitivity in adipose tissue, skeletal muscle, and liver.

ADVERSE EFFECTS — Serious: Hepatotoxicity, liver failure, heart failure exacerbation, resumption of ovulation, macular edema, fracture, bladder tumor, hypersensitivity, anaphylaxis, angioedema, pancreatitis. Frequent: Edema, wt gain, nasopharyngitis, HA, URI, myalgia.

PRANDIMET (repaglinide + metformin) ▶KL ♀C ▶? $$$

ADULT — DM, Type 2, initial therapy (drug-naive): Start 1/500 mg PO daily before meals; max 10/2500 mg daily or 4/1000 mg/meal. Inadequate control with metformin alone: Start 1/500 mg PO two times per day before meals. Inadequate control with repaglinide alone: Start 500 mg metformin component PO two times per day before meals. In patients taking repaglinide and metformin concomitantly: Start at current dose and titrate to achieve adequate response.

PEDS — Not approved in children.

FORMS — Trade: Tabs 1/500, 2/500 mg.

NOTES — May take dose immediately preceding meal to as long as 30 min before the meal. Patients should be advised to skip dose if skipping meal. Gemfibrozil and itraconazole increase blood repaglinide levels and may result in an increased risk of hypoglycemia. Do not use with NPH insulin.

MOA — Combination product that stimulates pancreatic beta-cell insulin release, decreases hepatic gluconeogenesis, and increases insulin sensitivity.

ADVERSE EFFECTS — Serious: Hypoglycemia, hypersensitivity, thrombocytopenia, leukopenia, increased serum transaminases, lactic acidosis, decreased serum vitamin B12. Frequent: Headache, diarrhea, arthralgia, N/V, flatulence, abdominal discomfort, weight loss, taste disturbance.

ENDOCRINE AND METABOLIC: Diabetes-Related—DPP-4 inhibitors

NOTE: No clinical studies have established conclusive evidence of decreased macrovascular outcomes with antidiabetic drugs. Not for use in Type 1 DM or DKA. When adding to sulfonylurea or insulin therapy, consider reducing dose of sulfonylurea or insulin to decrease risk of hypoglycemia. Monitor for pancreatitis at initiation of therapy and dosage increases; discontinue drug if occurs. Risk of pancreatitis increased if prior pancreatitis. Discontinue if signs of hypersensitivity, including anaphylaxis, angioedema and severe dermatologic reactions.

ALOGLIPTIN (*Nesina*) ▶K - ♀B ▶? $$$$$

ADULT — DM, Type 2: 25 mg PO daily. If CrCl 30 to 59 mL/min reduce dose to 12.5 mg daily; if CrCl less than 30 mL/min then 6.25 mg daily.

PEDS — Not approved in children.

FORMS — Trade only: Tabs 6.25, 12.5, 25 mg.

MOA — Dipeptidyl peptidase IV (DPP-IV) inhibitor that slows inactivation of incretin hormones, resulting in increased glucose-stimulated insulin secretion and decreased glucagon secretion.

ADVERSE EFFECTS — Serious: Hypersensitivity, anaphylaxis, angioedema, hepatic failure, pancreatitis. Frequent: nasopharyngitis, HA, URI.

LINAGLIPTIN (*Tradjenta*, ✦*Trajenta*) ▶L - ♀B ▶? $$$$$

ADULT — DM, Type 2: 5 mg PO once daily.

PEDS — Not approved in children

FORMS — Trade only: Tab 5 mg.

NOTES — Monitor for and discontinue if hypersensitivity reaction; reaction can occur early or late in therapy.

MOA — Dipeptidyl peptidase IV (DPP-IV) inhibitor that slows inactivation of incretin hormones, resulting in increased glucose-stimulated insulin secretion and decreased glucagon secretion.

ADVERSE EFFECTS — Serious: hypoglycemia, pancreatitis, hypersensitivity, urticaria, angioedema,

LINAGLIPTIN (*cont.*)

bronchial hyperreactivity. Frequent: nasopharyngitis, arthralgia, back pain, headache.

SAXAGLIPTIN (*Onglyza*) ▶LK ♀B ▶? $$$$$
WARNING — None
ADULT — DM, Type 2: 2.5 or 5 mg PO daily. If CrCl is 50 mL/min or less reduce dose to 2.5 mg daily.
PEDS — Not approved in children.
FORMS — Trade only: Tabs 2.5, 5 mg.
NOTES — Assess renal function periodically. Reduce dose when administered with strong CYP3A4/5 inhibitors such as ketoconazole.
MOA — Dipeptidyl peptidase IV (DPP-IV) inhibitor that slows inactivation of incretin hormones, resulting in increased glucose-stimulated insulin secretion and decreased glucagon secretion.
ADVERSE EFFECTS — Serious: hypersensitivity, angioedema, hypoglycemia, lymphopenia, pancreatitis. Frequent: URI, UTI, headache, GI, nasopharyngitis, peripheral edema.

SITAGLIPTIN (*Januvia*) ▶K ♀B ▶? $$$$$
ADULT — DM, Type 2: 100 mg PO daily. If CrCl 30 to 49 mL/min reduce dose to 50 mg daily; if CrCl less than 30 mL/min then 25 mg daily.
PEDS — Not approved in children.
FORMS — Trade only: Tabs 25, 50, 100 mg.
MOA — Dipeptidyl peptidase IV (DPP-IV) inhibitor that slows inactivation of incretin hormones, resulting in increased glucose-stimulated insulin secretion and decreased glucagon secretion.
ADVERSE EFFECTS — Serious: Hypersensitivity, anaphylaxis, angioedema, pancreatitis. Frequent: URI, nasopharyngitis, HA, increased serum transaminases, constipation, vomiting, arthralgia, myalgia, pain in extremity and back pain.

ENDOCRINE AND METABOLIC: Diabetes-Related—GLP-1 agonists

NOTE: No clinical studies have established conclusive evidence of decreased macrovascular outcomes with antidiabetic drugs. Start with low dose to increase GI tolerance. May promote slight wt loss. May give SC in upper arm, abdomen, or thigh. Take medications that require rapid GI absorption at least 1 h prior to exenatide immediate-release or liraglutide. Risk of hypoglycemia is higher when used with insulin or insulin secretagogue (sulfonylurea, meglitinides), therefore, consider reduction in sulfonylurea or insulin dose. Pancreatitis reported, monitor for signs and symptoms including abdominal pain and vomiting upon initiation and dose increases. Discontinue if pancreatitis occurs. : Thyroid C-cell tumors reported in animal studies. Contraindicated if history or family history of medullary thyroid cancer or in patients with multiple endocrine neoplasia syndrome type 2. Counsel patients on risk of thyroid tumors.

EXENATIDE (*Byetta, Bydureon*) ▶K ♀C ▶? $$$$$
ADULT — DM, Type 2, adjunctive therapy: Immediate-release: 5 mcg SC two times per day (within 1 h before the morning and evening meals, or 1 h before the two main meals of the day at least 6 h apart). May increase to 10 mcg SC two times per day after 1 month. Extended-release: 2 mg SC once weekly.
PEDS — Not approved in children.
FORMS — Trade only: Byetta, prefilled pen (60 doses each) 5 mcg/dose, 1.2 mL; 10 mcg/dose, 2.4 mL. Bydureon (extended-release): 2 mg/vial; 2 mg/prefilled pen (single-use).
NOTES — Protect from light. Prior to initial use, keep refrigerated. After initial use, store at temperature below 78°; do not freeze. Discard pen 30 days after first use. Avoid use if renal insufficiency (CrCl less than 30 mL/min). Caution recommended if increasing dose from 5 to 10 mcg in patients with CrCl 30 to 50 mL/min (immediate release). Monitor for kidney dysfunction. Not recommended in severe GI disease, including gastroparesis. Do not substitute for insulin in the insulin-dependent; concurrent use with prandial insulin has not been studied. Use with short or rapid acting insulins not recommended. May potentiate warfarin. Serious injection-site reactions (abcess, cellulitis, necrosis) may occur with extended-release; educate advise patients to seek attention if pain, swelling, blisters or open wounds.
MOA — Incretin analog that reduces fasting and postprandial glucose by increasing glucose-stimulated insulin secretion, decreasing glucagon secretion, slowing gastric emptying and reducing appetite.
ADVERSE EFFECTS — Serious: angioedema, hypersensitivity, anaphylaxis, pancreatitis, renal dysfunction, serious injection-site reactions (abcess, cellulitis, necrosis). Frequent: hypoglycemia, N/V, diarrhea, constipation, flatulence, dizziness, headache.

LIRAGLUTIDE (*Victoza*) ▶Endogenous ♀C ▶? $$$$$
ADULT — DM, Type 2: Start 0.6 mg SC daily for 1 week, then increase to 1.2 mg SC daily. May increase to 1.8 mg SC daily.
PEDS — Not approved in children.
FORMS — Trade only: Multidose pen (18 mg/3 mL) delivers doses of 0.6 mg, 1.2 mg or 1.8 mg.
NOTES — May be given any time of day, independent of meals. Use caution in patients with renal or hepatic impairment or history of pancreatitis. Concurrent use with insulin has not been studied. Not recommended as first line therapy or for use in DM, Type 1 or DKA.
MOA — Incretin analog that reduces fasting and postprandial glucose by increasing glucose-stimulated insulin secretion, decreasing glucagon secretion, slowing gastric emptying and reducing appetite.
ADVERSE EFFECTS — Serious: pancreatitis, hypersensitivity. Frequent: Headache, nausea, diarrhea, anti-liraglutide antibody formation, rash, pruritis.

ENDOCRINE AND METABOLIC: Diabetes-Related—Insulins

INJECTABLE INSULINS*

		Onset (h)	Peak (h)	duration (h)
Rapid-shortacting	Insulin aspart (NovoLog)	< 0.2	1–3	3–5
	Insulin glulisine (Apidra)	0.30–0.4	1	4–5
	Insulin lispro (Humalog)	0.25–0.5	0.5–2.5	≤5
	Regular (Novolin R, Humulin R)	0.5–1	2–3	3–6
Intermediate-/long acting	NPH (Novolin N, Humulin N)	2–4	4–10	10–16
	Insulin detemir (Levemir)	n.a.	flat action profile	up to 23
	Insulin glargine (Lantus)	2–4	peakless	24
Mixtures	Insulin aspart protamine susp/aspart (NovoLog Mix 70/30)	0.25	1–4 (biphasic)	up to 24
	Insulin lispro protamine susp/insulin lispro (Humalog Mix 75/25, Humalog Mix 50/50)	< 0.25	1–3 (biphasic)	10–20
	NPH/Reg (Humulin 70/30, Novolin 70/30)	0.5–1	2–10 (biphasic)	10–20

*These are general guidelines, as onset, peak, and duration of activity are affected by the site of injection, physical activity, body temperature, and blood supply.

†Dose-dependent duration of action, range from 6 to 23 h.

n.a. = not available.

NOTE: Adjust insulin dosing to achieve glycemic control. See table "diabetes numbers"; for goals. Administer rapid-acting insulin (Humalog, NovoLog, Apidra) within 15 min before or immediately after a meal. Administer regular insulin 30 min before meals. May mix NPH with aspart, lispro, glulisine or regular. Draw up rapid/short-acting insulin first. Do not mix Lantus (glargine) or Levemir (detemir) with other insulins. Pens for use by one person only.

INSULIN—INJECTABLE COMBINATIONS (*Humalog Mix 75/25, Humalog Mix 50/50, Humulin 70/30, Novolin 70/30, Novolog Mix 70/30*) ▶LK ♀B/C ▶+ $$$$
ADULT — Doses vary, but typically total insulin 0.3 to 1 unit/kg/day SC in divided doses (Type 1), and 0.5 to 1.5 unit/kg/day SC in divided doses (Type 2).
PEDS — Not approved in children.
UNAPPROVED PEDS — Diabetes: Maintenance: Total insulin 0.5 to 1 unit/kg/day SC, but doses vary.
FORMS — Trade only: Insulin lispro protamine susp/insulin lispro (Humalog Mix 75/25, Humalog Mix 50/50). Insulin aspart protamine/insulin aspart (NovoLog Mix 70/30,). NPH and regular mixtures (Humulin 70/30, Novolin 70/30). Insulin available in pen form: Novolin 70/30 InnoLet, NovoLog Mix 70/30 FlexPen, Humulin 70/30, Humalog Mix 75/25 KwikPen, Humalog Mix 50/50 KwikPen.
MOA — Stimulates peripheral glucose uptake, and inhibits hepatic gluconeogenesis.
ADVERSE EFFECTS — Serious: Hypoglycemia, allergic reaction, hypokalemia. Frequent: Weight gain, lipoatrophy, lipohypertrophy, injection site reaction.

INSULIN—INJECTABLE INTERMEDIATE/LONG-ACTING (*Novolin N, Humulin N, Lantus, Levemir*) ▶LK ♀B/C ▶+ $$$$
ADULT — Doses vary, but typically total insulin 0.3 to 0.5 unit/kg/day SC in divided doses (Type 1), and 1 to 1.5 unit/kg/day SC in divided doses (Type 2). Generally, 50 to 70% of insulin requirements are provided by rapid or short-acting insulin and the remainder from intermediate- or long-acting insulin. Lantus: Start 10 units SC daily (same time everyday) in insulin-naive patients, adjust to usual dose of 2 to 100 units/day. When transferring from twice a day NPH human insulin, the initial Lantus dose should be reduced by about 20% from the previous total daily NPH dose, then adjust dose based on patient response. Levemir, Type 2 DM (inadequately controlled on oral meds): Start 0.1 to 0.2 units/kg once a day; or 10 units SC one or two times per day. When transferring from basal insulin (Lantus, NPH) in type 1 or 2 DM, change on a unit-to-unit basis; more Levemir may be required than NPH insulin.
PEDS — Diabetes: Maintenance: Total insulin 0.5 to 1 unit/kg/day SC, but doses vary. Generally, 50 to 70% of insulin requirements are provided by rapid-acting insulin and the remainder from

INSULIN—INJECTABLE INTERMEDIATE/LONG-ACTING (cont.)

intermediate- or long-acting insulin. Age 6 to 15 yo (Lantus): Start 10 units SC daily (same time everyday) in insulin-naive patients, adjust to usual dose of 2 to 100 units/day. When transferring from twice a day NPH human insulin, the initial Lantus dose should be reduced by about 20% from the previous total daily NPH dose, then adjust dose based on patient response. Levemir (Type 1 DM): When transferring from NPH, change on a unit-to-unit basis; more Levemir may be required than NPH.

FORMS — Trade only: Injection NPH (Novolin N, Humulin N). Insulin glargine (Lantus). Insulin detemir (Levemir). Insulin available in pen form: Novolin N InnoLet, Humulin N Pen, Lantus SoloSTAR, Levemir FlexPen. Premixed preparations of NPH and regular insulin also available.

MOA — Stimulates peripheral glucose uptake, and inhibits hepatic gluconeogenesis.

ADVERSE EFFECTS — Serious: Hypoglycemia, allergic reaction, hypokalemia. Frequent: Weight gain, lipoatrophy, lipohypertrophy, injection site reaction.

INSULIN—INJECTABLE SHORT-RAPID-ACTING (Apidra, Novolin R, NovoLog, Humulin R, Humalog, ✷NovoRapid) ▶LK ♀B/C ▶+ $$$

ADULT — Doses vary, but typically total insulin 0.3 to 0.5 unit/kg/day SC in divided doses (Type 1), and 1 to 1.5 unit/kg/day SC in divided doses (Type 2). Generally, 50 to 70% of insulin requirements are provided by rapid or short-acting insulin and the remainder from intermediate- or long-acting insulin.

PEDS — Diabetes age older than 4 yo (Apidra), older than 3 yo (Humalog) or older than 2 yo (NovoLog): Doses vary, but typically total insulin maintenance dose 0.5 to 1 unit/kg/day SC in divided doses. Generally, 50 to 70% of insulin requirements are provided by rapid-acting insulin and the remainder from intermediate- or long-acting insulin.

UNAPPROVED ADULT — Severe hyperkalemia: 5 to 10 units regular insulin plus concurrent dextrose IV. Profound hyperglycemia (e.g., DKA): 0.1 unit/kg regular insulin IV bolus, then begin IV infusion 100 units in 100 mL NS (1 unit/mL) at 0.1 units/kg/h. 70 kg: 7 units/h (7 mL/h). Titrate to clinical effect.

UNAPPROVED PEDS — Profound hyperglycemia (e.g., DKA): 0.1 unit/kg regular insulin IV bolus, then IV infusion 100 units in 100 mL NS (1 unit/mL) at 0.1 units/kg/h. Titrate to clinical effect. Severe hyperkalemia: 0.1 units/kg regular insulin IV with glucose over 30 min. May repeat in 30 to 60 min or start 0.1 units/kg/h.

FORMS — Trade only: Injection regular 100 units/mL (Novolin R, Humulin R) Injection regular 500 units/mL (Humulin U-500, concentrated). Insulin glulisine (Apidra). Insulin lispro (Humalog). Insulin aspart (NovoLog). Insulin available in pen form: Novolin R InnoLet, Humulin R, Apidra SoloSTAR, Humalog KwikPen, NovoLog FlexPen.

NOTES — Apidra, Humalog and NovoLog approved for use by continuous subcutaneous infusion in insulin pump. Do not mix insulins in pump. Consult manufacturer instructions for frequency of reservoir change when used in pump. Caution: med errors have occurred when using concentrated Humulin R U-500, note strength 500 units/mL.

MOA — Stimulates peripheral glucose uptake, and inhibits hepatic gluconeogenesis.

ADVERSE EFFECTS — Serious: Hypoglycemia, allergic reaction, hypokalemia. Frequent: Weight gain, lipoatrophy, lipohypertrophy, injection site reaction.

ENDOCRINE AND METABOLIC: Diabetes-Related—Meglitinides

NOTE: No clinical studies have established conclusive evidence of decreased macrovascular outcomes with anti-diabetic drugs.

NATEGLINIDE (Starlix) ▶L ♀C ▶? $$$

ADULT — DM, Type 2, monotherapy or in combination with metformin or thiazolidinedione: 120 mg PO three times per day within 30 min before meals; use 60 mg PO three times per day in patients who are near goal A1C.

PEDS — Not approved in children.

FORMS — Generic/Trade: Tabs 60, 120 mg.

NOTES — Not to be used as monotherapy in patients inadequately controlled with glyburide or other anti-diabetic agents previously. Patients with severe renal impairment are at risk for hypoglycemic episodes.

MOA — Stimulates pancreatic beta-cell insulin release.

ADVERSE EFFECTS — Serious: Hypoglycemia, jaundice, cholestatic hepatitis, increased LFTs. Frequent: Arthralgia, upper respiratory tract infection, hypersensitivity.

REPAGLINIDE (Prandin, ✷Gluconorm) ▶L ♀C ▶? $$$

ADULT — DM, Type 2: 0.5 to 2 mg PO three times per day within 30 min before a meal. Allow 1 week between dosage adjustments. Usual range is 0.5 to 4 mg PO three to four times per day, max 16 mg/day.

PEDS — Not approved in children.

FORMS — Generic/Trade: Tabs 0.5, 1, 2 mg.

NOTES — May take dose immediately preceding meal to as long as 30 min before the meal. Gemfibrozil and itraconazole increase blood repaglinide levels and may result in an increased risk of hypoglycemia. Do not use with NPH insulin.

MOA — Stimulates pancreatic beta-cell insulin release.

ADVERSE EFFECTS — Serious: Hypoglycemia, hypersensitivity, thrombocytopenia, leukopenia, increased serum transaminases. Frequent: Diarrhea, arthralgia, upper respiratory tract infection.

ENDOCRINE AND METABOLIC: Diabetes-Related—SGLT2 Inhibitors

CANAGLIFLOZIN (Invokana) ▶LK - ♀C ▶? $$$$$
WARNING — No clinical studies have established conclusive evidence of decreased macrovascular outcomes with antidiabetic drugs.
ADULT — DM, Type 2: 100 mg PO daily before first meal of the day. If tolerated and needed for glycemic control, may increase to 300 mg PO daily if CrCl <60 mL/min.
PEDS — Not approved in children.
FORMS — Trade only: Tabs 100, 300 mg.
NOTES — Do not use if CrCl <45 mL/min. Check renal function prior to initiation and periodically. May cause hypotension, check volume status prior to use. May cause hyperkalemia; check K levels. Consider reducing dose of insulin prior to initiation to avoid hypoglycemia. Monitor for and treat genital fungal infections if occur. May increase LDL. Do not use in DM Type 1 or DKA. Do not monitor glycemic control with urine glucose tests due to potential for false positive.
MOA — Inhibitor of sodium-glucose cotransporter 2 (SGLT2) which blocks reabsorption of glucose from the kidney and increases glucose loss in the urine.
ADVERSE EFFECTS — Serious: hypotension, hyperkalemia, renal dysfunction, hypoglycemia, hypersensitivity. Frequent: genital fungal infections, urinary tract infections, increased urination, increased LDL.

DAPAGLIFLOZIN (Farxiga) ▶LK ♀C ▶– $$$$$
WARNING — No clinical studies have established conclusive evidence of decreased macrovascular outcomes with antidiabetic drugs.
ADULT — DM, Type 2: 5 mg PO daily in the morning, with or without food. If tolerated and needed for glycemic control, may increase to 10 mg PO daily.
FORMS — Trade only: Tabs 5, 10 mg
NOTES — Do not use if CrCl <60 mL/min. Check renal function prior to initiation and periodically. May cause hypotension, check volume status prior to use. May cause hyperkalemia, check K levels. Consider reducing dose of insulin or insulin secretagogue prior to initiation to avoid hypoglycemia. Monitor for and treat genital fungal infections if occur. May increase LDL. Do not use in DM Type 1 or DKA.
MOA — Inhibitor of sodium-glucose cotransporter 2 (SGLT2) which blocks reabsorption of glucose from the kidney and increases glucose loss in the urine.
ADVERSE EFFECTS — Serious: hypotension, hyperkalemia, renal dysfunction, hypoglycemia, hypersensitivity. Frequent: genital fungal infections, urinary tract infections, increased urination, increased LDL.

ENDOCRINE AND METABOLIC: Diabetes-Related—Sulfonylureas—1st Generation

NOTE: No clinical studies have established conclusive evidence of decreased macrovascular outcomes with antidiabetic drugs. Sulfonylureas can lead to hemolytic anemia in patients with G6PD deficiency; use caution or consider alternate agents.

CHLORPROPAMIDE (Diabinese) ▶LK ♀C ▶– $$
ADULT — DM, Type 2: Initiate therapy with 100 to 250 mg PO daily. Titrate after 5 to 7 days by increments of 50 to 125 mg at intervals of 3 to 5 days to obtain optimal control. Max 750 mg/day.
PEDS — Not approved in children.
FORMS — Generic/Trade: Tabs 100, 250 mg.
NOTES — Clinical use in the elderly has not been properly evaluated. Elderly are more prone to hypoglycemia and/or hyponatremia possibly from renal impairment or drug interactions. May cause disulfiram-like reaction with alcohol.
MOA — Stimulates pancreatic beta-cell insulin release.
ADVERSE EFFECTS — Serious: Hypoglycemia, hypersensitivity, SIADH, disulfiram-like reaction, cholestatic jaundice, hepatitis, hepatic porphyria, increased serum transaminases, aplastic anemia, hemolytic anemia, leukopenia, thrombocytopenia, agranulocytosis, pancytopenia, eosinophilia. Frequent: Weight gain, fatigue, diarrhea, nausea, dyspepsia, rash.

TOLAZAMIDE (Tolinase) ▶LK ♀C ▶? $
ADULT — DM, Type 2: Initiate therapy with 100 mg PO daily in patients with fasting blood glucose less than 200 mg/dL, and in patients who are malnourished, underweight, or elderly. Initiate therapy with 250 mg PO daily in patients with fasting blood glucose more than 200 mg/dL. Give with breakfast or the first main meal of the day. If daily doses exceed 500 mg, divide the dose two times per day. Max 1000 mg/day.
PEDS — Not approved in children.
FORMS — Generic only: Tabs 100, 250, 500 mg.
MOA — Stimulates pancreatic beta-cell insulin release.
ADVERSE EFFECTS — Serious: Hypoglycemia, hypersensitivity, SIADH, disulfiram-like reaction, cholestatic jaundice, aplastic anemia, hemolytic anemia, leukopenia, thrombocytopenia, agranulocytosis, pancytopenia, eosinophilia, hepatic porphyria, increased serum transaminases. Frequent: Weight gain, fatigue, diarrhea, nausea, dyspepsia, rash.

TOLBUTAMIDE ▶LK ♀C ▶+ $
ADULT — DM, Type 2: Start 1 g PO daily. Maintenance dose is usually 250 mg to 2 g PO daily. Total daily dose may be taken in the morning, divide doses if GI intolerance occurs. Max 3 g/day.
PEDS — Not approved in children.
FORMS — Generic only: Tabs 500 mg.
MOA — Stimulates pancreatic beta-cell insulin release.
ADVERSE EFFECTS — Serious: Hypoglycemia, hypersensitivity, SIADH, disulfiram-like reaction, cholestatic jaundice, aplastic anemia, hemolytic anemia, leukopenia, thrombocytopenia, agranulocytosis, pancytopenia, eosinophilia, hepatic porphyria, increased serum transaminases. Frequent: Weight gain, fatigue, diarrhea, nausea, dyspepsia, rash.

ENDOCRINE AND METABOLIC: Diabetes-Related—Sulfonylureas—2nd Generation

NOTE: No clinical studies have established conclusive evidence of decreased macrovascular outcomes with anti-diabetic drugs. Sulfonylureas can lead to hemolytic anemia in patients with G6PD deficiency; use caution or consider alternate agents.

GLICLAZIDE (✽Diamicron, Diamicron MR) ▶KL ♀C ▶? $

ADULT — Canada only, DM, Type 2: Immediate-release: Start 80 to 160 mg PO daily, max 320 mg PO daily (160 mg or more per day should be in divided doses). Modified-release: Start 30 mg PO daily, max 120 mg PO daily.

PEDS — Not approved in children.

FORMS — Generic/Trade: Tabs 80 mg (Diamicron). Trade only: Tabs, modified-release 30 mg (Diamicron MR).

NOTES — Immediate and modified-release not equipotent; 80 mg of immediate-release can be changed to 30 mg of modified-release.

MOA — Stimulates pancreatic beta-cell insulin release.

ADVERSE EFFECTS — Serious: Hypoglycemia, hypersensitivity, disulfiram-like reaction, cholestatic jaundice, aplastic anemia, hemolytic anemia, leukopenia, thrombocytopenia, agranulocytosis, pancytopenia, eosinophilia, hepatic porphyria, increased LFTs. Frequent: Weight gain, fatigue, diarrhea, nausea, dyspepsia, rash.

GLIMEPIRIDE (Amaryl) ▶LK ♀C ▶– $$

ADULT — DM, Type 2: Initiate therapy with 1 to 2 mg PO daily. Start with 1 mg PO daily in elderly, malnourished patients or those with renal or hepatic insufficiency. Give with breakfast or the first main meal of the day. Titrate in increments of 1 to 2 mg at 1 to 2 weeks intervals based on response. Usual maintenance dose is 1 to 4 mg PO daily, max 8 mg/day.

PEDS — Not approved in children.

FORMS — Generic/Trade: Tabs 1, 2, 4 mg. Generic only: Tabs 3, 6, 8 mg.

NOTES — Allergy may develop if allergic to other sulfonamide derivatives.

MOA — Stimulates pancreatic beta-cell insulin release.

ADVERSE EFFECTS — Serious: Hypoglycemia, hypersensitivity, SIADH, disulfiram-like reaction, cholestatic jaundice, aplastic anemia, hemolytic anemia, leukopenia, thrombocytopenia, agranulocytosis, pancytopenia, eosinophilia, hepatic porphyria, increased serum transaminases. Frequent: Weight gain, fatigue, diarrhea, nausea, dyspepsia, rash.

GLIPIZIDE (Glucotrol, Glucotrol XL) ▶LK ♀C ▶? $

ADULT — DM, Type 2: Initiate therapy with 5 mg PO daily. Give 2.5 mg PO daily to geriatric patients or those with liver disease. Adjust dose in increments of 2.5 to 5 mg to a usual maintenance dose of 10 to 20 mg/day, max 40 mg/day. Doses more than 15 mg should be divided two times per day. Extended-release (Glucotrol XL): Initiate therapy with 5 mg PO daily. Usual dose is 5 to 10 mg PO daily, max 20 mg/day.

PEDS — Not approved in children.

FORMS — Generic/Trade: Tabs 5, 10 mg; Extended-release tabs 2.5, 5, 10 mg.

NOTES — Maximum effective dose is generally 20 mg/day.

MOA — Stimulates pancreatic beta-cell insulin release.

ADVERSE EFFECTS — Serious: Hypoglycemia, hypersensitivity, SIADH, disulfiram-like reaction, cholestatic jaundice, hepatocellular injury, aplastic anemia, hemolytic anemia, leukopenia, thrombocytopenia, agranulocytosis, pancytopenia, eosinophilia, hepatic porphyria, increased serum transaminases. Frequent: Weight gain, fatigue, diarrhea, nausea, dyspepsia, rash.

GLYBURIDE (DiaBeta, Glynase PresTab, ✽Euglucon) ▶LK ♀B ▶? $

WARNING — Contraindicated with bosentan.

ADULT — DM, Type 2: Initiate therapy with 2.5 to 5 mg PO daily. Start with 1.25 mg PO daily in elderly or malnourished patients or those with renal or hepatic insufficiency. Give with breakfast or the first main meal of the day. Titrate in increments of no more than 2.5 mg at weekly intervals based on response. Usual maintenance dose is 1.25 to 20 mg PO daily or divided two times per day, max 20 mg/day. Micronized tabs: Initiate therapy with 1.5 to 3 mg PO daily. Start with 0.75 mg PO daily in elderly, malnourished patients or those with renal or hepatic insufficiency. Give with breakfast or the first main meal of the day. Titrate in increments of no more than 1.5 mg at weekly intervals based on response. Usual maintenance dose is 0.75 to 12 mg PO daily, max 12 mg/day. May divide dose two times per day if more than 6 mg/day.

PEDS — Not approved in children.

FORMS — Generic/Trade: Tabs (scored) 1.25, 2.5, 5 mg. Micronized Tabs (scored) 1.5, 3, 4.5, 6 mg.

NOTES — Maximum effective dose is generally 10 mg/day.

MOA — Stimulates pancreatic beta-cell insulin release.

ADVERSE EFFECTS — Serious: Hypoglycemia, hypersensitivity, SIADH, disulfiram-like reaction, cholestatic jaundice, hepatitis, liver failure, increased serum transaminases, aplastic anemia, hemolytic anemia, leukopenia, thrombocytopenia, agranulocytosis, pancytopenia, eosinophilia, hepatic porphyria. Frequent: Weight gain, fatigue, diarrhea, nausea, dyspepsia, rash.

ENDOCRINE AND METABOLIC: Diabetes-Related—Thiazolidinediones

NOTE: No clinical studies have established conclusive evidence of decreased macrovascular outcomes with antidiabetic drugs. May cause edema, wt gain, new heart failure, or exacerbate existing heart failure (contraindicated in NYHA Class III or IV), especially in combination with insulin. Monitor for signs of heart failure (rapid wt gain, dyspnea, edema) following initiation or dose increase. If occurs, manage fluid retention and consider discontinuation or dosage decrease. Avoid if liver disease or ALT greater than 2.5 times normal. Monitor LFTs before therapy and periodically thereafter. Discontinue if ALT greater than 3 times upper normal limit. Full effect may not be apparent for up to 12 weeks. May cause resumption of ovulation in premenopausal anovulatory women; recommend contraception use.

PIOGLITAZONE (Actos) ▶L ♀C ▶– $
ADULT — DM, Type 2: Start 15 to 30 mg PO daily, may adjust dose after 3 months to max 45 mg/day.
PEDS — Not approved nor recommended in children.
FORMS — Generic/Trade: Tabs 15, 30, 45 mg.
NOTES — Reports of fracture risk. Do not use in Type 1 DM or DKA. Urinary bladder tumors reported; advise patients to report macroscopic hematuria or dysuria.
MOA — Increases insulin sensitivity in adipose tissue, skeletal muscle, and liver.
ADVERSE EFFECTS — Serious: Hepatotoxicity, liver failure, heart failure exacerbation, resumption of ovulation, macular edema, fracture, bladder tumor. Frequent: Edema, wt gain, upper respiratory tract infection, headache, myalgia.

ROSIGLITAZONE (Avandia) ▶L ♀C ▶– $$$$
ADULT — DM, Type 2 monotherapy or in combination with metformin or sulfonylurea: Start 4 mg PO daily or divided two times per day, may increase after 8 to 12 weeks to max 8 mg/day.

PEDS — Not approved in children younger than 18 yo.
FORMS — Trade only (restricted access): Tabs 2, 4, 8 mg.
NOTES — Due to potential for elevated cardiovascular risks, restricted by FDA to use in patients where other medications cannot control Type 2 diabetes. In order to prescribe, providers must enroll in the Avandia-Rosiglitazone Medicines Access Program. Not recommended with nitrates or insulin, and its labeling includes boxed warning regarding increased risk of myocardial ischemic events and notes that studies are currently inconclusive. Reports of fracture risk.
MOA — Increases insulin sensitivity in adipose tissue, skeletal muscle, and liver.
ADVERSE EFFECTS — Serious: Potential hepatotoxicity, heart failure, resumption of ovulation, macular edema, fracture, myocardial infarction, hypersensitivity. Frequent: Edema, weight gain, upper respiratory tract infection, headache, back pain, dyslipidemia.

ENDOCRINE AND METABOLIC: Diabetes-Related—Other

DEXTROSE (Glutose, B-D Glucose, Insta-Glucose, Dex-4) ▶L ♀C ▶? $
ADULT — Hypoglycemia: 0.5 to 1 g/kg (1 to 2 mL/kg) up to 25 g (50 mL) of 50% soln by slow IV injection. Hypoglycemia in conscious diabetics: 10 to 20 g PO q 10 to 20 min prn.
PEDS — Hypoglycemia in neonates: 0.25 to 0.5 g/kg/dose (5 to 10 mL of 25% dextrose in a 5 kg infant). Severe hypoglycemia or older infants may require larger doses up to 3 g (12 mL of 25% dextrose) followed by a continuous IV infusion of 10% dextrose. Non-neonates may require 0.5 to 1 g/kg.
UNAPPROVED ADULT — Hypoglycemia: 15 to 20 g PO once, repeat in 15 minutes if continued hypoglycemia per self-monitoring
FORMS — OTC Generic/Trade: Chewable tabs 4 g (Dex-4), 5 g (Glutose). Trade only: Oral gel 40%.
NOTES — Do not exceed an infusion rate of 0.5 g/kg/h.
MOA — Elevates blood glucose.
ADVERSE EFFECTS — Serious: None. Frequent: Nausea.

GLUCAGON (GlucaGen) ▶LK ♀B ▶? $$$
ADULT — Hypoglycemia: 1 mg IV/IM/SC. If no response within 15 min, may repeat dose 1 to 2 times (preferred via IV for repeat). Diagnostic aid for GI tract radiography: 1 mg IV/IM/SC.

PEDS — Hypoglycemia in children wt greater 20 kg: Same as adults. Hypoglycemia in children wt less than 20 kg: 0.5 mg IV/IM/SC or 20 to 30 mcg/kg. If no response in 5 to 20 min, may repeat dose 1 to 2 times.
UNAPPROVED ADULT — The following indications are based upon limited data. Esophageal obstruction caused by food: 1 mg IV over 1 to 3 min. Symptomatic bradycardia/hypotension, especially with beta-blocker therapy: 3 to 10 mg IV bolus (0.05 mg/kg general recommendation) may repeat in 10 min; may be followed by continuous infusion of 1 to 5 mg/h or 0.07 mg/kg/h. Infusion rate should be titrated to the desired response.
FORMS — Trade only: Injection 1 mg.
NOTES — Should be reserved for refractory/severe cases or when IV dextrose cannot be administered. Advise patients to educate family members and co-workers how to administer a dose. Give supplemental carbohydrates when patient responds.
MOA — Inhibits glycogen synthesis, enhances glucose formation, and increases hepatic glycogenolysis; has relaxant effect on the GI tract; temporarily inhibits GI tract movement for diagnostic procedures.
ADVERSE EFFECTS — Serious: Generalized allergic reaction, hypotension. Frequent: N/V.

METFORMIN (*Glucophage, Glucophage XR, Glumetza, Fortamet, Riomet*) ▶K ♀B ▶? $

ADULT — DM, type 2: Immediate-release: Start 500 mg PO one to two times per day or 850 mg PO daily with meals. Increase by 500 mg q week or 850 mg q 2 weeks to a maximum of 2550 mg/day. Higher doses may be divided three times per day with meals. Extended-release: Glucophage XR: 500 mg PO daily with evening meal; increase by 500 mg q week to max 2000 mg/day (may divide two times per day). Glumetza: 1000 mg PO daily with evening meal; increase by 500 mg q week to max 2000 mg/day (may divide two times per day). Fortamet: 500 to 1000 mg daily with evening meal; increase by 500 mg q week to max 2500 mg/day. All products started at low doses to improve GI tolerability, gradually increase as tolerated.

PEDS — DM, Type 2, 10 yo or older: Start 500 mg PO one to two times per day (Glucophage) with meals, increase by 500 mg q week to max 2000 mg/day in divided doses (10 to 16 yo). Glucophage XR and Fortamet are indicated for age 17 yo or older.

UNAPPROVED ADULT — Polycystic ovary syndrome: 500 mg PO three times per day or 850 mg PO two times per day. Prevention/delay DM Type 2 (with lifestyle modifications): 850 mg PO daily for 1 month, then increase to 850 mg PO two times per day.

FORMS — Generic/Trade: Tabs 500, 850, 1000 mg, extended-release 500, 750 mg. Trade only, extended-release: Fortamet 500, 1000 mg; Glumetza 500, 1000 mg. Trade only: Oral soln 500 mg/5 mL (Riomet).

NOTES — May reduce the risk of progression to Type 2 diabetes in those with impaired glucose tolerance, but less effectively than intensive lifestyle modification. Metformin-containing products may cause life-threatening lactic acidosis, usually in setting of decreased tissue perfusion, hypoxia, hepatic dysfunction, unstable congestive heart failure or impaired renal clearance. Hold prior to IV contrast agents and for 48 h after. Avoid if ethanol abuse, hepatic or renal insufficiency (creatinine 1.4 mg/dL or greater in women, 1.5 mg/dL or greater in men), or hypoxic states (cardiogenic shock, septicemia, acute MI). No clinical studies have established conclusive evidence of decreased macrovascular outcomes with antidiabetic drugs.

MOA — Decreases hepatic gluconeogenesis and increases insulin sensitivity.

ADVERSE EFFECTS — Serious: Lactic acidosis, decreased serum vitamin B12. Frequent: Diarrhea, N/V, flatulence, abdominal discomfort, headache, weight loss, taste disturbance.

MIFEPRISTONE (*Korlym*) ▶L ♀X ▶— $$$$$

ADULT — Hyperglycemia in Cushing's syndrome (failed surgery or not surgical candidate): 300 mg PO once daily with meal. Titrate to max of 1200 mg daily as tolerated. Max 20 mg/kg/day. In renal impairment or mild-moderate hepatic impairment, max 600 mg/day.

PEDS — Not approved in peds.

FORMS — Trade only

NOTES — Contrainc gestational effects no pregnancy prior is interrupted for mc reproductive age. Do metrial hyperplasia o vaginal bleeding. Not unrelated to Cushing's and symptoms of adrer ...y.

MOA — Cortisol receptor blockade

ADVERSE EFFECTS — Serious: pregnancy termination, adrenal insufficiency, hypokelemia, vaginal bleeding, endometrial changes, QT interval prolongation. Frequent: N/V, fatigue, HA, arthralgia, edema, decreased appetite, dizziness, HTN.

PRAMLINTIDE (*Symlin, Symlinpen*) ▶K ♀C ▶? $$$$

WARNING — May cause severe insulin-induced hypoglycemia especially in Type 1 DM, usually within 3 h. Avoid if hypoglycemic unawareness, gastroparesis, GI motility medications, alpha-glucosidase inhibitors, A1C more than 9%, poor compliance, or hypersensitivity to the metacresol preservative. Appropriate patient selection, careful patient instruction, and insulin dose adjustments (reduction in premeal short-acting insulin of 50%) are critical for reducing the hypoglycemia risk.

ADULT — DM, Type 1 with mealtime insulin therapy: Initiate 15 mcg SC immediately before major meals and titrate by 15 mcg increments (if significant nausea has not occurred for at least 3 days) to maintenance 30 to 60 mcg as tolerated. If significant nausea, decrease to 30 mcg. DM, Type 2 with mealtime insulin therapy: Initiate 60 mcg SC immediately before major meals and increase to 120 mcg as tolerated (if significant nausea has not occurred for 3 to 7 days). If significant nausea, decrease dose to 60 mcg.

PEDS — Not approved in children.

FORMS — Trade only: 600 mcg/mL in 5 mL vials, 1000 mcg/mL pen injector (SymlinPen) 1.5, 2.7 mL.

NOTES — Keep unopened vials refrigerated. Opened vials can be kept at room temperature or refrigerated up to 28 days. May give SC in abdomen or thigh. Take medications that require rapid onset 1 h prior or 2 h after. Careful patient selection and skilled health care supervision are critical for safe and effective use. Monitor pre-/postmeal and bedtime glucose. Decrease initial premeal short-acting insulin doses by 50% including fixed-mix insulin (ie, 70/30). Do not mix with insulin. Use new needle and syringe for each dose.

MOA — Amylin analog that reduces postprandial hyperglycemia by slowing gastric emptying and decreasing postprandial glucagon secretion. It also decreases caloric intake by decreasing appetite.

ADVERSE EFFECTS — Serious: Severe hypoglycemia, systemic allergic reaction, pancreatitis. Frequent: N/V, headache, abdominal pain, hypoglycemia, injection site reactions.

ENDOCRINE AND METABOLIC: Diagnostic Agents

ICOTROPIN (*H.P. Acthar Gel*) ▶K ♀C ▶– $$$$$
ADULT — Diagnostic testing of adrenocortical function: 80 units IM or SC. Acute exacerbation of multiple sclerosis: 80 to 120 units IM daily IM for 2 to 3 weeks.
UNAPPROVED PEDS — Various dosing regimens have been used for infantile spasms.
NOTES — Limited therapeutic value in conditions responsive to corticosteroid therapy; corticosteroids should be the treatment of choice if responsive. Prolonged use in children may inhibit skeletal growth. Cosyntropin preferred for diagnostic testing as it is less allergenic and more potent.
MOA — Stimulates the adrenal cortex to secrete cortisol, corticosterone, aldosterone and weakly androgenic substances.
ADVERSE EFFECTS — Serious: Hypersensitivity, convulsions. Frequent: Electrolyte imbalances, menstrual irregularities.

COSYNTROPIN (*Cortrosyn*, *✦Synacthen*) ▶L ♀C ▶? $
ADULT — Rapid screen for adrenocortical insufficiency: 0.25 mg IM/IV over 2 min; measure serum cortisol before and 30 to 60 min after.
PEDS — Rapid screen for adrenocortical insufficiency: 0.25 mg (0.125 mg if age younger than 2 yo) IM/IV over 2 min; measure serum cortisol before and 30 to 60 min after.
MOA — Stimulates the adrenal cortex to produce and secrete hormones.

ADVERSE EFFECTS — Serious: Hypersensitivity. Frequent: None (since used diagnostically).
METYRAPONE (*Metopirone*) ▶KL ♀C ▶? $
WARNING — May cause acute adrenal insufficiency.
ADULT — Diagnostic aid for testing hypothalamic-pituitary adrenocorticotropic hormone (ACTH) function: Specialized single- and multiple-test dose available.
PEDS — (ACTH) function: Specialized single- and multiple-test dose available.
UNAPPROVED ADULT — Cushing's syndrome: Dosing varies.
FORMS — Trade only: Caps 250 mg. Only available from manufacturer due to limited supply: 1-800-988-7768.
NOTES — Ability of adrenals to respond to exogenous ACTH should be demonstrated before metyrapone is employed as a test. In the presence of hypo- or hyperthyroidism, response to the test may be subnormal. May suppress aldosterone synthesis. May cause dizziness and sedation.
MOA — Inhibits endogenous adrenal corticosteroid synthesis.
ADVERSE EFFECTS — Serious: Acute adrenal insufficiency, bone marrow suppression, neutropenia, hypotension. Frequent: Sedation, dizziness, headache, rash, abdominal discomfort, vomiting.

ENDOCRINE AND METABOLIC: Minerals

CALCIUM ACETATE (*PhosLo, Eliphos, Phoslyra*) ▶K ♀C ▶? $
ADULT — Phosphate binder to reduce serum phosphorous in end stage renal disease: Initially 2 tabs/caps or 10 mL of soln PO three times per day with each meal. Titrate dose gradually based on serum phosphorus. Usual dose 3 to 4 tabs/caps or 15 to 20 mL per meal.
PEDS — Not approved in children.
UNAPPROVED PEDS — Titrate to response.
FORMS — Generic/Trade: Gelcaps 667 mg (169 mg elem Ca). Tabs 667 mg (169 mg elem Ca). Trade only: Sol (Phoslyra): 667mg (169 mg elemental calcium)/5 mL.
NOTES — Avoid calcium supplements and antacids with calcium. Monitor serum calcium twice weekly initially and during dosage adjustment. Monitor for signs of hypercalcemia and discontinue if occurs. Consider decreasing or discontinuing vitamin D supplementation if mild hypercalcemia occurs. Maintain serum calcium-phosphorous product (Ca × P) less than 55. Hypercalcemia may aggrevate digoxin toxicity.
MOA — Binds with dietary phosphate to form a non-absorbable complex.
ADVERSE EFFECTS — Serious: Severe hypercalcemia (with confusion, delirium, stupor, coma), renal

calculi. Frequent: Mild hypercalcemia, constipation, anorexia, N/V.
CALCIUM CARBONATE (*Caltrate, Mylanta Children's, Os-Cal, Oyst-Cal, Tums, Surpass, Viactiv, ✦Calsan*) ▶K ♀+ (? 1st trimester) ▶? $
ADULT — Supplement: 1 to 2 g elem Ca/day or more PO with meals divided two to four times per day. Prevention of osteoporosis: 1000 to 1500 mg elem Ca/day PO divided two to three times per day with meals. The adequate intake in most adults is 1000 to 1200 mg elem Ca/day. Antacid: 1000 to 3000 mg (2 to 4 tab) PO q 2 h prn or 1 to 2 pieces gum chewed prn, max 7000 mg/day.
PEDS — Hypocalcemia: Neonates: 50 to 150 mg elem Ca/kg/day PO in 4 to 6 divided doses; Children: 45 to 65 mg elem Ca/kg/day PO divided four times per day. Adequate intake for children (in elem calcium): Age younger than 6 mo: 210 mg/day when fed human milk and 315 mg/day when fed cow's milk; 6 to 12 mo: 270 mg/day when fed human milk + solid food and 335 mg/day when fed cow's milk + solid food; 1 to 3 yo: 500 mg/day; 4 to 8 yo: 800 mg/day; 9 to 18 yo 1300 mg/day.
UNAPPROVED ADULT — May lower BP in patients with HTN. May reduce PMS symptoms such as fluid retention, pain, and negative affect.

CALCIUM CARBONATE (*cont.*)

FORMS — OTC Generic/Trade: Tabs 500, 650, 750, 1000, 1250, 1500 mg, Chewable tabs 400, 500, 750, 850, 1000, 1177, 1250 mg, Caps 1250 mg, Gum 300, 450 mg, Susp 1250 mg/5 mL. Calcium carbonate is 40% elem Ca and contains 20 mEq of elem Ca/g calcium carbonate. Not more than 500 to 600 mg elem Ca/dose. Available in combination with sodium fluoride, vitamin D and/or vitamin K. Trade examples: Caltrate 600 + D = 600 mg elemental Ca/200 units vitamin D, Os-Cal 500 + D = 500 mg elemental Ca/200 units vitamin D, Os-Cal Extra D = 500 mg elemental Ca/400 units vitamin D, Tums (regular strength) = 200 mg elemental Ca, Tums (ultra) = 400 mg elemental Ca, Viactiv (chewable) 500 mg elemental Ca+ 100 units vitamin D + 40 mcg vitamin K.

NOTES — Decreases absorption of levothyroxine, tetracycline, and fluoroquinolones.

MOA — Antacid, mineral supplement.

ADVERSE EFFECTS — Serious: Severe hypercalcemia (with confusion, delirium, stupor, coma), renal calculi. Frequent: Mild hypercalcemia, constipation, anorexia, N/V.

CALCIUM CHLORIDE ▸K ♀+ ▶+ $

ADULT — Hypocalcemia: 500 to 1000 mg slow IV q 1 to 3 days. Magnesium intoxication: 500 mg IV. Hyperkalemic ECG changes: Dose based on ECG.

PEDS — Hypocalcemia: 0.2 mL/kg IV up to 10 mL/day. Cardiac resuscitation: 0.2 mL/kg IV.

UNAPPROVED ADULT — Has been used in calcium channel blocker toxicity and to treat or prevent calcium channel blocker–induced hypotension.

UNAPPROVED PEDS — Has been used in calcium channel blocker toxicity.

FORMS — Generic only: Injectable 10% (1000 mg/10 mL) 10 mL ampules, vials, syringes.

NOTES — Calcium chloride contains 14.4 mEq Ca/g versus calcium gluconate 4.7 mEq Ca/g. For IV use only; do not administer IM or SC. Avoid extravasation. Administer no faster than 0.5 to 1 mL/min. Use cautiously in patients receiving digoxin; inotropic and toxic effects are synergistic and may cause arrhythmias. Usually not recommended for hypocalcemia associated with renal insufficiency because calcium chloride is an acidifying salt.

MOA — Antagonizes the cardiotoxic effects of hyperkalemia.

ADVERSE EFFECTS — Serious: Vasodilation, hypotension. Frequent: Irritation at infusion site.

CALCIUM CITRATE (*Citracal*) ▸K ♀+ ▶+ $

ADULT — 1 to 2 g elem Ca/day or more PO with meals divided two to four times per day. Prevention of osteoporosis: 1000 to 1500 mg elem Ca/day PO divided two to three times per day with meals. The adequate intake in most adults is 1000 to 1200 mg elem Ca/day.

PEDS — Not approved in children.

FORMS — OTC Trade/generic (mg elem Ca/units vitamin D): 200/250, 250/200, 315/250, 600/500 (slow release); some products available with magnesium

and/or phosphorus. Chewable gummies: 250 mg with 250 units vitamin D.

NOTES — Calcium citrate is 21% elem Ca. Not more than 500 to 600 mg elem Ca/dose. Decreases absorption of levothyroxine, tetracycline and fluoroquinolones. Acidic environment not needed for absorption; preferred calcium salt in patients on PPI or H2RA.

MOA — Essential mineral that maintains the nervous, muscular, and skeletal systems and cell membrane and capillary permeability.

ADVERSE EFFECTS — Serious: Severe hypercalcemia (with confusion, delirium, stupor, coma), renal calculi. Frequent: Mild hypercalcemia, constipation, anorexia, N/V.

CALCIUM GLUCONATE ▸K ♀+ ▶+ $

ADULT — Emergency correction of hypocalcemia: 7 to 14 mEq slow IV prn. Hypocalcemic tetany: 4.5 to 16 mEq IM prn. Hyperkalemia with cardiac toxicity: 2.25 to 14 mEq IV while monitoring ECG. May repeat after 1 to 2 min. Magnesium intoxication: 4.5 to 9 mEq IV, adjust dose based on patient response. If IV not possible, give 2 to 5 mEq IM. Exchange transfusions: 1.35 mEq calcium gluconate IV concurrent with each 100 mL of citrated blood. Oral calcium gluconate: 1 to 2 g elem Ca/day or more PO with meals divided two to four times per day. Prevention of osteoporosis: 1000 to 1500 mg elem Ca/day PO with meals in divided doses.

PEDS — Emergency correction of hypocalcemia: Children: 1 to 7 mEq IV prn. Infants: 1 mEq IV prn. Hypocalcemic tetany: Children: 0.5 to 0.7 mEq/kg IV three to four times per day. Neonates: 2.4 mEq/kg/day IV in divided doses. Exchange transfusions: Neonates: 0.45 mEq IV/100 mL of exchange transfusions. Oral calcium gluconate: Hypocalcemia: Neonates: 50 to 150 mg elem Ca/kg/day PO in 4 to 6 divided doses; children: 45 to 65 mg elem Ca/kg/day PO divided four times per day.

UNAPPROVED ADULT — Has been used in calcium channel blocker toxicity and to treat or prevent calcium channel blocker-induced hypotension.

UNAPPROVED PEDS — Has been used in calcium channel blocker toxicity.

FORMS — Generic only: Injectable 10% (1000 mg/10 mL, 4.65 mEq/10 mL) 1, 10, 50, 100, 200 mL. OTC Generic only: Tabs 50, 500, 650, 975, 1000 mg. Chewable tabs 650 mg.

NOTES — Calcium gluconate is 9.3% elem Ca and contains 4.6 mEq elem Ca/g calcium gluconate. Administer IV calcium gluconate not faster than 0.5 to 2 mL/min. Use cautiously in patients receiving digoxin; inotropic and toxic effects are synergistic and may cause arrhythmias.

MOA — Essential mineral that maintains the nervous, muscular, and skeletal systems and cell membrane and capillary permeability; antagonizes the cardiotoxic effects of hyperkalemia.

ADVERSE EFFECTS — Serious: Severe hypercalcemia (with confusion, delirium, stupor, coma), renal

(cont.)

CALCIUM GLUCONATE (cont.)

calculi; with IV: vasodilation, hypotension, arrhythmia, syncope and cardiac arrest. Frequent: Mild hypercalcemia, constipation, anorexia, N/V, irritation at infusion site (for IV).

COPPER GLUCONATE ▶L - ♀A ▶? $

ADULT — Supplementation: 2 to 5 mg PO daily. RDA: Adults: 900 mcg PO daily; pregnancy: 1000 mcg PO daily; Breastfeeding: 1300 mcg PO daily.

PEDS — RDA: 14 to 18 yo: 890 mcg PO daily; 9 to 13 yo: 700 mcg PO daily; 4 to 8 yo: 440 mcg PO daily; 1 to 3 yo: 340 mcg PO daily; 7 to 12 mo: 220 mcg PO daily; 0 to 6 mo: 200 mcg PO daily.

FORMS — OTC Generic: 2, 5 mg.

MOA — Essential element required for iron metabolism, CNS function and immune system activity.

ADVERSE EFFECTS — Serious: cirrhosis, hemoglobinuria. Common: arthralgias, myalgias, hypertension, dermatitis, N/V, diarrhea, abdominal pain, headache.

FERRIC CARBOXYMALTOSE (Injectafer) ▶NA ♀C ▶? $$$$$

ADULT — Iron deficiency anemia (unsatisfactory response to oral iron, non-dialysis dependent):If less than 50 kg: 15 mg/kg elemental iron IV for 2 doses, separated by at least 7 days. If 50 kg or greater: 750 mg elemental iron IV for 2 doses, separated by at least 7 days. Max: 1500 mg per course.

FORMS — Trade only: 750 mg iron/15 mL vial.

NOTES — Hypersensitivity reported, monitor during and at least 30 min following administration. Monitor for hypertension.

MOA — Essential mineral needed for hemoglobin, myoglobin, and enzymatic function.

ADVERSE EFFECTS — Serious: Hypersensitivity reactions, severe hypertension. Frequent: Nausea, hypertension, flushing, hypophosphatemia, dizziness.

FERRIC GLUCONATE COMPLEX (Ferrlecit) ▶KL ♀B ▶? $$$$$

WARNING — Potentially fatal hypersensitivity reactions rarely reported with sodium ferric gluconate complex. Facilities for CPR must be available during dosing.

ADULT — Iron deficiency in chronic hemodialysis patients: 125 mg elem iron IV over 10 min or diluted in 100 mL NS IV over 1 h. Most hemodialysis patients require 1 g of elem iron over 8 consecutive hemodialysis session.

PEDS — Iron deficiency in chronic hemodialysis age 6 yo or older: 1.5 mg/kg elem iron diluted in 25 mL NS and administered IV over 1 h at 8 sequential dialysis sessions. Max 125 mg/dose.

UNAPPROVED ADULT — Iron deficiency in cancer- and chemotherapy-induced anemia: 125 mg elem iron IV over 60 min, repeat weekly for 8 doses, or 200 mg IV over 3 to 4 h repeated q 3 weeks for 5 doses.

NOTES — Potentially fatal hypersensitivity reactions, including serious hypotension, reported with sodium ferric gluconate complex. Facilities for CPR must be available during dosing.

MOA — Essential mineral needed for hemoglobin, myoglobin, and enzymatic function.

ADVERSE EFFECTS — Serious: Anaphylactic reaction, chest pain, hypotension, shock, cardiac arrest, iron overdose. Frequent: Arthralgia, backache, chills, dizziness, fever, flushing, headache, infusion site reaction, malaise, myalgia, N/V.

FERROUS GLUCONATE (Fergon) ▶K ♀+ ▶+ $

WARNING — Severe iron toxicity possible in overdose, especially in children. Store out of reach of children and in child-resistant containers. Iron overdose is a leading cause of poisoning in children younger than 6 yo.

ADULT — Iron deficiency: 800 to 1600 mg ferrous gluconate (100 to 200 mg elem iron) PO divided three times per day. RDA (elem iron): 8 mg for adult males age 19 yo or older, 18 mg for adult premenopausal females age 19 to 50 yo, 8 mg for females age 51 yo or older, 27 mg during pregnancy, 10 mg during lactation if age 14 to 18 yo and 9 mg if age 19 to 50 yo. Upper limit: 45 mg/day.

PEDS — Mild to moderate iron deficiency: 3 mg/kg/day of elem iron PO in 1 to 2 divided doses. Severe iron deficiency: 4 to 6 mg/kg/day PO in 3 divided doses. RDA (elem iron): 0.27 mg for age younger than 6 mo, 11 mg for age 7 to 12 mo, 7 mg for age 1 to 3 yo, 10 mg for age 4 to 8 yo, 8 mg for age 9 to 13 yo, 11 mg for males age 14 to 18 yo,15 mg for females age 14 to 18 yo.

UNAPPROVED ADULT — Adjunct to epoetin to maximize hematologic response: 200 mg elem iron/day PO.

UNAPPROVED PEDS — Adjunct to epoetin to maximize hematologic response: 2 to 3 mg/kg elem iron/day PO.

FORMS — OTC Generic/Trade: Tabs (ferrous gluconate) 240 mg (27 mg elemental iron). Generic only: Tabs 324, 325 mg.

NOTES — Ferrous gluconate is 12% elem iron. For iron deficiency, 4 to 6 months of therapy generally necessary to replete stores even after hemoglobin has returned to normal. Do not take within 2 h of antacids, tetracyclines, levothyroxine or fluoroquinolones. May cause black stools, constipation or diarrhea.

MOA — Essential mineral needed for hemoglobin, myoglobin, and enzymatic function.

ADVERSE EFFECTS — Serious: Hypersensitivity, iron overdose. Frequent: Constipation, N/V, diarrhea, black stools.

FERROUS SULFATE (Fer-in-Sol, Feosol, Slow FE, ✷Ferodan, Slow-Fe) ▶K ♀+ ▶+ $

WARNING — Severe iron toxicity possible in overdose, especially in children. Store out of reach of children and in child-resistant containers. Iron overdose is a leading cause of poisoning in children younger than 6 yo.

ADULT — Iron deficiency: 500 to 1000 mg ferrous sulfate (100 to 200 mg elem iron) PO divided three times per day. For iron supplementation RDA see ferrous gluconate.

FERROUS SULFATE (*cont.*)

PEDS — Mild to moderate iron deficiency: 3 mg/kg/day of elem iron PO in 1 to 2 divided doses; Severe Iron deficiency: 4 to 6 mg/kg/day PO in 3 divided doses. For Iron supplementation RDA see ferrous gluconate.

UNAPPROVED ADULT — Adjunct to epoetin to maximize hematologic response: 200 mg elem iron/day PO.

FORMS — OTC Generic/Trade (mg ferrous sulfate): Tabs, extended-release 160 mg. Tabs 200, 324, 325 mg. OTC Generic only (mg ferrous sulfate): Soln 75 mg/0.6 mL. Elixir 220 mg/5 mL.

NOTES — Iron sulfate is 20% elem iron. For iron deficiency, 4 to 6 months of therapy generally necessary. Do not take within 2 h of antacids, tetracyclines, levothyroxine or fluoroquinolones. May cause black stools, constipation or diarrhea.

MOA — Essential mineral needed for hemoglobin, myoglobin, and enzymatic function.

ADVERSE EFFECTS — Serious: Hypersensitivity, iron overdose. Frequent: Constipation, N/V, diarrhea, black stools, tooth staining (liquid preparations).

FERUMOXYTOL (*Feraheme*) ▶KL ♀C ▶? $$$$$

ADULT — Iron deficiency in chronic kidney disease: Give 510 mg IV push, followed by 510 mg IV push for 1 dose given 3 to 8 days after initial injection. May re-administer if persistent/recurrent iron deficiency anemia.

PEDS — Not studied in pediatrics.

NOTES — Administer IV push undiluted up to 30 mg/sec. Monitor hemoglobin and iron studies at least 1 month following second injection. Observe for hypersensitivity for at least 30 min following injection, life-threatening hypersensitivity reported. May alter MRI imaging studies. Contraindicated in anemias not due to iron deficiency.

MOA — Superparamagnetic iron oxide to provide essential mineral needed for hemoglobin, myoglobin, and enzymatic function.

ADVERSE EFFECTS — Serious: Anaphylactic reaction, hypersensitivity, hypotension, iron overdose, syncope, cardiac arrest, arrhythmia, ischemic event, heart failure. Frequent: Diarrhea, nausea, dizziness, constipation, peripheral edema.

FLUORIDE (*Luride,* ✱*Fluor-A-Day*) ▶K ♀? ▶? $

ADULT — Prevention of dental cavities: 10 mL of topical rinse swish and spit daily.

PEDS — Prevention of dental caries: Dose based on age and fluoride concentrations in water. See table.

FLUORIDE SUPPLEMENTATION

Age	<0.3 ppm in drinking water	0.3–0.6 ppm in drinking water	>0.6 ppm in drinking water
0–6 mo	none	none	none
6 mo–3 yo	0.25 mg PO daily	none	none
3–6 yo	0.5 mg PO daily	0.25 mg PO daily	none
6–16 yo	1 mg PO daily	0.5 mg PO daily	none

JADA 2010;141:1480–1489

FORMS — Generic only: Chewable tabs 0.5, 1 mg; Tabs 1 mg, Gtts 0.125 mg, 0.25 mg, and 0.5 mg/dropperful. Lozenges 1 mg, Soln 0.2 mg/mL. Gel 0.1%, 0.5%, 1.23%. Rinse (sodium fluoride) 0.05, 0.1, 0.2%).

NOTES — In communities without fluoridated water, fluoride supplementation should be used until 13 to 16 yo. Chronic overdosage of fluorides may result in dental fluorosis (mottling of tooth enamel) and osseous changes. Use rinses and gels after brushing and flossing and before bedtime.

MOA — Trace element that promotes tooth remineralization and inhibits cariogenesis.

ADVERSE EFFECTS — Serious: Increased bone fracture, allergic rash. Frequent: Rash, eczema, gastric distress, headache, tooth staining (liquid preparations).

IRON DEXTRAN (*InFed, DexFerrum,* ✱*Dexiron, Infufer*) ▶KL ♀C ▶? $$$$

WARNING — Administer a test dose prior to 1st dose. Parenteral iron therapy has resulted in anaphylactic reactions, even with test dose and after uneventful test doses. Potentially fatal hypersensitivity reactions have been reported with iron dextran injection. Facilities for CPR must be available during dosing. Use only when clearly warranted.

ADULT — Iron deficiency: Dose based on patient wt and hemoglobin. Total dose (mL) = 0.0442 × (desired Hgb − observed Hgb) × wt (kg) + [0.26 × wt (kg)]. For wt, use lesser of lean body wt or actual body wt. Iron replacement for blood loss: Replacement iron (mg) = blood loss (mL) × hematocrit. Maximum daily IM dose 100 mg.

PEDS — Not recommended for infants younger than 4 mo. Iron deficiency in children greater than 5 kg: Dose based on patient wt and hemoglobin. Dose (mL) = 0.0442 × (desired Hgb− observed Hgb) × wt (kg) + [0.26 × wt (kg)]. For wt, use lesser of lean body wt or actual body wt. Iron replacement for blood loss: Replacement iron (mg) = blood loss (mL) × hematocrit. Maximum daily IM dose: Infant wt less than 5 kg give 25 mg; children 5 to 10 kg give 50 mg; children wt greater than 10 kg give 100 mg.

UNAPPROVED ADULT — Adjunct to epoetin to maximize hematologic response. Total dose (325 to 1500 mg) as a single, slow (6 mg/min) IV infusion has been used.

UNAPPROVED PEDS — Adjunct to epoetin to maximize hematologic response.

NOTES — A 0.5 mL IV test dose (0.25 mL in infants) over 30 sec or longer should be given at least 1 h before therapy. Infuse no faster than 50 mg/min. For IM administration, use Z-track technique.

MOA — Essential mineral needed for hemoglobin, myoglobin, and enzymatic function.

ADVERSE EFFECTS — Serious: Anaphylactic reaction, chest pain, hypotension, shock, cardiac arrest, iron overdose. Frequent: Arthralgia, backache, chills, dizziness, fever, flushing, headache, infusion site reaction, malaise, myalgia, N/V.

IRON POLYSACCHARIDE (*Niferex, Niferex-150, Nu-Iron 150, Ferrex 150*) ▶K ♀+ ▶+ $$
WARNING — Severe iron toxicity possible in overdose, especially in children. Store out of reach of children and in child-resistant containers. Iron overdose is a leading cause of poisoning in children younger than 6 yo.
ADULT — Iron deficiency: 50 to 200 mg PO divided one to three times per day. For iron supplementation RDA see ferrous gluconate.
PEDS — Mild-moderate iron deficiency: 3 mg/kg/day of elem iron PO in 1 to 2 divided doses. Severe iron deficiency: 4 to 6 mg/kg/day PO in 3 divided doses. For iron supplementation RDA see ferrous gluconate.
UNAPPROVED ADULT — Adjunct to epoetin to maximize hematologic response: 200 mg elem iron/day PO.
UNAPPROVED PEDS — Adjunct to epoetin to maximize hematologic response: 2 to 3 mg/kg elem iron/day PO.
FORMS — OTC Trade only: Caps 60 mg (Niferex). OTC Generic/Trade: Caps 150 mg (Niferex-150, Nu-Iron 150, Ferrex-150), Elixir 100 mg/5 mL (Niferex). 1 mg iron polysaccharide = 1 mg elemental iron.
NOTES — For iron deficiency, 4 to 6 months of therapy generally necessary. Do not take within 2 h of antacids, tetracyclines, levothyroxine, or fluoroquinolones. May cause black stools, constipation or diarrhea.
MOA — Essential mineral needed for hemoglobin, myoglobin, and enzymatic function.
ADVERSE EFFECTS — Serious: Hypersensitivity, iron overdose. Frequent: Constipation, N/V, diarrhea, black stools.

IRON SUCROSE (*Venofer*) ▶KL ♀B ▶? $$$$$
WARNING — Potentially fatal hypersensitivity reactions have been rarely reported with iron sucrose injection. Facilities for CPR must be available during dosing.
ADULT — Iron deficiency in chronic hemodialysis patients: 5 mL (100 mg elem iron) IV over 5 min or diluted in 100 mL NS IV over 15 min or longer. Iron deficiency in non-dialysis dependent chronic kidney disease patients: 10 mL (200 mg elem iron) IV over 5 min or 500 mg diluted in 250 mL NS IV over 4 h.
PEDS — Iron deficiency in chronic hemodialysis dependent or non-dialysis dependent chronic kidney disease (2 yo or older): 0.5 mg/kg slow IV injection or infusion. Max: 100 mg elemental iron. Give injection over 5 min or dilute in in 25 mL of NS and administer IV over 5 to 60 min.
UNAPPROVED ADULT — Iron deficiency: 5 mL (100 mg elem iron) IV over 5 min or diluted in 100 mL NS IV over 15 min or longer.
NOTES — Most hemodialysis patients require 1 g of elem iron over 10 consecutive hemodialysis sessions. Non-dialysis patients require 1 g of elemental iron divided and given over 14 days. Observe patients for at least 30 minutes following administration; anaphylaxis reported.
MOA — Essential mineral needed for hemoglobin, myoglobin, and enzymatic function.

ADVERSE EFFECTS — Serious: Anaphylaxis, chest pain, hypotension, shock, cardiac arrest, iron overdose. Frequent: Arthralgia, backache, chills, dizziness, fever, flushing, headache, infusion site reaction, malaise, myalgia, N/V.

MAGNESIUM CHLORIDE (*Slow-Mag*) ▶K ♀A ▶+ $
ADULT — Dietary supplement: 2 tabs PO daily. RDA (elem Mg): Adult males: 400 mg if 19 to 30 yo, 420 mg if older than 30 yo. Adult females: 310 mg if 19 to 30 yo, 320 mg if older than 30 yo.
PEDS — Not approved in children.
UNAPPROVED ADULT — Hypomagnesemia: 300 mg elem magnesium PO divided four times per day.
FORMS — OTC Trade only: Enteric coated tab 64 mg. 64 mg tab Slow-Mag = 64 mg elemental magnesium.
NOTES — May cause diarrhea. May accumulate in renal insufficiency.
MOA — Essential mineral needed for muscle function, organ function, potassium and calcium absorption.
ADVERSE EFFECTS — Serious: Potential magnesium intoxication. Frequent: Diarrhea, weakness, N/V.

MAGNESIUM GLUCONATE (*Almora, Magtrate, Maganate, ✲Maglucate*) ▶K ♀A ▶+ $
ADULT — Dietary supplement: 500 to 1000 mg/day PO divided three times per day. RDA (elem Mg): Adult males: 19 to 30 yo: 400 mg; older than 30 yo: 420 mg. Adult females: 19 to 30 yo: 310 mg; older than 30 yo: 320 mg.
PEDS — Not approved in children.
UNAPPROVED ADULT — Hypomagnesemia: 300 mg elem magnesium PO divided four times per day. Unproven efficacy for oral tocolysis following IV magnesium sulfate.
UNAPPROVED PEDS — Hypomagnesemia: 10 to 20 mg elem magnesium/kg/dose PO four times per day. RDA (elem Mg): Age 0 to 6 mo: 30 mg/day; age 7 to 12 mo: 75 mg/day; age 1 to 3 yo: 80 mg; age 4 to 8 yo: 130 mg; age 9 to 13 yo: 240 mg; age 14 to 18 yo (males): 410 mg; age 14 to 18 yo (females): 360 mg.
FORMS — OTC Generic only: Tabs 500 mg (27 mg elemental Mg), liquid 54 mg elemental Mg/5 mL.
NOTES — May cause diarrhea. Use caution in renal failure; may accumulate.
MOA — Essential mineral needed for muscle function, organ function, potassium and calcium absorption.
ADVERSE EFFECTS — Serious: Potential magnesium intoxication. Frequent: Diarrhea, weakness, N/V.

MAGNESIUM OXIDE (*Mag-200, Mag-Ox 400*) ▶K ♀A ▶+ $
ADULT — Dietary supplement: 400 to 800 mg PO daily. RDA (elem Mg): Adult males: 19 to 30 yo: 400 mg; older than 30 yo 420 mg. Adult females: 19 to 30 yo: 310 mg; older than 30 yo: 320 mg.
PEDS — Not approved in children.
UNAPPROVED ADULT — Hypomagnesemia: 300 mg elem magnesium PO four times per day. Has also been used as oral tocolysis following IV magnesium

MAGNESIUM OXIDE (*cont.*)

sulfate (unproven efficacy) and in the prevention of calcium-oxalate kidney stones.

FORMS — OTC Generic/Trade: Caps: 140 (84.5 mg elemental Mg), 250 (elemental), 400 (240 mg elemental Mg), 420 (253 mg elemental Mg), 500 mg (elemental).

NOTES — Take with food. Magnesium oxide is approximately 60% elemental magnesium. May accumulate in renal insufficiency.

MOA — Essential mineral needed for muscle function, organ function, potassium and calcium absorption.

ADVERSE EFFECTS — Serious: Potential magnesium intoxication. Frequent: Diarrhea, weakness, N/V.

MAGNESIUM SULFATE ▶K ♀D C/D ▶+ $

ADULT — Hypomagnesemia: Mild deficiency: 1 g IM q 6 h for 4 doses; severe deficiency: 2 g IV over 1 h (monitor for hypotension). Hyperalimentation: Maintenance requirements not precisely known; adults generally require 8 to 24 mEq/day. Seizure prevention in severe preeclampsia or eclampsia: ACOG Recommendations: 4 to 6 g IV loading dose, then 1 to 2 g/h IV continuous infusion for at least 24 h. Or per product information: total initial dose of 10 to 14 g administered via IV infusion and IM doses (4 g IV infusion with 5 g IM injections in each buttock). Initial dose is followed by 4 to 5 g IM into alternate buttocks q 4 h PRN or initial dose is followed by 1 to 2 g/hour constant IV infusion. Max: 30 to 40 g/24h.

PEDS — Not approved in children.

UNAPPROVED ADULT — Preterm labor: 6 g IV over 20 min, then 1 to 3 g/h titrated to decrease contractions. Has been used as an adjunctive bronchodilator in very severe acute asthma (2 g IV over 10 to 20 min), and in chronic fatigue syndrome. Torsades de pointes: 1 to 2 g IV in D5W over 5 to 60 min.

UNAPPROVED PEDS — Hypomagnesemia: 25 to 50 mg/kg IV/IM q 4 to 6 h for 3 to 4 doses, maximum single dose 2 g. Hyperalimentation: Maintenance requirements not precisely known; infants require 2 to 10 mEq/day. Acute nephritis: 20 to 40 mg/kg (in 20% soln) IM prn. Adjunctive bronchodilator in very severe acute asthma: 25 to 100 mg/kg IV over 10 to 20 min.

NOTES — 1000 mg magnesium sulfate contains 8 mEq elem magnesium. Do not give faster than 1.5 mL/min (of 10% soln) except in eclampsia or seizures. Use caution in renal insufficiency; may accumulate. Monitor urine output, patellar reflex, respiratory rate and serum magnesium level. Concomitant use with terbutaline may lead to fatal pulmonary edema. IM administration must be diluted to a 20% soln. If needed, may reverse toxicity with calcium gluconate 1 g IV. Continuous use in pregnancy beyond 5 to 7 days may cause fetal harm.

MOA — Essential mineral needed for muscle function, organ function, potassium and calcium absorption; blocks neuromuscular transmission to prevent or control convulsions.

ADVERSE EFFECTS — Serious: Magnesium intoxication (in recipient of drug or in newborn of pregnant woman receiving Mg), cardiac depression, CNS depression, respiratory paralysis, hypotension, stupor, hypothermia, circulatory collapse. Frequent: Flushing, sweating, depressed reflexes.

PHOSPHORUS (*Neutra-Phos, K-Phos*) ▶K ♀C ▶? $

ADULT — Dietary supplement: 1 cap/packet (Neutra-Phos) PO four times per day or 1 to 2 tab (K-Phos) PO four times per day after meals and at bedtime. Severe hypophosphatemia (less than 1 mg/dL): 0.08 to 0.16 mmol/kg IV over 6 h. In TPN, 310 to 465 mg/day (10 to 15 mM) IV is usually adequate, although higher amounts may be necessary in hypermetabolic states. RDA for adults is 800 mg.

PEDS — RDA (elem phosphorus): 0 to 6 mo: 100 mg; 6 to 12 mo: 275 mg; 1 to 3 yo: 460 mg; 4 to 8 yo: 500 mg; 9 to 18: 1250 mg. Severe hypophosphatemia (less than 1 mg/dL): 0.25 to 0.5 mmol/kg IV over 4 to 6 h. Infant TPN: 1.5 to 2 mmol/kg/day in TPN.

FORMS — OTC Trade only: (Neutra-Phos, Neutra-Phos K) tab/cap/packet 250 mg (8 mmol) phosphorus. Rx: Trade only: (K-Phos) tab 250 mg (8 mmol) phosphorus.

NOTES — Dissolve caps/tabs/powder in 75 mL water prior to ingestion.

MOA — Essential mineral needed for bone metabolism and enzymatic functions.

ADVERSE EFFECTS — Serious: Phosphate intoxication with reciprocal hypocalcemic tetany (with IV). Frequent: Laxative-like effect, nausea, abdominal pain, vomiting.

***POTASSIUM* (Cena-K)** ▶K ♀C ▶? $

ADULT — Hypokalemia: 20 to 40 mEq/day or more IV or immediate-release PO. Intermittent infusion: 10 to 20 mEq/dose IV over 1 to 2 h prn. Consider monitoring for infusions greater than 10 mEq/h. Prevention of hypokalemia: 20 to 40 mEq/day PO one to two times per day.

PEDS — Not approved in children.

UNAPPROVED ADULT — Diuretic-induced Hypokalemia: 20 to 60 mEq/day PO.

UNAPPROVED PEDS — Hypokalemia: 2.5 mEq/kg/day given IV/PO one to two times per day. Intermittent infusion: 0.5 to 1 mEq/kg/dose IV at 0.3 to 0.5 mEq/kg/h prn. Infusions faster than 0.5 mEq/kg/h require continuous monitoring.

FORMS — Injectable, many different products in a variety of salt forms (i.e., chloride, bicarbonate, citrate, acetate, gluconate), available in tabs, caps, liquids, effervescent tabs, packets. Potassium gluconate is available OTC. See table.

NOTES — Use potassium chloride for hypokalemia associated with alkalosis; use potassium bicarbonate, citrate, acetate, or gluconate when associated with acidosis.

(cont.)

POTASSIUM (cont.)

POTASSIUM (ORAL FORMS)*

Effervescent Granules	
20 mEq	Klorvess Effervescent, K-vescent

Effervescent Tabs	
10 mEq	Effer-K
20 mEq	Effer-K
25 mEq	Effer-K, K+Care ET, K-Lyte, K-Lyte/Cl, Klor-Con/EF
50 mEq	K-Lyte DS, K-Lyte/Cl 50

Liquids	
20 mEq/15 mL	Cena-K, Kaochlor S-F, K-G Elixir, Kaochlor 10%, Kay Ciel, Kaon, Kaylixir, Kolyum, Potasalan, Twin-K
30 mEq/15 mL	Rum-K
40 mEq/15 mL	Cena-K, Kaon-Cl 20%
45 mEq/15 mL	Tri-K

Powders	
15 mEq/pack	K+Care
20 mEq/pack	Gen-K, K+Care, Kay Ciel, K-Lor, Klor-Con
25 mEq/pack	K+Care, Klor-Con 25

Tabs/Caps	
8 mEq	K+8, Klor-Con 8, Slow-K, Micro-K
10 mEq	K+10, K-Norm, Kaon-Cl 10, Klor-Con M10 Klotrix, K-Tab, K-Dur 10, Micro-K 10
20 mEq	Klor-Con M20, K-Dur 20

MOA — Intracellular cation that participates in numerous essential physiological processes.

ADVERSE EFFECTS — Serious: Hyperkalemia, gastrointestinal toxicity (obstruction, bleed, ulcer, perforation, esophagitis). Frequent: N/V, diarrhea, abdominal pain, infusion site irritation (IV).

ZINC ACETATE (*Galzin*) ▶Minimal absorption ♀A ▶– $$$

ADULT — RDA (elemental Zn): Adult males: 11 mg daily. Adult females: 8 to 12 mg daily. Zinc deficiency: 25 to 50 mg (elemental) daily. Wilson's disease, previously treated with chelating agent: 25 to 50 mg (elemental) PO three times per day.

PEDS — RDA (elem Zn): Age 7 mo to 3 yo: 3 mg; 4 to 8 yo: 5 mg; 9 to 13 yo: 8 mg; 14 to 18 yo (males): 8 mg; 14 to 18 yo (females): 9 to 14 mg. Zinc deficiency: 0.5 to 1 mg elemental zinc mg/kg/day divided two to three times per day. Wilson's disease (age 10 yo or older): 25 to 50 mg (elemental) three times per day.

FORMS — Trade only: Caps 25, 50 mg elemental zinc.

NOTES — Poorly absorbed; take 1 h before or 2 to 3 h after meals. Decreases absorption of tetracycline and fluoroquinolones.

MOA — Nutritional supplement. Blocks intestinal absorption of copper.

ADVERSE EFFECTS — Serious: Sideroblastic anemia, pancreatitis. Frequent: N/V.

ZINC SULFATE (*Orazinc, Zincate*) ▶Minimal absorption ♀A ▶– $

ADULT — RDA (elemental Zn): Adult males: 11 mg daily. Adult females: 8 to 12 mg daily. Zinc deficiency: 25 to 50 mg (elemental) PO daily.

PEDS — RDA (elemental Zn): Age 7 mo to 3 yo: 3 mg; 4 to 8 yo: 5 mg; 9 to 13 yo: 8 mg; 14 to 18 yo (males): 8 mg; 14 to 18 yo (females): 9 to 14 mg. Zinc deficiency: 0.5 to 1 mg elemental zinc mg/kg/day PO divided two to three times per day.

UNAPPROVED ADULT — Wound healing in zinc deficiency: 200 mg PO three times per day.

FORMS — OTC Generic/Trade: Tabs 66, 110, 200 mg. Rx Generic/Trade: Caps 220 mg.

NOTES — Zinc sulfate is 23% elemental Zn. Decreases absorption of tetracycline and fluoroquinolones. Poorly absorbed; increased absorption on empty stomach; however, administration with food decreases GI upset.

MOA — Nutritional supplement.

ADVERSE EFFECTS — Serious: Sideroblastic anemia, pancreatitis. Frequent: N/V.

ENDOCRINE AND METABOLIC: Nutritionals

BANANA BAG ▶KL ♀+ ▶+ $

UNAPPROVED ADULT — Alcoholic malnutrition (example formula): Add thiamine 100 mg + folic acid 1 mg + IV multivitamins to 1 liter NS and infuse over 4 h. Magnesium sulfate 2 g may be added. "Banana bag" is jargon and not a valid drug order; also known as "rally pack"; specify individual components.

MOA — Mixture of vitamin supplements that mediates glucose utilization to prevent Wernicke-Korsakoff syndrome in alcoholism.

ADVERSE EFFECTS — Serious: Hypersensitivity, anaphylaxis, cyanosis, pulmonary edema, GI hemorrhage, cardiovascular shock. Frequent: Injection-site reaction, feeling of warmth, pruritus, sweating, N/V, restlessness, angioedema.

FAT EMULSION (*Intralipid, Liposyn*) ▶L ♀C ▶? $$$$$

WARNING — Deaths have occurred in preterm infants after infusion of IV fat emulsions. Autopsy results showed intravascular fat accumulation in the lungs. Strict adherence to total daily dose and administration rate is mandatory. Premature and small for gestational age infants have poor clearance of IV fat emulsion. Monitor infant's ability to eliminate fat (i.e., triglycerides or plasma free fatty acid levels).

ADULT — Calorie and essential fatty acids source: As part of TPN, fat emulsion should be no more than 60% of total calories; when correcting essential fatty acid deficiency, 8 to 10% of caloric intake should be supplied by lipids. Initial infusion rate 1 mL/min IV (10% fat emulsion) or 0.5 mL/min (20% fat emulsion) IV for first 15 to 30 min. If tolerated increase rate. If using 10% fat emulsion infuse no more than 500 mL 1st day and increase the next day. Maximum daily dose 2.5 g/kg. If using 20% fat emulsion, infuse up to 250 mL (Liposyn II) or up to 500 mL (Intralipid) first day and increase the next day. Maximum daily dose 2.5 g/kg.

PEDS — Calorie and essential fatty acids source: As part of TPN, fat emulsion should be no more than 60% of

FAT EMULSION (*cont.*)

total calories; when correcting essential fatty acid deficiency, 8 to 10% of caloric intake should be supplied by lipids. Initial infusion rate 0.1 mL/min IV (10% fat emulsion) or 0.05 mL/min (20% fat emulsion) for first 10 to 15 min. If tolerated increase rate up to 1 mL/kg/h (10% fat emulsion) or 0.5 mL/kg/h (20% fat emulsion). Max daily dose 3 g/kg. For premature infants, start at 0.5 g/kg/day and increase based on infant's ability to eliminate fat. Maximum infusion rate 1 g fat/kg in 4 h.

NOTES — Do not use in patients with severe egg allergy; contains egg yolk phospholipids. Use caution in severe liver disease, pulmonary disease, anemia, blood coagulation disorders, when there is the danger of fat embolism or in jaundiced or premature infants. Monitor CBC, blood coagulation, LFTs, plasma lipid profile and platelet count.

MOA — Treats or prevents nutritional deficiency by providing essential fatty acids.

ADVERSE EFFECTS — Serious: Intravascular fat accumulation in lungs (preterm infants), sepsis, hepatomegaly (long-term use). Frequent: Thrombophlebitis, hypertriglyceridemia, brown pigmentation (long-term use).

LEVOCARNITINE (*Carnitor*) ▶KL ♀B ▶? $$$$$

ADULT — Prevention of levocarnitine deficiency in dialysis patients: 10 to 20 mg/kg IV at each dialysis session. Titrate dose based on serum concentration.

PEDS — Prevention of deficiency in dialysis patients: 10 to 20 mg/kg IV at each dialysis session. Titrate dose based on serum concentration.

FORMS — Generic/Trade: Tabs 330 mg, Oral soln 1 g/10 mL.

NOTES — Adverse neurophysiologic effects may occur with long-term, high doses of oral levocarnitine in patients with renal dysfunction. Only the IV formulation is indicated in patients receiving hemodialysis.

MOA — Facilitates long-chain fatty acid utilization.

ADVERSE EFFECTS — Serious: Seizures. Frequent: N/V, body odor, mild myasthenia.

RALLY PACK ▶KL ♀C ▶– $

UNAPPROVED ADULT — See "Banana Bag". "Rally pack" is jargon and not a valid drug order; specify individual components.

MOA — Mixture of vitamin supplements that mediates glucose utilization to prevent Wernicke-Korsakoff syndrome in alcoholism.

ADVERSE EFFECTS — Serious: Hypersensitivity, anaphylaxis, cyanosis, pulmonary edema, GI hemorrhage, cardiovascular shock. Frequent: Injection-site reaction, feeling of warmth, pruritus, sweating, N/V, restlessness, angioedema.

ENDOCRINE AND METABOLIC: Phosphate Binders

LANTHANUM CARBONATE (*Fosrenol*) ▶Not absorbed ♀C ▶? $$$$$

ADULT — Treatment of hyperphosphatemia in end stage renal disease: Start 1500 mg/day PO in divided doses with meals. Titrate dose q 2 to 3 weeks in increments of 750 mg/day until acceptable serum phosphate is reached. Most will require 1500 to 3000 mg/day to reduce serum phosphate less than 6.0 mg/dL. Chew or crush tabs completely before swallowing; not to be swallowed whole.

PEDS — Not approved in children.

FORMS — Trade only: Chewable tabs 500, 750, 1000 mg.

NOTES — Divided doses up to 3750 mg/day have been used. Caution if acute peptic ulcer, ulcerative colitis, or Crohn's disease. Serious GI obstructions reported; contraindicated if pre-existing bowel obstruction, ileus, and fecal impaction. Avoid medications known to interact with antacids within 2 h. May be radiopaque enough to appear on abdominal x-ray.

MOA — Binds dietary phosphate forming highly insoluble complexes that are eliminated through the GI tract.

ADVERSE EFFECTS — Serious: Dialysis graft occlusion. Frequent: N/V, abdominal pain, diarrhea.

SEVELAMER (*Renagel, Renvela*) ▶Not absorbed ♀C ▶? $$$$$

ADULT — Hyperphosphatemia in kidney disease on dialysis: Start 800 to 1600 mg PO three times per day with meals, adjust according to serum phosphorus concentration.

PEDS — Not approved in children.

FORMS — Trade only (Renagel—sevelamer hydrochloride): Tabs 400, 800 mg. (Renvela—sevelamer carbonate): Tabs 800 mg. Powder: 800, 2400 mg packets.

NOTES — Titrate by 800 mg/meal at 2-week intervals to keep phosphorus less than 5.5 mg/dL; highest daily dose in studies: Renagel, 13 g; Renvela, 14 g. Decreases absorption of ciprofloxacin; may decrease absorption of antiarrhythmic and antiseizure medications; administer these meds 1 h before or 3 h. Caution in GI motility disorders, including severe constipation. Contraindicated if bowel obstruction. Dysphagia and esophageal tablet retention reported; consider susp form if history of swallowing difficulties.

MOA — Binds intestinal phosphate preventing absorption.

ADVERSE EFFECTS — Serious: Hypophosphatemia, intestinal obstruction, dysphagia, bowel perforation. Frequent: N/V, dyspepsia, diarrhea, flatulence, constipation.

SUCROFERRIC OXYHYDROXIDE (*Velphoro*) ▶not absorbed ♀B ▶+

ADULT — Hyperphosphatemia in kidney disease on dialysis: Start 1 tab (500 mg) PO three times daily with meals, adjust weekly according to serum phosphorus concentrations. Tablets must be chewed.

FORMS — Trade only: Tabs 500 mg.

(cont.)

SUCROFERRIC OXYHYDROXIDE (*cont.*)

NOTES — Titrate at weekly intervals to achieve serum phosphorous 5.5 mg/dL or less. Not studied in GI or hepatic disorders.

MOA — Binds intestinal phosphate preventing absorption.
ADVERSE EFFECTS — Common: discolored feces, diarrhea, nausea, altered taste.

ENDOCRINE AND METABOLIC: Thyroid Agents

LEVOTHYROXINE (*Levothroid, Levoxyl, Synthroid, Tirosint, Unithroid, T4, ✱Eltroxin, Euthyrox*) ▶L ♀A ▶+ $

WARNING — Do not use for obesity/wt loss; possible serious or life-threatening toxic effects when used in euthyroid patients.

ADULT — Hypothyroidism: Start 100 to 200 mcg PO daily (healthy adults) or 12.5 to 50 mcg PO daily (elderly or CV disease), increase by 12.5 to 25 mcg/day at 3 to 8 weeks intervals. Usual maintenance dose 100 to 200 mcg PO daily, max 300 mcg/day.

PEDS — Hypothyroidism: 0 to 6 mo: 8 to 10 mcg/kg/day PO; 6 to 12 mo: 6 to 8 mcg/kg/day PO; 1 to 5 yo: 5 to 6 mcg/kg/day PO; 6 to 12 yo: 4 to 5 mcg/kg/day PO; older than 12 yo: 2 to 3 mcg/kg/day PO, max 300 mcg/day.

UNAPPROVED ADULT — Hypothyroidism: 1.6 mcg/kg/day PO; start with lower doses (25 mcg PO daily) in elderly and patients with cardiac disease.

FORMS — Generic/Trade: Tabs 25, 50, 75, 88, 100, 112, 125, 137, 150, 175, 200, 300 mcg. Trade only: Caps (Tirosint): 13, 25, 50, 75, 88, 100, 112, 125, 137, 150 mcg.

NOTES — May crush tabs for infants and children. May give IV or IM at ½ oral dose in adults and ½ to ¾ oral dose in children; then adjust based on tolerance and therapeutic response. Generics are not necessarily bioequivalent to brand products; reevaluate thyroid function when switching.

MOA — Synthetic thyroid derivative that increases metabolic rate of body tissues.

ADVERSE EFFECTS — Serious: Hyperthyroidism (arrhythmia, heart failure, angina, cardiac arrest), pseudotumor cerebri. Frequent: Palpitations, tachycardia, tremor, headache, nervousness, insomnia, diarrhea, vomiting, weight loss, menstrual irregularity, sweating, heat intolerance.

LIOTHYRONINE (*T3, Cytomel, Triostat*) ▶L ♀A ▶? $$

WARNING — Do not use for obesity/weight loss; possible serious or life-threatening toxic effects when used in euthyroid patients.

ADULT — Mild hypothyroidism: 25 mcg PO daily, increase by 12.5 to 25 mcg/day at 1 to 2 weeks intervals to desired response. Usual maintenance dose 25 to 75 mcg PO daily. Goiter: 5 mcg PO daily, increase by 5 to 10 mcg/day at 1 to 2 weeks intervals. Usual maintenance dose 75 mcg PO daily. Myxedema: 5 mcg PO daily, increase by 5 to 10 mcg/day at 1 to 2 weeks intervals. Usual maintenance dose 50 to 100 mcg/day.

PEDS — Congenital hypothyroidism: 5 mcg PO daily, increase by 5 mcg/day at 3 to 4 days intervals to desired response.

FORMS — Generic/Trade: Tabs 5, 25, 50 mcg.

NOTES — Levothyroxine is preferred maintenance treatment for hypothyroidism. Start therapy at 5 mcg/day in children and elderly and increase by 5 mcg increments only. Rapidly absorbed from the GI tract. Monitor T3 and TSH. Elderly may need lower doses due to potential decreased renal function.

MOA — Synthetic thyroid derivative that increases metabolic rate of body tissues.

ADVERSE EFFECTS — Serious: Hyperthyroidism (arrhythmia, heart failure, angina, cardiac arrest), pseudotumor cerebri. Frequent: Palpitations, tachycardia, tremor, headache, nervousness, insomnia, diarrhea, vomiting, weight loss, menstrual irregularity, sweating, heat intolerance.

METHIMAZOLE (*Tapazole*) ▶L ♀D ▶+ $$$

ADULT — Hyperthyroidism. Mild: 5 mg PO three times per day. Moderate: 10 mg PO three times per day. Severe: 20 mg PO three times per day (q 8 h intervals). Maintenance dose is 5 to 30 mg/day.

PEDS — Hyperthyroidism: 0.4 mg/kg/day PO divided q 8 h. Maintenance dose is half of the initial dose, max 30 mg/day.

UNAPPROVED ADULT — Start 10 to 30 mg PO daily, then adjust.

FORMS — Generic/Trade: Tabs 5, 10. Generic only: Tabs 15, 20 mg.

NOTES — Check CBC for evidence of marrow suppression if fever, sore throat, or other signs of infection. Propylthiouracil preferred over methimazole in first trimester of pregnancy.

MOA — Inhibits synthesis of thyroid hormones.

ADVERSE EFFECTS — Serious: Agranulocytosis, granulocytopenia, thrombocytopenia, aplastic anemia, leukopenia, interstitial pneumonitis, dermatitis, hepatotoxicity, periarteritis, nephritis, hypoprothrombinemia. Frequent: N/V, rash, pruritus, headache, dizziness, vertigo, drowsiness, alopecia, constipation, paresthesia, neuritis, hyperpigmentation.

POTASSIUM IODIDE (*Iosat, SSKI, Thyrosafe, Thyroshield*) ▶L ♀D ▶– $

WARNING — Do not use for obesity.

ADULT — Thyroidectomy preparation: 50 to 250 mg PO three times per day for 10 to 14 days prior to surgery. Thyroid storm: 1 mL (Lugol's) PO three times per day at least 1 h after initial propylthiouracil or methimazole dose. Thyroid blocking in radiation emergency: 130 mg PO daily for 10 days or as directed by state health officials.

PEDS — Thyroid blocking in radiation emergency age 3 to 18 yo: 65 mg (½ of a 130 mg tab) PO daily, or 130 mg PO daily in adolescents greater than 70 kg. 1 mo to 3 yo: 32 mg (¼ of a 130 mg tab) PO daily. Birth to 1 mo: 16 mg (1/8 of a 130 mg tab) PO daily.

POTASSIUM IODIDE (*cont.*)

Duration is until risk of exposure to radioiodines no longer exists.

FORMS — OTC Trade only: Tabs 130 mg (Iosat). Trade only Rx: Soln 1 g/mL (30, 240 mL, SSKI). OTC Generic only: Tabs 65 mg (Thyrosafe), Soln 65 mg/mL (30 mL, Thyroshield).

MOA — Elemental substance used therapeutically to block thyroid uptake or suppress thyroid hormone synthesis and release.

ADVERSE EFFECTS — Serious: Agranulocytosis, granulocytopenia, thrombocytopenia, aplastic anemia, leukopenia, interstitial pneumonitis, exfoliative dermatitis, vasculitis, hepatotoxicity. Frequent: N/V, rash, pruritus, headache, dizziness, drowsiness, alopecia, constipation, paresthesia, neuritis, hyperpigmentation.

PROPYLTHIOURACIL (*PTU, ✦Propyl Thyracil*) ▶L ♀D (but preferred over methimazole in first trimester) ▶+ $

WARNING — Acute liver failure and severe liver injury reported, including fatal injury and need for liver transplantation. Use only if patient cannot tolerate methimazole or if not a candidate for radioactive iodine therapy or surgery.

ADULT — Hyperthyroidism: 100 to 150 mg PO three times per day. Severe hyperthyroidism and/or large goiters: 200 to 400 mg PO three times per day. Continue initial dose for approximately 2 months. Adjust dose to desired response. Usual maintenance dose 100 to 150 mg/day. Thyroid storm: 200 mg PO q 4 to 6 h once daily, decrease dose gradually to usual maintenance dose.

PEDS — Hyperthyroidism in children age 6 to 10 yo: 50 mg PO daily to three times per day. Children or older 10 yo: 50 to 100 mg PO three times per day. Continue initial dose for 2 months, then maintenance dose is one-third to two-thirds the initial dose.

UNAPPROVED PEDS — Hyperthyroidism in neonates: 5 to 10 mg/kg/day PO divided q 8 h. Children: 5 to 7 mg/kg/day PO divided q 8 h.

FORMS — Generic only: Tabs 50 mg.

NOTES — Monitor CBC for marrow suppression if fever, sore throat, or other signs of infection. Vasculitic syndrome with positive antineutrophilic icytoplasmic antibodies (ANCAs) reported requiring discontinuation. Propylthiouracil preferred over methimazole in first trimester of pregnancy.

MOA — Inhibits synthesis of thyroid hormones.

ADVERSE EFFECTS — Serious: Agranulocytosis, granulocytopenia, thrombocytopenia, aplastic anemia, leukopenia, interstitial pneumonitis, exfoliative dermatitis, vasculitis, hepatotoxicity. Frequent: N/V, rash, pruritus, headache, dizziness, drowsiness, alopecia, constipation, paresthesia, neuritis, hyperpigmentation.

SODIUM IODIDE I-131 (*Hicon, Iodotope*) ▶K ♀X ▶– $$$$$

ADULT — Specialized dosing for hyperthyroidism and thyroid carcinoma.

PEDS — Not approved in children.

FORMS — Generic/Trade: Caps Oral soln: Radioactivity range varies at the time of calibration. Hicon is a kit containing caps and a concentrated oral soln for dilution and cap preparation.

NOTES — Hazardous substance, handle with necessary precautions and use proper disposal. Avoid if preexisting vomiting or diarrhea. Discontinue antithyroid therapy at least 3 days before starting. Low serum chloride or nephrosis may increase uptake; renal insufficiency may decrease excretion and thus increase radiation exposure. Ensure adequate hydration before and after administration. Follow low-iodine diet for 1 to 2 weeks before treatment. Women should have negative pregnancy test prior to treatment and advise not to conceive for at least 6 months.

MOA — Radioactive iodide that is trapped by thyroid tissue; radiation exposure results in cell destruction.

ADVERSE EFFECTS — Serious: Hypersensitivity, bone marrow suppression (high doses), acute thyroid crises, chromosomal abnormalities, death, sialadenitis, hypoparathyroidism, solid cancers. Frequent: Hypothyroidism.

THYROID—DESICCATED (*Thyroid USP, Armour Thyroid*) ▶L ♀A ▶? $

WARNING — Do not use for wt loss; possible serious or life-threatening toxic effects when used in euthyroid patients.

ADULT — Obsolete; use levothyroxine instead. Hypothyroidism: Start 30 mg PO daily, increase by 15 mg/day at 2- to 3-week intervals to a maximum dose of 180 mg/day.

PEDS — Congenital hypothyroidism: 15 mg PO daily. Increase at 2-week intervals.

FORMS — Generic/Trade: Tabs 15, 30, 60, 90, 120, 180, 300 mg. Trade only: Tabs 240 mg.

NOTES — 60 mg thyroid desiccated is roughly equivalent to 100 mcg levothyroxine. Combination of levothyroxine (T4) and liothyronine (T3); content varies (range 2:1 to 5:1).

MOA — Thyroid hormones from animal thyroid gland that increases metabolic rate of body tissues.

ADVERSE EFFECTS — Serious: Hyperthyroidism (arrhythmia, heart failure, angina, cardiac arrest), pseudotumor cerebri, hypersensitivity. Frequent: Palpitations, tachycardia, tremor, headache, nervousness, insomnia, diarrhea, vomiting, weight loss, menstrual irregularity, sweating, heat intolerance.

THYROLAR, LIOTRIX (**levothyroxine + liothyronine**) ▶L ♀A ▶? $

WARNING — Do not use for wt loss; possible serious or life-threatening toxic effects when used in euthyroid patients.

ADULT — Hypothyroidism: 1 PO daily, starting with small doses initially (¼ to ½ strength), then increase at 2-week intervals.

PEDS — Not approved in children.

FORMS — Trade only: Tabs T4/T3 12.5 mcg/3.1 mcg (¼ strength), 25 mcg/6.25 mcg (half-strength),

(cont.)

THYROLAR, LIOTRIX (cont.)

50 mcg/12.5 mcg (#1), 100 mcg/25 mcg (#2), 150 mcg/37.5 mcg (#3).

NOTES — Combination of levothyroxine (T4) and liothyronine (T3).

MOA — Synthetic thyroid derivative that increases metabolic rate of body tissues.

ADVERSE EFFECTS — Serious: Hyperthyroidism (arrhythmia, heart failure, angina, cardiac arrest), pseudotumor cerebri. Frequent: Palpitations, tachycardia, tremor, headache, nervousness, insomnia, diarrhea, vomiting, weight loss, menstrual irregularity, sweating, heat intolerance.

ENDOCRINE AND METABOLIC: Vitamins

ASCORBIC ACID (*vitamin C, ✦Redoxon*) ▶K ♀C ▶? $

ADULT — Prevention of scurvy: 70 to 150 mg/day PO. Treatment of scurvy: 300 to 1000 mg/day PO. RDA females: 75 mg/day; males: 90 mg/day. Smokers: Add 35 mg/day more than nonsmokers.

PEDS — Prevention of scurvy: Infants: 30 mg/day PO. Treatment of scurvy: Infants: 100 to 300 mg/day PO. Adequate daily intake for infants 0 to 6 mo: 40 mg; 7 to 12 mo: 50 mg. RDA for children: 1 to 3 yo: 15 mg; 4 to 8 yo: 25 mg; 9 to 13 yo: 45 mg; 14 to 18 yo: 75 mg (males), 65 mg (females).

UNAPPROVED ADULT — Urinary acidification with methenamine: More than 2 g/day PO. Idiopathic methemoglobinemia: 150 mg/day or more PO. Wound healing: 300 to 500 mg/day or more PO for 7 to 10 days. Severe burns: 1 to 2 g/day PO.

FORMS — OTC Generic only: Tabs 25, 50, 100, 250, 500, 1000 mg. Chewable tabs 100, 250, 500 mg. Timed-release tabs 500, 1000, 1500 mg. Timed-release caps 500 mg. Lozenges 60 mg. Liquid 35 mg/0.6 mL. Oral soln 100 mg/mL. Syrup 500 mg/5 mL.

NOTES — Use IV/IM/SC ascorbic acid for acute deficiency or when oral absorption is uncertain. Avoid excessive doses in diabetics, patients prone to renal calculi, those undergoing stool occult blood tests (may cause false-negative), those on sodium restricted diets and those taking anticoagulants (may decrease INR). Doses in adults more than 2 g/day may cause osmotic diarrhea.

MOA — Water-soluble vitamin with antioxidant properties.

ADVERSE EFFECTS — Serious: Renal calculi, hypersensitivity. Frequent: Injection-site irritation (if IV).

CALCITRIOL (*Rocaltrol, Calcijex*) ▶L ♀C ▶? $$

ADULT — Hypocalcemia in chronic renal dialysis: Oral: 0.25 mcg PO daily, increase by 0.25 mcg q 4 to 8 weeks until normocalcemia achieved. Most hemodialysis patients require 0.5 to 1 mcg/day PO. Hypocalcemia and/or secondary hyperparathyroidism in chronic renal dialysis IV: 1 to 2 mcg, 3 times a week; increase dose by 0.5 to 1 mcg q 2 to 4 weeks. If PTH decreased less than 30% then increase dose; if PTH decreased 30 to 60% then maintain current dose; if PTH decreased more than 60% then decrease dose; if PTH 1.5 to 3 times the upper normal limit then maintain current dose. Hypoparathyroidism: 0.25 mcg PO q am; increase dose q 2 to 4 weeks if inadequate response. Most adults respond to 0.5 to 2 mcg/day PO. Secondary hyperparathyroidism in predialysis patients: 0.25 mcg PO q am; may increase dose to 0.5 mcg q am.

PEDS — Hypoparathyroidism 1 to 5 yo: 0.25 to 0.75 mcg PO q am. If age 6 yo or older then 0.25 mcg PO q am; increase dose in 2 to 4 weeks; usually respond to 0.5 to 2 mcg/day PO. Secondary hyperparathyroidism in predialysis patients age 3 yo or older: 0.25 mcg q am; may increase dose to 0.5 mcg q am. If younger than 3 yo: 0.01 to 0.015 mcg/kg/day PO.

UNAPPROVED ADULT — Psoriasis vulgaris: 0.5 mcg/day PO or 0.5 mcg/g petrolatum topically daily.

FORMS — Generic/Trade: Caps 0.25, 0.5 mcg. Oral soln 1 mcg/mL. Injection 1, 2 mcg/mL.

NOTES — Calcitriol is the activated form of vitamin D. During titration period, monitor serum calcium at least twice a week. Successful therapy requires an adequate daily calcium intake. Topical preparation must be compounded (not commercially available).

MOA — Vitamin D analogue that suppresses PTH secretion, bone resorption and increases gastrointestinal calcium absorption thus affecting bone homeostasis.

ADVERSE EFFECTS — Serious: Vitamin D toxicity/overdose, anaphylaxis, hypersensitivity, mild acidosis, renal toxicity, pancreatitis, arrhythmia, overt psychosis, elevated serum transaminases. Frequent: Weakness, headache, N/V, dry mouth, constipation, muscle pain, bone pain, metallic taste, irritability, weight loss, conjunctivitis, dyslipidemia, hypertension.

CYANOCOBALAMIN (*vitamin B12, CaloMist, Nascobal*) ▶K ♀C ▶+ $

ADULT — See also "unapproved adult" dosing. Maintenance of nutritional deficiency following IM correction: 500 mcg intranasal weekly (Nascobal: 1 spray 1 nostril once a week) or 50 to 100 mcg intranasal daily (CaloMist: 1 to 2 sprays each nostril daily). Pernicious anemia: 100 mcg IM/SC daily, for 6 to 7 days, then every other day for 7 doses, then q 3 to 4 days for 2 to 3 weeks, then q month. Other patients with vitamin B12 deficiency: 30 mcg IM daily for 5 to 10 days, then 100 to 200 mcg IM q month. RDA for adults is 2.4 mcg.

PEDS — Nutritional deficiency: 100 mcg/24 h deep IM/SC for 10 to 15 days then at least 60 mcg/month IM/deep SC. Pernicious anemia: 30 to 50 mcg/24 h for 14 days or more to total dose of 1000 to 5000 mcg deep IM/SC then 100 mcg/month deep IM/SC. Adequate daily intake for infants: 0 to 6 mo: 0.4

CYANOCOBALAMIN (*cont.*)

mcg; 7 to 11 mo: 0.5 mcg. RDA for children: 1 to 3 yo: 0.9 mcg; 4 to 8 yo: 1.2 mcg; 9 to 13 yo: 1.8 mcg; 14 to 18 yo: 2.4 mcg.

UNAPPROVED ADULT — Pernicious anemia and nutritional deficiency states: 1000 to 2000 mcg PO daily for 1 to 2 weeks, then 1000 mcg PO daily. Prevention and treatment of cyanide toxicity associated with nitroprusside.

UNAPPROVED PEDS — Prevention/treatment of nitroprusside-associated cyanide toxicity.

FORMS — OTC Generic only: Tabs 100, 500, 1000, 5000 mcg. Lozenges 100, 250, 500 mcg. Rx Trade only: Nasal spray 500 mcg/spray (Nascobal 2.3 mL), 25 mcg/spray (CaloMist, 18 mL).

NOTES — Prime nasal pump before use per package insert directions. Although official dose for deficiency states is 100 to 200 mcg IM q month, some give 1000 mcg IM periodically. Oral supplementation is safe and effective for B12 deficiency even when intrinsic factor is not present. Monitor B12, folate, iron and CBC.

MOA — Water-soluble vitamin required for purine nucleotides synthesis and amino acid metabolism.

ADVERSE EFFECTS — Serious: Anaphylaxis (IM), angioedema (IM). Frequent: Asthenia, dizziness, headache, infection, glossitis, nausea, paresthesia, rash, rhinitis (nasal), nasopharyngitis (nasal), nasal discomfort (nasal).

DOXERCALCIFEROL (*Hectorol*) ▶L ♀B ▶? $$$$$

ADULT — Secondary hyperparathyroidism on dialysis: Oral: If PTH greater than 400 pg/mL then start 10 mcg PO 3 times a week; if PTH greater than 300 pg/mL then increase by 2.5 mcg/dose q 8 weeks prn; if PTH 150 to 300 pg/mL then maintain current dose; if PTH less than 100 pg/mL then stop for 1 week, then resume at a dose at least 2.5 mcg lower. Max 60 mcg/week. IV: If PTH greater than 400 pg/mL then 4 mcg IV 3 times a week; if PTH decreased by less than 50% and greater than 300 pg/mL then increase by 1 to 2 mcg q 8 weeks as necessary; if PTH decreased by greater than 50% and greater than 300 pg/mL then maintain current dose; if PTH 150 to 300 pg/mL then maintain current dose; if PTH less than 100 pg/mL then stop for 1 week, then resume at a dose that is at least 1 mcg lower. Max 18 mcg/week. Secondary hyperparathyroidism not on dialysis: If PTH greater than 70 pg/mL (Stage 3) or greater than 110 pg/mL (Stage 4) then start 1 mcg PO daily; if PTH greater than 70 pg/mL (Stage 3) or greater than 110 pg/mL (Stage 4) then increase by 0.5 mcg/dose q 2 weeks; if PTH 35 to 70 pg/mL (Stage 3) or 70 to 110 pg/mL (Stage 4) then maintain current dose; if less than 35 pg/mL (Stage 3) or less than 70 pg/mL (Stage 4) then stop for 1 week, then resume at a dose that is at least 0.5 mcg lower. Max 3.5 mcg/day.

PEDS — Not approved in children.

FORMS — Generic/Trade: Caps 0.5, 1, 2.5 mcg.

NOTES — Monitor PTH, serum calcium and phosphorus weekly during dose titration; may need to monitor patients with hepatic insufficiency more closely.

MOA — Vitamin D analogue that suppresses PTH secretion and bone resorption thus affecting bone homeostasis.

ADVERSE EFFECTS — Serious: Vitamin D toxicity/overdose, hypersensitivity, mild acidosis, renal toxicity, pancreatitis, arrhythmia, overt psychosis, elevated serum transaminases. Frequent: Weakness, headache, N/V, dry mouth, constipation, muscle pain, bone pain, metallic taste, irritability, weight loss, conjunctivitis, dyslipidemia, hypertension.

ERGOCALCIFEROL (*vitamin D2, Calciferol, Drisdol, ✦Osteoforte*) ▶L ♀A (C if exceed RDA) ▶+ $

ADULT — Familial hypophosphatemia (Vitamin D Resistant Rickets): 12,000 to 500,000 units PO daily. Hypoparathyroidism: 50,000 to 200,000 units PO daily. Adequate daily intake: 18 to 70 yo: 600 units (15 mcg); older than 70 yo: 800 units (20 mcg).

PEDS — Adequate daily intake: 1 to 18 yo 600 units (15 mcg). Hypoparathyroidism: 1.25 to 5 mg PO daily.

UNAPPROVED ADULT — Osteoporosis prevention and treatment (age 50 or older): 800 to 1000 units PO daily with calcium supplements. Fanconi syndrome: 50,000 to 200,000 units PO daily. Osteomalacia: 1000 to 5000 units PO daily. Anticonvulsant-induced osteomalacia: 2000 to 50,000 units PO daily. Vitamin D deficiency: 50,000 units PO weekly or biweekly for 8 to 12 weeks.

UNAPPROVED PEDS — Familial hypophosphatemia: 400,000 to 800,000 units PO daily, increased by 10,000 to 20,000 units/day q 3 to 4 months as needed. Hypoparathyroidism: 50,000 to 200,000 units PO daily. Fanconi syndrome: 250 to 50,000 units PO daily.

FORMS — OTC Generic only: Caps 400, 1000, 5000 units. Soln 8000 units/mL (Calciferol). Rx Generic/Trade: Caps 50,000 units. Rx Generic only: Caps 25,000 units.

NOTES — 1 mcg ergocalciferol = 40 units vitamin D Sufficient level of 25(OH) Vitamin D is greater than 20 ng/mL, optimal is greater than 30 ng/mL. Vitamin D2 (ergocalciferol) is less effective than vitamin D3 (cholecalciferol) in maintaining 25-OH vitamin D levels; higher doses may be needed. IM or high-dose oral therapy may be necessary if malabsorption exists. Familial hypophosphatemia also requires phosphate supplementation; hypoparathyroidism also requires calcium supplementation.

MOA — Fat-soluble vitamin needed for calcium homeostasis (GI absorption, renal resorption, mobilization from bone).

ADVERSE EFFECTS — Serious: Vitamin D toxicity/overdose, hypersensitivity, mild acidosis, renal toxicity, pancreatitis, arrhythmia, overt psychosis, elevated serum transaminases. Frequent: Weakness, headache, N/V, dry mouth, constipation, muscle pain, bone pain, metallic taste, irritability, weight loss, conjunctivitis, dyslipidemia, hypertension.

FOLGARD (folic acid + cyanocobalamin + pyridoxine) ▶K ♀? ▶? $

ADULT — Nutritional supplement: 1 tab PO daily.

PEDS — Not approved in children.

FORMS — OTC Trade only: Folic acid 0.8 mg + cyanocobalamin 0.115 mg + pyridoxine 10 mg tab.

NOTES — Folic acid doses greater than 0.1 mg may obscure pernicious anemia, preventable with the concurrent cyanocobalamin.

MOA — Combination product containing 3 water-soluble vitamins that lowers plasma homocysteine.

ADVERSE EFFECTS — Serious: Masking pernicious anemia, sensory neuropathic syndromes. Frequent: Unstable gait, numb feet, awkwardness of the hands, perioral numbness, decreased sensations (touch, temperature, vibrations), paresthesia, photosensitivity, ataxia, asthenia, headache, infection, glossitis, nausea, rhinitis.

FOLGARD RX (folic acid + cyanocobalamin + pyridoxine) ▶K - ♀▶? $

ADULT — Nutritional supplement: 1 tab PO daily.

PEDS — Not approved in children.

FORMS — Trade only: Folic acid 2.2 mg + cyanocobalamin 1000 mcg + pyridoxine 25 mg tab.

NOTES — Folic acid doses greater than 0.1 mg may obscure pernicious anemia, preventable with the concurrent cyanocobalamin.

MOA — Combination product containing 3 water-soluble vitamins that lowers plasma homocysteine.

ADVERSE EFFECTS — Serious: Masking pernicious anemia, sensory neuropathic syndromes. Frequent: Unstable gait, numb feet, awkwardness of the hands, perioral numbness, decreased sensations (touch, temperature, vibrations), paresthesia, photosensitivity, ataxia, asthenia, headache, infection, glossitis, nausea, rhinitis.

FOLIC ACID (*folate, Folvite*) ▶K ♀A ▶+ $

ADULT — Megaloblastic anemia: 1 mg PO/IM/IV/SC daily. When symptoms subside and CBC normalizes, give maintenance dose of 0.4 mg PO daily and 0.8 mg PO daily in pregnant and lactating females. RDA for adults 0.4 mg, 0.6 mg for pregnant females, and 0.5 mg for lactating women. Max recommended daily dose 1 mg.

PEDS — Megaloblastic anemia: Infants: 0.05 mg PO daily, maintenance of 0.04 mg PO daily; Children: 0.5 to 1 mg PO daily, maintenance of 0.4 mg PO daily. Adequate daily intake for infants: 0 to 6 mo: 65 mcg; 7 to 12 mo: 80 mcg. RDA for children: 1 to 3 yo: 150 mcg; 4 to 8 yo: 200 mcg; 9 to 13 yo: 300 mcg, 14 to 18 yo: 400 mcg.

UNAPPROVED ADULT — Hyperhomocysteinemia: 0.5 to 1 mg PO daily.

FORMS — OTC Generic only: Tabs 0.4, 0.8 mg. Rx Generic 1 mg.

NOTES — Folic acid doses greater than 0.1 mg/day may obscure pernicious anemia. Prior to conception all women should receive 0.4 mg/day to reduce the risk of neural tube defects in infants. Consider high dose (up to 4 mg) in women with prior history of infant with neural tube defect.

Use oral route except in cases of severe intestinal absorption.

MOA — Water-soluble vitamin that stimulates red blood cell, white blood cell, and platelet production, and is a cofactor for transformylation reactions.

ADVERSE EFFECTS — Serious: Masking pernicious anemia. Frequent: None.

FOLTX (folic acid + cyanocobalamin + pyridoxine) ▶K ♀A ▶+ $$

ADULT — Nutritional supplement for end stage renal failure, dialysis, hyperhomocysteinemia, homocystinuria, nutrient malabsorption or inadequate dietary intake: 1 tab PO daily.

PEDS — Not approved in children.

FORMS — Trade only: Folic acid 2.5 mg/cyanocobalamin 2 mg/pyridoxine 25 mg tab.

NOTES — Folic acid doses greater than 0.1 mg may obscure pernicious anemia, preventable with the concurrent cyanocobalamin.

MOA — Combination product containing 3 water-soluble vitamins that lowers plasma homocysteine.

ADVERSE EFFECTS — Serious: Masking pernicious anemia, sensory neuropathic syndromes. Frequent: Unstable gait, numb feet, awkwardness of the hands, perioral numbness, decreased sensations (touch, temperature, vibrations), paresthesia, photosensitivity, ataxia, asthenia, headache, infection, glossitis, nausea, rhinitis.

MULTIVITAMINS (*MVI*) ▶LK ♀+ ▶+ $

WARNING — Severe iron toxicity possible in overdose, especially in children. Store out of reach of children and in child-resistant containers. Iron overdose is a leading cause of poisoning in children younger than 6 yo.

ADULT — Dietary supplement: Dose varies by product.

PEDS — Dietary supplement: Dose varies by product.

FORMS — OTC and Rx: Many different brands and forms available with and without iron (tabs, caps, chewable tabs, gtts, liquid).

NOTES — Do not take within 2 h of antacids, tetracyclines, levothyroxine, or fluoroquinolones.

MOA — Combination vitamin that usually contains vitamins A, D, E, B1, B2, B3, B5, B6, B12, and C, biotin and folic acid.

ADVERSE EFFECTS — Usually no adverse effects in recommended doses (see individual vitamins).

NEPHROCAP (ascorbic acid + folic acid + niacin + thiamine + riboflavin + pyridoxine + pantothenic acid + biotin + cyanocobalamin) ▶K ♀? ▶? $

ADULT — Nutritional supplement for chronic renal failure, uremia, impaired metabolic functions of the kidney and to maintain levels when the dietary intake of vitamins is inadequate or excretion and loss are excessive: 1 cap PO daily. If on dialysis, take after treatment.

PEDS — Not approved in children.

FORMS — Generic/Trade: Vitamin C 100 mg/folic acid 1 mg/niacin 20 mg/thiamine 1.5 mg/riboflavin 1.7 mg/pyridoxine 10 mg/pantothenic acid 5 mg/biotin 150 mcg/cyanocobalamin 6 mcg.

NEPHROCAP (cont.)

NOTES — Folic acid doses greater than 0.1 mg/day may obscure pernicious anemia (preventable with the concurrent cyanocobalamin).

MOA — Combination product containing water-soluble vitamins.

ADVERSE EFFECTS — Serious: Masking pernicious anemia. Frequent: Mild transient diarrhea.

NEPHROVITE (ascorbic acid + folic acid + niacin + thiamine + riboflavin + pyridoxine + pantothenic acid + biotin + cyanocobalamin) ▶K ♀? ▶? $

ADULT — Nutritional supplement for chronic renal failure, dialysis, hyperhomocysteinemia or inadequate dietary vitamin intake: 1 tab PO daily. If on dialysis, take after treatment.

PEDS — Not approved in children.

FORMS — Generic/Trade: Vitamin C 60 mg/folic acid 1 mg/niacin 20 mg/thiamine 1.5 mg/riboflavin 1.7 mg/pyridoxine 10 mg/pantothenic acid 10 mg/biotin 300 mcg/cyanocobalamin 6 mcg.

NOTES — Folic acid doses greater than 0.1 mg/day may obscure pernicious anemia (preventable with the concurrent cyanocobalamin).

MOA — Combination product containing water-soluble vitamins.

ADVERSE EFFECTS — Serious: Masking pernicious anemia. Frequent: Mild transient diarrhea.

NIACIN (vitamin B3, nicotinic acid, Niacor, Nicolar, Slo-Niacin, Niaspan) ▶K ♀C ▶? $

ADULT — Niacin deficiency: 100 mg PO daily. RDA: 16 mg for males, 14 mg for females. Hyperlipidemia: Start 50 to 100 mg PO two to three times per day with meals, increase slowly, usual maintenance range 1.5 to 3 g/day, max 6 g/day. Extended-release (Niaspan): Start 500 mg at bedtime with a low-fat snack for 4 weeks, increase prn q 4 weeks to max 2000 mg.

PEDS — Safety and efficacy not established for doses which exceed nutritional requirements. Adequate daily intake for infants: 0 to 6 mo: 2 mg; 7 to 12 mo: 3 mg. RDA for children: 1 to 3 yo: 6 mg; 48 yo: 8 mg; 9 to 13 yo: 12 mg; 14 to 18 yo: 16 mg (males) and 14 mg (females).

UNAPPROVED ADULT — Pellagra: 50 to 100 mg three to four times per day, up to 500 mg PO daily.

FORMS — OTC Generic only: Tabs 50, 100, 250, 500 mg. Timed-release cap 125, 250, 400 mg. Timed-release tab 250, 500 mg. Liquid 50 mg/5 mL. Tab only: 250, 500, 750 mg (Slo-Niacin). Rx: Generic/Trade: Timed-release tabs 500, 750, 1000 mg (Niaspan, $$$$). Trade only: Tabs 500 mg (Niacor).

NOTES — Start with low doses and increase slowly to minimize flushing; 325 mg aspirin (non-EC) 30 to 60 min prior to niacin ingestion will minimize flushing. Use caution in diabetics, patients with gout, peptic ulcer, liver, or gallbladder disease. Extended-release formulations may have greater hepatotoxicity.

MOA — Water-soluble vitamin that serves as a coenzyme for oxidation-reduction reactions. Decreases lipoproteins associated with high LDL-cholesterol and triglycerides and increases lipoproteins associated with low HDL-cholesterol.

ADVERSE EFFECTS — Serious: Hepatotoxicity, diabetes, peptic ulcer disease, gout, hypotension, myopathy, creatine kinase increase, hepatitis. Frequent: Flushing, dyspepsia, vomiting, abdominal pain, rash, burning paresthesias.

PARICALCITOL (Zemplar) ▶L ♀C ▶? $$$$$

ADULT — Prevention/treatment of secondary hyperparathyroidism with renal insufficiency: If PTH less than 500 pg/mL then start 1 mcg PO daily or 2 mcg PO three times per week. If PTH greater than 500 pg/mL then start 2 mcg PO daily or 4 mcg PO three times per week. Can increase PO dose by 1 mcg daily or 2 mcg three times per week based on PTH in 2- to 4-week intervals. Prevention/treatment of secondary hyperparathyroidism with renal failure (CrCl less than 15 mL/min): PO: To calculate initial dose divide baseline iPTH by 80 and then administer this dose in mcg three times per week. To titrate dose based on response, divide recent iPTH by 80 and then administer this dose in mcg three times per week. IV: Initially 0.04 to 0.1 mcg/kg (2.8 to 7 mcg) IV three times per week during dialysis. Can increase IV dose 2 to 4 mcg based on PTH in 2- to 4-week intervals. PO/IV: If PTH level decreased less than 30% then increase dose; if PTH level decreased 30 to 60% then maintain current dose; if PTH level decreased greater than 60% then decrease dose.

PEDS — Prevention/treatment of secondary hyperparathyroidism with renal failure (CrCl less than 15 mL/min): 0.04 to 0.1 mcg/kg (2.8 to 7 mcg) IV three times per week at dialysis; increase dose by 2 to 4 mcg or 0.04 mcg/kg q 2 to 4 weeks until desired PTH level is achieved. Max dose 0.24 mcg/kg (16.8 mcg).

FORMS — Generic/Trade: Caps 1, 2, 4 mcg.

NOTES — Monitor serum PTH, calcium, and phosphorus. IV doses up to 0.24 mcg/kg (16.8 mcg) have been administered. Do not initiate PO therapy in renal failure until calcium is 9.6 mg/dL or lower. Avoid prescription based doses of vitamin D and derivatives to minimize the risk of hypercalemia. Monitor closely (e.g., twice weekly) during dosage adjustment for acute hypercalcemia. Chronic hypercalemia may lead to vascular and soft tissue calcification. Do not administer with aluminum containing medications; risk of aluminum toxicity. Risk of digoxin toxicity if hypercalcemia.

MOA — Vitamin D analogue that suppresses PTH secretion and bone resorption thus affecting bone homeostasis.

ADVERSE EFFECTS — Serious: Vitamin D toxicity/overdose, hypersensitivity, mild acidosis, renal toxicity, pancreatitis, arrhythmia, overt psychosis, elevated serum transaminases, angioedema. Frequent: Weakness, headache, N/V, dry mouth, constipation, muscle pain, bone pain, metallic taste, irritability, weight loss, conjunctivitis, dyslipidemia, hypertension.

PHYTONADIONE (*vitamin K, Mephyton, AquaMephyton*)
▶L ♀C ▶+ $
WARNING — Severe reactions, including fatalities, have occurred during and immediately after IV injection, even with diluted injection and slow administration. Restrict IV use to situations where other routes of administration are not feasible.
ADULT — Excessive oral anticoagulation: Dose varies based on INR. INR 4.5-10: 2012 CHEST guidelines recommend AGAINST routine vitamin K administration; INR greater than 10 with no bleeding: 2012 CHEST guidelines recommend giving vitamin K, but do not specify a dose, 2008 guidelines previously recommended 5 to 10 mg PO; serious bleeding and elevated INR: 5 to 10 mg slow IV infusion. Hypoprothrombinemia due to other causes: 2.5 to 25 mg PO/IM/SC. Adequate daily intake: 120 mcg (males) and 90 mcg (females).
PEDS — Hemorrhagic disease of the newborn: Prophylaxis: 0.5 to 1 mg IM 1 h after birth; Treatment: 1 mg SC/IM.
UNAPPROVED PEDS — Nutritional deficiency: Children: 2.5 to 5 mg PO daily or 1 to 2 mg IM/SC/IV. Excessive oral anticoagulation: Infants: 1 to 2 mg IM/SC/IV q 4 to 8 h; Children: 2.5 to 10 mg PO/IM/SC/IV, may be repeated 12 to 48 h after PO dose or 6 to 8 h after IM/SC/IV dose.
FORMS — Trade only: Tabs 5 mg.
NOTES — Excessive doses of vitamin K in a patient receiving warfarin may cause warfarin resistance for up to a week. Avoid IM administration in patients with a high INR.
MOA — Fat-soluble vitamin that promotes formation of clotting factors.
ADVERSE EFFECTS — Serious: Anaphylactic reaction. Frequent: Injection-site reaction, flushing sensation, "peculiar" taste sensation.

PYRIDOXINE (*vitamin B6*) ▶K ♀A ▶+ $
ADULT — Dietary deficiency: 10 to 20 mg PO daily for 3 weeks. Prevention of deficiency due to isoniazid in high-risk patients: 10 to 25 mg PO daily. Treatment of neuropathies due to isoniazid: 50 to 200 mg PO daily. Isoniazid overdose (greater than 10 g): 4 g IV followed by 1 g IM over 30 min, repeat until total dose of 1 g for each g of isoniazid ingested. RDA for adults: 19 to 50 yo: 1.3 mg; older than 50 yo: 1.7 mg (males), 1.5 mg (females). Max recommended: 100 mg/day.
PEDS — Adequate daily intake for infants: 0 to 6 mo: 0.1 mg; 7 to 12 mo: 0.3 mg. RDA for children: 1 to 3 yo: 0.5 mg; 4 to 8 yo: 0.6 mg; 9 to 13 yo: 1 mg; 14 to 18 yo: 1.3 (boys) and 1.2 mg (girls).
UNAPPROVED ADULT — Premenstrual syndrome: 50 to 500 mg/day PO. Hyperoxaluria type I and oxalate kidney stones: 25 to 300 mg/day PO. Prevention of oral contraceptive-induced deficiency: 25 to 40 mg PO daily. Hyperemesis of pregnancy: 10 to 50 mg PO q 8 h. Has been used in hydrazine poisoning.
UNAPPROVED PEDS — Dietary deficiency: 5 to 10 mg PO daily for 3 weeks. Prevention of deficiency due to isoniazid: 1 to 2 mg/kg/day PO daily. Treatment of neuropathies due to isoniazid: 10 to 50 mg PO

daily. Pyridoxine-dependent epilepsy: Neonatal: 25 to 50 mg/dose IV; older infants and children: 100 mg/dose IV for 1 dose then 100 mg PO daily.
FORMS — OTC Generic only: Tabs 25, 50, 100 mg; Timed-release tab 100 mg.
MOA — Water-soluble vitamin that is a coenzyme involved in numerous metabolic transformations of proteins and amino acids.
ADVERSE EFFECTS — Serious: Sensory neuropathic syndromes. Frequent: Unstable gait, numb feet, awkwardness of the hands, perioral numbness, decreased sensations (touch, temperature, vibrations), paresthesia, photosensitivity, ataxia.

RIBOFLAVIN (*vitamin B2*) ▶K ♀A ▶+ $
ADULT — Deficiency: 5 to 25 mg/day PO. RDA for adults: 1.3 mg (males) and 1.1 mg (females), 1.4 mg for pregnant women, 1.6 mg for lactating women.
PEDS — Deficiency: 5 to 10 mg/day PO. Adequate daily intake for infants: 0 to 6 mo: 0.3 mg; 7 to 12 mo: 0.4 mg. RDA for children: 1 to 3 yo: 0.5 mg; 4 to 8 yo: 0.6 mg; 9 to 13 yo: 0.9 mg; 14 to 18 yo: 1.3 mg (males) and 1 mg (females).
UNAPPROVED ADULT — Prevention of migraine headaches: 400 mg PO daily.
FORMS — OTC Generic only: Tabs 25, 50, 100 mg.
NOTES — May cause yellow/orange discoloration of urine.
MOA — Water-soluble vitamin that catalyzes oxidative-reduction reactions.
ADVERSE EFFECTS — Serious: None. Frequent: Yellow discoloration of urine.

THIAMINE (*vitamin B1*) ▶K ♀A ▶+ $
ADULT — Beriberi: 10 to 20 mg IM 3 times per week for 2 weeks. Wet beriberi with MI: 10 to 30 mg IV three times per day. Wernicke encephalopathy: 50 to 100 mg IV and 50 to 100 mg IM for 1 dose then 50 to 100 mg IM daily until patient resumes normal diet. Give before starting glucose. RDA for adults: 1.2 mg (males) and 1.1 mg (females).
PEDS — Beriberi: 10 to 25 mg IM daily or 10 to 50 mg PO daily for 2 weeks then 5 to 10 mg PO daily for 1 month. Adequate daily intake infants: 0 to 6 mo: 0.2 mg; 7 to 12 mo: 0.3 mg. RDA for children: 1 to 3 yo: 0.5 mg; 4 to 8 yo: 0.6 mg; 9 to 13 yo: 0.9 mg; 14 to 18 yo: 1.2 mg (males), 1.0 mg (females).
FORMS — OTC Generic only: Tabs 50, 100, 250, 500 mg. Enteric-coated tab 20 mg.
MOA — Water-soluble vitamin needed for carbohydrate metabolism, normal growth maintenance, nerve impulse transmission, and acetylcholine synthesis.
ADVERSE EFFECTS — Serious: Hypersensitivity, anaphylaxis, cyanosis, pulmonary edema, GI hemorrhage, cardiovascular shock. Frequent: Injection site reaction, feeling of warmth, pruritus, sweating, N/V, restlessness, angioedema.

VITAMIN A ▶L ♀A (C if exceed RDA, X in high doses) ▶+ $
ADULT — Treatment of deficiency states: 100,000 units IM daily for 3 days, then 50,000 units IM daily for 2 weeks. RDA: 1000 mcg RE (males), 800 mcg RE (females). Max recommended daily dose in nondeficiency 3000 mcg (see notes).

VITAMIN A (cont.)

PEDS — Treatment of deficiency states: Infants: 7500 to 15,000 units IM daily for 10 days; children 1 to 8 yo: 17,500 to 35,000 units IM daily for 10 days. Kwashiorkor: 30 mg IM of water-soluble palmitate followed by 5000 to 10,000 units PO daily for 2 months. Xerophthalmia: Older than 1 yo: 110 mg retinyl palmitate PO or 55 mg IM plus 110 mg PO next day. Administer another 110 mg PO prior to discharge. Vitamin E (40 units) should be coadministered to increase efficacy of retinol. RDA for children: 0 to 6 mo: 400 mcg (adequate intake); 7 to 12 mo: 500 mcg; 1 to 3 yo: 300 mcg; 4 to 8 yo: 400 mcg; 9 to 13 yo: 600 mcg; 14 to 18 yo: 900 mcg (males), 700 mcg (females).

UNAPPROVED ADULT — Test for fat absorption: 7000 units/kg (2100 RE/kg) PO for 1 dose. Measure serum vitamin A concentrations at baseline and 4 h after ingestion. Dermatologic disorders such as follicularis keratosis: 50,000 to 500,000 units PO daily for several weeks.

UNAPPROVED PEDS — Has been tried in reduction of malaria episodes in children older than 12 mo and to reduce the mortality in HIV-infected children.

FORMS — OTC Generic only: Caps 10,000, 15,000 units. Trade only: Tabs 5000 units. Rx: Generic: 25,000 units. Trade only: Soln 50,000 units/mL.

NOTES — 1 RE (retinol equivalent) = 1 mcg retinol or 6 mcg beta-carotene. Continued Vitamin A/retinol intake of 2000 mcg/day or more may increase risk of hip fracture in postmenopausal women.

MOA — Fat-soluble vitamin needed for vision, dental development, growth, steroid synthesis, epithelial differentiation, embryonic development and reproduction.

ADVERSE EFFECTS — Serious: Vitamin A toxicity/overdose, hypersensitivity. Frequent: None.

VITAMIN D3 (cholecalciferol, DDrops) ▶L – ♀▶+ $

ADULT — Familial hypophosphatemia (vitamin D–resistant rickets): 12,000 to 500,000 units PO daily. Hypoparathyroidism: 50,000 to 200,000 units PO daily. Adequate daily intake adults: 1 to 70 yo: 600 units; older than 70 yo: 800 units. Max recommended daily dose in nondeficiency: 4000 units.

PEDS — Adequate daily intake: 1 to 18 yo 600 units. Hypoparathyroidism: 1.25 to 5 mg PO daily.

UNAPPROVED ADULT — Osteoporosis prevention and treatment (age 50 or older): 800 to 800 1000 units PO daily with calcium supplements.

UNAPPROVED PEDS — Familial hypophosphatemia: 400,000 to 800,000 units PO daily, increased by 10,000 to 20,000 units/day q 3 to 4 months as needed. Hypoparathyroidism: 50,000 to 200,000 units PO daily. Fanconi syndrome: 250 to 50,000 units PO daily.

FORMS — OTC Generic: 200 units, 400 units, 800 units, 1000 units, 2000 units (cap/tab). Trade only: Soln 400 units/drop, 1000 units/drop, 2000 units/drop.

NOTES — Sufficient level of 25(OH) Vitamin D is greater than 20 ng/mL, optimal is greater than 30 ng/mL.

MOA — Fat-soluble vitamin needed for calcium homeostasis (GI absorption, renal resorption, mobilization from bone).

ADVERSE EFFECTS — Serious: Vitamin D toxicity/overdose, hypersensitivity, mild acidosis, renal toxicity, pancreatitis, arrhythmia, overt psychosis, elevated serum transaminases. Frequent: Weakness, headache, N/V, dry mouth, constipation, muscle pain, bone pain, metallic taste, irritability, weight loss, conjunctivitis, dyslipidemia, hypertension.

VITAMIN E (tocopherol, ✚Aquasol E) ▶L ♀A ▶? $

ADULT — RDA: 22 units (natural, d-alpha-tocopherol) or 33 units (synthetic, d,l-alpha-tocopherol) or 15 mg (alpha-tocopherol). Max recommended 1000 mg (alpha-tocopherol).

PEDS — Adequate daily intake (alpha-tocopherol): Infants 0 to 6 mo: 4 mg; 7 to 12 mo: 6 mg. RDA for children (alpha-tocopherol): 1 to 3 yo: 6 mg; 4 to 8 yo: 7 mg; 9 to 13 yo: 11 mg; 14 to 18 yo: 15 mg.

UNAPPROVED PEDS — Nutritional deficiency: Neonates: 25 to 50 units PO daily; Children: 1 units/kg PO daily. Cystic fibrosis: 5 to 10 units/kg PO daily (use water soluble form), max 400 units/day.

FORMS — OTC Generic only: Tabs 200, 400 units. Caps 73.5, 100, 147, 165, 200, 330, 400, 500, 600, 1000 units. Gtts 50 mg/mL.

NOTES — 1 mg alpha-tocopherol equivalents equals ~1.5 units. Natural vitamin E (d-alpha-tocopherol) recommended over synthetic (d,l-alpha-tocopherol). Higher doses may increase risk of bleeding. Large randomized trials have failed to demonstrate cardioprotective effects.

MOA — Fat-soluble vitamin that protects cellular constituents from oxidation.

ADVERSE EFFECTS — Serious: Vitamin E toxicity/overdose. Frequent: None.

ENDOCRINE AND METABOLIC: Other

AMMONUL (sodium phenylacetate + sodium benzoate) ▶KL ♀C ▶? $$$$$

ADULT — Acute hyperammonemia with encephalopathy in urea cycle enzyme deficiency: 55 mL/m² IV over 90 to 120 min, followed by maintenance 55 mL/m² over 24 h. Stop when hyperammonemia resolved or oral nutrition and medications are tolerated.

PEDS — Acute hyperammonemia with encephalopathy in urea cycle enzyme deficiency: If wt 20 kg or less, then 2.5 mL/kg IV over 90 to 120 min, followed by maintenance 2.5 mL/kg over 24 h. If greater than 20 kg, then 55 mL/m² IV over 90 to 120 min, followed by maintenance 55 mL/m² over 24 h. Consider coadministration of arginine in hyperammonemic infants. Stop when hyperammonemia resolved or oral nutrition and medications are tolerated.

(cont.)

AMMONUL (cont.)

FORMS — Single-use vial 50 mL (10% sodium phenylacetate/10% sodium benzoate).

NOTES — Administer through a central line. Closely monitor if renal insufficiency. Monitor plasma ammonia level, neurological status, electrolytes, blood pH, blood pCO2 and clinical response. May cause hypokalemia. Consider coadministration of antiemetic. Penicillin and probenecid may affect renal secretion.

MOA — Serves an alternative to urea which effectively reduces waste nitrogen levels via hepatic conjugation and renal secretion.

ADVERSE EFFECTS — Serious: Neurotoxicity, brain edema, convulsions, pancytopenia, cardiac arrest, metabolic acidosis. Frequent: N/V, pyrexia, hyperglycemia, hypokalemia, hypotension, mental impairment.

BROMOCRIPTINE (*Cycloset, Parlodel*) ▶L ♀B ▶– $$$$$

ADULT — Type 2 DM: Start 0.8 mg PO q am, may increase by 0.8 weekly to max 4.8 mg. Hyperprolactinemia: Start 1.25 to 2.5 mg PO at bedtime, then increase q 3 to 7 days to usual effective dose of 2.5 to 15 mg/day, max 40 mg/day. Acromegaly: Usual effective dose is 20 to 30 mg/day, max 100 mg/day. Doses greater than 20 mg/day can be divided two times per day. Also approved for Parkinson's disease, but rarely used. Take with food to minimize dizziness and nausea.

PEDS — Not approved in children.

UNAPPROVED ADULT — Neuroleptic malignant syndrome: 2.5 to 5 mg PO 2 to 6 times per day. Hyperprolactinemia: 2.5 to 7.5 mg/day vaginally if GI intolerance occurs with PO dosing.

FORMS — Generic/Trade: Tabs 2.5 mg. Caps 5 mg. Trade only: Tabs 0.8 mg (Cycloset).

NOTES — Take with food to minimize dizziness and nausea. Ergots have been associated with potentially life-threatening fibrotic complications. Seizures, CVA, HTN, arrhythmias, and MI have been reported. Should not be used for postpartum lactation suppression. Contraindicated in Raynaud's syndrome. Avoid concomitant use of other ergot medications.

MOA — Dopamine agonist (ergot).

ADVERSE EFFECTS — Serious: Orthostatic hypotension, syncope, sleep attacks, shock, MI, stroke, arrhythmias, seizures, psychosis; retroperitoneal, pleural, pericardial, or cardiac valvular fibrosis, erythromelalgia, neutropenia and other blood dyscrasias, hemolytic anemia, adrenal insufficiency, hepatotoxicity, melanoma. Frequent: N/V, anorexia, diarrhea, constipation, abdominal pain, headache, dizziness, drowsiness, fatigue, confusion, orthostatic hypotension, edema, hallucinations, hypothyroidism, Parkinson's disease only: abnormal involuntary movements, urge to gamble, melanoma.

CABERGOLINE (*Dostinex*) ▶L ♀B ▶– $$$$$

ADULT — Hyperprolactinemia: Initiate therapy with 0.25 mg PO twice a week. Increase by 0.25 mg twice a week at 4-week intervals up to a maximum of 1 mg twice a week.

PEDS — Not approved in children.

UNAPPROVED ADULT — Acromegaly: 0.5 mg PO twice a week. Increase as needed up to 3.5 mg/week based on plasma IGF-1 levels.

FORMS — Generic/Trade: Tabs 0.5 mg.

NOTES — Monitor serum prolactin levels. Hepatically metabolized; use with caution in hepatic insufficiency. Contraindicated if cardiac vascular disease; perform pre-treament cardiovascular evaluation for valvular disease. Associated with valvular disease, especially during use for Parkinson's with higher doses and longer durations of use, but also reported with lower doses in hyperprolactinemia. Monitor for valvular disease via echocardiogram q 6 to 12 months or as clinically indicated. Discontinue if signs of valvular thickening, regurgitation or restriction. Postmarketing reports of pathological gambling, increased libido and hypersexuality. Reports of fibrosis. Monitor for signs of pleural fibrosis (dyspnea, shortness of breath, cough), retroperitoneal fibrosis (renal insufficiency, flank pain, abdominal mass) and cardiac fibrosis (cardiac failure).

MOA — Dopamine agonist that decreases prolactin secretion.

ADVERSE EFFECTS — Serious: Hypotension, pulmonary fibrosis, pleural fibrosis, retroperitoneal fibrosis, pericardial fibrosis, increased ESR, valvulopathy. Frequent: Nausea, headache, dizziness, fatigue, lightheadedness, vomiting, abdominal cramps, rhinorrhea.

CALCITONIN (*Miacalcin, Fortical, ✱Calcimar, Caltine*) ▶Plasma ♀C ▶? $$$$

ADULT — Osteoporosis: 100 units SC/IM every other day or 200 units (1 spray) intranasal daily (alternate nostrils). Paget's disease: 50 to 100 units SC/IM daily or 3 times per week. Hypercalcemia: 4 units/kg SC/IM q 12 h. May increase after 2 days to maximum of 8 units/kg q 6 h.

PEDS — Not approved in children.

UNAPPROVED ADULT — Acute osteoporotic vertebral fracture pain: 100 units SC/IM daily or 200 units intranasal daily (alternate nostrils).

UNAPPROVED PEDS — Osteogenesis imperfecta age 6 mo to 15 yo: 2 units/kg SC/IM 3 times per week with oral calcium supplements.

FORMS — Generic/Trade: Nasal spray 200 units/activation in 3.7 mL bottle (minimum of 30 doses/bottle).

NOTES — Skin test before using injectable product: 1 unit intradermally and observe for local reaction. Hypocalcemic effect diminishes in 2 to 7 days, therefore, only useful during acute short-term management of hypercalcemia.

MOA — Polypeptide hormone that decreases the rate of bone resorption.

ADVERSE EFFECTS — Serious: Antibody formation, hypersensitivity, anaphylaxis, bronchospasm, malignancy. Frequent: Nasal irritation, rhinitis,

CALCITONIN (*cont.*)

back pain, arthralgia, epistaxis, headache, sinusitis, dizziness, N/V, flushing, rash, abdominal pain, diarrhea, injection site irritation (for SC/IM), tremor.

CINACALCET (*Sensipar*) ▶LK ♀C ▶? $$$$$
ADULT — Treatment of secondary hyperparathyroidism in dialysis patients: 30 mg PO daily. May titrate q 2 to 4 weeks through sequential doses of 60, 90, 120, and 180 mg daily to target intact parathyroid hormone level of 150 to 300 pg/mL. Treatment of hypercalcemia in parathyroid carcinoma or primary hyperparathyroidism unable to undergo parathyroidectomy: 30 mg PO two times per day. May titrate q 2 to 4 weeks through sequential does of 60 mg two times per day, 90 mg two times per day, and 90 mg three to four times per day as necessary to normalize serum calcium levels.
PEDS — Not approved in children.
FORMS — Trade only: Tabs 30, 60, 90 mg.
NOTES — Monitor serum calcium and phosphorus 1 week after initiation or dose adjustment, then monthly after a maintenance dose has been established. Intact parathyroid hormone should be checked 1 to 4 weeks after initiation or dose adjustment, and then 1 to 3 months after a maintenance dose has been established. For parathyroid carcinoma, monitor serum calcium within 1 week after initiation or dose adjustment, then q 2 months after a maintenance dose has been established. Withhold if serum calcium falls below less than 7.5 mg/dL or if signs and symptoms of hypocalcemia. May restart when calcium level reaches 8.0 mg/dL or when signs and symptoms of hypocalcemia resolve. Re-initiate using the next lowest dose. Use calcium-containing phosphate binder and/or vitamin D to raise calcium if it falls between 7.5 to 8.4 mg/dL. Seizure threshold reduced if hypocalcemia. Reduce dose or discontinue if intact parathyroid hormone level is less than 150 to 300 pg/mL to prevent adynamic bone disease. Do not check parathyroid hormone levels within 12 h after administration of a dose. Inhibits metabolism by CYP2D6; may increase levels of flecainide, vinblastine, thioridazine, TCAs. Dose adjustment may be needed when initiating/discontinuing a strong CYP3A4 inhibitor (e.g., ketoconazole, erythromycin and itraconazole). Closely monitor parathyroid hormone and serum calcium if moderate to severe hepatic impairment.
MOA — Lowers parathyroid hormone levels and decreases serum calcium by increasing sensitivity of the calcium-sensing receptor to extracellular calcium.
ADVERSE EFFECTS — Serious: Seizures, adynamic bone disease, hypocalcemia, hypotension, worsening heart failure, arrhythmia, hypersensitivity. Frequent: N/V, diarrhea, myalgia, dizziness, rash.

CONIVAPTAN (*Vaprisol*) ▶LK ♀C ▶? $$$$$
ADULT — Euvolemic or hypervolemic hyponatremia: Loading dose of 20 mg IV over 30 min, then continuous infusion 20 mg over 24 h for 1 to 4 days. Titrate to desired serum sodium. Max dose 40 mg daily as continuous infusion.

PEDS — Not approved in children.
NOTES — No benefit expected in anuric patients. Avoid concurrent use of CYP3A4 inhibitors (ketoconazole, itraconazole, clarithromycin, ritonavir, indinavir). May increase digoxin levels. Discontinue if hypovolemia, hypotension, or rapid rise in serum sodium (greater than 12 mEq/L/24 h) occurs. Rapid correction of serum sodium may cause osmotic demyelination syndrome. Requires frequent monitoring of serum sodium, volume, and neurologic status. Administer through large veins and change infusion site daily to minimize irritation. Not approved for hyponatremia in heart failure. Increased exposure to conivaptan in renal or hepatic impairment. Not recommended if CrCl less than 30 mL/min.
MOA — Selective vasopressin V2-receptor antagonist that promotes free water excretion to raise sodium levels.
ADVERSE EFFECTS — Serious: hypotension, hypovolemia. Frequent: Infusion site reactions, constipation, nausea, diarrhea, vomiting, infection, electrolyte changes, polyuria, erythema, hypotension, hypertension.

DENOSUMAB (*Prolia*) ▶? ♀X ▶? $$$$
ADULT — Postmenopausal osteoporosis: 60 mg SC q6 months.
PEDS — Not approved in children
FORMS — Trade only: 60 mg/1 mL vial (Prolia), pre-filled syringe.
NOTES — Must correct hypocalcemia before administration, monitor calcium especially in renal insufficiency or dialysis. Elevations in PTH also noted in renal insufficiency. Administered by a health care professional SC in upper arm, upper thigh or abdomen. Give calcium 1000 mg and at least 400 IU vitamin D daily. Prolia contains same active ingredient (denosumab) as Xgeva; see oncology section for Xgeva indications.
MOA — RANK ligand (RANKL) inhibitor that decreases bone resorption.
ADVERSE EFFECTS — Serious: Hypocalcemia, serious infections, serious dermatologic reactions, cellulitis, osteonecrosis of the jaw, pancreatitis, hypersensitivity, anaphylaxis. Frequent: Dermatitis, rash, eczema, back pain, pain in extremity, hypercholesterlemia, musculoskeletal pain, cystitis, constipation.

DESMOPRESSIN (*DDAVP, Stimate, ✦Minirin, Octostim*) ▶LK ♀B ▶? $$$$
WARNING — Adjust fluid intake downward to decrease potential water intoxication and hyponatremia; use cautiously in those at risk.
ADULT — Diabetes insipidus: 10 to 40 mcg (0.1 to 0.4 mL) intranasally daily or divided two to three times per day or 0.05 to 1.2 mg PO daily or divided two to three times per day or 0.5 to 1 mL (2 to 4 mcg) SC/IV daily in 2 divided doses. Hemophilia A, von Willebrand's disease: 0.3 mcg/kg IV over 15 to 30 min; 300 mcg intranasally if wt 50 kg or more (1 spray in each nostril), 150 mcg intranasally if wt

(cont.)

DESMOPRESSIN (cont.)

less than 50 kg (single spray in 1 nostril). Primary nocturnal enuresis: 0.2 to 0.6 mg PO at bedtime.

PEDS — Diabetes insipidus 3 mo to 12 yo: 5 to 30 mcg (0.05 to 0.3 mL) intranasally once or twice daily or 0.05 mg PO daily. Hemophilia A, von Willebrand's disease (age 3 mo or older for IV, age 11 mo 12 yo for nasal spray): 0.3 mcg/kg IV over 15 to 30 min; 300 mcg intranasally if wt 50 kg or greater (1 spray in each nostril), 150 mcg intranasally if wt less than 50 kg (single spray in 1 nostril). Primary nocturnal enuresis age 6 yo or older: 0.2 to 0.6 mg PO at bedtime.

UNAPPROVED ADULT — Uremic bleeding: 0.3 mcg/kg IV single dose or q 12 h (onset 1 to 2 h; duration 6 to 8 h after single dose). Intranasal is 20 mcg/day (onset 24 to 72 h; duration 14 days during 14 days course).

UNAPPROVED PEDS — Hemophilia A and type 1 von Willebrand's disease: 2 to 4 mcg/kg intranasally or 0.2 to 0.4 mcg/kg IV over 15 to 30 min.

FORMS — Trade only: Stimate nasal spray 150 mcg/0.1 mL (1 spray), 2.5 mL bottle (25 sprays). Generic/Trade (DDAVP nasal spray): 10 mcg/0.1 mL (1 spray), 5 mL bottle (50 sprays). Note difference in concentration of nasal soln. Rhinal Tube: 2.5 mL bottle with 2 flexible plastic tube applicators with graduation marks for dosing. Generic only: Tabs 0.1, 0.2 mg.

NOTES — Monitor serum sodium and for sign/symptoms of hyponatremia including headache, wt gain, altered mental status, muscle weakness/cramps, seizure, coma or respiratory arrest. Restrict fluid intake 1 h before to 8 h after PO administration. Hold PO treatment for enuresis during acute illnesses that may cause fluid/electrolyte imbalances. Start at lowest dose with Diabetes insipidus. IV/SC doses are approximately 1/10 the intranasal dose. Anaphylaxis reported with both IV and intranasal forms. Do not give if type IIB von Willebrand's disease. Changes in nasal mucosa may impair absorption of nasal spray. Refrigerate nasal spray; stable for 3 weeks at room temperature. 10 mcg = 40 units desmopressin.

MOA — Synthetic vasopressin analogue with a rapid onset that promotes water resorption (anti-diuretic effect). Increases Factor VIII and von Willebrand's factor activity.

ADVERSE EFFECTS — Serious: Anaphylaxis, seizures (hyponatremia-associated), hyponatremia, fluid overload, chest pain, thrombotic events (rare). Frequent: Abdominal pain, flushing, headache, nasal congestion, nausea, rhinitis, agitation, balanitis, chills, increased blood pressure, sore throat, local irritation, epistaxis.

DIAZOXIDE (*Hyperstat, Proglycem*) ▶L ♀C ▶– $$$$$

ADULT — Hypoglycemia from hyperinsulinism: Initially 3 mg/kg/day PO divided equally q 8 h, usual maintenance dose 3 to 8 mg/kg/day divided equally q 8 to 12 h, max 10 to 15 mg/kg/day.

PEDS — Hypoglycemia from hyperinsulinism: Neonates and infants, initially 10 mg/kg/day divided equally q 8 h, usual maintenance dose 8 to 15 mg/kg/day divided equally q 8 to 12 h; children, same as adult.

FORMS — Trade only: Susp 50 mg/mL (30 mL).

NOTES — Close monitoring of blood glucose required. Consider reduced dose in renal impairment. Used for hyperinsulinism associated with islet cell adenoma, carcinoma, or hyperplasia; extrapancreatic malignancy, leucine sensitivity in children, nesidioblastosis. Avoid if hypersensitivity to thiazides or sulfonamide derivatives. Caution in gout; may increase uric acid. Monitor for edema and heart failure exacerbation during administration; diuretic therapy may be needed.

GALLIUM (*Ganite*) ▶K ♀C ▶? $$$$$

WARNING — Monitor creatinine (contraindicated if greater than 2.5 mg/dL), urine output, calcium and phosphorus. Avoid concurrent nephrotoxic drugs (e.g., aminoglycosides, amphotericin B). Establish urinary output of at least 2 L/day prior to treatment and maintain adequate hydration during therapy.

ADULT — Hypercalcemia of malignancy: 200 mg/m^2/day for 5 days. Shorten course if hypercalcemia is corrected. If mild hypercalcemia with few symptoms, consider 100 mg/m^2/day for 5 days. Administer as slow IV infusion over 24 h.

PEDS — Not approved in children.

NOTES — Monitor creatinine (contraindicated if greater than 2.5 mg/dL), urine output, calcium and phosphorus. Avoid concurrent nephrotoxic drugs (e.g., aminoglycosides, amphotericin B). Ensure adequate hydration prior to infusion.

MOA — Inhibits calcium resorption from bone; decreases serum calcium.

ADVERSE EFFECTS — Serious: Hypersensitivity, renal failure, optic neuritis. Frequent: Hypocalcemia, hypophosphatemia, decreased serum bicarbonate, anemia, hypotension.

SODIUM POLYSTYRENE SULFONATE (*Kayexalate*) ▶Fecal excretion ♀C ▶? $$$$

ADULT — Hyperkalemia: 15 g PO one to four times per day or 30 to 50 g retention enema (in sorbitol) q 6 h prn. Retain for 30 min to several h. Irrigate with tap water after enema to prevent necrosis.

PEDS — Hyperkalemia: 1 g/kg PO q 6 h.

UNAPPROVED PEDS — Hyperkalemia: 1 g/kg PR q 2 to 6 h.

FORMS — Generic only: Susp 15 g/60 mL. Powdered resin.

NOTES — 1 g binds approximately 1 mEq of potassium. Avoid in bowel obstruction, constipation, or abnormal bowel function, including patients without a bowel movement post-surgery. Avoid administration with sorbitol as intestinal necrosis has been reported. Discontinue use if constipation develops. Follow aspiration cautions during oral administration.

MOA — Cation exchange resin that reduces potassium in exchange for sodium.

SODIUM POLYSTYRENE SULFONATE (*cont.*)

ADVERSE EFFECTS — Serious: Hypokalemia, hypocalcemia, hypomagnesemia, intestinal obstruction, intestinal necrosis, serious GI events (bleeding, perforation). Frequent: Sodium and water retention, gastric irritation, anorexia, N/V, constipation.

SOMATROPIN (*human growth hormone, Genotropin, Humatrope, Norditropin, Norditropin NordiFlex, Norditropin FlexPro, Nutropin AQ, Nutropin Depot, Omnitrope, Protropin, Serostim, Serostim LQ, Saizen, Tev-Tropin, Valtropin, Zorbtive*) ▶LK ♀B/C ▶? $$$$$

WARNING — Avoid in patients with Prader-Willi syndrome who are severely obese, have severe respiratory impairment or sleep apnea, or unidentified respiratory infection; fatalities have been reported.

ADULT — Growth hormone deficiency (Genotropin, Humatrope, Nutropin, Nutropin AQ, Norditropin, Nutropin, Nutropin AQ, Omnitrope, Saizen, Valtropin): Doses vary according to product. AIDS wasting or cachexia (Serostim, Serostim LQ): 0.1 mg/kg SC daily, max 6 mg daily. Short bowel syndrome (Zorbtive): 0.1 mg/kg SC daily, max 8 mg daily.

PEDS — Growth hormone deficiency (Genotropin, Humatrope, Norditropin, Nutropin, Nutropin AQ, Nutropin Depot, Omnitrope, Tev-Tropin, Saizen): Doses vary according to product used. Turner syndrome (Genotropin, Humatrope, Norditropin, Nutropin, Nutropin AQ, Valtropin): Doses vary according to product used. Growth failure in Prader-Willi syndrome (Genotropin, Omnitrope): Individualized dosing. Idiopathic short stature (Genotropin, Humatrope): Individualized dosing. SHOX deficiency (Humatrope): Individualized dosing. Short stature in Noonan syndrome (Norditropin): Individualized dosing. Growth failure in chronic renal insufficiency (Nutropin, Nutropin AQ): Individualized dosing. Short stature in small for gestational age children (Humatrope, Norditropin, Omnitrope): Individualized dosing.

FORMS — Single-dose vials (powder for injection with diluent). Tev-Tropin: 5 mg vial (powder for injection with diluent, stable for 14 days when refrigerated). Genotropin: 1.5, 5.8, 13.8 mg cartridges. Humatrope: 6, 12, 24 mg pen cartridges; 5 mg vial (powder for injection with diluent, stable for 14 days when refrigerated). Nutropin AQ: 10 mg multidose vial, 5, 10, 20 mg/pen cartridges. Norditropin FlexPro: 5, 10, 15 mg prefilled pen. Norditropin NordiFlex: 30 mg prefilled pens. Omnitrope: 1.5, 5.8 mg vial (powder for injection with diluent). Saizen: Preassembled reconstitution device with autoinjector pen. Serostim: 4, 5, 6 mg single-dose vials; 4, 8.8 mg multidose vials; and 8.8 mg cartridges for autoinjector. Valtropin: 5 mg single-dose vials, 5 mg prefilled syringe. Zorbtive: 8.8 mg vial (powder for injection with diluent, stable for 14 days when refrigerated).

NOTES — Do not use in children with closed epiphyses. Contraindicated in active malignancy or acute

critical illness. Monitor glucose for insulin resistance; use with caution if diabetes or risk for diabetes. Transient and dose-dependent fluid retention may occur in adults. May cause hypothyroidism. Monitor thyroid function periodically. Evaluate patients with Prader-Willi syndrome for upper airway obstruction and sleep apnea prior to treatment; control wt and monitor for signs and symptoms of respiratory infection. Avoid if pre-proliferative or proliferative diabetic retinopathy. Perform funduscopic exam initially and then periodically. Monitor other hormonal replacement treatments closely in patients with hypopituitarism. Risk of pancreatitis may be greater in children, especially girls with Turner syndrome; consider pancreatitis if persistent abdominal pain.

MOA — Recombinantly derived human growth hormone that stimulates production of IGF-1.

ADVERSE EFFECTS — Serious: Diabetes, impaired glucose tolerance, antibody production, leukemia, pancreatitis, intracranial hypertension, dyspnea, malignancy. Frequent: Edema, increased nevi size, gynecomastia, headache, localized pain, weakness, hyperglycemia, injection-site pain, hypothyroidism, hypertension, sleep apnea.

TERIPARATIDE (*Forteo*) ▶LK ♀C ▶− $$$$$

WARNING — Osteosarcoma in animal studies; avoid in those at risk (e.g., Paget's disease, prior skeletal radiation).

ADULT — Treatment of postmenopausal osteoporosis, treatment of men and women with glucocorticoid-induced osteoporosis or to increase bone mass in men with primary or hypogonadal osteoporosis and high risk for fracture: 20 mcg SC daily in thigh or abdomen for no longer than 2 years.

PEDS — Not approved in children.

FORMS — Trade only: 28 dose pen injector (20 mcg/dose).

NOTES — Take with calcium and vitamin D. Pen-like delivery device requires education, and should be discarded 28 days after 1st injection even if not empty.

MOA — Parathyroid hormone analogue that stimulates trabecular and cortical bone formation.

ADVERSE EFFECTS — Serious: Orthostatic hypotension, HTN, angina, hypercalcemia, hyperuricemia. Frequent: Dizziness, leg cramps/spasms, back spasm, asthenia, arthralgia, depression, insomnia, dyspepsia.

TOLVAPTAN (*Samsca*) ▶K ♀C ▶? $$$$$

WARNING — Start and restart therapy in the hospital setting to closely monitor serum sodium. Avoid rapid correction of serum sodium (greater than 12 mEq/L/24 h); rapid correction may cause osmotic demyelination causing death or symptoms including dysarthria, dysphagia, lethargy, seizures, or coma. Slower correction advised in higher risk patients including malnutrition, alcoholism, or advanced liver disease.

ADULT — Euvolemic or hypervolemic hyponatremia (sodium less than 125 mEq/L): Start 15 mg PO

(cont.)

TOLVAPTAN (*cont.*)

daily. Titrate to desired serum sodium. If needed, increase q 24 h or more slowly to 30 mg PO daily; max dose 60 mg daily.

PEDS — Not approved in children.

FORMS — Trade only: Tabs 15, 30 mg.

NOTES — Avoid fluid restriction for first 24 h. May use for hyponatremia secondary to heart failure or SIADH. May use in hyponatremia with sodium greater than 125 mEq/L if resistant to fluid restriction and symptomatic. Do not use if urgent rise in serum sodium needed or serious neurologic symptoms. Requires frequent monitoring of serum sodium, volume, and neurologic status; monitor potassium if baseline K greater than 5 mEq/L. Avoid concurrent use of strong or moderate CYP3A4 inhibitors or inducers. Reports of liver injury, including fatal hepatotoxicity; do not use if underlying liver disease and limit use to 30 days.

MOA — Selective vasopressin V2-receptor antagonist that promotes free water excretion to raise sodium levels.

ADVERSE EFFECTS — Serious: Hypotension, hypovolemia, GI bleed (in cirrhosis), osmotic demyelination syndrome, hypernatremia, hepatotoxicity, hypersensitivity (anaphylactic shock). Frequent: Thirst, dry mouth, asthenia, constipation, polyuria, hyperglycemia.

VASOPRESSIN (*Pitressin, ADH, ✸Pressyn AR*) ▶LK ♀C ▶? $$$$$

ADULT — Diabetes insipidus: 5 to 10 units IM/SC two to four times per day prn.

PEDS — Not approved in children.

UNAPPROVED ADULT — Cardiac arrest: 40 units IV; may repeat if no response after 3 min. Septic shock: 0.01 to 0.1 units/min IV infusion, usual dose less than 0.04 units/min. Bleeding esophageal varices: 0.2 to 0.4 units/min initially (max 0.8 units/min).

UNAPPROVED PEDS — Diabetes insipidus: 2.5 to 10 units IM/SC two to four times per day prn. Bleeding esophageal varices: Start 0.002 to 0.005 units/kg/min IV, increase prn to 0.01 units/kg/min. Growth hormone and corticotropin provocative test: 0.3 units/kg IM, max 10 units.

NOTES — Monitor serum sodium. Injectable form may be given intranasally. May cause tissue necrosis with extravasation.

MOA — Promotes water resorption (antidiuretic effect) and smooth muscle contraction; stimulates vasoconstriction of arterioles and capillaries.

ADVERSE EFFECTS — Serious: Angina, arrhythmia, myocardial ischemia, peripheral vasoconstriction, hypersensitivity, anaphylaxis (rare), water intoxication, chronic nephritis, severe vasoconstriction with tissue necrosis (if infusion extravasates). Frequent: Abdominal cramps, dizziness, flatulence, N/V, tremor, sweating, headache.

ENT

ENT COMBINATIONS (SELECTED)

	Decongestant	Antihistamine	Antitussive	Typical Adult Doses
OTC				
Actifed Cold & Allergy	phenylephrine	chlorpheniramine	-	1 tab q 4–6 h
Actifed Cold & Sinus[‡]	pseudoephedrine	chlorpheniramine	-	2 tabs q 6 h
Allerfrim, Aprodine	pseudoephedrine	triprolidine	-	1 tab or 10 mL q 4–6 h
Benadryl Allergy/Coldt[‡]	phenylephrine	diphenhydramine	-	2 tabs q 4 h
Benadryl-D Allergy/Sinus Tablets	phenylephrine	diphenhydramine	-	1 tab q 4 h
Claritin-D 12-h, Alavert D-12	pseudoephedrine	loratadine	-	1 tab q 12 h
Claritin-D 24-h	pseudoephedrine	loratadine	-	1 tab daily
Dimetapp Cold & Allergy Elixir	phenylephrine	brompheniramine	-	20 mL q 4 h
Dimetapp DM Cold & Cough	phenylephrine	brompheniramine	dextromethorphan	20 mL q 4 h
Drixoral Cold & Allergy	pseudoephedrine	dexbrompheniramine	-	1 tab q 12 h
Mucinex-DM Extended-Release	-	-	guaifenesin, dextromethorphan	1-2 tabs q 12 h
Robitussin CF	phenylephrine	-	guaifenesin, dextromethorphan	10 mL q 4 h*
Robitussin DM, Mytussin DM	-	-	guaifenesin, dextromethorphan	10 mL q 4 h*
Robitussin PE, Guiatuss PE	phenylephrine	-	guaifenesin	10 mL q 4 h*
Triaminic Cold & Allergy	phenylephrine	chlorpheniramine	-	10 mL q 4 h*
Rx Only				
Allegra-D 12-h	pseudoephedrine	fexofenadine	-	1 tab q 12 h
Allegra-D 24-h	pseudoephedrine	fexofenadine	-	1 tab daily
Bromfenex	pseudoephedrine	brompheniramine	-	1 cap q 12 h
Clarinex-D 24-h	pseudoephedrinedesloratadine	desloratadine	-	1 tab daily
Deconamine	pseudoephedrine	chlorpheniramine	-	1 tab or 10 mL tid-qid
Deconamine SR, Chlordrine SR	pseudoephedrinechlorpheniramine	chlorpheniramine	-	1 tab q 12 h
Deconsal I	phenylephrine	-	guaifenesin	1-2 tabs q 12 h
Dimetane-DX	pseudoephedrine	brompheniramine	dextromethorphan	10 mL PO q 4 h
Duratuss	phenylephrine	-	guaifenesin	1 tab q 12 h
Duratuss HD©II	phenylephrine	-	guaifenesin, hydrocodone	5-10 mL q 4–6 h
Entex PSE, Guaifenex PSE 120	pseudoephedrine	-	guaifenesin	1 tab q 12 h
Histussin D ©II	pseudoephedrine	-	hydrocodone	5 mL qid
Histussin HC ©II	phenylephrine	chlorpheniramine	hydrocodone	10 mL q 4 h
Humibid DM	-	-	guaifenesin, dextromethorphan	1 tab q 12 h
Hycotuss ©II	-	-	guaifenesin, hydrocodone	5 mL after meals & at bedtime
Humibid DM	-	-	guaifenesin, dextromethorphan	1 tab q 12 h
Hycotuss ©II	-	-	guaifenesin, hydrocodone	5 mL after meals & at bedtime

(cont.)

ENT COMBINATIONS (SELECTED) (continued)

Phenergan/Dextromethorphan	promethazine	promethazine	dextromethorphan	5 mL q 4–6 h
Phenergan VC	phenylephrine	promethazine	-	5 mL q 4–6 h
Phenergan VC w/codeine ©V	phenylephrine	promethazine	codeine	5 mL q 4–6 h
Robitussin AC ©V (generic only)	-	-	guaifenesin, codeine	10 mL q 4 h*
Robitussin DAC ©V (generic only)	pseudoephedrine	-	guaifenesin, codeine	10 mL q 4 h*
Rondec Syrup	phenylephrine	chlorpheniramine	-	5 mL qid†
Rondec DM Syrup	phenylephrine	chlorpheniramine	dextromethorphan	5 mL qid†
Rondec Oral Drops	phenylephrine	chlorpheniramine	-	0.75 to 1 mL qid
Rondec DM Oral Drops	phenylephrine	chlorpheniramine	dextromethorphan	0.75 to 1 mL qid
Rynatan	phenylephrine	chlorpheniramine	-	1-2 tabs q 12 h
Rynatan-P Pediatric	phenylephrine	chlorpheniramine	-	2.5-5 mLq 12 h*
Semprex-D	pseudoephedrine	acrivastine	-	1 c ap q 4-6 h
Semprex-D	pseudoephedrine	acrivastine	-	1 c ap q 4-6 h
Tanafed (generic only)	pseudoephedrine	chlorpheniramine	-	10-20 mL q 12 h*
Tussionex ©II	-	chlorpheniramine	hydrocodone	5 mL q 12 h

tid=three times per day; qid=four times per day

*5 mL/dose if 6–11 yo. 2.5 mL if 2–5 yo.

†2.5 mL/dose if 6–11 yo. 1.25 mL if 2–5 yo.

‡Also contains acetaminophen.

ENT: Antihistamines—Non-Sedating

NOTE: Antihistamines ineffective when treating the common cold.

DESLORATADINE (*Clarinex*, *❖Aerius*) ▶LK ♀C ▶+ $$$$
ADULT — Allergic rhinitis/urticaria: 5 mg PO daily.
PEDS — Allergic rhinitis/urticaria: 2 mL (1 mg) PO daily for age 6 to 11 mo, ½ teaspoonful (1.25 mg) PO daily for age 12 mo to 5 yo, 1 teaspoonful (2.5 mg) PO daily for age 6 to 11 yo, 5 mg PO daily for age older than 12 yo.
FORMS — Generic/Trade: Tabs 5 mg. Orally disintegrating tabs 2.5, 5 mg. Trade only: Syrup 0.5 mg/mL.
NOTES — Increase dosing interval in liver or renal insufficiency to every other day. Use a measured dropper for syrup.
MOA — Antihistamine.
ADVERSE EFFECTS — Serious: None. Frequent: None.

FEXOFENADINE (*Allegra*) ▶LK ♀C ▶+ $$$
ADULT — Allergic rhinitis, urticaria: 60 mg PO two times per day or 180 mg PO daily. 60 mg PO daily if decreased renal function.
PEDS — Allergic rhinitis, urticaria: 30 mg PO two times per day or orally disintegrating tab two times per day for age 2 to 11 yo. Use adult dose for age older than 12 yo. 30 mg PO daily if decreased renal function. Urticaria: 15 mg (2.5 mL) twice daily for age 6 mo to younger than 2 yo. 15 mg PO daily if decreased renal function.

FORMS — OTC Generic/Trade: Tabs 30, 60, 180 mg. Caps 60 mg. Trade only: Susp 30 mg/5 mL. Orally disintegrating tab 30 mg.
NOTES — Avoid taking with fruit juice due to a large decrease in bioavailability. Do not remove orally disintegrating tab from its blister package until time of administration.
MOA — Antihistamine.
ADVERSE EFFECTS — Serious: None. Frequent: None.

LORATADINE (*Claritin, Claritin Hives Relief, Claritin RediTabs, Alavert, Tavist ND*) ▶LK ♀B ▶+ $
ADULT — Allergic rhinitis/urticaria: 10 mg PO daily.
PEDS — Allergic rhinitis/urticaria: 10 mg PO daily for age older than 6 yo, 5 mg PO daily (syrup) for age 2 to 5 yo.
FORMS — OTC Generic/Trade: Tabs 10 mg. Fast-dissolve tabs (Alavert, Claritin RediTabs) 5, 10 mg. Syrup 1 mg/mL. Rx Trade only (Claritin): Chewable tabs 5 mg, Liqui-gel caps 10 mg.
NOTES — Decrease dose in liver failure or renal insufficiency. Fast-dissolve tabs dissolve on tongue without water. ND indicates nondrowsy (Tavist).
MOA — Antihistamine.
ADVERSE EFFECTS — Serious: None. Frequent: None.

ENT: Antihistamines—Other

NOTE: Antihistamines ineffective when treating the common cold. Contraindicated in narrow-angle glaucoma, BPH, stenosing peptic ulcer disease, and bladder obstruction. Use half the normal dose in the elderly. May cause drowsiness and/or sedation, which may be enhanced with alcohol, sedatives, and other CNS depressants. Deaths have occurred in children younger than 2 yo attributed to toxicity from cough and cold medications; the FDA does not recommend their use in this age group.

CARBINOXAMINE (*Palgic, Karbinal ER*) ▶L ♀C ▶− $$$
ADULT — Allergic/vasomotor rhinitis/urticaria: 4 to 8 mg PO three to four times per day.
PEDS — Allergic/vasomotor rhinitis/urticaria: Give 2 mg PO three to four times per day for age 2 to 3 yo, give 2 to 4 mg PO three to four times per day for age 3 to 6 yo, give 4 to 6 mg PO three to four times per day for age 6 yo or older.
FORMS — Generic/Trade: Oral soln 4 mg/5 mL. Tab 4 mg. Trade only: Extended release suspension 4 mg/5 mL (Karbinal ER).
NOTES — Decrease dose in hepatic impairment.
MOA — Antihistamine.
ADVERSE EFFECTS — Serious: None. Frequent: Sedation, dizziness.

CETIRIZINE (*Zyrtec, ✲Reactine, Aller-Relief*) ▶LK ♀B ▶− $$$
ADULT — Allergic rhinitis/urticaria: 5 to 10 mg PO daily.
PEDS — Allergic rhinitis/urticaria: 5 to 10 mg PO daily for age older than 6 yo. Peds: Give 2.5 mg PO daily for age 6 to 23 mo, give 2.5 mg PO daily to two times per day or 5 mg PO daily for age 2 to 5 yo. If age older than 12 mo, may increase to 2.5 mg PO two times per day.
FORMS — OTC Generic/Trade: Tabs 5, 10 mg. Syrup 5 mg/5 mL. Chewable tabs, grape flavored 5, 10 mg.
NOTES — Decrease dose in renal or hepatic impairment.
MOA — Antihistamine.
ADVERSE EFFECTS — Serious: None. Frequent: Sedation in 14%.

CHLORPHENIRAMINE (*Chlor-Trimeton, Aller-Chlor*) ▶LK ♀B ▶− $
ADULT — Allergic rhinitis: 4 mg PO q 4 to 6 h. 8 mg PO q 8 to 12 h (timed-release) or 12 mg PO q 12 h (timed-release). Max 24 mg/day.
PEDS — Allergic rhinitis: 2 mg PO q 4 to 6 h (up to 12 mg/day) for age 6 to 11 yo, give adult dose for age 12 yo or older.
UNAPPROVED PEDS — Allergic rhinitis age 2 to 5 yo: 1 mg PO q 4 to 6 h (up to 6 mg/day). Timed release age 6 to 11 yo: 8 mg PO q 12 h prn.
FORMS — OTC Trade only: Tabs, extended-release 12 mg. Generic/Trade: Tabs 4 mg. Syrup 2 mg/5 mL. Tabs extended-release 8 mg.
MOA — Antihistamine.
ADVERSE EFFECTS — Serious: None. Frequent: Sedation.

CLEMASTINE (*Tavist-1*) ▶LK ♀B ▶− $
ADULT — Allergic rhinitis: 1.34 mg PO two times per day. Max 8.04 mg/day. Urticaria/angioedema: 2.68 mg PO one to three times per day. Max 8.04 mg/day.
PEDS — Allergic rhinitis: Give 0.67 mg PO two times per day. Max 4.02 mg/day for age 6 to 12 yo, give adult dose for age 12 yo or older. Urticaria/

angioedema: Give 1.34 mg PO two times per day (up to 4.02 mg/day) for age 6 to 12 yo, give adult dose for age 6 to 12 yo.
UNAPPROVED PEDS — Allergic rhinitis for age younger than 6 yo: 0.05 mg/kg/day (as clemastine base) PO divided two to three times per day. Max dose 1 mg/day.
FORMS — OTC Generic/Trade: Tabs 1.34 mg. Rx: Generic/Trade: Tabs 2.68 mg. Syrup 0.67 mg/5 mL. Rx: Generic only: Syrup 0.5 mg/5 mL.
NOTES — 1.34 mg is equivalent to 1 mg clemastine base.
MOA — Antihistamine.
ADVERSE EFFECTS — Serious: None. Frequent: Sedation, dry mouth.

CYPROHEPTADINE (*Periactin*) ▶LK ♀B ▶− $
ADULT — Allergic rhinitis/urticaria: Start 4 mg PO three times per day, usual effective dose is 12 to 16 mg/day. Max 32 mg/day.
PEDS — Allergic rhinitis/urticaria: Start 2 mg PO two to three times per day (up to 12 mg/day) for age 2 to 6 yo, Start 4 mg PO two to three times per day (up to 16 mg/day) for age 7 to 14 yo.
UNAPPROVED ADULT — Appetite stimulant: 2 to 4 mg PO three times per day 1 h before meals. Prevention of cluster headaches: 4 mg PO four times per day. Treatment of acute serotonin syndrome: 12 mg PO/NG followed by 2 mg q 2 h until symptoms clear, then 8 mg q 6 h maintenance while syndrome remains active.
FORMS — Generic only: Tabs 4 mg. Syrup 2 mg/5 mL.
MOA — Antihistamine/5-HT 2A antagonist.
ADVERSE EFFECTS — Serious: None. Frequent: Sedation.

DEXCHLORPHENIRAMINE (*Polaramine*) ▶LK ♀? ▶− $$
ADULT — Allergic rhinitis/urticaria: 2 mg PO q 4 to 6 h. Timed-release tabs: 4 or 6 mg PO at bedtime or q 8 to 10 h.
PEDS — Allergic rhinitis/urticaria: Immediate-release tabs and syrup: Give 0.5 mg PO q 4 to 6 h for age 2 to 5 yo, give 1 mg PO q 4 to 6 h for age 6 to 11 yo, give adult dose for age 12 yo or older. Timed-release tabs age 6 to 12 yo: 4 mg PO daily, preferably at at bedtime.
FORMS — Generic only: Tabs, immediate-release 2 mg; timed-release 4, 6 mg. Syrup 2 mg/5 mL.
MOA — Antihistamine.
ADVERSE EFFECTS — Serious: None. Frequent: Sedation.

DIPHENHYDRAMINE (*Benadryl, Banophen, Allermax, Diphen, Diphenhist, Dytan, Siladryl, Sominex, ✲Allerdryl, Nytol*) ▶LK ♀B ▶− $
ADULT — Allergic rhinitis, urticaria, hypersensitivity reactions: 25 to 50 mg PO/IM/IV q 4 to 6 h. Max

(cont.)

DIPHENHYDRAMINE (*cont.*)

300 to 400 mg/day. Motion sickness: 25 to 50 mg PO pre-exposure and q 4 to 6 h prn. Drug-induced parkinsonism: 10 to 50 mg IV/IM. Antitussive: 25 mg PO q 4 h. Max 100 mg/day. EPS: 25 to 50 mg PO three to four times per day or 10 to 50 mg IV/IM three to four times per day. Insomnia: 25 to 50 mg PO at bedtime.

PEDS — Hypersensitivity reactions: Give 12.5 to 25 mg PO q 4 to 6 h or 5 mg/kg/day PO/IV/IM divided four times per day for age 6 to 11 yo, give adult dose for age 12 yo or older. Max 150 mg/day. Antitussive (syrup): Give 6.25 mg PO q 4 h (up to 25 mg/day) for age 2 to 5 yo, give 12.5 mg PO q 4 h (up to 50 mg/day) for age 6 to 12 yo. EPS: 12.5 to 25 mg PO three to four times per day or 5 mg/kg/day IV/IM divided four times per day, max 300 mg/day. Insomnia age 12 yo or older: 25 to 50 mg PO at bedtime.

FORMS — OTC Trade only: Tabs 25, 50 mg. Chewable tabs 12.5 mg. OTC and Rx: Generic only: Caps 25, 50 mg. Softgel cap 25 mg. OTC Generic/Trade: Soln 6.25 or 12.5 mg per 5 mL. Rx: Trade only: (Dytan) Susp 25 mg/mL. Chewable tabs 25 mg.

NOTES — Anticholinergic side effects are enhanced in the elderly and may worsen dementia or delirium. Avoid use with donepezil, rivastigmine, galantamine, or tacrine.

MOA — Antihistamine.

ADVERSE EFFECTS — Serious: None. Frequent: Sedation, dry mouth.

HYDROXYZINE (*Atarax, Vistaril*) ▶L ♀C ▶– $$

ADULT — Pruritus: 25 to 100 mg IM/PO one to four times per day or prn.

PEDS — Pruritus: Give 50 mg/day PO divided four times per day for age younger than 6 yo, give 50 to 100 mg/day PO divided four times per day for age 6 or older.

FORMS — Generic only: Tabs 10, 25, 50, 100 mg. Caps 100 mg. Syrup 10 mg/5 mL. Generic/Trade: Caps 25, 50 mg. Susp 25 mg/5 mL (Vistaril). Caps = Vistaril; Tabs = Atarax.

NOTES — Atarax (hydrochloride salt), Vistaril (pamoate salt).

MOA — Antihistamine.

ADVERSE EFFECTS — Serious: None. Frequent: Sedation.

LEVOCETIRIZINE (*Xyzal*) ▶K ♀B ▶– $$$

ADULT — Allergic rhinitis/urticaria: 5 mg PO daily.

PEDS — Allergic rhinitis/urticaria: Give 2.5 mg PO daily for age 6 to 11 yo, give 5 mg PO daily for age 12 or older.

FORMS — Generic/Trade: Tabs, scored 5 mg. Oral soln 2.5 mg/5 mL (148 mL).

NOTES — Decrease dose in renal impairment.

MOA — Antihistamine.

ADVERSE EFFECTS — Serious: None. Frequent: Sedation.

MECLIZINE (*Antivert, Bonine, Medivert, Meclicot, Meni-D*) ▶L ♀B ▶? $

ADULT — Motion sickness: 25 to 50 mg PO 1 h prior to travel, then 25 to 50 mg PO daily.

PEDS — Not approved in children.

UNAPPROVED ADULT — Vertigo: 25 mg PO one to four times per day prn.

FORMS — Rx/OTC/Generic/Trade: Tabs 12.5, 25 mg. Chewable tabs 25 mg. Rx/Trade only: Tabs 50 mg.

NOTES — FDA classifies meclizine as "possibly effective" for vertigo. May cause dizziness and drowsiness.

MOA — Antihistamine.

ADVERSE EFFECTS — Serious: Tachycardia, confusion. Frequent: Dry mouth, constipation, drowsiness, dizziness, blurred vision, urinary retention, rash.

ENT: Antitussives / Expectorants

BENZONATATE (*Tessalon, Tessalon Perles*) ▶L ♀C ▶? $$

ADULT — Cough: 100 to 200 mg PO three times per day. Max 600 mg/day.

PEDS — Cough: give adult dose for age older than 10 yo.

FORMS — Generic/Trade: Softgel caps: 100, 200 mg.

NOTES — Swallow whole. Do not chew. Numbs mouth; possible choking hazard.

MOA — Local anesthetic.

ADVERSE EFFECTS — Serious: None. Frequent: None.

DEXTROMETHORPHAN (*Benylin, Delsym, DexAlone, Robitussin Cough, Vick's 44 Cough*) ▶L ♀+ ▶+ $

ADULT — Cough: 10 to 20 mg PO q 4 h or 30 mg PO q 6 to 8 h. 60 mg PO q 12 h (Delsym).

PEDS — Cough: Give either 2.5 to 5 mg PO q 4 h or 7.5 mg PO q 6 to 8 h of regular susp or 15 mg PO q 12 h of sustained action liquid for age 2 to 5 yo, give either 5 to 10 mg PO q 4 h or 15 mg PO q 6 to 8 h of regular susp, or 30 mg PO q 12 h of sustained action liquid for age 6 to 12 yo, give adult dose for age older than 12 yo.

FORMS — OTC Trade only: Caps 15 mg (Robitussin), 30 mg (DexAlone). Susp, extended-release 30 mg/5 mL (Delsym). Generic/Trade: Syrup 5, 7.5, 10, 15 mg/5 mL. Generic only: Lozenges 5, 10 mg.

NOTES — Contraindicated with MAOIs due to potential for serotonin syndrome.

MOA — Cough suppressant by depressing medullary cough center.

ADVERSE EFFECTS — Serious: None. Frequent: None.

GUAIFENESIN (*Robitussin, Hytuss, Guiatuss, Mucinex*) ▶L ♀C ▶+ $

ADULT — Expectorant: 100 to 400 mg PO q 4 h. 600 to 1200 mg PO q 12 h (extended-release). Max 2.4 g/day.

PEDS — Expectorant: 50 to 100 mg/dose for age 2 to 5 yo, give 100 to 200 mg/dose for age 6 to 11 yo, give adult dose for age 12 yo or older.

UNAPPROVED PEDS — Expectorant: Give 25 mg PO q 4 h (up to 150 mg/day) for age 6 to 11 mo, give

GUAIFENESIN (*cont.*)

50 mg po q 4 h (up to 300 mg/day) for age 12 to 23 mo.

FORMS — Rx Generic/Trade: Extended-release tabs 600, 1200 mg. OTC Generic/Trade: Liquid, Syrup 100 mg/5 mL. OTC Trade only: Caps 200 mg (Hytuss). Extended-release tabs 600 mg (Mucinex). OTC Generic only: Tabs 100, 200, 400 mg.

NOTES — Lack of convincing studies to document efficacy.

MOA — Expectorant.

ADVERSE EFFECTS — Serious: None. Frequent: None.

ENT: Combination Products—OTC

NOTE: Decongestants in some ENT combination products can increase BP, aggravate anxiety or cause insomnia (use caution). Some contain sedating antihistamines. Sedation can be enhanced by alcohol and other CNS depressants. Some states have restricted or ended OTC sale of pseudoephedrine and pseudoephedrine combination products or reclassified it as a scheduled drug due to the potential for diversion to methamphetamine labs. Deaths have occurred in children younger than 2 yo attributed to toxicity from cough and cold medications; the FDA does not recommend their use in this age group.

ACTIFED COLD AND ALLERGY (phenylephrine + chlorpheniramine) ▶L ♀C ▶+ $

ADULT — Allergic rhinitis/nasal congestion: 1 tab PO q 4 to 6 h. Max 4 tabs/day.

PEDS — Allergic rhinitis/nasal congestion: Give ½ tab PO q 4 to 6 h (up to 2 tabs/day) for age 6 to 12 yo, give adult dose for age older than 12 yo.

FORMS — OTC Trade only: Tabs 10 mg phenylephrine/4 mg chlorpheniramine.

MOA — Decongestant/antihistamine combination.

ADVERSE EFFECTS — Serious: None. Frequent: Insomnia, palpitations, sedation.

ACTIFED COLD AND SINUS (pseudoephedrine + chlorpheniramine + acetaminophen) ▶L ♀C ▶+ $$

ADULT — Allergic rhinitis/nasal congestion/headache: 2 caps PO q 6 h. Max 8 caps/day.

PEDS — Allergic rhinitis/nasal congestion/headache: Age older than 12 yo: Use adult dose.

FORMS — OTC Trade only: Tabs 30 mg pseudoephedrine/2 mg chlorpheniramine/500 mg acetaminophen.

MOA — Decongestant/antihistamine/analgesic combination.

ADVERSE EFFECTS — Serious: None. Frequent: Insomnia, palpitations, sedation.

ALAVERT D-12 (pseudoephedrine + loratadine) ▶LK ♀B ▶– $

ADULT — Allergic rhinitis/nasal congestion: 1 tab PO two times per day.

PEDS — Not approved in children.

FORMS — OTC Generic/Trade: Tabs, 12 h extended-release, 120 mg pseudoephedrine/5 mg loratadine.

NOTES — Decrease dose to 1 tab PO daily with CrCl less than 30 mL/min. Avoid in hepatic insufficiency.

MOA — Decongestant/antihistamine combination.

ADVERSE EFFECTS — Serious: None. Frequent: Insomnia, palpitations, sedation.

ALEVE COLD AND SINUS (naproxen + pseudoephedrine) ▶L ♀C (D in 3rd trimester) ▶+ $

ADULT — Nasal/sinus congestion, fever and pain: 1 cap PO q 12 h.

PEDS — Nasal/sinus congestion, fever and pain: Age older than 12 yo: Use adult dose.

FORMS — OTC Generic/Trade: Extended-release caps: 220 mg naproxen sodium/120 mg pseudoephedrine.

MOA — Decongestant/analgesic/antipyretic.

ADVERSE EFFECTS — Serious: Hypersensitivity, GI bleeding, nephrotoxicity. Frequent: Insomnia, palpitations.

ALLERFRIM (pseudoephedrine + triprolidine) ▶L ♀C ▶+ $

ADULT — Allergic rhinitis/nasal congestion: 1 tab or 10 mL PO q 4 to 6 h. Max 4 tabs/day or 40 mL/day.

PEDS — Allergic rhinitis/nasal congestion: Give ½ tab or 5 mL PO q 4 to 6 h (up to 2 tabs/day or 20 mL/day) for age 6 to 12 yo, give adult dose for age older than 12 yo.

FORMS — OTC Trade only: Tabs 60 mg pseudoephedrine/2.5 mg triprolidine. Syrup 30 mg pseudoephedrine/1.25 mg triprolidine/5 mL.

MOA — Decongestant/antihistamine combination.

ADVERSE EFFECTS — Serious: None. Frequent: Insomnia, palpitations, sedation.

APRODINE (pseudoephedrine + triprolidine) ▶L ♀C ▶+ $

ADULT — Allergic rhinitis/nasal congestion: 1 tab or 10 mL PO q 4 to 6 h. Max 4 tabs/day or 40 mL/day.

PEDS — Allergic rhinitis/nasal congestion: Age older than 12 yo: Use adult dose. 6 to 12 yo: ½ tab or 5 mL PO q 4 to 6 h. Max 2 tabs/day or 20 mL/day.

FORMS — OTC Trade only: Tabs 60 mg pseudoephedrine/2.5 mg triprolidine. Syrup 30 mg pseudoephedrine/1.25 mg triprolidine/5 mL.

MOA — Decongestant/antihistamine combination.

ADVERSE EFFECTS — Serious: None. Frequent: Insomnia, palpitations, sedation.

BENADRYL ALLERGY AND COLD (phenylephrine + diphenhydramine + acetaminophen) ▶L ♀C ▶– $

ADULT — Allergic rhinitis/nasal congestion/headache: 2 tabs PO q 4 h. Max 12 tabs/day.

PEDS — Allergic rhinitis/nasal congestion/headache: Give 1 tab PO q 4 h (up to 5 tabs/day) for age 6 to 12 yo, give adult dose for age older than 12 yo.

FORMS — OTC Trade only: Tabs 5/12.5/325 mg of phenylephrine/diphenhydramine/acetaminophen.

MOA — Decongestant/antihistamine/analgesic combination.

(cont.)

BENADRYL ALLERGY AND COLD (*cont.*)

ADVERSE EFFECTS — Serious: None. Frequent: Insomnia, palpitations, sedation.

BENADRYL-D ALLERGY AND SINUS (phenylephrine + diphenhydramine) ▶L ♀C ▶− $

ADULT — Allergic rhinitis/nasal congestion: 1 tab PO q 4 h. Max 6 tabs/day.

PEDS — Allergic rhinitis/nasal congestion: Age older than 12 yo: Use adult dose.

FORMS — OTC Trade only: Tabs 10/25 mg phenylephrine/diphenhydramine.

MOA — Decongestant/antihistamine combination.

ADVERSE EFFECTS — Serious: None. Frequent: Insomnia, palpitations, sedation.

CHERACOL D COUGH (guaifenesin + dextromethorphan) ▶L ♀C ▶? $

ADULT — Cough: 10 mL PO q 4 h.

PEDS — Cough: Give 2.5 mL PO q 4 h (up to 15 mL/day) for age 2 to 5 yo, give 5 mL PO q 4 h for age 6 to 11 yo, give adult dose for age 12 yo or older.

FORMS — OTC Generic/Trade: Syrup 100 mg guaifenesin/10 mg dextromethorphan/5 mL.

MOA — Expectorant/cough suppressant combination.

ADVERSE EFFECTS — Serious: None. Frequent: None.

CHILDREN'S ADVIL COLD (ibuprofen + pseudoephedrine) ▶L ♀C (D in 3rd trimester) ▶+ $

ADULT — Not approved for use in adults.

PEDS — Nasal congestion/sore throat/fever: Give 5 mL PO q 6 h for age 2 to 5 yo, give 10 mL PO q 6 h for age 6 to 11 yo.

FORMS — OTC Trade only: Susp: 100 mg ibuprofen/15 mg pseudoephedrine/5 mL. Grape flavor, alcohol-free.

NOTES — Shake well before using. Do not use for more than 7 days for cold, sinus, and flu symptoms.

MOA — Decongestant/anti-inflammatory/antipyretic combination.

ADVERSE EFFECTS — Serious: Allergic reactions. Frequent: Insomnia, palpitations.

CLARITIN-D 12 HR (pseudoephedrine + loratadine) ▶LK ♀B ▶+ $

ADULT — Allergic rhinitis/nasal congestion: 1 tab PO two times per day.

PEDS — Not approved in children.

FORMS — OTC Generic/Trade: Tabs, 12 h extended-release: 120 mg pseudoephedrine/5 mg loratadine.

NOTES — Decrease dose to 1 tab PO daily with CrCl less than 30 mL/min. Avoid in hepatic insufficiency.

MOA — Decongestant/antihistamine combination.

ADVERSE EFFECTS — Serious: None. Frequent: Insomnia, palpitations, sedation.

CLARITIN-D 24 HR (pseudoephedrine + loratadine) ▶LK ♀B ▶+ $

ADULT — Allergic rhinitis/nasal congestion: 1 tab PO daily.

PEDS — Not approved in children.

FORMS — OTC Generic/Trade: Tabs, 24 h extended-release: 240 mg pseudoephedrine/10 mg loratadine.

NOTES — Decrease dose to 1 tab PO every other day with CrCl less than 30 mL/min. Avoid in hepatic insufficiency.

MOA — Decongestant/antihistamine combination.

ADVERSE EFFECTS — Serious: None. Frequent: Insomnia, palpitations, sedation.

CORICIDIN HBP CONGESTION AND COUGH (guaifenesin + dextromethorphan) ▶LK ♀B ▶+ $$

ADULT — Productive cough: 1 to 2 softgels PO q 4 h. Max 12 softgels/day.

PEDS — Productive cough: Give adult dose for 12 yo or older.

FORMS — OTC Trade only: Softgels 200 mg guaifenesin/10 mg dextromethorphan.

MOA — Expectorant/cough suppressant combination.

ADVERSE EFFECTS — Serious: None. Frequent: None.

CORICIDIN HBP COUGH AND COLD (chlorpheniramine + dextromethorphan) ▶LK ♀B ▶+ $

ADULT — Rhinitis/cough: 1 tab q 6 h. Max 4 doses/day.

PEDS — Rhinitis/cough: Give adult dose for 12 yo or older.

FORMS — OTC Trade only: Tabs 4 mg chlorpheniramine/30 mg dextromethorphan.

MOA — Antihistamine/cough suppressant combination.

ADVERSE EFFECTS — Serious: None. Frequent: Sedation.

DIMETAPP COLD AND ALLERGY (phenylephrine + brompheniramine) ▶LK ♀C ▶− $

ADULT — Allergic rhinitis/nasal congestion: 20 mL PO q 4 h. Max 4 doses/day.

PEDS — Allergic rhinitis/nasal congestion: 10 mL PO q 4 h for age 6 to 11 yo, give adult dose for 12 yo or older.

FORMS — OTC Trade only: Liquid, Tabs 2.5 mg phenylephrine/1 mg brompheniramine per tab or 5 mL.

NOTES — Grape flavor, alcohol-free.

MOA — Decongestant/antihistamine combination.

ADVERSE EFFECTS — Serious: None. Frequent: Insomnia, palpitations, sedation.

DIMETAPP COLD AND COUGH (phenylephrine + brompheniramine + dextromethorphan) ▶LK ♀C ▶− $

ADULT — Nasal congestion/cough: 20 mL PO q 4 h. Max 6 doses/day.

PEDS — Nasal congestion/cough: Give 10 mL PO q 4 h (up to 6 doses/day) for age 6 to 11 yo, give adult dose for 12 yo or older.

FORMS — OTC Trade only: Liquid 2.5 mg phenylephrine/1 mg brompheniramine/5 mg dextromethorphan/5 mL.

NOTES — Red grape flavor, alcohol-free.

MOA — Decongestant/antihistamine/cough suppressant combination.

ADVERSE EFFECTS — Serious: None. Frequent: Insomnia, palpitations, sedation.

DIMETAPP NIGHTTIME COLD AND CONGESTION (phenylephrine + diphenhydramine) ▶LK ♀C ▶− $

ADULT — Nasal congestion/runny nose/fever/cough/sore throat: 20 mL PO q 4 h. Max 5 doses/day.

PEDS — Nasal congestion/runny nose/fever/cough/sore throat: Give 10 mL PO q 4 h (up to 5 doses/day) for age 6 to 11 yo, give adult dose for 12 yo or older.

FORMS — OTC Trade only: Syrup 2.5 mg phenylephrine and 6.25 mg diphenhydramine.

(cont.)

DIMETAPP NIGHTTIME COLD AND CONGESTION (cont.)

NOTES — Bubble gum flavor, alcohol-free.

MOA — Decongestant/antihistamine/cough suppressant/analgesic combination.

ADVERSE EFFECTS — Serious: Hepatotoxicity. Frequent: Insomnia, palpitations, sedation.

DRIXORAL COLD AND ALLERGY (pseudoephedrine + dexbrompheniramine) ▶LK ♀C ▶– $

ADULT — Allergic rhinitis/nasal congestion: 1 tab PO q 12 h.

PEDS — Allergic rhinitis/nasal congestion give adult dose for 12 yo or older.

FORMS — OTC Trade only: Tabs, sustained-action 120 mg pseudoephedrine/6 mg dexbrompheniramine.

MOA — Decongestant/antihistamine combination.

ADVERSE EFFECTS — Serious: None. Frequent: Insomnia, palpitations, sedation.

GUIATUSS PE (pseudoephedrine + guaifenesin) ▶L ♀C ▶– $

ADULT — Nasal congestion/cough: 10 mL PO q 4 h. Max 40 mL/day.

PEDS — Nasal congestion/cough: Give 2.5 mL PO q 4 h for age 2 to 5 yo, give 5 mL PO q 4 h for age 6 to 11 yo, give adult dose for 12 yo or older. Max 4 doses/day.

FORMS — OTC Trade only: Syrup 30 mg pseudoephedrine/100 mg guaifenesin/5 mL.

NOTES — PE indicates pseudoephedrine.

MOA — Decongestant/expectorant combination.

ADVERSE EFFECTS — Serious: None. Frequent: Insomnia, palpitations.

MUCINEX D (guaifenesin + pseudoephedrine) ▶L ♀C ▶? $

WARNING — Multiple strengths; write specific product on Rx.

ADULT — Cough/congestion: 2 tabs (600/60) PO q 12 h; max 4 tabs/24 h. 1 tab (1200/120) PO q 12 h; max 2 tabs/24 h.

PEDS — Cough: Give adult dose for 12 yo or older.

FORMS — OTC Trade only: Tabs, extended-release: 600/60, 1200/120 mg guaifenesin/pseudoephedrine.

NOTES — Do not crush, chew or break the tab. Take with a full glass of water.

MOA — Decongestant/expectorant combination.

ADVERSE EFFECTS — Serious: None. Frequent: Insomnia, palpitations.

MUCINEX DM (guaifenesin + dextromethorphan) ▶L ♀C ▶? $

WARNING — Multiple strengths; write specific product on Rx.

ADULT — Cough: 1 to 2 tabs (600/30) PO q 12 h; max 4 tabs/24 h. 1 tab (1200/60) PO q 12 h; max 2 tabs/24 h.

PEDS — Cough: Give adult dose for 12 yo or older.

FORMS — OTC Trade only: Tabs, extended-release: 600/30, 1200/60 mg guaifenesin/dextromethorphan.

NOTES — DM indicates dextromethorphan. Do not crush, chew or break the tab. Take with a full glass of water.

MOA — Expectorant/cough suppressant combination.

ADVERSE EFFECTS — Serious: None. Frequent: None.

ROBITUSSIN CF (phenylephrine + guaifenesin + dextromethorphan) ▶L ♀C ▶– $

ADULT — Nasal congestion/cough: 10 mL PO q 4 h.

PEDS — Nasal congestion/cough: Give 2.5 mL PO q 4 h for age 2 to 5 yo, give 5 mL PO q 4 h for age 6 to 11 yo, give adult dose for 12 yo or older.

FORMS — OTC Generic/Trade: Syrup 5 mg phenylephrine/100 mg guaifenesin/10 mg dextromethorphan/5 mL.

NOTES — CF indicates cough formula.

MOA — Decongestant/expectorant/cough suppressant combination.

ADVERSE EFFECTS — Serious: None. Frequent: Insomnia, palpitations.

ROBITUSSIN DM (guaifenesin + dextromethorphan) ▶L ♀C ▶+ $

ADULT — Cough: 10 mL PO q 4 h. Max 60 mL/day.

PEDS — Cough: Give 2.5 mL PO q 4 h (up to 15 mL/day) for age 2 to 5 yo, give 5 mL PO q 4 h (up to 30 mL/day) for age 6 to 11 yo, give adult dose for 12 yo or older.

FORMS — OTC Generic/Trade: Syrup 100 mg guaifenesin/10 mg dextromethorphan/5 mL.

NOTES — Alcohol-free. DM indicates dextromethorphan.

MOA — Expectorant/cough suppressant combination.

ADVERSE EFFECTS — Serious: None. Frequent: None.

TRIAMINIC CHEST AND NASAL CONGESTION (phenylephrine + guaifenesin) ▶LK ♀C ▶– $

ADULT — Child-only preparation.

PEDS — Chest/nasal congestion: Give 5 mL PO q 4 h (up to 6 doses/day) for age 2 to 6 yo, give 10 mL PO q 4 h (up to 6 doses/day) for age 6 to 12 yo.

FORMS — OTC Trade only, yellow label: Syrup 2.5 mg phenylephrine/50 mg guaifenesin/5 mL, tropical flavor.

MOA — Decongestant/expectorant combination.

ADVERSE EFFECTS — Serious: None. Frequent: Insomnia, palpitations.

TRIAMINIC COLD AND ALLERGY (phenylephrine + chlorpheniramine) ▶LK ♀C ▶– $

ADULT — Child-only preparation.

PEDS — Allergic rhinitis/nasal congestion: 10 mL PO q 4 h to max 6 doses/day for age 6 to 12 yo.

FORMS — OTC Trade only, orange label: Syrup 2.5 mg phenylephrine/1 mg chlorpheniramine/5 mL, orange flavor.

MOA — Decongestant/antihistamine combination.

ADVERSE EFFECTS — Serious: None. Frequent: Insomnia, palpitations, sedation.

TRIAMINIC COUGH AND SORE THROAT (dextromethorphan + acetaminophen) ▶LK ♀C ▶– $

ADULT — Child-only preparation.

PEDS — Cough/sore throat: Give PO q 4 h to max 5 doses/day: 5 mL or 1 softchew tab per dose for age 2 to 6 yo, give 10 mL or 2 softchew tabs per dose for age 7 to 12 yo.

FORMS — OTC Trade only, purple label: Syrup, Softchew tabs 5 mg dextromethorphan/160 mg acetaminophen/5 mL or tab, grape flavor.

MOA — Cough suppressant/analgesic combination.

ADVERSE EFFECTS — Serious: Hepatotoxicity. Frequent: Insomnia, palpitations.

TRIAMINIC DAY TIME COLD AND COUGH (phenylephrine + dextromethorphan) ▶LK ♀C ▶– $
ADULT — Child-only preparation.
PEDS — Nasal congestion/cough: Give PO q 4 h to max 6 doses/day: 5 mL or 1 strip per dose for age 2 to 6 yo, give 10 mL or 2 strips per dose for age 7 to 12 yo.
FORMS — OTC Trade only, red label: Syrup, thin strips 2.5 mg phenylephrine/5 mg dextromethorphan/5 mL, cherry flavor.
NOTES — Allow strips to dissolve on the tongue.
MOA — Decongestant/cough suppressant combination.
ADVERSE EFFECTS — Serious: None. Frequent: Insomnia, palpitations, sedation.

TRIAMINIC FLU COUGH AND FEVER (acetaminophen + chlorpheniramine + dextromethorphan) ▶LK ♀C ▶– $
ADULT — Child-only preparation.
PEDS — Fever/cough: 10 mL PO q 6 h to max 4 doses/day for age 6 to 12 yo.
FORMS — OTC Trade only, pink label: Syrup 160 mg acetaminophen/1 mg chlorpheniramine/7.5 mg dextromethorphan/5 mL, bubble gum flavor.
MOA — Analgesic/antihistamine/cough suppressant combination.
ADVERSE EFFECTS — Serious: None. Frequent: Insomnia, palpitations.

TRIAMINIC NIGHT TIME COLD AND COUGH (phenylephrine + diphenhydramine) ▶LK ♀C ▶– $
ADULT — Child-only preparation.
PEDS — Nasal congestion/cough: 10 mL PO q 4 h to max 6 doses/day for age 6 to 12 yo.
FORMS — OTC Trade only, blue label: Syrup 2.5 mg phenylephrine/6.25 mg diphenhydramine/5 mL, grape flavor.
MOA — Decongestant/antihistamine combination.
ADVERSE EFFECTS — Serious: None. Frequent: Insomnia, palpitations, sedation.

ENT: Combination Products—Rx Only

NOTE: Decongestants in some ENT combination products can increase BP, aggravate anxiety, or cause insomnia (use caution). Some contain sedating antihistamines. Sedation can be enhanced by alcohol and other CNS depressants. Deaths have occurred in children younger than 2 yo attributed to toxicity from cough and cold medications; the FDA does not recommend their use in this age group.

ALLEGRA-D 12-HOUR (fexofenadine + pseudoephedrine) ▶LK ♀C ▶+ $$$$
ADULT — Allergic rhinitis/nasal congestion: 1 tab PO q 12 h.
PEDS — Not approved in children.
FORMS — Trade only: Tabs, extended-release 60/120 mg fexofenadine/pseudoephedrine.
NOTES — Decrease dose to 1 tab PO daily with decreased renal function. Take on an empty stomach. Avoid taking with fruit juice due to a large decrease in bioavailability.
MOA — Decongestant/antihistamine combination.
ADVERSE EFFECTS — Serious: None. Frequent: Insomnia, palpitations.

ALLEGRA-D 24-HOUR (fexofenadine + pseudoephedrine) ▶LK ♀C ▶+ $$$$
ADULT — Allergic rhinitis/nasal congestion: 1 tab PO daily.
PEDS — Not approved in children.
FORMS — Trade only: Tabs, extended-release 180/240 mg fexofenadine/pseudoephedrine.
NOTES — Decrease dose to 1 tab PO every other day with decreased renal function. Take on an empty stomach. Avoid taking with fruit juice due to a large decrease in bioavailability.
MOA — Decongestant/antihistamine combination.
ADVERSE EFFECTS — Serious: None. Frequent: Insomnia, palpitations.

ALLERX (pseudoephedrine + methscopolamine + chlorpheniramine) ▶LK ♀C ▶– $$$
ADULT — Allergic rhinitis/vasomotor rhinitis/nasal congestion: 1 yellow am tab q am and 1 blue pm tab q pm.
PEDS — Allergic rhinitis/vasomotor rhinitis/nasal congestion: Use adult dose for age older than 12 yo.
FORMS — Trade only: Tabs, am (yellow): 120 mg pseudoephedrine/2.5 mg methscopolamine. pm (blue): 8 mg chlorpheniramine/2.5 mg methscopolamine.
NOTES — Contraindicated in severe HTN, CAD, MAOI therapy, narrow angle glaucoma, urinary retention, and peptic ulcer. Caution in elderly, hepatic and renal disease.
MOA — Decongestant/anticholinergic & antihistamine/anticholinergic combination.
ADVERSE EFFECTS — Serious: Arrhythmia. Frequent: Insomnia, palpitations, dizziness, dry mouth, blurred vision, urinary retention.

BROMFENEX (pseudoephedrine + brompheniramine) ▶LK ♀C ▶– $
ADULT — Allergic rhinitis/nasal congestion: 1 cap PO q 12 h. Max 2 caps/day.
PEDS — Allergic rhinitis/nasal congestion: Age older than 12 yo: Use adult dose. 6 to 11 yo: 1 cap PO daily.
FORMS — Generic/Trade: Caps, sustained-release 120 mg pseudoephedrine/12 mg brompheniramine.
MOA — Decongestant/antihistamine combination.
ADVERSE EFFECTS — Serious: None. Frequent: Insomnia, palpitations, sedation.

BROMFENEX PD (pseudoephedrine + brompheniramine) ▶LK ♀C ▶– $
ADULT — Allergic rhinitis/nasal congestion: 1 to 2 caps PO q 12 h. Max 4 caps/day.
PEDS — Allergic rhinitis/nasal congestion: Age older than 12 yo: 1 cap PO q 12 h. Max 2 caps/day.
FORMS — Generic/Trade: Caps, sustained-release 60 mg pseudoephedrine/6 mg brompheniramine.
NOTES — PD indicates pediatric.
MOA — Decongestant/antihistamine combination.
ADVERSE EFFECTS — Serious: None. Frequent: Insomnia, palpitations, sedation.

CARBODEC DM (pseudoephedrine + carbinoxamine + dextromethorphan) ▶L ♀C ▶– $
ADULT — Allergic rhinitis/nasal congestion/cough: 5 mL PO four times per day.
PEDS — Allergic rhinitis/nasal congestion/cough: Syrup give 2.5 mL PO four times per day for age 18 mo to 5 yo, give 5 mL PO four times per day for age older than 6 yo. Infant gtts: Give 0.25 mL PO four times per day for age 1 to 3 mo, give 0.5 mL PO four times per day for age 4 to 6 mo, give 0.75 mL PO four times per day for age 7 to 9 mo, give 1 mL PO four times per day for age10 mo to 17 mo.
FORMS — Generic only: Syrup, 60/4/15 mg pseudo-ephedrine/carbinoxamine/dextromethorphan/ 5 mL. Gtts, 25/2/4 mg/mL, grape flavor 30 mL with dropper, sugar-free.
NOTES — Carbinoxamine has potential for sedation similar to diphenhydramine. DM indicates dextromethorphan.
MOA — Decongestant/antihistamine/cough suppressant combination.
ADVERSE EFFECTS — Serious: None. Frequent: Insomnia, palpitations, sedation.

CHERATUSSIN AC (guaifenesin + codeine) ▶L ♀C ▶? ©V $
ADULT — Cough: 10 mL PO q 4 h. Max 60 mL/day.
PEDS — Cough: Give 1.25 to 2.5 mL PO q 4 h (up to 15 mL/day) for age 6 to 23 mo, give 2.5 to 5 mL PO q 4 h (up to 30 mL/day) for age 2 to 5 yo, give 5 mL PO q 4 h (up to 30 mL/day) for age 6 to 11 yo, give adult dose for age 12 or older.
FORMS — Generic/Trade: Syrup 100 mg guaifenesin/10 mg codeine/5 mL. Sugar-free.
MOA — Expectorant/cough suppressant combination.
ADVERSE EFFECTS — Serious: Respiratory depression/arrest. Frequent: N/V, constipation, sedation.

CHERATUSSIN DAC (pseudoephedrine + guaifenesin + codeine) ▶L ♀C ▶? ©V $
ADULT — Nasal congestion/cough: 10 mL PO q 4 h. Max 40 mL/day.
PEDS — Nasal congestion/cough: Give 5 mL PO q 4 h (up to 20 mL/day) for age 6 to 11 yo, give adult dose for 12 yo or older.
FORMS — Generic/Trade: Syrup 30 mg pseudoephedrine/100 mg guaifenesin/10 mg codeine/ 5 mL. Sugar-free.
NOTES — DAC indicates decongestant and codeine.
MOA — Decongestant/expectorant/cough suppressant combination.
ADVERSE EFFECTS — Serious: Respiratory depression/arrest. Frequent: N/V, constipation, sedation, insomnia, palpitations.

CHLORDRINE SR (pseudoephedrine + chlorpheniramine) ▶LK ♀C ▶– $
ADULT — Allergic rhinitis/nasal congestion: 1 cap PO q 12 h. Max 2 caps/day.
PEDS — Allergic rhinitis/nasal congestion: 1 cap PO daily for age 6 to 11 yo, use adult dose for age 12 yo or older.
FORMS — Generic only: Caps, sustained-release 120 mg pseudoephedrine/8 mg chlorpheniramine.

MOA — Decongestant/antihistamine combination.
ADVERSE EFFECTS — Serious: None. Frequent: Insomnia, palpitations, sedation.

CLARINEX-D 12 HOUR (pseudoephedrine + desloratadine) ▶LK ♀C ▶+ $$$$
ADULT — Allergic rhinitis: 1 tab PO q 12 h.
PEDS — Allergic rhinitis age 12 yo or older: Use adult dose.
FORMS — Trade only: Tabs, extended-release 120 mg pseudoephedrine/2.5 mg desloratadine.
NOTES — Swallow tabs whole. Avoid with hepatic or renal insufficiency.
MOA — Decongestant/antihistamine combination.
ADVERSE EFFECTS — Serious: None. Frequent: Insomnia, palpitations.

CLARINEX-D 24 HOUR (pseudoephedrine + desloratadine) ▶LK ♀C ▶+ $$$$
ADULT — Allergic rhinitis: 1 tab PO daily.
PEDS — Allergic rhinitis age 12 yo or older: Use adult dose.
FORMS — Trade only: Tabs, extended-release pseudoephedrine + desloratadine, 120/2.5, 240/5 mg.
NOTES — Instruct patients to swallow the tab whole. Increase dosing interval in renal insufficiency to every other day. Avoid with hepatic insufficiency.
MOA — Decongestant/antihistamine combination.
ADVERSE EFFECTS — Serious: None. Frequent: Insomnia, palpitations.

DECONAMINE (pseudoephedrine + chlorpheniramine) ▶LK ♀C ▶– $$
WARNING — Multiple strengths; write specific product on Rx.
ADULT — Allergic rhinitis/nasal congestion: 1 tab or 10 mL PO three to four times per day. Max 6 tabs or 60 mL/day. Sustained-release: 1 cap PO q 12 h. Max 2 caps/day.
PEDS — Allergic rhinitis/nasal congestion: Age older than 12 yo: Use adult dose. 6 to 11 yo: ½ tab or 5 mL PO three to four times per day. Max 3 tabs or 30 mL/day.
FORMS — Trade only: Tabs 60/4 mg pseudoephedrine/chlorpheniramine, scored. Syrup 30/2 mg per 5 mL. Chewable tabs 15/1 mg. Generic/Trade: Caps, sustained-release 120/8 mg (Deconamine SR).
MOA — Decongestant/antihistamine combination.
ADVERSE EFFECTS — Serious: None. Frequent: Insomnia, palpitations, sedation.

DECONSAL II (phenylephrine + guaifenesin) ▶L ♀C ▶– $$
ADULT — Nasal congestion/cough: 1 to 2 tabs PO q 12 h. Max 4 tabs/day.
PEDS — Nasal congestion/cough: Give ½ tab PO q 12 h (up to 1 tab/day) for age 2 to 5 yo, give 1 tab PO q 12 h up to tabs/day for 6 to 12 yo, give adult dose for age older than 12 yo.
FORMS — Trade only: Caps, sustained-release 20 mg phenylephrine/375 mg guaifenesin.
MOA — Decongestant/expectorant combination.
ADVERSE EFFECTS — Serious: None. Frequent: Insomnia, palpitations.

DICEL (pseudoephedrine + chlorpheniramine) ►L ♀C ►– $$

ADULT — Allergic rhinitis/nasal congestion: 10 to 20 mL PO q 12 h. Max 40 mL/day.

PEDS — Allergic rhinitis/nasal congestion: Give 2.5 to 5 mL (up to 10 mL/day) PO q 12 h for age 2 to 5 yo, give 5 to 10 mL PO q 12 h (up to 20 mL/day) for age 6 to 11 yo, give adult dose for age 12 yo or older.

FORMS — Generic/Trade: Susp 75 mg pseudoephedrine/4.5 mg chlorpheniramine/5 mL, strawberry-banana flavor.

MOA — Decongestant/antihistamine combination.

ADVERSE EFFECTS — Serious: None. Frequent: Insomnia, palpitations, sedation.

DIMETANE-DX COUGH SYRUP (pseudoephedrine + brompheniramine + dextromethorphan) ►L ♀C ►– $$$

ADULT — Nasal congestion/rhinitis/cough: 10 mL PO q 4 h prn.

PEDS — Nasal congestion/rhinitis/cough: Dose by wt: Give 1.25 mL PO four times per day prn for wt 12 to 22 kg, give 2.5 mL PO four times per day prn wt 23 to 40 kg. Dose by age: Give 2.5 mL PO q 4 h for age 2 to 5 yo, give 5 mL PO q 4 h for age 6 to 11 yo, give adult dosing for age older than 12 yo.

FORMS — Trade only: Liquid 30 mg pseudoephedrine/2 mg brompheniramine/10 mg dextromethorphan/5 mL, butterscotch flavor. Sugar-free.

MOA — Decongestant/antihistamine/cough suppressant combination.

ADVERSE EFFECTS — Serious: None. Frequent: Insomnia, palpitations, sedation.

DURATUSS (phenylephrine + guaifenesin) ►L ♀C ►– $

ADULT — Nasal congestion/cough: 1 tab PO q 12 h.

PEDS — Nasal congestion/cough: Give ½ tab PO q 12 h for age 6 to 12, use adult dosing for age older than 12 yo.

FORMS — Generic/Trade: Tabs, long-acting 25 mg phenylephrine/900 mg guaifenesin.

MOA — Decongestant/expectorant combination.

ADVERSE EFFECTS — Serious: None. Frequent: Insomnia, palpitations.

DURATUSS GP (phenylephrine + guaifenesin) ►L ♀C ►– $

ADULT — Nasal congestion/cough: 1 tab PO q 12 h.

PEDS — Not approved in children.

FORMS — Generic/Trade: Tabs, long-acting 25 mg phenylephrine/1200 mg guaifenesin.

MOA — Decongestant/expectorant combination.

ADVERSE EFFECTS — Serious: None. Frequent: Insomnia, palpitations.

DURATUSS HD (hydrocodone + phenylephrine + guaifenesin) ►L ♀C ►– ©II $$$

ADULT — Cough/nasal congestion: 10 mL PO q 4 to 6 h.

PEDS — Cough/nasal congestion: Give 5 mL PO q 4 to 6 h for age 6 to 12, use adult dosing for age older than 12 yo.

FORMS — Generic/Trade: Elixir 2.5 mg hydrocodone/10 mg phenylephrine/225 mg guaifenesin/5 mL. 5% alcohol.

MOA — Decongestant/expectorant/cough suppressant combination.

ADVERSE EFFECTS — Serious: Respiratory depression/arrest. Frequent: N/V, constipation, sedation, insomnia, palpitations.

ENTEX LA (phenylephrine + guaifenesin) ►L ♀C ►– $$

ADULT — Nasal congestion/cough: 1 tab PO q 12 h.

PEDS — Nasal congestion/cough: Give ½ tab PO q 12 h for age 6 to 11 yo, give adult dose for 12 yo or older.

FORMS — Generic/Trade: Tabs, long-acting 30/600 mg phenylephrine/guaifenesin. Caps, long-acting 30/400 mg.

NOTES — Do not crush or chew.

MOA — Decongestant/expectorant combination.

ADVERSE EFFECTS — Serious: None. Frequent: Insomnia, palpitations.

ENTEX LIQUID (phenylephrine + guaifenesin) ►L ♀C ►– $$$

ADULT — Nasal congestion/cough: 5 to 10 mL PO q 4 to 6 h. Max 40 mL/day.

PEDS — Nasal congestion/cough: Give 2.5 mL PO q 4 to 6 h (up 10 mL/day) for age 2 to 5 yo, give 5 mL PO q 4 to 6 h (up to 20 mL/day) for age 6 to 11 yo, give adult dose for age 12 yo or older.

FORMS — Generic/Trade: Liquid 7.5 mg phenylephrine/100 mg guaifenesin/5 mL. Punch flavor, alcohol-free.

MOA — Decongestant/expectorant combination.

ADVERSE EFFECTS — Serious: None. Frequent: Insomnia, palpitations.

ENTEX PSE (pseudoephedrine + guaifenesin) ►L ♀C ►– $

ADULT — Nasal congestion/cough: 1 tab PO q 12 h.

PEDS — Nasal congestion/cough: Give ½ tab PO q 12 h for age 6 to 12 yo, use adult dosing for age older than 12 yo.

FORMS — Generic/Trade: Tabs, long-acting 120 mg pseudoephedrine/600 mg guaifenesin, scored.

NOTES — PSE indicates pseudoephedrine.

MOA — Decongestant/expectorant combination.

ADVERSE EFFECTS — Serious: None. Frequent: Insomnia, palpitations.

GANI-TUSS NR (guaifenesin + codeine) ►L ♀C ►? ©V $

ADULT — Cough: 10 mL PO q 4 h. Max 60 mL/day.

PEDS — Cough: Give 1.25 to 2.5 mL PO q 4 h (up to 15 mL/day) for age 6 to 23 mo, give 2.5 to 5 mL PO q 4 h (up to 30 mL/day) for age 2 to 5 yo, give 5 mL PO q 4 h (up to 30 mL/day) for age 6 to 11 yo, give adult dosing for age 12 yo or older.

FORMS — Generic/Trade: Syrup 100 mg guaifenesin/10 mg codeine/5 mL. Sugar-free.

MOA — Expectorant/cough suppressant combination.

ADVERSE EFFECTS — Serious: Respiratory depression/arrest. Frequent: N/V, constipation, sedation.

GUAIFENEX DM (guaifenesin + dextromethorphan) ►L ♀C ►? $

ADULT — Cough: 1 to 2 tabs PO q 12 h. Max 4 tabs/day.

PEDS — Cough: Give ½ tab PO q 12 h (up to 1 tab/day) for age 2 to 6 yo, give 1 tab PO q 12 h (up to 2 tabs/day) for age 6 to 12 yo, give adult dose for age 12 yo or older.

GUAIFENEX DM (cont.)

FORMS — Generic/Trade: Tabs, sustained-release 600 mg guaifenesin/30 mg dextromethorphan, scored.
NOTES — DM indicates dextromethorphan.
MOA — Expectorant/cough suppressant combination.
ADVERSE EFFECTS — Serious: None. Frequent: None.

GUAIFENEX PSE (pseudoephedrine + guaifenesin) ▶L ♀C ▶– $
WARNING — Multiple strengths; write specific product on Rx.
ADULT — Nasal congestion/cough: PSE 60: 1 to 2 tabs PO q 12 h. Max 4 tabs/day. PSE 120: 1 tab PO q 12 h.
PEDS — Nasal congestion/cough: PSE 60: Give ½ tab PO q 12 h (up to 1 tab/day) for age 2 to 6 yo, give 1 tab PO q 12 h (up to 2 tabs/day) for age 6 to 12 yo, give adult dose for age 12 yo or older. PSE 120: ½ tab PO q 12 h for age 6 to 12 yo, give adult dose for age older than 12 yo.
FORMS — Generic/Trade: Tabs, extended-release 60/600 mg pseudoephedrine/guaifenesin, scored (Guaifenex PSE 60). Trade only: Tabs, extended-release 120/600 mg (Guaifenex PSE 120).
NOTES — PSE indicates pseudoephedrine.
MOA — Decongestant/expectorant combination.
ADVERSE EFFECTS — Serious: None. Frequent: Insomnia, palpitations.

GUAITEX II SR/PSE (pseudoephedrine + guaifenesin) ▶L ♀C ▶– $
WARNING — Multiple strengths; write specific product on Rx.
ADULT — Nasal congestion/cough: 1 to 2 tabs PO q 12 h. Max 4 tabs/day (Guaitex II SR). 1 tab PO q 12 h. Max 2 tabs/day (Guaitex PSE).
PEDS — Nasal congestion/cough: (Guaitex II SR) give ½ tab PO q 12 h (up to 1 tab/day) for age 2 to 6 yo, give 1 tab PO q 12 h (up to 2 tabs/day) for age 6 to 12 yo, give adult dose for age 12 yo or older. (Guaitex PSE): Give ½ tab PO q 12 h for age 6 to 12 yo, give adult dose for age older than 12 yo.
FORMS — Generic/Trade: Tabs, sustained-release 60 mg pseudoephedrine/600 mg guaifenesin (Guaitex II SR). Trade only: Tabs, long-acting 120 mg pseudoephedrine/600 mg guaifenesin (Guaitex PSE).
NOTES — PSE indicates pseudoephedrine.
MOA — Decongestant/expectorant combination.
ADVERSE EFFECTS — Serious: None. Frequent: Insomnia, palpitations.

GUIATUSS AC (guaifenesin + codeine) ▶L ♀C ▶? ©V $
ADULT — Cough: 10 mL PO q 4 h. Max 60 mL/day.
PEDS — Cough: Give 5 mL PO q 4 h (up to 30 mL/day) for age 6 to 11 yo, give adult dose for 12 yo or older.
FORMS — Generic/Trade: Syrup 100 mg guaifenesin/10 mg codeine/5 mL. Sugar-free.
NOTES — AC indicates before meals and codeine.
MOA — Expectorant/cough suppressant combination.
ADVERSE EFFECTS — Serious: Respiratory depression/arrest. Frequent: N/V, constipation, sedation.

GUIATUSSIN DAC (pseudoephedrine + guaifenesin + codeine) ▶L ♀C ▶– ©V $
ADULT — Nasal congestion/cough: 10 mL PO q 4 h. Max 40 mL/day.
PEDS — Nasal congestion/cough: Give 5 mL PO q 4 h (up to 20 mL/day) for age 6 to 11 yo, give adult dose for 12 yo or older.
FORMS — Generic/Trade: Syrup 30 mg pseudoephedrine/100 mg guaifenesin/10 mg codeine/5 mL. Sugar-free.
NOTES — DAC indicates decongestant and codeine.
MOA — Decongestant/expectorant/cough suppressant combination.
ADVERSE EFFECTS — Serious: Respiratory depression/arrest. Frequent: N/V, constipation, sedation, insomnia, palpitations.

HALOTUSSIN AC (guaifenesin + codeine) ▶L ♀C ▶? ©V $
ADULT — Cough: 10 mL PO q 4 h. Max 60 mL/day.
PEDS — Cough: Give 5 mL PO q 4 h (up to 30 mL/day) for age 6 to 11 yo, give adult dose for 12 yo or older.
FORMS — Generic/Trade: Syrup 100 mg guaifenesin/10 mg codeine/5 mL. Sugar-free.
NOTES — AC indicates before meals and codeine.
MOA — Expectorant/cough suppressant combination.
ADVERSE EFFECTS — Serious: Respiratory depression/arrest. Frequent: N/V, constipation, sedation.

HALOTUSSIN DAC (pseudoephedrine + guaifenesin + codeine) ▶L ♀C ▶– ©V $
ADULT — Nasal congestion/cough: 10 mL PO q 4 h. Max 40 mL/day.
PEDS — Nasal congestion/cough: Give 5 mL PO q 4 h (up to 20 mL/day) for age 6 to 11 yo, give adult dose for 12 yo or older.
FORMS — Generic/Trade: Syrup 30 mg pseudoephedrine/100 mg guaifenesin/10 mg codeine/5 mL. Sugar-free.
NOTES — DAC indicates decongestant and codeine.
MOA — Decongestant/expectorant/cough suppressant combination.
ADVERSE EFFECTS — Serious: Respiratory depression/arrest. Frequent: N/V, constipation, sedation, insomnia, palpitations.

HISTINEX HC (phenylephrine + chlorpheniramine + hydrocodone) ▶L ♀C ▶– ©II $
ADULT — Allergic rhinitis/congestion/cough: 10 mL PO q 4 h. Max 40 mL/day.
PEDS — Allergic rhinitis/congestion/cough: Give 5 mL PO q 4 h (up to 20 mL/day) for age 6 to 11 yo, give adult dose for 12 yo or older.
FORMS — Generic/Trade: Syrup 5 mg phenylephrine/2 mg chlorpheniramine/2.5 mg hydrocodone/5 mL. Alcohol- and sugar-free.
MOA — Decongestant/antihistamine/cough suppressant combination.
ADVERSE EFFECTS — Serious: Respiratory depression/arrest. Frequent: N/V, constipation, sedation, insomnia, palpitations.

HISTUSSIN D (pseudoephedrine + hydrocodone) ▶L ♀C ▶– ©ll $$
ADULT — Nasal congestion/cough: 5 mL PO four times per day prn.
PEDS — Nasal congestion/cough: Give 1.25 mL PO four times per day prn for wt 12 to 22 kg, give 2.5 mL PO four times per day prn for wt 22 to 40 kg.
FORMS — Generic/Trade: Liquid 60 mg pseudoephedrine/5 mg hydrocodone/5 mL, cherry/black raspberry flavor.
MOA — Decongestant/cough suppressant combination.
ADVERSE EFFECTS — Serious: Respiratory depression/arrest. Frequent: N/V, constipation, sedation, insomnia, palpitations.

HISTUSSIN HC (phenylephrine + dexbrompheniramine + hydrocodone) ▶L ♀C ▶– ©ll $$
ADULT — Allergic rhinitis/congestion/cough: 10 mL PO q 4 h. Max 40 mL/day.
PEDS — Allergic rhinitis/congestion/cough: Give 5 mL PO q 4 h (up to 20 mL/day) for age 6 to 11 yo, give adult dose for 12 yo or older.
FORMS — Generic/Trade: Syrup 5 mg phenylephrine/1 mg dexbrompheniramine/2.5 mg hydrocodone/5 mL.
MOA — Decongestant/antihistamine/cough suppressant combination.
ADVERSE EFFECTS — Serious: Respiratory depression/arrest. Frequent: N/V, constipation, sedation, insomnia, palpitations.

HUMIBID DM (guaifenesin + guaiacolsulfonate + dextromethorphan) ▶L ♀C ▶? $
ADULT — Cough: 1 cap PO q 12 h. Max 2 caps/day.
PEDS — Cough: Give 1 cap PO daily for age 6 to 12 yo, give adult dose for 12 yo or older.
FORMS — Trade only: Caps, sustained-release 400 mg guaifenesin/200 mg guaiacolsulfonate/50 mg dextromethorphan.
NOTES — DM indicates dextromethorphan.
MOA — Expectorant/cough suppressant combination.
ADVERSE EFFECTS — Serious: None. Frequent: None.

HUMIBID LA (guaifenesin + guaiacolsulfonate) ▶L ♀C ▶+ $
ADULT — Expectorant: 1 tab PO q 12 h (extended-release). Max 2 tabs/day.
PEDS — Expectorant age older than 12 yo: Use adult dose.
FORMS — Trade only: Tabs, extended-release 600 mg guaifenesin/300 mg guaiacolsulfonate.
MOA — Expectorant combination.
ADVERSE EFFECTS — Serious: None. Frequent: None.

HYCOCLEAR TUSS (hydrocodone + guaifenesin) ▶L ♀C ▶– ©ll $
ADULT — Cough: 5 mL PO after meals and at bedtime. Max 6 doses/day.
PEDS — Cough: Give 2.5 mL PO after meals and at bedtime (up to 6 doses/day) for age 6 to 12 yo, give adult dose for age older than 12 yo.
FORMS — Generic/Trade: Syrup 5 mg hydrocodone/100 mg guaifenesin/5 mL. Generic is alcohol- and sugar-free.
MOA — Expectorant/cough suppressant combination.
ADVERSE EFFECTS — Serious: Respiratory depression/arrest. Frequent: N/V, constipation, sedation.

HYCODAN (hydrocodone + homatropine) ▶L ♀C ▶– ©ll $
ADULT — Cough: 1 tab or 5 mL PO q 4 to 6 h. Max 6 doses/day.
PEDS — Cough: Give 2.5 mg (based on hydrocodone) PO q 4 to 6 h prn (up to 15 mg/day) for age 6 to 12 yo, give adult dose for age older than 12 yo.
FORMS — Generic/Trade: Syrup 5 mg hydrocodone/1.5 mg homatropine methylbromide/5 mL. Tabs 5/1.5 mg.
NOTES — May cause drowsiness/sedation. Dosing based on hydrocodone content.
MOA — Cough suppressant.
ADVERSE EFFECTS — Serious: Respiratory depression/arrest. Frequent: N/V, constipation, sedation.

HYCOTUSS (hydrocodone + guaifenesin) ▶L ♀C ▶– ©ll $
ADULT — Cough: 5 mL PO after meals and at bedtime. Max 6 doses/day.
PEDS — Cough: Give 2.5 mL PO after meals and at bedtime (up to 6 doses/day) for age 6 to 12 yo, give adult dose for age older than 12 yo.
FORMS — Generic/Trade: Syrup 5 mg hydrocodone/100 mg guaifenesin/5 mL. Generic is alcohol- and sugar-free.
MOA — Expectorant/cough suppressant combination.
ADVERSE EFFECTS — Serious: Respiratory depression/arrest. Frequent: N/V, constipation, sedation.

NOVAFED A (pseudoephedrine + chlorpheniramine) ▶LK ♀C ▶– $
ADULT — Allergic rhinitis/nasal congestion: 1 cap PO q 12 h. Max 2 caps/day.
PEDS — Allergic rhinitis/nasal congestion: 1 cap PO daily for age 6 to 12 yo, use adult dose for age older than 12 yo.
FORMS — Generic/Trade: Caps, sustained-release 120 mg pseudoephedrine/8 mg chlorpheniramine.
MOA — Decongestant/antihistamine combination.
ADVERSE EFFECTS — Serious: None. Frequent: Insomnia, palpitations, sedation.

PALGIC DS (pseudoephedrine + carbinoxamine) ▶L ♀C ▶– $$
ADULT — Allergic rhinitis/nasal congestion: 10 mL PO four times per day.
PEDS — Allergic rhinitis/nasal congestion: Give up to the following PO four times per day: 1.25 mL for age 1 to 3 mo, 2.5 mL for age 3 to 6 mo, 3.75 mL for age 6 to 9 mo, 3.75 to 5 mL for age 9 to 18 mo, 5 mL for age 18 mo to 6 yo, use adult dose for age older than 6 yo.
FORMS — Generic/Trade: Syrup, 25 mg pseudoephedrine/2 mg carbinoxamine/5 mL. Alcohol- and sugar-free.
NOTES — Carbinoxamine has potential for sedation similar to diphenhydramine.
MOA — Decongestant/antihistamine combination.
ADVERSE EFFECTS — Serious: None. Frequent: Insomnia, palpitations, sedation.

PHENERGAN VC (phenylephrine + promethazine) ▶LK ♀C ▶? $
WARNING — Promethazine contraindicated if age younger than 2 yo due to risk of fatal respiratory depression; caution in older children.
ADULT — Allergic rhinitis/congestion: 5 mL PO q 4 to 6 h. Max 30 mL/day.
PEDS — Allergic rhinitis/congestion: Give 1.25 to 2.5 mL PO q 4 to 6 h (up to 15 mL/day) for age 2 to 5 yo, give 2.5 to 5 mL PO q 4 to 6 h for age 6 to 12 yo (up to 20 mL/day), give adult dose for age 12 yo or older.
FORMS — Trade unavailable. Generic only: Syrup 6.25 mg promethazine/5 mg phenylephrine/ 5 mL.
NOTES — VC indicates vasoconstrictor.
MOA — Decongestant/antihistamine combination.
ADVERSE EFFECTS — Serious: None. Frequent: Insomnia, palpitations, sedation.

PHENERGAN VC W/CODEINE (phenylephrine + promethazine + codeine) ▶LK ♀C ▶? ©V $
WARNING — Promethazine contraindicated if younger than 2 yo due to risk of fatal respiratory depression; caution in older children.
ADULT — Allergic rhinitis/congestion/cough: 5 mL PO q 4 to 6 h. Max 30 mL/day.
PEDS — Allergic rhinitis/congestion/cough: Give 1.25 to 2.5 mL PO q 4 to 6 h (up to 10 mL/day) for age 2 to 5 yo, give 2.5 to 5 mL PO q 4 to 6 h for age 6 to 12 yo (up to 20 mL/day), give adult dose for age 12 yo or older.
FORMS — Trade unavailable. Generic only: Syrup 5 mg phenylephrine/6.25 mg promethazine/10 mg codeine/5 mL.
MOA — Decongestant/antihistamine/cough suppressant combination.
ADVERSE EFFECTS — Serious: Respiratory depression/arrest. Frequent: N/V, constipation, sedation, insomnia, palpitations.

PHENERGAN WITH CODEINE (promethazine + codeine) ▶LK ♀C ▶? ©V $
WARNING — Promethazine contraindicated if younger than 2 yo due to risk of fatal respiratory depression; caution in older children.
ADULT — Allergic rhinitis/cough: 5 mL PO q 4 to 6 h. Max 30 mL/day.
PEDS — Allergic rhinitis/cough: Give 1.25 to 2.5 mL PO q 4 to 6 h (up to 10 mL/day) for age 2 to 5 yo, give 2.5 to 5 mL PO q 4 to 6 h (up to 20 mL/day) for age 6 to 12 yo, give adult dose for age 12 yo or older.
FORMS — Trade unavailable. Generic only: Syrup 6.25 mg promethazine/10 mg codeine/5 mL.
MOA — Antihistamine/cough suppressant combination.
ADVERSE EFFECTS — Serious: Respiratory depression/arrest. Frequent: N/V, constipation, sedation.

PHENERGAN/DEXTROMETHORPHAN (promethazine + dextromethorphan) ▶LK ♀C ▶? $
WARNING — Promethazine contraindicated if younger than 2 yo due to risk of fatal respiratory depression; caution in older children.

ADULT — Allergic rhinitis/cough: 5 mL PO q 4 to 6 h. Max 30 mL/day.
PEDS — Allergic rhinitis/cough: Give 1.25 to 2.5 mL PO q 4 to 6 h (up to 10 mL/day) for age 2 to 5 yo, give 2.5 to 5 mL PO q 4 to 6 h (up to 20 mL/day) for age 6 to 12 yo, give adult dose for age 12 yo or older.
FORMS — Trade unavailable. Generic only: Syrup 6.25 mg promethazine/15 mg dextromethorphan/5 mL.
MOA — Decongestant/cough suppressant combination.
ADVERSE EFFECTS — Serious: None. Frequent: Sedation.

PSEUDO-CHLOR (pseudoephedrine + chlorpheniramine) ▶LK ♀C ▶– $
ADULT — Allergic rhinitis/nasal congestion: 1 cap PO q 12 h. Max 2 caps/day.
PEDS — Allergic rhinitis/nasal congestion: Age older than 12 yo: Use adult dose.
FORMS — Generic/Trade: Caps, sustained-release 120 mg pseudoephedrine/8 mg chlorpheniramine.
MOA — Decongestant/antihistamine combination.
ADVERSE EFFECTS — Serious: None. Frequent: Insomnia, palpitations, sedation.

REZIRA (hydrocodone + pseudoephedrine) ▶LK – ♀C ▶– ©II
ADULT — Nasal congestion/cough: 5 mL q 4 to 6 h. Max 20 mL/day.
PEDS — Not approved in children.
FORMS — Trade: Syrup 5 mg hydrocodone/60 mg pseudoephedrine/5 mL.
MOA — Decongestant/cough suppressant combination.
ADVERSE EFFECTS — Serious: respiratory depression. Common: sedation, insomnia, palpitations.

ROBITUSSIN AC (guaifenesin + codeine) ▶L ♀C ▶? ©V $
ADULT — The "Robitussin AC" brand is no longer produced; corresponding generics include Cheratussin AC, Gani-Tuss NR, Guiatuss AC, and Halotussin AC.
MOA — Expectorant/cough suppressant combination.
ADVERSE EFFECTS — Serious: Respiratory depression/arrest. Frequent: N/V, constipation, sedation.

ROBITUSSIN DAC (pseudoephedrine + guaifenesin + codeine) ▶L ♀C ▶– ©V $
ADULT — The "Robitussin DAC" brand is no longer produced; corresponding generics include Cheratussin DAC, Guiatuss DAC, and Halotussin DAC.
MOA — Decongestant/expectorant/cough suppressant combination.
ADVERSE EFFECTS — Serious: Respiratory depression/arrest. Frequent: N/V, constipation, sedation, insomnia, palpitations.

RONDEC (phenylephrine + chlorpheniramine) ▶L ♀C ▶– $$
ADULT — Allergic rhinitis/nasal congestion: 5 mL syrup PO four times per day.
PEDS — Allergic rhinitis/nasal congestion: Give 1.25 mL PO four times per day for age 2 to 5 yo, give 2.5 mL PO four times per day for age 6 to 12 yo, give adult dose for age older than 12 yo.

(cont.)

RONDEC (*cont.*)

FORMS — Trade only: Syrup 12.5 mg phenylephrine/4 mg chlorpheniramine/5 mL, bubble-gum flavor. Alcohol- and sugar-free.

MOA — Decongestant/antihistamine combination.

ADVERSE EFFECTS — Serious: None. Frequent: Insomnia, palpitations, sedation.

RONDEC DM (phenylephrine + chlorpheniramine + dextromethorphan) ▶L ♀C ▶– $$

ADULT — Allergic rhinitis/nasal congestion/cough: 5 mL syrup PO four times per day.

PEDS — Allergic rhinitis/nasal congestion/cough: Give 1.25 mL PO four times per day for age 2 to 5 yo, give 2.5 mL PO four times per day for age 6 to 12 yo, give adult dose for age older than 12 yo.

FORMS — Trade only: Syrup 12.5 mg phenylephrine/4 mg chlorpheniramine/15 mg dextromethorphan/5 mL, grape flavor. Alcohol- and sugar-free.

NOTES — DM indicates dextromethorphan.

MOA — Decongestant/antihistamine/cough suppressant combination.

ADVERSE EFFECTS — Serious: None. Frequent: Insomnia, palpitations, sedation.

RONDEC INFANT DROPS (phenylephrine + chlorpheniramine) ▶L ♀C ▶– $$

PEDS — Allergic rhinitis/nasal congestion: Give the following dose PO four times per day: 0.75 mL for age 6 to 12 mo, 1 mL for age 13 to 24 mo.

FORMS — Trade only: Gtts 3.5 mg phenylephrine/ 1 mg chlorpheniramine/mL, bubble-gum flavor, 30 mL. Alcohol- and sugar-free.

MOA — Decongestant/antihistamine combination.

ADVERSE EFFECTS — Serious: None. Frequent: Insomnia, palpitations, sedation.

RYNA-12 S (phenylephrine + pyrilamine) ▶L ♀C ▶– $$

PEDS — Nasal congestion, allergic rhinitis, sinusitis: Give 2.5 to 5 ML PO q 12 h for age 2 to 6 yo, give 5 to 10 mL PO q 12 h for age older than 6 yo.

FORMS — Generic/Trade: Susp 5 mg phenylephrine/30 mg pyrilamine/5 mL strawberry- currant flavor with graduated oral syringe.

MOA — Decongestant/antihistamine combination.

ADVERSE EFFECTS — Serious: None. Frequent: Insomnia, palpitations, sedation.

RYNATAN (phenylephrine + chlorpheniramine) ▶LK ♀C ▶– $$

ADULT — Allergic rhinitis/nasal congestion: 1 to 2 tabs PO q 12 h.

PEDS — Allergic rhinitis/nasal congestion age 12 yo or older: 1 tab PO q 12 h.

FORMS — Trade only: Tabs, extended-release: 25/9 mg phenylephrine/chlorpheniramine. Chewable tabs 5/4.5 mg.

MOA — Decongestant/antihistamine combination.

ADVERSE EFFECTS — Serious: None. Frequent: Insomnia, palpitations, sedation.

RYNATAN PEDIATRIC SUSPENSION (phenylephrine + chlorpheniramine) ▶L ♀C ▶– $$$

PEDS — Nasal congestion, allergic rhinitis, sinusitis: Give 2.5 to 5 mL PO q 12 h for age 2 to 6 yo, give 5 to 10 mL PO q 12 h for age older than 6 yo.

FORMS — Trade only: Susp 5 mg phenylephrine/4.5 mg chlorpheniramine/5 mL strawberry-currant flavor.

MOA — Decongestant/antihistamine combination.

ADVERSE EFFECTS — Serious: None. Frequent: Insomnia, palpitations, sedation.

SEMPREX-D (pseudoephedrine + acrivastine) ▶LK ♀C ▶– $$

ADULT — Allergic rhinitis/nasal congestion: 1 cap PO q 4 to 6 h. Max 4 caps/day.

PEDS — Not approved in children.

FORMS — Trade only: Caps 60 mg pseudoephedrine/8 mg acrivastine.

MOA — Decongestant/antihistamine combination.

ADVERSE EFFECTS — Serious: None. Frequent: Insomnia, palpitations, sedation.

TANAFED DMX (pseudoephedrine + dexchlorpheniramine + dextromethorphan) ▶L ♀C ▶– $$

ADULT — Allergic rhinitis/nasal congestion: 10 to 20 mL PO q 12 h. Max 40 mL/day.

PEDS — Allergic rhinitis/nasal congestion: Give 2.5 to 5 mL PO q 12 h (up to 10 mL/day) for 2 to 5 yo, give 5 to 10 mL PO q 12 h (up to 20 mL/day) for age 6 to 11 yo, give adult dose for age 12 yo or older.

FORMS — Generic/Trade: Susp 75 mg pseudoephedrine/2.5 mg dexchlorpheniramine/25 mg dextromethorphan/5 mL, strawberry-banana flavor.

MOA — Decongestant/antihistamine/cough suppressant combination.

ADVERSE EFFECTS — Serious: None. Frequent: Insomnia, palpitations, sedation.

TUSS-HC (phenylephrine + chlorpheniramine + hydrocodone) ▶L ♀C ▶– ©II $

ADULT — Allergic rhinitis/congestion/cough: 10 mL PO q 4 h. Max 40 mL/day.

PEDS — Allergic rhinitis/congestion/cough: Give 5 mL PO q 4 h (up to 20 mL/day) for age 6 to 12 yo, give adult dose for age older than 12 yo.

FORMS — Generic/Trade: Syrup 5 mg phenylephrine/2 mg chlorpheniramine/2.5 mg hydrocodone/5 mL.

MOA — Decongestant/antihistamine/cough suppressant combination.

ADVERSE EFFECTS — Serious: Respiratory depression/arrest. Frequent: N/V, constipation, sedation, insomnia, palpitations.

TUSSICAPS (chlorpheniramine + hydrocodone) ▶L ♀C ▶– ©II $$

ADULT — Allergic rhinitis/cough: 1 full-strength cap PO q 12 h. Max 2 caps/day.

PEDS — Allergic rhinitis/congestion/cough: Give half strength cap PO q 12 h (up to 2 caps/day) for age 6 to 12 yo, give adult dose for age older than 12 yo.

FORMS — Trade only: Caps, extended-release 4/5 mg (half-strength), 8/10 mg (full strength) chlorpheniramine/hydrocodone.

MOA — Antihistamine/cough suppressant combination.

ADVERSE EFFECTS — Serious: Respiratory depression/arrest. Frequent: N/V, constipation, sedation.

TUSSIONEX (chlorpheniramine + hydrocodone) ▶L ♀C ▶– ©II $$$
ADULT — Allergic rhinitis/cough: 5 mL PO q 12 h. Max 10 mL/day.
PEDS — Allergic rhinitis/cough: 2.5 mL PO q 12 h (up to 5 mL/day) for age 6 to 12 yo, give adult dose for age older than 12 yo.
FORMS — Generic/Trade: Extended-release susp 8 mg chlorpheniramine/10 mg hydrocodone/5 mL.
MOA — Antihistamine/cough suppressant combination.
ADVERSE EFFECTS — Serious: Respiratory depression/arrest. Frequent: N/V, constipation, sedation.

ZEPHREX-LA (pseudoephedrine + guaifenesin) ▶L ♀C ▶– $
ADULT — Nasal congestion/cough: 1 tab PO q 12 h.
PEDS — Nasal congestion/cough: Give ½ tab PO q 12 h for age 6 to 12 yo, give adult dosing for age older than 12 yo.
FORMS — Trade only: Tabs, extended-release 120 mg pseudoephedrine/600 mg guaifenesin.
MOA — Decongestant/expectorant combination.
ADVERSE EFFECTS — Serious: None. Frequent: Insomnia, palpitations.

ZUTRIPRO (hydrocodone + chlorpheniramine + pseudoephedrine) ▶LK – ♀C ▶– ©II
ADULT — Cough/nasal congestion/allergic rhinitis: 5 mL PO q 4 to 6 h . Max 20 mL/day.
PEDS — Not approved in children.
FORMS — Trade: Syrup 5 mg hydrocodone/4 mg chlorpheniramine/60 mg pseudoephedrine/5 mL.
MOA — Decongestant/antihistamine/cough suppressant combination.
ADVERSE EFFECTS — Serious: respiratory depression/arrest. Common: sedation, palpitations, insomnia.

ZYRTEC-D (cetirizine + pseudoephedrine) ▶LK ♀C ▶– $$
ADULT — Allergic rhinitis/nasal congestion: 1 tab PO q 12 h.
PEDS — Not approved in children.
FORMS — OTC Generic/Trade: Tabs, extended-release 5 mg cetirizine/120 mg pseudoephedrine.
NOTES — Decrease dose to 1 tab PO daily with decreased renal or hepatic function. Take on an empty stomach.
MOA — Decongestant/antihistamine combination.
ADVERSE EFFECTS — Serious: None. Frequent: Insomnia, palpitations, sedation.

ENT: Decongestants

NOTE: See ENT - Nasal Preparations for nasal spray decongestants (oxymetazoline, phenylephrine). Systemic decongestants are sympathomimetic and may aggravate HTN, anxiety, BPH, and insomnia. Use cautiously in such patients. Some states have restricted or ended OTC sale of pseudoephedrine or reclassified it as schedule III or V drug due to the potential for diversion to methamphetamine labs. Deaths have occurred in children younger than 2 yo attributed to toxicity from cough and cold medications; the FDA does not recommend their use in this age group.

PHENYLEPHRINE (*Sudafed PE*) ▶L ♀C ▶+ $
ADULT — Nasal congestion: 10 mg PO q 4 h prn. Max 6 doses/day.
PEDS — Nasal congestion, age older than 12 yo: Use adult dose.
FORMS — OTC Trade only: Tabs 10 mg.
NOTES — Avoid with MAOIs.
MOA — Decongestant.
ADVERSE EFFECTS — Serious: None. Frequent: Dizziness, anxiety, insomnia.

PSEUDOEPHEDRINE (*Sudafed, Sudafed 12 Hour, Efidac/24, Dimetapp Decongestant Infant Drops, PediaCare Infants' Decongestant Drops, Triaminic Oral Infant Drops*) ▶L ♀C ▶+ $
ADULT — Nasal congestion: 60 mg PO q 4 to 6 h. 120 mg PO q 12 h (extended-release). 240 mg PO daily (extended-release). Max 240 mg/day.

PEDS — Nasal congestion: give 15 mg PO q 4 to 6 h for age 2 to 5 yo, give: 30 mg PO q 4 to 6 h for age 6 to 12 yo, use adult dose for age older than 12 yo.
FORMS — OTC Generic/Trade: Tabs 30, 60 mg. Tabs, extended-release 120 mg (12 h). Soln 15, 30 mg/5 mL. Trade only: Chewable tabs 15 mg. Tabs, extended-release 240 mg (24 h). Rx only in some states.
NOTES — 12 to 24 h extended-release dosage forms may cause insomnia; use a shorter-acting form if this occurs.
MOA — Decongestant.
ADVERSE EFFECTS — Serious: None. Frequent: Insomnia, palpitations.

ENT: Ear Preparations

AURALGAN (benzocaine—otic + antipyrine) ▶Not absorbed ♀C ▶? $
ADULT — Otitis media, adjunct: Instill 2 to 4 gtts (or enough to fill the ear canal) three to four times per day or q 1 to 2 h prn. Cerumen removal: Instill 2 to 4 gtts (or enough to fill the ear canal) three times per day for 2 to 3 days to detach cerumen, then prn for

discomfort. Insert cotton plug moistened with soln after instillation.
PEDS — Otitis media, adjunct: Use adult dose. Cerumen removal: Use adult dose.
FORMS — Generic/Trade: Otic soln 10, 15 mL.
MOA — Local anesthetic/analgesic.
ADVERSE EFFECTS — Serious: None. Frequent: None.

CARBAMIDE PEROXIDE (*Debrox, Murine Ear*) ▶Not absorbed ♀? ▶? $
ADULT — Cerumen impaction: Instill 5 to 10 gtts into ear two times per day for 4 days.
PEDS — Not approved in children.
FORMS — OTC Generic/Trade: Otic soln 6.5%, 15, 30 mL.
NOTES — Drops should remain in ear more than 15 min. Do not use for more than 4 days. Remove excess wax by flushing with warm water using a rubber bulb ear syringe.
MOA — Emulsifies/disperses ear wax.
ADVERSE EFFECTS — Serious: None. Frequent: None.

CIPRO HC OTIC (ciprofloxacin—otic + hydrocortisone—otic) ▶Not absorbed ♀C ▶– $$$$
ADULT — Otitis externa: Instill 3 gtts into affected ear(s) two times per day for 7 days.
PEDS — Otitis externa age 1 yo or older: Use adult dose.
FORMS — Trade only: Otic susp 10 mL.
NOTES — Shake well. Contains benzyl alcohol.
MOA — Fluoroquinolone antibiotic/anti-inflammatory combination.
ADVERSE EFFECTS — Serious: None. Frequent: None.

CIPRODEX OTIC (ciprofloxacin—otic + dexamethasone—otic) ▶Not absorbed ♀C ▶– $$$$
ADULT — Otitis externa: Instill 4 gtts into affected ear(s) two times per day for 7 days.
PEDS — Otitis externa and otitis media with tympanostomy tubes, age 6 mo or older: Instill 4 gtts into affected ear(s) two times per day for 7 days.
FORMS — Trade only: Otic susp 5, 7.5 mL.
NOTES — Shake well. Warm susp by holding bottle in hands for 1 to 2 min before instilling.
MOA — Fluoroquinolone antibiotic/anti-inflammatory combination.
ADVERSE EFFECTS — Serious: None. Frequent: None.

CIPROFLOXACIN—OTIC (*Cetraxal*) ▶Not absorbed ♀C ▶– $$$$
ADULT — Otitis externa: Instill 1 single-use container into affected ear(s) twice per day for 7 days.
PEDS — Otitis externa age 1 yo or older: Use adult dose.
FORMS — Trade only: 0.25 mL single-use containers with 0.2% ciprofloxacin soln, #14.
NOTES — Protect from light.
MOA — Fluoroquinolone antibiotic.
ADVERSE EFFECTS — Serious: None. Frequent: None.

CORTISPORIN OTIC (hydrocortisone—otic + polymyxin—otic + neomycin--otic) ▶Not absorbed ♀? ▶? $
ADULT — Otitis externa: Instill 4 gtts in affected ear(s) three to four times per day up to 10 days.
PEDS — Otitis externa: Instill 3 gtts in affected ear(s) three to four times per day up to 10 days.
FORMS — Generic only: Otic soln or susp 7.5, 10 mL.
NOTES — Caveats with perforated TMs or tympanostomy tubes: (1) Risk of neomycin ototoxicity, especially if use prolonged or repeated; (2) Use susp rather than acidic soln.
MOA — Antibiotic/anti-inflammatory combination.
ADVERSE EFFECTS — Serious: Ototoxicity. Frequent: None.

CORTISPORIN TC OTIC (hydrocortisone—otic + neomycin—otic + thonzonium + colistin) ▶Not absorbed ♀? ▶? $$$
ADULT — Otitis externa: Instill 5 gtts in affected ear(s) three to four times per day up to 10 days.
PEDS — Otitis externa: Instill 4 gtts in affected ear(s) three to four times per day up to 10 days.
FORMS — Trade only: Otic susp, 10 mL.
MOA — Antibiotic/anti-inflammatory combination.
ADVERSE EFFECTS — Serious: None. Frequent: None.

DOMEBORO OTIC (acetic acid + aluminum acetate) ▶Not absorbed ♀? ▶? $
ADULT — Otitis externa: Instill 4 to 6 gtts in affected ear(s) q 2 to 3 h.
PEDS — Otitis externa: Instill 2 to 3 gtts in affected ear(s) q 3 to 4 h.
FORMS — Generic only: Otic soln 60 mL.
NOTES — Insert a saturated wick. Keep moist for 24 h.
MOA — Antibacterial.
ADVERSE EFFECTS — Serious: None. Frequent: None.

FLUOCINOLONE–OTIC (*DermOtic*) ▶L ♀C ▶? $$
ADULT — Chronic eczematous external otitis: Instill 5 gtts in affected ear(s) two times per day for 7 to 14 days.
PEDS — Chronic eczematous external otitis: Age 2 yo or older: Use adult dose.
FORMS — Trade only: Otic oil 0.01% 20 mL.
NOTES — Contains peanut oil.
MOA — Anti-inflammatory.
ADVERSE EFFECTS — Serious: None. Frequent: Burning, itching, irritation.

OFLOXACIN—OTIC (*Floxin Otic*) ▶Not absorbed ♀C ▶– $$$
ADULT — Otitis externa: Instill 10 gtts in affected ear(s) daily for 7 days. Chronic suppurative otitis media: Instill 10 gtts in affected ear(s) two times per day for 14 days.
PEDS — Otitis externa: Instill 5 gtts in affected ear(s) daily for 7 days for age 1 to 12 yo, use adult dose for age 12 yo or older. Chronic suppurative otitis media for age older than 12 yo: Use adult dose. Acute otitis media with tympanostomy tubes age 1 to 12 yo: Instill 5 gtts in affected ear(s) two times per day for 10 days.
FORMS — Generic/Trade: Otic soln 0.3% 5, 10 mL. Trade only: "Singles": Single-dispensing containers 0.25 mL (5 gtts), 2 per foil pouch.
MOA — Fluoroquinolone antibiotic.
ADVERSE EFFECTS — Serious: None. Frequent: None.

SWIM-EAR (isopropyl alcohol + anhydrous glycerins) ▶Not absorbed ♀? ▶? $
ADULT — Otitis externa, prophylaxis: Instill 4 to 5 gtts in ears after swimming, showering, or bathing.
PEDS — Otitis externa, prophylaxis: Use adult dose.
FORMS — OTC Trade only: Otic soln 30 mL.
MOA — Drying agent.
ADVERSE EFFECTS — Serious: None. Frequent: None.

VOSOL HC (acetic acid + propylene glycol + hydrocortisone) ▶Not absorbed ♀? ▶? $
ADULT — Otitis externa: Instill 5 gtts in affected ear(s) three to four times per day. Insert cotton plug moistened with 3 to 5 gtts q 4 to 6 h for the 1st 24 h.
PEDS — Otitis externa age older than 3 yo: Instill 3 to 4 gtts in affected ear(s) three to four times per day.

Insert cotton plug moistened with 3 to 4 gtts q 4 to 6 h for the 1st 24 h.
FORMS — Generic/Trade: Otic soln 2%/3%/1% 10 mL.
MOA — Antibacterial.
ADVERSE EFFECTS — Serious: None. Frequent: None.

ENT: Mouth and Lip Preparations

AMLEXANOX (Aphthasol, OraDisc A) ▶LK ♀B ▶? $
ADULT — Aphthous ulcers: Apply ¼ inch paste or mucoadhesive patch to ulcer in mouth four times per day after oral hygiene for up to 10 days.
PEDS — Aphthous ulcers age older than 12 yo: Use adult dose.
FORMS — Trade only: Oral paste 5% (Aphthasol), 3, 5 g tube. Mucoadhesive patch (OraDisc) 2 mg, #20.
NOTES — Mucoadhesive patch should be applied at least 80 min before bedtime to ensure its erosion before sleep. Up to 3 patches may be applied at one time. Avoid food or liquid for 1 h after application.
MOA — Anti-inflammatory.
ADVERSE EFFECTS — Serious: None. Frequent: Pain or burning at the site.

CEVIMELINE (Evoxac) ▶L ♀C ▶— $$$$$
WARNING — May alter cardiac conduction/heart rate; caution in heart disease. May worsen bronchospasm in asthma/COPD.
ADULT — Dry mouth due to Sjögren's syndrome: 30 mg PO three times per day.
PEDS — Not approved in children.
FORMS — Generic/Trade: Caps 30 mg.
NOTES — Contraindicated in narrow-angle glaucoma, acute iritis and severe asthma. May potentiate beta-blockers.
MOA — Cholinergic stimulant.
ADVERSE EFFECTS — Serious: AV block, arrhythmias, brady/tachycardia, pulmonary edema, bronchospasm, blurred vision, cholecystitis. Frequent: Sweating, nausea, rhinitis, flushing.

CHLORHEXIDINE GLUCONATE (Peridex, Periogard) ▶Fecal excretion ♀B ▶? $
ADULT — Gingivitis: Twice per day as an oral rinse, morning and evening after brushing teeth. Rinse with 15 mL of undiluted soln for 30 sec. Do not swallow. Spit after rinsing.
PEDS — Not approved in children.
FORMS — Generic/Trade: Oral rinse 0.12% 473 to 480 mL bottles.
MOA — Antibacterial.
ADVERSE EFFECTS — Serious: Hypersensitivity. Frequent: Staining of teeth, calculus formation, and altered taste.

DEBACTEROL (sulfuric acid + sulfonated phenolics) ▶Not absorbed ♀C ▶+ $$
ADULT — Aphthous stomatitis, mucositis: Apply to dry ulcer. Rinse with water.
PEDS — Not approved in children younger than 12 yo.
FORMS — Trade only: 1 mL prefilled, single-use applicator.

NOTES — 1 application per ulcer treatment. Dry ulcer area with cotton swab. Apply to ulcer and ring of normal mucosa around it for 5 to 10 sec. Rinse and spit. Return of ulcer pain right after rinsing indicates incomplete application; can be reapplied immediately once. Avoid eye contact. If excess irritation, rinse with dilute bicarbonate soln.
MOA — Topical analgesic + cauterizing agent.
ADVERSE EFFECTS — Serious: None. Frequent: Brief stinging during application.

GELCLAIR (maltodextrin + propylene glycol) ▶Not absorbed ♀+ ▶+ $$$
ADULT — Aphthous ulcers, mucositis, stomatitis: Rinse mouth with 1 packet three times per day or prn.
PEDS — Not approved in children.
FORMS — Trade only: 21 packets/box.
NOTES — Mix packet with 3 tablespoons of water. Swish for 1 min, then spit. Do not eat or drink for 1 h after treatment.
MOA — Protective barrier.
ADVERSE EFFECTS — Serious: None. Frequent: None.

LIDOCAINE—VISCOUS (Xylocaine) ▶LK ♀B ▶+ $
WARNING — Avoid swallowing during oral or labial use due to GI absorption and toxicity. Measure dose exactly. May apply to small areas in mouth with a cotton-tipped applicator.
ADULT — Mouth or lip pain: 15 to 20 mL topically or swish and spit q 3 h. Max 8 doses/day.
PEDS — Use with extreme caution, as therapeutic doses approach potentially toxic levels. Use the lowest effective dose. Mouth or lip pain age older than 3 yo: 3.75 to 5 mL topically or swish and spit up to q 3 h.
FORMS — Generic/Trade: Soln 2%, 20 mL unit dose, 100 mL bottle.
NOTES — High risk of adverse effects and overdose in children. Consider benzocaine as a safer alternative. Clearly communicate the amount, frequency, max daily dose, and mode of administration (eg, cotton pledget to individual lesions, ½ dropper to each cheek q 4 h, or 20 min before meals). Do not prescribe on a "prn" basis without specified dosing intervals.
MOA — Local anesthetic.
ADVERSE EFFECTS — Serious: Hypersensitivity. Frequent: Burning, stinging.

MAGIC MOUTHWASH (diphenhydramine + Mylanta + sucralfate) ▶LK ♀ ▶— $$$
ADULT — See components.
PEDS — Not approved in children.
UNAPPROVED ADULT — Stomatitis: 5 mL PO swish and spit or swish and swallow three times per day before meals and prn.

(cont.)

MAGIC MOUTHWASH (cont.)

UNAPPROVED PEDS — Stomatitis: Apply small amounts to lesions prn.

FORMS — Compounded susp. A standard mixture is 30 mL diphenhydramine liquid (12.5 mg/5 mL)/60 mL Mylanta or Maalox/4 g Carafate.

NOTES — Variations of this formulation are available. The dose and decision to swish and spit or swallow may vary with the indication and/or ingredient. Some preparations may contain: Kaopectate, nystatin, tetracycline, hydrocortisone, 2% lidocaine, cherry syrup (for children). Check local pharmacies for customized formulations. Avoid diphenhydramine formulations that contain alcohol: May cause stinging of mouth sores.

MOA — Antihistamine/antacid/antiulcer combination.

ADVERSE EFFECTS — Serious: None. Frequent: Sedation, constipation, diarrhea.

PILOCARPINE (*Salagen*) ▶L ♀C ▶– $$$$

ADULT — Dry mouth due to radiation of head and neck: 5 mg PO three times per day. May increase to 10 mg PO three times per day. Dry mouth due to Sjögren's syndrome: 5 mg PO four times per day. Hepatic dysfunction: 5 mg PO two times per day.

PEDS — Not approved in children.

UNAPPROVED ADULT — Dry mouth due to Sjögren's syndrome: 2% pilocarpine eye gtts: Swish and swallow 4 gtts diluted in water three times per day ($).

FORMS — Generic/Trade: Tabs 5, 7.5 mg.

NOTES — Contraindicated in narrow-angle glaucoma, acute iritis and severe asthma. May potentiate beta-blockers.

MOA — Cholinergic stimulant.

ADVERSE EFFECTS — Serious: AV block, arrhythmias, brady/tachycardia, pulmonary edema, bronchospasm, blurred vision. Frequent: Sweating, urinary frequency, nausea, diarrhea, flushing, dizziness.

ENT: Nasal Preparations—Corticosteroids

NOTE: Decrease to the lowest effective dose for maintenance therapy. Tell patients to prime pump before first use and shake well before each subsequent use.

BECLOMETHASONE—NASAL (*Beconase AQ, Qnasl*) ▶L ♀C ▶? $$$$

ADULT — Allergic rhinitis/nasal polyp prophylaxis: Vancenase: 1 spray in each nostril two to four times per day. Beconase AQ: 1 to 2 spray(s) in each nostril two times per day. Vancenase AQ Double Strength: 1 to 2 spray(s) in each nostril daily. Allergic rhinitis: Qnasl 1 to 2 spray(s) in each nostril daily.

PEDS — Allergic rhinitis/nasal polyp prophylaxis: 1 spray in each nostril three times per day for age 6 to 12 yo, give adult dose for age older than 12 yo. Beconase AQ: 1 to 2 spray(s) in each nostril two times per day for age older than 6 yo. Vancenase AQ Double Strength: 1 to 2 spray(s) in each nostril daily for age older than 6 yo. Allergic rhinitis: Qnasl 1 to 2 spray(s) in each nostril once daily for age 12 and over.

FORMS — Trade only: Beconase AQ 42 mcg/spray, 200 sprays/bottle. Qnasl: 80 mcg/spray, 120 sprays/bottle.

NOTES — AQ (aqueous) formulation may cause less stinging.

MOA — Steroidal anti-inflammatory.

ADVERSE EFFECTS — Serious: Hypersensitivity, anaphylactoid reactions, urticaria, angioedema, bronchospasm, rash. Frequent: Nasal irritation.

BUDESONIDE—NASAL (*Rhinocort Aqua*) ▶L ♀B ▶? $$$$

ADULT — Allergic rhinitis: 1 to 4 sprays per nostril daily.

PEDS — Allergic rhinitis age 6 yo or older: 1 to 2 sprays per nostril daily.

FORMS — Generic/Trade: Nasal inhaler 120 sprays/bottle.

NOTES — CYP3A4 inhibitors such as ketoconazole, erythromycin, ritonavir, etc., significantly increase systemic concentrations, possibly causing adrenal suppression.

MOA — Steroidal anti-inflammatory.

ADVERSE EFFECTS — Serious: Hypersensitivity. Frequent: Nasal irritation.

CICLESONIDE—NASAL (*Omnaris, Zetonna*) ▶L ♀C ▶? $$$

ADULT — Allergic rhinitis: Omnaris: 2 sprays per nostril daily. Zetonna: 1 actuation per nostril daily.

PEDS — Allergic rhinitis, seasonal: Omnaris: give adult dose for age 6 yo or older. Zetonna: give adult dose for age 12 yo or older. Allergic rhinitis, perennial: Omnaris and Zetonna: give adult dose for age 12 yo or older.

FORMS — Trade only: Nasal spray, 50 mcg/spray, 120 sprays/bottle (Omnaris). Nasal aerosol, 37 mcg/actuation, 60 actuations/canister (Zetonna).

MOA — Steroidal anti-inflammatory.

ADVERSE EFFECTS — Serious: None. Frequent: Epistaxis, headache.

FLUNISOLIDE—NASAL (*Nasalide, *Rhinalar*) ▶L ♀C ▶? $$$

ADULT — Allergic rhinitis: 2 sprays per nostril two times per day, may increase to three times per day. Max 8 sprays/nostril/day.

PEDS — Allergic rhinitis age 6 to 14 yo: 1 spray per nostril three times per day or 2 sprays per nostril two times per day. Max 4 sprays/nostril/day.

FORMS — Generic only: Nasal soln 0.025%

MOA — Steroidal anti-inflammatory.

ADVERSE EFFECTS — Serious: Hypersensitivity. Frequent: Nasal irritation.

FLUTICASONE—NASAL (*Flonase, Veramyst*) ▶L ♀C ▶? $$$

ADULT — Allergic rhinitis: 2 sprays per nostril daily or 1 spray per nostril two times per day, decrease to 1 spray per nostril daily when appropriate. Seasonal

(cont.)

FLUTICASONE—NASAL (*cont.*)

allergic rhinitis alternative: 2 sprays per nostril daily prn.
PEDS — Allergic rhinitis for age older than 4 yo: 1 to 2 sprays per nostril daily. Max 2 sprays/nostril/day. Seasonal allergic rhinitis alternative for age older than 12 yo: 2 sprays per nostril daily prn.
FORMS — Generic/Trade: Flonase: Nasal spray 0.05%, 120 sprays/bottle. Trade only: (Veramyst): Nasal spray susp: 27.5 mcg/spray, 120 sprays/bottle.
NOTES — CYP3A4 inhibitors such as ketoconazole, erythromycin, ritonavir, etc., significantly increase systemic concentrations, possibly causing adrenal suppression.
MOA — Steroidal anti-inflammatory.
ADVERSE EFFECTS — Serious: Hypersensitivity. Frequent: Nasal irritation.

MOMETASONE—NASAL (*Nasonex*) ▶L ♀C ▶? $$$$

ADULT — Prevention or treatment of symptoms of allergic rhinitis: 2 sprays per nostril daily. Treatment of nasal polyps: 2 sprays per nostril two times per day (once daily may also be effective).
PEDS — Prevention or treatment of symptoms of allergic rhinitis age 12 yo or older: Use adult dose. 2 to 11 yo: 1 spray per nostril daily.

FORMS — Trade only: Nasal spray, 120 sprays/bottle.
MOA — Steroidal anti-inflammatory.
ADVERSE EFFECTS — Serious: Hypersensitivity. Frequent: Nasal irritation.

TRIAMCINOLONE—NASAL (*Nasacort AQ, Nasacort HFA, Tri-Nasal, AllerNaze*) ▶L ♀C ▶– $$$$

ADULT — Allergic rhinitis: Nasacort HFA, Tri-Nasal, AllerNaze: Start 2 sprays per nostril daily, may increase to 2 sprays/nostril two times per day. Max 4 sprays/nostril/day. Nasacort AQ: 2 sprays per nostril daily.
PEDS — Allergic rhinitis: Nasacort and Nasacort AQ: 1 to 2 sprays per nostril daily for age 6 to 12 yo, give adult dose for age older than 12 yo. Nasacort AQ: 1 spray in each nostril once daily for age 2 to 5 yo.
FORMS — Trade only: Nasal inhaler 55 mcg/spray, 100 sprays/bottle (Nasacort HFA). Nasal spray, 55 mcg/spray, 120 sprays/bottle (Nasacort AQ). Nasal spray 50 mcg/spray, 120 sprays/bottle (Tri-Nasal, AllerNaze).
NOTES — AQ (aqueous) formulation may cause less stinging. Decrease to lowest effective dose after allergy symptom improvement.
MOA — Steroidal anti-inflammatory.
ADVERSE EFFECTS — Serious: Hypersensitivity. Frequent: Nasal irritation.

ENT: Nasal Preparations—Other

NOTE: For ALL nasal sprays except saline, oxymetazoline, and phenylephrine, tell patients to prime pump before first use and shake well before each subsequent use.

AZELASTINE—NASAL (*Astelin, Astepro*) ▶L ♀C ▶? $$$$

ADULT — Allergic/vasomotor rhinitis: 1 to 2 sprays/nostril two times per day.
PEDS — Allergic rhinitis: 1 spray/nostril two times per day for age 5 to 11 yo, give adult dose for 12 yo or older. Vasomotor rhinitis give adult dose for 12 yo or older.
FORMS — Generic/Trade: Nasal spray, 200 sprays/bottle. Trade only: Astepro 0.15% nasal spray 200 sprays/bottle.
MOA — Antihistamine.
ADVERSE EFFECTS — Serious: Atrial fibrillation. Frequent: Bitter taste, sedation.

CETACAINE (**benzocaine + tetracaine + butamben**) ▶LK ♀C ▶? $$

WARNING — Do not use on the eyes. Hypersensitivity (rare). Methemoglobinemia (rare).
ADULT — Topical anesthesia of mucous membranes: Spray: Apply for 1 sec or less. Liquid or gel: Apply with cotton applicator directly to site.
PEDS — Use adult dose.
FORMS — Trade only: (14%/2%/2%) Spray 56 mL. Topical liquid 56 mL. Topical gel 5, 29 g.
NOTES — Do not hold cotton applicator in position for extended time due to increased risk of local reactions. Do not use multiple applications. Maximum anesthesia occurs 1 min after application; duration 30 min. May result in potentially

dangerous methemoglobinemia; use minimum amount needed.
MOA — Local anesthetic combination.
ADVERSE EFFECTS — Serious: Hypersensitivity, methemoglobinemia. Frequent: Erythema, pruritus.

CROMOLYN—NASAL (*NasalCrom*) ▶LK ♀B ▶+ $

ADULT — Allergic rhinitis: 1 spray per nostril three to four times per day up to 6 times per day.
PEDS — Allergic rhinitis for age 2 yo or older: Use adult dose.
FORMS — OTC Generic/Trade: Nasal inhaler 200 sprays/bottle 13, 26 mL.
NOTES — Therapeutic effects may not be seen for 1 to 2 weeks.
MOA — Anti-inflammatory mast-cell stabilizer.
ADVERSE EFFECTS — Serious: None. Frequent: None.

DYMISTA (**azelastine—nasal + fluticasone—nasal**) ▶L – ♀C ▶? $$$$

ADULT — Seasonal allergic rhinitis: 1 spray per nostril 2 times per day.
PEDS — Seasonal allergic rhinitis: give adult dose for 12 yo or older.
FORMS — Trade only: Nasal spray: 137 mcg astelazine/50 mcg fluticasone/spray, 120 sprays/bottle.
NOTES — CYP3A4 inhibitors such as ketoconazole, erythromycin, ritonavir, etc., significantly increase systemic concentrations of fluticasone, possibly causing adrenal suppression.

(cont.)

DYMISTA (cont.)

MOA — Intranasal antihistamine/anti-inflammatory steroid combination.

ADVERSE EFFECTS — Serious: Atrial fibrillation, hypersensitivity. Frequent: Bitter taste, sedation, nasal irritation.

IPRATROPIUM—NASAL (*Atrovent Nasal Spray*) ▶L ♀B ▶? $$

ADULT — Rhinorrhea due to allergic/nonallergic rhinitis: 2 sprays (0.03%) per nostril two to three times per day or 2 sprays (0.06%) per nostril four times per day. Rhinorrhea due to common cold: 2 sprays (0.06%) per nostril three to four times per day.

PEDS — Rhinorrhea due to allergic/nonallergic rhinitis: Give adult dose (0.03% strength) for age 6 yo or older, give adult dose (0.06% strength) for age 5 yo or older. Rhinorrhea due to common cold: 2 sprays (0.06% strength) per nostril three times per day for age 5 yo or older.

UNAPPROVED ADULT — Vasomotor rhinitis: 2 sprays (0.06%) in each nostril three to four times per day.

FORMS — Generic/Trade: Nasal spray 0.03%, 345 sprays/bottle, 0.06%, 165 sprays/bottle.

MOA — Anticholinergic.

ADVERSE EFFECTS — Serious: Hypersensitivity. Frequent: Nasal irritation, epistaxis.

LEVOCABASTINE—NASAL (✱*Livostin*) ▶L (but minimal absorption) ♀C ▶– $$

ADULT — Canada only. Allergic rhinitis: 2 sprays per nostril two times oer day; increase prn to 2 sprays per nostril three to four times per day.

PEDS — Not approved in children younger than 12 yo.

FORMS — Trade only: Nasal spray 0.5 mg/mL, plastic bottles of 15 mL. 50 mcg/spray.

NOTES — Nasal spray is devoid of CNS effects. Safety/efficacy in patients older than 65 yo has not been established.

MOA — Antihistamine.

ADVERSE EFFECTS — Frequent: Nasal irritation.

OLOPATADINE—NASAL (*Patanase*) ▶L ♀C ▶? $$$

ADULT — Allergic rhinitis: 2 sprays/nostril two times per day.

PEDS — Allergic rhinitis age 12 yo or older: Use adult dose. For age 6 to 11 yo: 1 spray/nostril two times per day.

FORMS — Trade only: Nasal spray, 240 sprays/bottle.

MOA — Antihistamine.

ADVERSE EFFECTS — Serious: None. Frequent: Epistaxis, nasal irritation, bitter taste, sedation.

OXYMETAZOLINE (*Afrin, Dristan 12 Hr Nasal, Nostrilla, Vicks Sinex 12 Hr*) ▶L ♀C ▶? $

ADULT — Nasal congestion: 2 to 3 sprays or gtts (0.05%) per nostril two times per day for no more than 3 days.

PEDS — Nasal congestion: Give 2 to 3 gtts (0.025%) per nostril two times per day no more than 3 days for age 2 to 5 yo, give 2 to 3 sprays or gtts (0.05%) per nostril two times per day not more than 3 days.

FORMS — OTC Generic/Trade: Nasal spray 0.05% 15, 30 mL; Nose gtts 0.025%, 0.05% 20 mL with dropper.

NOTES — Overuse (more than 3 to 5 days) may lead to rebound congestion. If this occurs, taper to use in 1 nostril only, alternating sides, then discontinue. Substituting an oral decongestant or nasal steroid may also be useful.

MOA — Decongestant.

ADVERSE EFFECTS — Serious: None. Frequent: Stinging, rebound congestion.

PHENYLEPHRINE—NASAL (*Neo-Synephrine, Vicks Sinex*) ▶L ♀C ▶? $

ADULT — Nasal congestion: 2 to 3 sprays or gtts (0.25 or 0.5%) per nostril q 4 h prn for 3 days. Use 1% soln for severe congestion.

PEDS — Nasal congestion: Give 1 to 2 gtts (0.125% or 0.16%) per nostril q 4 h prn for 3 days for age 6 to 11 mo, give 2 to 3 gtts (0.125% or 0.16%) per nostril q 4 h prn for 3 days for age 1 to 5 yo, give 2 to 3 gtts or sprays (0.25%) per nostril q 4 h prn for 3 days for age 6 to 12 yo, give adult dose for age older than 12 yo.

FORMS — OTC Generic/Trade: Nasal gtts/spray 0.25, 0.5, 1% (15 mL).

NOTES — Overuse (more 3 to 5 days) may lead to rebound congestion. If this occurs, taper to use in 1 nostril only, alternating sides, then discontinue. Substituting an oral decongestant or nasal steroid may also be useful.

MOA — Decongestant.

ADVERSE EFFECTS — Serious: None. Frequent: Stinging, rebound congestion.

SALINE NASAL SPRAY (*SeaMist, Entsol, Pretz, NaSal, Ocean,* ✱*HydraSense*) ▶Not metabolized ♀A ▶+ $

ADULT — Nasal dryness: 1 to 3 sprays per nostril prn.

PEDS — Nasal dryness: 1 to 3 gtts per nostril prn.

FORMS — Generic/Trade: Nasal spray 0.4, 0.5, 0.65, 0.75%. Nasal gtts 0.4, 0.65%. Trade only: Preservative-free nasal spray 3% (Entsol).

NOTES — May be prepared at home by combining: ¼ teaspoon salt with 8 ounces (1 cup) warm water. Add ¼ teaspoon baking soda (optional) and put in spray bottle, ear syringe, neti pot, or any container with a small spout. Discard after 1 week.

MOA — Moisturizer.

ADVERSE EFFECTS — Serious: None. Frequent: None.

GASTROENTEROLOGY

HELICOBACTER PYLORI THERAPY

- Triple therapy PO for 10 to 14 days: clarithromycin 500 mg two times per day plus amoxicillin 1 g two times per day (or metronidazole 500 mg two times per day) plus PPI*

- Quadruple therapy PO for 14 days: bismuth subsalicylate 525 mg (or 30 mL) three to four times per day plus metronidazole 500 mg three to four times per day plus tetracycline 500 mg three to four times per day plus a PPI* or an H2 blocker†

- PPI or H2 blocker may need to be continued past 14 days to heal the ulcer.

*PPIs include esomeprazole 40 mg daily, lansoprazole 30 mg two times per day, omeprazole 20 mg two times per day, pantoprazole 40 mg two times per day, rabeprazole 20 mg two times per day.

†H2 blockers include cimetidine 400 mg two times per day, famotidine 20 mg two times per day, nizatidine 150 mg two times per day, ranitidine 150 mg two times per day. Adapted from Medical Letter Treatment Guidelines 2008:55.

GASTROENTEROLOGY: Antidiarrheals

BISMUTH SUBSALICYLATE (*Pepto-Bismol, Kaopectate*) ▶K ♀D ▶? $

WARNING — Avoid in children and teenagers with chickenpox or flu due to possible association with Reye's syndrome.

ADULT — Diarrhea: 2 tabs or 30 mL (262 mg/15 mL) PO q 30 to 60 min up to 8 doses/day for up to 2 days.

PEDS — Diarrhea: 100 mg/kg/day divided into 5 doses or ⅓ tab, chew tab, or 5 mL (262 mg/15 mL) q 30 to 60 min prn up to 8 doses/day for age 3 to 6 yo, ⅔ tab, chew tab, or 10 mL (262 mg/15 mL) q 30 to 60 min prn up to 8 doses/day for age 7 to 9 yo, 1 tab or chew tab or 15 mL (262 mg/15 mL) q 30 to 60 min prn up to 8 doses/day for age 10 to 12 yo. Do not take for more than 2 days.

UNAPPROVED ADULT — Prevention of traveler's diarrhea: 2.1 g/day or 2 tab four times per day before meals and at bedtime. Has been used as part of a multidrug regimen for Helicobacter pylori.

UNAPPROVED PEDS — Chronic infantile diarrhea: 2.5 mL (262 mg/15 mL) PO q 4 h for age 2 to 24 mo, 5 mL (262 mg/15 mL) PO q 4 h for age 25 to 48 mo, 10 mL (262 mg/15 mL) PO q 4 h for age 49 to 70 mo.

FORMS — OTC Generic/Trade: Chewable tabs 262 mg. Susp 262, 525, 750 mg/15 mL. OTC Trade only: Caplets 262 mg (Pepto-Bismol). Susp 87 mg/5 mL (Kaopectate Children's Liquid).

NOTES — Use with caution in patients already taking salicylates or warfarin, children recovering from chickenpox or flu. Decreases absorption of tetracycline. May darken stools or tongue. Children's Pepto-Bismol contains calcium carbonate.

MOA — Antidiarrheal.

ADVERSE EFFECTS — Frequent: None.

IMODIUM MULTI-SYMPTOM RELIEF (loperamide + simethicone) ▶L ♀C ▶– $

ADULT — Diarrhea: 2 tabs/caps PO initially, then 1 tab/cap PO after each unformed stool to a max of 4 tabs/caps/day.

PEDS — Diarrhea: 1 cap PO initially, then ½ tab/cap PO after each unformed stool (up to 2 tabs/caps/day for age 6 to 8 yo or wt 48 to 59 lbs, up to 3 tabs/caps/day for age 9 to 11 yo or wt 60 to 95 lbs).

FORMS — OTC Generic/Trade: Caplets, Chewable tabs 2 mg loperamide/125 mg simethicone.

NOTES — Not for C. difficile–associated diarrhea, toxigenic bacterial diarrhea, or most childhood diarrhea (difficult to exclude toxigenic).

MOA — Antidiarrheal, inhibits peristalsis of intestinal muscles.

ADVERSE EFFECTS — Frequent: Sedation in children.

LOMOTIL (diphenoxylate + atropine) ▶L ♀C ▶– ©V $

ADULT — Diarrhea: 2 tabs or 10 mL PO four times per day.

PEDS — Diarrhea: 0.3 to 0.4 mg diphenoxylate/kg/24 h in 4 divided doses. Max daily dose 20 mg. Not recommended for younger than 2 yo, 1.5 to 3 mL PO four times per day for age 2 yo or wt 11 to 14 kg; 2 to 3 mL PO four times per day for age 3 yo or wt 12 to 16 kg; 2 to 4 mL PO four times per day for age 4 yo or wt 14 to 20 kg; 2.5 to 4.5 mL PO four times per day for age 5 yo or wt 16 to 23 kg; 2.5 to 5 mL PO four times per day for age 6 to 8 yo or wt 17 to 32 kg; 3.5 to 5 mL PO four times per day for 9 to 12 yo or wt 23 to 55 kg.

FORMS — Generic/Trade: Oral soln or tab 2.5 mg/0.025 mg diphenoxylate/atropine per 5 mL or tab.

NOTES — Give with food to decrease GI upset. May cause atropinism in children, especially with Down syndrome, even at recommended doses. Can cause delayed toxicity. Has been reported to cause severe respiratory depression, coma, brain damage, death after overdose in children. Naloxone reverses toxicity. Do not use for C. difficile–associated diarrhea, toxigenic bacterial diarrhea, or most childhood diarrhea (difficult to exclude toxigenic).

LOMOTIL (*cont.*)

MOA — Antidiarrheal, inhibits peristalsis of intestinal muscles.

ADVERSE EFFECTS — Frequent: Nervousness, dizziness, headache, depression, restlessness.

LOPERAMIDE (*Imodium, Imodium AD, ✦Loperacap, Diarr-eze*) ▶L ♀C ▶+ $

WARNING — Discontinue if abdominal distention or ileus. Caution in children due to variable response.

ADULT — Diarrhea: 4 mg PO initially, then 2 mg after each unformed stool to max 16 mg/day.

PEDS — Diarrhea: First dose: 1 mg PO three times per day for age 2 to 5 yo or wt 13 to 20 kg, 2 mg PO two times per day for age 6 to 8 yo or wt 21 to 30 kg, 2 mg PO three times per day for age 9 to 12 yo or wt greater than 30 kg. After 1st day: give 0.1 mg/kg PO after each loose stool; daily dose not to exceed daily dose of 1st day.

UNAPPROVED ADULT — Chronic diarrhea or ileostomy drainage: 4 mg initially then 2 mg after each stool until symptoms are controlled, then reduce dose for maintenance treatment, average adult maintenance dose 4 to 8 mg daily as a single dose or in divided doses.

UNAPPROVED PEDS — Chronic diarrhea: Limited information. Average doses of 0.08 to 0.24 mg/kg/day PO in 2 to 3 divided doses. Max 2 mg/dose. Max 16 mg/day.

FORMS — OTC Generic/Trade: Tabs 2 mg. Oral soln 1 mg/5 mL. Oral soln 1 mg/7.5 mL.

NOTES — Not for C. difficile–associated diarrhea, toxigenic bacterial diarrhea, or most childhood diarrhea (difficult to exclude toxigenic). Doses greater than 16 mg/day have been used.

MOA — Antidiarrheal, inhibits peristalsis of intestinal muscles.

ADVERSE EFFECTS — Frequent: Sedation in children.

MOTOFEN (**difenoxin + atropine**) ▶L ♀C ▶– ©IV $$

ADULT — Diarrhea: 2 tabs PO initially, then 1 after each loose stool q 3 to 4 h prn (up to 8 tabs/day).

PEDS — Not approved in children. Contraindicated younger than 2 yo.

FORMS — Trade only: Tabs difenoxin 1 mg + atropine 0.025 mg.

NOTES — Do not use for C. difficile–associated diarrhea, toxigenic bacterial diarrhea, or most childhood diarrhea (difficult to exclude toxigenic). May cause atropinism in children, especially with Down syndrome, even at recommended doses. Can cause delayed toxicity. Has been reported to cause severe respiratory depression, coma, brain damage, death after overdose in children. Difenoxin is the primary metabolite of diphenoxylate.

MOA — Antidiarrheal, inhibits peristalsis of intestinal muscles.

ADVERSE EFFECTS — Frequent: Anticholinergic effects, nervousness, dizziness, headache, depression, restlessness.

OPIUM (*opium tincture, paregoric*) ▶L ♀B (D with long-term use) ▶? ©II (opium tincture), III (paregoric) $$

ADULT — Diarrhea: Paregoric: 5 to 10 mL PO daily (up to four times). Opium tincture: 0.6 mL (range 0.3 to 1 mL) PO q 2 to 6 h, prn, to a max of 6 mL per day.

PEDS — Diarrhea: 0.25 to 0.5 mL/kg paregoric PO daily (up to four times per day) or 0.005 to 0.01 mL/kg PO opium tincture q 3 to 4 h (up to 6 doses/day).

FORMS — Trade only: Opium tincture 10% (deodorized opium tincture, 10 mg morphine equivalent/mL). Generic only: Paregoric (camphorated opium tincture, 2 mg morphine equivalent/5 mL).

NOTES — Opium tincture contains 25 times more morphine than paregoric. Do not use for C. difficile–associated diarrhea, toxigenic bacterial diarrhea, or most childhood diarrhea.

MOA — Antidiarrheal, inhibits peristalsis of intestinal muscles.

ADVERSE EFFECTS — Frequent: Palpitations, hypotension, bradycardia, dizziness, drowsiness, weakness, urinary retention. Severe: Possible biliary tract spasm.

GASTROENTEROLOGY: Antiemetics—5-HT3 Receptor Antagonists

DOLASETRON (*Anzemet*) ▶LK ♀B ▶? $$$

ADULT — Prevention of N/V with chemo: 100 mg PO single dose 60 min before chemo.

PEDS — Prevention of N/V with chemo: 1.8 mg/kg up to 100 mg PO single dose 60 min before chemo for age 2 to 16 yo.

UNAPPROVED ADULT — N/V due to radiotherapy: 0.3 mg/kg IV as a single dose.

FORMS — Trade only: Tabs 50, 100 mg. Injectable no longer available in Canada.

NOTES — Use caution in patients of any age who have or may develop prolongation of QT interval (ie, hypokalemia, hypomagnesemia, concomitant antiarrhythmic therapy, cumulative high-dose anthracycline therapy). Cimetidine may increase serum concentrations, rifampin may reduce serum concentrations.

MOA — Antiemetic, serotonin antagonist blocking chemoreceptor trigger zone.

ADVERSE EFFECTS — Frequent: None. Severe: Prolongation of cardiac conduction intervals, particularly QTc, ventricular tachycardia, ventricular fibrillation.

GRANISETRON (*Sancuso*) ▶L ♀B ▶? $$$$

ADULT — Prevention of N/V with chemo: Transdermal (Sancuso): 1 patch to upper outer arm at least 24 h (but up to 48 h) before chemotherapy. Remove 24 h after completion of chemotherapy. Can be worn up to 7 days depending on the duration of chemo.

PEDS — Not approved for use in children.

FORMS — Trade only: Transdermal patch (Sancuso) 34.3 mg of granisetron delivering 3.1 mg/24 h.

MOA — Antiemetic, serotonin antagonist blocking chemoreceptor trigger zone.

GRANISETRON *(cont.)*

ADVERSE EFFECTS — Frequent: Headache. Severe: Arrhythmias, QT prolongation.

ONDANSETRON *(Zofran, Zuplenz)* ▶L ♀B ▶? $$$$$

WARNING — Avoid in patients with congenital long QT syndrome. ECG monitoring is recommended in patients with electrolyte abnormalities, CHF, brady-arrhythmias or patients taking other medications that can prolong QT interval.

ADULT — Prevention of N/V with chemo: 0.15 mg/kg IV (max 16 mg) 30 min prior to chemo and repeated at 4 and 8 h after 1st dose. Alternatively, 8 mg PO 30 min before moderately emetogenic chemo and 8 h later. Can be given q 12 h for 1 to 2 days after completion of chemo. For single-day highly emeto-genic chemo, 24 mg PO 30 min before chemo. Prevention of post-op nausea: 4 mg IV over 2 to 5 min or 4 mg IM or 16 mg PO 1 h before anesthesia. Prevention of N/V associated with radiotherapy: 8 mg PO three times per day.

PEDS — Prevention of N/V with chemo: IV: 0.15 mg/kg (max 16 mg) 30 min prior to chemo and repeated at 4 and 8 h after 1st dose for age older than than 6 mo. PO: Give 4 mg 30 minutes prior to chemo and repeat at 4 and 8 h after 1st dose for age 4 to 11 yo. Can be given q 8 h PO for 1 to 2 days after completion of chemo. Give 8 mg PO 30 min before chemo and 8 h later for age 12 yo or older. Prevention of post-op N/V: 0.1 mg/kg IV over 2 to 5 min for age 1 mo to 12 yo if wt 40 kg or less; give 4 mg IV over 2 to 5 min if wt greater than 40 kg.

UNAPPROVED ADULT — Has been used in hypereme-sis associated with pregnancy.

UNAPPROVED PEDS — Use with caution if younger than 4 yo. Dosing based on BSA: give 1 mg PO three times per day for BSA less than 0.3 m², give 2 mg PO three times per day for BSA 0.3 to 0.6 m², give 3 mg PO three times per day for BSA 0.6 to 1 m², give 4 mg PO three times per day for BSA greater than 1 m². Use caution in infants younger than 6 mo of age.

FORMS — Generic/Trade: Tabs 4, 8, 24 mg. Orally disintegrating tab 4, 8 mg. Oral soln 4 mg/5 mL. Trade only: Oral film (Zuplenz) 4, 8 mg.

NOTES — Can prolong QT interval. Maximum oral dose if severe liver disease is 8 mg/day. Maximum IV dos is 16 mg. Use following abdominal surgery or in those receiving chemotherapy may mask a progres-sive ileus or gastric distension. Contraindicated with apomorphine; concomitant use can lead to hypotension and loss of consiousness.

MOA — Antiemetic, serotonin antagonist blocking chemoreceptor trigger zone.

ADVERSE EFFECTS — Frequent: Headache, fever, diarrhea, constipation, transient increases in LFTs. Severe: Transient blindness, especially with IV, arrhythmia, QT prolongation, Stevens-Johnson syn-drome and toxic epidermal necrolysis.

PALONOSETRON *(Aloxi)* ▶L ♀B ▶? $$$$$

ADULT — Prevention of N/V with chemo: 0.25 mg IV over 30 sec, 30 min prior to chemo. Prevention of postop N/V: 0.075 mg IV over 10 sec just prior to anesthesia.

PEDS — Prevention of N/V with chemo (1 month to 17 years): 20 mcg/kg (max 1.5 mg) over 15 min-utes, 30 minutes prior to chemo.

UNAPPROVED PEDS — Limited information suggests 3 mcg/kg (maximum 0.25 mg) IV is effective and safe in children older than 2 yo.

FORMS — Trade only: injectable.

MOA — Antiemetic, serotonin antagonist blocking chemoreceptor trigger zone.

ADVERSE EFFECTS — Frequent: Headache, constipa-tion. Severe: Arrhythmia, QT prolongation.

GASTROENTEROLOGY: Antiemetics—Other

APREPITANT *(Emend, fosaprepitant)* ▶L ♀B ▶? $$$$$

ADULT — Prevention of N/V with moderately to highly emetogenic chemo, in combination with a cortico-steroid and a 5-HT3 antagonist: 125 mg PO on day 1 (1 h prior to chemo), then 80 mg PO q am on days 2 and 3. Alternative for 1st dose only is 115 mg IV (fosaprepitant form) over 15 min given 30 min prior to chemo. Prevention of postop N/V: 40 mg PO within 3 h prior to anesthesia.

PEDS — Not approved in children.

FORMS — Trade only (aprepitant): Caps 40, 80, 125 mg. IV prodrug form is fosaprepitant.

NOTES — Use caution with other medications metabo-lized by CYP3A4 hepatic enzyme system and an inducer of the CYP2C9 hepatic enzyme system. Contraindicated with pimozide. May decrease efficacy of oral contraceptives; women should use alternate/back-up method. Monitor INR in patients receiving warfarin. Fosaprepitant is a prodrug of aprepitant.

MOA — Antiemetic, substance P/neurokinin-1 recep-tor antagonist.

ADVERSE EFFECTS — Frequent: Fatigue, diar-rhea, constipation, muscular weakness, hic-cups. Severe: Hypersensitivity and anaphylactic reactions.

DICLEGIS (doxylamine + pyridoxine, *✦Diclectin*) ▶LK − ♀A ▶− $$$$$

ADULT — N/V due to pregnancy: 2 tablets PO at bed-time. If not controlled, can increase to a maximum of 4 tablets daily (2 tablet PO qam, 1 tablet PO mid-afternoon, 2 tablets PO at bedtime).

PEDS — Not indicated for children.

FORMS — Trade: doxylamine 10 mg and pyridoxine 10 mg.

MOA — Unknown.

ADVERSE EFFECTS — Frequent: drowsiness, somnolence.

DIMENHYDRINATE *(Dramamine, ✦Gravol)* ▶LK ♀B ▶− $

ADULT — Nausea: 50 to 100 mg/dose PO/IM/IV q 4 to 6 h prn. Maximum PO dose 400 mg/24 h, maximum IV/IM dose 600 mg/24 h. Canada only: 50 to 100 mg/dose PR q 4 to 6 h prn.

(cont.)

DIMENHYDRINATE (cont.)

PEDS — Nausea: Not recommended for age younger than 2 yo. Give 12.5 to 25 mg PO q 6 to 8 h or 5 mg/kg/day (up to 75 mg/day) PO divided q 6 h for age 2 to 5 yo, give 25 to 50 mg (up to 150 mg/day) PO q 6 to 8 h or for age 6 to 12 yo.

FORMS — OTC Generic/Trade: Tabs 50 mg. Trade only: Chewable tabs 25, 50 mg. Generic only: Oral soln 12.5 mg/5 mL. Canada only: Supp 25, 50, 100 mg.

NOTES — May cause drowsiness. Use with caution in conditions that may be aggravated by anticholinergic effects (ie, prostatic hypertrophy, asthma, narrow-angle glaucoma). Available as suppositories in Canada.

MOA — Antihistamine.

ADVERSE EFFECTS — Frequent: Blurred vision, dry mouth, dizziness. Severe: Hallucinations, psychosis.

DOMPERIDONE ▸L ♀? ▶ $$

ADULT — Canada only. Postprandial dyspepsia: 10 to 20 mg PO three to four times per day, 30 min before a meal. N/V: 20 mg PO three to four times per day.

PEDS — Not approved in children.

UNAPPROVED ADULT — Has been used for diabetic gastroparesis, chemotherapy/radiation-induced N/V. Has also been used to increase milk production in lactating mothers although this is not currently recommended due to safety concerns.

UNAPPROVED PEDS — Use in children generally not recommended except for chemotherapy- or radiation-induced N/V: 200 to 400 mcg/kg PO q 4 to 8 h.

FORMS — Canada only. Trade/generic: Tabs 10, 20 mg.

NOTES — Similar in efficacy to metoclopramide but less likely to cause EPS.

MOA — Dopamine antagonist at GI muscle receptors and chemoreceptor trigger zone, resulting in improved gastric emptying.

ADVERSE EFFECTS — Serious: Cardiac dysrhythmia. Frequent: galactorrhea, gynecomastia.

DOXYLAMINE (Unisom Nighttime Sleep Aid, others) ▸L ♀A ▶? $

PEDS — Not approved in children younger than 12 yo.

UNAPPROVED ADULT — Nausea and vomiting associated with pregnancy: 12.5 mg PO two to four times per day; often used in combination with pyridoxine.

FORMS — OTC, Generic/Trade: Tabs 25 mg.

MOA — Anticholinergic and sedative.

ADVERSE EFFECTS — Frequent: None.

DRONABINOL (Marinol) ▸L ♀C ▶– ©III $$$$$

ADULT — Nausea with chemo: 5 mg/m² PO 1 to 3 h before chemo then 5 mg/m²/dose q 2 to 4 h after chemo for 4 to 6 doses/day. Dose can be increased to max 15 mg/m². Anorexia associated with AIDS: Initially 2.5 mg PO two times per day before lunch and dinner. If indicated and tolerated, increase to 20 mg/day.

PEDS — Nausea with chemo: 5 mg/m² PO 1 to 3 h before chemo then 5 mg/m²/dose PO q 2 to 4 h after chemo (up to 4 to 6 doses/day). Dose can

be increased to max 15 mg/m². Not approved for anorexia associated with AIDS in children.

UNAPPROVED ADULT — Appetitie stimulant: 2.5 mg PO twice daily.

UNAPPROVED PEDS — Nausea with chemo: 5 mg/m² PO 1 to 3 h before chemo then 5 mg/m²/dose PO q 2 to 4 h after chemo (up to 4 to 6 doses/day). Dose can be increased to max 15 mg/m².

FORMS — Generic/Trade: Caps 2.5, 5, 10 mg.

NOTES — Patient response varies; individualize dosing (start with low doses in elderly). Additive CNS effects with alcohol, sedatives, hypnotics, psychomimetics. Caution if history of seizures.

MOA — Unknown.

ADVERSE EFFECTS — Frequent: Drowsiness, dizziness, anxiety, detachment, mood changes, anorexia. Severe: Syncope.

DROPERIDOL (Inapsine) ▸L ♀C ▶? $

WARNING — Cases of fatal QT prolongation and/or torsades des pointes have occurred in patients receiving droperidol at or below recommended doses (some without risk factors for QT prolongation). Reserve for nonresponse to other treatments, and perform 12-lead ECG prior to administration and continue ECG monitoring 2 to 3 h after treatment. Avoid if prolonged baseline QT.

ADULT — Antiemetic premedication: 0.625 to 2.5 mg IV or 2.5 mg IM then 1.25 mg prn.

PEDS — Pre-op: 0.088 to 0.165 mg/kg IV for age 2 to 12 yo. Children older than 12 yo: 2.5 mg IM/IV, additional doses of 1.25 mg can be given with caution. Post-op antiemetic: 0.01 to 0.03 mg/kg/dose IV q 6 to 8 h prn. Usual dose 0.05 to 0.06 mg/kg/dose (up to 0.1 mg/kg/dose).

UNAPPROVED ADULT — Chemo-induced nausea: 2.5 to 5 mg IV/IM q 3 to 4 h prn.

UNAPPROVED PEDS — Chemo-induced nausea: 0.05 to 0.06 mg/kg/dose IV/IM q 4 to 6 h prn.

NOTES — Has no analgesic or amnestic effects. Consider lower doses in geriatric, debilitated, or high-risk patients such as those receiving other CNS depressants. May cause hypotension or tachycardia, extrapyramidal reactions, drowsiness.

MOA — Alters action of dopamine to sedate and reduce emesis.

ADVERSE EFFECTS — Frequent: QTc prolongatioon, restlessness, anxiety, dystonic reactions. Severe: Cardiac arrest, sedation, hypotension, seizures, extrapyramidal reactions.

METOCLOPRAMIDE (Reglan, Metozolv ODT, ✱Maxeran) ▸K ♀B ▶? $

WARNING — Irreversible tardive dyskinesia with high dose or long-term (greater than 3 months) use.

ADULT — Gastroesophageal reflux: 10 to 15 mg PO four times per day 30 min before meals and at bedtime. Diabetic gastroparesis: 10 mg PO/IV/IM 30 min before meals and at bedtime. Prevention of chemo-induced emesis: 1 to 2 mg/kg PO/IV/IM 30 min before chemo and then q 2 h for 2 doses then q 3 h for 3 doses prn. Prevention of postop nausea: 10

METOCLOPRAMIDE (*cont.*)

to 20 mg IM/IV near end of surgical procedure, may repeat q 3 to 4 h prn. Intubation of small intestine: 10 mg IV. Radiographic exam of upper GI tract: 10 mg IV.

PEDS — Intubation of small intestine: 0.1 mg/kg IV for age younger than 6 yo; 2.5 to 5 mg IV for age 6 to 14 yo. Radiographic exam of upper GI tract: 0.1 mg/kg IV for age younger than 6 yo; 2.5 to 5 mg IV for age 6 to 14 yo.

UNAPPROVED ADULT — Prevention/treatment of chemo-induced emesis: 3 mg/kg IV over 1 h followed by continuous IV infusion of 0.5 mg/kg/h for 12 h. Migraine treatment: 10 mg IV. Migraine adjunct: 10 mg PO 5 to 10 min before ergotamine/analgesic/sedative.

UNAPPROVED PEDS — Gastroesophageal reflux: 0.4 to 0.8 mg/kg/day in 4 divided doses. Prevention of chemo-induced emesis: 1 to 2 mg/kg 30 min before chemo and then q 3 h prn (up to 5 doses/day or 5 to 10 mg/kg/day).

FORMS — Generic/Trade: Tabs 5, 10 mg. Trade: Orally disintegrating tabs 5, 10 mg (Metozolv). Generic only: Oral soln 5 mg/5 mL.

NOTES — To reduce incidence and severity of akathisia, consider giving IV doses over 15 min. If extrapyramidal reactions occur (especially with high IV doses) give diphenhydramine IM/IV. Adjust dose in renal dysfunction. Irreversible tardive dyskinesia with high dose or long-term (greater than 12 weeks) use. Avoid use greater than 12 weeks except in rare cases where benefit outweighs risk of tardive dyskinesia. May cause drowsiness, agitation, seizures, hallucinations, galactorrhea, hyperprolactinemia, constipation, diarrhea. Increases cyclosporine and ethanol absorption. Do not use if bowel perforation or mechanical obstruction present. Levodopa decreases metoclopramide effects.

MOA — Dopamine blockade; inhibits chemoreceptor trigger zone.

ADVERSE EFFECTS — Frequent: Restlessness, drowsiness, diarrhea, asthenia.

NABILONE (*Cesamet*) ▶L ♀C ▶– ©II $$$$$

ADULT — N/V in cancer chemotherapy patients with poor response to other agents: 1 to 2 mg PO two times per day, 1 to 3 h before chemotherapy. Max dose 6 mg/day in 3 divided doses.

PEDS — Not approved in children.

UNAPPROVED PEDS — Children 4 yo or older: wt less than 18 kg: 0.5 mg PO two times per day, wt 18 to 30 kg: 1 mg PO two times per day, wt 30 kg or greater: 1 mg PO three times per day.

FORMS — Trade only: Caps 1 mg.

NOTES — Contraindicated in known sensitivity to marijuana or other cannabinoids. Use with caution with current or past psychiatric reactions. Additive CNS effects with alcohol, sedatives, hypnotics, psychomimetics. Additive cardiac effects with amphetamines, antihistamines, anticholinergic medications.

MOA — Synthetic cannabinoid with antiemetic properties.

ADVERSE EFFECTS — Frequent: Drowsiness, vertigo, dry mouth, euphoria, ataxia, headache, impaired concentration. Serious: Psychotic reactions, seizures, hallucinations.

PHOSPHORATED CARBOHYDRATES (*Emetrol*) ▶L ♀A ▶+ $

ADULT — Nausea: 15 to 30 mL PO q 15 min until nausea subsides or up to 5 doses.

PEDS — Nausea: 2 to 12 yo: 5 to 10 mL q 15 min until nausea subsides or up to 5 doses.

UNAPPROVED ADULT — Morning sickness: 15 to 30 mL PO upon rising, repeat q 3 h prn. Motion sickness or nausea due to drug therapy or anesthesia: 15 mL/dose.

UNAPPROVED PEDS — Regurgitation in infants: 5 to 10 mL PO 10 to 15 min prior to each feeding. Motion sickness or nausea due to drug therapy or anesthesia: 5 mL/dose.

FORMS — OTC Generic/Trade: Soln containing dextrose, fructose, and phosphoric acid.

NOTES — Do not dilute. Do not ingest fluids before or for 15 min after dose. Monitor blood glucose in diabetic patients.

MOA — Hyperosmolar effect on GI wall to reduce contraction.

ADVERSE EFFECTS — Frequent: Abdominal pain, diarrhea (in high doses).

PROCHLORPERAZINE (*Compazine*, ✦*Stemetil*) ▶LK ♀C ▶? $

ADULT — Nausea and vomiting: 5 to 10 mg PO/IM three to four times per day (up to 40 mg/day); Sustained release: 10 mg PO q 12 h or 15 mg PO q am; Suppository: 25 mg PR q 12 h; IV/IM: 5 to 10 mg IV over at least 2 min q 3 to 4 h prn (up to 40 mg/day); 5 to 10 mg IM q 3 to 4 h prn (up to 40 mg/day).

PEDS — Nausea and vomiting: Not recommended in age younger than 2 yo or wt less than 10 kg, 0.4 mg/kg/day PO/PR in 3 to 4 divided doses for age older than 2 yo; 0.1 to 0.15 mg/kg/dose IM; IV not recommended in children.

UNAPPROVED ADULT — Migraine: 10 mg IV/IM or 25 mg PR single dose for acute headache.

UNAPPROVED PEDS — N/V during surgery: 5 to 10 mg IM 1 to 2 h before anesthesia induction, may repeat in 30 min; 5 to 10 mg IV 15 to 30 min before anesthesia induction, may repeat once.

FORMS — Generic only: Tabs 5, 10, 25 mg. Supp 25 mg.

NOTES — May cause extrapyramidal reactions (especially in elderly), hypotension (with IV), arrhythmias, sedation, seizures, hyperprolactinemia, gynecomastia, dry mouth, constipation, urinary retention, leukopenia, thrombocytopenia. Elderly more prone to adverse effects. Brand name Compazine no longer available.

MOA — Blocks post-synaptic dopaminergic receptors.

ADVERSE EFFECTS — Frequent: None. Severe: Cardiac arrest, hypotension, extrapyramidal signs.

PROMETHAZINE (*Phenergan*) ▶LK ♀C ▶– $
WARNING — Contraindicated if age younger than 2 yo due to risk of fatal respiratory depression; caution in older children. Risks of severe tissue injury associated with IV administration including gangrene. Preferred route of administration is deep IM injection, subcutaneous injection is contraindicated.
ADULT — N/V: 12.5 to 25 mg q 4 to 6 h PO/IM/PR prn. Motion sickness: 25 mg PO/PR 30 to 60 min prior to departure and q 12 h prn. Hypersensitivity reactions: 25 mg IM/IV, may repeat in 2 h. Allergic conditions: 12.5 mg PO/PR/IM/IV four times per day or 25 mg PO/PR at bedtime.
PEDS — N/V: 0.25 to 1 mg/kg/dose PO/IM/PR (up to 25 mg/dose) q 4 to 6 h prn for age 2 yo or older. Motion sickness: 0.5 mg/kg (up to 25 mg/dose) PO 30 to 60 min prior to departure and q 12 h prn. Hypersensitivity reactions: 6.25 to 12.5 mg PO/PR/IM/IV q 6 h prn for age older than 2 yo.
UNAPPROVED ADULT — N/V: 12.5 to 25 mg IV q 4 h prn.
UNAPPROVED PEDS — N/V: 0.25 mg/kg/dose IV q 4 h prn for age 2 yo or older.
FORMS — Generic only: Tabs/Supp 12.5, 25, 50 mg. Syrup 6.25 mg/5 mL.
NOTES — May cause sedation, extrapyramidal reactions (especially with high IV doses), hypotension with rapid IV administration, anticholinergic side effects, e.g., dry mouth, blurred vision. Brand name Phenergan no longer available.
MOA — Antihistamine; blocks post-synaptic dopaminergic receptors.
ADVERSE EFFECTS — Frequent: Sedation, dry mouth. Severe: Cardiac arrest, hypotension, extrapyramidal signs, cholestatic jaundice.

SCOPOLAMINE (*Transderm-Scop, Scopace,* ✸*Transderm-V*) ▶L ♀C ▶+ $$
ADULT — Motion sickness: 1 disc behind ear at least 4 h before travel and q 3 days prn or 0.4 to 0.8 mg PO 1 h before travel and q 8 h prn. Prevention of postop N/V: Apply patch behind ear 4 h before surgery, remove 24 h after surgery. Spastic states, postencephalitic parkinsonism: 0.4 to 0.8 mg PO q 8 h prn.
PEDS — Not approved for age younger than 12 yo.
UNAPPROVED PEDS — Preop and antiemetic: 6 mcg/kg/dose IM/IV/SC (max dose 0.3 mg/dose). May repeat q 6 to 8 h. Has also been used in severe drooling.
FORMS — Trade only: Topical disc 1.5 mg/72 h, box of 4. Oral tab 0.4 mg.
NOTES — Dry mouth common. Also causes drowsiness, blurred vision.
MOA — Acetylcholine blockage at parasympathetic sites.
ADVERSE EFFECTS — Frequent: Blurred vision, photophobia.

TRIMETHOBENZAMIDE (*Tigan*) ▶LK ♀C ▶? $
ADULT — N/V: 300 mg PO q 6 to 8 h, 200 mg IM q 6 to 8 h.
PEDS — Not approved for use in children.
UNAPPROVED PEDS — 100 to 200 mg PO q 6 to 8 h if wt 13.6 to 40.9 kg.
FORMS — Generic/Trade: Cap 300 mg.
NOTES — Not for IV use. May cause sedation. Reduce starting dose in the elderly or if reduced renal function to minimize risk of adverse effects.
MOA — Inhibits chemoreceptor trigger zone.
ADVERSE EFFECTS — Frequent: Drowsiness. Severe: EPS.

GASTROENTEROLOGY: Antiulcer—Antacids

ALKA-SELTZER (acetylsalicylic acid + citrate + bicarbonate) ▶LK ♀? (– 3rd trimester) ▶? $
ADULT — Relief of upset stomach: 2 regular-strength tabs in 4 oz water q 4 h PO prn (up to 8 tabs daily for age younger than 60 yo, up to 4 tabs daily for age 60 yo or older) or 2 extra-strength tabs in 4 oz water q 6 h PO prn (up to 7 tabs daily for age younger than 60 yo, up to 3 tabs daily for age 60 yo or older).
PEDS — Not approved in children.
FORMS — OTC Trade only: Regular-strength, original: aspirin 325 mg + citric acid 1000 mg + sodium bicarbonate 1916 mg. Regular-strength lemon lime and cherry: 325 mg + 1000 mg + 1700 mg. Extra-strength: 500 mg + 1000 mg + 1985 mg. Not all forms of Alka-Seltzer contain aspirin (e.g., Alka-Seltzer Heartburn Relief).
NOTES — Avoid aspirin-containing forms in children and teenagers due to risk of Reye's syndrome.
MOA — Antacid.
ADVERSE EFFECTS — Frequent: None. Serious: Sodium content may worsen BP or heart failure; peptic ulcer.

ALUMINUM HYDROXIDE (*Alternagel, Amphojel, Alu-Tab, Alu-Cap,* ✸*Basaljel, Mucaine*) ▶K ♀C ▶? $
ADULT — Hyperphosphatemia in chronic renal failure (short-term treatment only to avoid aluminum accumulation): 300 to 600 mg PO with meals. Titrate prn. Upset stomach, indigestion: 5 to 10 mL or 300 to 600 mg PO 6 times per day, between meals and at bedtime and prn.
PEDS — Not approved in children.
UNAPPROVED ADULT — Symptomatic reflux: 15 to 30 mL PO q 30 to 60 min. Long-term management of reflux disease: 15 to 30 mL PO 1 and 3 h after meals and at bedtime prn. Peptic ulcer disease: 15 to 45 mL or 1 to 3 tab PO 1 and 3 h after meals and at bedtime. Prophylaxis against GI bleeding (titrate dose to maintain gastric pH greater than 3.5): 30 to 60 mL or 2 to 4 tab PO q 1 to 2 h.
UNAPPROVED PEDS — Peptic ulcer disease: 5 to 15 mL PO 1 and 3 h after meals and at bedtime. Prophylaxis against GI bleeding (titrate dose to maintain gastric pH greater than 3.5): Neonates 0.5 to 1 mL/kg/dose PO q 4 h. Infants 2 to 5 mL PO q 1 to 2 h. Child: 5 to 15 mL PO q 1 to 2 h.

(cont.)

ALUMINUM HYDROXIDE (cont.)

FORMS — OTC Generic/Trade: Susp 320, 600 mg/ 5 mL.

NOTES — For concentrated suspensions, use ½ the recommended dose. May cause constipation. Avoid administration with tetracyclines, digoxin, iron, isoniazid, buffered/enteric aspirin, diazepam, fluoroquinolones.

MOA — Antacid.

ADVERSE EFFECTS — Frequent: Constipation, chalky taste, stomach cramps, fecal impaction.

GAVISCON (aluminum hydroxide + magnesium carbonate) ▸K♀? ▶? $

ADULT — 2 to 4 tabs or 15 to 30 mL (regular-strength) or 10 mL (extra-strength) PO four times per day prn.

PEDS — Not approved in children.

UNAPPROVED PEDS — Peptic ulcer disease: 5 to 15 mL PO after meals and at bedtime.

FORMS — OTC Trade only: Tabs: Regular-strength (Al hydroxide 80 mg + magnesium carbonate 20 mg), Extra-strength (Al hydroxide 160 mg + magnesium carbonate 105 mg). Liquid: Regular-strength (Al hydroxide 95 mg + magnesium carbonate 358 mg per 15 mL), Extra-strength (Al hydroxide 254 mg + magnesium carbonate 237.5 mg per 5 mL).

NOTES — Contains alginic acid or sodium alginate, which is considered an "inactive" ingredient. Alginic acid forms foam barrier which floats in stomach to minimize esophageal contact with acid. Chronic use may cause metabolic alkalosis. Contains sodium.

MOA — Antacid, "foam barrier" in stomach to minimize esophageal contact with acid (alginic acid).

ADVERSE EFFECTS — Frequent: Diarrhea, constipation. Serious: Sodium content may worsen BP or heart failure.

MAALOX (aluminum hydroxide + magnesium hydroxide) ▸K♀C ▶? $

ADULT — Heartburn/indigestion: 10 to 20 mL or 1 to 2 tab PO four times per day, after meals and at bedtime and prn.

PEDS — Not approved in children.

UNAPPROVED ADULT — Peptic ulcer disease: 15 to 45 mL PO 1 and 3 h after meals and at bedtime. Symptomatic reflux: 15 to 30 mL PO q 30 to 60 min prn. Long-term management of reflux disease: 15 to 30 mL PO 1 and 3 h after meals and at bedtime prn. Prophylaxis against GI bleeding (titrate dose to maintain gastric pH greater than 3.5): 30 to 60 mL PO q 1 to 2 h.

UNAPPROVED PEDS — Peptic ulcer disease: 5 to 15 mL PO 1 and 3 h after meals and at bedtime. Prophylaxis against GI bleeding (titrate dose to maintain gastric pH greater than 3.5): Neonates 1 mL/kg/dose PO q 4 h. Infants 2 to 5 mL PO q 1 to 2 h. Child: 5 to 15 mL PO q 1 to 2 h.

FORMS — OTC Generic/Trade: Regular-strength chewable tabs (Al hydroxide + magnesium hydroxide 200/200 mg). Susp (225/200 mg per 5 mL). Other strengths available.

NOTES — Maalox Extra Strength and Maalox TC are more concentrated than Maalox. Maalox Plus has added simethicone. May cause constipation or diarrhea. Avoid concomitant administration with tetracyclines, digoxin, iron, isoniazid, buffered/enteric aspirin, diazepam, fluoroquinolones. Avoid chronic use in patients with renal dysfunction due to potential for magnesium accumulation.

MOA — Antacid.

ADVERSE EFFECTS — Frequent: None.

MAGALDRATE (Riopan) ▸K♀C ▶? $

ADULT — Relief of upset stomach: 5 to 10 mL between meals and at bedtime and prn.

PEDS — Younger than 12 yo: not approved. 12 yo or older: 5 to 10 mL between meals and at bedtime and prn.

UNAPPROVED PEDS — Peptic ulcer disease: 5 to 10 mL PO 1 and 3 h after meals and at bedtime.

FORMS — OTC generic: Riopan susp 540/20 mg/5 mL.

NOTES — Avoid concomitant administration with tetracyclines, fluoroquinolones, digoxin, iron, isoniazid, buffered/enteric aspirin, diazepam. Avoid chronic use in patients with renal failure. Brand name Riopan no longer available.

MOA — Antacid.

ADVERSE EFFECTS — Frequent: None.

MYLANTA (aluminum hydroxide + magnesium hydroxide + simethicone) ▸K♀C ▶? $

ADULT — Heartburn/indigestion: 10 to 20 mL between meals and at bedtime.

PEDS — Safe dosing has not been established.

UNAPPROVED ADULT — Peptic ulcer disease: 15 to 45 mL PO 1 and 3 h after meals and at bedtime. Symptomatic reflux: 15 to 30 mL PO q 30 to 60 min. Long-term management of reflux: 15 to 30 mL PO 1 and 3 h postprandially and at bedtime prn.

UNAPPROVED PEDS — Peptic ulcer disease: 5 to 15 mL PO or 0.5 to 2 mL/kg/dose (max 15 mL/dose) after meals and and at bedtime.

FORMS — OTC Generic/Trade: Liquid (various concentrations, e.g., regular-strength, maximum-strength, supreme, etc.).

NOTES — May cause constipation or diarrhea. Avoid concomitant administration with tetracyclines, fluoroquinolones, digoxin, iron, isoniazid, buffered/enteric aspirin, diazepam. Avoid chronic use in renal dysfunction.

MOA — Antacid.

ADVERSE EFFECTS — Frequent: None.

ROLAIDS (calcium carbonate + magnesium hydroxide) ▸K♀? ▶? $

ADULT — 2 to 4 tabs PO q 1 h prn, max 12 tabs/day (regular-strength) or 10 tabs/day (extra-strength).

PEDS — Not approved in children.

FORMS — OTC Trade only: Tabs regular-strength (Ca carbonate 550 mg, magnesium hydroxide 110 mg), extra-strength (Ca carbonate 675 mg, magnesium hydroxide 135 mg).

NOTES — Chronic use may cause metabolic alkalosis.

MOA — Antacid.

ADVERSE EFFECTS — Frequent: None. Serious: None.

GASTROENTEROLOGY: Antiulcer—H2 Antagonists

CIMETIDINE (*Tagamet, Tagamet HB*) ▶LK ♀B ▶+ $

ADULT — Treatment of duodenal or gastric ulcer: 800 mg PO at bedtime or 300 mg PO four times per day with meals and at bedtime or 400 mg PO two times per day. Prevention of duodenal ulcer: 400 mg PO at bedtime. Erosive esophagitis: 800 mg PO two times per day or 400 mg PO four times per day. Prevention or treatment of heartburn (OTC product only approved for this indication): 200 mg PO prn max 400 mg/day for up to 14 days. Hypersecretory conditions: 300 mg PO four times per day with meals and at bedtime. Patients unable to take oral medications: 300 mg IV/IM q 6 to 8 h or 37.5 mg/h continuous IV infusion. Prevention of upper GI bleeding in critically ill patients: 50 mg/h continuous infusion.

PEDS — 16 yo and older: Duodenal ulcer/benign gastric ulcer: 300 mg IV/IM q 6 to 8 h. GI bleed: 50 mg/h IV. Pathological hypersecretory: 300 mg IV/IM q 6 to 8 h.

UNAPPROVED ADULT — Prevention of aspiration pneumonitis during surgery: 300 to 600 mg PO or 200 to 400 mg IV 60 to 90 min prior to anesthesia. Has been used as adjunctive therapy with H1 antagonist for severe allergic reactions.

UNAPPROVED PEDS — Treatment of duodenal or gastric ulcers, erosive esophagitis, hypersecretory conditions: Neonates: 5 to 10 mg/kg/day PO/IV/IM divided q 8 to 12 h. Infants: 10 to 20 mg/kg/day PO/IV/IM divided q 6 h. Children: 20 to 40 mg/kg/day PO/IV/IM divided q 6 h. Chronic viral warts in children: 25 to 40 mg/kg/day PO in divided doses.

FORMS — Tabs 200, 300, 400, 800 mg. Rx Generic only: Oral soln 300 mg/5 mL. OTC Generic/Trade: Tabs 200 mg.

NOTES — May cause dizziness, drowsiness, headache, diarrhea, nausea. Decreased absorption of ketoconazole, itraconazole. Increased levels of carbamazepine, cyclosporine, diazepam, labetalol, lidocaine, theophylline, phenytoin, procainamide, quinidine, propranolol, TCAs, valproic acid, warfarin. Stagger doses of cimetidine and antacids. Decrease dose with CrCl less than 30 mL/min.

MOA — Histamine-2 receptor blocker.

ADVERSE EFFECTS — Frequent: Drowsiness, dizziness, agitation, diarrhea, N/V.

FAMOTIDINE (*Pepcid, Pepcid AC, Maximum Strength Pepcid AC*) ▶LK ♀B ▶? $

ADULT — Treatment of duodenal ulcer: 40 mg PO at bedtime or 20 mg PO two times per day. Maintenance of duodenal ulcer: 20 mg PO at bedtime. Treatment of gastric ulcer: 40 mg PO at bedtime. GERD: 20 mg PO two times per day. Treatment or prevention of heartburn: (OTC product only approved for this indication) 10 to 20 mg PO prn, up to 2 tabs per day. Hypersecretory conditions: 20 mg PO q 6 h. Patients unable to take oral medications: 20 mg IV q 12 h.

PEDS — GERD: 0.5 mg/kg/day PO daily for up to 8 weeks for age younger than 3 mo; 0.5 mg/kg PO two times per day for age 3 to 12 mo; 1 mg/kg/day PO divided two times per day or 2 mg/kg/day PO daily, max 40 mg PO two times per day for age 1 to 16 yo. Peptic ulcer: 0.5 mg/kg/day PO at bedtime or divided two times per day up to 40 mg/day.

UNAPPROVED ADULT — Prevention of aspiration pneumonitis during surgery: 40 mg PO prior to anesthesia. Upper GI bleeding: 20 mg IV q 12 h. Has been used as adjunctive therapy with H1 antagonist for severe allergic reactions.

UNAPPROVED PEDS — Treatment of hypersecretory conditions: 0.25 mg/kg IV q 12 h (max 40 mg daily) or 1 to 1.2 mg/kg/day PO in 2 to 3 divided doses, max 40 mg/day.

FORMS — Generic/Trade: Tabs 10 mg (OTC, Pepcid AC Acid Controller), 20 mg (Rx and OTC, Maximum Strength Pepcid AC), 40 mg. Rx Generic/Trade: Susp 40 mg/5 mL.

NOTES — May cause dizziness, headache, constipation, diarrhea. Decreased absorption of ketoconazole, itraconazole. Adjust dose in patients with CrCl < 50 mL/min.

MOA — Histamine-2 receptor blocker.

ADVERSE EFFECTS — Frequent: Dizziness, headache, nausea. Severe: Convulsion in renal impairment, interstitial pneumonia, Stevens-Johnson syndrome, rhabdomyolysis.

NIZATIDINE (*Axid, Axid AR*) ▶K ♀B ▶? $$$$

ADULT — Treatment of duodenal or gastric ulcer: 300 mg PO at bedtime or 150 mg PO two times per day. Maintenance of duodenal ulcer: 150 mg PO at bedtime. GERD: 150 mg PO two times per day. Treatment or prevention of heartburn: (OTC product only approved for this indication) 75 mg PO prn, max 150 mg/day.

PEDS — Esophagitis, GERD: 150 mg PO two times per day for age 12 yo or older.

UNAPPROVED ADULT — Has been used as adjunctive therapy with H1 antagonist for severe allergic reactions.

UNAPPROVED PEDS — 6 mo to 11 yo (limited data): 5 to 10 mg/kg/day PO in 2 divided doses.

FORMS — OTC (Axid AR): Tabs 75 mg. Rx Generic: Caps 150 mg. Oral soln 15 mg/mL (120, 480 mL). Caps 300 mg.

NOTES — May cause dizziness, headache, constipation, diarrhea. Decrease absorption of ketoconazole, itraconazole. Adjust dose if CrCl less than 50 mL/min.

MOA — Histamine-2 receptor blocker.

ADVERSE EFFECTS — Frequent: Dizziness, headache, nausea, constipation.

PEPCID COMPLETE (**famotidine + calcium carbonate + magnesium hydroxide**) ▶LK ♀B ▶? $

ADULT — Treatment of heartburn: 1 tab PO prn. Max 2 tabs/day.

PEDS — Not approved in children younger than 12 yo. In children 12 yo or older, use adult dosing for OTC product.

FORMS — OTC trade/generic: Chewable tab, famotidine 10 mg with calcium carbonate 800 mg and magnesium hydroxide 165 mg.

PEPCID COMPLETE *(cont.)*

MOA — Histamine-2 receptor blocker, antacid.

ADVERSE EFFECTS — Frequent: Dizziness, headache, nausea.

RANITIDINE (*Zantac, Zantac Efferdose, Zantac 75, Zantac 150, Peptic Relief*) ▸K ♀B ▶? $$$

ADULT — Treatment of duodenal ulcer: 150 mg PO two times per day or 300 mg at bedtime. Treatment of gastric ulcer or GERD: 150 mg PO two times per day. Maintenance of duodenal or gastric ulcer: 150 mg PO at bedtime. Treatment of erosive esophagitis: 150 mg PO four times per day. Maintenance of erosive esophagitis: 150 mg PO two times per day. Prevention/treatment of heartburn: (OTC product only approved for this indication) 75 to 150 mg PO prn, max 300 mg/day. Hypersecretory conditions: 150 mg PO two times per day. Patients unable to take oral meds: 50 mg IV/IM q 6 to 8 h or 6.25 mg/h continuous IV infusion.

PEDS — Treatment of duodenal or gastric ulcers: 2 to 4 mg/kg PO two times per day (max 300 mg) or 2 to 4 mg/kg/day IV q 6 to 8 h for ages 1 mo to 16 yo. GERD, erosive esophagitis: 2.5 to 5 mg/kg PO two times per day (max 200 mg/day) or 2 to 4 mg/kg/day IV divided q 6 to 8 h (max 200 mg/day). Maintenance of duodenal or gastric ulcers: 2 to 4 mg/kg/day PO daily (max 150 mg).

UNAPPROVED ADULT — Prevention of upper GI bleeding in critically ill patients: 6.25 mg/h continuous IV infusion (150 mg/day). Has been used as adjunctive therapy with H1 antagonist for severe allergic reactions.

UNAPPROVED PEDS — Treatment of duodenal or gastric ulcers, GERD, hypersecretory conditions: Premature and term infants younger than 2 weeks of age: 1 mg/kg/day PO two times per day or 1.5 mg/kg IV for one dose then 12 h later 0.75 to 1 mg/kg IV q 12 h. Continuous infusion 1.5 mg/kg for 1 dose then 0.04 to 0.08 mg/kg/h infusion. Neonates: 1 to 2 mg/kg PO two times per day or 2 mg/kg/24 h IV divided q 12 h. Infants and children: 2 to 4 mg/kg/24 h IV/IM divided q 6 to 12 h or 1 mg/kg IV loading dose followed by 0.08 to 0.17 mg/kg/h continuous IV infusion.

FORMS — Generic/Trade: Tabs 75 mg (OTC: Zantac 75), 150 mg (OTC and Rx: Zantac 150), 300 mg. Syrup 75 mg/5 mL. Rx Trade only: Effervescent tabs 25 mg. Rx Generic only: Caps 150, 300 mg.

NOTES — May cause dizziness, sedation, headache, drowsiness, rash, nausea, constipation, diarrhea. Elevations in SGPT have been observed when H2-antagonists have been administered IV greater-than-recommended dosages for 5 days or longer. Bradycardia can occur if the IV form is injected too rapidly. Variable effects on warfarin, decreased absorption of ketoconazole, itraconazole. Dissolve effervescent tabs in water. Stagger doses of ranitidine and antacids. Adjust dose in patients with CrCl less than 50 mL/min.

MOA — Histamine-2 receptor blocker.

ADVERSE EFFECTS — Frequent: Dizziness, headache, nausea, constipation, taste changes, stool or tongue darkening.

GASTROENTEROLOGY: Antiulcer—Helicobacter pylori Treatment

PREVPAC (lansoprazole + amoxicillin + clarithromycin, *★HP-Pac*) ▸LK ♀C ▶? $$$$$

ADULT — Active duodenal ulcer associated with H. pylori: 1 dose PO two times per day for 10 to 14 days.

PEDS — Not approved in children.

FORMS — Generic/Trade: Each dose consists of lansoprazole 30 mg cap + amoxicillin 1 g (2 × 500 mg cap), + clarithromycin 500 mg tab.

NOTES — See components.

MOA — Antimicrobial treatment for Helicobacter pylori.

ADVERSE EFFECTS — See components. Frequent: Diarrhea, headache, altered taste. Severe: Colitis, hypersensitivity reactions such as serum-sickness-like reactions, erythema multiforme, Stevens-Johnson syndrome, and exfoliative dermatitis, hepatic dysfunction, hemolytic anemia.

PYLERA (bismuth subcitrate potassium + metronidazole + tetracycline) ▸LK ♀D ▶– $$$$$

ADULT — Duodenal ulcer associated with H. pylori: 3 caps PO four times per day (after meals and at bedtime) for 10 days. To be given with omeprazole 20 mg PO two times per day.

PEDS — Not approved in children.

FORMS — Trade only: Each cap contains bismuth subcitrate potassium 140 mg + metronidazole 125 mg + tetracycline 125 mg.

NOTES — See components.

MOA — Antimicrobial treatment for Helicobacter pylori.

ADVERSE EFFECTS — Frequent: Diarrhea, headache, altered taste. Severe: Colitis, hypersensitivity reactions such as serum-sickness, erythema multiforme, Stevens-Johnson syndrome, and exfoliative dermatitis; hepatic dysfunction, hemolytic anemia.

GASTROENTEROLOGY: Antiulcer—Proton Pump Inhibitors

DEXLANSOPRAZOLE (*Dexilant*) ▸L ♀B ▶-

ADULT — Healing of erosive esophagitis: 60 mg PO once daily for up to 8 weeks. Maintenance of erosive esophagitis: 30 mg PO once daily for up to 6 months. Symptomatic non-erosive GERD: 30 mg PO once daily for 4 weeks.

PEDS — Not approved in children younger than 18 years.

FORMS — Rx: Cap 30 mg, 60 mg.

NOTES — Take without regard tp meals. Many drug interactions. Capsule can be opened and mixed with applesauce or water.

(cont.)

DEXLANSOPRAZOLE (cont.)

MOA — Na-K-ATPase inhibitor

ADVERSE EFFECTS — Frequent: diarrhea, abdominal pain, nausea, upper respiratory tract infection, vomiting, and flatulence.. Severe: Pancreatitis, severe skin reactions, hypersensitivity.

ESOMEPRAZOLE (Nexium) ▶L ♀B ▪? $$$$$

ADULT — Erosive esophagitis: 20 to 40 mg PO daily for 4 to 8 weeks. Maintenance of erosive esophagitis: 20 mg PO daily. Zollinger-Ellison: 40 mg PO two times per day. GERD: 20 mg PO daily for 4 weeks. Prevention of NSAID–associated gastric ulcer: 20 to 40 mg PO daily for up to 6 months. H. pylori eradication: 40 mg PO daily with amoxicillin 1000 mg PO two times per day and clarithromycin 500 mg PO two times per day for 10 days.

PEDS — GERD: wt less than 20 kg: 10 mg PO daily; wt 20 kg or more: 10 to 20 mg daily. Alternatively, 2.5 mg (for 3 kg to 5 kg), 5 mg (for 5.1 kg to 7.5 kg), or 10 mg (for 7.6 kg to 12 kg) PO once daily for up to 6 weeks for ages 1 month to less than 1 year, 10 to 20 mg PO daily for up to 8 weeks for age 1 to 11 yo, 20 to 40 mg PO daily for up to 8 weeks for age 12 to 17 yo.

FORMS — Rx/Trade only: Caps, delayed-release 20, 40 mg. Delayed-release granules for oral susp 2.5, 5, 10, 40 mg per packet. OTC/Trade: Caps, delayed-release 20 mg.

NOTES — Concomitant administration with voriconazole, an inhibitor of CYP2C19 and CYP3A4 may lead to a more than doubling of esomeprazole exposure. Esomeprazole may reduce the efficacy of clopidogrel. Use caution with high dose methotrexate. May increase serum chromogranin A levels iwhich may cause false positive results in diagnostic investigations for neuroendocrine tumors.

MOA — H-K ATPase proton pump inhibitor.

ADVERSE EFFECTS — Frequent: Headache, dizziness, rash, diarrhea, N/V, taste perversion. Severe: Anaphylaxis, toxic epidermal necrolysis, Stevens-Johnson syndrome, erythema multiforme, pancreatitis, hepatitis.

LANSOPRAZOLE (Prevacid) ▶L ♀B ▪? $$$$

ADULT — Heartburn: 15 mg PO daily. Erosive esophagitis: 30 mg PO daily for 4 weeks or 30 mg IV daily for 7 days or until taking PO. Maintenance therapy following healing of erosive esophagitis: 15 mg PO daily. NSAID–induced gastric ulcer: 30 mg PO daily for 8 weeks (treatment), 15 mg PO daily for up to 12 weeks (prevention). GERD: 15 mg PO daily for up to 8 weeks. Duodenal ulcer treatment and maintenance: 15 mg PO daily. Gastric ulcer: 30 mg PO daily for up to 8 weeks. Part of a multidrug regimen for H. pylori eradication: 30 mg PO two times per day with amoxicillin 1000 mg PO two times per day and clarithromycin 500 mg PO two times per day for 10 to 14 days (see table) or 30 mg PO three times per day with amoxicillin 1000 mg PO three times per day for 14 days. Hypersecretory conditions: 60 mg PO daily.

PEDS — Not effective in patients with symptomatic GERD age 1 mo to younger than 1 year of age. Esophagitis and GERD: 1 to 11 years, less than 30 kg: 15 mg PO daily up to 12 weeks; 12 to 17 years, 30 kg or greater: 30 mg PO daily up to 12 weeks.

FORMS — OTC Generic/Trade: Caps 15 mg. Rx Generic/Trade: 15, 30 mg. Rx Trade only: Orally disintegrating tab 15, 30 mg.

NOTES — Take before meals. Potential for PPIs to reduce the response to clopidogrel. Evaluate the need for a PPI in clopidogrel-treated patients and consider H2-blocker/antacid. Orally disintegrating tabs can be dissolved water (15 mg tab in 4 mL, 30 mg tab in 10 mL) and administered via an oral syringe or nasogastric tube at least 8 French within 15 min. Delayed-release orally disintegrating tabs should not be broken or cut.

MOA — H-K ATPase proton pump inhibitor.

ADVERSE EFFECTS — Frequent: fatigue, dizziness, headache, abdominal pain, diarrhea, nausea, increased appetite. Severe: Pancreatitis, severe skin reactions, myositis, interstitial nephritis.

OMEPRAZOLE (Prilosec, ✦Losec) ▶L ♀C ▪? OTC $, Rx $$$$

WARNING — Serum chromogranin A levels increase and may cause false positive results in diagnostic investigations for neuroendocrine tumors.

ADULT — GERD, duodenal ulcer, erosive esophagitis: 20 mg PO daily. Heartburn (OTC): 20 mg PO daily for 14 days. Gastric ulcer: 40 mg PO daily. Hypersecretory conditions: 60 mg PO daily. Part of a multidrug regimen for H. pylori eradication: 20 mg PO two times per day with amoxicillin 1000 mg PO two times per day and clarithromycin 500 mg PO two times per day for 10 day, with additional 18 days of omeprazole 20 mg PO daily if ulcer present (see table). Or 40 mg PO daily with clarithromycin 500 mg PO three times per day for 14 days, with additional 14 days of omeprazole 20 mg PO daily if ulcer present.

PEDS — GERD, acid-related disorders, maintenance of healing erosive esophagitis in children 1-16 yo: 5 mg PO daily for wt 5 to 9 kg, 10 mg PO daily for wt 10 to 19 kg, give 20 mg PO daily for wt 20 kg or greater.

UNAPPROVED PEDS — Gastric or duodenal ulcers, hypersecretory states: 0.2 to 3.5 mg/kg/dose PO daily. GERD: 1 mg/kg/day PO one or two times per day.

FORMS — Rx Generic/Trade: Caps 10, 20, 40 mg. Trade only: Granules for oral susp 2.5 mg, 10 mg. OTC Trade only: Cap 20 mg.

NOTES — Take before meals. Caps contain enteric-coated granules; do not chew. Caps may be opened and administered in acidic liquid (e.g., apple juice) or 1 tablespoon of applesauce. May increase levels of diazepam, warfarin, and phenytoin. May decrease absorption of ketoconazole, itraconazole, iron, ampicillin, and digoxin. Reduces plasma levels of atazanavir. Concomitant administration with voriconazole, an inhibitor of

OMEPRAZOLE (cont.)

CYP2C19 and CYP3A4 may lead to a more than doubling of omeprazole exposure. Avoid administration with sucralfate. Use caution with high dose methotrexate. Omeprazole may reduce the efficacy of clopidogrel.

MOA — H-K ATPase proton pump inhibitor.

ADVERSE EFFECTS — Frequent: Headache, dizziness, rash, diarrhea, N/V, taste perversion. Severe: Stevens-Johnson syndrome, erythema multiforme, stomatitis, agitation, pancytopenia, agranulocytosis, other blood dyscrasias, pancreatitis, psychiatric disturbances.

PANTOPRAZOLE (Protonix, ✦Pantoloc, Tecta) ▶L ♀B ▶? $

ADULT — Treatment of erosive esophagitis associated with GERD: 40 mg PO daily for 8 to 16 weeks. Maintenance of erosive esophagitis: 40 mg PO once daily. Zollinger-Ellison syndrome and other hypersecretory conditions: 40 mg PO twice daily or 80 mg IV q 8 to 12 h for 7 days until taking PO.

PEDS — Erosive esophagitis associated with GERD, 5 years or older: 15 kg to less than 40 kg: 20 mg PO daily for up to 8 weeks. 40 kg or greater: 40 mg PO daily for up to 8 weeks.

UNAPPROVED ADULT — Has been studied as part of various multidrug regimens for H. pylori eradication. Reduce peptic ulcer re-bleeding after hemostasis: 80 mg IV bolus, then 8 mg/h continuous IV infusion for 3 days, followed by oral therapy (or 40 mg IV q 12 h for 4 to 7 days if unable to tolerate PO).

UNAPPROVED PEDS — GERD associated with a history of erosive esophagitis: 0.5 to 1 mg/kg/day (max 40 mg/day).

FORMS — Generic/Trade: Tabs 20, 40 mg. Trade only: Granules for susp 40 mg/packet.

NOTES — Use caution with high dose methotrexate. Do not co-administer with atazanavir or nelfinavir. Concomitant warfarin use may require monitoring. May interfere with the absorption of drugs where gastric pH is important for bioavailability.

MOA — H-K ATPase proton pump inhibitor.

ADVERSE EFFECTS — Frequent: Headache. Serious: rhabdomyolysis, anaphylaxis, angioedema, severe dermatologic reactions, hepatocellular damage, interstitial nephritis, pancreatitis, pancytopenia, agranulocytosis.

RABEPRAZOLE (AcipHex, ✦Pariet) ▶L ♀B ▶? $$$$

ADULT — GERD: 20 mg PO daily for 4 to 16 weeks. Duodenal ulcers: 20 mg PO daily for 4 weeks. Zollinger-Ellison syndrome: 60 mg PO daily, may increase up to 100 mg daily or 60 mg two times per day. Part of a multidrug regimen for H. pylori eradication: 20 mg PO two times per day, with amoxicillin 1000 mg PO two times per day and clarithromycin 500 mg PO two times per day for 7 days.

PEDS — GERD: Children 1 yo to 11 yo: less than 15 kg: 5 mg PO once daily, may increase to 10 mg; 15 kg or greater: 10 mg PO once daily. Children 12 yo or older: 20 mg PO daily up to 8 weeks.

FORMS — Generic/Trade: Tabs 20 mg. Trade only: Sprinkle caps (open and sprinkle on soft food or liquid) 5 mg and 10 mg.

NOTES — Does not appear to interact with clopidogrel.

MOA — H-K ATPase proton pump inhibitor.

ADVERSE EFFECTS — Frequent: Headache. Serious: rhabdomyolysis, anaphylaxis, angioedema, severe dermatologic reactions, hepatocellular damage, interstitial nephritis, pancreatitis, pancytopenia.

ZEGERID (omeprazole + bicarbonate) ▶L ♀C ▶? $$$$$

ADULT — Duodenal ulcer, GERD, erosive esophagitis: 20 mg PO daily for 4 to 8 weeks. Gastric ulcer: 40 mg PO once daily for 4 to 8 weeks. Reduction of risk of upper GI bleed in critically ill (susp only): 40 mg PO, then 40 mg 6 to 8 h later, then 40 mg once daily thereafter for up to 14 days.

PEDS — Not approved in children.

FORMS — OTC Trade only: omeprazole/sodium bicarbonate caps 20 mg/1.1 g. Rx Generic/Trade: caps 20 mg/1.1 g and 40 mg/1.1 g. Trade only: powder packets for susp 20 mg/1.1 g and 40 mg/1.68 g.

NOTES — Omeprazole may reduce the efficacy of clopidogrel. Serum chromogranin A levels increase and may cause false positive results in diagnostic investigations for neuroendocrine tumors.

MOA — H-K ATPase proton pump inhibitor plus antacid combination.

ADVERSE EFFECTS — Frequent: Headache, dizziness, rash, diarrhea, N/V, taste perversion. Severe: Stevens-Johnson syndrome, erythema multiforme, stomatitis, agitation, pancytopenia, agranulocytosis, other blood dyscrasias, pancreatitis, psychiatric disturbances.

GASTROENTEROLOGY: Antiulcer—Other

DICYCLOMINE (Bentyl, ✦Bentylol) ▶LK ♀B ▶– $

WARNING — May cause psychosis or delirium, especially in elderly or those with pre-existing psychiatric disease.

ADULT — Treatment of functional bowel/irritable bowel syndrome (irritable colon, spastic colon, mucous colon): Initiate with 20 mg PO four times per day and increase to 40 mg PO four times per day, if tolerated. Patients who are unable to take oral medications: 20 mg IM q 6 h.

PEDS — Not approved in children.

UNAPPROVED PEDS — Treatment of functional/irritable bowel syndrome: Infants 6 mo or older: 5 mg PO three to four times per day. Children: 10 mg PO three to four times per day.

FORMS — Generic/Trade: Tabs 20 mg. Caps 10 mg.

NOTES — Although some use lower doses (i.e., 10 to 20 mg PO four times per day), the only adult oral dose proven to be effective is 160 mg/day.

MOA — Inhibits effect of acetylcholine at parasympathetic receptors.

(cont.)

DICYCLOMINE (*cont.*)

ADVERSE EFFECTS — Frequent: None specific but generally similar to other anticholinergic drugs.

DONNATAL (**phenobarbital + hyoscyamine + atropine + scopolamine**) ▶LK ♀C ▶– $$$

ADULT — Adjunctive therapy of irritable bowel syndrome or adjunctive treatment of duodenal ulcers: 1 to 2 tabs/caps or 5 to 10 mL PO three to four times per day or 1 extended-release tab PO q 8 to 12 h.

PEDS — Adjunctive therapy of irritable bowel syndrome, adjunctive treatment of duodenal ulcers: 0.1 mL/kg/dose q 4 h, max 5 mL. Alternative dosing regimen: Give 0.5 mL PO q 4 h or 0.75 mL PO q 6 h for wt 4.5 kg, give 1 mL PO q 4 h or 1.5 mL PO q 6 h for wt 9.1 kg, give 1.5 mL PO q 4 h or 2 mL PO q 6 h for wt 13.6 kg, give 2.5 mL PO q 4 h or 3.75 mL PO q 6 h for wt 22.7 kg, give 3.75 mL PO q 4 h or 5 mL PO q 6 h for wt 34 kg, give 5 mL PO q 4 h or 7.5 mL PO q 6 h for wt 45 kg or greater.

FORMS — Generic/trade: Phenobarbital 16.2 mg + hyoscyamine 0.1 mg + atropine 0.02 mg + scopolamine 6.5 mcg in each tab or 5 mL. Trade only: Extended-release tab, 48.6 + 0.3111 + 0.0582 + 0.0195 mg.

NOTES — The FDA has classified Donnatal as "possibly effective" for treatment of irritable bowel syndrome and duodenal ulcer. Heat stroke may occur in hot weather. Can cause anticholinergic side effects; use caution in narrow-angle glaucoma, BPH, etc.

MOA — Anticonvulsant, inhibits effect of acetylcholine at parasympathetic receptors.

ADVERSE EFFECTS — Frequent: xerostomia, blurred vision, urinary retention and hesitancy, N/V, dizziness.

GI COCKTAIL (***green goddess***) ▶LK ♀See individual ▶See individual $

ADULT — See components.

PEDS — Not approved in children.

UNAPPROVED ADULT — Acute GI upset: Mixture of Maalox/Mylanta 30 mL + viscous lidocaine (2%) 10 mL + Donnatal 10 mL administered PO in a single dose.

NOTES — Avoid repeat dosing due to risk of lidocaine toxicity.

MOA — Antacid, anesthetic, anti-spasmodic.

ADVERSE EFFECTS — Frequent: None. Severe: Lidocaine toxicity with repeat dosing.

HYOSCINE (✱*Buscopan*) ▶LK ♀C ▶? $$

ADULT — Canada: GI or bladder spasm: 10 to 20 mg PO/IV up to 60 mg daily (PO) or 100 mg daily (IV).

PEDS — Not approved in children.

FORMS — Canada Trade only: Tabs 10 mg.

NOTES — May cause dizziness, drowsiness, blurred vision, dry mouth, N/V, urinary retention. Contraindicated in glaucoma, obstructive conditions (e.g., pyloric, duodenal or other intestinal obstructive lesions, ileus, and obstructive uropathies), and myasthenia gravis.

MOA — Anticholinergic that counteracts urinary and GI smooth muscle contraction.

ADVERSE EFFECTS — Serious: Heat stroke, paralytic ileus, increased ocular pressure, psychosis, anaphylaxis. Frequent: Dry mouth, urinary retention, constipation, headache, dizziness, drowsiness, fever, weakness, impotence, suppressed lactation, confusion, blurred vision, tachycardia, palpitations, anhidrosis, mydriasis, cycloplegia, loss of taste.

HYOSCYAMINE (*Anaspaz, A-spaz, Cystospaz, ED Spaz, Hyosol, Hyospaz, Levbid, Levsin, Levsinex, Medispaz, NuLev, Spacol, Spasdel, Symax*) ▶LK ♀C ▶– $

ADULT — Bladder spasm, control gastric secretion, GI hypermotility, irritable bowel syndrome: 0.125 to 0.25 mg PO/SL q 4 h or prn. Extended-release 0.375 to 0.75 mg PO q 12 h. Max 1.5 mg/day.

PEDS — Bladder spasm: Use adult dosing in age older than 12 yo. To control gastric secretion, GI hypermotility, irritable bowel syndrome, and others: Initial oral dose by wt for age younger than 2 yo: give 12.5 mcg for 2.3 kg, give 16.7 mcg for 3.4 kg, give 20.8 mcg for 5 kg, give 25 mcg for 7 kg, give 31.3 to 33.3 mcg for 10 kg, give 45.8 mcg for 15 kg. Alternatively, if age younger than 2 yo: 3 gtts for wt 2.3 kg, give 4 gtts for 3.4 kg, give 5 gtts for 5 kg, give 6 gtts for 7 kg, give 8 gtts for 10 kg, give 11 gtts for 15 kg. Doses can be repeated q 4 h prn, but maximum daily dose is six times initial dose. Initial oral dose by wt for age 2 to 12 yo: give 31.3 to 33.3 mcg for 10 kg, give 62.5 mcg for 20 kg, give 93.8 mcg for 40 kg, and give 125 mcg for 50 kg. Doses may be repeated q 4 h, but maximum daily dose should not exceed 750 mcg.

FORMS — Generic/Trade: Tabs 0.125. Sublingual tabs 0.125 mg. Chewable tabs 0.125 mg. Extended-release tabs 0.375 mg. Elixir 0.125 mg/5 mL. Gtts 0.125 mg/1 mL.

NOTES — May cause dizziness, drowsiness, blurred vision, dry mouth, N/V, urinary retention. Contraindicated in glaucoma, obstructive conditions (e.g., pyloric, duodenal or other intestinal obstructive lesions, ileus, achalasia, GI hemorrhage, and obstructive uropathies), unstable cardiovascular status, and myasthenia gravis.

MOA — Anticholinergic that counteracts urinary and GI smooth muscle contraction.

ADVERSE EFFECTS — Serious: Heat stroke, paralytic ileus, increased ocular pressure, psychosis. Frequent: Dry mouth, urinary retention, constipation, headache, dizziness, drowsiness, fever, weakness, impotence, suppressed lactation, confusion, blurred vision, tachycardia, palpitations, anhidrosis, mydriasis, cycloplegia, loss of taste.

MEPENZOLATE (*Cantil*) ▶K + gut ♀B ▶? $$$$$

ADULT — Adjunctive therapy in peptic ulcer disease: 25 to 50 mg PO four times per day, with meals and at bedtime.

PEDS — Not approved in children.

(cont.)

MEPENZOLATE (*cont.*)

FORMS — Trade only: Tabs 25 mg.

NOTES — Contraindicated in glaucoma, obstructive uropathy, paralytic ileus, toxic megacolon, obstructive diseases of GI tract, intestinal atony in elderly/debilitated, myasthenia gravis, unstable CV status, acute GI bleed.

MOA — Post-ganglionic parasympathetic inhibitor.

ADVERSE EFFECTS — Frequent: Drowsiness, blurred vision, constipation, headache, dry mouth, urinary retention, tachycardia.

MISOPROSTOL (*PGE1, Cytotec*) ▶LK ♀X ▶– $$$$

WARNING — Contraindicated in desired early or pre-term pregnancy due to its abortifacient property. Pregnant women should avoid contact/exposure to the tabs. Uterine rupture reported with use for labor induction and medical abortion.

ADULT — Prevention of NSAID–induced gastric ulcers: 200 mcg PO four times per day. If not tolerated, use 100 mcg PO four times per day.

PEDS — Not approved in children.

UNAPPROVED ADULT — Cervical ripening and labor induction: 25 mcg intravaginally q 3 to 6 h (or 50 mcg q 6 h). First-trimester pregnancy failure: 800 mcg intravaginally, repeat on day 3 if expulsion incomplete. Medical abortion 63 days gestation or less: With mifepristone, see mifepristone; with methotrexate: 800 mcg intravaginally 5 to 7 days after 50 mg/m² IM methotrexate. Pre-op cervical ripening: 400 mcg intravaginally 3 to 4 h before mechanical cervical dilation. Postpartum hemorrhage: 400 mcg to 600 mcg PO or PR single dose. Treatment of duodenal ulcers: 100 mcg to 200 mcg PO four times per day. Alternatively, 400 mcg PO twice daily has been tried.

UNAPPROVED PEDS — Improvement in fat absorption in cystic fibrosis in children 8 to 16 yo: 100 mcg PO four times per day.

FORMS — Generic/Trade: Oral tabs 100, 200 mcg.

NOTES — Contraindicated with prior C-section. Oral tabs can be inserted into the vagina for labor induction/cervical ripening. Monitor for uterine hyperstimulation and abnormal fetal heart rate. Risk factors for uterine rupture: Prior uterine surgery and 5 previous pregnancies or more.

MOA — Prostaglandin E1 analog, uterine stimulant.

ADVERSE EFFECTS — Serious: Uterine hyperstimulation, uterine rupture. Frequent: Diarrhea, abdominal pain.

PROPANTHELINE (*Pro-Banthine*) ▶LK ♀C ▶– $$$

ADULT — Adjunctive therapy in peptic ulcer disease: 7.5 to 15 mg PO 30 min before meals and 30 mg at bedtime.

PEDS — Not approved in children.

UNAPPROVED ADULT — Irritable bowel, pancreatitis, urinary bladder spasms: 7.5 to 15 mg PO three times per day and 30 mg at bedtime.

UNAPPROVED PEDS — Antisecretory effects: 1 to 2 mg/kg/day PO in 3 to 4 divided doses. Antispasmodic

effects: 2 to 3 mg/kg/day PO divided q 4 to 6 h and at bedtime.

FORMS — Generic only: Tabs 15 mg.

NOTES — For elderly adults and those with small stature use 7.5 mg dose. May cause constipation, dry mucous membranes.

MOA — Antispasmodic.

ADVERSE EFFECTS — Frequent: None

SIMETHICONE (*Mylicon, Gas-X, Phazyme, ✱Ovol*) ▶not absorbed ♀C but + ▶? $

ADULT — Excessive gas in GI tract: 40 to 360 mg PO after meals and at bedtime prn, max 500 mg/day.

PEDS — Excessive gas in GI tract: 20 mg PO four times per day prn, max 240 mg/day for age younger than 2 yo, 40 mg PO four times per day prn for age 2 to 12 yo (max 500 mg/day).

UNAPPROVED PEDS — Although used to treat infant colic (in approved dose for gas), several studies suggest no benefit.

FORMS — OTC Generic/Trade: Chewable tabs 80, 125 mg. Gtts 40 mg/0.6 mL. Trade only: Softgels 166 mg (Gas-X) 180 mg (Phazyme). Strips, oral (Gas-X) 62.5 mg (adults), 40 mg (children).

NOTES — For administration to infants, may mix dose in 30 mL of liquid. Chewable tabs should be chewed thoroughly.

MOA — Theoretically, relieves gas pressure and bloating.

ADVERSE EFFECTS — Frequent: None.

SUCRALFATE (*Carafate, ✱Sulcrate*) ▶not absorbed ♀B ▶? $$

ADULT — Duodenal ulcer: 1 g PO four times per day, 1 h before meals and at bedtime. Maintenance therapy of duodenal ulcer: 1 g PO two times per day.

PEDS — Not approved in children.

UNAPPROVED ADULT — Gastric ulcer, reflux esophagitis, NSAID–induced GI symptoms, stress ulcer prophylaxis: 1 g PO four times per day 1 h before meals and at bedtime. Oral and esophageal ulcers due to radiation/chemo/sclerotherapy: (susp only) 5 to 10 mL swish and spit/swallow four times per day.

UNAPPROVED PEDS — Reflux esophagitis, gastric or duodenal ulcer, stress ulcer prophylaxis: 40 to 80 mg/kg/day PO divided q 6 h. Alternative dosing: 500 mg PO four times per day for age younger than 6 yo, give 1 g PO four times per day for age 6 yo or older.

FORMS — Generic/Trade: Tabs 1 g. Susp 1 g/10 mL.

NOTES — May cause constipation. May reduce the absorption of cimetidine, ciprofloxacin, digoxin, ketoconazole, levothyroxine, itraconazole, norfloxacin, phenytoin, ranitidine, tetracycline, theophylline and warfarin; separate doses by at least 2 h. Antacids should be separated by at least 30 min. Hyperglycemia has been reported in patients with diabetes.

MOA — Forms synthetic barrier against peptic acid.

ADVERSE EFFECTS — Frequent: Constipation. Severe: hypersensitivity reactions.

GASTROENTEROLOGY: Laxatives—Bulk-Forming

METHYLCELLULOSE (*Citrucel*) ▶not absorbed ♀+ ▶? $
ADULT —Laxative: 1 heaping tablespoon in 8 oz cold water PO daily (up to three times per day).
PEDS —Laxative: Age 6 to 12 yo: 1½ heaping teaspoons in 4 oz cold water daily (up to three times per day) PO prn.
FORMS — OTC Trade only: Regular and sugar-free packets and multiple-use canisters, Clear-mix soln, Caplets 500 mg.
NOTES — Must be taken with water to avoid esophageal obstruction or choking.
MOA — Osmotic effect in intestinal lumen.
ADVERSE EFFECTS — Frequent: None.
POLYCARBOPHIL (*FiberCon, Konsyl Fiber, Equalactin*) ▶not absorbed ♀+ ▶? $
ADULT —Laxative: 2 tabs (1250 mg) PO four times per day prn.
PEDS —Laxative: 6 to 12 years: 625 mg PO up to four times per day prn; 12 years or older: 2 tabs (1250 mg) PO four times per day prn.
UNAPPROVED ADULT — Diarrhea: 2 tabs (1250 mg) PO q 30 min prn. Max daily dose 6 g.
UNAPPROVED PEDS —Diarrhea: 500 mg PO q 30 min prn (up to 1 g polycarbophil/day for age 3 to 5 yo, and 2 g/day for age older than 6 yo).
FORMS — OTC Generic/Trade: Tabs/Caps 625 mg. OTC Trade only: Chewable tabs 625 mg (Equalactin).
NOTES — When used as a laxative, take dose with at least 8 oz of fluid. Do not administer concomitantly with tetracycline; separate by at least 2 h.

MOA — Bulk-forming laxatives.
ADVERSE EFFECTS — Frequent: None. Severe: Esophageal obstruction, hypersensitivity.
PSYLLIUM (*Metamucil, Fiberall, Konsyl, Hydrocil*) ▶not absorbed ♀+ ▶? $
ADULT —Laxative: 1 rounded tsp in liquid, 1 packet in liquid or 1 wafer with liquid PO daily (up to three times per day).
PEDS —Laxative (children 6 to 11 yo): ½ to 1 rounded tsp in liquid, ½ to 1 packet in liquid or 1 wafer with liquid PO daily (up to three times per day).
UNAPPROVED ADULT — Reduction in cholesterol: 1 rounded tsp in liquid, 1 packet in liquid or 1 to 2 wafers with liquid PO three times per day. Prevention of GI side effects with orlistat: 6 g in liquid with each orlistat dose or 12 g in liquid at bedtime.
FORMS — OTC Generic/Trade: Regular and sugar-free powder, Granules, Caps, Wafers, including various flavors and various amounts of psyllium.
NOTES — Powders and granules must be mixed with 8 oz water/liquid prior to ingestion. Start with 1 dose/day and gradually increase to minimize gas and bloating. Can bind with warfarin, digoxin, potassium-sparing diuretics, salicylates, tetracycline and nitrofurantoin; space at least 3 h apart.
MOA — Adsorbs water to bulk stool.
ADVERSE EFFECTS — Frequent: None. Severe: Bronchospasm, anaphylaxis.

GASTROENTEROLOGY: Laxatives—Osmotic

GLYCERIN (*Fleet*) ▶not absorbed ♀C ▶? $
ADULT — Constipation: 1 adult suppository or 5 mL to 15 mL as an enema PR prn.
PEDS — Constipation: 0.5 mL/kg/dose as an enema PR prn in neonates, 1 infant suppository or 2 to 5 mL rectal soln as an enema PR prn for age younger than 6 yo, 1 adult suppository or 5 to 15 mL of rectal soln as enema PR prn for age 6 yo or older.
FORMS — OTC Generic/Trade: Supp, infant and adult. Soln (Fleet Babylax) 4 mL/applicator.
MOA — Softens and lubricates stool.
ADVERSE EFFECTS — Frequent: None.
LACTULOSE (*Enulose, Kristalose*) ▶not absorbed ♀B ▶? $$
ADULT — Constipation: 15 to 30 mL (syrup) or 10 to 20 g (powder for oral soln) PO daily. Evacuation of barium following barium procedures: 15 to 30 mL (syrup) PO daily, may increase to 60 mL. Acute hepatic encephalopathy: 30 to 45 mL syrup/dose PO q 1 h until laxative effect observed or 300 mL in 700 mL water or saline PR as a retention enema q 4 to 6 h. Prevention of encephalopathy: 30 to 45 mL syrup PO three to four times per day.
PEDS — Prevention or treatment of encephalopathy: Infants: 2.5 to 10 mL/day (syrup) PO in 3 to 4

divided doses. Children/adolescents: 40 to 90 mL/day (syrup) PO in 3 to 4 divided doses.
UNAPPROVED ADULT — Restoration of bowel movements in hemorrhoidectomy patients: 15 mL syrup PO two times per day on days before surgery and for 5 days following surgery.
UNAPPROVED PEDS —Constipation: 7.5 mL syrup PO daily, after breakfast.
FORMS — Generic/Trade: Syrup 10 g/15 mL. Trade only (Kristalose): 10, 20 g packets for oral soln.
NOTES — May be mixed in water, juice, or milk to improve palatability. Packets for oral soln should be mixed in 4 oz of water or juice. Titrate dose to produce 2 to 3 soft stools/day.
MOA — Converts NH3 to NH4+ to prevent rediffusion into plasma.
ADVERSE EFFECTS — Frequent: Flatulence, diarrhea.
MAGNESIUM CITRATE ▶K ♀B ▶? $
ADULT —Evacuate bowel prior to procedure: 150 to 300 mL PO once or in divided doses.
PEDS — Evacuate bowel prior to procedure: 2 to 4 mL/kg PO once or in divided doses for age younger than 6 yo. 100 to 150 mL PO once or in divided doses for age 6 to 12 yo.
FORMS — OTC Generic only: Soln 300 mL/bottle. Low-sodium and sugar-free available.

(cont.)

MAGNESIUM CITRATE (*cont.*)

NOTES — Use caution with impaired renal function. May decrease absorption of phenytoin, ciprofloxacin, benzodiazepines, and glyburide. May cause additive CNS depression with CNS depressants. Chill to improve palatability.
MOA — Osmotic effect in intestinal lumen.
ADVERSE EFFECTS — Frequent: None. Severe: Electrolyte disturbances, CNS depression.

MAGNESIUM HYDROXIDE (*Milk of Magnesia*) ▶K ♀+ ▶? $

ADULT — Laxative: 30 to 60 mL regular strength (400 mg per 5 mL), 15 to 30 mL (800 mg per 5 mL strength) or 10 to 20 mL (1200 mg per 5 mL) PO as a single dose or divided doses. Antacid: 5 to 15 mL/dose PO four times per day prn or 622 to 1244 mg PO four times per day prn.
PEDS — Laxative: 0.5 mL/kg regular strength (400 mg per 5 mL) PO as a single dose or in divided doses for age younger than 2 yo, 5 to 15 mL/day PO as a single dose or in divided doses for age 2 to 5 yo, 15 to 30 mL PO in a single dose or in divided doses for age 6 to 11 yo. Antacid: 5 to 15 mL/dose regular strength (400 mg per 5 mL) PO four times per day prn for age older than 12 yo.
FORMS — OTC Generic/Trade: Susp 400 mg/5 mL. Trade only: Chewable tabs 311, 400 mg. Generic only: Susp 800 mg/5 mL, (concentrated) 1200 mg/5 mL, sugar-free 400 mg/5 mL.
NOTES — Use caution with impaired renal function.
MOA — Osmotic effect in intestinal lumen.
ADVERSE EFFECTS — Frequent: Diarrhea.

POLYETHYLENE GLYCOL (*MiraLax, GlycoLax*) ▶not absorbed ♀C ▶? $

ADULT — Constipation: 17 g (1 heaping tablespoon) in 4 to 8 oz water, juice, soda, coffee, or tea PO daily.
PEDS — Not approved in children.
UNAPPROVED PEDS — Children older than 6 months: 0.5 to 1.5 g/kg/day PO, maximum 17 g/day.
FORMS — OTC Generic/Trade: Powder for oral soln 17 g/scoop, 17 g packets. Rx Generic/Trade: Powder for oral soln 17 g/scoop.
NOTES — Takes 1 to 3 days to produce bowel movement. Indicated for up to 14 days.
MOA — Osmotic laxative.
ADVERSE EFFECTS — Frequent: Nausea, fullness, bloating. Serious: Risk of aspiration in children.

POLYETHYLENE GLYCOL WITH ELECTROLYTES (*GoLytely, Colyte, Suclear, Suprep, TriLyte, NuLytely, Moviprep, HalfLytely, ✚Klean-Prep, Electropeg, Peg-Lyte*) ▶not absorbed ♀C ▶? $

ADULT — Bowel cleansing prior to GI examination: 240 mL PO q 10 min or 20 to 30 mL/min NG until 4 L are consumed or rectal effluent is clear. MoviPrep: 240 mL q 15 min for 4 doses (over 1 h) the night before plus additional clear liquid and 240 mL q 15 min for 4 doses (over 1 h) plus additional clear liquid on the morning of the colonoscopy. Alternatively, 240 mL q 15 min for 4 doses (over 1 h) at 6 pm on the evening before the colonoscopy and then 1.5 h later, 240 mL q 15 min for 4 doses (over 1 h) plus additional clear liquid on the evening before the colonoscopy (MoviPrep only). Suclear: Dose 1 PO evening before and dose 2 PO morning of colonoscopy with additional liquid after each dose. Alternatively, Dose 1 PO early evening before and Dose 2 PO 2 h after starting Dose 1 on evening before colonoscopy with additional liquid with each dose. Suprep: One diluted bottle PO evening before and morning of (at least 2 h before colonoscopy) colonoscopy. Additional water after each dose.
PEDS — Bowel prep: (NuLYTELY, TriLyte): 25 mL/kg/h PO/NG, until rectal effluent is clear, maximum 4 L for age older than 6 mo.
UNAPPROVED ADULT — Chronic constipation: 125 to 500 mL/day PO daily (up to two times per day). Whole bowel irrigation in iron overdose: 1500 to 2000 mL/h.
UNAPPROVED PEDS — Bowel cleansing prior to GI examination: 25 to 40 mL/kg/h PO/NG for 4 to 10 h or until rectal effluent is clear or 20 to 30 mL/min NG until 4 L are consumed or rectal effluent is clear. Whole bowel irrigation in iron overdose: 9 mo to 6 yo: 500 mL/h; 6 yo to 12 yo 1000 mL/h; older than 12 yo, use adult dose.
FORMS — Generic/Trade: Powder for oral soln in disposable jug 4 L or 2 L (MoviPrep). Trade only: GoLYTELY Packet for oral soln to make 3.785 L. Suclear: Dose 1 (16 oz) and Dose 2 (2 L bottle) for reconstitution. Suprep: two 6 oz bottles.
NOTES — Solid food should not be given within 2 h of soln. Effects should occur within 1 to 2 h. Chilling improves palatability.
MOA — Osmotic and cathartic effect in intestinal lumen.
ADVERSE EFFECTS — Frequent: Nausea, fullness, bloating. Severe: Hypersensitivity reactions, ischemic colitis, electrolyte and fluid imbalances, anaphylaxis, fever, chills, dehydration.

***PREPOPIK* (sodium picosulfate)** ▶minimal absorption ♀B ▶? $

ADULT — Bowel cleansing prior to colonoscopy: Preferred method: 1 packet (diluted) evening before the colonoscopy and second packet (diluted) morning prior to colonoscopy. Alternatively, first dose during afternoon or early evening before the colonoscopy and second dose 6 h later in evening before colonoscopy. Additional clear liquids should be consumed.
PEDS — Not approved for use in children.
FORMS — Trade: 2 packets of 16 g powder for reconstitution.
NOTES — Use caution in patients with renal dysfunction and in patients at risk for aspiration.
MOA — Osmotic and cathartic effect in intestinal lumen.
ADVERSE EFFECTS — Frequent: nausea, headache, vomiting, abdominal bloating, pain and cramping, watery diarrhea.

SODIUM PHOSPHATE (*Fleet enema, Fleet Phospho-Soda, Fleet EZ-Prep, Accu-Prep, Osmoprep, Visicol, ✚Enemol, Phoslax*) ▶not absorbed ♀C ▶? $

WARNING — Phosphate-containing bowel cleansing regimens have been reported to cause acute phosphate nephropathy. Risk factors include advanced age, kidney disease or decreased intravascular volume, bowel obstruction or active colitis, and medications that

(cont.)

SODIUM PHOSPHATE (*cont.*)

affect renal perfusion or function such as diuretics, ACE inhibitors, ARBs, and maybe NSAIDs. Use extreme caution in bowel cleansing. Also associated with ischemic colitis and electrolyte and fluid imbalances.

ADULT — Constipation: 1 adult or pediatric enema PR or 20 to 30 mL of oral soln PO prn (max 45 mL/24 h). Prep prior to colonoscopy: Visicol: Evening before colonoscopy: 3 tabs with 8 oz clear liquid q 15 min until 20 tabs are consumed. Day of colonoscopy: Starting 3 to 5 h before procedure, 3 tabs with 8 oz clear liquid q 15 min until 20 tabs are consumed. Osmoprep: 32 tabs PO with total of 2 quarts clear liquids as follows: evening before procedure: 4 tabs PO with 8 oz of clear liquids q 15 min for a total of 20 tabs; day of procedure: 3 to 5 h before procedure, 4 tabs with 8 oz of clear liquids q 15 min for a total of 12 tabs.

PEDS — Laxative: 2 to 11 yo: one pediatric enema (67.5 mL) PR prn or 5 to 9 yo: 5 mL of oral soln PO prn. 10 to 12 yo: 10 mL of oral soln PO prn.

UNAPPROVED ADULT — Visicol: Evening before colonoscopy: 3 tabs with 8 oz clear liquid q 15 min until 20 tabs are consumed. Day of colonoscopy: Starting 3 to 5 h before procedure, 3 tabs with 8 oz clear liquid q 15 min until 8 to 12 tabs are consumed.

FORMS — OTC Generic/Trade: Adult enema, oral soln. OTC Trade only: Pediatric enema, bowel prep. Rx Trade only: Visicol, OsmoPrep tab ($$$$) 1.5 g.

NOTES — Taking the last 2 doses of Visicol with ginger ale appears to minimize residue. Excessive doses (more than 45 mL/24 h) of oral products may lead to serious electrolyte disturbances. Use with caution in severe renal impairment.

MOA — Osmotic and cathartic effect in intestinal lumen.

ADVERSE EFFECTS — Frequent: Bloating, nausea, abdominal pain, and vomiting. Severe: Electrolyte and fluid imbalances, ischemic colitis, arrhythmias, seizures, aspiration.

SORBITOL ▶not absorbed ♀C ▶? $

ADULT — Laxative: 30 to 150 mL (of 70% soln) PO or 120 mL (of 25 to 30% soln) PR. Cathartic: 4.3 mL/kg PO.

PEDS — Laxative: Children 2 to 11 yo: 2 mL/kg (of 70% soln) PO or 30 to 60 mL (of 25 to 30% soln) PR.

UNAPPROVED PEDS — Cathartic: 4.3 mL/kg of 35% soln (diluted from 70% soln) PO single dose.

FORMS — Generic only: Soln 70%.

NOTES — When used as a cathartic, can be given with activated charcoal to improve taste and decrease gastric transit time of charcoal. May precipitate electrolyte changes.

MOA — Osmotic and cathartic effect in intestinal lumen.

ADVERSE EFFECTS — Serious: Pulmonary congestion, angina-like pain, acidosis, electrolyte loss, convulsions. Frequent: Hyperglycemia, diarrhea, tachycardia, diuresis, urinary retention, blurred vision, dry mouth, thirst, dehydration, edema, N/V, rhinitis, chills, vertigo, headache, urticaria.

SUPREP (sodium sulfate + potassium sulfate + magnesium sulfate) ▶not absorbed ♀C ▶? $

ADULT — Evening before colonoscopy: Dilute 1 bottle to 16 oz with water and drink, then drink 32 oz water over next hour. Next morning, repeat both steps. Compete 1 h before colonoscopy.

PEDS — Not approved in children.

FORMS — Trade: Two 6 oz bottles for dilution.

MOA — osmotic

ADVERSE EFFECTS — Frequent: discomfort, abdominal fullness, nausea, cramping, vomiting.

GASTROENTEROLOGY: Laxatives—Other or Combinations

LUBIPROSTONE (*Amitiza*) ▶gut ♀C ▶? $$$$$

WARNING — Avoid if symptoms or history of mechanical GI obstruction.

ADULT — Chronic idiopathic constipation: 24 mcg PO two times per day with food and water. Irritable bowel syndrome with constipation in age 18 yo or older: 8 mcg PO two times per day. Opioid-induced constipation in adults with chronic, non-cancer pain: 24 mcg PO two times per day with food and water.

PEDS — Not approved in children.

FORMS — Trade only: Cap 8, 24 mcg.

NOTES — Reduce dose with moderate to severe hepatic dysfunction. Has not been studied with diphenylheptane opioids such as methadone-induced constipation. Swallow capsules whole.

MOA — Chloride channel activator which enhances intestinal fluid secretion, thereby increasing intestinal motility.

ADVERSE EFFECTS — Frequent: Nausea, diarrhea, headache, abdominal pain/distension, flatulence.

MINERAL OIL (*Kondremul, Fleet Mineral Oil Enema, Liqui-Doss, ✸Lansoyl*) ▶not absorbed ♀C ▶? $

ADULT — Laxative: 15 to 45 mL PO in a single dose or in divided doses, 60 to 150 mL PR.

PEDS — Laxative: Children 6 to 11 yo: 5 to 15 mL PO in a single dose or in divided doses. Children 2 to 11 yo: 30 to 60 mL PR.

FORMS — OTC Generic/Trade: Oil (30, 480 mL), Enema (Fleet). OTC Trade only: Oral liquid (Liqui-Doss) 13.5 mg/15 mL. Oral microemulsion (Kondremul) 2.5 mg/5 mL.

NOTES — Use with caution in children younger than 4 yo and elderly or debilitated patients due to concerns for aspiration pneumonitis. Although usual directions for plain mineral oil are to administer at bedtime, this increases risk of lipid pneumonitis. Mineral oil emulsions may be administered with meals.

MOA — Softens and lubricates stool.

ADVERSE EFFECTS — Frequent: None.

PERI-COLACE (docusate + sennosides) ▶L ♀C ▶? $

ADULT — Constipation: 2 to 4 tabs PO once daily or in divided doses prn.

PEDS — Constipation 6 to 12 yo: 1 to 2 tabs PO daily prn. 2 to 6 yo: Up to 1 tab PO daily prn.

FORMS — OTC Generic/Trade: Tabs 50 mg docusate + 8.6 mg sennosides.

NOTES — Chronic use of stimulant laxatives (casanthranol) may be habit forming.

PERI-COLACE (cont.)

MOA — Softens stool.

ADVERSE EFFECTS — Frequent: Abdominal cramping.

SENOKOT-S (**senna + docusate**) ▶L ♀C ▶+ $

ADULT — 2 tabs PO daily, maximum 4 tabs two times per day.

PEDS — 6 to 12 yo: 1 tab PO daily, max 2 tabs two times per day. 2 to 6 yo: ½ tab PO daily, max 1 tab two times per day.

FORMS — OTC Generic/Trade: Tabs 8.6 mg senna concentrate + 50 mg docusate.

NOTES — Effects occur 6 to 12 h after oral administration. Use caution in renal dysfunction. Chronic use of stimulant laxatives may be habit forming.

MOA — Natural product; enhances GI motility and softens stool.

ADVERSE EFFECTS — Frequent: None.

GASTROENTEROLOGY: Laxatives—Stimulant

BISACODYL (**Correctol, Dulcolax, Feen-a-Mint, Fleet**) ▶L ♀C ▶? $

ADULT — Constipation/colonic evacuation prior to a procedure: 5 to 15 mg PO daily prn, 10 mg PR daily prn.

PEDS — Constipation/colonic evacuation prior to a procedure: 0.3 mg/kg/day PO daily prn. Children younger than 2 yo, 5 mg PR prn; 2 to 11 yo, 5 to 10 mg PO or PR prn; 12 yo or older: 10 mg PO or PR prn.

FORMS — OTC Generic/Trade: Tabs 5 mg, suppository 10 mg. OTC Trade only: Enema, 10 mg/30 mL.

NOTES — Oral tab has onset of 6 to 10 h. Onset of action of suppository is approximately 15 to 60 min. Do not chew tabs, swallow whole. Do not give within 1 h of antacids or dairy products. Chronic use of stimulant laxatives may be habit forming.

MOA — Direct colonic stimulant.

ADVERSE EFFECTS — Frequent: None.

CASCARA ▶L ♀C ▶+ $

ADULT — Constipation: 5 mL/day of aromatic fluid extract PO at bedtime prn.

PEDS — Constipation: Infants: 1.25 mL/day of aromatic fluid extract PO daily prn. Children 2 to 11 yo: 2.5 mL/day of aromatic fluid extract PO daily prn.

FORMS — Rx Generic only: Lliquid aromatic fluid extract.

NOTES — Cascara sagrada fluid extract is 5 times more potent than cascara sagrada aromatic fluid extract. Chronic use of stimulant laxatives may be habit forming.

MOA — Direct irritation of intestinal mucosa.

ADVERSE EFFECTS — Frequent: Lightheadedness, fluid/electrolyte imbalance, abdominal cramps, nausea, diarrhea, discoloration of urine.

CASTOR OIL ▶Not absorbed ♀– ▶? $

ADULT — Constipation: 15 to 60 mL PO daily prn. Colonic evacuation prior to procedure: 15 to 60 mL of castor oil or 30 to 60 mL emulsified castor oil PO as a single dose 16 h prior to procedure.

PEDS — Colonic evacuation prior to procedure: 1 to 5 mL of castor oil or 2.5 to 7.5 mL emulsified castor oil PO as a single dose 16 h prior to procedure for age younger than 2 yo. 5 to 15 mL of castor oil or 7.5 to 30 mL of emulsified castor oil PO as a single dose 16 h prior to procedure for age 2 to 11 yo.

FORMS — OTC Generic only: Oil 60, 120, 180, 480 mL.

NOTES — Emulsions somewhat mask the bad taste. Onset of action approximately 2 to 6 h. Do not give at bedtime. Chill or administer with juice to improve taste.

MOA — Softens and lubricates stool.

ADVERSE EFFECTS — Frequent: None.

SENNA (**Senokot, SenokotXTRA, Ex-Lax, Fletcher's Castoria**) ▶L ♀C ▶+ $

ADULT — Laxative or evacuation of the colon for bowel or rectal examinations: 1 tsp granules in water or 10 to 15 mL or 2 tabs PO at bedtime. Max daily dose 4 tsp of granules, 30 mL of syrup or 8 tabs.

PEDS — Laxative: 10 to 20 mg/kg/dose PO at bedtime. Alternative regimen: 1 mo to 2 yo: 1.25 to 2.5 mL syrup PO at bedtime, max 5 mL/day; 2 to 5 yo: 2.5 to 3.75 mL syrup PO at bedtime, max 7.5 mL/day; 6 to 12 yo: 5 to 7.5 mL syrup PO at bedtime, max 15 mL/day.

FORMS — OTC Generic/Trade (All dosing is based on sennosides content; 1 mg sennosides is equivalent to 21.7 mg standardized senna concentrate): Syrup 8.8 mg/5 mL. Liquid 33.3 mg senna concentrate/mL (Fletcher's Castoria). Tabs 8.6, 15, 17, 25 mg. Chewable tabs 10, 15 mg.

NOTES — Effects occur 6 to 24 h after oral administration. Use caution in renal dysfunction. Chronic use of stimulant laxatives may be habit forming.

MOA — Enhances GI motility.

ADVERSE EFFECTS — Frequent: Potential for severe diaper rash in children wearing diapers.

GASTROENTEROLOGY: Laxatives—Stool Softener

DOCUSATE (**Colace, Docu-Soft, DOK, Dulcolax, Docu-Liquid, Enemeez, Fleet Sof-Lax, Octycine, Silace**) ▶L ♀C ▶? $

ADULT — Constipation: Docusate calcium: 240 mg PO daily. Docusate sodium: 50 to 500 mg/day PO in 1 to 4 divided doses.

PEDS — Constipation: Docusate sodium: 10 to 40 mg/day for age younger than 3 yo, 20 to 60 mg/day for age 3 to 6 yo, 40 to 150 mg/day for age 6 to 12 yo. In all cases doses are divided up to four times per day.

UNAPPROVED ADULT — Docusate sodium, Constipation: Can be given as a retention enema: Mix 50 to 100 mg docusate liquid with saline or water retention enema for rectal use. Cerumen removal: Instill 1 mL liquid (not syrup) in affected

(cont.)

DOCUSATE (*cont.*)

ear; allow to remain for 10 to 15 min, then irrigate with 50 mL lukewarm NS if necessary.
UNAPPROVED PEDS — Docusate sodium: Cerumen removal: Instill 1 mL liquid (not syrup) in affected ear; allow to remain for 10 to 15 min, then irrigate with 50 mL lukewarm NS if necessary.

FORMS — Docusate calcium OTC Generic/Trade: Caps 240 mg. Docusate sodium OTC Generic/Trade: Caps 50, 100, 250 mg. Liquid 50 mg/5 mL. Syrup 20 mg/5 mL. Docusate sodium OTC Trade only (Enemeez): Enema, rectal 283 mg/5 mL.
NOTES — Takes 1 to 3 days to notably soften stools.
MOA — Softens stool, cerumen.
ADVERSE EFFECTS — Frequent: Abdominal cramping.

GASTROENTEROLOGY: Ulcerative Colitis

BALSALAZIDE (*Colazal, Giazo*) ▶minimal absorption ♀B ▶? $$$$$
ADULT — Ulcerative colitis: 2.25 g PO three times per day (Colazal) for 8 to 12 weeks or 1.1 g PO twice per day (Giazo) for 8 weeks.
PEDS — 5 to 17 yo (Colazal): Mild to moderately active ulcerative colitis: 2.25 g PO three times per day for 8 weeks. Alternatively, 750 mg PO three times per day for 8 weeks.
FORMS — Generic/Trade (Colazal): Caps 750 mg. Trade (Giazo): Tabs 1.1 g.
NOTES — Contraindicated in salicylate allergy. Caution with renal insufficiency.
MOA — Mesalamine prodrug, inhibits cyclooxygenase pathways.
ADVERSE EFFECTS — Frequent: Headache, abdominal pain, nausea, diarrhea, vomiting, respiratory infection, arthralgias. Severe: Cholestatic jaundice, cirrhosis, liver failure, hypersensitivity, pericarditis.

MESALAMINE (*5-aminosalicylic acid, Apriso, 5-Aspirin, Lialda, Pentasa, Canasa, Rowasa, Delzicol, ✦Mesasal, Salofalk*) ▶gut ♀C ▶? $$$$$
ADULT — Ulcerative colitis: Delzicol: 800 mg PO three times a day (treatment) or 800 mg PO twice a day (maintenance). Pentasa: 1 g PO four times per day. Lialda: 2.4 to 4.8 g PO daily with a meal for 8 weeks. Rectal susp: 4 g (60 mL) PR retained for 8 h at bedtime. Maintenance of remission of ulcerative colitis: Apriso: 1.5 g (4 caps) PO q am. Lialda: 2.4 g PO daily. Ulcerative proctitis: Canasa suppository: 500 mg PR two to three times per day or 1000 mg PR at bedtime.
PEDS — Active ulcerative colitis 5 yo and older: 17 kg to 32 kg: 36 to 71 mg/kg/day (max 1.2 g/day); 33 kg to 53 kg: 37 to 61 mg/kg/day (max 2.0 g/day); 54 kg to 90 kg: 27 to 44 mg/kg/day (max 2.4 g/day).
UNAPPROVED ADULT — Active Crohn's: 0.4 to 4.8 g/day PO in divided doses. Maintenance of remission of Crohn's: 2.4 g/day in divided doses.
FORMS — Trade only: Delayed-release cap (Delzicol) 400 mg. Controlled-release cap 250, 500 mg (Pentasa). Delayed-release tab 1200 mg (Lialda). Rectal suppository 1000 mg (Canasa). Controlled-release cap 0.375 g (Apriso). Generic/Trade: Rectal susp 4 g/60 mL (Rowasa).
NOTES — Avoid in salicylate sensitivity or hepatic dysfunction. Reports of hepatic failure in patients with pre-existing liver disease. May decrease digoxin levels. May discolor urine yellow-brown.

Most common adverse effects include headache, abdominal pain, fever, rash. Two Delzicol are not bioequivalent to Asacol HD. The coating of Asacol and Asacol HD contain the inactive chemical, dibutyl phthalate (DBP) In animal studies at doses more than 190 times the human dose, maternal DBP was associated with external and skeletal malformations and adverse effects on the male reproductive system. Use may cause false elevations of urinary normetanephrine concentrations.
MOA — Unknown.
ADVERSE EFFECTS — Frequent: Headache, malaise, abdominal pain, cramps, flatulence, gas, hair loss. Severe: Cytopenias, myo- and pericarditis, hepatitis, pneumonitis, nephritis, anaphylactic reaction, Steven-Johnson syndrome, drug reaction with eosinophilia and systematic symptoms (DRESS).

OLSALAZINE (*Dipentum*) ▶L ♀C ▶– $$$$$
ADULT — Maintenance of remission of ulcerative colitis in patients intolerant to sulfasalazine: 500 mg PO two times per day with food.
PEDS — Not approved in children.
UNAPPROVED ADULT — Crohn's: 1.5 to 3 g/day PO in divided doses with food.
FORMS — Trade only: Caps 250 mg.
NOTES — Diarrhea in up to 17%. Avoid in salicylate sensitivity.
MOA — Unknown.
ADVERSE EFFECTS — Frequent: Diarrhea, cramps, abdominal pain.

SULFASALAZINE—GASTROENTEROLOGY (*Azulfidine, Azulfidine EN-tabs, ✦Salazopyrin En-tabs*) ▶L ♀B ▶? $$
WARNING — Beware of hypersensitivity, marrow suppression, renal and liver damage, central nervous system effects, irreversible neuromuscular and CNS changes, fibrosing alveolitis.
ADULT — Induction of remission, ulcerative colitis: Initial dose of 500 to 1000 mg PO four times per day. Maintenance of remission: 500 mg PO four times per day.
PEDS — Induction of remission, ulcerative colitis, age 6 yo or older: Initially 40 to 60 mg/kg/day PO divided into 3 to 6 doses. Maximum 75 mg/kg/day. Maintenance of remission: 30 mg/kg/day PO divided into 4 doses.
FORMS — Generic/Trade: Tabs 500 mg, scored. Enteric-coated, delayed-release (EN-tabs) 500 mg.

SULFASALAZINE—GASTROENTEROLOGY (cont.)

NOTES — Contraindicated in children younger than 2 yo. Avoid with hepatic or renal dysfunction, intestinal or urinary obstruction, porphyria, or sulfonamide or salicylate sensitivity. Monitor CBC q 2 to 4 weeks for 3 months then q 3 months. Monitor LFTs, CBC, and renal function. Oligospermia and infertility, and photosensitivity may occur. May decrease folic acid, digoxin, cyclosporine, and iron levels. May turn body fluids, contact lenses, or skin orange-yellow. Enteric-coated (Azulfidine EN, Salazopyrin EN) tabs may cause fewer GI adverse effects. Supplement with folic acid during pregnancy. Reports of bloody stools or diarrhea in breast-fed infants of mothers taking sulfasalazine.

MOA — Colonic antiinflammatoru, immunosuppressant.

ADVERSE EFFECTS — Serious: Agranulocytosis, hemolytic anemia, nephro/hepatotoxicity, hepatic failure, drug rash and other severe skin reactions, hypersensitivity, anaphylaxis, angioedema, neural tube defect, reversible male infertility, infections associated with myelosuppression and severe hypersensitivity reactions. Frequent: Nausea, dyspepsia, rash.

GASTROENTEROLOGY: Other GI Agents

ALOSETRON (Lotronex) ▶L ♀B ▷? $$$$$

WARNING — Can cause severe constipation and ischemic colitis. Concomitant use with fluvoxamine, a potent CYP1A2 inhibitor, is contraindicated. Use caution with moderate CYP1A2 inhibitors such as quinolone antibiotics and cimetidine. Use caution with strong inhibitors of CYP3A4 such as ketoconazole, clarithromycin, protease inhibitors, voriconazole, and itraconazole. Can be prescribed only by drug company authorized clinicians using special sticker and written informed consent.

ADULT — Diarrhea-predominant irritable bowel syndrome in women who have failed conventional therapy: 0.5 mg PO twice a day for 4 weeks; discontinue in patients who become constipated. If well tolerated and symptoms not controlled after 4 weeks, may increase to 1 mg PO two times per day. Discontinue if symptoms not controlled in 4 weeks on 1 mg PO two times per day.

PEDS — Not approved in children.

FORMS — Trade only: Tabs 0.5, 1 mg.

NOTES — Specific medication guide must be distributed with prescriptions.

MOA — Selective 5-HT3 receptor antagonist.

ADVERSE EFFECTS — Frequent: Constipation, nausea, abdominal pain. Severe: Severe constipation, ischemic colitis.

ALPHA-GALACTOSIDASE (Beano) ▶minimal absorption ♀? ▷? $

ADULT — 5 gtts or 1 tab per ½ cup gassy food, 2 to 3 tabs PO (chew, swallow, or crumble) or 1 melt-away tab or 10 to 15 gtts per typical meal.

PEDS — Not approved in age younger than 12 yo.

FORMS — OTC Trade only: Oral gtts, tabs, melt-away tabs.

NOTES — Beano produces 2 to 6 g of carbohydrates for every 100 g of food treated by Beano; may increase glucose levels.

MOA — Enzyme that breaks down complex sugars in gassy foods making them more digestible.

ADVERSE EFFECTS — Frequent: None. Severe: None.

ALVIMOPAN (Entereg) ▶intestinal flora ♀B ▷? ?

WARNING — Increased risk of myocardial infarction in a clinical trial of patients taking alvimopan long-term. Only available through a restricted program for short-term use (15 doses).

ADULT — To accelerate time to upper and lower gastrointestinal recovery following partial bowel resection with primary anastomosis, short-term (up to 15 doses) only: 12 mg PO 30 min to 5 h prior to surgery, then 12 mg PO two times per day starting the day after surgery for up to 7 days.

PEDS — Not approved in children.

FORMS — Trade only: Caps 12 mg.

NOTES — Only available to hospitals who are authorized to use the medication (requires hospital DEA number to be dispensed). Contraindicated in patients who have taken therapeutic doses of opioids for more than 7 consecutive days. Not for use in those with severe hepatic or renal disease, or for gastric primary pancreatic anastomosis. Serum concentrations in patients of Japanese descent may be up to 2-fold greater than Caucasian subjects with same dose. Monitor Japanese patients for adverse events.

MOA — Peripherally acting mu-opioid receptor antagonist used for post operative ileus.

ADVERSE EFFECTS — Frequent: Anemia, dyspepsia, hypokalemia, back pain, urinary retention. Severe: Myocardial infarction.

BUDESONIDE (Entocort EC, Uceris) ▶L ♀C ▷? $$$$$

ADULT — Mild to moderate Crohn's, induction of remission: 9 mg PO daily for up to 8 weeks. May repeat 8 week course for recurring episodes. Maintenance: 6 mg PO daily for 3 months (Entocort only). Mild to moderate ulcerative colitis, induction of remission: 9 mg PO q am for up to 8 weeks.

PEDS — Not approved in children.

UNAPPROVED PEDS — Mild to moderate Crohn's: 0.45 mg/kg up to 9 mg PO daily for 8 to 12 weeks for age 9 yo or older.

FORMS — Generic/Trade: Caps 3 mg. Trade only: Extended-Release Tabs (Uceris) 9 mg. (Uceris for ulcerative colitis, only).

NOTES — May taper dose to 6 mg for 2 weeks prior to discontinuation.

MOA — Affects cell motility and protein synthesis; anti-inflammatory.

ADVERSE EFFECTS — Frequent: Palpitations, nervousness, dizziness, headache, pruritus, rash, GI irritation, nausea, bitter taste, hyperglycemia, increased infection rate. Severe: Anaphylaxis.

CHLORDIAZEPOXIDE–CLIDINIUM ▶K ♀D ▶– $$$
ADULT — Irritable bowel syndrome: 1 cap PO three to four times per day.
PEDS — Not approved in children.
FORMS — Generic: Caps, chlordiazepoxide 5 mg + clidinium 2.5 mg.
NOTES — May cause drowsiness. After prolonged use, gradually taper to avoid withdrawal symptoms. Contains ingredients formerly contained in Librax.
MOA — Anticholinergic/benzodiazepine.
ADVERSE EFFECTS — Frequent: Dry mouth, drowsiness, ataxia, memory impairment, rash, decreased libido, xerostomia, changes in appetite, micturation difficulties. Severe: CNS, respiratory depression.

CROFELEMER (Fulyzaq) ▶minimal absorption ♀C ▶? $$$$$
ADULT — Noninfectious AIDS diarrhea: 125 mg PO twice daily.
PEDS — Not approved in children younger than 18 yo.
FORMS — Trade: Delayed-release tab 125 mg.
NOTES — Rule out infectious causes of diarrhea before initiating.
MOA — Inhibits cAMP-stimulated cystic fibrosis transmembrane conductance regulator chloride ion channel, and calcium-activated Cl channels at the luminal membrane of enterocytes
ADVERSE EFFECTS — Common: flatulence, bronchitis, cough.

GLYCOPYRROLATE (Robinul, Robinul Forte, Cuvposa) ▶K ♀B ▶? $$$$
ADULT — Peptic ulcer disease: 1 to 2 mg PO two to three times per day. Preop/intraoperative respiratory antisecretory: 0.1 mg IV/IM prn.
PEDS — Chronic drooling in children 3 to 16 yo (Cuvposa): 0.02 mg/kg three times per day, 1 h before or 2 h after meals. Increase by 0.02 mg/kg q 5 to 7 days.
UNAPPROVED ADULT — Drooling: 0.1 mg/kg PO two to three times per day, max 8 mg/day.
FORMS — Trade: Solution 1 mg/5 mL (480 mL, Cuvposa). Generic/Trade: Tabs 1, 2 mg.
NOTES — Contraindicated in glaucoma, obstructive uropathy, paralytic ileus or GI obstruction, myasthenia gravis, severe ulcerative colitis, toxic megacolon, and unstable cardiovascular status in acute hemorrhage.
MOA — Inhibits effects of acetylcholine.
ADVERSE EFFECTS — Frequent: Dry skin, dry mouth/throat, constipation, vomiting, flushing, nasal congestion, urinary retention, dry nose, local irritation.

LACTASE (Lactaid) ▶not absorbed ♀+ ▶+ $
ADULT — Swallow or chew 3 caps (Original-strength), 2 caps (Extra-strength), 1 caplet (Ultra) with first bite of dairy foods. Adjust dose based on response.
PEDS — Titrate dose based on response.
FORMS — OTC Generic/Trade: Caplets, Chewable tabs.
MOA — Replenish lactase enzymes.
ADVERSE EFFECTS — Frequent: None.

LINACLOTIDE (Linzess, ✦Constella) ▶gut – ♀C ▶? $$$$$
WARNING — Contraindicated in children 6 yo or younger. Avoid use in children 6 yo to 17 yo.
ADULT — IBS: 290 mcg PO daily. Chronic idiopathic constipation: 145 mcg PO once daily.
PEDS — Not approved in children younger than 18 yo.
FORMS — Trade: Cap 145, 290 mcg.
NOTES — Take on empty stomach, 30 minutes before food. Do not use in patients with mechanical GI obstruction.
MOA — guanylate cyclase-C (GC-C) agonist.
ADVERSE EFFECTS — Frequent: diarrhea, abdominal pain, flatulence, abdominal distension.

LORCASERIN (Belviq) ▶L ♀X ▶– $$$
WARNING — Contraindicated in pregnancy.
ADULT — Obesity or ooverweight with comorbidities: 10 mg PO twice a day. Discontinue if 5% wt loss not achieved by 12 weeks.
PEDS — Not approved for use in children.
FORMS — Trade: Tab 10 mg.
NOTES — Can cause serotonin syndrome when given with other serotonergic or antidopaminergic agent. Monitor for signs or symptoms of valvular heart disease. Can cause cognitive impairment. May be associated with psychiatric diseases. May cause priapism.
MOA — Selective serotonin 2C receptor agonist
ADVERSE EFFECTS — Frequent: headache, dizziness, fatigue, nausea, dry mouth, constipation, hypoglycemia in diabetic patients. Severe: serotonin syndrome, valvular heart disease.

METHYLNALTREXONE (Relistor) ▶unchanged ♀B ▶? $$$$$
ADULT — Opioid-induced constipation in patients with advanced illness who are receiving palliative care, when response to laxative therapy has not been sufficient: Less than 38 kg: 0.15 mg/kg SC every other day; 38 kg to 61 kg: 8 mg SC every other day; 62 kg to 114 kg: 12 mg SC every other day: 115 kg or greater: 0.15 mg/kg SC every other day.
PEDS — Not approved in children.
FORMS — Single-use vial 12 mg/0.6 mL and 8 mg/0.4 mL solution for subcutaneous injection; single-use pre-filled syringe 12 mg/0.6 mL solution for subcutaneous injection.
NOTES — Do not use with GI obstruction or lesions of GI tract. If severe or persistent diarrhea develops stop medication and consult physician. Usual dose every other day, but no more frequently than once dail. For CrCl < 30 mL/min reduce dose by one half
MOA — Peripherally acting opioid antagonist
ADVERSE EFFECTS — Frequent: Abdominal pain, flatulence, nausea, dizziness, diarrhea, hyperhidrosis. Severe: GI perforation

NEOMYCIN—ORAL (Neo-Fradin) ▶minimal absorption ♀D ▶? $$$
ADULT — Suppression of intestinal bacteria (given with erythromycin): 1 g PO at 19 h, 18 h, and 9 h prior to procedure (i.e., 1 pm, 2 pm, 11 pm on prior day). Alternative regimen 1 g PO q 1 h for 4 doses then 1 g PO q 4 h for 5 doses. Hepatic encephalopathy: 4 to 12 g/day PO divided q 4 to 6 h for 5 to 6 days. Diarrhea caused by enteropathogenic E. coli: 3 g/day PO divided q 6 h.

NEOMYCIN–ORAL (cont.)

PEDS — Suppression of intestinal bacteria (given with erythromycin): 25 mg/kg PO at 19 h, 18 h and 9 h prior to procedure (i.e., 1 pm, 2 pm, 11 pm on prior day). Alternative regimen 90 mg/kg/day PO divided q 4 h for 2 days. Hepatic encephalopathy: 50 to 100 mg/kg/day PO divided q 6 to 8 h for 5 to 6 days. Diarrhea caused by enteropathogenic E. coli: 50 mg/kg/day PO divided q 6 h for 2 to 3 days.

FORMS — Generic only: Tabs 500 mg. Trade only: Soln 125 mg/5 mL.

NOTES — Increased INR with warfarin, decreased levels of digoxin, methotrexate.

MOA — Inhibits bacterial protein synthesis.

ADVERSE EFFECTS — Frequent: None.

OCTREOTIDE (Sandostatin, Sandostatin LAR) ▶LK ♀B ▶? $$$$$

ADULT — Diarrhea associated with carcinoid tumors: 100 to 600 mcg/day SC/IV in 2 to 4 divided doses for 2 weeks or 20 mg IM (Sandostatin LAR) q 4 weeks for 2 months. Adjust dose based on response. Diarrhea associated with vasoactive intestinal peptide-secreting tumors: 200 to 300 mcg/day SC/IV in 2 to 4 divided doses for 2 weeks or 20 mg IM (Sandostatin LAR) q 4 weeks for 2 months. Adjust dose based on response.

PEDS — Not approved in children.

UNAPPROVED ADULT — Variceal bleeding: Bolus 25 to 50 mcg IV followed by 25 to 50 mcg/h continuous IV infusion. AIDS diarrhea: 25 to 250 mcg SC three times per day, max 500 mcg SC q 8 h. Irritable bowel syndrome: 100 mcg as a single dose to 125 mcg SC two times per day. GI and pancreatic fistulas: 50 to 200 mcg SC/IV q 8 h.

UNAPPROVED PEDS — Diarrhea: Initially 1 to 10 mcg/kg SC/IV q 12 h. Congenital hyperinsulinism: 1 to 40 mcg/kg SC daily. Hypothalamic obesity in children 6 to 17 yo: 40 mg IM q 4 weeks (Sandostatin LAR) or 5 to 15 mcg/kg SC daily.

FORMS — Generic/Trade: Injection vials 0.05, 0.1, 0.2, 0.5, 1 mg. Trade only: Long-acting injectable susp (Sandostatin LAR) 10, 20, 30 mg.

NOTES — For the treatment of variceal bleeding, most studies treat for 3 to 5 days. Individualize dose based on response. Dosage reduction often necessary in elderly. May cause hypoglycemia, hyperglycemia; caution especially in diabetes. May cause hypothyroidism, cardiac arrhythmias. Increases bioavailability of bromocriptine. Sandostatin LAR only indicated for patients who are stabilized on Sandostatin.

MOA — Mimics natural somatostatin.

ADVERSE EFFECTS — Frequent: Sinus bradycardia, chest pain, fatigue, headache, malaise, fever, dizziness, pruritis, hyperglycemia, abdominal pain, nausea, diarrhea. Severe: Hepatitis, progressive abdominal distension, severe epigastric pain.

ORLISTAT (Alli, Xenical) ▶gut ♀X ▶? $$$

ADULT — Weight loss and wt management: 60 mg to 120 mg PO three times per day with meals or up to 1 h after meals.

PEDS — Children 12 to 16 yo: 60 mg to 120 mg PO three times per day with meals. Not approved in age younger than 12 yo.

FORMS — OTC Trade only (Alli): Caps 60 mg. Rx Trade only (Xenical): Caps 120 mg.

NOTES — All patients should take a vitamin containing fat-soluble vitamins (A, E, D, K, beta carotene). May cause fatty stools, fecal urgency, flatus with discharge and oily spotting in more than 20% of patients. GI adverse effects greater when taken with high-fat diet. Has been associated with liver damage. Can reduce the effect of levothyroxine or increase the effects of warfarin. Administer orlistat and levothyroxine at least 4 h apart. Administer cyclosporine 3 h after orlistat. Monitor INR and antiepileptic serum concentrations.

MOA — Inhibits gastric and pancreatic lipases.

ADVERSE EFFECTS — Frequent: CNS effects, oily stool, fecal incontinence, flatus with discharge Severe: Cholelithiasis, nephrolithiasis, nephropathy, pancreatitis, severe liver injury with hepatocellular necrosis or acute hepatic failure.

PANCREATIN (Creon, Ku-Zyme, ✦Entozyme) ▶gut ♀C ▶? $$$

ADULT — Enzyme replacement (initial dose): 8000 to 24,000 units lipase (1 to 2 caps/tabs) PO with meals and snacks.

PEDS — Enzyme replacement (initial dose): 2000 units lipase PO with meals for age younger than 1 yo, 4000 to 8000 units lipase PO with meals or 4000 units lipase with snacks for age 1 to 6 yo, 4000 to 12,000 units lipase PO with meals and snacks for age 7 to 12 yo.

FORMS — Tabs, Caps with varying amounts of lipase, amylase, and protease.

NOTES — Titrate dose to stool fat content. Products are not interchangeable. Avoid concomitant calcium carbonate and magnesium hydroxide since these may affect the enteric coating. Do not crush/chew microspheres or tabs. Possible association of colonic strictures and high doses of lipase (greater than 16,000 units/kg/meal) in pediatric patients.

MOA — Replaces endogenous enzymes.

ADVERSE EFFECTS — Frequent: None.

PANCRELIPASE (Creon, Pancreaze, Pancrecarb, Cotazym, Ku-Zyme HP, Ultresa, Viokace, Zenpep) ▶gut ♀C ▶? $$$

ADULT — Enzyme replacement (initial dose): 500 lipase units/kg per meal, max 2500 lipase units/kg per meal.

PEDS — Enzyme replacement (initial dose, varies by wt): Infants (up to 12 mo): 2000 to 4000 lipase units per 120 mL of formula or per breastfeeding. 12 mo or older to younger than 4 yo: 1000 lipase units/kg, max 2500 lipase units/kg per meal. 4 yo or older: 500 lipase units/kg per meal, max 2500 lipase units/kg per meal.

FORMS — Tabs, Caps, Powder with varying amounts of lipase, amylase, and protease.

NOTES — Titrate dose to stool fat content. Products are not interchangeable. Avoid concomitant

(cont.)

PANCRELIPASE (*cont.*)

calcium carbonate and magnesium hydroxide since these may affect the enteric coating. Do not crush/chew. Possible association of colonic strictures and high doses of lipase (greater than 16,000 units/kg/meal) in pediatric patients.

MOA — Replaces endogenous enzymes.

ADVERSE EFFECTS — Frequent: None.

PINAVERIUM (*Dicetel*) ▶? ♀C ▶– $$$

ADULT — Canada only. Irritable bowel syndrome: 50 mg PO three times per day, may increase to maximum of 100 mg three times per day.

PEDS — Not for children.

FORMS — Trade only: tabs 50, 100 mg.

NOTES — Take with a full glass of water during meal or snack.

MOA — Calcium antagonist; blocks voltage-dependent calcium channels at the smooth muscle cell level; highly selective for intestinal smooth muscle.

ADVERSE EFFECTS — Frequent: Epigastric pain, nausea, constipation.

QSYMIA (**phentermine + topiramate**) ▶KL ♀X ▶– ©IV $$$$

WARNING — Contraindicated in pregnancy glaucoma, hyperthyroidism, and during 14 days after MAO inhibitor.

ADULT — Obesity or overweight with comorbidities: 3.75 mg/23 mg PO once daily for 14 days, then increase to 7.5 mg/46 mg PO once daily. Can increase dose if 3% wt loss not achieved after 12 weeks. Max dose 15 mg/92 mg PO daily. Discontinue if 5% wt loss not achieved on max dose for 12 weeks.

PEDS — Not approved for use in children.

FORMS — Trade: Tab 3.75/23, 7.5/46, 11.25/69, 15/92 mg (phentermine/topiramate).

NOTES — Do not exceed 7.5 mg/46 mg in moderate to severe renal impairment or moderate hepatic impairment. May increase heart rate, Monitor for suicidal thoughts or depression. Measure creatinine and electrolytes before and during treatment. Monitor for hypoglycemia in patients with diabetes.

MOA — See components.

ADVERSE EFFECTS — See components.

RECTIV (*nitroglycerin—rectal*) ▶L ♀C ▶? $$$$$

ADULT — Chronic anal fisures: Apply 1 inch intra-anally q 12 for up to 3 weeks.

PEDS — Not approved in children younger than 18 yo.

FORMS — Ointment 0.4% 30 g.

NOTES — Use within 8 weeks of opening. Do not use with PDE5 inhibitors.

MOA — Relaxation of the internal anal sphincter muscle

ADVERSE EFFECTS — Frequent: headache, dizziness.

SECRETIN (*SecreFlo, ChiRhoStim*) ▶serum ♀C ▶? $$$$$

ADULT — Stimulation of pancreatic secretions, to aid in diagnosis of exocrine pancreas dysfunction: Test dose 0.2 mcg IV. If tolerated, 0.2 mcg/kg IV over 1 min. Stimulation of gastrin to aid in diagnosis of gastrinoma: Test dose 0.2 mcg IV. If tolerated, 0.4

mcg/kg IV over 1 min. Identification of ampulla of Vater and accessory papilla during ERCP: 0.2 mcg/kg IV over 1 min.

PEDS — Not approved in children.

UNAPPROVED PEDS — Has been tried in autism, but does not appear to be effective.

NOTES — Previously known as SecreFlo. Contraindicated in acute pancreatitis.

MOA — Increases volume and bicarbonate content of secreted pancreatic juices.

ADVERSE EFFECTS — Frequent: Abdominal discomfort, hypotension, diaphoresis, flushing, nausea.

TEDUGLUTIDE (*Gattex*) ▶endrogeneous ♀B ▶? $$$$$

WARNING — May accelerate neoplastic growth, May cause intestinal obstruction or fluid overload or pancreatic and biliary disease.

ADULT — Short bowel syndrome patients receiving IV TPN: 0.05 mg/kg (max 3.8 mg) SC daily.

PEDS — Not approved in children.

FORMS — Trade Only: 5 mg/vial - powder for reconstitution.

MOA — glucagon-like peptide-2

ADVERSE EFFECTS — Frequent: abdominal pain, injection site reactions, nausea, headache, abdominal distension, vomiting. Severe: neoplastic growth, intestinal obstruction, biliary and pancreatic disease, fluid overload.

URSODIOL (*Actigall, URSO, URSO Forte*) ▶bile ♀B ▶? $$$$

ADULT — Radiolucent gallstone dissolution (Actigall): 8 to 10 mg/kg/day PO divided in 2 to 3 doses. Prevention of gallstones associated with rapid wt loss (Actigall): 300 mg PO two times per day. Primary biliary cirrhosis (URSO): 13 to 15 mg/kg/day PO divided in 2 to 4 doses.

PEDS — Not approved in children.

UNAPPROVED ADULT — Cholestasis of pregnancy: 300 to 600 mg PO two times per day.

UNAPPROVED PEDS — Biliary atresia: 10 to 15 mg/kg/day PO once daily. Cystic fibrosis with liver disease: 15 to 30 mg/kg/day PO divided two times per day. TPN-induced cholestasis: 30 mg/kg/day PO divided three times per day.

FORMS — Generic/Trade: Caps 300 mg, Tabs 250, 500 mg.

NOTES — Do not use in patients with complete biliary obstruction. Gallstone dissolution requires months of therapy. Complete dissolution does not occur in all patients and 5-year recurrence up to 50%. Does not dissolve calcified cholesterol stones, radiopaque stones, or radiolucent bile pigment stones. Monitor LFTs and bilirubin. Avoid concomitant antacids, cholestyramine, colestipol, estrogen, oral contraceptives.

MOA — Decreases cholesterol content of bile and bile stones.

ADVERSE EFFECTS — Frequent: Diarrhea, constipation, nausea, vomiting, dizziness. Serious: Thrombocytopenia, hypersensitivity reactions.

HEMATOLOGY ANTICOAGULANTS

HEMATOLOGY/ANTICOAGULANTS: Anticoagulants - Direct Thrombin Inhibitors

ARGATROBAN ▶L ♀B ▶– $$$$$

ADULT — Prevention/treatment of thrombosis in HIT: Start 2 mcg/kg/min IV infusion. Get PTT at baseline and 2 h after starting infusion. Adjust dose (up to 10 mcg/kg/min) until PTT is 1.5 to 3 times baseline (but not more than 100 sec). Percutaneous coronary intervention in those with or at risk for HIT: Bolus 350 mcg/kg IV over 3 to 5 min then 25 mcg/kg/min infusion. Target activated clotting time (ACT): 300 to 450 sec. If ACT less than 300 sec, give 150 mcg/kg bolus and increase infusion rate to 30 mcg/kg/min. If ACT more than 450 sec, reduce infusion rate to 15 mcg/kg/min. Maintain ACT 300 to 450 sec for the duration of the procedure.

PEDS — Not approved in children.

NOTES — ACCP recommends starting max of 2 mcg/kg/min with lower doses of 0.5 to 1.2 mcg/kg/min in patients with heart failure, multiorgan failure, anasarca, or postcardiac surgery. Argatroban prolongs INR with warfarin; discontinue when INR greater than 4 on combined therapy, recheck INR in 4 to 6 h and restart argatroban if INR subtherapeutic. Dosage reduction recommended in liver dysfunction.

MOA — Direct thrombin inhibitor, synthetic derivative of L-arginine.

ADVERSE EFFECTS — Serious: Major bleeding, hypotension. Frequent: Fever, diarrhea.

BIVALIRUDIN (*Angiomax*) ▶proteolysis/K ♀B ▶? $$$$$

ADULT — Anticoagulation in patients undergoing PCI (including patients with or at risk of HIT or HIT and thrombosis syndrome): 0.75 mg/kg IV bolus prior to intervention, then 1.75 mg/kg/h for duration of procedure (with provisional Gp IIb/IIIa inhibition) and optionally up to 4 h postprocedure. For CrCl less than 30 mL/min, reduce infusion dose to 1 mg/kg/h after bolus. For patients on dialysis, reduce infusion dose to 0.25 mg/kg/h after bolus. Use with aspirin 300 to 325 mg PO daily. Additional bolus of 0.3 mg/kg if activated clotting time less than 225 sec. Can additionally infuse 0.2 mg/kg/h for up to 20 h more.

PEDS — Not approved in children.

UNAPPROVED ADULT — Acute coronary syndrome (with or without Gp IIb/IIIa inhibition): 0.1 mg/kg bolus followed by 0.25 mg/kg/h. If PCI, then additional bolus 0.5 mg/kg then 1.75 mg/kg/h. Use with aspirin.

NOTES — Contraindicated in active major bleeding. Monitor activated clotting time. Former trade name Hirulog.

MOA — Direct thrombin inhibitor (reversible).

ADVERSE EFFECTS — Serious: Major bleeding. Frequent: Back pain, nausea.

DABIGATRAN (*Pradaxa*) ▶K ♀C ▶? $$$$$

WARNING — Increased risk of thrombotic event, including stroke, when discontinued. Consider coverage with alternative anticoagulant unless discontinuing due to life-threatening bleeding.

ADULT — Stroke prevention in atrial fibrillation: CrCl greater than 30 mL/min with no interacting medications: 150 mg PO two times per day; CrCL between 30 to 50 mL/min with p-glycoprotein inhibitors (dronedarone and ketoconazole) or CrCL between 15 to 30 mL/min without interacting medications: 75 mg PO two times per day; CrCl less than 15 mL/min or CrCl between 15 to 30 mL/min with p-glycoprotein: contraindicated. Per ACCP CHEST guidelines, not recommended if CrCl is less than 30 mL/min. Treatment of DVT/PE and reduction in risk of recurrence: CrCl greater than 30 mL/min: 150 mg PO two times per day after 5 to 10 days of parenteral anticoagulation.

PEDS — Not approved in children.

UNAPPROVED ADULT — VTE prevention in knee replacement: start 110 mg for one dose given 1 to 4 h after surgery or start 220 mg once if started on postop day 1, then 220 mg daily for 10 days. VTE prevention in hip replacement: 110 mg for one dose given 1 to 4 h after surgery or start 220 mg once if started on postop day 1, then 220 mg daily for 28 to 35 days. Start only after hemostasis has been achieved. Note: 110 mg dose not available in U.S.

FORMS — Trade only: caps 75, 150 mg.

NOTES — Do not break, open, or chew capsules; administer with a full glass of water. Must be stored in original container and used within 4 months or discarded; protect from moisture. Check renal function at baseline and periodically to dose adjust appropriately. May cause gastritis. Avoid use with p-glycoprotein inducers, including rifampin. Potent p-glycoprotein inhibitors may increase exposure and risk of bleeding, particularly if renal dysfunction; see dose adjustment in adult FDA dosing for concomittant use with dronedarone and ketoconazole. Discontinue 1 to 2 days (if CrCl ≥50 mL/min) or 3 to 5 days (if CrCl < 50 mL/min) before invasive procedures. When transitioning from warfarin, stop warfarin and start dabigatran when INR < 2. When transitioning from heparin/LMWH, timing of initiation depends on renal function, see prescribing information. Serious, sometimes fatal, bleeding has been reported. Contraindicated for use in prosthetic heart valves. Removed by hemodialysis, but experience limited for use during bleeding. Minimize lapses in therapy, including those for temporary discontinuation for procedures, to decrease risk of stroke.

MOA — Direct thrombin inhibitor

ADVERSE EFFECTS — Serious: bleeding, hypersensitivity (anaphylaxis, angioedema), thrombotic event (stroke), thrombocytopenia, esophageal ulcers. Frequent: dyspepsia, gastritis, hypersensitivity (urticaria, rash, and pruritus).

DESIRUDIN (*Iprivask*) ▶K ♀C ▶? $$$$$
WARNING — Contraindicated in active major bleeding. High risk of spinal/epidural hematoma if spinal puncture or neuraxial anesthesia before/during treatment. Risk increased by drugs that affect hemostasis including NSAIDs, antiplatelets, and other anticoagulants. Risk also increased by use of indweling catheters, history of trauma or repeated epidural punctures, spinal deformity, or spinal surgery.
ADULT — DVT prophylaxis (hip replacement surgery): 15 mg SC q 12 h. (If CrCl is 31 to 60 mL/min give 5 mg SC q 12 h; if CrCl less than 31 mL/min give 1.7 mg SC q 12 h.)

PEDS — Not approved in children.
NOTES — ACCP guidelines recommend against use if CrCl less than 30 mL/min and against repeated use due to risk of anaphylaxis. Severe anaphylactic reactions resulting in death have been reported upon initial or re-exposure.
MOA — Direct thrombin inhibitor.
ADVERSE EFFECTS — Serious: Anaphylaxis, major hemorrhage (including fatal, intracranial, intraspinal, intraocular), hypotension. Frequent: Injection site reactions, hematoma, minor bleeding, nausea.

HEMATOLOGY/ANTICOAGULANTS: Anticoagulants-Factor Xa Inhibitors

NOTE: See cardiovascular section for antiplatelet drugs and thrombolytics. Contraindicated in active major bleeding. High risk of spinal/epidural hematoma if spinal puncture or neuraxial anesthesia before/during treatment (see Reg Anesth Pain Med 2010;35:64-101.); optimal timing between administration and neuraxial procedures unknown. Risk of bleeding increased by oral anticoagulants, aspirin, dipyridamole, dextran, glycoprotein IIb/IIIA inhibitors, NSAIDs (including ketorolac), ticlopidine, clopidogrel, and thrombolytics. Monitor platelets, Hb, stool for occult blood.

APIXABAN (*Eliquis*) ▶LK ♀B ▶? $$$$$
WARNING — Discontinuation increases risk of thrombotic events, including stroke. If discontinued for a reason other than bleeding, strongly consider coverage with alternative anticoagulant during periods of interruption.
ADULT — Nonvalvular atrial fibrillation: 5 mg PO two times per day. If at least two of the following characteristics: age 80 years or older, wt 60 kg or less, serum creatinine 1.5 mg/dL or greater, then decrease dose to 2.5 mg PO two times daily. In ESRD on hemodialysis: 5 mg PO two times per day; if at least one of the following characteristics: age 80 years or older, wt 60 kg or less, then decrease dose to 2.5 mg PO two times daily. DVT prophylaxis in hip or knee replacement: 2.5 mg PO two times per day. Treatment of DVT/PE: 10 mg PO two times daily for 7 days, then 5 mg PO two times daily. Reduction in risk of recurrence of DVT/PE: 2.5 mg PO two times daily after initial therapy for treatment (minimum 6 months).
PEDS — Not approved in children.
FORMS — Trade only: Tabs 2.5, 5 mg.
NOTES — For atrial fibrillation, when transitioning from warfarin, start apixaban when INR below 2.0. When transitioning from apixaban to warfarin, note that apixaban impacts INR and the effect is highly variable. Therefore, labeling recommends discontinuing apixaban and starting a parenteral anticoagulant with warfarin at the time the next apixaban dose is due. Avoid concomittant use with strong inducers of CYP3A4 and p-glycoprotein or strong dual inhibitors of CYP3A4 and p-glycoprotein.
MOA — Direct Factor Xa inhibitor
ADVERSE EFFECTS — Serious: Major bleeding (GI, intracranial, intraocular, fatal). Common: minor bleeding (bruising, nosebleeds), nausea, anemia.

FONDAPARINUX (*Arixtra*) ▶K ♀B ▶? $$$$$
ADULT — DVT prophylaxis, hip/knee replacement or hip fracture surgery, abdominal surgery: 2.5 mg SC daily starting 6 to 8 h postop (giving earlier increases risk of bleeding). Usual duration is 5 to 9 days; extend prophylaxis up to 24 additional days (max 32 days) in hip fracture surgery. DVT/PE treatment based on wt: wt less than 50 kg: 5 mg SC daily; wt between 50 and 100 kg: 7.5 mg SC daily; wt greater than 100 kg: 10 mg SC daily for at least 5 days and therapeutic oral anticoagulation.
PEDS — Not approved in children. Since risk for bleeding is increased if wt less than 50 kg, bleeding may be a particular concern in pediatrics.
UNAPPROVED ADULT — Unstable angina or non-ST-elevation MI: 2.5 mg SC daily until hospital discharge or for up to 8 days. ST-elevation MI and creatinine < 3 mg/dL: 2.5 mg IV loading dose, then 2.5 mg SC daily until hospital discharge or for up to 8 days. Heparin-induced thrombocytopenia with thrombosis: 5 mg SC daily if < 50 kg; 7.5 mg SC daily if 50-100 kg; 10 mg SC daily if > 100 kg.
FORMS — Generic/Trade: Prefilled syringes 2.5 mg/0.5 mL, 5 mg/0.4 mL, 7.5 mg/0.6 mL, 10 mg/0.8 mL.
NOTES — May cause thrombocytopenia; however, lacks in vitro cross-reactivity with heparin-induced thrombocytopenia antibodies. Risk of major bleeding increased in elderly. Contraindicated if CrCl < 30 mL/min due to increased bleeding risk. Caution advised if CrCl 30 to 50 mL/min. Monitor renal function in all patients; discontinue if severely impaired or labile. In DVT prophylaxis, contraindicated if body wt less than 50 kg. Protamine ineffective for reversing anticoagulant effect. Factor VIIa partially reverses anticoagulant effect in small studies. Risk of catheter thrombosis in PCI; use in conjunction

FONDAPARINUX (*cont.*)

with anticoagulant with anti-IIa activity. Store at room temperature.

MOA — Synthetic pentasaccharide sequence of heparin that binds with antithrombin III to inactivate factor Xa.

ADVERSE EFFECTS — Serious: Major bleeding (especially in elderly, low body weight, or renal dysfunction), thrombocytopenia (rare), spinal/epidural hematomas associated with neuraxial anesthesia/spinal punctures before/during treatment, anaphylaxis. Frequent: None.

RIVAROXABAN (*Xarelto*) ▶K - ♀C ▶? $$$$$

WARNING — Premature discontinuation without alternative anticoagulation increases risk of thrombotic events. If discontinued for a reason other than bleeding, strongly consider coverage with alternative anticoagulant during periods of interruption. Not studied for anticoagulation for prosthetic heart valves. Do not use for acute PE if hemodynamically unstable or planned thrombolysis or pulmonary embolectomy. Spinal or epidural hematomas reported; consider risk/benefit if neuraxial intervention required. Avoid use with combined p-glycoprotein and strong CYP3A4 inhibitors/inducers.

ADULT — DVT prophylaxis in knee or hip replacement: 10 mg PO daily, if CrCl < 30 mL/min avoid use. Start at least 6 to 10 h post-surgery after hemostasis. Continue for 35 days in hip replacement and 12 days in knee replacement. Nonvalvular atrial fibrillation: 20 mg PO daily with the evening meal if CrCl > 50 mL/min; reduce dose to 15 mg PO daily with the evening meal if CrCl 15 to 50 mL/min, avoid use if CrCl <15 mL/min. DVT/PE treatment and to reduce risk of DVT/PE recurrence: 15 mg PO two times daily with food for 21 days, then 20 mg PO daily with food. If CrCl 30 to 49 mL/min: 15 mg PO twice daily with food for 3 weeks, then 15 mg PO daily with food.

FORMS — Trade only: Tabs 10, 15, 20 mg.

NOTES — Concomitant use with anticoagulants, clopidogrel NSAIDs and other drugs impacting hemostasis may increase risk of bleeding. Avoid use with combined p-glycoprotein and strong CYP3A4 inhibitors or inducers. For DVT prophylaxis, DVT/PE treatment and to reduce the risk of recurrence of DVT/PE, avoid if CrCl less than 30 mL/min. For DVT prophylaxis, caution if CrCl 30 to 50 mL/min due to increased rivaroxaban exposure. For atrial fibrillation, when transitioning from warfarin, start rivaroxaban when INR below 3.0. Rivaroxaban affects INR, initial measurements of INR during transition may be unreliable. When transitioning from LMWH or other oral anticoagulant, start rivaroxaban 0 to 2 h before next scheduled evening administration of the anticoagulant. When transitioning from heparin, start rivaroxaban when heparin drip infusion is discontinued.

MOA — Direct Factor Xa inhibitor

ADVERSE EFFECTS — Serious: major bleeding, thrombocytopenia, agranulocytosis, jaundice, cholestasis, hypersensitivity, anaphylactic shock, Stevens-Johnson syndrome, syncope. Frequent: wound secretion, pain in extremity, muscle spasm, pruritus, blister, transaminase elevations.

HEMATOLOGY/ANTICOAGULANTS: Anticoagulants—Low Molecular Weight Heparins (LWMH)

NOTE: Contraindicated in active major bleeding. High risk of spinal/epidural hematoma if spinal puncture or neuraxial anesthesia before/during treatment (see Reg Anesth Pain Med. 2010;35(1):64-101.); optimal timing between LMWH administration and neuraxial procedures is unknown, see product information for some guidance. Risk of bleeding increased by oral anticoagulants, aspirin, dipyridamole, dextran, glycoprotein IIb/IIIA inhibitors, NSAIDs (including ketorolac), ticlopidine, clopidogrel, and thrombolytics. Monitor platelets, Hb, stool for occult blood. Use caution and consider monitoring anti-Xa levels if CrCl less than 30 mL/min, pregnancy, morbidly obese, underweight, or abnormal coagulation/bleeding. Contraindicated in patients with heparin or pork allergy, history of heparin-induced thrombocytopenia. Drug effect can be partially reversed with protamine.

DALTEPARIN (*Fragmin*) ▶KL ♀B ▶+ $$$$$

ADULT — DVT prophylaxis, acute medical illness with restricted mobility: 5000 units SC daily for 12 to 14 days. DVT prophylaxis, abdominal surgery: 2500 units SC 1 to 2 h preop and daily postop for 5 to 10 days. DVT prophylaxis, abdominal surgery in patients with malignancy: 5000 units SC evening before surgery and daily postop for 5 to 10 days. Alternatively, 2500 units SC 1 to 2 h preop and 12 h later, then 5000 units SC daily for 5 to 10 days. DVT prophylaxis, hip replacement: Give SC for up to 14 days. Preop start (day of surgery): 2500 units 2 h preop and 4 to 8 h postop, then 5000 units daily starting at least 6 h after second dose. Preop start (evening before surgery): 5000 units SC given evening before surgery then 5000 units daily starting at least 4 to 8 h postop (approximately 24 h between doses). Postop start regimen: 2500 units 4 to 8 h postop, then 5000 units daily starting at least 6 h after first dose. Treatment of DVT/PE in cancer: 200 units/kg SC daily for 1 month, then 150 units/kg SC daily for 5 months. Max 18,000 units/day, round to nearest commercially available syringe dose (if CrCl < 30 mL/min then target therapeutic anti-Xa level of 0.5 to 1.5 units/mL; recheck 4 to 6 h after dose following at least 3 to 4 doses.). Unstable angina or non-Q-wave MI: 120 units/kg up to 10,000 units SC q 12 h with aspirin (75 to 165 mg/day PO) until clinically stable.

PEDS — Not approved in children.

(cont.)

DALTEPARIN (*cont.*)

UNAPPROVED ADULT — Therapeutic anticoagulation: 200 units/kg SC daily or 100 to 120 units/kg SC two times per day. Venous thromboembolism in pregnancy. Prevention: 5000 units SC daily. Treatment: 100 units/kg SC q 12 h or 200 units/kg SC daily. To avoid unwanted anticoagulation during delivery, stop LMWH 24 h before elective induction of labor.

FORMS — Trade only: Single-dose syringes 2500, 5000 units/0.2 mL, 7500 units/0.3 mL, 10,000 units/1 mL, 12,500 units/0.5 mL, 15,000 units/0.6 mL, 18,000 units/0.72 mL; multidose vial 10,000 units/mL, 9.5 mL and 25,000 units/mL, 3.8 mL.

NOTES — Longer prophylaxis may be warranted based on individual thromboembolic risk. ACCP recommendations suggest that patients with total hip or knee replacement or hip fracture surgery receive prophylaxis for at least 10 days; consider extended prophylaxis (28 to 35 days) in hip replacement or hip fracture surgery.

MOA — Low molecular weight heparin, antithrombin activator that preferentially inhibits factor Xa and inhibits factor IIa.

ADVERSE EFFECTS — Serious: Major bleeding, HIT (rare), spinal/epidural hematomas associated with neuraxial anesthesia/spinal punctures before/during treatment. Frequent: Asymptomatic increase in hepatic transaminases, injection site pain.

ENOXAPARIN (*Lovenox*) ▶KL ♀B ▶+ $$$$$

ADULT —See table.

PEDS — Not approved in children.

UNAPPROVED ADULT — DVT prophylaxis after major trauma: 30 mg SC q 12 h starting 12 to 36 h postinjury if hemostasis achieved. DVT prophylaxis in acute spinal cord injury: 30 mg SC q 12 h. Venous thromboembolism in pregnancy: Prevention: 40 mg SC daily. Treatment: 1 mg/kg SC q 12 h. To avoid unwanted anticoagulation during delivery, stop LMWH 24 h before elective induction of labor.

UNAPPROVED PEDS — Therapeutic anticoagulation: Age younger than 2 mo: 1.5 mg/kg/dose SC q 12 h titrated to anti-Xa level of 0.5 to 1 units/mL. Age 2 mo or older: 1 mg/kg/dose SC q 12 h titrated to anti-Xa level of 0.5 to 1 units/mL. DVT prophylaxis: Age younger than 2 mo: 0.75 mg/kg/dose q 12 h. Age 2 mo or older: 0.5 mg/kg/dose q 12 h.

FORMS — Generic/Trade: Syringes 30, 40 mg; graduated syringes 60, 80, 100, 120, 150 mg. Concentration is 100 mg/mL except for 120, 150 mg, which are 150 mg/mL. All strengths also available preservative free. Trade only: Multidose vial 300 mg.

ENOXAPARIN ADULT DOSING

Indication	Dose	Dosing in Renal Impairment (CrCl less than 30 mL/min)*
DVT prophylaxis		
Abdominal surgery	40 mg SC once daily	30 mg SC once daily
Knee replacement	30 mg SC q 12 h	30 mg SC once daily
Hip replacement	30 mg SC q 12 h or 40 mg SC once daily	30 mg SC once daily
Medical patients	40 mg SC once daily	30 mg SC once daily
Acute DVT		
Inpatient treatment with or without PE	1 mg/kg SC q 12 h or 1.5 mg/kg SC once daily	1 mg/kg SC once daily
Outpatient treatment without PE	1 mg/kg SC q 12 h	1 mg/kg SC once daily
Acute coronary syndrome		
Unstable angina and non-Q-wave MI with aspirin	1 mg/kg SC q 12 h with aspirin	1 mg/kg SC once daily
Acute STEMI in patients younger than 75 yo with aspirin†	30 mg IV bolus with 1 mg/kg SC dose, then 1 mg/kg SC q 12 h (max 100 mg/dose for the 1st two doses)	30 mg IV bolus with 1 mg/kg SC dose, then 1 mg/kg SC once daily
Acute STEMI in patients 75 yo or older with aspirin†	No IV bolus, 0.75 mg/kg SC q 12 h (max 75 mg/dose for the 1st two doses)	No IV bolus, 1 mg/kg SC once daily

DVT = Deep vein thrombosis, PE = pulmonary embolism.

*Not FDA-approved in dialysis.

†If used with thrombolytics, SC dose should be started between 15 min before and 30 min after thrombolytic dose.

NOTES — Longer prophylaxis may be warranted based on individual thromboembolic risk. ACCP recommendations suggest that patients with total hip or knee replacement or hip fracture surgery receive prophylaxis for at least 10 days; consider extended prophylaxis (28 to 35 days) in hip replacement or hip fracture surgery. In PCI, if last enoxaparin administration was more than 8 h before balloon inflation, give 0.3 mg/kg IV bolus. Use caution in mechanical heart valves, especially in pregnancy; reports of valve thrombosis (maternal and fetal deaths reported). Congenital anomalies linked to enoxaparin use during pregnancy; causality unclear. Multidose formulation contains benzyl alcohol, which can cause hypersensitivity and cross placenta in pregnancy.

MOA — Low molecular weight heparin, antithrombin activator that preferentially inhibits factor Xa and inhibits factor IIa.

ADVERSE EFFECTS — Serious: Major bleeding, thrombocytopenia (rare), hemorrhagic anemia, eosinophilia, hepatocellular/cholestatic liver injury, osteoporosis with long-term therapy, spinal/epidural hematomas associated with neuraxial anesthesia/spinal punctures before/during treatment. Reports of valve thrombosis when used for thromboprophylaxis in patients with prosthetic heart valves, especially pregnant women (maternal and fetal deaths reported). Frequent: Asymptomatic increase in hepatic transaminases, injection site reactions, peripheral edema.

HEMATOLOGY/ANTICOAGULANTS: Anticoagulants—Other

HEPARIN DOSING FOR ACUTE CORONARY SYNDROME (ACS)

ST elevation myocardial infarction (STEMI)	Adjunct to thrombolytics: For use with alteplase, reteplase, or tenecteplase: Bolus 60 units/kg IV load (max 4000 units), then initial infusion 12 units/kg/h (max 1000 units/h) adjusted to achieve target PTT 1.5 to 2 times control.
Unstable angina/non-ST elevation myocardial infarction (UA/NSTEMI)	Initial treatment: Bolus 60 units/kg IV load (max 4000 units), then initiate infusion at 12 to 15 units/kg/h (max 1000 units) and adjusted to achieve target PTT 1.5 to 2.5 times control.
Percutaneous coronary intervention (PCI)	With prior anticoagulant therapy but *without* concurrent GPIIb/IIIa inhibitor planned: Additional heparin as needed (2000 to 5000 units) to achieve target ACT 250–300 seconds for HemoTec or 300–350 seconds for Hemochron.
	With prior anticoagulant therapy but *with* planned concurrent GPIIb/IIIa inhibitor: Additional heparin as needed (2000 to 5000 units) to achieve target 200–250 seconds.
	Without prior anticoagulant therapy but *without* concurrent GPIIb/IIIa inhibitor planned: Bolus 70–100 units/kg with target ACT 250–300 seconds for HemoTec or 300–350 seconds for Hemochron.
	Without prior anticoagulant therapy but *with* planned concurrent GPIIb/IIIa inhibitor: Bolus 50–70 units/kg with target ACT 200–250 seconds.

References: *J Am Coll Cardiol* 2011;57:1946. *Circulation* 2011;124:e608. *Circulation* 2004;110:e82–292. *J Am Coll Cardiol* 2009;54:2235.

WEIGHT-BASED HEPARIN DOSING FOR DVT/PE*

Initial dose	80 units/kg IV bolus, then 18 units/kg/h; check PTT in 6 h
PTT less than 35 sec (less than 1.2 x control)	80 units/kg IV bolus, then increase infusion rate by 4 units/kg/h
PTT 35–45 sec (1.2–1.5 x control)	40 units/kg IV bolus, then increase infusion by 2 units/kg/h
PTT 46–70 sec (1.5–2.3 x control)	No change
PTT 71–90 sec (2.3–3 x control)	Decrease infusion rate by 2 units/kg/h
PTT greater than 90 sec (greater than 3 x control)	Hold infusion for 1 h, then decrease infusion rate by 3 units/kg/h

*PTT = Activated partial thromboplastin time. Reagent-specific target PTT may differ; use institutional nomogram when available. Consider establishing a max bolus dose/max initial infusion rate or use an adjusted body wt in obesity. Monitor PTT 6 h after heparin initiation and 6 h after each dosage adjustment. When PTT is stable within therapeutic range, monitor every morning. Therapeutic PTT range corresponds to anti-factor Xa activity of 0.3–0.7 units/mL. Check platelets between days 3 and 5. Can begin warfarin on 1 day of heparin; continue heparin for at least 4 to 5 days of combined therapy. Adapted from *Ann Intern Med* 1993;119;874. *Chest* 2012;141:e28S, e154S. *Circulation* 2001;103:2994.

THERAPEUTIC GOALS FOR ANTICOAGULATION WITH WARFARIN

INR Range*	Indication
2.0–3.0	Atrial fibrillation, deep venous thrombosis, pulmonary embolism, bioprosthetic heart valve (mitral position), mechanical prosthetic heart valve (aortic position)
2.5–3.5	Mechanical prosthetic heart valve (mitral position)

*Aim for an INR in the middle of the INR range (eg, 2.5 for range of 2 to 3 and 3.0 for range of 2.5 to 3.5). Adapted from: *Chest* 2012; 141:e422S, e425S, e533S, e578S; see these guidelines for additional information and other indications.

HEPARIN ▶Reticuloendothelial system ♀C but + ▶+ $$

ADULT — Venous thrombosis/pulmonary embolus treatment: Load 80 units/kg IV, then initiate infusion at 18 units/kg/h. Adjust based on coagulation testing (PTT)—see Table. DVT prophylaxis: 5000 units SC q 8 to 12 h. Prevention of thromboembolism in pregnancy: 5000 to 10,000 units SC q 12 h. Treatment of thromboembolism in pregnancy: 80 units/kg IV load, then infuse 18 units/kg/h with dose titrated to achieve full anticoagulation for at least 5 days. Then continue via SC route with at least 10,000 units SC q 8 to 12 h adjusted to achieve PTT of 1.5 to 2.5× control. To avoid unwanted anticoagulation during delivery, stop SC heparin 24 h before elective induction of labor.

PEDS — Venous thrombosis/pulmonary embolus treatment: Load 50 units/kg IV, then 25 units/kg/h infusion.

UNAPPROVED ADULT — Venous thrombosis/pulmonary embolus treatment (unmonitored): Load 333 units/kg SC, then 250 units/kg SC q 12 h based on max 100 kg wt. Venous thrombosis/pulmonary embolus treatment (monitored): initial dose 17,500 units or 250 units/kg SC twice daily with dose adjustment to achieve and maintain an APTT prolongation that corresponds to plasma heparin levels of 0.3 to 0.7 units/mL anti-Xa activity when measured 6 h after injection. Acute coronary syndromes with or without PCI: 60 units/kg IV, then 12 units/kg/h infusion, adjust according to aPTT or antiXa. See Table.

UNAPPROVED PEDS — Venous thrombosis/pulmonary embolus treatment: Load 75 units/kg IV over 10 min, then 28 units/kg/h if age younger than 1 yo, 20 units/kg/h if age 1 yo or older.

FORMS — Generic only: 1000, 5000, 10,000, 20,000 units/mL in various vial and syringe sizes.

NOTES — Beware of HIT, which may present as a serious thrombotic event. When HIT suspected/diagnosed, discontinue all heparin sources and use alternative anticoagulant. HIT can occur up to several weeks after heparin discontinued. Monitor for elevated LFTs, hyperkalemia/hypoaldosteronism. Osteoporosis with long-term use. Bleeding risk increased by high dose; concomitant thrombolytic or platelet GPIIb/IIIa receptor inhibitor; recent surgery, trauma, or invasive procedure; concomitant hemostatic defect. Monitor platelets, Hb, stool for occult blood. Anti-Xa is an alternative to PTT for monitoring. Drug effect can be reversed with protamine. Do not administer heparin preserved with benzyl alcohol to neonates, infants, or pregnant or lactating women. Do not use Heparin Sodium Injection product as a "catheter lock flush", fatal medication errors have occurred.

MOA — Antithrombin activator that inhibits factors Xa and IIa.

ADVERSE EFFECTS — Serious: Major bleeding, HIT, elevated LFTs, hyperkalemia/hypoaldosteronism, osteoporosis (with long-term use). Frequent: None.

WARFARIN (*Coumadin, Jantoven*) ▶L ♀X, (D for mechanical heart valve replacement) ▶+ $

WARNING — Major or fatal bleeding possible. Higher risk during initiation and when INR elevated. Additional risk factors include: High intensity of anticoagulation (INR greater than 4.0), age 65 yo or older, highly variable INRs, history of GI bleed, hypertension, cerebrovascular disease, heart disease, anemia, malignancy, trauma, renal insufficiency, and long duration of therapy. Regular monitoring of INR needed; monitor those at higher risk more frequently. Educate patients about signs and symptoms of bleeding, measures to reduce risk, and how to manage/seek treatment if bleeding occurs. Many important drug interactions that increase/decrease INR, see table.

ADULT — Oral anticoagulation for prophylaxis/treatment of DVT/PE, thromboembolic complications associated with A-fib, mechanical and bioprosthetic heart valves: Individualize dosing. Start 2 to 5 mg PO daily for 1 to 2 days, then adjust dose to maintain therapeutic PT/INR. Consider using an initial dose of less than 5 mg/day if elderly, malnourished, liver disease, or high bleeding risk. For healthy outpatients, 2012 ACCP CHEST guidelines recommend starting at 10 mg PO daily for 2 days, then adjust dose to maintain therapeutic INR. See product information if CYP2C9 or VKOR1C genotypes are known. Target INR of 2 to 3 for most indications, 2.5 to 3.5 for mechanical mitral heart valve. See table for specific target INR.

PEDS — Not approved in children.

FORMS — Generic/Trade: Tabs 1, 2, 2.5, 3, 4, 5, 6, 7.5, 10 mg.

WARFARIN (*cont.*)

NOTES — Clinical factors that may affect maintenance dose needed to achieve target PT/INR include age, race, wt, sex, medications, and comorbidities. Many important drug interactions that increase/decrease INR, see table for significant drug interactions. Warfarin onset of action is within 24 h, peak effect delayed by 3 to 4 days. Most patients can begin warfarin at the same time as injectable (heparin/LMWH/fondaparinux) therapy. Continue injectable therapy until the INR has been in the therapeutic range for 24 h. Tissue necrosis in protein C or S deficiency. See phytonadione (vitamin K) entry for management of abnormally high INR.

MOA — Inhibits vitamin K-dependent coagulation factors II, VII, IX, X. Also inhibits biologic anticoagulant proteins C&S.

ADVERSE EFFECTS — Serious: Major bleeding, tissue necrosis in protein C or S deficiency (rare), systemic cholesterol microembolization, purple toe syndrome. Frequent: Bruising.

HEMATOLOGY/ANTICOAGULANTS: Antihemophilic Agents

ANTI-INHIBITOR COAGULANT COMPLEX (*Feiba VH, Feiba NF, ✱Feiba VH Immuno*) ▶L ♀C ▶? $$$$$

ADULT — Hemophilia A or B with factor VIII inhibitors, XI and XII (if surgery or active bleeding): 50 to 100 units/kg IV; specific dose and frequency based on site of bleeding, max 200 units/kg/day.

PEDS — Not approved in children.

FORMS — Trade only: Single-dose vials 500, 1000, 2500 units/vial.

NOTES — Contraindicated if normal coagulation. Human plasma product, thus risk of infectious agent transmission. Avoid in active or impending disseminated intravascular coagulation (DIC).

MOA — Coagulation factors II, IX, X and activated factor VII with factor VIII inhibitor bypassing activity that shortens the APTT of plasma containing factor VIII inhibitor.

ADVERSE EFFECTS — Serious: DIC, thromboembolic events, myocardial infarction, anaphylaxis, infectious agent transmission. Frequent: Hypersensitivity (rash, urticaria), anamnestic response (increase in factor VIII inhibitor titer).

FACTOR IX (*AlphaNine SD, Benefix, Mononine, ✱Immunine VH*) ▶L ♀C ▶? $$$$$

ADULT — Hemophilia B: Individualize factor IX dose.

PEDS — Hemophilia B: Individualize factor IX dose.

FORMS — Specific formulation usually chosen by specialist in Hemophilia Treatment Center.

NOTES — Risk of HIV/hepatitis transmission varies by product. Products that contain factors II, VII, and X may cause thrombosis in at-risk patients. Stop infusion if signs of DIC.

MOA — Coagulation factor in the intrinsic coagulation pathway. Activated factor IXa in combination with Factor VIII:C activates Factor X to Xa.

ADVERSE EFFECTS — Serious: HIV/hepatitis transmission (risk varies by product). Products that contain factors II, VII, & X may cause thrombosis in at-risk patients. Frequent: Infusion-related fever, chills, flushing, nausea, IV-site discomfort.

FACTOR VIIA (*NovoSeven, NovoSeven RT, ✱Niastase*) ▶L ♀C ▶? $$$$$

WARNING — Serious thrombotic events reported when used outside of labeled indications, including fatal arterial and venous events. Thrombotic events also reported when used for labeled uses. Monitor all patients for thrombosis. Patients with DIC, advanced atherosclerotic disease, crush injury, or septicemia may be at increased risk for thrombosis. Use with caution in those with thromboembolic risk factors. If DIC or thrombosis confirmed, reduce dose or stop treatment depending on symptoms.

ADULT — Hemophilia A or B: Individualize factor VIIa dose.

PEDS — Hemophilia A or B: Individualize factor VIIa dose.

UNAPPROVED ADULT — Serious bleeding with INR elevation or life-threatening bleeding (ACCP guidelines): Varying doses have been shown effective (10 mcg/kg to max cumulative dose 400 mcg/kg). Factor VIIa has a short half-life; monitor for desired effect. Intracerebral hemorrhage (within 4 h of symptom onset): 40 to 160 mcg/kg IV over 1 to 2 min. Perioperative blood loss in retropubic prostatectomy: 20 or 40 mcg/kg IV bolus.

FORMS — Trade only: NovoSeven: 1200, 2400, 4800 mcg/vial. NovoSeven RT: 1, 2, 5, 8 mg/vial.

NOTES — Caution if hypersensitivity to mouse, hamster or bovine proteins.

MOA — Coagulation factor that acts as a cofactor in extrinsic pathway of coagulation by conversion of Factor IX to IXa and X to Xa.

ADVERSE EFFECTS — Serious: DIC, hemorrhage, hemarthrosis, arterial and venous thromboembolic events. Frequent: Fever, plasma fibrinogen decrease, hyper/hypotension, allergic reactions, infusion site reactions.

FACTOR VIII (*Advate, Alphanate, Helixate, Hemofil M, Humate P, Koate, Kogenate, Monoclate P, Monarc-M, Recombinate, ReFacto, Xyntha*) ▶L ♀C ▶? $$$$$

ADULT — Hemophilia A: Individualize factor VIII dose. Surgical procedures in patients with von Willebrand disease (Alphanate, Humate P): Individualized dosing. Bleeding in patients with von Willebrand disease (Humate P): Individualized dosing.

PEDS — Hemophilia A: Individualize factor VIII dose.

FORMS — Specific formulation usually chosen by specialist in Hemophilia Treatment Center. Recombinant formulations: Advate, Helixate, Kogenate, Recombinate, ReFacto, Xyntha. Human

(cont.)

FACTOR VIII (*cont.*)

plasma-derived formulations: Alphanate, Hemofil M, Humate P, Koate, Monoclate P, Monarc-M.

NOTES — Risk of HIV/hepatitis transmission varies by product; no such risk with recombinant product. Reduced response with development of factor VIII inhibitors. Hemolysis with large/repeated doses in patients with A, B, AB blood type.

MOA — Coagulation factor in the intrinsic coagulation pathway, activated factor VIII acts as a cofactor for conversion of Factor X to Xa.

ADVERSE EFFECTS — Serious: HIV/hepatitis transmission (risk varies by product; no such risk if recombinant). Reduced response with development of factor VIII inhibitors (antibodies). Hemolysis with large/repeated doses in patients with A, B, AB blood type. Frequent: Allergic reactions, infusion site reactions.

HEMATOLOGY/ANTICOAGULANTS: Colony-Stimulating Factors

DARBEPOETIN (*Aranesp, NESP*) ▶cellular sialidases, L ♀C ▶? $$$$$

WARNING — Increased risk of death and serious cardiovascular events, including arterial and venous thrombotic events; may shorten time to tumor progression in cancer patients. To minimize risks in cancer patients, use lowest effective dose. To minimize risks in chronic renal failure, individualize dosing to maintain Hb 10 to 12 g/dL; risks have not been excluded with targeted Hb less than 12 g/dL. Consider antithrombotic DVT prophylaxis, especially in peri-operative period. Not approved for use in cancer patients unless anemia is caused by concurrent myelosuppressive chemotherapy; discontinue when chemotherapy completed. Not for patients receiving myelosuppressive chemotherapy in whom anticipated outcome is cure.

ADULT — Anemia of chronic renal failure: 0.45 mcg/kg IV/SC q week, or 0.75 mcg/kg SC q 2 weeks for some nondialysis patients. Maintenance dose may be lower in predialysis patients than dialysis patients. Initiate when Hb less than 10 g/dL, decrease dose or discontinue when Hb approaches or exceeds 11 g/dL if on dialysis or 10 g/dL if not on dialysis. Anemia in cancer chemo patients: Initially 2.25 mcg/kg SC q week, or 500 mcg SC q 3 weeks. For weekly administration, max 4.5 mcg/kg/dose. Adjust dose based on Hb to maintain lowest level to avoid transfusion. Weekly dose conversion to darbepoetin (D) from erythropoietin (E): 6.25 mcg D for less than 2500 units E; 12.5 mcg D for 2500 to 4999 units E; 25 mcg D for 5000 to 10,999 units E; 40 mcg D for 11,000 to 17,999 units E; 60 mcg D for 18,000 to 33,999 units E; 100 mcg D for 34,000 to 89,999 units E; 200 mcg D for 90,000 units E or greater. Give D once a week for patients taking E 2 to 3 times per week; give D once q 2 weeks for patients taking E once a week. Monitor Hb weekly until stable, then at least monthly.

PEDS — Not approved in children.

UNAPPROVED ADULT — Chemotherapy-induced anemia: 3 mcg/kg or 200 mcg SC q 2 weeks.

FORMS — Trade only: All forms are available with or without albumin. Single-dose vials: 25, 40, 60, 100, 200, 300, 500 mcg/1 mL, and 150 mcg/0.75 mL. Single-dose prefilled syringes or autoinjectors: 25 mcg/0.42 mL, 40 mcg/0.4 mL, 60 mcg/0.3 mL, 100 mcg/0.5 mL, 150 mcg/0.3 mL, 200 mcg/0.4 mL, 300 mcg/0.6 mL, 500 mcg/1 mL.

NOTES — May exacerbate HTN; contraindicated if uncontrolled HTN. Not for immediate correction of anemia. Evaluate iron stores before and during treatment; most patients eventually require iron supplements. Consider other causes of anemia if no response. Use only 1 dose per vial/syringe; discard any unused portion. Do not shake. Protect from light.

MOA — Long-acting form of erythropoietin that gains its increased serum half-life and biologic activity from increased sialic acid content; stimulates erythroid progenitor cells to increase RBC production.

ADVERSE EFFECTS — Serious: Hypertension, seizures, pure red cell aplasia, thrombotic events, severe anemia secondary to antibodies. Frequent: Iatrogenic iron deficiency, myalgia/arthralgia, headache, edema, GI complaints.

EPOETIN ALFA (*Epogen, Procrit, erythropoietin alpha,Eprex*) ▶L ♀C ▶? $$$$$

WARNING — Increased risk of death and serious cardiovascular events, including myocardial infarction, stroke, venous thromboembolism and vascular access thrombosis; in controlled trials, these events were demonstrated when Hb of greater than 11 g/dL was targeted. May shorten time to tumor progression in cancer patients. To minimize risks, use lowest effective dose. Consider antithrombotic DVT prophylaxis, especially in the peri-operative period. Not approved for use in cancer patients unless anemia is caused by concurrent myelosuppressive chemotherapy; discontinue when chemotherapy completed. Not for patients receiving myelosuppressive chemotherapy in whom anticipated outcome is cure.

ADULT — Anemia of chronic renal failure: Initial dose 50 to 100 units/kg IV/SC 3 times per week. Initiate when Hb less than 10 g/dL, decrease dose or discontinue when Hb approaches or exceeds 11 g/dL if on dialysis or 10 g/dL if not on dialysis. Maintain lowest level to avoid transfusion. Zidovudine-induced anemia in HIV-infected patients: 100 to 300 units/kg IV/SC 3 times per week. Anemia in cancer chemo patients: 150 to 300 units/kg SC 3 times per week or 40,000 units SC once a week. Start only if Hb less than 10 g/dL and two additional months of myelosuppression therapy planned. Adjust dose based on Hb to maintain lowest level to avoid transfusion. Reduction of

EPOETIN ALFA (cont.)

allogeneic blood transfusion in surgical patients: 300 units/kg/day SC for 10 days preop, on the day of surgery, and 4 days postop. Or 600 units/kg SC once a week starting 21 days preop and ending on day of surgery (4 doses).

PEDS — Anemia in cancer chemo: 600 Units/kg IV qweek until completion of chemo.

UNAPPROVED PEDS — Anemia of chronic renal failure: Initial dose 50 to 100 units/kg IV/SC 3 times per week. Zidovudine-induced anemia in HIV-infected patients: 100 units/kg SC 3 times per week; max of 300 units/kg/dose.

FORMS — Trade only: Single-dose 1-mL vials 2000, 3000, 4000, 10,000, 40,000 units/mL. Multidose vials 10,000 units/mL 2 mL, 20,000 units/mL 1 mL.

NOTES — May exacerbate HTN; contraindicated if uncontrolled HTN. Not for immediate correction of anemia. Evaluate iron stores before and during treatment; most patients eventually require iron supplements. Consider other causes of anemia if no response. Single-dose vials contain no preservatives. Use 1 dose per vial; do not re-enter vial. Discard unused portion.

MOA — Stimulates erythroid progenitor cells to increase red blood cell production.

ADVERSE EFFECTS — Serious: Hypertension in patients with chronic renal failure, seizures, pure red cell aplasia, thrombotic events, severe anemia secondary to antibodies. Frequent: Iatrogenic iron deficiency, headache, arthralgia, fever.

FILGRASTIM (G-CSF, Neupogen, Granix) ▶L ♀C ▶? $$$$$

ADULT — Neutropenia from myelosuppressive chemotherapy: 5 mcg/kg/day SC/IV until postnadir ANC is at least 10,000/mm^3 for no more than 2 weeks. Can increase by 5 mcg/kg/day with each cycle prn. Bone marrow transplant: 10 mcg/kg/day IV infusion over 4 to 24 h or 24-h SC infusion. Administer 1st dose at least 24 h after cytotoxic chemotherapy and at least 24 h after bone marrow. Adjust to neutrophil response (see prescribing information). Peripheral blood progenitor cell collection: 10 mcg/kg/day in donors for at least 4 days (usually 6 to 7 days) before the 1st leukapheresis and continued until the final leukapheresis. Consider decreased dose if WBC greater than 100,000/mm^3. Severe chronic neutropenia (congenital): Start 6 mcg/kg SC two times per day. Severe chronic neutropenia (idiopathic or cyclic): Start 5 mcg/kg SC daily.

PEDS — Neutropenia from myelosuppressive chemotherapy: 5 mcg/kg/day SC/IV for no more than 2 weeks until postnadir ANC is at least 10,000/mm^3. 10,000/mm^3 for no more than 2 weeks. Can increase by 5 mcg/kg/day with each cycle prn. Bone marrow transplant: 10 mcg/kg/day IV infusion over 4 to 24 h or 24 h SC infusion. Administer 1st dose at least 24 h after cytotoxic chemotherapy and at least 24 h after bone marrow. Adjust to neutrophil response (see product information). Peripheral blood progenitor cell collection: 10 mcg/kg/day in donors for

at least 4 days (usually 6 to 7 days) before the first leukapheresis and continued until the final leukapheresis. Consider decreased dose if WBC greater than 100,000/mm^3. Severe chronic neutropenia (congenital): Start 6 mcg/kg SC two times per day. Severe chronic neutropenia (idiopathic or cyclic): Start 5 mcg/kg SC daily.

UNAPPROVED ADULT — AIDS: 0.3 to 3.6 mcg/kg/day.

FORMS — Trade only: Single-dose vials: 300 mcg/1 mL, 480 mcg/1.6 mL. Single-dose syringes: 300 mcg/0.5 mL, 480 mcg/0.8 mL (Neupogen, Granix).

NOTES — Allergic-type reactions, bone pain, cutaneous vasculitis. Do not give within 24 h before/after cytotoxic chemotherapy. Store in refrigerator; use within 24 h when kept at room temperature.

MOA — Granulocyte colony-stimulating factor, a colony-stimulating factor that stimulates neutrophil production.

ADVERSE EFFECTS — Serious: Allergic-type reactions, cutaneous vasculitis, osteoporosis, thrombocytopenia, splenomegaly. Frequent: Bone pain, increased levels of LDH and alkaline phosphatase.

OPRELVEKIN (Neumega) ▶K ♀C ▶? $$$$$

WARNING — Risk of allergic reactions and anaphylaxis.

ADULT — Prevention of severe thrombocytopenia after chemo for nonmyeloid malignancies: 50 mcg/kg SC daily starting 6 to 24 h after chemo and continuing until postnadir platelet count is at least 50,000 cells/mcL (usual duration 10 to 21 days).

PEDS — Not approved in children. Safe and effective dose not established. Papilledema with 100 mcg/kg; 50 mcg/kg ineffective.

FORMS — Trade only: 5 mg single-dose vials with diluent.

NOTES — Fluid retention: Monitor fluid and electrolyte balance. Transient atrial arrhythmias, visual blurring, papilledema.

MOA — Interleukin-11, thrombopoietic growth factor that increases platelet production.

ADVERSE EFFECTS — Serious: Anaphylaxis, allergy, papilledema. Frequent: Edema, dyspnea, pleural effusions, transient atrial arrhythmias, transient visual blurring, conjunctival injection, thrush, asthenia.

PEGFILGRASTIM (Neulasta) ▶Plasma ♀C ▶? $$$$$

ADULT — To reduce febrile neutropenia after chemo for nonmyeloid malignancies: 6 mg SC once each chemo cycle.

PEDS — Not approved in children.

FORMS — Trade only: Single-dose syringes 6 mg/0.6 mL.

NOTES — Do not use if wt less than 45 kg. Bone pain common. Do not give in the time period between 14 days prior to and 24 h after cytotoxic chemo. Store in refrigerator. Stable at room temperature for no more than 48 h. Protect from light.

MOA — Long-acting form of filgrastim that is conjugated to polyethylene glycol (pegylated).

(cont.)

PEGFILGRASTIM (cont.)

ADVERSE EFFECTS — Serious: cutaneous vasculitis. Frequent: Bone pain, reversible increases in LDH, alkaline phosphatase, uric acid.

SARGRAMOSTIM (GM-CSF, Leukine) ▶L ♀C ▶? $$$$$

ADULT — Specialized dosing for leukemia, bone marrow transplantation.

PEDS — Not approved in children.

MOA — Granulocyte-macrophage colony-stimulating factor, a colony-stimulating factor that stimulates the production of neutrophils, monocytes, and eosinophils.

ADVERSE EFFECTS — Serious: Capillary leak syndrome, dyspnea due to sequestration of WBCs in lungs (rare). Frequent: Fluid retention, fever, asthenia, headache, bone pain, chills, myalgia.

HEMATOLOGY/ANTICOAGULANTS: Other Hematological Agents

AMINOCAPROIC ACID (Amicar) ▶K ♀D ▶? $ IV $$$$$

Oral

ADULT — To improve hemostasis when fibrinolysis contributes to bleeding: 4 to 5 g IV/PO over 1 h, then 1 g/h for 8 h or until bleeding controlled.

PEDS — Not approved in children.

UNAPPROVED ADULT — Prevention of recurrent subarachnoid hemorrhage: 6 g IV/PO q 4 h (6 doses/day). Reduction of postop bleeding after cardiopulmonary bypass: 5 g IV, then 1 g/h for 6 to 8 h.

UNAPPROVED PEDS — To improve hemostasis when fibrinolysis contributes to bleeding: 100 mg/kg or 3 g/m² IV infusion during 1st h, then continuous infusion of 33.3 mg/kg/h or 1 g/m²/h. Max dose of 18 g/m2/day. IV prep contains benzyl alcohol; do not use in newborns.

FORMS — Generic/Trade: Syrup 250 mg/mL, Tabs 500 mg. Trade only: Tabs 1000 mg.

NOTES — Contraindicated in active intravascular clotting. Do not use in DIC without heparin. Can cause intrarenal thrombosis, hyperkalemia. Skeletal muscle weakness, necrosis with prolonged use; monitor CPK. Use with estrogen/oral contraceptives can cause hypercoagulability. Rapid IV administration can cause hypotension, bradycardia, arrhythmia.

MOA — Inhibits fibrinolysis.

ADVERSE EFFECTS — Serious: Skeletal muscle weakness and necrosis with prolonged use. Rapid IV administration can cause hypotension, bradycardia, arrhythmia. Frequent: None.

ANAGRELIDE (Agrylin) ▶LK ♀C ▶? $$$$$

ADULT — Thrombocythemia due to myeloproliferative disorders (including essential thrombocythemia): Start 0.5 mg PO four times per day or 1 mg PO two times per day, then after 1 week adjust to lowest effective dose that maintains platelet count less than 600,000/mcL. Max 10 mg/day or 2.5 mg as a single dose. Usual dose 1.5 to 3 mg/day.

PEDS — Limited data. Thrombocythemia due to myeloproliferative disorders (including essential thrombocythemia): Start 0.5 mg PO daily, then after 1 week adjust to lowest effective dose that maintains platelet count less than 600,000/mcL. Max 10 mg/day or 2.5 mg as a single dose. Usual dose 1.5 to 3 mg/day.

FORMS — Generic/Trade: Caps 0.5 mg. Generic only: Caps 1 mg.

NOTES — Caution with heart disease, may cause hypotension, vasodilation, tachycardia, palpitations,

heart failure, QTc prolongation, torsades; obtain baseline ECG and consider periodic monitoring. Contraindicated in severe hepatic impairment, use with caution in mild to moderate hepatic impairment. Monitor LFTs baseline and during therapy. Caution in lung disease and renal insufficiency. Dosage should be increased by not more than 0.5 mg/day in any 1 week.

MOA — Unknown; a decrease in megakaryocyte hypermaturation may decrease platelet production.

ADVERSE EFFECTS — Serious: May cause cardiovascular events including hypotension, vasodilation, tachycardia, palpitations, heart failure, QTc prolongation and torsades, renal failure, tubulointerstitial nephritis, pulmonary disorders, hepatotoxicity. Frequent: Headache, diarrhea, edema, palpitation, abdominal pain.

DEFERASIROX (Exjade) ▶L ♀B ▶? $$$$$

WARNING — Monitor renal and hepatic function closely. Renal impairment, including failure and death, has been reported; assess serum creatinine and creatinine clearance twice before therapy and monthly thereafter. Fatal hepatic failure has been reported; monitor LFTs and bilirubin baseline, q 2 weeks for 1 month, then monthly. Gastrointestinal bleeding reported, especially if thrombocytopenia or advanced hematologic malignancies. Severe skin reactions reported, monitor for and discontinue if Stevens-Johnson Syndrome or erythema multiforme suspected.

ADULT — Chronic iron overload due to blood transfusions: 20 mg/kg PO daily; adjust dose q 3 to 6 months based on ferritin trends. Max 40 mg/kg/day. Chronic iron overload in non-transfusion-dependent thalassemia syndromes: 10mg/kg PO daily; adjust dose based on ferritin and liver iron concentration. Max 20 mg/kg/day.

PEDS — Chronic iron overload due to blood transfusions, age 2 yo or older: 20 mg/kg PO daily; adjust dose q 3 to 6 months based on ferritin trends. Max 40 mg/kg/day. Chronic iron overload in non-transfusion-dependent thalassemia syndromes, age 10 yo or older: 10mg/kg PO daily; adjust dose based on ferritin and liver iron concentration. Max 20 mg/kg/day.

FORMS — Trade only: Tabs for dissolving into oral susp 125, 250, 500 mg.

NOTES — Do not use if CrCl < 40 mL/min, serum creatinine greater than twice upper limit of normal. Do not use if severe (Child-Pugh C) hepatic

DEFERASIROX (*cont.*)

impairment. Reduce starting dose by 50% in moderate (Child-Pugh B) hepatic impairment or in renal impairment (CrCl 40 to 60 ml/min). Closely monitor patients with mild hepatic impairment. Contraindicated if high-risk for myelodysplastic syndrome, advanced malignancy, poor performance status or platelet count < 50 x 10^9/L. Give on an empty stomach, 30 min or more before food. Reports of fatal cytopenias, monitor CBC regularly. Perform auditory and ophthalmic testing before initiation of therapy and yearly thereafter. Do not take with aluminum-containing antacids. May decrease serum ferritin and liver iron concentrations. See product information for detailed information regarding criteria of iron overload.

MOA — Chelates free serum iron.

ADVERSE EFFECTS — Serious: Renal failure, tubulointerstitial nephritis, hepatic failure, hearing disturbance/loss, ocular disturbances, optic neuritis, neutropenia, thrombocytopenia, GI hemorrhage/ulcer, erythema multiforme, Stevens-Johnson Syndrome Frequent: Fever, headache, abdominal pain, cough, diarrhea, creatinine increase, N/V, rash, arthralgia, fatigue.

ECULIZUMAB (*Soliris*) ▶Serum ♀C ▶? $$$$$

WARNING — Increased risk of meningococcal infections. Administer meningococcal vaccine at least 2 weeks prior to therapy and revaccinate according to current guidelines. Monitor patients for early signs of meningococcal infections, evaluate and treat with antibiotics as necessary.

ADULT — Reduction of hemolysis in paroxysmal nocturnal hemoglobinuria: 600 mg IV infusion q 7 days for 4 weeks, then 900 mg for fifth dose 7 days later, then 900 mg q 14 days. Atypical hemolytic uremic syndrome: 900 mg IV infusion weekly for 4 weeks, then 1200 mg for fifth dose 1 week later, then 1200 mg q 14 days. Administer infusion over 35 minutes.

PEDS — Not approved in children.

NOTES — Contraindicated if active meningococcal infection or without current meningococcal vaccination. Increases risk of infection with encapsulated bacteria, including Streptococcus pneumoniae and Haemophilus influenzae type b (Hib). Consider appropriate immunization. Caution if systemic infection. Dose may be given within 2 days of scheduled dosing date. Give supplemental dose after plasmapheresis, plasma exchange or fresh frozen plasma infusion; see product information for dosing. Monitor LDH (if used for paroxysmal nocturnal hemoglobinuria) or LDH, platelets and serum creatinine (if used for atypical hemolytic uremic syndrome) during therapy. Monitor following discontinuation for hemolysis for 8 weeks (if used for paroxysmal nocturnal hemoglobinuria) or thrombotic microangiopathy for 12 weeks (if used for atypical hemolytic uremic syndrome).

MOA — Recombinant humanized monoclonal antibody that inhibits complement mediated intravascular hemolysis.

ADVERSE EFFECTS — Serious: meningococcal infections, serious infection. Frequent: Hypersensitivity, infusion reaction, headache, nasopharyngitis, back pain, nausea.

ELTROMBOPAG (*Promacta,* ✦*Revolade*) ▶LK ♀C ▶? $$$$$

WARNING — Hepatotoxicity; may increase risk of hepatic decompensation in patients with chronic hepatitis C in combination with interferon and ribavirin. Obtain serum transaminases and bilirubin at baseline and q 2 weeks during dose adjustment, then monthly. If abnormal, repeat LFTs within 3 to 5 days. If LFTs remain abnormal, monitor weekly until LFTs return to baseline, stabilize or resolve. Discontinue if ALT is 3 or more times upper limit of normal and increasing, persistent for at least 4 weeks, hepatotoxicity symptoms or with increased direct bilirubin.

ADULT — Thrombocytopenia in ITP (unresponsive to steroids, immunoglobulins, or splenectomy): Start 50 mg PO daily. In hepatic insufficiency or East Asian ancestry, start 25 mg daily. Adjust to achieve platelet count of 50,000; max 75 mg daily. Discontinuation may worsen thrombocytopenia, monitor CBC weekly for 4 weeks after discontinuation. Thrombocytopenia in patients with chronic hepatitis C (to allow the initiation and maintenance of interferon-based therapy): 25 mg PO daily. Adjust every 2 weeks to achieve a platelet count which allows antiviral therapy, max 100 mg daily.

PEDS — Not approved in children.

FORMS — Trade only: Tabs,12.5, 25, 50, 75, 100 mg.

NOTES — Available through restricted access program. Give on empty stomach (1 h before or 2 h after meal); separate from medications and food containing iron, Ca, Mg, selenium, and zinc with an interval of at least 4 h. Monitor CBC weekly until platelet counts stabilize, then monthly. In ITP, discontinue if no response after 4 weeks on 75 mg daily. Not for use to normalize platelet count; goal is increase platelet count to a level that reduces bleeding or allows antiviral therapy. Monitor peripheral blood for signs of marrow fibrosis. Portal vein thrombosis reported in patients with chronic liver disease.

MOA — thrombopoietin receptor agonist

ADVERSE EFFECTS — Serious: hepatotoxicity, marrow fibrosis, thromboembolism. Frequent: nausea, vomiting, menorrhagia, myalgia, paresthesia, cataract, dyspepsia, ecchymosis, increased serum transaminases, conjunctival hemorrhage.

HYDROXYUREA (*Hydrea, Droxia*) ▶LK ♀D ▶— $ varies by therapy

WARNING — Mutagenic and clastogenic; may cause secondary leukemia. Instruct patients to report promptly fever, sore throat, signs of local infection, bleeding from any site, or symptoms suggestive of anemia. Cutaneous vasculitic toxicities, including vasculitic ulcerations and gangrene, have been reported most often in patients on interferon therapy.

(cont.)

HYDROXYUREA (*cont.*)

ADULT — Sickle cell anemia (Droxia): Start 15 mg/kg PO daily while monitoring CBC q 2 weeks. If WBC is 2500/mm^3 or greater, platelet count is 95,000/mm^3 or greater, and Hb is above 5.3 g/dL, then increase dose q 12 weeks by 5 mg/kg/day (max 35 mg/kg/day). Solid tumors (Hydrea): Intermittent dose: 80 mg/kg PO for a single dose q 3 days. Continuous therapy: 20 to 30 mg/kg PO daily. Head and neck cancer with radiation (Hydrea): 80 mg/kg PO for a single dose q 3 days. Resistant chronic myelocytic leukemia: 20 to 30 mg/kg PO daily. Give concomitant folic acid.

PEDS — Not approved in children.

UNAPPROVED ADULT — Essential thrombocythemia at high risk for thrombosis: 0.5 to 1 g PO daily adjusted to keep platelets < 400/mm^3. Also has been used for HIV, psoriasis, polycythemia vera.

UNAPPROVED PEDS — Sickle cell anemia.

FORMS — Generic/Trade: Caps 500 mg. Trade only: (Droxia) Caps 200, 300, 400 mg.

NOTES — Reliable contraception is recommended. Monitor CBC and renal function. Elderly may need lower doses. Minimize exposure to the drug by wearing gloves during handling.

MOA — Antimetabolite.

ADVERSE EFFECTS — Serious: Bone marrow suppression, nephrotoxicity. Frequent: Bone marrow suppression, erythropoiesis, mucositis, rash.

PLERIXAFOR (*Mozobil*) ▶K ♀D ▶? $$$$$

ADULT — Hematopoietic stem cell mobilization with G-CSF for autologous transplantation in non-Hodgkin's lymphoma and multiple myeloma: 0.24 mg/kg (actual body wt) SC once daily for up to 4 days, max 40 mg/day.

PEDS — Not approved in children.

FORMS — Trade only: Single-dose vials 20 mg/mL, 1.2 mL vial.

NOTES — Use with G-CSF; initiate after patient has received G-CSF daily for 4 days. Administer 11 h prior to apheresis. If CrCl less than 50 mL/min, decrease dose to 0.16 mg/kg. Do not use in leukemia. Monitor CBC, may increase WBC and decrease platelets. May mobilize tumor cells from marrow. Evaluate for splenic rupture if left upper abdominal, scapular, or shoulder pain. Risk of anaphylaxis; administer in health care setting and monitor for at least 30 minutes.

MOA — CXCR4 chemokine antagonist.

ADVERSE EFFECTS — Serious: Leukocytosis, thrombocytopenia, splenic rupture, anaphylactic shock. Frequent: Diarrhea, nausea, fatigue, injection site reactions, headache, arthralgia, dizziness, vomiting.

PROTAMINE ▶Plasma ♀C ▶? $

WARNING — Hypotension, cardiovascular collapse, pulmonary edema/vasoconstriction/hypertension may occur. May be more common with higher doses, overdose or repeated doses, including previous exposure to protamine or protamine-containing drugs (including insulin). Other risk factors include fish allergy, vasectomy, LV dysfunction, and pulmonary hemodynamic instability.

ADULT — Heparin overdose: Within 30 minutes of IV heparin: 1 mg antagonizes about 100 units heparin. If greater than 30 minutes since heparin: 0.5 mg antagonizes about 100 units heparin. Due to short half-life of heparin (60 to 90 min), use IV heparin doses only from last several hours to calculate dose of protamine. SC heparin may require prolonged administration of protamine. Give IV over 10 min in doses of no greater than 50 mg.

PEDS — Not approved in children.

UNAPPROVED ADULT — Reversal of low-molecular-weight heparin: If within 8 h of LMWH dose: give 1 mg protamine per 100 anti-Xa units of dalteparin or 1 mg protamine per 1 mg enoxaparin. Smaller doses advised if greater than 8 h since LMWH administration. Give additional 0.5 mg protamine per 100 anti-Xa units of dalteparin or 0.5 mg protamine per 1 mg enoxaparin if aPTT remains prolonged 2 to 4 h after first infusion of protamine.

UNAPPROVED PEDS — Heparin overdose: Within 30 min of last heparin dose, give 1 mg protamine per 100 units of heparin received; between 30 to 60 min since last heparin dose, give 0.5 to 0.75 mg protamine per 100 units of heparin received; between 60 to 120 min since last heparin dose, give 0.375 to 0.5 mg protamine per 100 units of heparin; more than 120 min since last heparin dose, give 0.25 to 0.375 mg protamine per 100 units of heparin.

NOTES — Severe hypotension/anaphylactoid reaction possible with too rapid administration. Additional doses of protamine may be required in some situations (neutralization of SC heparin, heparin rebound after cardiac surgery). Monitor aPTT to confirm. Incomplete neutralization of LMWHs.

MOA — Binds with and neutralizes heparin and partially reverses LMWHs.

ADVERSE EFFECTS — Serious: Severe hypotension/anaphylactoid reaction with too rapid administration, allergic reactions in patients with fish allergy, previous exposure to protamine (including insulin), pulmonary edema, circulatory collapse. Frequent: Back pain, transient flushing.

PROTEIN C CONCENTRATE (*Ceprotin*) ▶Serum ♀C ▶? $$$$$

ADULT — Severe congenital protein C deficiency (prevention and treatment of venous thrombosis and purpura fulminans): Individualized dosing.

PEDS — Severe congenital protein C deficiency (prevention and treatment of venous thrombosis and purpura fulminans): Individualized dosing.

NOTES — Product contains heparin; do not use if history of heparin induced thrombocytopenia. Check platelets and discontinue if heparin induced thrombocytopenia suspected. Product contains sodium. Made from pooled human plasma, may transmit infectious agents.

PROTEIN C CONCENTRATE (cont.)

MOA — Concentrated protein C from human blood donors that controls the coagulation system to prevent excessive procoagulant responses to activating stimuli.

ADVERSE EFFECTS — Serious: Hypersensitivity, hemothorax, hypotension, thrombocytopenia. Frequent: Rash, itching, lightheadedness.

ROMIPLOSTIM (Nplate) ▶L ♀C ▶? $$$$$

ADULT — Chronic immune idiopathic thrombocytopenic purpura: 1 mcg/kg SC weekly. Adjust by 1 mcg/kg weekly to achieve and maintain platelet count at least 50,000 cells/mcL; max 10 mcg/kg weekly. Hold dose if platelet count is 400,000 cells/mcL or greater.

PEDS — Not approved in children.

NOTES — Use only for chronic ITP; do not use if low platelets from other causes. Use only if increased risk of bleeding and insufficient response to corticosteroids, immunoglobulins, or splenectomy. Do not use to normalize platelet counts; excessive therapy may increase risk of thrombosis. May increase risk for fibrous deposits in bone marrow. Monitor CBC (platelets and peripheral blood smears) weekly until stable dose; then monthly. Platelet counts may drop below baseline following discontinuation; monitor CBC for 2 weeks following cessation of therapy. May increase risk of hematologic malignancies, especially if myelodysplastic syndrome. Available only through restricted distribution program. To minimize errors, follow specific administration instructions in product information.

MOA — Throbopoietin receptor agonist.

ADVERSE EFFECTS — Serious: Thrombosis, bone marrow fibrosis, hypersensitivity, angioedema. Frequent: Headache, arthralgia, dizziness, insomnia, myalgia, pain in extremity, shoulder pain, dyspepsia, paresthesia.

THROMBIN—TOPICAL (Evithrom, Recothrom, Thrombin-JMI) ▶? ♀C ▶? $$$

WARNING — The bovine form (Thrombin-JMI) has been associated with rare but potentially fatal abnormalities in hemostasis ranging from asymptomatic alterations in PT and/or aPTT to severe bleeding or thrombosis. Hemostatic abnormalities are likely due to antibody formation, may cause factor V deficiency, and are more likely with repeated applications.

Consult hematologist if abnormal coagulation, bleeding, or thrombosis after topical thrombin use.

ADULT — Hemostatic aid for minor bleeding: Apply topically to site of bleeding; dose depends on area to be treated.

PEDS — Hemostatic aid for minor bleeding (Evithrom): Apply topically to site of bleeding; dose depends on area to be treated. Recothrom/Thrombin-JMI not approved in children.

NOTES — Do not inject; for topical use only. Do not use for severe or brisk arterial bleeding. Thaw Evithrom prior to use. Reconstitute Recothrom and Thrombin-JMI prior to use. Evithrom is human-derived and carries risk of viral transmission. Recothrom is a recombinant product; risk of allergic reaction in known hypersensitivity to snake proteins; contraindicated in hypersensitivity to hamster proteins. Thrombin-JMI is a bovine origin product; contraindicated in hypersensitivity to products of bovine origin.

MOA — Promotes clot formation by activating platelets and catalyzing the conversion of fibrinogen to fibrin.

ADVERSE EFFECTS — Serious: Anaphylaxis, antibody development, hemostatic abnormalities, thrombosis, severe bleeding. Frequent: Pruritus, incision/procedure site complications.

TRANEXAMIC ACID (Cyklokapron, Lysteda) ▶K ♀B ▶– $$$$

WARNING — Do not use with combined hormonal contraceptives; risk of thromboembolism.

ADULT — Prophylaxis/reduction of bleeding during tooth extraction in hemophilia patients: 10 mg/kg IV immediately before surgery, then 10 mg/kg PO 3 to 4 times per day for 2 to 8 days following surgery. Heavy menstrual bleeding (Lysteda): 1300 mg PO three times per day for up to 5 days during menstruation.

PEDS — Not approved in children.

FORMS — Generic/Trade (Lysteda, PO): oral tab 650 mg. Generic/Trade (Cyklokapron, IV): 100 mg/mL, 10 mL vial.

NOTES — Dose adjust in renal impairment.

MOA — Competitively inhibits plasminogen activator and noncompetitively plasmin (at higher doses).

ADVERSE EFFECTS — Severe: Hypotension (infusion rate limiting), DVT, PE, vision abnormalities, convulsions. Frequent: N/V, diarrhea, giddiness, menstrual discomfort.

HERBAL AND ALTERNATIVE THERAPIES

NOTE: In the United States, herbal and alternative therapy products are regulated as dietary supplements, not drugs. Premarketing evaluation and FDA approval are not required unless specific therapeutic claims are made. Because these products are not required to demonstrate efficacy, it is unclear whether many of them have health benefits. In addition, there may be considerable variability in content from lot to lot or between products. See www.tarascon.com/herbals for the evidence-based efficacy ratings used by Tarascon editorial staff.

CHAMOMILE (*Matricaria recutita–German chamomile, Anthemis nobilis–Roman chamomile*) ▶? ♀– ▶? $
UNAPPROVED ADULT — Oral extract: Modest benefit in study for generalized anxiety disorder, but little to no benefit in study for primary chronic insomnia. Topical: Efficacy unclear for skin infections or inflammation. Does not appear to reduce mucositis caused by 5-fluorouracil or radiation.
UNAPPROVED PEDS — Supplements not for use in children. Efficacy and safety unclear for treatment of infant colic with multi-ingredient teas/extracts of chamomile, fennel, and lemon balm.
FORMS — Not by prescription.
NOTES — Theoretical concern (no clinical evidence) for interactions due to increased sedation, increased risk of bleeding (contains coumarin derivatives), delayed GI absorption of other drugs (due to antispasmodic effect). Increased INR with warfarin attributed to chamomile in single case report.
MOA — Contains compounds with antispasmodic, antiinflammatory, antimicrobial, and mild sedative effects in animal and in vitro studies.
ADVERSE EFFECTS — Rare allergic reactions including anaphylaxis, contact dermatitis. Cross-hypersensitivity with other plants in Compositae family, including arnica, chrysanthemum, echinacea, feverfew, ragweed, Artemisia. Topical application to the eye can cause conjunctivitis.

MILK THISTLE (*Silybum marianum, Legalon, silymarin, Thisiylin*) ▶LK ♀– ▶– $
UNAPPROVED ADULT — Hepatic cirrhosis (efficacy unclear): 100 to 200 mg PO three times per day of standardized extract with 70 to 80% silymarin. Guidelines for management of alcoholic liver disease recommend against use. Hepatitis C: Does not appear to improve viral load, serum transaminases, or liver histology; the American Gastroenterological Association recommends against use. Amatoxin-containing mushroom poisoning (possibly effective): IV silibinin (Legalon SIL) available from NIH study by calling 1-866-520-4412; oral milk thistle has been used when IV silibinin is not available.
UNAPPROVED PEDS — Not for use in children.
FORMS — Not by prescription.
NOTES — May inhibit CYP2C9. May decrease blood glucose in patients with cirrhosis and diabetes.
MOA — Hepatoprotectant with antioxidant, membrane-stabilizing, liver cell regeneration properties.

Silibinin inhibits OATP 1B3 and NTCP transport of amatoxin into hepatocytes.
ADVERSE EFFECTS — Serious: Anaphylaxis. Other: GI distress, headache, skin reactions, arthralgias.

ALOE VERA (*acemannan, burn plant*) ▶LK ♀oral– topical+? ▶oral — topical + ? $
UNAPPROVED ADULT — Topical: Efficacy unclear for seborrheic dermatitis, psoriasis, genital herpes, partial-thickness skin burns. Does not prevent radiation-induced skin injury. Do not apply to surgical incisions; impaired healing reported. Oral: Efficacy unclear for active ulcerative colitis or type 2 diabetes.
UNAPPROVED PEDS — Not for use in children.
FORMS — Not by prescription.
NOTES — OTC laxatives containing aloe latex were removed from the US market due to concerns about increased risk of colon cancer. Cases of Henoch-Schonlein purpura and hepatotoxicity reported with oral administration.
MOA — Topical: Constituents of gel from within leaves have skin-moisturizing, immunomodulatory, anti-inflammatory, and antiviral activity in vitro. Oral: Aloe latex contains anthraquinone glycosides (stimulant laxative). Pancreatic beta cell stimulation in vitro.
ADVERSE EFFECTS — Topical: Contact dermatitis, pruritus. Oral: Abdominal cramping, diarrhea. Potassium depletion or electrolyte imbalance possible with chronic administration. Hepatotoxicity (hypersensitivity probable mechanism). Henoch-Schonlein purpura (several case reports).

ALPHA LIPOIC ACID (*lipoic acid, thioctic acid, ALA*) ▶intracellular ♀C ▶? $
UNAPPROVED ADULT — Diabetic peripheral neuropathy (possibly effective): 600 mg PO daily. American Academy of Neurology found evidence insufficent to support or refute use to treat painful diabetic neuropathy. May lower blood sugar and is used as adjunct in patients with diabetes at doses of 600 to 1200 mg daily. Does not appear effective for burning mouth syndrome.
UNAPPROVED PEDS — Not for use in children
FORMS — Not by prescription
NOTES — Considered an essential nutrient, but has not been studied as a supplement in pregnancy, lactation, and children.
MOA — Antioxidant.
ADVERSE EFFECTS — Rash, N/V (dose-related), vertigo (dose-related), low blood sugar, urine odor. Case report of acute cholestatic hepatitis.

ANDROSTENEDIONE (*andro*) ▶L, peripheral conversion to estrogens and androgens ♀–▶– $

UNAPPROVED ADULT — Was marketed as anabolic steroid to enhance athletic performance. Advise patients against use because of potential for androgenic (primarily in women) and estrogenic (primarily in men) side effects.

UNAPPROVED PEDS — Not for use in children.

FORMS — Not by prescription.

NOTES — Banned as dietary supplement by FDA. Also banned by many athletic organizations. In theory, chronic use may increase risk of hormone-related cancers (prostate, breast, endometrial, ovarian). Increase in androgen levels could exacerbate hyperlipidemia.

MOA — Anabolic steroid precursor; converted to estrogen and testosterone.

ADVERSE EFFECTS — Potential long-term effects include: Testicular atrophy, impotence, and gynecomastia in men; acne, male pattern baldness, deep voice, hirsutism, clitoral enlargement, abnormal menstrual cycles, and thromboembolism in women; premature puberty and short stature in children/adolescents. May exacerbate hyperlipidemia. Case report of priapism.

ARISTOLOCHIC ACID (*Aristolochia, Asarum, Bragantia, Mu Tong, Fangchi*) ▶? ♀–▶– $

UNAPPROVED ADULT — Do not use due to well-documented risk of nephrotoxicity. Was promoted for wt loss.

UNAPPROVED PEDS — Do not use.

FORMS — Not by prescription.

NOTES — Banned by FDA due to risk of nephrotoxicity and cancer. Possible adulterant in other Chinese herbal products like Akebia, Clematis, Stephania, and others. Rule out aristolochic acid nephrotoxicity in cases of unexplained renal failure.

MOA — Nephrotoxic (causes interstitial renal fibrosis). Also caused lymphoma and kidney, bladder, stomach, and lung cancer in animal studies.

ADVERSE EFFECTS — Serious: End-stage renal disease and urothelial carcinoma reported in humans.

ARNICA (*Arnica montana, leopard's bane, wolf's bane*) ▶? ♀– ▶– $

UNAPPROVED ADULT — Toxic if taken by mouth. Topical preparations promoted for treatment of bruises, aches, and sprains; but insufficient data to assess efficacy. Do not use on open wounds.

UNAPPROVED PEDS — Not for use in children.

FORMS — Not by prescription.

NOTES — Repeated topical application can cause skin reactions.

MOA — Contains derivatives of thymol. Thymol is a subcutanuos vasodilator, may have anti-inflammatory and analgesic effects. Helenalin in the product is a GI toxin.

ADVERSE EFFECTS — Repeated topical application can cause skin reactions. Contact dermatitis; cross-hypersensitivity possible with other plants in Compositae family, including chamomile, chrysanthemum, echinacea, feverfew, ragweed, Artemisia.

If ingested, may cause gastroenteritis and GI bleeding.

ARTICHOKE LEAF EXTRACT (*Cynara scolymus*) ▶? ♀? ▶? $

UNAPPROVED ADULT — May reduce total cholesterol, but clinical significance is unclear. Possibly effective for functional dyspepsia. Does not appear to prevent alcohol-induced hangover.

UNAPPROVED PEDS — Not for use in children.

FORMS — Not by prescription.

NOTES — Advise against use by patients with bile duct obstruction or gallstones.

MOA — Contains cynarine, a choleretic that increases bile secretion.

ADVERSE EFFECTS — Contact dermatitis (rare).

ASTRAGALUS (*Astragalus membranaceus, huang qi, Jin Fu Kang, vetch*) ▶? ♀? ▶? $

UNAPPROVED ADULT — Used in combination with other herbs in traditional Chinese medicine for CHD, CHF, chronic kidney disease, viral infections, upper respiratory tract infections. Early studies suggested that astragalus might improve efficacy of platinum-based chemotherapy for non-small-cell lung cancer. However, an astragalus-based herbal formula (Jinfukang) did not affect survival in phase II study of non-small cell lung cancer.

UNAPPROVED PEDS — Not for use in children.

FORMS — Not by prescription.

NOTES — Not used for more than 3 weeks without close follow-up in traditional Chinese medicine. In theory, may enhance activity of drugs for diabetes, HTN, and anticoagulation.

MOA — Has immunostimulant properties. Contains saponins, astragalosides, high-weight polysaccharides, amino acids, and trace minerals.

ADVERSE EFFECTS — GI discomfort, facial flushing, low blood pressure reported with IV administration.

BILBERRY (*Vaccinium myrtillus, huckleberry, Tegens, VMA extract*) ▶Bile, K ♀–▶– $

UNAPPROVED ADULT — Insufficient data to evaluate efficacy for macular degeneration or cataracts. Does not appear to improve night vision.

UNAPPROVED PEDS — Supplements not for use in children.

FORMS — Not by prescription.

NOTES — High doses may impair platelet aggregation, affect clotting time, and cause GI distress.

MOA — Contains bioflavonoids (antioxidants) and anthocyanosides (stabilize collagen).

ADVERSE EFFECTS — GI distress, rash. High doses may impair platelet aggregation and affect clotting time.

BITTER MELON (*Momordica charantia, ampalaya, karela*) ▶? ♀–▶– $$

UNAPPROVED ADULT — Efficacy unclear for type 2 diabetes.

UNAPPROVED PEDS — Not for use in children. Two cases of hypoglycemic coma in children ingesting bitter melon tea.

FORMS — Not by prescription.

(cont.)

BITTER MELON (*cont.*)

MOA — Mechanism of hypoglycemic action unknown but contains insulin-like peptide. MAP30 protein in seeds has in vitro antiviral and antineoplastic activity.

ADVERSE EFFECTS — Two cases of hypoglycemic coma in children ingesting bitter melon tea. Seeds can cause hemolytic anemia in G6PD deficiency. Can cause diarrhea and abdominal pain.

BITTER ORANGE (*Citrus aurantium, Seville orange*) ▶K ♀– ▶– $

UNAPPROVED ADULT — Marketed as substitute for ephedra in weight-loss dietary supplements; safety and efficacy not established.

UNAPPROVED PEDS — Not for use in children.

FORMS — Not by prescription.

NOTES — Contains sympathomimetics including synephrine and octopamine. Synephrine banned by some sports organizations. Do not use within 14 days of an MAOI. Juice may inhibit intestinal CYP3A4.

MOA — Contains sympathomimetics, including synephrine (similar to phenylephrine) and octopamine. May increase blood pressure and heart rate. Juice contains furocoumarin which inhibits CYP3A4.

ADVERSE EFFECTS — Treatment-resistant hypertension. Supplements containing synephrine linked to reports of rhabdomyolysis, MI, stroke, ischemic colitis, and ventricular tachycardia. Ephedra, a related compound, was banned from US market due to similar adverse effects. Bitter orange peel oil may be phototoxic.

BLACK COHOSH (*Cimicifuga racemosa, Remifemin, Menofem*) ▶Bile + Feces ♀– ▶– $

UNAPPROVED ADULT — Ineffective for relief of menopausal symptoms.

UNAPPROVED PEDS — Not for use in children.

FORMS — Not by prescription.

NOTES — US Pharmacopoeia concluded black cohosh is possible cause of hepatotoxicity in 30 case reports. Does not alter vaginal epithelium, endometrium, or estradiol levels in postmenopausal women.

MOA — Contains triterpene glycosides. Mechanism of action unknown, but does not appear to interact directly with estrogen receptors.

ADVERSE EFFECTS — GI distress, rash. United States Pharmacopoeia determined black cohosh to be possible cause of hepatotoxicity in 30 case reports.

BUTTERBUR (*Petasites hybridus, Petadolex*) ▶? ♀– ▶– $$

UNAPPROVED ADULT — Migraine prophylaxis (effective): Petadolex 50 to 75 mg PO two times per day. Am Acad Neurology and Am Headache Society recommend for migraine prophylaxis. Allergic rhinitis prophylaxis (possibly effective): Petadolex 50 mg PO two times per day. Efficacy unclear for asthma.

UNAPPROVED PEDS — Not for use in children.

FORMS — Not by prescription. Standardized pyrrolizidine-free extracts: Petadolex tabs 50, 75 mg.

NOTES — Do not use raw butterbur; it may contain hepatotoxic pyrrolizidine alkaloids which are removed by processing. Butterbur is related to Asteraceae and Compositae; consider the potential for cross-allergenicity between plants in these families.

MOA — Cerebrovascular smooth muscle relaxant and inhibitor of leukotriene synthesis.

ADVERSE EFFECTS — Serious: None reported. Frequent: Nausea, burping, stomach pain. No long-term safety data.

CESIUM CHLORIDE ▶K ♀– ▶– $$$

UNAPPROVED ADULT — Health Canada and FDA are taking action against Internet sellers promoting cesium chloride as alternative treatment of late-stage cancer. Evidence for benefit as cancer treatment is lacking.

FORMS — Not by prescription.

NOTES — Can prolong QT interval and cause torsades de pointes. Toxicity can be prolonged due to extremely long half-life (approximately 200 days to reach steady-state). Prussian blue has been used to speed cesium chloride elimination.

MOA — Cesium chloride is a non-radioactive alkali metal (not to be confused with radioactive cesium-137). Claims that cesium kills tumor cells by increasing intracellular pH are unproven. Cesium prolongs QT interval by blocking potassium channels; effect is so reproducible that it is used in animal model of long-QT syndrome.

ADVERSE EFFECTS — Syncope, QT interval prolongation, torsades de pointes, hypokalemia, diarrhea, paresthesias.

CHASTEBERRY (*Vitex agnus castus fruit extract, Femaprin*) ▶? ♀– ▶– $

UNAPPROVED ADULT — Premenstrual syndrome (possibly effective): 20 mg PO daily of extract ZE 440 (ratio 6–12:1; standardized for casticin).

UNAPPROVED PEDS — Not for use in children.

FORMS — Not by prescription.

NOTES — Liquid formulations may contain alcohol. Avoid concomitant dopamine antagonists such as haloperidol or metoclopramide.

MOA — Higher doses may reduce prolactin levels by binding to dopamine D2 receptors in the pituitary. Low doses may increase serum prolactin levels.

ADVERSE EFFECTS — Rash, acne, GI upset, intermenstrual bleeding.

CHONDROITIN ▶K ♀? ▶? $

UNAPPROVED ADULT — Does not appear effective for relief of OA pain overall. Chondroitin 400 mg PO three times per day + glucosamine may improve pain in subgroup of patients with moderate to severe knee OA.

UNAPPROVED PEDS — Not for use in children.

FORMS — Not by prescription.

NOTES — Chondroitin content not standardized and known to vary. Cosamin DS contains 3 mg manganese/cap; tolerable upper limit of manganese is 11 mg/day. Some products made from bovine cartilage. Case reports of increased INR/

CHONDROITIN (cont.)

bleeding with warfarin in patient taking chondroitin + glucosamine.

MOA — Glycosaminoglycan that may stimulate production of cartilage matrix.

ADVERSE EFFECTS — GI distress, allergic reactions. Adverse effects appear minor and infrequent. Rare case reports of increased serum transaminases and hepatotoxicity with glucosamine + chondroitin.

CINNAMON (*Cinnamomum cassia, Cinnamomum aromaticum*) ▶? ♀+ in food, - in supplements ▶+ in food, - in supplements $

UNAPPROVED ADULT — Doses of 1 to 6 g/day do not appear to substantially reduce HgA1c, fasting glucose, or lipids in type 2 diabetes.

UNAPPROVED PEDS — Does not appear to improve glycemic control in adolescents with type 1 diabetes.

FORMS — Not by prescription.

NOTES — A ½ teaspoon of powdered cinnamon from grocery store is approximately 1 g. Warn against ingesting cinnamon powder in "cinnamon challenge" due to risk of choking and aspiration; collapsed lung reported.

MOA — Increases insulin sensitivity via stimulation of insulin receptor.

ADVERSE EFFECTS — Hypersensitivity reactions including allergic contact stomatitis; nausea; abdominal pain. Collapsed lung reported from ingestion of cinnamon powder in "cinnamon challenge".

COENZYME Q10 (*CoQ-10, ubiquinone*) ▶Bile ♀- ▶- $

UNAPPROVED ADULT — Heart failure: 100 mg/day PO divided two to three times per day (conflicting clinical trials; may reduce hospitalization, dyspnea, edema, but AHA does not recommend). Statin-induced myalgia: 100 to 200 mg PO daily (efficacy unclear; conflicting clinical trials). Study for progression of Huntington's disease was inconclusive. Prevention of migraine (possibly effective): 100 mg PO three times per day. May be considered for migraine prevention per Am Academy Neurology and Am Headache Society. Efficacy unclear for hypertension, and improving athletic performance. Appears ineffective for diabetes, amyotrophic lateral sclerosis. Did not improve cancer-related fatigue or quality of life in RCT of women with breast cancer. Does not slow functional decline in early Parkinson disease.

UNAPPROVED PEDS — Not for use in children.

FORMS — Not by prescription.

NOTES — Case reports of increased INR with warfarin; but a crossover study did not find an interaction.

MOA — Coenzyme in mitochondrial metabolism; also an antioxidant.

ADVERSE EFFECTS — Mild insomnia, increased LFTs, rash, GI distress.

CRANBERRY (*Cranactin, Vaccinium macrocarpon*) ▶? ♀+ in food, - in supplements ▶+ in food, - in supplements $

UNAPPROVED ADULT — Prevention of UTI (possibly ineffective): 300 mL/day PO cranberry juice cocktail.

Usual dose of cranberry juice extract caps/tabs is 300 to 400 mg PO two times per day. Insufficient data to assess efficacy for treatment of UTI. Does not appear to prevent UTI in spinal cord injury; IDSA advises against routine use to reduce bacteriuria/UTI in neurogenic bladder managed with intermittent/indwelling catheter.

UNAPPROVED PEDS — Insufficient data to assess efficacy for prevention/treatment of UTI in children. Does not appear to prevent UTI in spinal cord injury; IDSA advises against routine use to reduce bacteriuria/UTI in neurogenic bladder managed with intermittent/indwelling catheter.

FORMS — Not by prescription.

NOTES — Numerous case reports of increased INRs and bleeding with warfarin. However, most clinical trials did not find an increase in the INR with cranberry. Approximately 100 calories/6 oz of cranberry juice cocktail. Advise diabetics that some products have high sugar content. Increases urinary oxalate excretion; may increase risk of oxalate kidney stones.

MOA — Proanthocyanidin or fructose appears to block adhesion of bacteria to uroepithelial cells. Although cranberry juice is acidic, it does not appear to significantly change urine pH.

ADVERSE EFFECTS — GI distress and diarrhea with more than 3 L/day.

CREATINE ▶LK ♀- ▶- $

UNAPPROVED ADULT — Promoted to enhance athletic performance. No benefit for endurance exercise, but modest benefit for intense anaerobic tasks lasting less than 30 sec. Usually taken as loading dose of 10 to 20 g/day PO for 4 to 7 days, then 2 to 5 g/day divided 2 times per day. Possibly effective for increasing muscle strength in Duchenne muscular dystrophy, polymyositis/ dermatomyositis. Does not appear effective for myotonic dystrophy Type 1, amyotrophic lateral sclerosis. Research ongoing in Huntington's disease, and Parkinson's disease.

UNAPPROVED PEDS — Not usually for use in children. The AAP strongly discourages performance-enhancing substances by athletes. Possibly effective for increasing muscle strength in Duchenne muscular dystrophy.

FORMS — Not by prescription.

NOTES — Caffeine may antagonize the ergogenic effects of creatine. Creatine is metabolized to creatinine. In young healthy adults, large doses can increase serum creatinine slightly without affecting CrCl. The effect in elderly is unknown.

MOA — Endogenous product converted in muscle to creatine phosphate which may increase ATP levels and increase the force of muscle contraction. Improved mitochondrial function and antioxidant activity are proposed mechanism in Parkinson's disease.

ADVERSE EFFECTS — Single case of lone atrial fibrillation (causality unclear). Manic switch reported in two patients in pilot study of bipolar depression. Anecdotal reports of GI distress and myalgia.

(cont.)

CREATINE (*cont.*)

Diarrhea with doses at least 10 g. Creatine is metabolized to creatinine. Supplements slightly increase serum creatinine in young healthy adults; effect in elderly is unknown. Infrequent reports of renal impairment are unconfirmed. Creatine, especially when taken with protein supplements, has led to misdiagnosis of chronic kidney disease.

DANSHEN (*Salvia miltiorrhiza*) ▶? ♀? ▶? $

UNAPPROVED ADULT — Used for treatment of cardiovascular diseases in traditional Chinese medicine.

UNAPPROVED PEDS — Not for use in children.

FORMS — Not by prescription.

NOTES — Case reports of increased INR with warfarin.

MOA — Tanoshionones may cause coronary artery vasodilation. Fatty acids in danshen may inhibit thromboxane formation and platelet aggregation/adhesion.

ADVERSE EFFECTS — May increase INR with warfarin.

DEHYDROEPIANDROSTERONE (*DHEA, Aslera, Fidelin, Prasterone*) ▶Peripheral conversion to estrogens and androgens ♀– ▶– $

UNAPPROVED ADULT — To improve well-being in women with adrenal insufficiency: 50 mg PO daily (possibly effective; conflicting clinical trials). Does not improve cognition, quality of life, or sexual function in elderly. Not recommended as androgen replacement in late-onset male hypogonadism. Used by athletes as a substitute for anabolic steroids; but no convincing evidence of enhanced athletic performance or increased muscle mass. Banned by many sports organizations.

UNAPPROVED PEDS — Not for use in children.

FORMS — Not by prescription.

NOTES — In theory, chronic use may increase risk of hormone-related cancers (prostate, breast, ovarian). But epidemiologic studies found no link between sex hormone serum levels and prostate cancer.

MOA — Adrenal steroid precursor for estrogen and testosterone. Physiologic doses increase androgen and estrogen levels in women, and estrogen levels in men. May increase insulin sensitivity.

ADVERSE EFFECTS — Acne, hirsutism, and decreased HDL with 100-200 mg/day in women. Case reports of mania induction.

DEVIL'S CLAW (*Harpagophytum procumbens, Doloteffin, Harpadol*) ▶? ♀– ▶– $

UNAPPROVED ADULT — OA, acute exacerbation of chronic low-back pain (possibly effective): 2400 mg extract/day (50 to 100 mg harpagoside/day) PO divided two to three times per day.

UNAPPROVED PEDS — Not for use in children.

FORMS — Not by prescription. Extracts standardized to harpagoside (iridoid glycoside) content.

MOA — Contains harpagoside and other iridoid glycosides with antiinflammatory and analgesic effects. Appears to inhibit COX-2 (but not COX-1), and nitric oxide synthetase. May increase gastric acid secretion. May decrease heart rate and contractility.

ADVERSE EFFECTS — Serious: Bradycardia. Frequent: Dyspepsia, diarrhea. No long-term safety data.

DONG QUAI (*Angelica sinensis*) ▶? ♀– ▶– $

UNAPPROVED ADULT — Appears ineffective for postmenopausal symptoms; North American Menopause Society recommends against use. Used with other herbs for treatment and prevention of dysmenorrhea, TIA, CVA, PAD, and cardiovascular conditions in traditional Chinese medicine.

UNAPPROVED PEDS — Not for use in children.

FORMS — Not by prescription.

NOTES — Increased risk of bleeding with warfarin with/without increase in INR; avoid concurrent use.

MOA — Unknown. In vitro evidence of platelet antagonism; contains natural coumarins.

ADVERSE EFFECTS — Photosensitivity possible. A case of subarachnoid hemorrhage attributed to supplement containing Siberian ginseng, dong quai, red clover.

ECHINACEA (*E. purpurea, E. angustifolia, E. pallida, cone flower, EchinaGuard, Echinacin Madaus*) ▶L ♀– ▶– $

UNAPPROVED ADULT — Promoted as immune stimulant. Conflicting clinical trials for prevention or treatment of upper respiratory infections. Does not appear effective for treatment of common cold.

UNAPPROVED PEDS — Not for use in children. Appears ineffective for treatment of upper respiratory tract infections in children. Risk of rash and allergic reactions outweighs any benefit in children <12 yo.

FORMS — Not by prescription.

NOTES — Single case reports of eosinophilia, precipitation of thrombotic thrombocytopenic purpura, and exacerbation of pemphigus vulgaris; causality unclear. Rare allergic reactions including anaphylaxis. Cross-hypersensitivity possible with other plants in Compositae family. Photosensitivity possible. Could interact with immunosuppressants due to immunomodulating effects. Some experts limit use to no more than 8 weeks and recommend against use in patients with autoimmune disorders.

MOA — May have immunomodulating and/or antiviral effects.

ADVERSE EFFECTS — Serious: Rare allergic reactions including anaphylaxis (may be more common in atopic individuals), photosensitivity possible. Single case reports of eosinophilia, precipitation of thrombotic thrombocytopenic purpura and exacerbation of pemphigus vulgaris; causality unclear. Other: GI complaints. Frequent: Rash in children.

ELDERBERRY (*Sambucus nigra, Rubini, Sambucol*) ▶LK ♀– ▶– $

UNAPPROVED ADULT — Efficacy unclear for influenza, sinusitis, and bronchitis.

UNAPPROVED PEDS — Not for use in children.

FORMS — Not by prescription.

NOTES — Sinupret and Sambucol also contain other ingredients. Eating uncooked elderberries may cause nausea or cyanide toxicity.

MOA — Stimulates cytokine production and inhibits influenza virus replication in vitro. Flowers and

ELDERBERRY (cont.)

berries contain flavonoids and antioxidant with immunomodulating activity. Also reported to have diuretic and hypoglycemic effects.

ADVERSE EFFECTS — Eating uncooked elderberries may cause nausea or cyanide toxicity.

EPHEDRA (*Ephedra sinica, ma huang*) ▶K ♀– ▶– $

UNAPPROVED ADULT — Little evidence of efficacy for obesity, other than modest short-term wt loss. Traditional use as a bronchodilator.

UNAPPROVED PEDS — Not for use in children.

FORMS — Not by prescription.

NOTES — FDA banned ephedra supplements in 2004 because of link to CVA, MI, sudden death, HTN, palpitations, tachycardia, seizures. Risk of serious reactions may increase with dose, strenuous exercise, or concomitant use of other stimulants like caffeine. Country mallow (Sida cordifolia) contains ephedrine.

MOA — Contains sympathomimetics, ephedrine and pseudoephedrine, which cause CNS stimulation, bronchodilation, hypertension, and chronotropic and inotropic effects.

ADVERSE EFFECTS — Serious: Linked to stroke, myocardial infarction, sudden death, HTN, tachycardia, seizures, psychiatric symptoms. Case reports of ephedra kidney stones. Frequent: N/V, palpitations, tremor, insomnia.

EVENING PRIMROSE OIL (*Oenothera biennis*) ▶? ♀? ▶? $

UNAPPROVED ADULT — Appears ineffective for premenstrual syndrome, postmenopausal symptoms, atopic dermatitis. Inadequate data to evaluate efficacy for cervical ripening.

UNAPPROVED PEDS — Not for use in children.

FORMS — Not by prescription.

MOA — Contains gamma linolenic acid and linoleic acid, precursors of arachidonic acid and other eicosanoids. Promoted to have anti-inflammatory properties.

ADVERSE EFFECTS — No significant health hazards identified other than mild nausea, diarrhea, headache.

FENUGREEK (*Trigonelle foenum-graecum*) ▶? ♀– ▶? $$

UNAPPROVED ADULT — Efficacy unclear for diabetes or hyperlipidemia. Insufficient data to evaluate efficacy as galactagogue.

UNAPPROVED PEDS — Not for use in children.

FORMS — Not by prescription.

NOTES — Case report of increased INR with warfarin possibly related to fenugreek. Can cause maple syrup-like body odor. Fiber content could decrease GI absorption of some drugs.

MOA — A legume that is a good source of fiber. Hydroxyisoleucine may increase glucose-mediated insulin release. Sapogenins may increase biliary cholesterol excretion.

ADVERSE EFFECTS — Abdominal pain, flatulence, diarrhea. Generally regarded as safe as food by FDA.

FEVERFEW (*Chrysanthemum parthenium, MigreLief, Tanacetum parthenium L.*) ▶? ♀– ▶– $

UNAPPROVED ADULT — Prevention of migraine (probably effective): 50 to 100 mg extract PO daily; 2 to 3 fresh leaves PO daily; 50 to 125 mg freeze-dried leaf PO daily. Take either leaf form with or after meals. Benefit of alcoholic extract questioned. May take 1 to 2 months to be effective. Inadequate data to evaluate efficacy for acute migraine. Should be considered for migraine prevention per Am Academy Neurology and Am Headache Society.

UNAPPROVED PEDS — Not for use in children.

FORMS — Not by prescription.

NOTES — May cause uterine contractions; avoid in pregnancy. MigraLief contains feverfew, riboflavin and magnesium. MigraSpray and Gelstat are homeopathic products that are unlikely to be beneficial.

MOA — Parthenolide may inhibit prostaglandin synthesis or act as serotonin antagonist. Inhibition of platelet aggregation in vitro, but not in humans. Leaves contain tiny amount of melatonin.

ADVERSE EFFECTS — Mouth and lip irritation after chewing fresh leaves. Mild GI complaints. Rebound headache reported after chronic use. Cross-hypersensitivity possible with other composite flowers (arnica, chamomile, echinacea, ragweed, marigolds, chrysanthemums, daisies).

FLAVOCOXID (*Limbrel*) ▶L ♀– ▶– $$$

UNAPPROVED ADULT — OA (efficacy unclear): 250 to 500 mg PO two times per day. Max 2000 mg/day short-term. Taking 1 h before or after meals may increase absorption.

UNAPPROVED PEDS — Not for use in children.

FORMS — Caps 250, 500 mg. Marketed as medical food by prescription only (not all medical foods require a prescription).

NOTES — Hepatotoxicity reported. Be alert for confusion between the brand names, Limbrel and Enbrel, as well as misidentification of flavocoxid as a COX-2 inhibitor. Baicalin, a component of Limbrel, may reduce exposure to rosuvastatin in some patients. Each cap contains 10 mg elemental zinc.

MOA — Contains flavonoids (baicalin, catechin) from Scutellaria baicalensis and Acacia catechu that may inhibit the production of inflammatory prostaglandins and leukotrienes in the arachidonic acid pathway. Flavonoids may also act as antioxidants. Flavocoxid is not a COX-2 inhibitor.

ADVERSE EFFECTS — Rash, synovitis, hypersensitivity, hypersensitivity pneumonitis, increased LFTs, hepatotoxicity. Frequent: Nausea, diarrhea, flatulence.

GARCINIA (*Garcinia cambogia, Citri Lean*) ▶? ♀– ▶– $

UNAPPROVED ADULT — Appears ineffective for wt loss.

UNAPPROVED PEDS — Not for use in children.

FORMS — Not by prescription.

MOA — Contains hydroxycitric acid which may inhibit lipogenesis.

(cont.)

GARCINIA (*cont.*)

ADVERSE EFFECTS — Case reports of hepatotoxicity and rhabdomyolysis with multi-ingredient wt loss supplements containing Garcinia.

GARLIC SUPPLEMENTS (*Allium sativum, Kwai, Kyolic*) ▶LK ♀– ▶– $

UNAPPROVED ADULT — Ineffective for hyperlipidemia; American College of Cardiology does not recommend for this indication. Small reduction in BP, but efficacy in HTN unclear. Does not appear effective for diabetes. Efficacy unclear for prevention of common cold.

UNAPPROVED PEDS — Not for use in children.

FORMS — Not by prescription.

NOTES — Topical application of garlic can cause burn/rash. Significantly decreases saquinavir levels; may also interact with other protease inhibitors. May increase bleeding risk with warfarin with/without increase in INR. However, Kyolic (aged garlic extract) and enteric-coated garlic did not affect the INR in clinical studies.

MOA — May inhibit HMG-CoA reductase; may inhibit platelet aggregation and enhances fibrinolytic activity; may have antioxidant activity; may cause vasodilation.

ADVERSE EFFECTS — GI irritation, bad breath, rash. Topical application can cause burns. Case reports of anaphylaxis to raw garlic, and garlic-induced eosinophilic esophagitis.

GINGER (*Zingiber officinale*) ▶bile ♀? ▶? $

UNAPPROVED ADULT — American Congress of Obstetricians and Gynecologists considers ginger 250 mg PO four times per day a nonpharmacologic option for N/V in pregnancy. Some experts advise pregnant women to limit dose to usual dietary amount (no more than 1 g/day). Acute chemotherapy-induced nausea (efficacy unclear as adjunct to standard antiemetics): 250 to 500 mg PO two times per day for 6 days, starting 3 days before chemo. No benefit for chemo-induced acute vomiting, or delayed N/V. American Society of Clinical Oncology and National Comprehensive Cancer Network guidelines do not support use for chemo-induced N/V. Possibly ineffective for prevention of motion sickness. Does not appear effective for postoperative N/V. Efficacy unclear for relief of OA pain.

UNAPPROVED PEDS — Not for use in children.

FORMS — Not by prescription.

NOTES — Increased INR attributed to ginger in a phenprocoumon-treated patient, but study in healthy volunteers found no effect of ginger on INR or pharmacokinetics of warfarin. Some European countries advise pregnant women to avoid ginger in supplements because it is cytotoxic in vitro. A ½ teaspoon of ground ginger is about 1 g of ginger.

MOA — Gingerols and shogaols may increase rate of gastric emptying. Ginger is cytotoxic in vitro, raising concern about use by pregnant women.

ADVERSE EFFECTS — Heartburn; bruising/flushing; rash. GI irritation possible at high doses.

GINKGO BILOBA (*EGb 761, Ginkgold, Ginkoba*) ▶K ♀– ▶– $

UNAPPROVED ADULT — Dementia (efficacy unclear): 40 mg PO three times per day of standardized extract containing 24% ginkgo flavone glycosides and 6% terpene lactones. American Psychiatric Association and others find evidence too weak to recommend for Alzheimer's or other dementias. Does not prevent dementia in elderly with normal or mildly impaired cognitive function. Does not improve cognition in healthy younger people. Does not appear effective for prevention of acute altitude sickness. Ineffective for intermittent claudication, tinnitus.

UNAPPROVED PEDS — Not for use in children.

FORMS — Not by prescription.

NOTES — Possible increased risk of stroke. Case reports of intracerebral, subdural, and ocular bleeding; but no increase in major bleeding in large clinical trial. Does not appear to increase INR with warfarin, but monitoring for bleeding is advised. May reduce efficacy of efavirenz. Ginkgo seeds contain a neurotoxin. A few reports attributing exacerbation or precipitation of seizures to ginkgo supplements have raised concern about possible contamination with the neurotoxin. Some experts advise caution or avoidance of ginkgo by those with seizures or taking drugs that lower the seizure threshold.

MOA — May decrease capillary fragility or blood viscosity, cause vasodilation, increase peripheral blood flow, affect neurotransmitters, and act as antioxidant.

ADVERSE EFFECTS — Serious: Seizures possible (rare), intracerebral, subdural, ocular bleeding (rare). Higher risk of stroke in clinical trial of ginkgo for prevention of cognitive decline in elderly. Other: GI complaints, headache, allergy, anxiety/restlessness, sleep disturbances.

GINSENG—SIBERIAN (*Eleutherococcus senticosus, Ci-wu-jia*) ▶? ♀– ▶– $

UNAPPROVED ADULT — Does not appear to improve athletic endurance. Did not appear effective in single clinical trial for chronic fatigue syndrome.

UNAPPROVED PEDS — Not for use in children.

FORMS — Not by prescription.

NOTES — May interfere with some digoxin assays. A case report of thalamic CVA attributed to Siberian ginseng plus caffeine.

MOA — Considered an adaptogen. Vasodilatory and antiviral activity reported. Not related to Asian or American ginseng (Panax ginseng or quinquefolius).

ADVERSE EFFECTS — A case of thalamic stroke attributed to Siberian ginseng plus caffeine. A case of subarachnoid hemorrhage attributed to supplement containing Siberian ginseng, dong quai, red clover. Hypertension and dysrhythmia also reported.

GINSENG—AMERICAN (*Panax quinquefolius L., Cold-fX*) ▶K ♀– ▶– $

UNAPPROVED ADULT — Reduction of postprandial glucose in type 2 diabetes (possibly effective): 3 g PO taken with or up to 2 h before meal. Cold-fX (1 cap PO two times per day) may modestly reduce

GINSENG—AMERICAN (cont.)

the frequency of colds/flu; approved in Canada to strengthen immune system. Cancer-related fatigue (possibly effective): 1000 mg PO two times per day in am and midafternoon.

UNAPPROVED PEDS — Usually not for use in children. Cold-fX (1 cap PO two times per day) may modestly reduce the frequency of colds/flu; approved in Canada for children 12 yo and older to strengthen immune system.

FORMS — Not by prescription.

NOTES — Ginseng content varies widely and some products are mislabeled or adulterated with caffeine. American, Asian, and Siberian ginseng are often misidentified. Decreased INR with warfarin.

MOA — Ginsenosides may increase insulin sensitivity or secretion. Polysaccharides in Cold-fX may have immunomodulating effect; it does not contain ginsenosides.

ADVERSE EFFECTS — None found.

GINSENG—ASIAN (*Panax ginseng, Ginsana, G115, Korean red ginseng*) ▶? ♀– ▶– $

UNAPPROVED ADULT — Promoted to improve vitality and well-being: 200 mg PO daily. Ginsana: 2 caps PO daily or 1 cap PO two times per day. Preliminary evidence of efficacy for erectile dysfunction. Efficacy unclear for improving physical or psychomotor performance, diabetes, herpes simplex infections, cognitive or immune function. American Congress of Obstetricians and Gynecologists and North American Menopause Society recommend against use for postmenopausal hot flashes.

UNAPPROVED PEDS — Not for use in children.

FORMS — Not by prescription.

NOTES — Some formulations may contain up to 34% alcohol. Reports of an interaction with the MAOI, phenelzine. May decrease INR with warfarin. Ginseng content varies widely and some products are mislabeled or adulterated with caffeine. American, Asian, and Siberian ginseng are often misidentified. May interfere with some digoxin assays.

MOA — Unknown. Considered an adaptogen.

ADVERSE EFFECTS — Hypertension, headache, restlessness, estrogenic effects (swollen breasts, menstrual bleeding), a case report of mania, case report of QT interval prolongation, a case report of hypertensive crisis and TIA, a case report of gynecomastia in adolescent boy.

GLUCOSAMINE (*Cosamin DS, Dona*) ▶L ♀– ▶– $

UNAPPROVED ADULT — OA: Glucosamine HCl 500 mg PO three times per day or glucosamine sulfate (Dona $$) 1500 mg PO once daily. Appears ineffective overall for OA pain, but glucosamine plus chondroitin may improve pain in moderate to severe knee OA.

UNAPPROVED PEDS — Not for use in children.

FORMS — Not by prescription.

NOTES — Use cautiously or avoid in patients with shellfish allergy. Case reports of increased INR/

bleeding with warfarin in patient taking chondroitin + glucosamine.

MOA — May stimulate production of cartilage matrix.

ADVERSE EFFECTS — GI complaints, allergic skin reactions (rare). Well-tolerated in the GAIT study. Rare case reports of increased serum transaminases and hepatotoxicity with glucosamine + chondroitin. Increased intraocular pressure reported with glucosamine.

GOLDENSEAL (*Hydrastis canadensis*) ▶? ♀– ▶– $

UNAPPROVED ADULT — Often used in attempts to achieve false-negative urine test for illicit drug use (efficacy unclear). Often combined with echinacea in cold remedies; but insufficient data to assess efficacy of goldenseal for the common cold or URIs.

UNAPPROVED PEDS — Not for use in children.

FORMS — Not by prescription.

NOTES — Alkaloids in goldenseal with antibacterial activity not well absorbed orally. Oral use contraindicated in pregnancy (may cause uterine contractions), newborns (may cause kernicterus), and HTN (high doses may cause peripheral vasoconstriction). Adding goldenseal directly to urine turns it brown. May inhibit CYP2D6 and 3A4. Berberine, a component of goldenseal, may increase cyclosporine levels.

MOA — Contains isoquinoline alkaloids (berberine and others) with antimicrobial activity.

ADVERSE EFFECTS — Oral use contraindicated in pregnancy (may cause uterine contractions), newborns (may cause kernicterus), and hypertension (high doses may cause peripheral vasoconstriction). Berberine doses more than 500 mg may be toxic; may cause ventricular arrhythmias in patients with heart failure. Possible exacerbation of severe hypernatremia reported in child with type I diabetes.

GRAPE SEED EXTRACT (*Vitis vinifera L., procyanidolic oligomers*) ▶? ♀? ▶? $

UNAPPROVED ADULT — Small clinical trials suggest benefit in chronic venous insufficiency. No benefit in single study of seasonal allergic rhinitis. Insufficient evidence to evaluate for treatment of hypertension.

UNAPPROVED PEDS — Not for use in children.

FORMS — Not by prescription.

NOTES — Pine bark (pycnogenol) and grape seed extract are often confused; they both contain oligomeric proanthocyanidins.

MOA — Contains oligomeric proanthocyanidins (OPC/PCO) with antioxidant properties. May inhibit platelet aggregation or reactivity.

ADVERSE EFFECTS — None.

GREEN TEA (*Camellia sinensis, Polyphenon E*) ▶LK ♀+ in moderate amount in food, – in supplements ▶+ in moderate amount in food, -- in supplements $

UNAPPROVED ADULT — Some population studies suggest a reduction in adenomatous polyps and chronic atrophic gastritis in green tea drinkers. Efficacy unclear for cancer prevention, hypercholesterolemia. Efficacy for short-term weight loss is minimal. Green tea catechins (polyphenon E) under

(cont.)

GREEN TEA (cont.)

evaluation for chronic lymphocytic leukemia and prevention of prostate cancer in men with high-grade prostate intraepithelial neoplasia.

UNAPPROVED PEDS — Not for children.

FORMS — Not by prescription. Green tea extract available in caps standardized to polyphenol content.

NOTES — Case report of decreased INR with warfarin attributed to drinking large amounts of green tea (due to vitamin K content). The vitamin K content of green tea is low with usual consumption. Can decrease nadolol exposure; avoid coadministration. May contain caffeine. Case reports of hepatotoxicity with supplements (not tea).

MOA — May contain caffeine (approximately 50 mg/cup of tea), catechins, polyphenols including (–)-epigallocatechin-3-gallate (ECGC; primary catechin in polyphenon E), trace elements, vitamins. Has antioxidant activity.

ADVERSE EFFECTS — Case reports of hepatotoxicity with supplements (not tea). N/V, insomnia, fatigue, diarrhea, abdominal pain, and confusion reported in clinical trials.

GUARANA (Paullinia cupana) ▶? ♀+ in food, – in supplements ▶+ in food, - in supplements $

UNAPPROVED ADULT — Marketed as a source of caffeine in weight-loss dietary supplements. Guarana in weight-loss dietary supplements may provide high doses of caffeine.

UNAPPROVED PEDS — Not for use in children.

FORMS — Not by prescription.

MOA — Stimulant effects. Contains caffeine.

ADVERSE EFFECTS — Sympathomimetic effect may increase the risk of serious cardiovascular adverse effects. Case reports of rhabdomyolysis and seizures possibly related to caffeine intoxication from sports drinks containing caffeine, guarana, garcinia, and other ingredients.

GUGGULIPID (Commiphora mukul extract, guggul) ▶? ♀– ▶– $$

UNAPPROVED ADULT — Does not appear effective for hyperlipidemia with doses up to 2000 mg PO three times per day.

UNAPPROVED PEDS — Not for use in children.

FORMS — Not by prescription.

NOTES — May decrease levels of propranolol and diltiazem. A randomized controlled trial conducted in the United States with 1000 mg or 2000 mg PO three times per day reported no change in total cholesterol, triglycerides, or HDL, and a small increase in LDL. Earlier studies of weaker design reported reductions in total cholesterol of up to 27%.

MOA — Resin from the mukul mirth tree traditionally used in Ayurvedic medicine. Contains E and Z guggalsterones which may facilitate cholesterol catabolism via FXR receptor. May reduce C-reactive protein and improve insulin sensitivity at high doses.

ADVERSE EFFECTS — GI distress, headache, and rash. Allergic contact dermatitis reported with guggulipid anticellulite cream.

HAWTHORN (Crataegus laevigata, monogyna, oxyacantha, Crataegutt, HeartCare) ▶? ♀– ▶– $

UNAPPROVED ADULT — Symptomatic improvement of mild CHF (NYHA I–II; possibly effective): 80 mg PO two times per day to 160 mg PO three times per day of standardized extract (19% oligomeric procyanidins; HeartCare 80 mg tabs); doses as high as 900 to 1800 mg/day have been studied. Initial presentation of SPICE study found no benefit for primary outcome (composite of cardiac death/hospitalization) but possible reduction of sudden cardiac death for LVEF 25 to 35%. American College of Cardiology found evidence insufficient to recommend for mild heart failure. Does not appear effective for HTN.

UNAPPROVED PEDS — Not for use in children.

FORMS — Not by prescription.

NOTES — Unclear whether hawthorn and digoxin should be used together; mechanisms of action may be similar.

MOA — Contains oligomeric procyanidins and flavonoids with positive inotropic and vasodilatory properties, and possible antioxidant activity. May have anti-ischemic activity.

ADVERSE EFFECTS — GI distress, dizziness, palpitations (rare). Some inotropic agents increase mortality in heart failure. Initial presentation of SPICE study did not report increased mortality; hawthorn was safe in combo with other heart failure meds.

HONEY (Medihoney) ▶? ♀+ ▶+ $ for oral $$$ for Medihoney

ADULT — Topical for burn/wound care (including pressure ulcers, 1st and 2nd degree partial thickness burns, donor sites, surgical/traumatic wounds): Apply Medihoney to wound for 12 to 24 h/day.

PEDS — Topical for burn/wound care (including pressure ulcers, 1st- and 2nd-degree partial thickness burns, donor sites, surgical/traumatic wounds): Apply Medihoney to wound for 12 to 24 h/day.

UNAPPROVED ADULT — Constipation (efficacy unclear): 1 to 2 tbsp (30 to 60 g) PO in glass of water. Efficacy of topical honey unclear for prevention of dialysis catheter infections.

UNAPPROVED PEDS — Do not feed honey to children younger than 1 yo due to risk of infant botulism. Nocturnal cough due to upper RTI in children (effective): Give PO within 30 min before sleep. Give ½ tsp for 2 to 5 yo, 1 tsp for 6 to 11 yo, 2 tsp for 12 to 18 yo. WHO considers honey a cheap, popular, and safe demulcent for children.

FORMS — Mostly not by prescription. Medihoney is FDA approved.

NOTES — Honey may contain trace amounts of antimicrobials used to treat infection in honeybee hives. Medihoney sterile dressings contain Leptospermum (Manuka) honey that is irradiated to inactivate C. botulinum spores.

HONEY (*cont.*)

MOA — Topical: Antimicrobial due to hygroscopic property, low pH, generation of hydrogen peroxide. May also have anti-inflammatory activity. Leptospermum honey may have unique antimicrobial properties. Oral: May act as a demulcent. Laxative effect due to unabsorbed fructose.

ADVERSE EFFECTS — Serious: Botulism from ingestion of honey by infants younger than 1 yo; anaphylaxis reported after honey ingestion in patient with history of Compositae pollen allergy. Topical: Stinging sensation after application in ~5% of patients; local atopic reaction in atopic patients. Oral: Well-tolerated, diarrhea.

HORSE CHESTNUT SEED EXTRACT (*Aesculus hippocastanum, buckeye, Venastat*) ▶? ♀– ▶– $

UNAPPROVED ADULT — Chronic venous insufficiency (effective): 1 cap Venastat PO two times per day with water before meals. Response within 1 month. Venastat is 16% escin in standardized extract. American College of Cardiology found evidence insufficient to recommend for peripheral arterial disease.

UNAPPROVED PEDS — Not for use in children.

FORMS — Not by prescription.

NOTES — Venastat does not contain aesculin, a toxin in horse chestnuts.

MOA — Escin increases venous pressure; may prevent leukocyte activation or inhibit elastase and hyaluronidase.

ADVERSE EFFECTS — Mild and infrequent GI distress, dizziness, headache.

KAVA (*Piper methysticum*) ▶K ♀– ▶– $

UNAPPROVED ADULT — Promoted as anxiolytic (possibly effective) or sedative; recommend against use due to hepatotoxicity.

UNAPPROVED PEDS — Not for use in children.

FORMS — Not by prescription.

NOTES — Reports of severe hepatotoxicity leading to liver transplantation. May potentiate CNS effects of benzodiazepines and other sedatives, including alcohol. Reversible yellow skin discoloration with long-term use.

MOA — Anxiolytic and sedative effects.

ADVERSE EFFECTS — Serious: Reports of severe hepatotoxicity leading to death or liver transplantation. Most cases used kava products prepared by ethanol or acetone extraction methods. Reversible yellow skin discoloration with long-term use. Case report of rhabdomyolysis.

KOMBUCHA TEA (*Manchurian or Kargasok tea*) ▶? ♀– ▶– $

UNAPPROVED ADULT — Promoted for many indications, but no scientific evidence to support benefit for any condition. FDA advises caution due to a case of fatal acidosis.

UNAPPROVED PEDS — Not for use in children.

FORMS — Not by prescription.

NOTES — Acidic fermented drink made from addition of bacterial and yeast culture to sweetened black or green tea. It may contain alcohol, ethyl acetate, acetic acid, and lactate.

MOA — Culture of bacteria and yeast that is very acidic after preparation.

ADVERSE EFFECTS — Serious: Fatal acidosis, hepatic dysfunction.

LICORICE (*Cankermelt, Glycyrrhiza glabra, Glycyrrhiza uralensis*) ▶bile ♀– ▶– $

UNAPPROVED ADULT — Prevention of post-operative sore throat (possibly effective): Licorice 0.5 g in 30 mL water gargled 5 minutes before anesthesia. Aphthous ulcers (efficacy unclear): Apply CankerMelt oral patch to ulcer for 16 h/day until healed. Insufficient data to assess efficacy for postmenopausal vasomotor symptoms.

UNAPPROVED PEDS — Not for use in children.

FORMS — Not by prescription.

NOTES — Chronic high doses can cause pseudo-primary aldosteronism (with hypertension, edema, hypokalemia). Case reports of myopathy. Diuretics or stimulant laxatives could potentiate licorice-induced hypokalemia. In the United States, "licorice" candy usually does not contain licorice. Deglycyrrhizinated licorice does not have mineralocorticoid effects.

MOA — Has in vitro antioxidant, antimicrobial, antiviral, and anti-inflammatory activity. Glycyrrhizin has mineralocorticoid activity (not present in deglycyrrhizinated licorice), and antitussive and expectorant properties. Mucilage also sooths cough.

ADVERSE EFFECTS — Pseudo-primary aldosteronism (with hypertension, edema, hypokalemia) possible with chronic high doses. Licorice-induced hypokalemia led to metabolic alkalosis and rhabdomyolysis in case reports. Case reports of myopathy. Transient visual loss.

MELATONIN (*N-acetyl-5-methoxytryptamine*) ▶L ♀– ▶– $

UNAPPROVED ADULT — To reduce jet lag after flights across more than 5 time zones (effective; especially traveling East; may also help for 2 to 4 time zones): 0.5 to 5 mg PO at bedtime (10 pm to midnight) for 3 to 6 nights starting on day of arrival. Faster onset and better sleep quality with 5 mg. No benefit with use before departure or slow-release formulations. Do not take earlier in day (may cause drowsiness and delay adaptation to local time). To promote daytime sleep in night shift workers: 1.8 to 3 mg PO prior to daytime sleep. Delayed sleep phase disorder: 0.3 to 5 mg PO 1.5 to 6 h before habitual bedtime. Orphan drug for treatment of circadian rhythm-related sleep disorders in blind patients with no light perception. Possibly effective for difficulty falling asleep but not for staying asleep. American Academy of Sleep Medicine does not recommend for chronic insomnia but does recommend for jet lag.

UNAPPROVED PEDS — Not usually used in children. Sleep-onset insomnia in ADHD, age 6 yo or older (possibly effective): 3 to 6 mg PO at bedtime. Insomnia in autism (possibly effective for improving

(cont.)

MELATONIN (cont.)

sleep latency and duration): Initial dose of 0.5 to 1 mg PO given 30 to 45 minutes before bedtime, increasing the dose in 1 mg increments every 1 to 3 weeks to a maximum of 10 mg/dose. Orphan drug treatment of circadian rhythm-related sleep disorders in blind patients with no light perception.

FORMS — Not by prescription.

NOTES — High melatonin levels linked to nocturnal asthma; some experts advise patients with nocturnal asthma to avoid melatonin supplements until more data available.

MOA — Pineal hormone related to 5-hydroxytryptamine. Synthesis is controlled by environmental factors including light. Melatonin helps to regulate circadian rhythms, induces pigment lightening of skin cells, and suppresses ovarian function at high doses. May reset endogenous circadian pacemaker.

ADVERSE EFFECTS — Occasional short-term use appears safe. May cause drowsiness for 4-5 h after the dose; warn against hazardous tasks. May increase withdrawn behavior in elderly patients with dementia.

METHYLSULFONYLMETHANE (*MSM, dimethyl sulfone, crystalline DMSO2*) ▶? ♀− ▶− $

UNAPPROVED ADULT — Insufficient data to assess efficacy of oral and topical MSM for arthritis pain.

UNAPPROVED PEDS — Not for use in children.

FORMS — Not by prescription.

NOTES — Can cause nausea, diarrhea, headache. DMSO metabolite promoted as a source of sulfur without odor.

MOA — DMSO metabolite promoted as a source of sulfur without odor.

ADVERSE EFFECTS — Nausea, diarrhea, headache.

NETTLE ROOT (*stinging nettle, Urtica dioica radix*) ▶? ♀− ▶− $

UNAPPROVED ADULT — Efficacy unclear for treatment of BPH or OA.

UNAPPROVED PEDS — Not for use in children.

FORMS — Not by prescription.

NOTES — Can cause allergic skin reactions, mild GI upset, sweating. Case reports of gynecomastia in a man and galactorrhea in a woman.

MOA — May have anti-inflammatory effects. Contains phytosterols.

ADVERSE EFFECTS — Allergic skin reactions, mild GI upset, sweating. Case reports of gynecomastia in a man and galactorrhea in a woman.

NONI (*Morinda citrifolia*) ▶? ♀− ▶− $$$

UNAPPROVED ADULT — Promoted for many medical disorders; but insufficient data to assess efficacy.

UNAPPROVED PEDS — Supplements not for use in children.

FORMS — Not by prescription.

NOTES — Potassium content comparable to orange juice. Hyperkalemia reported in a patient with chronic renal failure. Case reports of hepatotoxicity.

MOA — Antineoplastic, anthelmintic, and immunostimulant activity in vitro and in animal studies.

ADVERSE EFFECTS — Hyperkalemia reported in a patient with chronic renal failure. Case reports of hepatotoxicity.

PEPPERMINT OIL (*Mentha x piperita oil*) ▶LK ♀+ in food, ? in supplements ▶+ in food, ? in supplements $

UNAPPROVED ADULT — Irritable bowel syndrome (possibly effective): 0.2 to 0.4 mL enteric-coated caps PO three times per day before meals. Efficacy of peppermint oil plus caraway seed is unclear for dyspepsia.

UNAPPROVED PEDS — Irritable bowel syndrome, age 8 yo or older (possibly effective): 0.1 to 0.2 mL enteric-coated capsules PO three times per day before meals.

FORMS — Not by prescription.

NOTES — Generally regarded as safe as food by FDA. May exacerbate GERD. For irritable bowel syndrome, use enteric-coated caps that deliver peppermint oil to lower GI tract. Drugs that increase gastric pH (antacids, H2 blockers, proton pump inhibitors) may dissolve enteric-coated capsules too soon, causing heart burn and reducing benefit. Separate peppermint oil and antacid doses by at least 2 h.

MOA — Antispasmotic activity.

ADVERSE EFFECTS — Perianal burning, nausea.

POLICOSANOL (*CholeRx*) ▶? ♀− ▶− $

UNAPPROVED ADULT — Ineffective for hyperlipidemia. A Cuban formulation (unavailable in the United States) 5 mg two times per day reduced LDL cholesterol in studies by a single group of researchers, but studies by other groups found no benefit. Clinical study of a US formulation also found no benefit.

UNAPPROVED PEDS — Not for use in children.

FORMS — Not by prescription.

MOA — Mixture of aliphatic alcohols extracted from sugar cane wax (octacosanol); may inhibit platelet aggregation and anitoxidants. Mechanism of action in hyperlipidemia unknown.

ADVERSE EFFECTS — Serious: None reported.

PROBIOTICS (*Acidophilus, Align, Bacid, Bifantis, Bifidobacteria, BioGaia, Culturelle, Florastor, Gerber Soothe Colic drops, Intestinex, Lactobacillus, Power-Dophilus, Primadophilus, Saccharomyces boulardii, VSL#3*) ▶? ♀+ ▶+ $

ADULT — VSL#3 approved as medical food. Ulcerative colitis, maintenance (effective); 1 to 2 sachets PO per day; ½ to 1 DS sachets PO per day. Active ulcerative colitis, mild to moderate (effective): 4 to 8 sachets PO per day; 2 to 4 DS sachets per day. Pouchitis (effective): 2 to 4 sachets PO per day; 1 to 2 DS sachets PO per day. Dosage range of caps for ulcerative colitis: 4 to 8 caps PO per day. Irritable bowel syndrome (may relieve gas and bloating): ½ to 1 packet PO daily or 2 to 4 caps daily. Mix powder from packets with at least 4 oz of cold water before taking.

PEDS — VSL#3 approved as medical food for ulcerative colitis (effective) and irritable bowel syndrome: Dose based on age. See http://www.vsl3

PROBIOTICS (*cont.*)

.com/.Mix powder with at least 4 oz of cold water before taking.

UNAPPROVED ADULT — Antibiotic-associated diarrhea (effective): Saccharomyces boulardii 500 mg PO two times per day (Florastor 2 caps PO two times per day). IDSA recommends against probiotics to prevent C. difficile–associated diarrhea; safety and efficacy is unclear. Probiotics may reduce GI side effects of H. pylori eradication regimens. Bifidobacterium and some combo products improve abdominal pain and bloating in irritable bowel syndrome. (e.g., Align 1 cap PO once daily), but Lactobacillus alone did not improve symptoms. Efficacy of probiotics unclear for traveler's diarrhea (conflicting evidence), Crohn's disease, H. pylori, radiation enteritis. Lactobacillus GG appears ineffective for prevention of post-antibiotic vulvovaginitis.

UNAPPROVED PEDS — Prevention of antibiotic-associated diarrhea (effective): Lactobacillus GG 10 to 20 billion cells/day PO given 2 h before/after antibiotic or S. boulardii 250 mg PO two times per day (Floraster 1 cap/packet PO two times per day). IDSA recommends against probiotics to prevent C. difficile–associated diarrhea; safety and efficacy is unclear. Acute gastroenteritis, adjunct to rehydration therapy (effective): Lactobacillus GG at least 10 billion (10^{10}) colony forming units per day for 5 to 7 days or Saccharomyces boulardii 250 to 750 mg per day for 5 to 7 days. Infant colic (efficacy unclear; conflicting study results): 5 drops of L reuteri DMS 17938 (Gerber Soothe Colic drops) once daily for 21 days. Efficacy of probiotics unclear for radiation enteritis. Lactobacillus GG does not appear effective for Crohn's disease in children. Research ongoing for prevention and treatment of atopic dermatitis.

FORMS — Mostly not by prescription. Culturelle Kids contains Lactobacillus GG 5 billion cells per powder packet/chewable tab. Culturelle Digestive Health contains Lactobacillus GG 10 billion cells per cap/ chewable tab (also contains inulin). Culturelle Health & Wellness contains Lactobacillus GG 15 billion cells/cap. Florastor and Florastor Kids contain Saccharomyces boulardii 250 mg per cap/ powder packet (contains lactose). VSL#3 (nonprescription medical food) contains 225 billion cells/ Junior packet; 450 billion cells/sachet, 900 billion cells/DS sachet (Rx only); 225 billion cells/2 caps (Bifidobacterium breve, B. longum, B. infantis; Lactobacillus acidophilus, L. plantarum, L. casei, L. bulgaricus; Streptococcus thermophilus). Align contains Bifidobacterium infantis 35624, 1 billion cells/cap. Gerber Soothe Colic drops contains Lactobacillus reuteri DSM 17938 100 million cells per 5 drops. BioGaia ProTectis chew tabs and straws containLactobacillus reuteri DSM 17938 100 million cells per tab/straw.

NOTES — Do not use probiotics in patients with acute pancreatitis; increased mortality and bowel ischemia reported in clinical trial. Acquired infection possible, especially in immunocompromised or critically ill patients; bacteremia, endocarditis, abscess reported, with possible contamination of central venous access port in some cases. Microbial type and content varies by product. Pick yogurt products labeled "Live and active cultures." Refrigerate packets of VSL#3; can store at room temp for 1 week.

MOA — Lactobacillus bacteria and Saccharomyces boulardii, a nonpathogenic yeast, are part of gut normal flora. They inhibit pathogen attachment in colon, modulate intestinal inflammation, reduce colonic permeability, and may enhance barrier function. Bifidobacterium infantis may reduce gut transit time.

ADVERSE EFFECTS — Serious: Acquired infection possible, especially in immunocompromised or critically ill patients; bacteremia, endocarditis, abscess reported, with possible contamination of central venous access port in some cases. Increased risk of bowel ischemia and death in clinical trial evaluting probiotics for acute pancreatitis.

PYCNOGENOL (*French maritime pine tree bark*) ▶L ♀? ▶? $

UNAPPROVED ADULT — Promoted for many medical disorders, but efficacy unclear for chronic venous insufficiency, sperm dysfunction, melasma, OA, HTN, type 2 diabetes, diabetic retinopathy, and ADHD.

UNAPPROVED PEDS — Not for use in children.

FORMS — Not by prescription.

NOTES — Pine bark (pycnogenol) and grape seed extract are often confused; they both contain oligomeric proanthocyanidins.

MOA — Antioxidant. Contains oligomeric proanthocyanidins and bioflavonoids.

ADVERSE EFFECTS — GI distress.

PYGEUM AFRICANUM (*African plum tree*) ▶? ♀– ▶– $

UNAPPROVED ADULT — Benign prostatic hypertrophy (may have modest efficacy): 50 to 100 mg PO two times per day or 100 mg PO daily of standardized extract containing 14% triterpenes.

UNAPPROVED PEDS — Not for use in children.

FORMS — Not by prescription.

NOTES — Appears well-tolerated. Self-treatment could delay diagnosis of prostate cancer.

MOA — Unknown, but may inhibit 5-alpha reductase.

ADVERSE EFFECTS — Well-tolerated, GI distress.

RED CLOVER (*red clover isoflavone extract, Trifolium pratense, trefoil, Promensil, Trinovin*) ▶Gut, L, K ♀– ▶– $$

UNAPPROVED ADULT — Promensil (1 tab PO one to two times per day with meals) marketed for menopausal symptoms; Trinovin (1 tab PO daily) for maintaining prostate health and urinary function in men. Conflicting evidence of efficacy for postmenopausal vasomotor symptoms. Does not appear effective overall, but may have modest benefit for severe symptoms. Efficacy unclear for prevention of osteoporosis and treatment of hyperlipidemia in postmenopausal women, and for BPH symptoms in men.

(cont.)

RED CLOVER (*cont.*)

UNAPPROVED PEDS — Not for use in children.

FORMS — Not by prescription. Isoflavone content (genistein, daidzein, biochanin, formononetin) is 40 mg/tab in Promensil and Trinovin.

NOTES — Does not appear to stimulate endometrium. Effect on breast cancer risk is unclear; some experts recommend against use of isoflavone supplements by women with breast cancer. No effect on breast density in women with Wolfe P2 or DY mammographic breast density patterns. H2 blockers, proton pump inhibitors, and antibiotics may decrease metabolic activation of isoflavones in GI tract. Ingesting large amounts of red clover can cause bleeding in cattle; bleeding risk of supplements in humans is theoretical.

MOA — Contains isoflavone phytoestrogens (biochanin, formononetin, genistein, daidzein), which may act as selective estrogen receptor modulators. Biochanin and formononetin metabolized to genistein and daidzein.

ADVERSE EFFECTS — Appears well tolerated. May increase hepatic transaminases. Safety of isoflavone supplements unclear in women with breast cancer. A case of subarachnoid hemorrhage attributed to supplement containing Siberian ginseng, dong quai, red clover.

RED YEAST RICE (*Monascus purpureus, Xuezhikang, Zhibituo, Hypocol*) ▶L ♀– ▶– $$

UNAPPROVED ADULT — Hyperlipidemia: Usual dose is 1200 mg PO two times per day. Efficacy for hyperlipidemia depends on whether formulation contains lovastatin or other statins. In the United States, red yeast rice should not contain more than trace amounts of statins, but some products contain up to 10 mg lovastatin per cap. Some clinicians consider red yeast rice an alternative for patients who develop myalgia with prescription statins. In China, red yeast rice was effective for secondary prevention of CAD events.

UNAPPROVED PEDS — Not for use in children.

FORMS — Not by prescription. Xuezhikang marketed in Asia, Norway (HypoCol).

NOTES — In 1997, a red yeast rice product called Cholestin was marketed in the United States as a cholesterol-lowering supplement. It was removed from the market in 2001 after a judge ruled it an unapproved drug because it contained lovastatin. Cholestin later returned to the market; it now contains policosanol (ineffective for hyperlipidemia). Current red yeast rice products should not contain more than trace amounts of statins, but tests show they may contain up to 10 mg lovastatin per capsule. Can cause myopathy. Case reports of hepatotoxicity. Consider the potential for lovastatin drug interactions.

MOA — Fermentation product of red yeast (Monascus purpureus) grown on rice; it contains some statins (monacolins) and sterols, including lovastatin (Monocolin K).

ADVERSE EFFECTS — Case reports of myopathy, including rhabdomyolysis in a transplant patient treated with cyclosporine. Case reports of hepatotoxicity, peripheral neuropathy. A potential nephrotoxin, citrinin, can be produced with improper fermentation of red yeast rice and has been found in some products in the United States. Usual adverse effects of Xuezhikang/Zibituo: Dizziness, stomach ache, abdominal distension, nausea, diarrhea.

S-ADENOSYLMETHIONINE (*SAM-e*) ▶L ♀? ▶? $$$

UNAPPROVED ADULT — Mild to moderate depression (effective): 800 to 1600 mg/day PO in divided doses with meals. Efficacy unclear for OA and alcoholic liver disease.

UNAPPROVED PEDS — Not for use in children.

FORMS — Not by prescription.

NOTES — Serotonin syndrome possible when co-administered with SSRIs. Do not use within 2 weeks of an MAOI or in bipolar disorder.

MOA — Acts as a methyl group donor in methylation reactions. Mechanism of action in depression and osteoarthritis unknown.

ADVERSE EFFECTS — Anxiety, headache, insomnia, nausea, induction of mania in bipolar disorder.

SAW PALMETTO (*Serenoa repens*) ▶? ♀– ▶– $

UNAPPROVED ADULT — Ineffective for BPH symptoms.

UNAPPROVED PEDS — Not for use in children.

FORMS — Not by prescription.

NOTES — Not for use by women of childbearing potential. Does not interfere with PSA test. Self-treatment could delay diagnosis of prostate cancer.

MOA — May have anti-androgenic, anti-estrogenic, and estrogenic effects.

ADVERSE EFFECTS — Adverse reactions are mild and infrequent. May cause nausea, diarrhea, abdominal pain. Single case reports of intraoperative hemorrhage and acute pancreatitis.

SHARK CARTILAGE (*Cartilade*) ▶? ♀– ▶– $$$$$

UNAPPROVED ADULT — Appears ineffective for palliative care of advanced cancer. A derivative of shark cartilage was ineffective in a phase 3 clinical trial for non-small-cell lung cancer.

UNAPPROVED PEDS — Not for use in children.

FORMS — Not by prescription.

NOTES — Case reports of hypercalcemia linked to high calcium content (up to 600 to 780 mg/day elemental calcium in BeneFin or Cartilade). Contamination with Salmonella was reported in some shark cartilage caps.

MOA — Contains proteins, glycoproteins, and glycosaminoglycans (chondroitin). Inhibits tumor angiogenesis in animal models.

ADVERSE EFFECTS — Hypercalcemia (has high calcium content; up to 600–780 mg/day elemental calcium in Cartilade), hyperglycemia, GI distress, constipation, hypotension.

SILVER—COLLOIDAL ▶tissues ♀– ▶– $

UNAPPROVED ADULT — The FDA does not recognize OTC colloidal silver products as safe or effective for any use.

SILVER—COLLOIDAL (*cont.*)

UNAPPROVED PEDS — Not for use in children.

FORMS — Not by prescription. May come as silver chloride, cyanide, iodide, oxide, or phosphate.

NOTES — Silver accumulates in skin (leads to permanent grey tint), conjunctiva, and internal organs with chronic use.

MOA — Suspension of silver particles in a colloidal (gelatinous) base. Silver has antimicrobial effects.

ADVERSE EFFECTS — Serious: Silver accumulates in skin (leads to gray tint), conjunctiva, and internal organs with chronic use.

SOUR CHERRY (*Prunus cerasus, tart cherry, Montmorency cherry*) ▶LK ♀+ for moderate amount in food, — in supplements ▶+ for moderate amount in food, — in supplements $$

UNAPPROVED ADULT — OA (efficacy unclear): 240 mL juice (~45 to 100 Montmorency cherries/dose) PO two times per day. Prevention of gout (efficacy unclear): 15 mL concentrate (~45 to 60 cherries/dose) PO two times per day. Insomnia (possibly effective): 240 mL juice (~50 Montmorency cherries/dose) or 30 mL concentrate (~90 to 100 Montmorency cherries) PO two times per day. Prevention of exercise-induced muscle damage/pain after strenuous exercise (efficacy unclear): 240 mL or 360 mL juice (~50 to 60 Montmorency cherries/dose) or 30 mL concentrate (~90 Montmorency cherries/dose) PO two times per day. Dilute concentrate before drinking.

FORMS — Not by prescription.

MOA — Contains anthocyanins with antioxidant and anti-inflammatory activit (in vitro inhibitor of COX-1 and -2). Some cultivars contain melatonin.

ADVERSE EFFECTS — Serious: Anaphylaxis. Case report of acute reversible renal failure.

SOY (*Genisoy, Healthy Woman, Novasoy, Phyto soya, Supro*) ▶Gut, L, K ♀+ for food, ? for supplements ▶+ for food, ? for supplements $

UNAPPROVED ADULT — Soy protein or isoflavone supplements do not substantially reduce hyperlipidemia or HTN. Postmenopausal vasomotor symptoms (modest benefit): Per North Am Menopause Society, consider 50 mg/day or more of soy isoflavones for at least 12 weeks. There is not enough data to make recommendations about soy or isoflavone consumption by breast cancer survivors. Conflicting clinical trials for reducing postmenopausal bone loss. AHA recommends against isoflavone supplements for treatment or prevention of hyperlipidemia, or breast, endometrial, or prostate cancer.

UNAPPROVED PEDS — Soy foods are regarded as safe for children.

FORMS — Not by prescription.

NOTES — Effect of soy supplements on breast cancer risk is unclear. Per North Am Menopause Society, there is not enough data to make recommendations about soy or isoflavone consumption by breast cancer survivors. Some experts recommend against use of isoflavone or phytoestrogen supplements by women with endometrial or breast cancer

(esp. estrogen receptor-positive tumor or receiving tamoxifen). Case report of decreased INR with ingestion of soy milk by patient taking warfarin. Report of decreased levothyroxine absorption with soy protein.

MOA — Contains isoflavone phytoestrogens (genistein, daidzein), which may act as estrogen receptor agonists or antagonists. In 30-50% of the population, gut microbes convert daidzein to equol, a nonsteroidal estrogen. Benefit for postmenopausal symptoms may be limited to equol producers. Soy foods are low in saturated fat and high in fiber, vitamins, and minerals.

ADVERSE EFFECTS — Soy is generally regarded as safe as a food. Protein powder may cause GI complaints. High doses (150 mg/day isoflavones) may cause endometrial hyperplasia.

ST. JOHN'S WORT (*Hypericum perforatum*) ▶L ♀– ▶– $

UNAPPROVED ADULT — Mild to moderate depression (effective): 300 mg PO three times per day of standardized extract (0.3% hypericin).

UNAPPROVED PEDS — Not for use in children. Does not appear effective for ADHD.

FORMS — Not by prescription.

NOTES — Photosensitivity possible with more than 1800 mg/day. Inducer of hepatic CYP3A4, CYP2C9, CYP2C19, and p-glycoprotein. May decrease efficacy of drugs with hepatic metabolism including alprazolam, cyclosporine, methadone, non-nucleoside reverse transcriptase inhibitors, omeprazole, oral contraceptives, oxycodone, protease inhibitors, statins, tacrolimus, voriconazole, zolpidem. May need increased dose of digoxin, theophylline, TCAs. Decreased INR with warfarin. Administration with SSRIs, SNRIs, triptans may cause serotonin syndrome. Do not use within 14 days of a MAOI.

MOA — May inhibit uptake of serotonin, dopamine, norepinephrine, GABA, or L-glutamate.

ADVERSE EFFECTS — Serious: Induction of mania/hypomania, serotonin syndrome. Other: Photosensitivity possible with more than 1800 mg/day, dry mouth, dizziness, GI symptoms, fatigue, headache. Better tolerated than paroxetine in short-term trial for depression.

STEVIA (*Stevia rebaudiana*) ▶L ♀– ▶? $

ADULT — Rebaudioside A (a component of stevia) is FDA approved as a general purpose sweetener.

PEDS — Rebaudioside A (a component of stevia) is FDA approved as a general purpose sweetener.

UNAPPROVED ADULT — Leaves traditionally used as a sweetener but not enough safety data for FDA approval as such. WHO acceptable daily intake of up to 4 mg/kg/day of steviol glycosides. Health Canada advises a max of 280 mg/day of stevia leaf powder in adults.

UNAPPROVED PEDS — Stevia leaves not for use in children.

FORMS — Not by prescription. Rebaudioside A available as Rebiana, Truvia, PureVia.

NOTES — Unrefined stevia is available as a dietary supplement in the United States, but is not FDA

(cont.)

STEVIA (cont.)

approved as a food sweetener. Rebaudioside A (FDA approved as sweetner) lacks bitter aftertaste of unrefined stevia. Canadian labeling advises against use by pregnant women, children, or those with low BP.

MOA — Leaves of stevia plant contain glycosides (stevioside and rebaudioside). Stevioside is 100-fold sweeter than sucrose; rebaudioside A is even sweeter. Stevia may stimulate insulin secretion by pancreatic beta cells at high glucose levels.

ADVERSE EFFECTS — No effect of rebaudioside A on blood pressure or glycemic control in type 2 diabetes.

TEA TREE OIL (melaleuca oil, Melaleuca alternifolia) ▶? ♀– ▶– $

UNAPPROVED ADULT — Not for oral use; CNS toxicity reported. Limited evidence for topical treatment of onychomycosis, tinea pedis, acne vulgaris, dandruff, pediculosis.

UNAPPROVED PEDS — Not for use in children.

FORMS — Not by prescription.

NOTES — Can cause allergic contact dermatitis, especially with concentration of 2% or greater.

MOA — Antimicrobial, scabicidal, and antifungal effects in vitro. Weak estrogenic and antiandrogenic activity in vitro. Oil is distilled from leaves of Melaleuca alternifolia.

ADVERSE EFFECTS — Allergic contact dermatitis; products with concentration of 2% or greater linked to skin reactions. Single case reports of immediate hypersensitivity reaction, and gynecomastia in prepubertal boy.

TRIBULUS TERRESTRIS ▶? - ♀- ▶? $$

UNAPPROVED ADULT — Ineffective for erectile dysfunction in a single clinical trial. Does not increase testosterone levels. Studies in athletes do not show an ergogenic effect.

UNAPPROVED PEDS — Not for use in children.

FORMS — Capsules with 625 mg extract standardized to 125 mg of saponins.

ADVERSE EFFECTS — Toxic to sheep. No adverse effects yet identified in humans.

VALERIAN (Valeriana officinalis, Alluna) ▶? ♀– ▶– $

UNAPPROVED ADULT — Insomnia (possibly modestly effective; conflicting clinical trials): 400 to 900 mg of standardized extract PO 30 min before bedtime. Response reported in 2 to 4 weeks. Alluna (valerian + hops): 2 tabs PO 1 h before bedtime. American Academy of Sleep Medicine does not recommend for chronic insomnia due to inadequate safety and efficacy data.

UNAPPROVED PEDS — Not for use in children.

FORMS — Not by prescription.

NOTES — Do not combine with CNS depressants. Withdrawal symptoms reported after long-term use. Some products have unpleasant smell.

MOA — Valerenic acid inhibits breakdown of GABA in CNS.

ADVERSE EFFECTS — Headache. Some products have unpleasant smell. Withdrawal symptoms

reported after long-term use. Serious: Case reports of possible hepatotoxicity.

WILD YAM (Dioscorea villosa) ▶L ♀? ▶? $

UNAPPROVED ADULT — Ineffective as topical "natural progestin."

UNAPPROVED PEDS — Not for use in children.

FORMS — Not by prescription.

MOA — Contains diosgenin which is structurally similar to cholesterol. Was used historically to synthesize progestins, cortisone, and androgens; it is not converted to them or DHEA in the body.

ADVERSE EFFECTS — None known.

WILLOW BARK EXTRACT (Salix alba, Salicis cortex, salicin) ▶K ♀– ▶– $

UNAPPROVED ADULT — OA, low-back pain (possibly effective): 60 to 240 mg/day salicin PO divided two to three times per day. Onset of pain relief is approximately 2 h. Often included in multi-ingredient wt-loss supplements based on preliminary research suggesting that aspirin increases thermogenesis.

UNAPPROVED PEDS — Not for use in children.

FORMS — Not by prescription. Some products standardized to 15% salicin content.

NOTES — Contraindicated in 3rd trimester of pregnancy and in patients with intolerance or allergy to aspirin or other NSAIDs. Consider contraindications and precautions that apply to other salicylates. Avoid concomitant use of NSAIDs.

MOA — Antipyretic, anti-inflammatory, and analgesic activity. Inhibits prostaglandin synthesis. Salicin, the primary component, is a prodrug that is metabolized to salicylic acid. Salicin does not irreversibly inhibit platelet aggregation like aspirin. The pharmacologic activity of willow is not due solely to salicin.

ADVERSE EFFECTS — Serious: Anaphylactic reactions possible in patients with a history of aspirin hypersensitivity; risk of gastrointestinal bleeding unclear. Frequent: Dose-related tinnitus; GI complaints.

YOHIMBE (Corynanthe yohimbe, Pausinystalia yohimbe) ▶L ♀– ▶– $

UNAPPROVED ADULT — Promoted for impotence and as aphrodisiac, but some products contain little yohimbine (active constituent). FDA considers yohimbe bark in herbal remedies an unsafe herb.

UNAPPROVED PEDS — Not for use in children.

FORMS — Not by prescription.

NOTES — Can cause CNS stimulation. High doses of yohimbine have MAOI activity and can increase BP. Avoid in patients with hypotension, diabetes, heart, liver or kidney disease. Reports of renal failure, seizures, death in patients taking products containing yohimbe.

MOA — Yohimbine is the primary alkaloid in the bark of the yohimbe tree. Yohimbine is an alpha 2-adrenergic receptor blocker.

ADVERSE EFFECTS — High doses can increase blood pressure. Can also cause tachycardia, GI distress, and anxiety/agitation. Case report of priapism.

IMMUNOLOGY

ADULT IMMUNIZATION SCHEDULE*

Tetanus, diphtheria (Td): For all ages, 1 dose booster q 10 years.

Pertussis: Consider single dose of pertussis in adults younger than 65 yo (as part of Tdap), at least 10 years since last tetanus dose. If patient has never received a pertussis booster, use Boostrix if 10 to 18 yo, Adacel if 11 to 64 yo.

Influenza: 1 yearly dose if age 50 yo or older. If younger than 50 yo, then 1 yearly dose if healthcare worker, pregnant, chronic underlying illness, household contact of person with chronic underlying illness or household contact with children younger than 5 yo, or those who request vaccination. Intranasal vaccine indicated for healthy adults younger than 50 yo.

Pneumococcal (polysaccharide): 1 dose if age 65 yo or older. If younger than 65 yo, consider immunizing if chronic underlying illness, nursing home resident. Consider revaccination 5 years later if high risk or if age 65 yo or older and received primary dose before age 65 yo. CDC recommends conjugate vaccine (Prevnar) for certain high-risk adults.

Hepatitis A: For all ages with clotting factor disorders, chronic liver disease, or exposure risk (travel to endemic areas, illegal drug use, men having sex with men), 2 doses (0, 6 to 12 months).

Hepatitis B: For all ages with medical (hemodialysis, clotting factor recipients, chronic liver disease), occupational (healthcare or public safety workers with blood exposure), behavioral (illegal drug use, multiple sex partners, those seeking evaluation or treatment of sexually transmitted disease, men having sex with men), or other (household/sex contacts of those with chronic HBV or HIV infections, clients/staff of developmentally disabled, more than 6 months of travel to high-risk areas, inmates of correctional facilities) indications, 3 doses (0, 1–2, 4–6 months). Hemodialysis patients require 4 doses and higher dose (40 mcg). Consider conjugate vaccine in high-risk adults.

Measles, mumps, rubella (MMR): If born during or after 1957 and immunity in doubt, see www.cdc.gov.

Varicella: For all ages if immunity in doubt, age 13 yo or older, 2 doses separated by 4 to 8 weeks.

Meningococcal (conjugate vaccine is preferred for 55yo or younger): For all ages with medical indications (complement deficiency, anatomic or functional asplenia) or other indications (travel to endemic regions, college dormitory residents, military recruits), administer 1 dose. Consider revaccination in 3 to 5 years if high risk.

Human papillomavirus: Consider HPV vaccine in women 9 to 26 yo at 0, 2, and 6 months. Can be used in males 9 to 26 yo to decrease risk of genital warts.

Herpes zoster: Consider single dose of HZ vaccine in individuals for 60yo or older.

Haemophilus influezae type b (Hib): 1 dose in high-risk adults (sickle cell, leukemia, HIV, splenectomy), if not previously immunized.

*2013 schedule from the CDC, ACIP, & AAFP, see: www.cdc.gov/vaccines/schedules.

CHILDHOOD IMMUNIZATION SCHEDULE*

Title	Months								Years		
Age	Birth	1	2	4	6	12	15	18	2	4–6	11–12
Hepatitis B	HB	HB				HB					
Rotavirus			Rota	Rota	Rota®						
DTP***			DTaP	DTaP	DTaP		DTaP			DTaP	
H influenzae bˣ			Hib	Hib	Hibˣ	Hibˣ					
Pneumococci**			PCV	PCV	PCV	PCV					
Polio#			IPV	IPV		IPV				IPV#	
Influenza†					Influenza (yearly)†						
MMR						MMR				MMR	
Varicella						Varicella				Varicella	

(cont.)

CHILDHOOD IMMUNIZATION SCHEDULE* (*continued*)

Hepatitis A[¶]						Hep A × 2[¶]					
Papillomavirus[§,¶]										HPV × 3[§]	
Meningococcal[^]										MCV[^]	

*2014 schedule from the CDC, ACIP, AAP, & AAFP, see CDC website (www.cdc.gov).

**Administer first dose Prevnar 13 to all healthy children 24 to 59 mo having an incomplete schedule.

***When immunizing adolescents 10 yo or older, consider DTaP if patient has never received a pertussis booster (Boostrix if 10 yo or older, Adacel if 11 to 64 yo).

[@]If using Rotarix, give at 2 and 4 mo (no earlier than 6 weeks). Give at 2, 4, and 6 mo if using Rotateq. Max age for final dose is 8 mo.

[#]Last IPV on or after 4th birthday, and at least 6 months since last dose.

[×]If using PedvaxHib or Comvax, dose at 6 mo not necessary, but booster at 12 to 15 mo indicated.

[†] For healthy patients age 2 yo or older can use intranasal form. If age younger than 9 yo and receiving for 1 time, administer 2 doses 4 or more weeks apart for injected form and 6 or more weeks apart for intranasal form. FluLaval, Fluarix, and single-dose Fluzone syringe not indicated in younger than 3 years. Fluvirin not indicated in younger than 4 years. Do not use Afluria in younger than 9 years. Do not use Flucelvax, Fluzone ID or Fluzone HD in children.

[¶]Two doses 6 to 18 months apart.

[§]Second and third doses 2 and 6 months after 1 dose. Also approved (Gardasil only) for males 9 to 18 yo to reduce risk of genital warts.

[^]Vaccinate all children at age 11 to 12 years with a single dose of Menactra or Menveo, with a booster dose at age 16. For high-risk younger children, refer to CDC for recommendations.

TETANUS WOUND CARE (www.cdc.gov)

Title Cell	Unknown or less than 3 prior tetanus immunizations	3 or more prior teta n immunizations
Non-tetanus-prone wound (eg, clean and minor)	Td (DT age younger than 7 yo)	Td if more than 10 years since last dose
Tetanus-prone wound (eg, dirt, contamination, punctures, crush components)	Td (DT age younger than 7 yo), tetanus immune globulin 250 units IM at site other than Td	Td if more than 5 years since last dose

If patient age 10 yo or older has never received a pertussis booster consider DTaP (Boostrix if 10 yo or older, Adacel if 11–64 yo).

IMMUNOLOGY: Immunizations

NOTE: For vaccine info see CDC website (www.cdc.gov).

BCG VACCINE ▶immune system ♀C ▶? $$$$
WARNING — BCG infections reported in healthcare workers following exposure from accidental needle sticks or skin lacerations. Nosocomial infections reported in patients receiving parenteral drugs that were prepared in areas in which BCG was reconstituted. Serious infections, including fatal infections, have been reported in patients receiving intravesical BCG.
ADULT — 0.2 to 0.3 mL percutaneously (using 1 mL sterile water for reconstitution).
PEDS — Decrease concentration by 50% using 2 mL sterile water for reconstitution, then 0.2 to 0.3 mL percutaneously for age younger than 1 mo. May revaccinate with full dose (adult dose) after 1 yo if necessary. Use adult dose for age older than 1 mo.
MOA — Active immunity, stimulates antibody production.
ADVERSE EFFECTS — Frequent: None.

COMVAX **(haemophilus B vaccine + hepatitis B vaccine)** ▶immune system ♀C ▶? $$$
ADULT — Do not use in adults.
PEDS — Infants born of HBsAg (−) mothers: 0.5 mL IM for 3 doses at 2, 4, and 12 to 15 mo.
NOTES — Combination is made of PedvaxHIB (haemophilus b vaccine) + Recombivax HB (hepatitis B vaccine). For infants 8 weeks of age or older.
MOA — Active immunity, stimulates antibody production.
ADVERSE EFFECTS — Frequent: Acute febrile reaction.

DIPHTHERIA TETANUS AND ACELLULAR PERTUSSIS VACCINE (***DTaP, Tdap, Infanrix, Daptacel, Boostrix, Adacel,*** ✚***Tripacel***) ▶immune system ♀C ▶– $$
ADULT — 0.5 mL IM in deltoid as a single dose, 2 to 5 years since last tetanus dose one time only. ACIP recommends DTaP in every pregnancy, preferably between 27 and 35 weeks of gestation.
PEDS — Check immunization history: DTaP is preferred for all DTP doses. Give 1st dose of 0.5 mL IM at approximately 2 mo, 2nd dose at 4 mo, 3rd dose at 6 mo, 4th dose at 15 to 18 mo, and 5th dose (booster) at 4 to 6 yo. Use Boostrix only if 10 yo or older, and at least 2 to 5 years after the last

DIPHTHERIA TETANUS (*cont.*)

childhood dose of DTaP. Use Adacel only in 11 to 64 yo and at least 2 to 5 years after last childhood dose of DTaP or Td.

NOTES — When feasible, use same brand for first 3 doses. Do not give if prior DTaP vaccination caused anaphylaxis or encephalopathy within 7 days. Avoid Tripedia in thimerosal-allergic patients. Do not use Boostrix or Adacel for primary childhood vaccination series, if prior DTaP vaccination caused anaphylaxis or encephalopathy, or if progressive neurologic disorders (eg, encephalopathy) or uncontrolled epilepsy. For adolescents and adults, only 1 dose should be given, at least 2 to 5 years after last tetanus dose. Specify Adacel/Boostrix vaccine for adolescent and adult booster as pediatric formulations have increased pertussis concentrations and may increase local reaction. No information available on repeat doses in adolescents or adults.

MOA — Active immunity, stimulates antibody production.

ADVERSE EFFECTS — Frequent: Agitation, drowsiness, pain, redness and swelling at injection site, headache, fatigue.

DIPHTHERIA-TETANUS TOXOID (*Td, DT, ✦D2T5*) ▸immune system ♀C ▶? $

ADULT — 0.5 mL IM, 2nd dose 4 to 8 weeks later, and 3rd dose 6 to 12 months later. Give 0.5 mL booster dose at 10 year intervals. Use adult formulation (Td) for adults and children at least 7 yo.

PEDS — 0.5 mL IM for age 6 weeks to 6 yo, 2nd dose 4 to 8 weeks later, and 3rd dose 6 to 12 months later using DT for pediatric use. If immunization of infants begins in the first year of life using DT rather than DTP (ie, pertussis is contraindicated), give three 0.5 mL doses 4 to 8 weeks apart, followed by a fourth dose 6 to 12 months later.

FORMS — Injection DT (Peds: 6 weeks to 6 yo). Td (adult and children at least 7 yo).

NOTES — DTaP is preferred for most children age less than 7 yo. Td is preferred for adults and children at least 7 yo. Avoid in thimerosal allergy.

MOA — Active immunity, stimulates antibody production.

ADVERSE EFFECTS — Frequent: Agitation, drowsiness.

HAEMOPHILUS B VACCINE (*ActHIB, Hiberix, PedvaxHIB*) ▸immune system ♀C ▶? $$

PEDS — Doses vary depending on formulation used and age at first dose. ActHIB: Give 0.5 mL IM for 3 doses at 2-month intervals for age 2 to 6 mo, give 0.5 mL IM for 2 doses at 2-month intervals for age 7 to 11 mo, give 0.5 mL IM for 1 dose for age 12 to 14 mo. A single 0.5 mL IM booster dose is given to previously immunized children at least 15 mo, and at least 2 months after the previous injection. For children age 15 mo to 5 yo at age of 1st dose, give 0.5 mL IM for 1 dose (no booster). PedvaxHIB: 0.5 mL IM for 2 doses at 2-month intervals for age 2 to 14 mo. If the 2 doses are given before 12 mo of age, a 3rd 0.5 mL IM (booster) dose is given at least

2 months after the 2nd dose. 0.5 mL IM for 1 dose (no booster) for age 15 mo to 5 yo.

UNAPPROVED ADULT — Asplenia, at least 14 days prior to elective splenectomy, or immunodeficiency: 0.5 mL IM for 1 dose of any Hib conjugate vaccine.

UNAPPROVED PEDS — Asplenia, at least 14 days prior to elective splenectomy, or immunodeficiency age 5 yo or older: 0.5 mL IM for 1 dose of any Hib vaccine.

NOTES — Not for IV use. No data on interchangeability between brands; AAP and ACIP recommend use of any product in children age 12 to 15 mo.

MOA — Active immunity, stimulates antibody production.

ADVERSE EFFECTS — Frequent: Acute febrile reaction, soreness and redness at injection site.

HEPATITIS A VACCINE (*Havrix, Vaqta, ✦Avaxim, Epaxal*) ▸immune system ♀C ▶+ $$$

ADULT — Havrix: 1 mL (1440 ELU) IM, then 1 mL (1440 ELU) IM booster dose 6 to 12 months later. Vaqta: 1 mL (50 units) IM, then 1 mL (50 units) IM booster 6 months later for age 18 yo or older.

PEDS — Havrix: 0.5 mL (720 ELU) IM for 1 dose, then 0.5 mL (720 ELU) IM booster 6 to 12 months after 1st dose for age 1 to 18 yo. Vaqta: 0.5 mL (25 units) IM for 1 dose, then 0.5 mL (25 units) IM booster 6 to 18 months later for age 1 to 18 yo.

FORMS — Single-dose vial (specify pediatric or adult).

NOTES — Do not inject IV, SC, or ID. Brands may be used interchangeably. Need for boosters is unclear. Postexposure prophylaxis with hepatitis A vaccine alone is not recommended. Should be given 4 weeks prior to travel to endemic area. May be given at the same time as immune globulin, but preferably at different site.

MOA — Active immunity, stimulates antibody production.

ADVERSE EFFECTS — Frequent: Headache, pain, tenderness, warmth, soreness and redness at injection site.

HEPATITIS B VACCINE (*Engerix-B, Recombivax HB*) ▸immune system ♀C ▶+ $$$

ADULT — Engerix-B: 1 mL (20 mcg) IM, repeat in 1 and 6 months for age 20 yo or older. Hemodialysis: Give 2 mL (40 mcg) IM, repeat in 1, 2, and 6 months. Give 2 mL (40 mcg) IM booster when antibody levels decline to less than 10 mIU/mL. Recombivax HB: 1 mL (10 mcg) IM, repeat in 1 and 6 months. Hemodialysis: 1 mL (40 mcg) IM, repeat in 1 and 6 months. Give 1 mL (40 mcg) IM booster when antibody levels decline to less than 10 mIU/mL. Patients with diabetes: ACIP recommends hepatitis B vaccine for all previously unvaccinated diabetics aged 19 through 59 years, vaccinate as soon as possible after diabetes diagnosis.

PEDS — Dosing based on age and maternal HBsAg status. Engerix-B 10 mcg (0.5 mL) IM 0, 1, 6 months for infants of hepatitis B negative and positive mothers and children age 15 to 20 yo. Recombivax 5 mcg (0.5 mL) IM 0, 1, 6 months for infants of

(cont.)

HEPATITIS B VACCINE (cont.)

hepatitis B negative and positive mothers and children age 15 to 20 yo. A 2-dose schedule can be used (Recombivax HB) 10 mcg (1 mL) IM at 0 and 4 to 6 months for age 11 to 15 yo.

NOTES — Infants born to hepatitis B positive mothers should also receive hepatitis B immune globulin and hepatitis B vaccine within 12 h of birth. Not for IV or ID use. May interchange products. Recombivax HB Dialysis Formulation is intended for adults only. Avoid if yeast allergy.

MOA — Active immunity, stimulates antibody production.

ADVERSE EFFECTS — Frequent: Dizziness, malaise, pain and tenderness at injection site.

HUMAN PAPILLOMAVIRUS RECOMBINANT VACCINE (Cervarix, Gardasil) ▶immune system ♀B ▶? $$$$$

ADULT — Prevention of cervical cancer, vulvar and vaginal cancer in females 9 to 26 yo: 0.5 mL IM at time 0, 2 and 6 months. Prevention of anal cancer, genital warts, anal intraepithelial neoplasia in males 9 to 26 yo (Gardasil only): 0.5 mL IM at time 0, 2, and 6 months.

PEDS — Prevention of cervical cancer, vulvar and vaginal cancer in females 9 to 26 yo: 0.5 mL IM at time 0, 2, and 6 months. Prevention of anal cancer, genital warts, anal intraepithelial neoplasia in males 9 to 26 yo (Gardasil only): 0.5 mL IM at time 0, 2, and 6 months.

NOTES — Patients must be counseled to continue to use condoms. Immunosuppression may reduce response. Fainting and falling may occur after vaccination; observe patient for 15 min after vaccination. Cervarix not approved for use in males.

MOA — Active immunity, stimulates antibody production.

ADVERSE EFFECTS — Frequent: Pain, tenderness, pruritus and erythema at injection site, fainting.

INFLUENZA VACCINE—INACTIVATED INJECTION (Afluria, Fluarix, FluLaval, Fluzone, Fluvirin, Flucelvax, Flublok, *Fluviral, Vaxigrip) ▶immune system ♀C ▶+ $

ADULT — 0.5 mL IM or ID (Fluzone ID). Fluarix, FluLaval not indicated in children younger than 3 years. Fluvirin not indicated in children younger than 4 years. Afluria not indicated in children younger than 9 years. Flublok for 18 to 49 years. Flucelvax for 18 years and older. Fluzone ID for 18 to 64 years. Fluzone HD for 65 years and older.

PEDS — Give 0.25 mL IM for age 6 to 35 mo (Fluzone only), repeat dose after 4 weeks if previously unvaccinated. Give 0.5 mL IM for age 3 to 8 yo (Fluzone,Fluarix,FluLaval if 3 years or older, FLuvirin if 4 years or older) repeat dose after 4 weeks if previously unvaccinated. Give 0.5 mL IM once a year for age 9 to 12 yo.

NOTES — Fluarix, FluLaval not indicated in children younger than 3 years. Fluvirin not indicated in children younger than 4 years. Afluria not indicated in children younger than 9 years. Flucelvax for 18 years and older. Fluzone ID for 18 to 64 years;

lower amount of antigen, lower immunogenicity and higher rate of local reactions compared with standard IM injections. Fluzone HD for 65 years; clinically greater flu prevention, but may be assocaited with increase rate of local reactions. Thimerosal-free products available. Optimal administration October to November. FluBlok is egg-free product for those 18 to 49 years with egg allergy.

MOA — Active immunity, stimulates antibody production.

ADVERSE EFFECTS — Frequent: Fever, malaise, pain, tenderness and erythema at injection site. Severe: Allergic or anaphylactoid reactions in egg-allergic persons, Guillain-Barré syndrome, angioedema.

INFLUENZA VACCINE—LIVE INTRANASAL (FluMist) ▶immune system ♀C ▶+ $

ADULT — 1 dose (0.2 mL) intranasally once a year for healthy adults age 18 to 49 yo.

PEDS — 1 dose (0.2 mL) intranasally for healthy children age 2 to 17 yo, repeat dose after 4 weeks if previously unvaccinated and age 2 to 8 yo. If available, live, intranasal vaccine should be preferentially used for healthy children aged 2 through 8 years who have no contraindications or precautions.

NOTES — Avoid in Guillain-Barré syndrome, chicken egg allergy, aspirin therapy in children (Reye's risk), pregnancy, chronic illness that could increase vulnerability to influenza complications (CHF, asthma, diabetes, renal failure), recurrent wheezing and in children younger than 2 yo. Optimal administration October to November. Since FluMist is a live vaccine, do not use with immune deficiencies (eg, HIV, malignancy, etc.) or altered immune status (eg, taking systemic corticosteroids, chemotherapy, radiation, etc.).

MOA — Active immunity, stimulates antibody production.

ADVERSE EFFECTS — Frequent: Fever, malaise. Severe: Allergic or anaphylactoid reactions in egg-allergic persons, Guillain-Barré syndrome, angioedema.

JAPANESE ENCEPHALITIS VACCINE (Ixiaro) ▶immune system ♀C ▶? $$$$

ADULT — 1 mL SC for 3 doses on day 0, 7, and 30.

PEDS — 0.5 mL SC for 3 doses on day 0, 7, and 30 for age 1 to 3 yo. Give 1 mL SC for 3 doses on days 0, 7, and 30 for age 3 yo or older.

NOTES — Give at least 10 days before travel to endemic areas. An abbreviated schedule on days 0, 7, and 14 can be given if time limits. A booster dose may be given after 2 years. Avoid in thimerosal allergy.

MOA — Active immunity, stimulates antibody production.

ADVERSE EFFECTS — Frequent: Tenderness, redness and swelling at injection site. Severe: Anaphylactic reaction, angioedema, dyspnea, encephalitis, encephalopathy, erythema nodosum, erythema multiforme, peripheral neuropathy, seizures.

MEASLES, MUMPS, & RUBELLA VACCINE (M-M-R II, *Priorix) ▶immune system ♀C ▶+ $$$

ADULT — 0.5 mL (1 vial) SC.

PEDS — 0.5 mL (1 vial) SC for age 12 to 15 mo. Revaccinate prior to elementary and/or middle

MEASLES, MUMPS, & RUBELLA VACCINE (*cont.*)

school according to local health guidelines. If measles outbreak, may immunize infants 6 to 12 mo with 0.5 mL SC; then start 2-dose regimen between 12 to 15 mo.

NOTES — Do not inject IV. Contraindicated in pregnancy. Advise women to avoid pregnancy for 4 weeks following vaccination. Live virus, contraindicated in immunocompromised patients. Avoid if allergic to neomycin or gelatin; caution in egg allergy.

MOA — Active immunity, stimulates antibody production.

ADVERSE EFFECTS — Frequent: Fever, burning, induration, rash. Severe: Allergic reactions, encephalitis, convulsions, erythema multiforme, prolonged high fever, Guillain-Barré syndrome, thrombocytopenia.

MENINGOCOCCAL VACCINE (*Menveo, Menomune-A/C/Y/W-135, Menactra, ✱Menjugate*) ▶immune system ♀C ▶? $$$$

WARNING — Reports of associated Guillain-Barré syndrome; avoid if prior history of this condition.

ADULT — 0.5 mL SC (Menomune) or IM (Menactra, Menveo) in high risk indivduals (aspelnia, etc), repeat in 2 months.

PEDS — Menveo: Four-dose series starting at 2 mo old at 2, 4, 6, and 12 months. Menactra: Vaccinate all children 11 to 12 years, and 16 years. One dose only if between 13 years and 18 years and previously unvaccinated.

UNAPPROVED PEDS — 0.5 mL SC for 2 doses separated by 3 months for age 3 to 18 mo.

NOTES — Give 2 weeks before elective splenectomy or travel to endemic areas. May consider revaccination q 3 to 5 years in high-risk patients. Do not inject IV. Contraindicated in pregnancy. Vaccinate all 1st-year college students living in dormitories who are unvaccinated. Avoid in thimerosal allergy (except Menactra which is thimerosal-free).

MOA — Active immunity, stimulates antibody production.

ADVERSE EFFECTS — Frequent: Pain, erythema, induration, tenderness. Severe: Guillain-Barré syndrome.

PEDIARIX (diphtheria tetanus and acellular pertussis vaccine + hepatitis B vaccine + polio vaccine) ▶immune system ♀C ▶? $$$

PEDS — 0.5 mL at 2, 4, 6 mo IM.

NOTES — Do not administer before 6 weeks of age.

MOA — Active immunity, stimulates antibody production.

ADVERSE EFFECTS — Frequent: Local injection site reactions (pain, swelling, redness), fever, fussiness. Severe: Convulsions, encephalopathy.

PLAGUE VACCINE ▶Immune system ♀C ▶+ $

ADULT — 1 mL IM for 1 dose, then 0.2 mL IM 1 to 3 months after the 1st injection, then 0.2 mL IM 5 to 6 months after the 2nd injection for age 18 to 61 yo.

PEDS — Not approved in children.

NOTES — Up to 3 booster doses (0.2 mL) may be administered at 6-month intervals in high-risk patients. Jet injector gun may be used for IM administration.

MOA — Active immunity, stimulates antibody production.

ADVERSE EFFECTS — Frequent: Malaise, fever, headache, tenderness, nausea.

PNEUMOCOCCAL 13-VALENT CONJUGATE VACCINE (*Prevnar 13*) ▶immune system ♀C ▶? $$$

ADULT — Not approved in most adults. May be indicated for some high-risk adults.

PEDS — 0.5 mL IM for 3 doses at 2 months old, 4 months old, and 6 months old, followed by a fourth dose of 0.5 mL IM at 12 to 15 months of age. For previously unvaccinated older infants and children age 7 to 11 months old: 0.5 mL for 2 doses 4 weeks apart, followed by a third dose of 0.5 mL at 12 to 15 months of age. For previously unvaccinated older infants and children age 12 to 23 months old: Give 0.5 mL for 2 doses 8 weeks apart. For previously unvaccinated children 24 months old to 5 years old, give a single 0.5 mL dose IM before the 6th birthday.

NOTES — For IM use only; do not inject IV. Shake susp vigorously prior to administration.

MOA — Active immunity, stimulates antibody production.

ADVERSE EFFECTS — Frequent: Erythema, induration, tenderness. Severe: Component hypersensitivity.

PNEUMOCOCCAL 23-VALENT VACCINE (*Pneumovax, ✱Pneumo 23*) ▶immune system ♀C ▶+ $$

ADULT — All adults 65 yo or older: 0.5 mL IM/SC for 1 dose. Vaccination also recommended for high-risk individuals younger than age 65 yo. Routine revaccination in immunocompetent patients is not recommended. Consider revaccination once in patients age 65 yo or older who were vaccinated before the age of 65 or patients at high risk of developing serious pneumococcal infection if more than 5 years from initial vaccine.

PEDS — 0.5 mL IM/SC for age 2 yo or older. Consider revaccination once in patients at high risk of developing serious pneumococcal infection after 3 to 5 years from initial vaccine in patients who would be 10 yo or younger at time of revaccination.

NOTES — Do not give IV or ID. May be given in conjunction with influenza virus vaccine at different site. OK for high-risk children at least 2 yo who received Prevnar series already to provide additional serotype coverage. Consult CC guidelines for intervals between PCV13 and PPSV23 pneumococcal vaccines.

MOA — Active immunity, stimulates antibody production.

ADVERSE EFFECTS — Frequent: Induration and soreness at the injection site. Severe: Anaphylaxis, Guillain-Barré syndrome,

POLIO VACCINE (*IPOL*) ▶immune system ♀C ▶? $$

ADULT — Previously unvaccinated adults at increased risk of exposure should receive a complete primary immunization series of 3 doses (2 doses at intervals of 4 to 8 weeks; a third dose at 6 to 12 months after the second dose). Accelerated

(cont.)

POLIO VACCINE (*cont.*)

schedules are available. Travelers to endemic areas who have received primary immunization should receive a single booster in adulthood.

PEDS — 0.5 mL IM/SC at age 2 mo, with second dose at 4 mo, third dose at 6 to 18 mo, and fourth dose at 4 to 6 yo.

NOTES — Oral polio vaccine no longer available.

MOA — Active immunity, stimulates antibody production.

ADVERSE EFFECTS — Frequent; Fever, erythema, induration, pain, irritability, sleepiness, fussiness, crying.

PROQUAD (measles mumps & rubella vaccine + varicella vaccine) ▸immune system ♀C ▶? $$$$

ADULT — Not indicated in adults.

PEDS — 0.5 mL (1 vial) SC for age 12 mo to 12 yo.

NOTES — Give at least 1 month after a MMR-containing vaccine and at least 3 months after a varicella-containing vaccine. Do not inject IV. Contraindicated in pregnancy. Following vaccination avoid pregnancy for 3 months and aspirin/salicylates for 6 weeks. Live virus, contraindicated in immunocompromise or untreated TB. Avoid if allergic to neomycin; caution with egg allergies.

MOA — Active immunity, stimulates antibody production.

ADVERSE EFFECTS — Frequent: Fever, pain, tenderness, soreness, swelling, rash. Severe: Allergic reactions, encephalitis, convulsions, erythema multiforme, prolonged high fever, Guillain-Barré syndrome, thrombocytopenia.

RABIES VACCINE (*RabAvert, Imovax Rabies, BioRab, Rabies Vaccine Adsorbed*) ▸immune system ♀C ▶? $$$$$

ADULT — Postexposure prophylaxis: Give rabies immune globulin (20 international units/kg) immediately after exposure, then give rabies vaccine 1 mL IM in deltoid region on days 0, 3, 7, 14, and 28. If patients have received pre-exposure immunization, give 1 mL IM rabies vaccine on day 0 and 3 only, without rabies immune globulin. Preexposure immunization: 1 mL IM rabies vaccine on days 0, 7, and between days 21 and 28. Or 0.1 mL ID on days 0, 7, and between days 21 and 28. (Imovax Rabies ID vaccine formula only). Repeat q 2 to 5 years based on antibody titer.

PEDS — Same as adults.

NOTES — Do not use ID preparation for postexposure prophylaxis.

MOA — Active immunity, stimulates antibody production.

ADVERSE EFFECTS — Frequent: Pain, swelling, erythema, pruritus. Severe: Immune-complex like reactions, Guillain-Barré syndrome.

ROTAVIRUS VACCINE (*RotaTeq, Rotarix*) ▸immune system ♀ Not applicable ▶? $$$$$

ADULT — Not recommended.

PEDS — RotaTeq: Give the first dose (2 mL PO) between 6 to 12 weeks of age, and then the second and third doses at 4- to 10-week intervals thereafter (last dose no later than 32 weeks). Rotarix: Give first dose (1 mL) at 6 weeks of age, and second dose (1 mL) at least 4 weeks later, and prior to 24 weeks of age.

FORMS — Trade only: Oral susp 2 mL (RotaTeq), 1 mL (Rotarix).

NOTES — Live vaccine so potential for transmission, especially to immunodeficient close contacts. Safety unclear in immunocompromised infants.

MOA — Active immunity, stimulates antibody production.

ADVERSE EFFECTS — Frequent: Diarrhea, vomiting.

SMALLPOX VACCINE (*ACAM 2000, vaccinia vaccine*) ▸immune system ♀C ▶– Not available to civilians.

ADULT — Prevention of smallpox or monkeypox: Specialized administration using bifurcated needle SC for 1 dose.

PEDS — Specialized administration using bifurcated needle SC for 1 dose for children older than 1 yo.

NOTES — Caution in polymyxin, neomycin, tetracycline, or streptomycin allergy. Avoid in those (or household contacts of those) with eczema or a history of eczema, those with a rash due to other causes (eg, burns, zoster, impetigo, psoriasis), immunocompromised, or pregnancy. Persons with known cardiac disease or at least 3 risk factors for cardiac disease should not be vaccinated.

MOA — Active immunity, stimulates antibody production.

ADVERSE EFFECTS — Frequent: Fever, malaise, swelling/tenderness of regional lymph nodes. Severe: Generalized vaccinia, encephalitis, encephalopathy, eczema vaccinatum, myopericarditis, myocardial infarction, angina, death.

TETANUS TOXOID ▸immune system ♀C ▶+ $$

WARNING — Td is preferred in adults and children age 7 yo or older. DTaP is preferred in children younger than 7 yo. Use fluid tetanus toxoid in assessing cell-mediated immunity only.

ADULT — 0.5 mL IM (adsorbed) for 2 doses 4 to 8 weeks apart. Give third dose 6 to 12 months after second injection. Give booster q 10 years. Assess cell-mediated immunity: 0.1 mL of 1:100 diluted skin-test reagent or 0.02 mL of 1:10 diluted skin-test reagent injected intradermally.

PEDS — 0.5 mL IM (adsorbed) for 2 doses 4 to 8 weeks apart. Give third dose 6 to 12 months after second injection. Give booster q 10 years.

NOTES — May use tetanus toxoid fluid for active immunization in patients hypersensitive to the aluminum adjuvant of the adsorbed formulation: 0.5 mL IM or SC for 3 doses at 4- to 8-week intervals. Give fourth dose 6 to 12 months after third injection. Give booster dose q 10 years. Avoid in thimerosal allergy.

MOA — Active immunity, stimulates antibody production.

ADVERSE EFFECTS — Frequent: Local induration at the injection site, chills, fever. Severe: Hypersensitivity reactions, fever (>103 F), neurological disturbances.

TWINRIX (hepatitis A vaccine + hepatitis B vaccine) ▸immune system ♀C ▶? $$$$
ADULT — 1 mL IM in deltoid only for age 18 yo or older, repeat at 1 and 6 months. Accelerated dosing schedule: 0, 7, 21, and 30 days and booster dose at 12 months.
PEDS — Not approved in children.
NOTES — Not for IV or ID use. 1 mL is equivalent to 720 ELU inactivated hepatitis A + 20 mcg hepatitis B surface antigen. Due to lower antigen dose of hepatitis A in Twinrix product compared with standard 2-dose hep A vaccine, all three doses must be given for hepatitis A immunity in adults.
MOA — Active immunity, stimulates antibody production.
ADVERSE EFFECTS — Frequent: Headache, local pain, tenderness, warmth, dizziness, malaise, urticaria, rash, erythema. Severe: Angioedema, anaphylaxis.
TYPHOID VACCINE—INACTIVATED INJECTION (*Typhim Vi, ✹Typherix*) ▸immune system ♀C ▶? $$
ADULT — 0.5 mL IM for 1 dose given at least 2 weeks prior to potential exposure. May consider revaccination q 2 years in high-risk patients.
PEDS — Same as adult dose for age 2 yo or older.
NOTES — Recommended for travel to endemic areas.
MOA — Active immunity, stimulates antibody production.
ADVERSE EFFECTS — Frequent: Headache, fever, local tenderness at site, erythema, induration, myalgia.
TYPHOID VACCINE—LIVE ORAL (*Vivotif Berna*) ▸immune system ♀C ▶? $$
ADULT — 1 cap 1 h before a meal with cold or lukewarm drink every other day for 4 doses to be completed at least 1 week prior to potential exposure. May consider revaccination q 5 years in high-risk patients.
PEDS — Give adult dose for age 6 yo or older.
FORMS — Trade only: Caps.
NOTES — Recommended for travel to endemic areas. Oral vaccine may be inactivated by antibiotics, including antimalarials.
MOA — Active immunity, stimulates antibody production.
ADVERSE EFFECTS — Frequent (oral): Rash, abdominal pain, diarrhea, N/V.
VARICELLA VACCINE (*Varivax, ✹Varilrix*) ▸immune system ♀C ▶+ $$$$
ADULT — 0.5 mL SC. Repeat 4 to 8 weeks later.

PEDS — 0.5 mL SC for 1 dose for age 1 to 12 yo. Repeat at ages 4 yo to 6 yo. Use adult dose for age 13 yo or older. Not recommended for infants younger than 1 yo.
UNAPPROVED PEDS — Postexposure prophylaxis: 0.5 mL SC within 3 to 5 days of exposure.
NOTES — Do not inject IV. Following vaccination avoid pregnancy for 3 months and aspirin/salicylates for 6 weeks. This live vaccine is contraindicated in immunocompromised.
MOA — Active immunity, stimulates antibody production.
ADVERSE EFFECTS — Frequent: Fever, inflammation at the injection site.
YELLOW FEVER VACCINE (*YF-Vax*) ▸immune system ♀C ▶+ $$$
ADULT — 0.5 mL SC.
PEDS — 0.5 mL SC into thigh (6 mo to 3 yo) or deltoid region for age 3 yo or older.
NOTES — Must be accredited site to administer vaccination. International Certificate of Vaccination obligatory for some travel destinations. Consult CDC traveler's health website for accredited sites or to apply for accreditation. A booster dose (0.5 mL) may be administered q 10 years.
MOA—Active immunity, stimulates antibody production.
ADVERSE EFFECTS — Frequent: Fever, malaise, headache, myalgia.
ZOSTER VACCINE—LIVE (*Zostavax*) ▸immune system ♀C ▶? $$$$
ADULT — 0.65 mL SC for 1 dose for age 50 yo or older. However, ACIP recommends immunizing those 60 years and older.
PEDS — Not approved in children.
NOTES — Avoid if history of anaphylactic/anaphylactoid reaction to gelatin or neomycin, if primary or acquired immunodeficiency states, or if taking immunosuppressives. Do not administer if active untreated TB or in possible pregnancy. Theoretically possible to transmit to pregnant household contact who has not had varicella infection or immunocompromised contact. Do not substitute for Varivax in children.
MOA — Active immunity, boosts pre-existing immunity on individuals who have a history of varicella disease.
ADVERSE EFFECTS — Frequent: Pain, tenderness, pruritus and erythema at injection site.

IMMUNOLOGY: Immunoglobulins

NOTE: Adult IM injections should be given in the deltoid region; injection in the gluteal region may result in suboptimal response.

ANTIVENIN–CROTALIDAE IMMUNE FAB OVINE POLYVALENT (*CroFab*) ▸? ♀C ▶? $$$$$
ADULT — Rattlesnake envenomation: Give 4 to 6 vials IV infusion over 60 min, within 6 h of bite if possible. Administer 4 to 6 additional vials if no initial control of envenomation syndrome, then 2 vials q 6 h for up to 18 h (3 doses) after initial control has been established.

PEDS — Same as adults, although specific studies in children have not been conducted.
NOTES — Contraindicated in allergy to papaya or papain. Start IV infusion slowly over the first 10 min at 25 to 50 mL/h and observe for allergic reaction, then increase to full rate of 250 mL/h.
MOA — Antivenom.
ADVERSE EFFECTS — Frequent: None,

ANTIVENIN—CROTALIDAE POLYVALENT ▶L ♀C ▶? $$$$$
ADULT — Pit viper envenomation: 20 to 40 mL (2 to 4 vials) IV infusion for minimal envenomation, 50 to 90 mL (5 to 9 vials) IV infusion for moderate envenomation; give at least 100 to 150 mL (10 to 15 vials) IV infusion for severe envenomation. Administer within 4 h of bite, less effective after 8 h, and of questionable value after 12 h. May give additional 10 to 50 mL (1 to 5 vials) IV infusion based on clinical assessment and response to initial dose.
PEDS — Larger relative doses of antivenin are needed in children and small adults because of small volume of body fluid to dilute the venom. The dose is not based on wt.
NOTES — Test first for sensitivity to horse serum. Serum sickness may occur 5 to 24 days after dose. IV route is preferred. May give IM.
MOA — Antivenom.
ADVERSE EFFECTS — Frequent: None.
ANTIVENIN—LATRODECTUS MACTANS ▶L ♀C ▶? $$
ADULT — Specialized dosing for black widow spider toxicity; consult poison center.
PEDS — Specialized dosing for black widow spider toxicity; consult poison center.
NOTES — Test first for horse serum sensitivity. Serum sickness may occur 5 to 24 days after dose.
MOA — Antivenom.
ADVERSE EFFECTS — Frequent: None.
BOTULISM IMMUNE GLOBULIN (*BabyBIG*) ▶L ♀? ▶? $$$$$
ADULT — Not approved in age 1 yo or older.
PEDS — Infant botulism: 1 mL (50 mg)/kg IV for age younger than 1 yo.
MOA — Passive immunity.
ADVERSE EFFECTS — Frequent: Mild, transient erythematous rash of face or trunk. Severe: Anaphylaxis, angioedema, urticaria, renal dysfunction/failure.
CYTOMEGALOVIRUS IMMUNE GLOBULIN HUMAN (*Cytogam*) ▶L ♀C ▶? $$$$$
ADULT — Specialized dosing based on indication and time since transplant.
PEDS — Specialized dosing based on indication and time since transplant.
MOA — Passive immunity.
ADVERSE EFFECTS — Frequent: Flushing, fever, pain, N/V. Severe: Anaphylaxis.
HEPATITIS B IMMUNE GLOBULIN (*H-BIG, HyperHep B, HepaGam B, NABI-HB*) ▶L ♀C ▶? $$$
ADULT — Postexposure prophylaxis for needlestick, ocular, mucosal exposure: 0.06 mL/kg IM (usual dose 3 to 5 mL) within 24 h of exposure. Initiate hepatitis B vaccine series within 7 days. Consider a second dose of hepatitis B immune globulin (HBIG) 1 month later if patient refuses hepatitis B vaccine series. Postexposure prophylaxis for sexual exposure: 0.06 mL/kg IM within 14 days of sexual contact. Initiate hepatitis B vaccine series. Prevention of hepatitis B recurrence following liver transplantation in HBsAg-positive (HepaGam B): first dose given during transplantation surgery. Subsequent doses daily for 7 days, then biweekly

up to 3 months and monthly thereafter. Doses adjusted based on regular monitoring of HBsAg, HBV-DNA, HBeAg, and anti-HBs antibody levels.
PEDS — Prophylaxis of infants born to HBsAg (+) mothers: 0.5 mL IM within 12 h of birth. Initiate hepatitis B vaccine series within 7 days. If hepatitis B vaccine series is refused, repeat HBIG dose at 3 and 6 mo. Household exposure age younger than 12 mo: give 0.5 mL IM within 14 days of exposure. Initiate hepatitis B vaccine series.
NOTES — HBIG may be administered at the same time or up to 1 month prior to hepatitis B vaccine without impairing the active immune response from hepatitis B vaccine.
MOA — Passive immunity.
ADVERSE EFFECTS — Frequent: Pain at injection site. Severe: Anaphylaxis, angioedema, urticaria.
IMMUNE GLOBULIN—INTRAMUSCULAR (*Baygam,* ✱*Gamastan*) ▶L ♀C ▶? $$$$
ADULT — Hepatitis A postexposure prophylaxis for household or institutional contacts: 0.02 mL/kg IM within 2 weeks of exposure. Hepatitis A pre-exposure prophylaxis (ie, travel to endemic area): give 0.02 mL/kg IM for length of stay less than 3 months, give 0.06 mL/kg IM and repeat q 4 to 6 months for length of stay longer than 3 months. Measles: 0.2 to 0.25 mL/kg IM within 6 days of exposure, max 15 mL. Varicella zoster: 0.6 to 1.2 mL/kg IM. Rubella exposure in pregnant, susceptible women: 0.55 mL/kg IM. Immunoglobulin deficiency: 0.66 mL/kg IM q 3 to 4 weeks.
PEDS — Not approved in children.
UNAPPROVED PEDS — Measles: 0.2 to 0.25 mL/kg IM within 6 days of exposure. In susceptible immunocompromised children use 0.5 mL/kg IM (max 15 mL) immediately after exposure. Varicella zoster: 0.6 to 1.2 mL/kg IM.
NOTES — Human-derived product, increased infection risk. Hepatitis A vaccine preferred over immune globulin for age 2 yo or older who plan to travel to high-risk areas repeatedly or for long periods of time.
MOA — Passive immunity.
ADVERSE EFFECTS — Frequent: Pain at injection site, tenderness, muscle stiffness, HA. Severe: Anaphylaxis, angioedema, urticaria, nephrotic syndrome.
IMMUNE GLOBULIN—INTRAVENOUS (*Carimune, Flebogamma, Gammagard, Gammaplex, Gamunex, Octagam, Privigen*) ▶L ♀C ▶? $$$$$
WARNING — Renal dysfunction, acute renal failure, osmotic nephrosis, and death may be associated with IV immune globulins, especially those containing sucrose. Administer at the minimum concentration available and the minimum practical infusion rate.
ADULT — Idiopathic thrombocytopenic purpura (induction): 400 mg/kg IV daily for 5 days (or 1 g/kg IV daily for 1 to 2 days). Bone marrow transplant: 500 mg/kg IV daily, given 7 and 2 days before transplant, and then weekly until 90 days post transplant for age older than 20 yo. Primary

IMMUNE GLOBULIN—INTRAVENOUS (*cont.*)

humoral immunodeficiency: 200 to 300 mg/kg IV each month; increase prn to max 400 to 800 mg/kg/month. B-cell chronic lymphocytic leukemia: Specialized dosing. Chronic inflammatory demyelinating polyneuropathy (CIDP): (Gamunex) 2 g/kg IV loading dose followed by 1 g/kg IV q 3 weeks.

PEDS — Pediatric HIV: 400 mg/kg IV q 28 days. Idiopathic thrombocytopenic purpura (induction): 400 mg/kg IV daily for 5 days (or 1 g/kg IV daily for 1 to 2 days). Kawasaki syndrome (acute): 400 mg/kg IV daily for 4 days (or 2 g/kg IV for 1 dose over 10 h). Primary humoral immunodeficiency: 200 to 300 mg/kg IV each month; increase prn to max 400 to 800 mg/kg/month.

UNAPPROVED ADULT — First-line therapy in severe Guillain-Barré syndrome, chronic inflammatory demyelinating polyneuropathy, multifocal motor neuropathy, severe posttransfusion purpura, inclusion body myositis, fetomaternal alloimmune thrombocytopenia; 2nd-line therapy in stiff-person syndrome, dermatomyositis, myasthenia gravis, and Lambert-Eaton myasthenic syndrome. Various dosing regimens have been used; a common one is myasthenia gravis (induction): 400 mg/kg IV daily for 5 days (total 2 g/kg). Has been used in multiple sclerosis and inflammatory myositis (polymyositis and dermatomyositis), renal transplant rejection, systemic lupus erythematosus, toxic epidermal necrolysis and Stevens-Johnson syndrome, Clostridium difficile colitis, Graves' ophthalmopathy, pemphigus, Wegener's granulomatosis, Churg-Strauss syndrome, and Duchenne muscular dystrophy.

UNAPPROVED PEDS — Myasthenia gravis (induction): 400 mg/kg IV daily for 5 days. Other dosing regimens have been used.

NOTES — Indications and doses vary by product. Follow LFTs, renal function, vital signs, and urine output closely. Contraindicated in IgA deficiency. Use caution (and lower infusion rates) if risk factors for thrombosis, heart failure, or renal insufficiency. Use slower infusion rates for initial doses. Consider pretreatment with acetaminophen and/or diphenhydramine to minimize some infusion-related adverse effects. Human-derived product; although donors are carefully screened there is risk of transmission of infectious agents.

MOA — Immunomodulatory effects through exogenous immunoglobulins.

ADVERSE EFFECTS — Serious: Acute renal failure, noncardiogenic pulmonary edema, hemolysis, heart failure, stroke, MI, DVT, aseptic meningitis, anaphylaxis. Frequent: Infusion reactions, HA, vomiting, fever, chills, hypotension, rash, back pain, reversible neutropenia, pain at injection site.

IMMUNE GLOBULIN—SUBCUTANEOUS (*Vivaglobulin, Hizentra*) ▶L ♀C ▶? $$$$$

ADULT — Primary immune deficiency: 100 to 200 mg/kg SC weekly. In patients already receiving IV immune globulin: SC dose is equivalent to (previous IV dose × 1.37) divided by frequency of IV regimen in week.

PEDS — Limited information. Dosing appears to be same as in adults.

NOTES — Do not administer IV. Contraindicated in IgA deficiency. Human-derived product, increased infection risk.

MOA — Passive immunity.

ADVERSE EFFECTS — Serious: Acute hypersensitivity reactions, anaphylaxis. Frequent: Injection site reactions, HA, nausea/vomiting, fever, rash, pain, diarrhea, sore throat.

LYMPHOCYTE IMMUNE GLOBULIN (*Atgam*) ▶L ♀C ▶? $$$$$

ADULT — Renal allograft recipients: 10 to 30 mg/kg IV daily. Delaying onset of allograft rejection: 15 mg/kg IV daily for 14 days, then every other day for 14 days. Treatment of renal transplant rejection: 10 to 15 mg/kg IV for 14 days. Aplastic anemia: 10 to 20 mg/kg IV daily for 8 to 14 days, then every other day, prn, up to 21 total doses.

PEDS — Limited experience. Has been safely administered to a limited number of children with renal transplant and aplastic anemia at doses comparable to adults.

NOTES — Equine product. Doses should be administered over at least 4 h.

MOA — Lymphocyte-specific immunosuppressant.

ADVERSE EFFECTS — Frequent: Fever, chills, skin reactions, systemic infections, abnormal renal function, serum-sickness-like reactions, dyspnea, arthralgia, chest, back, flank pain, diarrhea, N/V. Severe: Anaphylaxis, hemolysis, thrombocytopenia, leukopenia.

RABIES IMMUNE GLOBULIN HUMAN (*Imogam Rabies-HT, HyperRAB S/D*) ▶L ♀C ▶? $$$$$

ADULT — Postexposure prophylaxis: 20 units/kg (0.133 mL/kg), with as much as possible infiltrated around the bite and the rest given IM. Give as soon as possible after exposure. Administer with the first dose of vaccine, but in a different extremity.

PEDS — Not approved in children.

UNAPPROVED PEDS — Use adult dosing.

NOTES — Do not repeat dose once rabies vaccine series begins. Do not give to patients who have been completely immunized with rabies vaccine. Do not administer IV.

MOA — Passive immunity.

ADVERSE EFFECTS — Frequent: Pain at injection site, sensitization. Severe: Anaphylaxis, angioedema, skin rash, nephrotic syndrome.

RSV IMMUNE GLOBULIN (*RespiGam*) ▶Plasma ♀C ▶? $$$$$

PEDS — RSV prophylaxis: 1.5 mL/kg/h for 15 min for age younger than 24 mo. Increase rate as clinical condition permits to 3 mL/kg/h for 15 min, then to a maximum rate of 6 mL/kg/h. Max total dose/month is 750 mg/kg.

NOTES — May cause fluid overload; monitor vital signs frequently during IV infusion. RSV season is typically November through April.

RSV IMMUNE GLOBULIN (cont.)

MOA — Passive immunity.

ADVERSE EFFECTS — Frequent: Rash, fever, tachycardia, hypotension, hypertension, vomiting, diarrhea, gastroenteritis.

TETANUS IMMUNE GLOBULIN (BayTet) ▶L ♀C ▶? $$$$

ADULT — See tetanus wound management table. Postexposure prophylaxis in tetanus-prone wounds for age 7 yo or older: if less than 3 doses of tetanus vaccine have been administered or if history is uncertain, give 250 units IM for 1 dose along with dT. If at least 3 doses of tetanus vaccine have been administered in the past, do not give tetanus

immune globulin. Tetanus treatment: 3000 to 6000 units IM in combination with other therapies.

PEDS — 4 units/kg IM or 250 units IM for age younger than 7 yo. Initiate tetanus toxoid vaccine (DTP or DT).

NOTES — Do not give tetanus immune globulin for clean, minor wounds. May be given at the same time as tetanus toxoid active immunization. Do not inject IV.

MOA — Passive immunity.

ADVERSE EFFECTS — Frequent: Pain at injection site, sensitization. Severe: Anaphylaxis, angioedema, skin rash, nephrotic syndrome.

IMMUNOLOGY: Immunosuppression

BASILIXIMAB (Simulect) ▶plasma ♀B ▶? $$$$$

WARNING — To be used only by trained physicians. To be given only in facility with adequate laboratory and supportive medical resources.

ADULT — Specialized dosing for organ transplantation.

PEDS — Specialized dosing for organ transplantation.

MOA — Immunosuppressant, prophylaxis of acute organ rejection.

ADVERSE EFFECTS — Frequent: Administration did not increase the incidence or severity of adverse events over placebo in immunosuppressed patients.

BELATACEPT (Nulojix) ▶serum ♀C ▶– $$$$$

WARNING — Should only be prescribed by physicians who are knowledgable about the drug. Serious adverse effects have been reported.

ADULT — Specialized dosing for organ transplantation. PEDS — Not approved in children.

MOA — T-cell blocker.

ADVERSE EFFECTS — many

CYCLOSPORINE (Sandimmune, Neoral, Gengraf) ▶L ♀C ▶– $$$$$

WARNING — Should only be prescribed by physicians who are knowledgeable about the drug. Many drug interactions. Serious adverse effects can occur. Monitor closely in those with renal or hepatic impairment

ADULT — Specialized dosing for organ transplantation, RA, and psoriasis.

PEDS — Not approved in children.

UNAPPROVED ADULT — Specialized dosing for autoimmune eye disorders, vasculitis, inflammatory myopathies, Behcet's disease, psoriatic arthritis, chronic refractory idiopathic thrombocytopenia.

UNAPPROVED PEDS — Specialized dosing for organ transplantation, chronic refractory idiopathic thrombocytopenia.

FORMS — Generic/Trade: Microemulsion Caps 25, 100 mg. Generic/Trade: Caps (Sandimmune) 25, 100 mg. Soln (Sandimmune) 100 mg/mL. Microemulsion soln (Neoral, Gengraf) 100 mg/mL.

NOTES — Monitor cyclosporine blood concentrations closely. Many drug interactions including atorvastatin, azithromycin, lovastatin, oral contraceptives, rosuvastatin, simvastatin, sirolimus, terbinafine, voriconazole,

HIV protease inhibitors, grapefruit juice and others. Use caution when combining with methotrexate or potassium sparing drugs such as ACE inhibitors. Reduce dose in renal dysfunction. Monitor BP and renal function closely. Avoid excess UV light exposure. Monitor patients closely when switching from Sandimmune to microemulsion formulations.

MOA — Immunosuppressant, prophylaxis of acute organ rejection.

ADVERSE EFFECTS — Frequent: Hypertension, hirsutism, hypomagnesemia, hypokalemia, gingival hypertrophy, tremor, nephrotoxicity. Severe: Anaphylaxis, infection and increased risk of lymphoma and other malignancies, especially those of the skin, risk, optic disc edema, benign intracranial hypertension, papilledema, visual impairment, thrombotic microangiopathy, hepatotoxicity, polyoma virus infection, neurotoxicty .

EVEROLIMUS (Zortress) ▶L - ♀C ▶– $$$$$

WARNING — Increased risk of infection and malignancies. Increased risk of kidney graft thrombosis, Increased mortality in heart transplant trials so not recommended in heart transplant patients. reduce dose of cyclosporine to reduce nephrotoxicity.

ADULT — Specialized dosing for organ transplantation.

PEDS — Not approved for use in children.

FORMS — Trade: tab 0.25, 0.,5, 0.75 mg.

NOTES — Reduce dose in renal dysfunction, Monitor BP and real function closely. Many drug interactions. Increased risk of infections/malignancy.

MOA — Immunosuppressant, prophylaxis of acute organ rejection

ADVERSE EFFECTS — Severe: delayed wound healing, fluid accumulation, interstitial lung disease, bon-infectious pneumonitis, proteinuria, thrombotic microangiopathy, thrombotic thrombocytopenic purpura, hemolytic uremic syndrome, new onset diabetes, male infertility.

MYCOPHENOLATE MOFETIL (Cellcept, Myfortic) ▶? ♀D ▶– $$

WARNING — Has been associated with embryofetal toxicity, lymphoma, malignancy, increased risk of infection, and progressive multifocal leukoencephalopathy (PML).

MYCOPHENOLATE MOFETIL (*cont.*)

ADULT — Specialized dosing for organ transplantation. Take 1 hr before or 2 h after food.

PEDS — Not approved in children.

UNAPPROVED ADULT — Lupus nephritis: 1000 mg PO two times per day. Has been used in pemphigus, bullous pemphigoid, and refractory uveitis.

UNAPPROVED PEDS — Specialized dosing for organ transplantation.

FORMS — Generic/Trade: Caps 250 mg. Tabs 500 mg. Tabs extended-release (Myfortic): 180, 360 mg. Trade only (CellCept): Susp 200 mg/mL (160 mL).

NOTES — Avoid live vaccine administration. Increased risk of 1st trimester pregnancy loss and increased risk of congenital malformations, especially external ear and facial abnormalities. Counsel women regarding pregnancy prevention and planning.

MOA — Immunosuppressant, prophylaxis of acute organ rejection.

ADVERSE EFFECTS — Frequent: GI upset, thrombophlebitis, thrombosis (with IV administration). Severe: Infection, GI bleeding, nephrotic syndrome, bone marrow suppression, leukopenia, lymphoma, malignancy, progressive multifocal leukoencephalopathy, pure red cell aplasia.

SIROLIMUS (*Rapamune*) ▶L ♀C ▶– $$$$$

WARNING — Increased risk of infection and lymphoma. Combination of sirolimus plus cyclosporine or tacrolimus is associated with hepatic artery thrombosis in liver transplant patients. Combination with tacrolimus and corticosteroids in lung transplant patients may cause bronchial anastomotic dehiscence. Possible increased mortality in stable liver transplant patients after conversion from a calcineurin inhibitor (CNI)-based immunosuppressive regimen to sirolimus. Can cause hypersensitivity reactions including anaphylactic and/or anaphylactoid reactions, angioedema, vasculitis. Many drug interactions. Avoid with strong inhibitors of CYP3A4 and/or p-glycoprotein (ketoconazole, voriconazole, itraconazole, erythromycin, clarithromycin) or strong inducers CYP3A4 and/or p-glycoprotein (rifampin, rifabutin). Monitor level if cyclosporine is discontinued or has dose markedly changed.

ADULT — Specialized dosing for organ transplantation.

PEDS — Not approved in children.

UNAPPROVED PEDS — Specialized dosing for organ transplantation.

FORMS — Generic/Trade: Tabs 0.5 mg. Trade only: Soln 1 mg/mL (60 mL). Tabs 1, 2 mg.

NOTES — Wear protective clothing and sunscreen when exposed to sunlight to reduce the risk of skin cancer. Be aware of site-specific assay method, as this may affect reported serum concentrations. Adjust dose by $^1/_3$ to ½ in liver dysfunction. Monitor trough levels, particularly in patients likely to have altered drug metabolism, age 13 yo or older with wt less than 40 kg, hepatic impairment, when changing doses or with interacting medications. Do not adjust dose more frequently than q 1 to 2 weeks. Oral soln and tabs are clinically equivalent from a dosing standpoint at the 2 mg level; however, this is unknown at higher doses.

MOA — Immunosuppressant, prophylaxis of acute organ rejection in solid organ transplant.

ADVERSE EFFECTS — Frequent: Hypertension, edema, chest pain, fever, headache, pain, insomnia, rash, abdominal pain, renal dysfunction, nausea, diarrhea, anemia, thrombocytopenia, arthralgia, dyspnea. Hyperlipidemia in up to 90% of patients. Severe: Hepatic artery thrombosis in liver transplant patients, hypersensitivity reactions, progressive multifocal leukoencephalopathy, nephrotic syndrome, exfoliative dermatitis, impaired wound healing, angioedema, vasculitis, interstitial lung disease, hemolytic uremic syndrome/thrombotic thrombocytopenic purpura/thrombotic microangiopathy, increased risk of infections such as tuberculosis, especially when used with calcineurin inhibitor.

TACROLIMUS (*Astagraf XL, Hecoria, Prograf, FK 506*) ▶L ♀C ▶– $$$$$

ADULT — Specialized dosing for organ transplantation.

PEDS — Specialized dosing for organ transplantation.

UNAPPROVED ADULT — RA (approved in Canada), active vasculitis, systemic lupus erythematosus nephritis, and vasculitis.

FORMS — Generic/Trade: Caps 0.5, 1, 5 mg. Trade only: Extended-release caps (Astagraf XL) 0.5, 1, 5 mg.

NOTES — Reduce dose in renal dysfunction. Monitor BP and renal function closely. Neurotoxic, especially in high doses. Many drug interactions. Increased risk of infections, QT prolongation, gastrointestinal perforation.

MOA — Immunosuppressant, prophylaxis of acute organ rejection.

ADVERSE EFFECTS — Frequent: Hypertension, peripheral edema, headache, insomnia, pain, fever, pruritus, N/V, diarrhea, abdominal pain, tremors, paresthesias. Severe: Anaphylaxis, edema, hypertrophic cardiomyopathy, gastrointestinal perforation, myocardial hypertrophy, ECG abnormalities including QT prolongation and Torsades de Pointes, paralysis, stroke, hemolytic uremic syndrome, nephrotoxicity, secondary malignancy.

IMMUNOLOGY: Other

HYMENOPTERA VENOM ▶Serum ♀C ▶? $$$$

ADULT — Specialized desensitization dosing protocol.

PEDS — Specialized desensitization dosing protocol.

NOTES — Venom products available: Honey bee (Apis mellifera) and yellow jacket (Vespula sp.), yellow hornet (Dolichovespula arenaria), white-faced hornet

(cont.)

HYMENOPTERA VENOM (*cont.*)

(D. maculata) and wasp (Polistes sp.). Mixed vespid venom protein (yellow jacket, yellow hornet and white-faced hornet) is also available.

MOA — Desensitization protein.

ADVERSE EFFECTS — Frequent: Erythema, swelling, pruritus, burning. Severe: Systemic reactions, anaphylaxis, death.

RILONACEPT (*Arcalyst*) ▶? ♀? ▶? $$$$$

ADULT — Familial cold auto-inflammatory syndrome (FCAS) and Muckle-Wells syndrome (MWS): Begin therapy with a loading dose of 320 mg (160 mg SC on the same day at two different sites), then 160 mg SC once weekly.

PEDS — Familial cold auto-inflammatory syndrome (FCAS) and Muckle-Wells syndrome (MWS): Begin therapy with a loading dose of 4.4 mg/kg (to a maximum of 320 mg) SC in one or two doses, then 2.2 mg/kg (to a max of 160 mg) SC once weekly.

NOTES — Increased risk of infections.

MOA — interleukin 1 blocker

ADVERSE EFFECTS — Frequent: injection site reactions.

TUBERCULIN PPD (*Aplisol, Tubersol, Mantoux, PPD*) ▶L ♀C ▶+ $

ADULT — 5 tuberculin unites (0.1 mL) intradermally.

PEDS — Same as adult dose. AAP recommends screening at 12 mo, 4 to 6 yo, and 14 to 16 yo.

NOTES — Avoid SC injection. Read 48 to 72 h after intradermal injection. Repeat testing in patients with known prior positive PPD; may cause scarring at injection site.

MOA — Skin test for diagnosis of tuberculosis.

ADVERSE EFFECTS — Frequent: Ulceration, necrosis, vesiculation.

NEUROLOGY

Dermatomes

MOTOR FUNCTION BY NERVE ROOTS

Level	Motor Function
C3/C4/C5	Diaphragm
C5/C6	Deltoid/biceps
C7/C8	Triceps
C8/T1	Finger flexion/ intrinsics
T1–T12	Intercostal/ abd muscles
L2/L3	Hip flexion
L2/L3/L4	Hip adductor/quads
L4/L5	Ankle dorsiflexion
S1/S2	Ankle plantarflexion
S2/S3/S4	Rectal tone

LUMBOSACRAL NERVE ROOT COMPRESSIONS	Root	Motor	Sensory	Reflex
	L4	quadriceps	medial foot	knee-jerk
	L5	dorsiflexors	dorsum of foot	medial hamstring
	S1	plantarflexors	lateral foot	ankle-jerk

GLASGOW COMA SCALE

Eye Opening	Verbal Activity	Motor Activity
4. Spontaneous	5. Oriented	6. Obeys commands
3. To command	4. Confused	5. Localizes pain
2. To pain	3. Inappropriate	4. Withdraws to pain
1. None	2. Incomprehensible	3. Flexion to pain
	1. None	2. Extension to pain
		1. None

NEUROLOGY: Alzheimer's Disease—Cholinesterase Inhibitors

NOTE: Avoid concurrent use of anticholinergic agents. Use caution in asthma/COPD. May be coadministered with memantine.

DONEPEZIL (*Aricept*) ▶LK ♀C ▶? $$$$
ADULT — Alzheimer's disease: Start 5 mg PO at bedtime. May increase to 10 mg PO at bedtime in 4 to 6 weeks. Max 10 mg/day for mild to moderate disease. For moderate to severe disease (MMSE 10 or less), may increase after 3 months to 23 mg/ day.
PEDS — Not approved in children.
UNAPPROVED ADULT — Dementia in Parkinson's disease: 5 to 10 mg/day.
FORMS — Generic/Trade: Tabs 5, 10 mg, Orally disintegrating tabs 5, 10 mg. Trade only: Tab 23 mg.
NOTES — Some clinicians start with 5 mg PO every other day to minimize GI side effects.
MOA — Reversible acetylcholinesterase inhibitor.
ADVERSE EFFECTS — Serious: Cholinergic crisis, seizures, bradycardia, syncope, hypotension, respiratory depression. Frequent: N/V, diarrhea, anorexia, insomnia, muscle cramps, fatigue, ecchymosis.

GALANTAMINE (*Razadyne, Razadyne ER, ✹Reminyl*)
▶LK ♀B ▶? $$$$
ADULT — Alzheimer's disease: Extended-release: Start 8 mg PO q am with food; increase to 16 mg q am after 4 weeks. May increase to 24 mg q am after another 4 weeks. Immediate-release: Start 4 mg PO two times per day with food; increase to 8 mg two times per day after 4 weeks. May increase to 12 mg PO two times per day after another 4 weeks.
PEDS — Not approved in children.
UNAPPROVED ADULT — Dementia in Parkinson's disease: 4 to 8 mg PO two times per day (immediate-release).
FORMS — Generic/Trade: Tabs 4, 8, 12 mg. Extended-release caps 8, 16, 24 mg. Oral soln 4 mg/mL. Prior to April 2005 was called Reminyl in the US.
NOTES — Do not exceed 16 mg/day in renal or hepatic impairment. Use caution with CYP3A4 and CYP2D6 inhibitors. Avoid abrupt discontinuation. If therapy

(cont.)

GALANTAMINE (*cont.*)

has been interrupted for several days or more, then restart at the lowest dose.

MOA — Reversible acetylcholinesterase inhibitor.

ADVERSE EFFECTS — Serious: Cholinergic crisis, seizures, bradycardia, syncope, hypotension. Frequent: N/V, diarrhea, anorexia, weight loss, muscle cramps.

RIVASTIGMINE (*Exelon, Exelon Patch*) ►K ♀B ▶? $$$$$

ADULT — Alzheimer's disease: Start 1.5 mg PO two times per day with food. Increase to 3 mg two times per day after 2 weeks. Usual effective dose is 6 to 12 mg/day. Max 12 mg/day. Patch: Start 4.6 mg/24 h once daily; may increase after 1 month or more to recommended dose of 9.5 mg/24 h, max 13.3 mg/24 h. Rotate sites. Dementia in Parkinson's disease: Start 1.5 mg PO two times per day with food. Increase by 3 mg/day at intervals more than 4 weeks to max 12 mg/day. Patch: Use dosing for Alzheimer's disease.

PEDS — Not approved in children.

FORMS — Generic/Trade: Caps 1.5, 3, 4.5, 6 mg. Trade only: Transdermal patch: 4.6 mg/24 h, 9.5 mg/24 h, 13.3 mg/24 h

NOTES — Restart treatment with the lowest daily dose (ie, 1.5 mg PO two times per day) if discontinued for several days to reduce the risk of severe vomiting. When changing from PO to patch, patients taking less than 6 mg/day can be placed on 4.6 mg/24 h patch. For those taking 6 to 12 mg/day, may start with 9.5 mg/24 h patch. Have patient start the day after stopping oral dosing. Rotate application sites and do not apply to same spot for 14 days. Patches have been associated with contact dermatitis.

MOA — Reversible acetylcholinesterase inhibitor.

ADVERSE EFFECTS — Serious: Cholinergic crisis, seizures, bradycardia, syncope, hypotension, respiratory depression. Frequent: N/V, diarrhea, dyspepsia, anorexia, weight loss, muscle cramps, headache, dizziness, asthenia.

NEUROLOGY: Alzheimer's Disease—NMDA Receptor Antagonists

MEMANTINE (*Namenda, Namenda XR, ✳Ebixa*) ►KL ♀B ▶? $$$$$

ADULT — Alzheimer's disease (moderate to severe): Start 5 mg PO daily. Increase by 5 mg/day at weekly intervals to max 20 mg/day. Doses greater than 5 mg/day should be divided two times per day. Extended-release: Start 7 mg once daily. Increase at weekly intervals to target dose of 28 mg/day. Reduce to 14 mg/day in renal impairment.

PEDS — Not approved in children.

FORMS — Trade only: Tabs 5, 10 mg. Oral soln 2 mg/mL. Extended-release caps 7, 14, 21, 28 mg.

NOTES — May be used in combination with acetylcholinesterase inhibitors. Reduce target dose to 5 mg PO two times per day in severe renal impairment (CrCl 5 to 29 mL/min). No dosage adjustment needed for mild–moderate renal impairment. When switching to extended-release caps patients taking 10 mg two times per day can be changed to 28 mg/day of ER after last regular dose. Patients switched from 5 mg two times per day can be changed to 14 mg/day of ER.

MOA — N-methyl-D-aspartate (NMDA) receptor antagonist.

ADVERSE EFFECTS — Serious: None. Frequent: Hypertension, dizziness, headache, constipation, confusion.

NEUROLOGY: Anticonvulsants

NOTE: Avoid rapid discontinuation of anticonvulsants, since this can precipitate seizures or other withdrawal symptoms. Recent data suggest an increased risk of suicidal ideation or behaviors with antiepileptic drugs. Monitor closely for signs of depression, anxiety, hostility, hypomania/mania, or suicidality. Symptoms may develop within 1 week of initiation, and risk continues for at least 24 weeks.

CARBAMAZEPINE (*Tegretol, Tegretol XR, Carbatrol, Epitol, Equetro*) ►LK ♀D ▶+ $$

WARNING — Risk of aplastic anemia, agranulocytosis, and hyponatremia; contraindicated if prior bone marrow depression. Monitor CBC and serum sodium at baseline and periodically.

ADULT — Epilepsy: Start 200 mg PO twice per day. Increase by 200 mg/day at weekly intervals, divided into three or four doses per day (immediate-release), or two times per day (extended-release), or four times per day (susp) to max 1600 mg/day. Trigeminal neuralgia: Start 100 mg PO twice per day or 50 mg PO four times per day (susp); increase by 200 mg/day until pain relief. Max 1200 mg/day. Bipolar disorder, acute manic/mixed episodes (Equetro): Start 200 mg PO two times per day; increase by 200 mg/day to max 1600 mg/day. See "unapproved adult" section for alternative bipolar dosing.

PEDS — Epilepsy, Age 13 yo and above use adult dosing. Age 6-12 yo: Start 100 mg PO twice daily (immediate-release or extended-release) or 1/2 teaspoon (50 mg) suspension four times daily. Increase by 100 mg/day at weekly intervals divided into three or four daily doses (immediate-release tabs or suspension) or two times per day (extended-release). Max 1,000 mg/day. Age younger than 6 yo: Start 10 to 20 mg/kg/day PO divided into two to three doses per day (immediate-release tabs) or four times per day (susp). Increase weekly prn. Max 35 mg/kg/day.

UNAPPROVED ADULT — Neuropathic pain: Start 100 mg PO two times per day; usual effective dose is 200 mg PO two to four times per day. Max 1200 mg/day. Mania (American Psychiatric Association guidelines): Start 200 to 600 mg/day divided into three or four doses per day (standard-release) or

CARBAMAZEPINE (*cont.*)

two times per day (extended-release), then increase by 200 mg/day q 2 to 4 days. Mean effective dose is 1000 mg/day. Max 1600 mg/day.

UNAPPROVED PEDS — Bipolar disorder (manic or mixed phase): Start 100 to 200 mg PO daily or two times per day; titrate to usual effective dose of 200 to 600 mg/day for children and up to 1200 mg/day for adolescents.

FORMS — Generic/Trade: Tabs 200 mg, Chewable tabs 100 mg, Susp 100 mg/5 mL. Extended-release tabs (Tegretol XR) 100, 200, 400 mg. Extended-release caps (Carbatrol): 100, 200, 300 mg. Trade only: Extended-release caps (Equetro): 100, 200, 300 mg.

NOTES — Usual therapeutic level is 4 to 12 mcg/mL. Stevens-Johnson syndrome, hepatitis, aplastic anemia, and hyponatremia may occur. Monitor CBC and LFTs. Many drug interactions. Should not be used for absence or atypical absence seizures. Dangerous and possibly fatal skin reactions are more common with the HLA-B*1502 allele (most common in people of Asian and Indian ancestry); screen new patients for this allele prior to starting therapy. The HLA-A*3101 allele may also be associated with increased risk of cutaneous reactions.

MOA — Anticonvulsant, sodium channel blocker.

ADVERSE EFFECTS — Serious: Aplastic anemia and other blood dyscrasias, hepatotoxicity, SIADH/hyponatremia, rash, Stevens-Johnson syndrome, toxic epidermal necrolysis, hypersensitivity reactions, suicidality, vanishing bile duct syndrome. Frequent: Drowsiness, ataxia, dizziness, confusion, N/V, blurred vision, nystagmus.

CLOBAZAM (***ONFI, ✦FRISIUM***) ▶L ♀C ▶− ©IV $$$$$

WARNING — Use caution in the elderly; may accumulate and cause side effects such as psychomotor impairment.

ADULT — Epilepsy (Lennox-Gastaut syndrome), adjunctive: Weight greater than 30 kg: Start 5 mg PO twice per day. Increase to 10 mg PO twice daily after 1 week then to 20 mg PO twice daily after 2 weeks. Weight 30 kg or less: Start 5 mg PO daily. Increase to 5 mg PO twice per day after 1 week, then 10 mg PO twice per day after 2 weeks. Canada, Epilepsy (Lennox-Gastaut syndrome), adjunctive: Start 5 to 15 mg PO daily. Gradually increase prn to max 80 mg/day.

PEDS — US, Epilepsy (Lennox-Gastaut syndrome), adjunctive. Children 2 yrs and older, weight greater than 30 kg: Start 5 mg PO twice per day. Increase to 10 mg PO twice daily after 1 week then to 20 mg PO twice daily after 2 weeks. Weight 30 kg or less: Start 5 mg PO daily. Increase to 5 mg PO twice per day after 1 week, then 10 mg PO twice per day after 2 weeks. Canada, Epilepsy, adjunctive: Start 0.5 to 1 mg/kg PO daily for age younger than 2 yo or 5 mg daily for age 2 to 16 yo: Then may increase prn to max 40 mg/day.

FORMS — Trade only: Tabs 5, 10, 20 mg. Oral susp 2.5 mg/mL.

NOTES — Reduce dose in hepatic or renal dysfunction. Only use the oral dosing syringe supplied with the suspension.

MOA — Benzodiazepine; potentiates GABA-ergic transmission.

ADVERSE EFFECTS — Serious: Respiratory and CNS depression, tolerance, dependence, suicidality, Stevens-Johnson syndrome, toxic epidermal necrolysis. Frequent: Drowsiness, dizziness, fatigue, orthostatic hypotension.

ESLICARBAZEPINE (***Aptiom***) ▶L ♀C ▶? Enters breast-milk

ADULT — Partial seizures, adjunct: Start: 400 mg PO once daily. Increase after one week to recommended maintenance dose of 800 mg PO once daily. May increase at weekly intervals to max 1200 mg/day. May initiate at 800 mg/day if need for seizure control outweighs increase risk of ADRs. Do not use with oxcabazepine.

PEDS — Not approved for children and adolescents.

FORMS — Trade only: Tabs 200, 400, 600, 800 mg.

NOTES — May reduce efficacy of oral contraceptives. Enzyme inducing or inhibiting drugs may affect serum concentrations. See package insert for dosing recommendations. Reduce dose if creatinine clearance less than 50 mL/min.

MOA — Inhibition of voltage gated sodium channels.

ADVERSE EFFECTS — Serious: Stevens-Johnson syndrome, toxic epidermal necrolysis, drug reaaction with eosinophilia and systemic symptoms (DRESS), hypersensitivity, hyponatremia, cognitive dysfunction, elevated LFTs. Frequent: dizziness, nausea, vomiting, ataxia, diplopia, somnolence, headache, blurred vision, asthenia, fatigue, rash, dysarthria, tremor.

ETHOSUXIMIDE (***Zarontin***) ▶LK ♀C ▶+ $$$$

ADULT — Absence seizures: Start 500 mg PO given once daily or divided twice per day. Increase by 250 mg/day q 4 to 7 days prn. Max 1.5 g/day.

PEDS — Absence seizures: Start 250 mg PO daily or divided two times per day (up to 500 mg/day) for age 3 to 6 yo. Use adult dosing for age older than 6 yo.

UNAPPROVED PEDS — Absence seizures, age younger than 3 yo: Start 15 mg/kg/day PO divided two times per day. Increase q 4 to 7 days prn. Usual effective dose is 15 to 40 mg/kg/day divided two times per day. Max 500 mg/day.

FORMS — Generic/Trade: Caps 250 mg. Syrup 250 mg/5 mL.

NOTES — Usual therapeutic level is 40 to 100 mcg/mL. Monitor CBC for blood dyscrasias. Use caution in hepatic and renal impairment. May increase the risk of grand mal seizures in some patients.

MOA — Increases seizure threshold by reducing current in T-type calcium channels.

ADVERSE EFFECTS — Serious: Blood dyscrasias, hepatotoxicity, Stevens-Johnson syndrome, drug-induced lupus, suicidality, drug reaction with eosinophilia and systemic symptoms (DRESS). Frequent: N/V, anorexia, weight loss, abdominal pain, rash, drowsiness, irritability, headache, fatigue, ataxia, euphoria.

ETHOTOIN (***Peganone***) ▶L ♀C ▶+ $$$$

ADULT — Generalized tonic/clonic or complex partial seizures: Start 1 g or less per day given in 4 to 6 divided doses. Usual effective dose is 2 to 3 g/day.

(cont.)

ETHOTOIN (*cont.*)

PEDS — Generalized tonic/clonic or complex partial seizures: Star 750 mg/day or less in 4 to 6 divided doses. Usual effective dose is 0.5 to 1 g/day. Max 2 to 3 g/day.

FORMS — Trade only: Tabs 250 mg.

NOTES — Usual therapeutic level is 15 to 50 mcg/mL. Doses less than 2 g/day are usually ineffective in adults. Give after food to reduce GI side effects.

MOA — Increases seizure threshold through modulation of sodium and calcium channels.

ADVERSE EFFECTS — Serious: lymphadenopathy, drug-induced lupus, suicidality. Frequent: ataxia, diplopia, dizziness, fatigue, fever, headache, N/V, nystagmus, rash.

EZOGABINE (*POTIGA*) ▶KL - ♀C ▶?

WARNING — Associated with retinal abnormalities with fundoscopic features similar to retinal pigment dystrophies, which can affect visual acuity, and may cause retinal damage and vision loss. Ophthalmic exams should be done every 6 months including visual acuity and dilated fundus photography. Discontinue if pigment abnormalities or visual changes occur unless no other options for seizure control.

ADULT — Partial-onset seizures, adjunctive: Start 100 mg PO three times per day. Increase weekly by no more than 50 mg three times daily to usual maintenance dose of 200-400 mg PO three times daily or max of 250 mg three times daily if older than 65 yrs.

PEDS — Not approved for use in children or adolescents.

FORMS — Trade: Tabs 50, 200, 300, 400 mg.

NOTES — Taper dose over at least 3 weeks when discontinuing. Reduce dose to max of 200 mg three times daily for CrCl less than 50 mL/min or severe hepatic impairment, or 250 mg three times daily for moderate hepatic impairment.

MOA — Enhances transmembrane potassium currents

ADVERSE EFFECTS — Serious: urinary retention, confusion, psychosis, prolonged QT interval, suicidal ideation. Frequent: dizziness, somnolence, fatigue, tremor, diplopia, memory impairment, asthenia, blurred vision.

FELBAMATE (*Felbatol*) ▶KL ♀C ▶- $$$$$

WARNING — Aplastic anemia and fatal hepatic failure have occurred.

ADULT — Severe, refractory epilepsy: Start 400 mg PO three times per day. Increase by 600 mg/day q 2 weeks to max 3600 mg/day.

PEDS — Lennox-Gastaut syndrome, adjunctive therapy, age 2 to 14 yo: Start 15 mg/kg/day PO in 3 to 4 divided doses. Increase by 15 mg/kg/day at weekly intervals to max 45 mg/kg/day.

FORMS — Generic/Trade: Tabs 400, 600 mg. Oral susp 600 mg/5 mL.

NOTES — Not a first-line agent. Use only after discussing the risks and obtaining written informed consent. Many drug interactions.

MOA — Increases seizure threshold by blocking glycine binding to NMDA receptors.

ADVERSE EFFECTS — Serious: Aplastic anemia, hepatotoxicity, liver failure, purpura, maculopapular rash, suicidality. Frequent: Insomnia, headache, anxiety, N/V, diarrhea, constipation, rhinitis.

FOSPHENYTOIN (*Cerebyx*) ▶L ♀D ▶+ $$$$$

ADULT — Status epilepticus: Load 15 to 20 mg "phenytoin equivalents" (PE) per kg IV no faster than 100 to 150 mg PE/min. Nonemergent loading dose: 10 to 20 mg PE/kg IM/IV at rate no greater than 150 mg/min. Maintenance: 4 to 6 mg PE/kg/day.

PEDS — Not approved in children.

UNAPPROVED PEDS — Status epilepticus: 15 to 20 mg PE/kg IV at a rate less than 2 mg PE/kg/min. Nonemergent use age older than 7 yo: 4 to 6 mg PE/kg/24 h IV/IM no faster than 100 to 150 mg PE/min.

NOTES — Fosphenytoin is dosed in "phenytoin equivalents" (PE). Use beyond 5 days has not been systematically studied. Monitor ECG and vital signs continuously during and after infusion. Contraindicated in cardiac conduction block. Many drug interactions. Usual therapeutic level is 10 to 20 mcg/mL in normal hepatorenal function. Renal/hepatic disease may change protein binding and levels. Low albumin levels may increase free fraction.

MOA — Prodrug for phenytoin. Increases seizure threshold by modulating sodium and calcium channels.

ADVERSE EFFECTS — Serious: Cardiovascular collapse, CNS depression, hypotension, arrhythmias, hypersensitivity reactions, drug reaction with eosinophilia syndrome and systemic symptoms (DRESS)/multiorgan hypersensitivity syndrome, Stevens-Johnson syndrome, blood dyscrasias, hepatotoxicity, suicidality. Frequent: Nystagmus, dizziness, pruritus, paresthesia, headache, drowsiness, ataxia.

GABAPENTIN (*Neurontin, Horizant, Gralise*) ▶K ♀C ▶? $$$$

ADULT — Partial seizures, adjunctive therapy: Start 300 mg PO at bedtime. Increase gradually to usual effective dose of 300 to 600 mg PO three times per day. Max 3600 mg/day divided three times per day. Partial seizures, initial monotherapy: Titrate as above. Usual effective dose is 900 to 1800 mg/day. Postherpetic neuralgia, immediate-release tabs: Start 300 mg PO on day 1. Increase to 300 mg twice per day on day 2, and to 300 mg three times per day on day 3. Max 1800 mg/day divided three times per day. Postherpetic neuralgia (Gralise): start 300 mg PO once daily with evening meal. Increase to 600 mg on day 2, 900 mg on days 3 to 6, 1200 mg on days 7 to 10, 1500 mg on days 11 to 14, and 1800 mg on day 15. Max 1800 mg/day. Postherpetic neuralgia (Horizant): Start 600 mg PO q am for 3 days, then increase to 600 mg PO twice per day. Max 1200 mg/day. Restless legs syndrome (Horizant): 600 mg PO once daily around 5 pm taken with food.

PEDS — Partial seizures, adjunctive therapy: Start 10 to 15 mg/kg/day PO divided three times per day for age 3 to 12 yo. Titrate over 3 days to usual effective dose of 25 to 40 mg/kg/day divided three times per day. Max 50 mg/kg/day. Use adult dosing for age older than 12 yo.

(cont.)

GABAPENTIN *(cont.)*

UNAPPROVED ADULT — Neuropathic pain: 300 mg PO three times per day, max 3600 mg/day in 3 to 4 divided doses. Migraine prophylaxis: Start 300 mg PO daily, then gradually increase to 1200 to 2400 mg/day in 3 to 4 divided doses. Restless legs syndrome: Start 300 mg PO at bedtime. Max 3600 mg/day divided three times per day. Hot flashes: 300 mg PO three times per day.

UNAPPROVED PEDS — Neuropathic pain: Start 5 mg/kg PO at bedtime. Increase to 5 mg/kg twice per day on day 2 and 5 mg/kg three times per day on day 3. Titrate to usual effective level of 8 to 35 mg/kg/24 h.

FORMS — Generic only: Tabs 100, 300, 400 mg. Generic/Trade: Caps 100, 300, 400 mg. Tabs, scored 600, 800 mg. Soln 50 mg/mL. Trade only: Tabs, extended-release 600 mg (gabapentin enacarbil, Horizant). Trade only (Gralise): Tabs 300, 600 mg.

NOTES — Reduce dose in renal impairment (CrCl less than 60 mL/min); table in prescribing information. Discontinue gradually over 1 week or longer. Do not substitute other brands for Gralise because of bioavailability differences.

MOA — Unknown. Does not appear to be a GABA analog.

ADVERSE EFFECTS — Serious: Leukopenia, rhabdomyolysis. Frequent: Fatigue, drowsiness, dizziness, ataxia, nystagmus, tremor, peripheral edema, weight gain, suicidality. Peds only: Emotional lability, hostility, hyperactivity.

LACOSAMIDE (*Vimpat*) ▶KL ♀C ▶? $$$$$

ADULT — Partial onset seizures, adjunctive (17 yo and older): Start 50 mg PO/IV twice per day. Increase by 50 mg twice per day to recommended dose of 100 to 200 mg twice per day. Max 600 mg/day (max 300 mg/day in mild/mod hepatic failure or severe renal impairment with CrCl < 30 mL/min).

PEDS — Not approved in children.

FORMS — Trade only: Tabs 50, 100, 150, 200 mg.

NOTES — Use caution in patients with cardiac conduction problems or taking drugs that increase the PR interval.

MOA — Enhances slow inactivation of voltage-gated sodium channels.

ADVERSE EFFECTS — Severe: Increased PR interval, AV block, suicidality, syncope, agranulocytosis. Frequent: Dizziness, ataxia, nausea/vomiting, diplopia, vertigo, blurred vision, headache.

LAMOTRIGINE (*Lamictal, Lamictal CD, Lamictal ODT, Lamictal XR*) ▶LK ♀C (see notes) ▶- $$$$

WARNING — Potentially life-threatening rashes (e.g., Stevens-Johnson syndrome) have been reported in 0.3% of adults and 0.8% of children, usually within 2 to 8 weeks of initiation; discontinue at first sign of rash. Drug interaction with valproate; see adjusted dosing guidelines. Life-threatening drug reaction with eosinophilia and systemic symptoms (DRESS) has been reported.

ADULT — Partial seizures, Lennox-Gastaut syndrome, or generalized tonic-clonic seizures, adjunctive therapy with an enzyme-inducing anticonvulsant (age older than 12 yo): Immediate-release: Start 50 mg PO daily for 2 weeks, then 50 mg PO twice per day for 2 weeks. Increase by 100 mg/day q 1 to 2 weeks to usual maintenance dose of 150 to 250 mg PO twice per day. Extended-release: Start 50 mg PO daily for weeks 1-2, then increase to 100 mg PO daily for weeks 3-4. Then increase by 100 mg/day at weekly intervals to target dose of 400-600 mg/day. Partial seizures, conversion to monotherapy from adjunctive therapy with a single enzyme-inducing anticonvulsant (immediate-release) (age 16 yo and older): Use above guidelines to gradually increase the dose to 250 mg PO twice per day; then taper the enzyme-inducing anticonvulsant by 20% per week over 4 weeks. Extended-release: Achieve dose of 500 mg/day then begin to reduce the enzyme-inducing AED by 20% decrements weekly over a 4 week period. Two weeks after the enzyme-inducing AED is discontinued Lamictal XR can be decreased no faster than 100 mg/day each week to the target dose of 250-350 mg/day. Partial seizures, Lennox-Gastaut syndrome, or generalized tonic-clonic seizures, adjunctive therapy with valproate (age older than 12 yo): Start 25 mg PO every other day for 2 weeks, then 25 mg PO daily for 2 weeks. Increase by 25 to 50 mg/day q 1 to 2 weeks to usual maintenance dose of 100 to 400 mg/day (when used with valproate + other anticonvulsants) or 100 to 200 mg/day (when used with valproate alone) given once daily or divided twice per day. Extended-release: Start 25 mg PO every other day for weeks 1-2, then increase to 25 mg/day for weeks 3-4. Then increase to 50 mg/day on week five and increase weekly by 50 mg/day to target dose of 200-250 mg/day. Partial seizures, conversion to monotherapy from adjunctive therapy with valproate (immediate-release) (age 16 yo and older): Use above guidelines to gradually increase the dose to 200 mg/day PO given daily or divided twice per day; then decrease valproate weekly in increments less than or equal to 500 mg/day to an initial goal of 500 mg/day. After 1 week at these doses, increase lamotrigine to 300 mg/day and decrease valproate to 250 mg/day divided twice per day. A week later, discontinue valproate; then increase lamotrigine weekly by 100 mg/day to usual maintenance dose of 500 mg/day. Extended-release: Achieve a dose of 150 mg/day of Lamictal XR and maintain valproate dose. Then decrease valproate by nor more than 500 mg/day/week to 500 mg/day and maintain for one week. Then increase lamictal XR to 200 mg/day at the same time as decreasing valproate to 250 mg/day for one week. then increase Lamictal XR to 250-300 mg/day while discontinuing valproate. Partial seizures, conversion to monotherapy from other AEDs (not valproate or enzyme-inducers, Extended-release): Achieve a dose of 250-300 mg/day of Lamictal XR then begin to withdraw the other AED by 20% decrements weekly over a 4-week period. Partial seizures, Lennox-Gastaut syndrome, or generalized tonic-clonic seizures, adjunctive therapy with other anticonvulsants (not valproate or enzyme inducers) (age older than 12 yo): Start 25 mg PO daily for 2 weeks, the 50 mg PO daily for 2

LAMOTRIGINE (*cont.*)

weeks. Increase by 50 mg/day q 1 to 2 weeks to usual maintenance dose of 225 to 375 mg/day divided twice per day. Extended-release: Start 25 mg PO daily for weeks 1-2, then increase to 50 mg/day for weeks 3-4. Increase to 100 mg/day on week then then increase weekly by 50 mg/day to target dose of 300-400 mg/day. See psychiatry section for bipolar disorder dosing.

PEDS — Partial seizures, Lennox-Gastaut syndrome or generalized tonic-clonic seizures, adjunctive therapy with an enzyme-inducing anticonvulsant, age 2 to 12 yo: Start 0.6 mg/kg/day PO divided twice per day for 2 weeks, then 1.2 mg/kg/day PO divided twice per day for 2 weeks. Increase q 1 to 2 weeks by 1.2 mg/kg/day (rounded down to the nearest whole tab) to usual maintenance dose of 5 to 15 mg/kg/day. Max 400 mg/day. Partial seizures, Lennox-Gastaut syndrome, or generalized tonic-clonic seizures, adjunctive therapy with valproate, age 2 to 12 yo: Start 0.15 mg/kg/day PO (given daily or divided twice per day) for 2 weeks, then 0.3 mg/kg/day PO (given daily or divided twice per day) for 2 weeks. Increase q 1 to 2 weeks by 0.3 mg/kg/day (rounded down to nearest whole tab) to usual maintenance dose of 1 to 5 mg/kg/day (lamotrigine + valproate and other anticonvulsants) or 1 to 3 mg/kg/day if used with valproate alone. Max 200 mg/day. Partial seizures, Lennox-Gastaut syndrome, or generalized tonic-clonic seizures, adjunctive therapy with other anticonvulsants (not valproate or enzyme inducers), age 2 to 12 yo: Start 0.3 mg/kg/day (given daily or divided twice per day) for 2 weeks, then 0.6 mg/kg/day for 2 weeks. Increase q 1 to 2 weeks by 0.6 mg/kg/day (rounded down to nearest whole tab) to usual maintenance dose of 4.5 to 7.5 mg/kg/day. Max 300 mg/day. Age older than 12 yo: Use adult dosing for all of the above indications including for Lamictal XR.

UNAPPROVED ADULT — Initial monotherapy for partial seizures: Start 25 mg PO daily. Usual maintenance dose is 100 to 300 mg/day divided twice per day. Max 500 mg/day.

UNAPPROVED PEDS — Initial monotherapy for partial seizures: Start 0.5 mg/kg/day given daily or divided twice per day. Max 10 mg/kg/day. Newly diagnosed absence seizures: Titrate as above. Usual effective dose is 2 to 15 mg/kg/day.

FORMS — Generic/Trade: Tabs, 25, 100, 150, 200 mg. Chewable dispersible tabs (Lamictal CD) 5, 25 mg. Extended release tabs (Lamictal XR) 25, 50, 100, 200, 250, 300 mg. Trade only: Orally disintegrating tabs (Lamictal ODT) 25, 50, 100, 200 mg. Trade only: Chewable dispersible tabs 2 mg (Lamictal CD) may not be available in all pharmacies; obtain through manufacturer representative, or by calling 888-825-5249.

NOTES — Drug interactions with valproate and enzyme-inducing antiepileptic drugs (i.e., carbamazepine, phenobarbital, phenytoin, primidone); may need to adjust dose. May increase carbamazepine toxicity. Women taking estrogen-containing oral contraceptives without an enzyme-inducing anticonvulsant will generally require an increase of the lamotrigine maintenance dose by up to 2-fold. Consider increasing the lamotrigine dose when the contraceptive is started. Taper lamotrigine by 25% or less of daily dose q week over a 2-week period if the contraceptive is stopped. Preliminary evidence suggests that exposure during the first trimester of pregnancy is associated with a risk of cleft palate and/or cleft lip.

MOA — Blocks sodium channels and inhibits the release of glutamate.

ADVERSE EFFECTS — Serious: Stevens-Johnson syndrome, toxic epidermal necrolysis, hypersensitivity reactions, drug reaction with eosinophilia and systemic symptoms (DRESS), blood dyscrasias, multiorgan failure, suicidality, aseptic meningitis. Frequent: Rash, dizziness, diplopia, ataxia, drowsiness, headache, blurred vision, N/V, somnolence, insomnia.

LEVETIRACETAM (*Keppra, Keppra XR*) ▸K ♀C ▶? $$$

ADULT — Partial seizures, juvenile myoclonic epilepsy (JME), or primary generalized tonic-clonic seizures (GTC), adjunctive therapy: Start 500 mg PO/IV twice per day (Keppra, IV route not approved for GTC) or 1000 mg PO daily (Keppra XR, partial seizures only); increase by 1000 mg/day q 2 weeks prn to max 3000 mg/day (partial seizures) or to target dose of 3000 mg/day (JME or GTC).

PEDS — Partial seizures, adjunctive therapy for age older than 4 yo: Start 20 mg/kg/day PO (or IV if 16 yo or older) divided twice per day. Increase q 2 weeks as tolerated to target dose of 60 mg/kg/day. Juvenile myoclonic epilepsy, adjunctive therapy, age 12 yo or older: See adult dosing (IV approved for 16 yo or older only). Primary generalized tonic-clonic seizures (GTC), adjunctive therapy, age 6 to 15 yo: Start 20 mg/kg/day PO (or IV if 16 yo or older) divided twice per day. Increase by 20 mg/kg/day q 2 weeks to target dose of 60 mg/kg/day.

UNAPPROVED ADULT — Myoclonus: Start 500 to 1000 mg/day in divided doses. May increase to max 1500 to 3000 mg/day or 50 mg/kg/day.

FORMS — Generic/Trade: Tabs 250, 500, 750, 1000 mg. Oral soln 100 mg/mL. Tabs, extended-release 500, 750 mg.

NOTES — Drug interactions unlikely. Decrease dose in renal dysfunction (CrCl < 80 mL/min). Emotional lability, hostility, and depression may occur. Use same dose when switching between IV and PO forms.

MOA — Unknown but may involve opposition of negative modulators of GABA and glycine-gated currents and inhibition of N-type calcium currents.

ADVERSE EFFECTS — Serious: Pancytopenia, pancreatitis, psychosis, depression, panic attacks, suicidality. Frequent: Drowsiness, dizziness, fatigue, asthenia, nervousness, emotional lability, hostility, ataxia.

METHSUXIMIDE (*Celontin*) ▸L ♀C ▶? $$$

ADULT — Refractory absence seizures: Start 300 mg PO daily; increase weekly by 300 mg/day. Max 1200 mg/day.

PEDS — Refractory absence seizures: Start 10 to 15 mg/kg/day PO in 3 to 4 divided doses; increase weekly prn. Max 30 mg/kg/day.

FORMS — Trade only: Caps 150, 300 mg.

NOTES — Monitor CBC, UA, and LFTs.

METHSUXIMIDE (cont.)

MOA — Inhibits low threshold calcium (T) currents.
ADVERSE EFFECTS — Serious: pancytopenia and other blood dyscrasias, drug-induced lupus, Stevens-Johnson syndrome, suicidality. Frequent: N/V, weight loss, anorexia, constipation, drowsiness, ataxia, dizziness.

OXCARBAZEPINE (Trileptal, Oxtellar XR) ▶LK ♀C ▶– $$$$$

WARNING — Serious multiorgan hypersensitivity reactions and life-threatening rashes (e.g., Stevens-Johnson syndrome, toxic epidermal necrolysis) have occurred, with some fatalities. Consider discontinuation if skin reactions occur.
ADULT — Partial seizures, monotherapy: Start 300 mg PO two times per day. Increase by 300 mg/day q 3 day to usual effective dose of 1200 mg/day. Max 2400 mg/day. Partial seizures, adjunctive: Immediate-release: Start 300 mg PO two times per day. Increase by no more than 600 mg/day at weekly intervals to usual effective dose of 1200 mg/day. Max 2400 mg/day. Extended-release, adjunctive: Start 600 mg PO daily. Increase by 600 mg/day weekly if needed, max 2400 mg/day.
PEDS — Partial seizures, adjunctive, age 2 to 16 yo: Start 8 to 10 mg/kg/day PO divided two times per day (max starting dose 600 mg/day). Titrate to max 60 mg/kg/day for age 2 to less than 4 yo, titrate to max 900 mg/day for wt 20 to 29 kg, titrate to max 1200 mg/day for wt 29.1 to 39 kg, titrate to max 1800 mg/day for wt greater than 39 kg. Consider using a starting dose of 16 to 20 mg/kg for children age 2 to younger than 4 yo who weigh less than 20 kg to account for more rapid clearance. Extended-release (adjunctive for 6 to 17 yo): Start 8 mg/kg to 10 mg/kg PO once daily not to exceed 600 mg/day. May increase weekly by 8 mg/kg to 10 mg/kg once daily if needed to max based on wt of 900 mg/day (20-29 kg), 1200 mg/day (29.1-39 kg), or 1800 mg/day (greater than 39 kg). Partial seizures, initial monotherapy, age 4 to 16 yo: Start 8 to 10 mg/kg/day divided two times per day. Increase by 5 mg/kg/day q 3 days to recommended dose (in mg/day based on wt rounded to nearest 5 kg) as follows: 600 to 900 for wt 20 kg, 900 to 1200 for wt 25 and 30 kg, 900 to 1500 for wt 35 and 40 kg, 1200 to 1500 for wt 45 kg, 1200 to 1800 for wt 50 and 55 kg, 1200 to 2100 for wt 60 and 65 kg, 1500 to 2100 for wt 70 kg. Partial seizures, conversion to monotherapy, age 4 to 16 yo: Start 8 to 10 mg/kg/day divided two times per day. Increase at weekly intervals by no more than 10 mg/kg/day to target dose listed for initial monotherapy.
FORMS — Generic/Trade: Tabs (scored) 150, 300, 600 mg. Oral susp 300 mg/5 mL. Trade only: Extended-release tabs (Oxtellar XR) 150, 300, 600mg
NOTES — Monitor serum sodium. Decrease initial dose by ½ in renal dysfunction (CrCl less than 30 mL/min). Inhibits CYP2C19 and induces CYP3A4/5. Interactions with other antiepileptic drugs, oral contraceptives, and dihydropyridine calcium channel blockers.
MOA — Unknown. May inhibit sodium channels, increase potassium conductance, and modulate calcium channels.

ADVERSE EFFECTS — Serious: Stevens-Johnson syndrome, toxic epidermal necrolysis, hyponatremia/SIADH, bone marrow depression, leukopenia, agranulocytosis, aplastic anemia, angioedema, suicidality. Frequent: Dizziness, drowsiness, fatigue, headache, ataxia, diplopia, nystagmus, gait disturbance, tremor, N/V, abdominal pain.

PERAMPANEL (Fycompa, ✦Fycompa) ▶L ♀C ▶? ©III

ADULT — Partial seizures with or without secondary generalization, without enzyme inducing drugs: Start 2 mg PO once daily at bedtime. increase weekly by 2 mg/day to usual range of 8-12 mg/day. Max 12 mg/day. With enzyme inducing drugs: Start 4 mg PO once daily at bedtime. Increase weekly to usual range of 8-12 mg/day. Max 12 mg/day.
PEDS — Ages 12-17 years old: use adult dosing.
FORMS — Tabs: 2, 4, 6, 8, 10, 12 mg.
NOTES — May reduce efficacy of levonorgestrel-containing oral contraceptives. Avoid with strong CYP3A inducers.
MOA — Non-competitive antagonist of the AMPA glutamate receptor on postsynaptic neurons.
ADVERSE EFFECTS — Severe: Suicidal thoughts and behavior, aggression, hostility, anger, homicidal ideation/threats. Frequent: Dizziness, gait disturbances, falls, somnolence, blurred vision, ataxia, weight gain.

PHENOBARBITAL (Luminal) ▶L ♀D ▶– ©IV $

ADULT — Epilepsy: 100 to 300 mg/day PO divided one to two times per day. Status epilepticus: 20 mg/kg IV at rate no faster than 60 mg/min.
PEDS — Epilepsy: 3 to 5 mg/kg/day PO divided two to three times per day. Status epilepticus: 20 mg/kg IV at rate no faster than 60 mg/min.
UNAPPROVED ADULT — Status epilepticus: May give up to a total dose of 30 mg/kg IV.
UNAPPROVED PEDS — Status epilepticus: 15 to 20 mg/kg IV load; may give additional 5 mg/kg doses q 15 to 30 mins to max total dose of 30 mg/kg. Epilepsy: Give 3 to 5 mg/kg/day given once daily or divided two times per day for neonates, give 5 to 6 mg/kg/day once daily or divided two times per day for infants, give 6 to 8 mg/kg/day given once daily or divided two times per day for age 1 to 5 yo, give 4 to 6 mg/kg/day once daily or divided two times per day for age 6 to 12 yo, give 1 to 3 mg/kg/day once daily or divided two times per day for age older than 12 yo.
FORMS — Generic only: Tabs 15, 16.2, 30, 32.4, 60, 100 mg. Elixir 20 mg/5 mL.
NOTES — Usual therapeutic level is 15 to 40 mcg/mL. Monitor cardiopulmonary function closely when administering IV. Decrease dose in renal or hepatic dysfunction. Many drug interactions.
MOA — Nonselective CNS depressant.
ADVERSE EFFECTS — Serious: Respiratory and CNS depression, blood dyscrasias, anemia, thrombocytopenia, Stevens-Johnson syndrome, angioedema, suicidality. Frequent: Drowsiness, fatigue, N/V, bradycardia, ataxia, nystagmus, dizziness, cognitive symptoms, paradoxical CNS excitation.

PHENYTOIN (*Dilantin, Phenytek*) ▶L ♀D ▶+ $$

ADULT — Status epilepticus: 15 to 20 mg/kg IV at rate no faster than 50 mg/min, then 100 mg IV/PO q 6 to 8 h. Epilepsy, oral loading dose: 400 mg PO initially, then 300 mg in 2 h and 4 h. Epilepsy, maintenance dose: 300 mg/day PO given once daily (extended release) or divided three times per day (susp and chew tabs) and titrated to a therapeutic level.

PEDS — Epilepsy, age older than 6 yo: 5 mg/kg/day PO divided two to three times per day, to max 300 mg/day. Status epilepticus: 15 to 20 mg/kg IV at a rate no faster than 1 mg/kg/min.

FORMS — Generic/Trade: Extended-release caps 100 mg (Dilantin). Susp 125 mg/5 mL. Extended-release caps 200, 300 mg (Phenytek). Chewable tabs 50 mg (Dilantin Infatabs). Trade only: Extended-release caps 30 mg (Dilantin)

NOTES — Usual therapeutic level is 10 to 20 mcg/mL. Limit dose increases to 10% or less due to saturable metabolism. Monitor ECG and vital signs when administering IV. Many drug interactions. Monitor serum levels closely when switching between forms (free acid vs. sodium salt). The free fraction may be increased in patients with low albumin levels. IV loading doses of 15 to 20 mg/kg have also been recommended. May need to reduce loading dose if patient is already on phenytoin. Avoid in patients known to be positive for HLA-B*1502 due to possible increased risk of Stevens-Johnson syndrome.

MOA — Increases seizure threshold through modulation of sodium and calcium channels.

ADVERSE EFFECTS — Serious: Arrhythmias, blood dyscrasias, Stevens-Johnson syndrome, toxic epidermal necrolysis, hypotension, cardiovascular collapse, thrombocytopenia, anemia, hypersensitivity, local skin necrosis (IV only), suicidality. Frequent: Rash, nystagmus, tremor, ataxia, dizziness, vertigo, sedation, lymphadenopathy. Frequent (chronic use): gingival hyperplasia, osteomalacia, coarse facies.

PREGABALIN (*Lyrica*) ▶K ♀C ▶? ©V $$$$$

ADULT — Painful diabetic peripheral neuropathy: Start 50 mg PO three times per day; may increase within 1 week to max 100 mg PO three times per day. Postherpetic neuralgia: Start 150 mg/day PO divided two to three times per day; may increase within 1 week to 300 mg/day divided two to three times per day; max 600 mg/day. Partial seizures (adjunctive): Start 150 mg/day PO divided two to three times per day; may increase prn to max 600 mg/day divided two to three times per day. Fibromyalgia: Start 75 mg PO two times per day; may increase to 150 mg two times per day within 1 week; max 225 mg two times per day. Neuropathic pain associated with spinal cord injury: Start 75 mg PO two times per day; may increase to 150 mg two times per day within 1 week and then to 300 mg two times per day after 2-3 weeks if tolerated.

PEDS — Not approved in children.

FORMS — Trade only: Caps 25, 50, 75, 100, 150, 200, 225, 300 mg. Oral soln 20 mg/mL (480 mL).

NOTES — Adjust dose if CrCl less than 60 mL/min; refer to prescribing information. Warn patients to report changes in visual acuity and muscle pain. May increase creatine kinase. Must taper if discontinuing to avoid withdrawal symptoms. Increased risk of peripheral edema when used in conjunction with thiazolidinedione antidiabetic agents.

MOA — Unknown. Binds to alpha-2-delta subunit of voltage-gated calcium channels and reduces neurotransmitter release.

ADVERSE EFFECTS — Serious: Visual field changes, reduced visual acuity, thrombocytopenia, suicidality. Frequent: Dizziness, somnolence, dry mouth, decreased concentration/attention, blurred vision, peripheral edema, weight gain, ataxia, withdrawal reactions.

PRIMIDONE (*Mysoline*) ▶LK ♀D ▶– $$$$

ADULT — Epilepsy: Start 100 to 125 mg PO at bedtime. Increase over 10 days to usual maintenance dose of 250 mg PO three to four time per day. Max 2 g/day.

PEDS — Epilepsy, age younger than 8 yo: Start 50 mg PO at bedtime. Increase over 10 days to usual maintenance dose of 125 to 250 mg PO three times per day or 10 to 25 mg/kg/day.

UNAPPROVED ADULT — Essential tremor: Start 12.5 to 25 mg PO at bedtime. May increase weekly prn by 50 mg/day to 250 mg/day given once daily or in divided doses. Max 750 mg/day.

FORMS — Generic/Trade: Tabs 50, 250 mg.

NOTES — Usual therapeutic level is 5 to 12 mcg/mL. Metabolized to phenobarbital.

MOA — Converted to phenobarbital and PEMA. Nonselective CNS depressant.

ADVERSE EFFECTS — Serious: Respiratory and CNS depression, anemia, thrombocytopenia, suicidality. Frequent: Drowsiness, ataxia, vertigo, lethargy, irritability, emotional lability, nystagmus, rash, N/V, paradoxical CNS excitation.

RUFINAMIDE (*Banzel*) ▶K ♀C ▶? $$$$$

ADULT — Epilepsy, Lennox-Gastaut syndrome (adjunctive): Start 400 to 800 mg/day PO divided two times per day. Increase by 400 to 800 mg/day q 2 days to max 3200 mg/day divided two times per day.

PEDS — Epilepsy, Lennox-Gastaut syndrome (adjunctive) age 4 yo or older: Start 10 mg/kg/day PO given two times per day. Increase by 10 mg/kg every other day to target of 45 mg/kg/day or 3200 mg/day divided two times per day.

FORMS — Trade only: Tabs 200, 400 mg. Susp 40 mg/mL.

NOTES — Give with food. Use caution for patients with mild to moderate hepatic impairment and avoid in severe hepatic impairment and short QT syndrome.

MOA — Modulates activity of sodium channels.

ADVERSE EFFECTS — Serious: Suicidality, multiorgan hypersensitivity. Frequent: Headache, dizziness, fatigue, somnolence, nausea.

TIAGABINE (*Gabitril*) ▶L ♀C ▶? $$$$$

WARNING — New onset-seizures and status epilepticus may occur when used in patients without epilepsy, particularly when combined with other medications that lower the seizure threshold. Avoid off-label use.

ADULT — Partial seizures, adjunctive therapy with an enzyme-inducing anticonvulsant: Start 4 mg PO

TIAGABINE (*cont.*)

daily. Increase by 4 to 8 mg/day prn at weekly intervals to max 56 mg/day divided two to four times per day.

PEDS — Partial seizures, adjunctive therapy with an enzyme-inducing anticonvulsant (age 12 to 18 yo): Start 4 mg PO daily. Increase by 4 mg/day prn q 1 to 2 weeks to max 32 mg/day divided two to four times per day.

FORMS — Trade only: Tabs 2, 4, 12, 16 mg.

NOTES — Take with food. Dosing is for patients on enzyme-inducing anticonvulsants such as carbamazepine, phenobarbital, phenytoin, or primidone. Reduce dosage in patients who are not taking enzyme-inducing medications, and in those with liver dysfunction.

MOA — Inhibits presynaptic reuptake of GABA.

ADVERSE EFFECTS — Serious: Stevens-Johnson syndrome, generalized weakness, status epilepticus (with overdose); new onset seizures or status epilepticus (with off-label use), suicidality. Frequent: Dizziness, lightheadedness, asthenia, sedation, tremor, confusion, ataxia, nervousness, depression, decreased concentration, N/V, diarrhea.

TOPIRAMATE (*Qudexy XR, Topamax, Trokendi XR*) ▶K ♀D ▶? $$$$$

ADULT — Partial seizures or primary generalized tonic-clonic seizures, monotherapy (standard tablets): Start 25 mg PO two times per day (week 1), 50 mg two times per day (week 2), 75 mg two times per day (week 3), 100 mg two times per day (week 4), 150 mg two times per day (week 5), then 200 mg two times per day as tolerated. Extended release (Trokendi XR and Quedexy XR: Start 50 mg PO daily. Increase weekly by 50 mg/day for 4 weeks then by 100 mg/day for weeks 5 and 6 to recommended dose of 400 mg oce daily. Partial seizures, primary generalized tonic-clonic seizures, or Lennox-Gastaut syndrome, adjunctive therapy: Start 25 to 50 mg PO at bedtime. Increase weekly by 25 to 50 mg each day to usual effective dose of 100-200 mg PO two times per day (partial seizures and LGS) or 200 mg PO two times per day (generalized tonic-clonic seizures). Doses greater than 400 mg per day not shown to be more effective. Extended-release (Trokendi XR and Quedexy XR): Start 25-50 mg PO once daily. Increase weekly by 25 to 50 mg/day to effective dose. Recommended dose 200-400 mg/day for partial seizures or Lennox-Gastaut syndrome or 400 mg/day for generalized tonic-clonic seizures. Migraine prophylaxis: Start 25 mg PO at bedtime (week 1), then 25 mg two times per day (week 2), then 25 mg q am and 50 mg q pm (week 3), then 50 mg two times per day (week 4 and thereafter).

PEDS — Partial seizures or primary generalized tonic-clonic seizures, monotherapy age older than 10 yo: Use adult dosing. Ages 2 to less than 10 yrs: Start 25 mg PO nightly (week 1), 25 mg two times daily (week 2), then increase by 25 to 50 mg/day weekly as tolerated to maintenance range based on weight of 75 to 125 mg twice daily (weight up to 11 kg), 100 to 150 mg twice daily (12 to 22 kg), 100 to 175 mg twice

daily (23 to 31 kg), 125-175 mg twice daily (32 to 38 kg), or 125 to 200 mg twice daily (greater than 38 kg). Extended-release (Trokendi XR and Quedexy XR) ages 10 years and older: Use adult dosing. Partial seizures, primary generalized tonic-clonic seizures, or Lennox-Gastaut syndrome, adjunctive therapy age 2 to 16 yo: Start 1 to 3 mg/kg (max 25 mg) PO at bedtime. Increase by 1 to 3 mg/kg/day q 1 to 2 weeks to usual effective dose of 5 to 9 mg/kg/day divided twice a day. Extended-release (Trokendi XR for 6 years and older) or (Quedexy XR for 2 years and older): Start 25 mg PO once daily at night for one week (or 1 mg/kg to 3 mg/kg once nightly). Increase at 1 to 2 week intervals by increments of 1 mg/kg to 3 mg/kg daily to recommended dose of 5 mg/kg to 9 mg/kg given once daily. Migraine prophylaxis (adolescents 12 yo and older: Use adult dosing.

UNAPPROVED ADULT — Essential tremor: Start 25 mg PO daily. Increase by 25 mg/day at weekly intervals to 100 mg/day; max 400 mg/day. Bipolar disorder: Start 25 to 50 mg PO daily. Titrate prn to max 400 mg/day. Alcohol dependence: Start 25 mg PO q day; increase by 25 mg/day at weekly intervals as tolerated to 300 mg/day for up to 14 weeks total.

FORMS — Generic/Trade: Tabs 25, 50, 100, 200 mg. Sprinkle caps 15, 25 mg. Trade only: Extended-release caps (Trokendi XR and Qudexy XR) 25, 50, 100, 200 mg and (Qudexy XR) 150 mg.

NOTES — Give ½ usual adult dose in renal impairment (CrCl less than 70 mL/min). Confusion, nephrolithiasis, glaucoma, and wt loss may occur. Risk of oligohidrosis and hyperthermia, particularly in children; use caution in warm ambient temperatures and/or with vigorous physical activity. Hyperchloremic, non-anion gap metabolic acidosis may occur; monitor serum bicarbonate and either reduce dose or taper off entirely if this occurs. Max dose tested was 1600 mg/day. Use during pregnancy associated with cleft palate/lip. Report fetal exposure to North American Antiepileptic Drug Pregnancy Registry (888-233-2334). May increase the risk of hyperammonemia if used with valproic acid.

MOA — Unknown. May modulate sodium channels and enhance GABA action.

ADVERSE EFFECTS — Serious: Acute angle-closure glaucoma, visual field defects, nephrolithiasis, oligohidrosis, hyperthermia, metabolic acidosis, suicidality, hyperammonemia. Frequent: Somnolence, fatigue, ataxia, psychomotor slowing, cognitive symptoms, confusion, diplopia, nystagmus, dizziness, depression, nervousness, weight loss, paresthesia.

VALPROIC ACID (*Depakene, Depakote, Depakote ER, Depacon, Stavzor*, divalproex, sodium valproate, *✲Epival, Deproic*) ▶L ♀D ▶+ $$$$

WARNING — Fatal hepatic failure has occurred; monitor LFTs during first 6 months of treatment. Should not be used in children under 2 yo. Life-threatening pancreatitis has been reported after initial or prolonged use. Evaluate for abdominal pain, N/V, and/or anorexia. Discontinue if pancreatitis occurs. May be more teratogenic than other anticonvulsants

(cont.)

VALPROIC ACID (cont.)

(eg, carbamazepine, lamotrigine, and phenytoin). Hepatic failure and clotting disorders have occurred when used during pregnancy. Life-threatening pancreatitis has been reported.

ADULT — Epilepsy: 10 to 15 mg/kg/day (for absence seizures start 15 mg/kg/day) PO or IV infusion over 60 min (rate no faster than 20 mg/min) divided two to four times per day (standard-release, delayed-release, or IV) or given once daily (Depakote ER). Increase dose by 5 to 10 mg/kg/day at weekly intervals to max 60 mg/kg/day. Migraine prophylaxis: Start 250 mg PO two times per day (Depakote or Stavzor) or 500 mg PO daily (Depakote ER) for 1 week, then increase to max 1000 mg/day PO divided two times per day (Depakote or Stavzor) or given once daily (Depakote ER). Simple and complex absence seizures: Start 15 mg/kg/day and increase as needed by 5-10 mg/kg/day to max dose 60 mg/kg/day. Doses above 250 mg/day should be divided in two to three doses.

PEDS — Seizures, age older than 2 yo: 10 to 15 mg/kg/day PO or IV infusion over 60 min (rate no faster than 20 mg/min). Increase dose by 5 to 10 mg/kg/day at weekly intervals to max 60 mg/kg/day. Divide doses greater than 250 mg/day into two to four times per day; may give once daily (Depakote ER) if age older than 10 yo. Complex partial seizures: Stavzor can be used for ages 10 yo or older. Use adult dosing. Simple and complex absence seizures (ages 10 yo and older):Start 15 mg/kg/day and increase as needed by 5-10 mg/kg/day to max dose 60 mg/kg/day. Doses above 250 mg/day should be divided in two to three doses.

UNAPPROVED ADULT — Status epilepticus (not first line): Load 20 to 40 mg/kg IV (rate no faster than 6 mg/kg/min), then continue 4 to 8 mg/kg IV three times per day to achieve therapeutic level. May use lower loading dose if already on valproate.

UNAPPROVED PEDS — Status epilepticus, age older than 2 yo (not first line): Load 20 to 40 mg/kg IV over 1 to 5 min, then 5 mg/kg/h adjusted to achieve therapeutic level. May use lower loading dose if already on valproate.

FORMS — Generic/Trade: Immediate-release caps 250 mg (Depakene), syrup (Depakene, valproic acid) 250 mg/5 mL. Delayed-release tabs (Depakote) 125, 250, 500 mg. Extended-release tabs (Depakote ER) 250, 500 mg. Delayed-release sprinkle caps (Depakote) 125 mg. Trade only (Stavzor): Delayed-release caps 125, 250, 500 mg.

NOTES — Contraindicated in urea cycle disorders or hepatic dysfunction. Usual therapeutic trough level is 50 to 100 mcg/mL. Depakote and Depakote ER are not interchangeable. Depakote ER is approximately 10% less bioavailable than Depakote. Depakote-releases divalproex sodium over 8 to 12 h (daily to four times per day dosing); Depakote ER-releases divalproex sodium over 18 to 24 h (daily dosing). Many drug interactions. Patients receiving other anticonvulsants may require higher doses of valproic acid. Reduce dose in the elderly. Hyperammonemia, GI irritation, or thrombocytopenia may occur. Concurrent use of topiramate may increase risk of hyperammonemia. Contraindicated for migraine prophylaxis in pregnant women. Contraindicated in patients with genetic mutations in mitochondrial DNA polymerase gamma.

MOA — May increase GABA levels and modulate sodium channels.

ADVERSE EFFECTS — Serious: Hepatotoxicity, anaphylaxis, polycystic ovarian syndrome, bone marrow suppression, thrombocytopenia, pancreatitis, SIADH, Stevens-Johnson syndrome, hyperammonemia, suicidality. Frequent: N/V, diarrhea, weight gain, CNS depression, drowsiness, tremor, alopecia, rash, nystagmus, asthenia.

VIGABATRIN (Sabril) ▶K ♀C ▶− $$$$$

WARNING — Ophthalmologic abnormalities including permanent vision constriction and loss have been reported. Visual field testing should be performed prior to treatment and q 3 months thereafter. Continue testing for 3-6 months after drug is discontinued. Once visual loss occurs, it is not reversible. Given the limitations of visual field testing in children younger than 9 yo, vigabatrin should be used in this age group only if clearly indicated. Do not use with other retinotoxic drugs.

ADULT — Refractory complex partial seizures (adjunctive treatment): Start: 500 mg PO twice daily. May increase in 500 mg increments weekly to usual recommended dose of 1500 mg twice daily.

PEDS — Refractory complex partial seizures (adjunctive treatment 10-16 yrs old): Start: 250 mg PO twice daily. May increase weekly to maintenance dose of 1000 mg PO twice daily. Patients > 60 kg should be dosed using adult guidelines. Infantile spasms (monotherapy): Start: 50 mg/kg/day PO divided twice daily. May increase in increments of 25 mg/kg/day to 50 mg/kg/day every 3 days to a max of 150 mg/kg/day in 2 divided doses.

FORMS — Trade only: Tabs 500 mg. Oral powder 500 mg/packet.

NOTES — Due to possible vision loss the drug is only available in a restricted distribution program called SHARE, and patients must be enrolled by calling 1-888-45-SHARE. See package insert for dosing with renal insufficiency.

MOA — Irreversible inhibitor of GABA-transaminase; increases CNS levels of GABA.

ADVERSE EFFECTS — Serious: Ophthalmologic abnormalities: Retinal atrophy, optic neuritis, optic atrophy, peripheral neuropathy, suicidality. Frequent: Drowsiness, dizziness, headache.

ZONISAMIDE (Zonegran) ▶LK ♀C ▶? $$$$

ADULT — Partial seizures, adjunctive: Start 100 mg PO daily for 2 weeks, then increase to 200 mg PO daily. May increase prn q 2 weeks to 300 to 400 mg/day, given once daily or divided two times per day. Max 600 mg/day.

PEDS — Not approved in children.

FORMS — Generic/Trade: Caps 25, 50, 100 mg.

ZONISAMIDE (*cont.*)

NOTES — This is a sulfonamide; contraindicated in sulfa allergy. Fatalities and severe reactions including Stevens-Johnson syndrome, toxic epidermal necrolysis, fulminant hepatic necrosis, and blood dyscrasias have occurred with sulfonamides. Clearance is affected by CYP3A4 inhibitors or inducers such as phenytoin, carbamazepine, phenobarbital, and valproic acid. Nephrolithiasis may occur. Oligohidrosis and hyperthermia may occur, and are more common in children. Patients with renal disease may require slower titration.

MOA — Unknown. May involve inhibition of sodium and calcium channels.

ADVERSE EFFECTS — Serious: Toxic epidermal necrolysis, Stevens-Johnson syndrome, hepatic necrosis, agranulocytosis, aplastic anemia, hypersensitivity, nephrolithiasis, psychosis, suicidality, oligohidrosis, hyperthermia. Frequent: Abdominal pain, headache, somnolence, fatigue, N/V, anorexia, dizziness, drowsiness, cognitive symptoms, ataxia, diplopia, confusion, depression, irritability, agitation, insomnia, weight loss.

NEUROLOGY: Migraine Therapy—Triptans (5-HT1 Receptor Agonists)

NOTE: May cause vasospasm. Avoid in ischemic or vasospastic heart disease, cerebrovascular syndromes, peripheral arterial disease, uncontrolled HTN, and hemiplegic or basilar migraine. Do not use within 24 h of ergots or other triptans. Risk of serotonin syndrome if used with SSRIs or MAOIs. May be associated with medication overuse headaches if used 10 or more days per month.

ALMOTRIPTAN (*Axert*) ▶LK ♀C ▶? $$

ADULT — Migraine treatment: 6.25 to 12.5 mg PO. May repeat in 2 h prn. Max 25 mg/day.

PEDS — Migraine treatment: for age older than 12 yo same dose as adult

FORMS — Trade only: Tabs 6.25, 12.5 mg.

NOTES — MAOIs inhibit almotriptan metabolism; use together only with extreme caution. Use lower doses (6.25 mg) in renal and/or hepatic dysfunction. Use with caution in patients with known hypersensitivity to sulfonamides.

MOA — Serotonin 5-HT1B/D agonist.

ADVERSE EFFECTS — Serious: Chest pain/tightness, coronary vasospasm, acute MI, arrhythmias, peripheral ischemia, stroke. Frequent: N/V, headache, paresthesias, sedation, dry mouth.

ELETRIPTAN (*Relpax*) ▶LK ♀C ▶? $$$

ADULT — Migraine treatment: 20 to 40 mg PO at onset. May repeat after 2 h prn. Max 40 mg/dose or 80 mg/day.

PEDS — Not approved in children.

FORMS — Trade only: Tabs 20, 40 mg.

NOTES — Do not use within 72 h of potent CYP3A4 inhibitors such as ketoconazole, itraconazole, nefazodone, troleandomycin, clarithromycin, ritonavir, or nelfinavir.

MOA — Serotonin 5-HT1B/D agonist.

ADVERSE EFFECTS — Serious: Chest pain/tightness, coronary vasospasm, acute MI, arrhythmias, peripheral ischemia, stroke, HTN, seizures. Frequent: Dizziness, somnolence, nausea, asthenia, chest tightness.

FROVATRIPTAN (*Frova*) ▶LK ♀C ▶? $

ADULT — Migraine treatment: 2.5 mg PO. May repeat in 2 h prn. Max 7.5 mg/24 h.

PEDS — Not approved in children.

FORMS — Trade only: Tabs 2.5 mg.

MOA — Serotonin 5-HT1B/D agonist.

ADVERSE EFFECTS — Serious: Chest pain/tightness, coronary vasospasm, acute MI, arrhythmias, peripheral ischemia, stroke, HTN. Frequent: N/V, headache, paresthesias, sedation, dizziness, fatigue, dry mouth.

NARATRIPTAN (*Amerge*) ▶KL ♀C ▶? $$$

ADULT — Migraine treatment: 1 to 2.5 mg PO. May repeat in 4 h prn. Max 5 mg/24 h.

PEDS — Not approved in children.

FORMS — Generic/Trade: Tabs 1, 2.5 mg.

NOTES — Contraindicated in severe renal or hepatic impairment.

MOA — Serotonin 5-HT1B/D agonist.

ADVERSE EFFECTS — Serious: Chest pain/tightness, coronary vasospasm, acute MI, arrhythmias, peripheral ischemia, stroke, HTN. Frequent: Paresthesia, dizziness, drowsiness, malaise, fatigue.

RIZATRIPTAN (*Maxalt, Maxalt MLT*) ▶LK ♀C ▶? $$$

ADULT — Migraine treatment: 5 to 10 mg PO; May repeat in 2 h prn. Max 30 mg/24 h.

PEDS — Migraine treatment: Children 6-17 yo, 5 mg PO if less 40 kg and 10 mg PO for 40 kg and above. Do not give more than one dose in 24 h.

FORMS — Generic/Trade: Tabs 5, 10 mg. Orally disintegrating tabs 5, 10 mg.

NOTES — Should not be combined with MAOIs. MLT form dissolves on tongue without liquids. Adult patients receiving propranolol should only receive 5 mg dose and not more than 3 doses per 24 h. For pediatric patients taking propranolol and weighing more than 40 kg only a 5 mg dose one time in 24 h should be used. Do not give to children weighing less than 40 kg and taking propranolol.

MOA — Serotonin 5-HT1B/D agonist.

ADVERSE EFFECTS — Serious: Chest pain/tightness, coronary vasospasm, acute MI, arrhythmias, peripheral ischemia, stroke, HTN. Frequent: Asthenia, fatigue, drowsiness, pain/pressure sensation, dizziness, paresthesia.

SUMATRIPTAN (*Imitrex, Alsuma, Sumavel, Zecuity*) ▶LK ♀C ▶+ $

ADULT — Migraine treatment: 4 to 6 mg SC. May repeat in 1 h prn. Max 12 mg/24 h. Tabs: 25 to 100 mg PO (50 mg most common). May repeat q 2 h prn with 25

SUMATRIPTAN (*cont.*)

to 100 mg doses. Max 200 mg/24 h. Intranasal spray: 5 to 20 mg. May repeat q 2 h prn. Max 40 mg/24 h. Transdermal: one patch topically, max two patches/24 hours with no less than 2 hours before second application. No evidence of increased benefit with second patch. Cluster headache treatment: 6 mg SC. May repeat after 1 h or longer prn. Max 12 mg/24 h. Initial oral dose of 50 mg appears to be more effective than 25 mg. If HA returns after initial SC injection, then tabs may be used q 2 h prn, max 100 mg/24 h.

PEDS — Not approved in children.

UNAPPROVED PEDS — Acute migraine, intranasal spray, for age 8 to 17 yo: Give 20 mg for wt 40 kg or greater or 10 mg for wt 20 to 39 kg intranasally at headache onset. May repeat after 2 h prn.

FORMS — Generic/Trade: Tabs 25, 50, 100 mg. Injection (STATdose System) 4-, 6-mg prefilled cartridges. Trade only: Nasal spray (Imitrex Nasal) 5 mg and 20 mg (box of #6). Alsuma, Sumavel: Injection 6-mg prefilled cartridge. Zecuity Transdermal Patch: 6.5 mg/4 hours. Generic only: Nasal spray 5 mg and 20 mg (box of #6)

NOTES — Should not be combined with MAOIs. Avoid IM/IV route.

MOA — Serotonin 5-HT1B/D agonist.

ADVERSE EFFECTS — Serious: Chest pain/tightness, coronary vasospasm, acute MI, arrhythmias, peripheral ischemia, stroke, seizures, HTN. Frequent: Dizziness, lightheadedness, weakness, myalgias, muscle cramps, N/V, fatigue, drowsiness, flushing, pain/pressure sensation.

TREXIMET (sumatriptan + naproxen) ▶LK ♀C ▶– $$

WARNING — Risk of GI bleeding and perforation. Do not use ergots within 24 h of Treximet.

ADULT — Migraine treatment: 1 tab PO at onset. Efficacy of more than one tablet not established. Max 2 tabs/24 h separated by at least 2 hours.

PEDS — Not approved in children.

FORMS — Trade only: Tabs 85 mg sumatriptan + 500 mg naproxen sodium.

NOTES — Avoid if CrCl less than 30 mL/min, hepatic impairment, cerebrovascular, cardiovascular, or peripheral vascular disease, uncontrolled HTN. Contraindicated with MAOIs.

MOA — Combination of serotonin 5-HT1B/D agonist and anti-inflammatory/analgesic.

ADVERSE EFFECTS — Serious: Serotonin syndrome, renal toxicity, anaphylactic reactions, chest pain/tightness, coronary vasospasm, acute MI, arrhythmias, peripheral ischemia, stroke, seizures, HTN, gastrointestinal bleeding/ulceration. Frequent: Dizziness, lightheadedness, weakness, myalgias, muscle cramps, N/V, fatigue, drowsiness, flushing, pain/pressure sensation.

ZOLMITRIPTAN (*Zomig, Zomig ZMT*) ▶L ♀C ▶? $$$$

ADULT — Migraine treatment: Tabs: 1.25 to 2.5 mg PO q 2 h. Max 10 mg/24 h. Orally disintegrating tabs (ZMT): 2.5 mg PO. May repeat in 2 h prn. Max 10 mg/24 h. Nasal spray: 5 mg (1 spray) in 1 nostril. May repeat in 2 h prn. Max 10 mg/24 h.

PEDS — Not approved in children.

FORMS — Generic/Trade: Tabs 2.5, 5 mg. Orally disintegrating tabs (ZMT) 2.5, 5 mg. Trade only: Nasal spray 5 mg/spray.

NOTES — Use lower doses (less than 2.5 mg) in hepatic dysfunction. May break 2.5 mg tabs in half and reduce max to 5 mg/day.

MOA — Serotonin 5-HT1B/D agonist.

ADVERSE EFFECTS — Serious: Chest pain/tightness, coronary vasospasm, acute MI, arrhythmia, peripheral and splenic ischemia, stroke, HTN. Frequent: Asthenia, pain/pressure, diaphoresis, dizziness, drowsiness, dyspepsia, flushing, paresthesia, dysgeusia (nasal spray only).

NEUROLOGY: Migraine Therapy—Other

CAFERGOT (ergotamine + caffeine) ▶L ♀X ▶– $

WARNING — Contraindicated with concomitant use of potent CYP3A4 inhibitors (eg, macrolides, protease inhibitors) due to risk of serious/life-threatening peripheral ischemia. Ergots have been associated with potentially life-threatening fibrotic complications.

ADULT — Migraine and cluster headache treatment: 2 tabs PO at onset, then 1 tab q 30 min prn to max 6 tabs/attack or 10 tabs/week.

PEDS — Not approved in children.

UNAPPROVED PEDS — Migraine treatment: 1 tab PO at onset, then 1 tab q 30 min prn to max 3 tabs/attack.

FORMS — Trade only: Tabs 1/100 mg ergotamine/caffeine.

NOTES — Contraindicated in sepsis, CAD, peripheral arterial disease, HTN, impaired hepatic or renal function, malnutrition, or severe pruritus.

MOA — Vasoconstrictor. Partial agonist/antagonist at alpha-adrenergic and serotonin receptors (ergotamine).

ADVERSE EFFECTS — Serious: Coronary vasospasm, coronary or peripheral ischemia, arrhythmias, HTN; retroperitoneal, pleural, pericardial, or cardiac valvular fibrosis. Frequent: N/V, dry mouth, abdominal pain, localized edema and pruritus, myalgias, leg weakness, peripheral ischemia, paresthesias, asthenia

DIHYDROERGOTAMINE (*D.H.E. 45, Migranal*) ▶L ♀X ▶– $$

WARNING — Contraindicated with concomitant use of potent CYP3A4 inhibitors (eg, macrolides, protease inhibitors) due to risk of serious/life-threatening peripheral ischemia. Ergots have been associated with potentially life-threatening fibrotic complications.

ADULT — Migraine treatment: Soln (DHE 45): 1 mg IV/IM/SC; may repeat q 1 h prn to max 2 mg (IV)

(cont.)

DIHYDROERGOTAMINE (*cont.*)

or 3 mg (IM/SC) per 24 h. Nasal spray (Migranal): 1 spray (0.5 mg) in each nostril; may repeat in 15 min prn to max 6 sprays (3 mg)/24 h or 8 sprays (4 mg)/week.

PEDS — Not approved in children.

FORMS — Trade only: Nasal spray 0.5 mg/spray (Migranal). Self-injecting soln (D.H.E 45): 1 mg/mL.

NOTES — Contraindicated in basilar or hemiplegic migraine, sepsis, ischemic or vasospastic cardiac disease, peripheral vascular disease, vascular surgery, impaired hepatic or renal function, or uncontrolled HTN. Avoid concurrent ergotamine, methysergide, or triptan use.

MOA — Serotonin 5-HT1D receptor agonist.

ADVERSE EFFECTS — Serious: Coronary vasoconstriction, MI, ventricular arrhythmias, stroke, HTN, peripheral ischemia; retroperitoneal, pleural, pericardial, or cardiac valvular fibrosis. Frequent: N/V, diarrhea, paresthesia, chest pain. Rhinitis and dysgeusia (nasal spray only).

ERGOTAMINE (*Ergomar*) ▶L ♀X ▶– $$

ADULT — Vascular headache: Start 2 mg SL; may repeat q 30 min to max 6 mg/24 h. Drug interactions. Fibrotic complications.

PEDS — Not approved in children.

FORMS — Trade only: Sublingual tabs (ergotamine tartrate) 2 mg.

NOTES — Avoid use with potent CYP3A4 inhibitors (eg, ritonavir, nelfinavir, indinavir, erythromycin, clarithromycin, troleandomycin); severe peripheral vasoconstriction may result.

MOA — Vasoconstrictor. Partial agonist/antagonist at alpha-adrenergic and serotonin receptors (ergotamine).

ADVERSE EFFECTS — Serious: coronary vasospasm, coronary or peripheral ischemia, arrhythmias, HTN; retroperitoneal, pleural, pericardial, or cardiac valvular

fibrosis. Frequent: N/V, dry mouth, abdominal pain, localized edema and pruritus, myalgias, leg weakness, peripheral ischemia, paresthesia, asthenia.

FLUNARIZINE ▶L ♀C ▶– $$

ADULT — Canada only. Migraine prophylaxis: 10 mg PO at bedtime; if side effects occur, then reduce dose to 5 mg at bedtime. Safety of long-term use (more than 4 months) has not been established.

PEDS — Not approved in children.

FORMS — Generic/Trade: Caps 5 mg.

NOTES — Gradual onset of benefit, over 6 to 8 weeks. Not for acute therapy. Contraindicated if history of depression or extrapyramidal disorders.

MOA — Selective calcium channel blocker.

ADVERSE EFFECTS — Serious: Depression, extrapyramidal symptoms, tardive syndromes. Frequent: Drowsiness, weight gain.

ISOMETHEPTENE + DICHLORALPHENAZONE + ACETAMINOPHEN) ▶L ♀? ▶? ©IV $

ADULT — Tension and vascular headache treatment: 1 to 2 caps PO q 4 h, to max of 8 caps/day. Migraine treatment: 2 caps PO single dose, then 1 cap q 1 h prn to max 5 caps within 12 h.

PEDS — Not approved in children.

FORMS — Generic only: Caps (isometheptene/dichloralphenazone/acetaminophen) 65/100/325 mg.

NOTES — Midrin brand no longer available. FDA has classified as possibly effective for migraine treatment; however, products containing this combination are not FDA approved. Contraindicated in glaucoma, severe renal disease, heart disease, hepatic disease, or concurrent MAOI use. Use caution in HTN, peripheral arterial disease, or recent MI.

MOA — Combination sympathomimetic (vasoconstrictor), CNS depressant, and analgesic.

ADVERSE EFFECTS — Serious: Hepatotoxicity, renal tubular necrosis, chronic analgesic nephropathy. Frequent: Rash, dizziness.

NEUROLOGY: Multiple sclerosis

DALFAMPRIDINE (*Ampyra★Fampyra*) ▶K– ♀C ▶? $$$$$

WARNING — Risk of drug-induced seizures.

ADULT — Multiple sclerosis: 10 mg PO two times per day.

PEDS — Not approved for use in children or adolescents

FORMS — Trade: Extended-release tabs 10 mg.

NOTES — Contraindicated with moderate to severe renal impairment (ClCr < 50 ml/min) and history of seizures. Obtained from a specialty pharmacy (Ampyra Patient Support Service 888-883-3053). Do not exceed recommended dose. Do not combine with other forms of 4-aminopyridine.

MOA — Broad spectrum potassium channel blocker.

ADVERSE EFFECTS — Serious: Seizures. Frequent: Urinary tract infection, insomnia, dizziness, headache, nausea, asthenia, back pain, balance disorder, multiple sclerosis relapse, paresthesia, nasopharyngitis, constipation, dyspepsia, pharyngolaryngeal pain.

DIMETHYL FUMARATE (*Tecfidera*) ▶esterases - ♀C ▶?

ADULT — Multiple sclerosis (relapsing): Start 120 mg PO twice per day. Increase to maintenance dose of 240 mg tiwce per day after 7 days.

PEDS — Not approved for use in children.

FORMS — Delayed-release capsules: 120, 240 mg.

NOTES — Obtain complete blood count prior to initiation of treatment. Administration with food may reduce flushing.

MOA — Unknown but may activate the Nuclear factor (Nrf2) pathway.

ADVERSE EFFECTS — Serious: Lymphopenia. Frequent: flushing, abdominal pain, diarrhea, nausea.

FINGOLIMOD (*Gilenya*) ▶L– ♀C ▶?

ADULT — Relapsing multiple sclerosis: 0.5 mg PO once daily.

PEDS — Not approved for use in children or adolescents.

FORMS — Trade only: Caps 0.5 mg.

FINGOLIMOD (*cont.*)

NOTES — Do not use within 6 months of MI, stroke/TIA, unstable angina, AV block, decompensated or Class III or IV heart failure. Observe all patients for bradycardia for 6 h after the first dose. Obtain baseline ECG for patients on drugs such as beta blockers and antiarrhythmics that can cause bradycardia. Contraindicated if QTc > 500 msec or treatment with antiarrhythmics. Obtain CBC prior to initiation. Monitor for infection and consider stopping if a serious infection occurs. Obtain baseline ophthalmic exam and after 3 to 4 months of therapy to monitor for macular edema. Obtain baseline LFTs. Use effective contraception during and for 2 months following therapy. Avoid live attenuated vaccines during and for 2 months following therapy. Avoid use with ketoconazole.

MOA — Sphingosine 1-phosphate receptor modulator reducing lymphocyte egress from lymph nodes

ADVERSE EFFECTS — Serious: bradycardia, AV block, leukopenia, macular edema, posterior reversible encephalopathy syndrome. Frequent: headache, influenza, diarrhea, increased liver enzymes, cough, back pain

GLATIRAMER (*Copaxone*) ▶tissues Local hydrolysis ♀B ▶? $$$$$

ADULT — Multiple sclerosis (relapsing-remitting): Copaxone 20 mg/mL: 20 mg SC daily. Copaxone 40 mg/mL: 40 mg SC thre times weekly.

PEDS — Not approved in children.

FORMS — Trade only: Pre-filled syringes 20, 40 mg per mL for injection. Not interchangeable.

NOTES — Do not inject IV. Patients my experience immediate post-injection reaction that includes flushing, chest pain, palpitations, anxiety, dyspnea, tightness of the throat, and urticaria. It is usually self-limited and does not require treatment. Patients should be told to report unusual or prolonged chest pain.

MOA — Immunomodulator.

ADVERSE EFFECTS — Serious: Anaphylaxis. Frequent: Injection site reactions, flu-like symptoms, flushing, dyspnea, chest pain, anxiety, palpitations, asthenia, pain, N/V, arthralgia.

INTERFERON BETA-1A (*Avonex, Rebif*) ▶L ♀C ▶? $$$$$

WARNING — Risk of severe hepatic injury and failure, possibly greater when used with other hepatotoxic drugs. Monitor LFTs. Suicidality risk; use caution in depression.

ADULT — Multiple sclerosis (relapsing forms): Avonex 30 mcg (6 million units) IM q week. Rebif , for 22 mcg maintenance dose start 4.4 SC mcg three times weekly for two weeks, then increase to 11 mcg three times weekly for two weeks, then increase to 22 mcg three times weekly. For 44 mcg maintenance dose start 8.8 mcg SC three times weekly for two weeks, then increase to 22 mcg three times weekly for two weeks, then increase to 44 mcg three times weekly.

PEDS — Not approved in children.

FORMS — Trade only (Avonex): Injection 30 mcg single-dose vial with or without albumin. Prefilled syringe 30 mcg. Trade only (Rebif): Starter kit 20 mcg prefilled syringe. Prefilled syringe 22, 44 mcg.

NOTES — Use caution in patients with depression, seizure disorders, or cardiac disease. Follow LFTs and CBC. Avonex: Indicated for the first attack of MS. Rebif: Give same dose 3 days each week, with at least 48 h between doses.

MOA — Immunomodulator.

ADVERSE EFFECTS — Serious: Depression, suicidal ideation, psychosis, hepatotoxicity, anaphylaxis, autoimmune disorders (idiopathic thrombocytopenia, hyper- and hypothyroidism, hepatitis), cytopenias, seizures, cardiomyopathy, cardiac failure, Steven's Johnson Syndrome, thrombotic thrombocytopenic purpura, SLE. Frequent: Injection site reactions, headache, fever, chills, N/V, diarrhea, flu-like symptoms, fatigue, muscle pain.

INTERFERON BETA-1B (*Betaseron*) ▶L ♀C ▶? $$$$$

ADULT — Multiple sclerosis (relapsing-remitting): Start 0.0625 mg SC every other day; titrate over 6 weeks to 0.25 mg (8 million units) SC every other day.

PEDS — Not approved in children.

FORMS — Trade only: Injection 0.3 mg (9.6 million units) single-dose vial.

NOTES — Suicidality risk; use caution in depression. Check LFTs after 1, 3, and 6 months and then periodically. Product can be stored at room temp until reconstituted; then refrigerate and use within 3 h.

MOA — Immunomodulator.

ADVERSE EFFECTS — Serious: Depression, suicidality, autoimmune hepatitis, hepatic failure, hypersensitivity, leukopenia, injection site necrosis, hypertension. Frequent: Injection site reactions, headache, fever, chills, N/V, diarrhea, constipation, abdominal pain, edema, flu-like symptoms, myalgia, palpitations, dizziness, somnolence, increased LFTs, abnormal menses.

NATALIZUMAB (*Tysabri*) ▶Serum ♀C ▶? $$$$$

WARNING — May cause progressive multifocal leukoencephalopathy; avoid concomitant use of other immunomodulators. Risk of severe hepatotoxicity; discontinue if jaundice or evidence of liver injury. Risk of anaphylaxis or other hypersensitivity reactions; permanently discontinue if they occur. Risk factors include prior use of immunosuppressants, duration of therapy, and the presence of anti-JCV antibodies.

ADULT — Refractory, relapsing multiple sclerosis (monotherapy) and Crohn's disease: 300 mg IV infusion over 1 h q 4 weeks.

PEDS — Not approved in children.

NOTES — Not first line; recommended only when there has been an inadequate response or failure to tolerate other therapies. Available only through the MS-TOUCH or CD-TOUCH prescribing programs at 800-456-2255. Observe closely for infusion reactions. Avoid other immunosuppressants when using for Crohn's disease; discontinue if no response by 12 weeks. For patients on steroids, taper them as soon as a benefit is noted and discontinue natalizumab if steroids cannot be tapered off within 6 months. Consider stopping natalizumab in patients who require steroids more than 3 months/year.

MOA — Specific mechanism unknown. Monoclonal antibody that blocks interaction of alpha-4-beta

NATALIZUMAB (*cont.*)

1-integrin expressed inflammatory cells to vascular endothelium and parenchymal cells in the brain.
ADVERSE EFFECTS — Serious: Progressive multifocal leukoencephalopathy, cholelithiasis, hepatotoxicity, depression, suicidality, anaphylaxis, hypersensitivity reactions, infection. Frequent: Infusion reactions, headache, fatigue, arthralgia, urinary urgency/frequency, abdominal discomfort, diarrhea, rash, irregular menstruation/dysmenorrhea.

TERIFLUNOMIDE (*Aubagio*) ▶bile ♀X ▶?
WARNING — Severe, potentially fatal hepatotoxicity has been seen with a related drug leflunomide, and it may occur with teriflunomide. Obtain baseline liver function tests within 6 months of initiation, and then monitor ALT at least monthly for 6 months. Discontinue at first sign of liver toxicity and employ methods to accelerate drug elimination such as cholestyramine or charcoal.

Teriflunomide is a known teratogen. Patients must use reliable contraception during use, and pregnancy should be avoided while using this drug.
ADULT — Multiple sclerosis, relapsing forms: Recommended dose 7 mg or 14 mg PO once daily.
PEDS — Not approved for use by children or adolescents.
FORMS — Trade only: Tabs 7 and 14 mg.
NOTES — Obtain liver function tests including bilirubin and a CBC prior to initation of therapy. Screen patients for TB prior to initiation.
MOA — Immunomodulator/pyrimidine synthesis inhibitor
ADVERSE EFFECTS — Serious: hepatotoxicity, teratogenicity, bone marrow suppression, peripheral neuropathy, acute renal failure, Steven's Johnson syndrome, toxic epidermal necrolysis, hypertension, interstitial lung disease. Frequent: alopecia, diarrhea, influenza, paresthesia, nausea.

NEUROLOGY: Myasthenia Gravis

EDROPHONIUM (*Tensilon, Enlon*) ▶Plasma ♀C ▶? $
ADULT — Evaluation for myasthenia gravis (diagnostic purposes only): 2 mg IV over 15 to 30 sec (test dose) while on cardiac monitor, then 8 mg IV after 45 sec. Reversal of neuromuscular blockade: 10 mg IV over 30 to 45 sec; repeat prn to max 40 mg.
PEDS — Evaluation for myasthenia gravis (diagnostic purposes only): Give 1 mg IV (test dose), then 1 mg IV q 30 to 45 sec to max 5 mg for wt 34 kg or less, give 2 mg IV (test dose), then 2 mg IV q 30 to 45 sec to max 10 mg for wt greater than 34 kg.
UNAPPROVED ADULT — Reversal of nondepolarizing neuromuscular blocking agents: 0.5 to 1 mg/kg IV together with atropine 0.007 to 0.014 mg/kg.
FORMS — 10 mg/mL MDV vial.
NOTES — Not for maintenance therapy of myasthenia gravis because of short duration of action (5 to 10 min). May give IM. Monitor cardiac function. Atropine should be readily available in case of cholinergic reaction. Contraindicated in mechanical urinary or intestinal obstruction.
MOA — Reversible cholinesterase inhibitor.
ADVERSE EFFECTS — Serious: Arrhythmias, bradycardia, respiratory paralysis, cholinergic toxicity, dysphagia, seizures. Frequent: N/V, abdominal cramping, diarrhea, miosis, lacrimation, diplopia, fasciculations.

PYRIDOSTIGMINE (*Mestinon, Mestinon Timespan, Regonol*) ▶Plasma, K ♀C ▶+ $$
ADULT — Myasthenia gravis, Standard-release tabs: Start 60 mg PO three times per day; gradually increase to usual therapeutic dose of 200 mg PO three times per day. Extended-release tabs: Start 180 mg PO daily or divided two times per day. Max 1500 mg/day. May give 2 mg IM or slow IV injection q 2 to 3 h.
PEDS — Not approved in children.
UNAPPROVED PEDS — Myasthenia gravis, neonates: 5 mg PO q 4 to 6 h or 0.05 to 0.15 mg/kg IM/IV q 4 to 6 h. Myasthenia gravis, children: 7 mg/kg/day PO in 5 to 6 divided doses, or 0.05 to 0.15 mg/kg/dose IM/IV q 4 to 6 h. Max 10 mg IM/IV single dose.
FORMS — Generic/Trade: Tabs 60 mg. Trade only: Extended-release tabs 180 mg. Syrup 60 mg/ 5 mL.
NOTES — Give injection at 1/30th of oral dose when oral therapy is not possible.
MOA — Reversible cholinesterase inhibitor.
ADVERSE EFFECTS — Serious: Cholinergic toxicity, bronchospasm, respiratory paralysis, bradycardia, arrhythmias, cardiac arrest. Frequent: N/V, diarrhea, abdominal cramps/pain, muscle cramps/weakness, fasciculation, miosis, hypersalivation, increased bronchial secretions.

NEUROLOGY: Parkinsonian Agents—Anticholinergics

NOTE: Anticholinergic medications may cause memory loss, delirium, or psychosis, particularly in elderly patients or those with baseline cognitive impairment. Contraindicated in narrow angle glaucoma, bowel obstruction, and megacolon.

BENZTROPINE MESYLATE (*Cogentin*) ▶LK ♀C ▶? $
ADULT — Parkinsonism: Start 0.5 to 2 mg/day PO/IM/IV. Increase in 0.5 mg increments at weekly intervals to max 6 mg/day. May divide doses one to four times

per day. Drug-induced extrapyramidal disorders: 1 to 4 mg PO/IM/IV given once daily or divided two times per day.
PEDS — Not approved in children.

BENZTROPINE MESYLATE (*cont.*)

UNAPPROVED PEDS — Parkinsonism in age older than 3 yo: 0.02 to 0.05 mg/kg/dose given once daily or divided two times per day. Use caution; potential for undesired anticholinergic effects.

FORMS — Generic only: Tabs 0.5, 1, 2 mg.

NOTES — Contraindicated in narrow-angle glaucoma. Avoid concomitant use of donepezil, rivastigmine, galantamine, or tacrine. Brand name Cogentin discontinued.

MOA — Anticholinergic.

ADVERSE EFFECTS — Serious: Tachycardia, anticholinergic toxicity, psychosis, delirium. Frequent: Dry mouth, constipation, urinary retention, blurred vision, drowsiness, dizziness, headache, rash, N/V, memory problems.

BIPERIDEN (*Akineton*) ▶LK ♀C ▶? $$$

ADULT — Parkinsonism: 2 mg PO three to four times per day. Titrate to max 16 mg/day. Drug-induced extrapyramidal disorders: 2 mg PO daily to three times per day to max 8 mg/24 h.

PEDS — Not approved in children.

FORMS — Trade only: Tabs 2 mg.

NOTES — Contraindicated in narrow-angle glaucoma, bowel obstruction, and megacolon.

MOA — Anticholinergic.

ADVERSE EFFECTS — Serious: Tachycardia, anticholinergic toxicity, psychosis, delirium. Frequent: Dry mouth, constipation, urinary retention, blurred vision, drowsiness, dizziness, headache, rash, N/V, memory problems, delirium.

TRIHEXYPHENIDYL (*Artane*) ▶LK ♀C ▶? $

ADULT — Parkinsonism: 1 mg PO daily. Increase by 2 mg/day at 3- to 5-day intervals to usual therapeutic dose of 6 to 10 mg/day divided three times per day with meals. Max 15 mg/day.

PEDS — Not approved in children.

FORMS — Generic only: Tabs 2, 5 mg. Elixir 2 mg/5 mL.

MOA — Anticholinergic.

ADVERSE EFFECTS — Serious: Tachycardia, anticholinergic toxicity, psychosis, delirium. Frequent: Dry mouth, constipation, urinary retention, blurred vision, drowsiness, dizziness, headache, rash, N/V, memory problems.

NEUROLOGY: Parkinsonian Agents—COMT Inhibitors

ENTACAPONE (*Comtan*) ▶L ♀C ▶? $$$$$

ADULT — Parkinson's disease, adjunctive: Start 200 mg PO with each dose of carbidopa/levodopa. Max 8 tabs (1600 mg)/day.

PEDS — Not approved in children.

FORMS — Generic/Trade: Tabs 200 mg.

NOTES — Adjunct to carbidopa/levodopa in patients who have end-of-dose "wearing off." Has no antiparkinsonian effect on its own. Avoid concomitant use of nonselective MAOIs. Use caution in hepatobiliary dysfunction. Avoid rapid withdrawal, which may precipitate neuroleptic malignant syndrome. Use caution if using medications metabolized by COMT such as isoproterenol, epinephrine, norepinephrine, dopamine, and dobutamine becuase an exaggerated response is possible. Use may be associated with abruptly falling asleep from the drug's impact on L-dopa.

MOA — Blocks dopamine breakdown by inhibiting catechol-o-methyltransferase.

ADVERSE EFFECTS — Serious: Orthostatic hypotension, rhabdomyolysis, hallucinations, delirium, severe diarrhea, impulse control disorders. Frequent: Dyskinesia, hyperkinesia, N/V, abdominal pain, diarrhea, urine discoloration.

TOLCAPONE (*Tasmar*) ▶LK ♀C ▶? $$$$$

WARNING — Fatal hepatic failure has occurred. Use only in patients on carbidopa/levodopa who fail alternative therapies and provide written informed consent. Monitor LFTs at baseline, q 2 to 4 weeks for 6 months, and then periodically. Discontinue if LFT elevation is more than 2 times upper limit of normal or if there is no clinical benefit after 3 weeks of therapy.

ADULT — Parkinson's disease, adjunctive (not first line): Start 100 mg PO three times per day. Increase to 200 mg PO three times per day only if expected benefit justifies the risk. Max 600 mg/day. Only effective when used in combination with carbidopa/levodopa.

PEDS — Not approved in children.

FORMS — Trade only: Tabs 100, 200 mg.

NOTES — Adjunct to carbidopa-levodopa in patients who have refractory end-of-dose "wearing off." Has no antiparkinsonian effect on its own. Contraindicated in hepatic dysfunction. Monitor LFTs. Avoid concomitant use of non-selective MAOIs. Avoid rapid withdrawal, which may precipitate neuroleptic malignant syndrome. Informed consent forms are available from the manufacturer (www.tasmar.com).

MOA — Blocks dopamine breakdown by inhibiting catechol-o-methyltransferase

ADVERSE EFFECTS — Serious: fulminant hepatotoxicity, orthostatic hypotension, hallucinations, severe diarrhea, impulse control disorders. Frequent: dyskinesia, dystonia, anorexia, N/V, diarrhea, constipation, confusion, sleep disorders.

NEUROLOGY: Parkinsonian Agents—Dopaminergic Agents and Combinations

NOTE: Dopaminergic medications may cause hallucinations, particularly when used in combination. They have also been associated with sudden-onset episodes of sleep without warning ("sleep attacks"), and with the development of impulse control disorders such as compulsive gambling, hypersexuality, and hyperphagia. This is more common with dopamine agonists than L-dopa. Avoid rapid discontinuation, which may precipitate neuroleptic malignant syndrome.

APOMORPHINE (*Apokyn*) ▸L ♀C ▶? $$$$$

WARNING — Never administer IV due to risk of severe adverse effects including pulmonary embolism.

ADULT — Acute, intermittent treatment of hypomobility ("off episodes") in Parkinson's disease: Start 0.2 mL SC test dose in the presence of medical personnel. May increase dose by 0.1 mL every few days as tolerated. Max 0.6 mL/dose or 2 mL/day. Monitor for orthostatic hypotension after initial dose and with dose escalation. Potent emetic; pretreat with trimethobenzamide 300 mg PO three times per day (or domperidone 20 mg PO three times per day) starting 3 days prior to use, and continue for at least 6 weeks before weaning.

PEDS — Not approved in children.

FORMS — Trade only: Cartridges (for injector pen, 10 mg/mL) 3 mL. Ampules (10 mg/mL) 2 mL.

NOTES — Write doses exclusively in mL rather than mg to avoid errors. Most effective when administered at (or just prior to) the onset of an "off" episode. Avoid concomitant use of 5HT3 antagonists (eg, ondansetron, granisetron, dolasetron, palonosetron, alosetron), which can precipitate severe hypotension and loss of consciousness. Inform patients that the dosing pen is labeled in mL (not mg), and that it is possible to dial in a dose of medication even if the cartridge does not contain sufficient drug. Rotate injection sites. Restart at 0.2 mL/day if treatment is interrupted for 1 week or more. Use cautiously with hepatic impairment. Reduce starting dose to 0.1 mL in patients with mild or moderate renal failure. Contains sulfites.

MOA — Dopamine agonist (non-ergot).

ADVERSE EFFECTS — Serious: Syncope, orthostatic hypotension, QT prolongation, arrhythmias, myocardial infarction, anaphylaxis, sleep attacks, priapism, inappropriate sexual behavior, impulse control disorders. Frequent: N/V, yawning, chest pain, confusion, hallucinations, sedation, drowsiness, dyskinesia, dizziness, rhinorrhea, peripheral edema, injection site reactions.

CARBIDOPA (*Lodosyn*) ▸LK ♀C ▶? $$$

ADULT — Parkinson's disease, adjunct to carbidopa/levodopa: Start 25 mg PO daily with 1st daily dose of carbidopa/levodopa. May give an additional 12.5 to 25 mg with each dose of carbidopa/levodopa prn. Max 200 mg/day.

PEDS — Not approved in children.

FORMS — Trade only: Tabs 25 mg.

NOTES — Adjunct to carbidopa/levodopa to reduce peripheral side-effects such as nausea. Also increases the CNS availability of levodopa. Monitor for CNS side effects such as dyskinesias and hallucinations when initiating therapy, and reduce the dose of levodopa as necessary.

MOA — Blocks the peripheral conversion of levodopa to dopamine.

ADVERSE EFFECTS — Serious: melanoma. Frequent: None. The adverse effects of carbidopa/levodopa are due to the levodopa component.

CARBIDOPA/LEVODOPA (*Sinemet, Sinemet CR, Parcopa*) ▸L ♀C ▶— $$$$

ADULT — Parkinsonism: Standard-release and orally disintegrating tab: Start 1 tab (25/100 mg) PO three times per day. Increase by 1 tab/day q 1 to 2 days prn. Use 1 tab (25/250 mg) PO three times per day to four times per day when higher levodopa doses are needed. Sustained-release: Start 1 tab (50/200 mg) PO twice per day; separate doses by at least 4 h. Increase prn at intervals of 3 days or more. Typical max dose is 1600 to 2000 mg/day of levodopa, but higher doses have been used.

PEDS — Not approved in children.

UNAPPROVED ADULT — Restless legs syndrome: Start ½ tab (25/100 mg) PO at bedtime; increase q 3 to 4 days to max 50/200 mg (two 25/100 tabs) at bedtime. If symptoms recur during the night, then a combination of standard-release (25/100 mg, 1 to 2 tabs at bedtime) and sustained-release (25/100 or 50/200 mg at bedtime) tabs may be used. Dopa-responsive dystonia: Start 1 tab (25/100) PO daily and titrate to max 1000 mg of levodopa daily.

FORMS — Generic/Trade: Tabs (carbidopa/levodopa) 10/100, 25/100, 25/250 mg. Tabs, sustained-release (Sinemet CR, carbidopa-levodopa ER) 25/100, 50/200 mg. Trade only: Orally disintegrating tab (Parcopa) 10/100, 25/100, 25/250 mg.

NOTES — Motor fluctuations and dyskinesias may occur. The 25/100 mg tabs are preferred as initial therapy, since most patients require at least 70 to 100 mg/day of carbidopa to reduce the risk of N/V. The 10/100 mg tabs have limited clinical utility. Extended-release formulations have a lower bioavailability than conventional preparations. Do not use within 2 weeks of a nonselective MAOI. When used for restless legs syndrome, may precipitate rebound (recurrence of symptoms during the night) or augmentation (earlier daily onset of symptoms). Orally disintegrating tab is placed on top of the tongue and does not require water or swallowing, but is absorbed through the GI tract (not sublingually). Use caution in patients with undiagnosed skin lesions or a history of melanoma. Intense urges (gambling and sexual for example) have been reported. Consider discontinuing the medication or reducing the dose if these occur.

MOA — Levodopa is a dopamine precursor. Carbidopa blocks the peripheral conversion of levodopa to dopamine.

ADVERSE EFFECTS — Serious: Orthostatic hypotension, psychosis, agranulocytosis, leukopenia, hepatotoxicity, thrombocytopenia, pathologic gambling, sudden onset of sleep. Frequent: Dyskinesia, dystonia, orthostatic hypotension, N/V, abdominal cramps, confusion, hallucinations.

PRAMIPEXOLE (*Mirapex, Mirapex ER*) ▸K ♀C ▶? $$$$$

ADULT — Parkinson's disease: Start 0.125 mg PO three times per day for 1 week, then 0.25 mg for 1 week; after that, increase by 0.75 mg/week divided three times per day. Usual effective dose is 0.5 to 1.5 mg

PRAMIPEXOLE (*cont.*)

PO three times per day. Extended release: Start 0.375 mg daily. May increase after 5 to 7 days to 0.75 mg/day then by 0.75 mg/day increments q 5 to 7 days to max 4.5 mg/day. Restless legs syndrome: Start 0.125 mg PO 2 to 3 h prior to bedtime. May increase q 4 to 7 days to 0.25 mg then 0.5 mg if needed.

PEDS — Not approved in children.

FORMS — Generic/Trade: Tabs 0.125, 0.25, 0.5, 0.75, 1, 1.5 mg. Trade only: Tabs, extended-release 0.375, 0.75, 1.5, 2.25, 3, 3.75, 4.5 mg.

NOTES — Decrease dose in renal impairment. Titrate slowly. May change to extended-release tabs at same daily dose as regular tabs overnight.

MOA — Dopamine agonist (non-ergot).

ADVERSE EFFECTS — Serious: Sleep attacks, orthostatic hypotension, psychosis, impulse control disorders, SIADH. Frequent: Edema, N/V, dizziness, drowsiness, insomnia, constipation, dry mouth, orthostatic hypotension, dyskinesia, dystonia, hallucinations.

ROPINIROLE (*Requip, Requip XL*) ▶L ♀C ▶? $$$

ADULT — Parkinson's disease: Start 0.25 mg PO three times per day. Increase by 0.25 mg/dose (0.75 mg/day) at weekly intervals to 1 mg PO three times daily. If needed after week 4 may increase dose by 1.5 mg/day weekly up to 9 mg/day and then 3 mg/day weekly to max 24 mg/day. Extended-release: Start 2 mg PO daily, then increase by 2 mg daily at weekly or longer intervals. Max 24 mg/day. Restless legs syndrome: Start 0.25 mg PO 1 to 3 h before bedtime for 2 days, then increase to 0.5 mg/day on days 3 to 7. Increase by 0.5 mg/day at weekly intervals prn to max 4 mg/day given 1 to 3 h before bedtime.

PEDS — Not approved in children.

FORMS — Generic/Trade: Tabs, immediate-release 0.25, 0.5, 1, 2, 3, 4, 5 mg. Tabs, extended-release 2, 4, 6, 8, 12 mg.

NOTES — Retitrate if significant interruption of therapy occurs.

MOA — Dopamine agonist (non-ergot).

ADVERSE EFFECTS — Serious: Sleep attacks, atrial fibrillation, syncope, orthostatic hypotension, HTN, psychosis, impulse control disorders. Frequent: N/V, dizziness, syncope, drowsiness, fatigue, asthenia, headache, dyspepsia, constipation, abdominal pain, dyskinesia, dystonia, pain, edema, diaphoresis, dry mouth, confusion, hallucinations, visual changes.

ROTIGOTINE (*Neupro*) ▶L - ♀C ▶?

ADULT — Early stage Parkinson's disease: Start 2 mg/24 h patch daily; may increase by 2 mg/24 h at weekly intervals to max 6 mg/24 h. Advanced-stage Parkinson's disease: Start 4 mg/24 h patch daily; may increase by 2 mg/24 h at weekly intervals

to max 8 mg/24 h. Restless legs syndrome: Start 1 mg/24 h patch daily; may be increased by 1 mg/24 h at weekly intervals to max 3 mg/24 h.

PEDS — Not approved for use in children.

FORMS — Trade: Transdermal patch 1, 2, 3, 4, 6, 8 mg/24 h.

NOTES — Contains sulfites. Remove prior to MRI or cardioversion to avoid burns. Apply to clean, dry intact skin of the abdomen, thigh, flank, shoulder, or upper arm and hold in place for 20-30 seconds. Rotate application sites daily, and wash skin after removal. Taper by 2 mg/24 h every other day when discontinuing.

MOA — Dopamine agonist, non-ergot

ADVERSE EFFECTS — Serious: sleep attacks, orthostatic hypotension, psychosis, syncope, HTN, impulse control disorder. Frequent: N/V, application site reactions, weight gain, fluid retention, dyskinesia, somnolence, dizziness, headache, insomnia, constipation.

STALEVO (**carbidopa + levodopa + entacapone**) ▶L ♀C ▶– $$$$$

ADULT — Parkinson's disease (conversion from carbidopa/levodopa with or without entacapone): Start Stalevo tab that contains the same amount of carbidopa/levodopa as the patient was previously taking, and titrate to desired response. May need to lower the dose of levodopa in patients not already taking entacapone. Max 1600 mg/day of entacapone or 1600 to 2000 mg/day of levodopa.

PEDS — Not approved in children.

FORMS — Trade/generic: Tabs (carbidopa/levodopa/entacapone): Stalevo 50 (12.5/50/200 mg), Stalevo 75 (18.75/75/200 mg), Stalevo 100 (25/100/200 mg), Stalevo 125 (31.25/125/200 mg), Stalevo 150 (37.5/150/200 mg), Stalevo 200 (50/200/200 mg).

NOTES — Patients who are not currently taking entacapone may benefit from titration of the individual components of this medication before conversion to this fixed-dose preparation. Avoid concomitant use of nonselective MAOIs. Use caution in hepatobiliary dysfunction. Motor fluctuations and dyskinesias may occur.

MOA — Levodopa is a dopamine precursor. Carbidopa blocks the peripheral conversion of levodopa to dopamine. Entacapone blocks the peripheral metabolism of dopamine by inhibiting catechol-o-methyltransferase.

ADVERSE EFFECTS — Serious: Orthostatic hypotension, psychosis, agranulocytosis, leukopenia, hepatotoxicity, thrombocytopenia, rhabdomyolysis, severe diarrhea, colitis. Frequent: Dyskinesia, hyperkinesia, dystonia, orthostatic hypotension, N/V, abdominal cramps, diarrhea, confusion, hallucinations, urine discoloration.

NEUROLOGY: Parkinsonian Agents—Monoamine Oxidase Inhibitors (MAOIs)

RASAGILINE (*Azilect*) ▶L ♀C ▶? $$$$$

ADULT — Parkinson's disease, monotherapy: 1 mg PO q am. Parkinson's disease, adjunctive: 0.5 mg PO q am. Max 1 mg/day.

PEDS — Not approved in children.

FORMS — Trade only: Tabs 0.5, 1 mg.

NOTES — Requires an MAOI diet that avoids foods very high in tyramine content. Contraindicated (risk

(cont.)

RASAGILINE (*cont.*)

of hypertensive crisis) with meperidine, methadone, tramadol, propoxyphene, dextromethorphan, sympathomimetic amines (e.g., pseudoephedrine, phenylephrine, ephedrine), antidepressants, other MAOIs, cyclobenzaprine, and general anesthesia. Discontinue at least 14 days before liberalizing diet, starting one of these medications, or proceeding with elective surgery that requires general anesthesia. May need to reduce levodopa dose when used in combination. Reduce dose to 0.5 mg when used with CYP1A2 inhibitors (e.g., ciprofloxacin) and in mild hepatic impairment. Do not use in moderate or severe liver disease. Parkinson's disease and drugs used to treat it have been associated with an increased risk of melanoma. Consider periodic skin exams for melanoma.

MOA — Irreversible MAO inhibitor.

ADVERSE EFFECTS — Serious: Hypertensive crisis with food/drug interactions, psychosis, orthostatic hypotension, injury/falls, melanoma, sudden sleep onset. Frequent: Worsening of levodopa-induced dyskinesias, anorexia, N/V, constipation, abdominal pain, weight loss, hallucinations, arthralgia, dry mouth, rash, ecchymosis, somnolence, paresthesia.

SELEGILINE (*Eldepryl, Zelapar*) ▶LK ♀C ▶? $$$$

ADULT — Parkinsonism (adjunct to levodopa): 5 mg PO q am and q noon; max 10 mg/day. Zelapar ODT: Start 1.25 mg sublingual q am for at least 6 weeks, then increase prn to max 2.5 mg q am.

PEDS — Not approved in children.

UNAPPROVED ADULT — Parkinsonism (monotherapy): 5 mg PO q am and q noon; max 10 mg/day.

FORMS — Generic/Trade: Caps 5 mg. Tabs 5 mg. Trade only: Orally disintegrating tabs (Zelapar ODT) 1.25 mg.

NOTES — Should not be combined with meperidine or other opioids. Do not exceed max recommended dose; risk of nonselective MAO inhibition. Zelapar should be taken in the morning before food and without water. Intense urges (gambling and sexual for example) have been reported. Consider discontinuing the medication or reducing the dose if these occur. Parkinson's disease and drugs used to treat it have been associated with an increased risk of melanoma.

MOA — Selective MAO-B inhibitor.

ADVERSE EFFECTS — Serious: Angina, syncope, mood lability, psychosis, orthostatic hypotension, impulse control disorders. Frequent: N/V, confusion, depression, ataxia, insomnia, orthostatic hypotension, hallucinations.

NEUROLOGY: Other Agents

ABOBOTULINUM TOXIN A (*DYSPORT*) ▶ ♀C ▶?

WARNING — Symptoms of systemic botulism have been reported, particularly in children treated for spasticity due to cerebral palsy.

ADULT — Cervical dystonia: 500 units IM total dose divided among affected muscles. May repeat q 12 weeks or longer. Max dose 1000 units per treatment. Glabellar line (age younger than 65 yo): 50 units IM total dose divided into 10 unit injections at 5 sites (see prescribing information). May repeat q 12 weeks or longer.

PEDS — Not approved for use in children.

FORMS — Trade: vials 300, 500 units for reconstitution.

NOTES — Refer to prescribing information for injection sites and technique. Use caution in peripheral motor neuropathic diseases, amyotrophic lateral sclerosis, or neuromuscular junction disorders (eg, myasthenia gravis or Lambert-Eaton syndrome) and monitor closely when given botulinum toxin due to increased risk of severe dysphagia or respiratory compromise. Contains trace amounts of cow's milk protein: Do not use in patients allergic to milk. Use cautiously with neuromuscular blocking drugs (eg, aminoglycosides and curare-like drugs).

MOA — Acetylcholine release inhibitor and neuromuscular blocking agent

ADVERSE EFFECTS — Serious: dysphagia, respiratory failure, systemic spread of effect, hypersensitivity. Frequent: muscular weakness, dysphagia, dry mouth, injection site discomfort, fatigue, headache, neck pain, musculoskeletal pain, dysphonia, injection site pain, eyelid ptosis and edema.

BETAHISTINE (*✶Serc*) ▶LK ♀? ▶? $

ADULT — Canada only. Vertigo of Meniere's disease: 8 to 16 mg PO three times per day.

PEDS — Not approved in children.

FORMS — Trade only: Tabs 8, 16 mg.

NOTES — Contraindicated in peptic ulcer disease and pheochromocytoma; use caution in asthmatics.

MOA — Histamine H1-receptor agonist

ADVERSE EFFECTS — Frequent: Urticaria, pruritus, gastrointestinal upset, nausea, headache.

BOTULINUM TOXIN TYPE B (*Myobloc*) ▶Not significantly absorbed ♀+ ▶? $$$$$

WARNING — Symptoms of systemic botulism have been reported, particularly in children treated for spasticity due to cerebral palsy.

ADULT — Cervical dystonia: Start 2500 to 5000 units IM in affected muscles. Use lower initial dose if no prior history of botulinum toxin therapy. Benefits usually last for 12 to 16 weeks when a total dose of 5000 to 10,000 units has been administered. Titrate to effective dose. Give treatments at least 3 months apart to decrease the risk of producing neutralizing antibodies.

PEDS — Not approved in children.

NOTES — Low systemic concentrations are expected with IM injection; monitor closely for dysphagia. Contraindicated in peripheral motor neuropathic disease (eg, ALS, motor neuropathy), neuromuscular junction disease (eg, myasthenia gravis, Lambert-Eaton syndrome due to an increased risk

BOTULINUM TOXIN TYPE B (cont.)

of systemic effects) and with other drugs that block neuromuscular function (eg, aminoglycosides, curare-like compounds).

MOA — Neuromuscular transmission blockade; inhibits presynaptic acetylcholine release.

ADVERSE EFFECTS — Serious: Systemic botulism, dysphagia, respiratory compromise, hypersensitivity. Frequent: Dry mouth, dyspepsia/nausea, injection site pain, flu-like syndrome, arthralgia, back pain, cough, myasthenia, asthenia, dizziness.

DEXTROMETHORPHAN/QUINIDINE (Nuedexta) ▶LK - ♀C ▶?

ADULT — Pseudobulbar affect: Start 1 cap PO daily. Increase after 7 days to maintenance dose of 1 cap two times per day.

PEDS — Not approved for use in children.

FORMS — Trade only: cap 10 mg dextromethorphan plus 20 mg quinidine.

NOTES — Contraindicated with prolonged QT interval, a history of torsades de pointes, with drugs that prolong the QT interval and metabolized by CYP2D6, or with MAOIs. Contraindicated with complete AV block. Obtain ECG at baseline and at 4-hours post-dose to evaluate effect on QT in the presence of CYP3A4 inhibitors, or patients with left ventricular hypertrophy or left ventricular dysfunction. May cause serotonin syndrome if used with serotonergic drugs. Clinical trials were only conducted in patients with PBA secondary to Alzheimer's disease. Response in other subgroups has not been assessed.

MOA — Dextromethorphan: sigma-1 agonist and uncompetitive NMDA antagonist. Quinidine: included to increase DM concentrations by CYP2D6 inhibition.

ADVERSE EFFECTS — Serious: thrombocytopenia, hypersensitivity, lupus-like syndrome, respiratory failure, muscle spasticity. Frequent: diarrhea, dizziness, cough, vomiting, asthenia, peripheral edema.

INCOBOTULINUMTOXIN A (Xeomin) ▶not absorbed - ♀C ▶?

WARNING — Symptoms of systemic botulism have been reported.

ADULT — Cervical dystonia: Total of 120 units IM divided among the sternocleidomastoid, levator scapulae, splenis capitis, scalenus, and trapezius muscles as indicated. Repeat at intervals of at least 12 weeks with dose individualized according to response. Blepharospasm in patients previously treated with Botox: Start with same dose as Botox used before. If prior Botox dose unknown start with 1.25 to 2.5 units per injection site. Usual number of injections is 6 per eye. Average dose 33 units/eye. Do not exceed initial dose of 35 units/eye. May repeat at intervals of at least 12 weeks.

PEDS — Not approved for use in children or adolescents.

FORMS — Trade only: 50 and 100 unit single use vials.

NOTES — Cannot convert units of Xeomin to other botulinum toxins. The max dose in trials for blepharospasm was 50 units/eye. Toxin effects may become systemic and produce asthenia, muscle weakness, diplopia, ptosis, dysphagia, dysphonia, urinary incontinence, and breathing difficulties.

MOA — Cholinergic neuromuscular blocker. Inhibits presynaptic release of acetylcholine.

ADVERSE EFFECTS — Serious: hypersensitivity. Frequent: dysphagia, neck pain, muscle weakness and pain, injection site pain, dry eye, dry mouth, diarrhea, visual impairment, dypnea, nasopharyngitis, flu-like symptoms.

MANNITOL (Osmitrol, Resectisol) ▶K ♀C ▶? $$

ADULT — Intracranial HTN: 0.25 to 2 g/kg IV over 30 to 60 min as a 15, 20, or 25% soln.

PEDS — Not approved in children.

UNAPPROVED ADULT — Increased ICP or Head trauma: 0.25 to 1 g/kg IV push over 20 min. Repeat q 4 to 6 h prn.

UNAPPROVED PEDS — Increased ICP/Cerebral edema: 0.25 to 1 g/kg/dose IV push over 20 to 30 min, then 0.25 to 0.5 g/kg/dose IV q 4 to 6 h prn.

NOTES — Monitor fluid and electrolyte balance and cardiac function. Filter IV solns with concentrations at least 20%; crystals may be present.

MOA — Osmotic diuretic.

ADVERSE EFFECTS — Serious: Congestive heart failure, pulmonary edema, seizures, electrolyte changes, CNS depression, acute renal failure. Frequent: Headache, dizziness, N/V, polydipsia.

MILNACIPRAN (Savella) ▶KL ♀C ▶? $$$$

ADULT — Fibromyalgia: Start day 1: 12.5 mg PO once, then days 2 to 3: 12.5 mg two times per day. Days 4 to 7: 25 mg two times per day. After that: 50 mg two times per day. Max 200 mg/day.

PEDS — Not approved for use in children.

FORMS — Trade only: Tabs 12.5, 25, 50, 100 mg.

NOTES — Reduce dose by 50% for severe renal impairment with CrCl less than 30 mL/min. Taper if discontinued.

MOA — Selective serotonin/norepinephrine reuptake inhibitor.

ADVERSE EFFECTS — Severe: Worsening of psychiatric symptoms including depression, suicidality, aggression, hostility, anger, serotonin syndrome, hypertension, tachycardia, seizures, hepatotoxicity, abnormal bleeding, hyponatremia. Frequent: Nausea/vomiting, headache, dizziness, insomnia, hot flushes, hyperhidrosis, palpitations, dry mouth.

NIMODIPINE (Nimotop, Nymalize) ▶L ♀C ▶– $$$$$

ADULT — Subarachnoid hemorrhage: 60 mg PO q 4 h for 21 days.

PEDS — Not approved in children.

FORMS — Generic only: Caps 30 mg. Trade only: 60 mg/20 mL oral solution (Nymalize)

NOTES — Begin therapy within 96 h. Give 1 h before or 2 h after meals. May give cap contents SL or via NG tube. Reduce dose in hepatic dysfunction.

MOA — Calcium channel blocker.

ADVERSE EFFECTS — Serious: Heart failure, disseminated intravascular coagulation, deep vein thrombosis, neurological deterioration. Frequent:

NIMODIPINE (*cont.*)

Hypotension, N/V, diarrhea, flushing, edema, headache.

ONABOTULINUM TOXIN TYPE A (*Botox, Botox Cosmetic*)
▶Not absorbed ♀C ▶? $$$$$
WARNING — Symptoms of systemic botulism have been reported, particularly in children treated for spasticity due to cerebral palsy.
ADULT — Moderate to severe glabellar lines in patients no older than age 65 yo: Inject 0.1 mL into each of 5 sites. Blepharospasm: 1.25 to 5 units IM into each of several sites in the orbicularis oculi of upper and lower lids q 3 months; use lower doses at initial visit. Strabismus: 1.25 to 5 units depending on diagnosis, injected into extraocular muscles. Cervical dystonia: 15 to 100 units IM (with or without EMG guidance) into affected muscles q 3 months (e.g., splenius capitis/cervicis, sternocleidomastoid, levator scapulae, trapezius, semispinalis, scalene, longissimus); usual total dose is 200 to 300 units/treatment. Primary axillary hyperhidrosis: 50 units/axilla intradermally, divided over 10 to 15 sites. Upper limb spasticity: Biceps brachii, 100 to 200 units IM divided into 4 sites (with or without EMG guidance) q 3 months; flexor carpi radialis, 12.5 to 50 units IM in 1 site; flexor carpi ulnaris, 12.5 to 50 units IM in 1 site; flexor digitorum profundus, 30 to 50 units IM in 1 site; flexor digitorum sublimis, 30 to 50 units IM in 1 site. Chronic migraine headache: Dilute to 5 units/0.1 mL then inject 155 units total as a series of 0.1 mL (5 units) IM injections at 7 specific head/neck sites. Refer to prescribing information for locations of injections and amount per site. Repeat q 12 weeks. Botulinum toxin products are not interchangeable. Overactive bladder: 100 units IM into detrusor divided into 20 injections of 0.5 mL each (total volume 10 mL). May repeat no sooner than 12 weeks later if needed. Detrusor overactivity associated with neurological conditions: 200 units IM into detrusor divided into 30 injections of 1 mL each (total volume 30 mL). May repeat no sooner 12 weeks later if needed.
PEDS — Not approved in children younger than 12 yo for blepharospasm and strabismus, younger than 16 yo for cervical dystonia, or younger than 18 yo for hyperhidrosis, spasticity, or chronic migraine headahce.
UNAPPROVED ADULT — Hemifacial spasm: 1.25 to 2.5 units IM into affected muscles q 3 to 4 months (e.g., corrugator, orbicularis oculi, zygomaticus major, buccinator, depressor anguli oris, platysma); usual total dose is 10 to 34 units/treatment.
FORMS — Trade only: 100 unit single-use vials.
NOTES — Clinical benefit occurs within 2 weeks (2 to 3 days for facial injections), peaks at 1 to 6 weeks, and wears off in approximately 3 months. Contraindicated in peripheral motor neuropathic disease (e.g., ALS, motor neuropathy) or neuromuscular junction disease (e.g., myasthenia gravis, Lambert-Eaton syndrome). The use of lower doses and longer dosing intervals may decrease the risk of producing neutralizing antibodies. Increased risk of dysphagia when more than 100 units are injected into the sternocleidomastoid or with bilateral sternocleidomastoid injections. Potency units of Botox cannot be interchanged with other products. For chronic migraine headache the amount injected varies by muscle site. Refer to prescribing information for specific amounts to inject at each stie.
MOA — Neuromuscular transmission blockade; inhibits presynaptic acetylcholine release.
ADVERSE EFFECTS — Severe: Anaphylaxis, dysphagia, arrhythmias, myocardial infarction, systemic botulism, death. Frequent: Rash, urticaria, pruritus, flu-like symptoms, excessive weakness, upper respiratory tract infection, neck pain, headache. Periorbital injections may cause ptosis, dry eyes, superficial keratosis, or lacrimation; injections of facial muscles may cause facial asymmetry.

OXYBATE (*Xyrem, GHB, gamma hydroxybutyrate*) ▶L ♀B ▶? ©III $$$$$
WARNING — CNS depressant with abuse potential; avoid concurrent alcohol or sedative use.
ADULT — Cataplexy or excessive daytime sleepiness in narcolepsy: 2.25 g PO at bedtime. Repeat in 2.5 to 4 h. May increase by 1.5 g/day at 2-week intervals to max 9 g/day. Dilute each dose in 60 mL water.
PEDS — Not approved in children.
FORMS — Trade only: Soln 180 mL (500 mg/mL) supplied with measuring device and child-proof dosing cups.
NOTES — Available only through the Xyrem Success Program centralized pharmacy (866-997-3688). Adjust dose in hepatic dysfunction. Prepare doses just prior to bedtime, and use within 24 h. May need an alarm to signal 2nd dose. Contraindicated with sedative-hypnotics. Do not use with alcohol.
MOA — Unknown.
ADVERSE EFFECTS — Serious: Abuse and dependence, depression, syncope, seizures, CNS and respiratory depression, coma. Frequent: Headache, nausea, dizziness, pain, somnolence, pharyngitis, infection, flu-like symptoms, accidental injury, diarrhea, urinary incontinence, confusion, sleepwalking.

RILUZOLE (*Rilutek*) ▶LK ♀C ▶— $$$$$
ADULT — ALS: 50 mg PO q 12 h.
PEDS — Not approved in children.
FORMS — Generic/Trade: Tabs 50 mg.
NOTES — Take 1 h before or 2 h after meals. Monitor LFTs.
MOA — Glutamate antagonist.
ADVERSE EFFECTS — Serious: Tachycardia, hypertension, hepatotoxicity, neutropenia, interstitial lung disease. Frequent: Asthenia, N/V, diarrhea, abdominal pain, pneumonia, dizziness, paresthesia, drowsiness.

TETRABENAZINE (*Xenazine, ✚Nitoman*) ▶L ♀C ▶? $$$$$
WARNING — Contraindicated with untreated or inadequately responding depression or suicidality; monitor closely and discontinue at the first signs thereof.

(cont.)

TETRABENAZINE *(cont.)*

ADULT — Chorea associated with Huntington's disease: Start 12.5 mg PO q am. Increase after 1 week to 12.5 mg PO two times per day. May increase by 12.5 mg/day weekly. For doses greater than 37.5 to 50 mg/day divide doses three times per day. For doses greater than 50 mg/day genotype the patient for CYP2D6 activity, titrate by 12.5 mg/day weekly and divide doses three times per day to max 37.5 mg/dose and 100 mg/day (extensive/intermediate metabolizers) or 25 mg/dose and 50 mg/day (poor metabolizers).

PEDS — Not approved in children.

UNAPPROVED ADULT — Hyperkinetic movement disorders such as tic disorders (including Tourette's syndrome), tardive syndromes, hemiballismus, dystonia, and other choreas (approved dosing in Canada): Start 12.5 mg PO two to three times per day. May increase by 12.5 mg/day q 3 to 5 days to usual dose of 25 mg PO three times per day. Max 200 mg/day, but most patients do not tolerate more than 75 mg/day. Discontinue if there is no benefit after 7 days of treatment at max tolerated dose.

UNAPPROVED PEDS — Limited data suggest that ½ of the adult dose may be used and titrated as tolerated.

FORMS — Trade only: Tabs 12.5, 25 mg.

NOTES — Contraindicated in hepatic impairment, suicidality, untreated/inadequately responding depression, and with MAOIs. Reduce dose by 50% if used with potent CYP2D6 inhibitors. Monitor patient for depression, akathisia, sedation/somnolence, and parkinsonism, which may respond to dose reduction. Retitrate dose if interrupted longer than 5 days. Use caution when combined with antipsychotics and other dopamine receptor blocking agents. May attenuate the effects of levodopa and antidepressants. Increases QTc by approximately 8 msec.

MOA — Depletes monoamines from storage sites.

ADVERSE EFFECTS — Serious: Parkinsonism, cognitive decline, orthostatic hypotension, depression, suicidality, neuroleptic malignant syndrome. Frequent: Drowsiness, fatigue, weakness, anxiety, insomnia, akathisia, sialorrhea, irritability, agitation, N/V, epigastric pain, confusion, disorientation, dizziness.

OB/GYN

EMERGENCY CONTRACEPTION

Emergency contraception within 72 h of unprotected sex.
Progestin-only methods (causes less nausea and may be more effective. Available OTC with no age restriction) : Fallback Solo, Plan B One-Step (levonorgestrel 1.5 mg tab): Take 1 pill. Next Choice (levonorgestrel 0.75 mg): Take 1 tab ASAP and 2nd dose 12 h later.
Progestin and estrogen method : Dose is defined as 2 pills of Ogestrel, 4 pills of Cryselle, Enpresse*, Jolessa, Levora, Lo/Ovral, Low-Ogestrel, Nordette, Portia, Quasense, Seasonale, Seasonique, Solia, or Trivora*, or 5 pills of Aviane, Lessina, LoSeasonique, Lutera, or Sronyx: Take 1 dose ASAP and 2nd dose 12 h later. If vomiting occurs within 1 h of taking dose, consider repeating that dose with an antiemetic 1 h prior.
Emergency contraception within 120 h of unprotected sex. Ella (ulipristal 30 mg): Take 1 pill. More info at: www.not-2-late.com.

*Use 0.125 mg levonorgestrel/30 mcg ethinyl estradiol tabs.

ORAL CONTRACEPTIVES* ▸ L CX

	Estrogen (mcg)	Progestin (mg)
Monophasic		
Lo Loestrin Fe, Lo Minastrin Fe	10 ethinyl estradiol	1 norethindrone
Beyaz, Loryna, Nikki, *Yaz*		3 drospirenone
Aviane, Falmina, Lessina, Lutera, Orsythia, Sronyx		0.1 levonorgestrel
Gildess Fe 1/20, Junel 1/20, Junel Fe 1/20, Larin Fe 1/20, *Loestrin-21 1/20*, Loestrin Fe 1/20, Loestrin-24 Fe, Microgestin 1/20, Microgestin Fe 1/20, Minastrin 24 Fe	20 ethinyl estradiol	1 norethindrone
Generess Fe chewable (generic only)	25 ethinyl estradiol	0.8 norethindrone
Desogen, Emoquette, *Enskyce, Ortho-Cept*		0.15 desogestrel
Safyral, Syeda, *Yasmin*		3 drospirenone
Altavera, Kurvelo, Levora, Marlissa, *Nordette*, Portia	30 ethinyl estradiol	0.15 levonorgestrel
Gildess Fe 1.5/30, 1.5/30, Junel 1.5/30, Junel 1.5/30 Fe, Larin Fe 1.5/30, *Loestrin 1.5/30, Loestrin Fe 1.5/30*, Microgestin 1.5/30, Microgestin Fe 1.5/30		1.5 norethindrone
Cryselle, Elinest, Lo/Ovral		0.3 norgestrel

(cont.)

ORAL CONTRACEPTIVES* ▶ L CX (*continued*)

Kelnor 1/35, *Zovia 1/35E*	35 ethinyl estradiol	1 ethynodiol
Balziva, Briellyn, Femcon Fe, Gildagia, *Ovcon-35*, Philith, Vyfemla		0.4 norethindrone
Brevicon, *Modicon*, Nortrel 0.5/35, Wera		0.5 norethindrone
Alyacen 1/35, Cyclafem 1/35, Dasetta 1/35, Norinyl 1+35, Nortrel 1/35, Norethin 1/35, *Ortho-Novum 1/35*, Pirmella 1/35		1 norethindrone
Estarylla, Mono-Linyah, *Ortho-Cyclen*, Previfem, Sprintec		0.25 norgestimate
Zovia 1/50E	50 ethinyl estradiol	1 ethynodiol
Ogestrel		0.5 norgestrel
Norinyl 1+50	50 mestranol	1 norethindrone
Progestin only		
Camila, Errin, Heather, Jencycla, *Micronor*, Nor-Q.D.	None	0.35 norethindrone
Biphasic (estrogen and progestin contents vary)		
Kariva, *Mircette*, Pimtrea, Viorele	20/10 ethinyl estradiol	0.15 desogestrel
Triphasic (estrogen and progestin contents vary)		
Estrostep Fe, Tri-Legest, Tri-Legest Fe	20/30/35 ethinyl estradiol	1 norethindrone
Cyclessa, Velivet	25 ethinyl estradiol	0.1/0.125/0.150 desogestrel
Ortho Tri-Cyclen Lo		0.18/0.215/0.25 norgestimate
Enpresse, Levonest, Myzilra, *Trivora-28*	30/40/30 ethinyl estradiol	0.5/0.75/0.125 levonorgestrel
Alyacen 7/7/7, Cyclafem 7/7/7, Dasetta 7/7/7, Nortrel 7/7/7, *Ortho-Novum 7/7/7*, Primella 7/7/7	35 ethinyl estradiol	0.5/0.75/1 norethindrone
Aranelle, *Tri-Norinyi*		0.5/1/0.5 norethindrone
Ortho Tri-Cyclen, Tri-Estarylla, Tri- Linyah, Tri-Previfem, Tri-Sprintec		0.18/0.215/0.25 norgestimate
Quadphasic		
Natazia	3 mg/2 mg estradiol valerate	2/3/1 dienogest

ORAL CONTRACEPTIVES* ▶ L CX (*continued*)

Extended Cycle		
Lybrel[†]	20 ethinyl estradiol	0.09 levonorgestrel
LoSeasonique[††]	20/10 ethinyl estradiol	0.1 levonorgestrel
Quartette[††]	20/25/30/10 ethinyl estradiol	0.15 levonorgestrel
Introvale, Quasense, *Seasonale*	30 ethinyl estradiol	
Daysee, Seasonique[††]	30/10 ethinyl estradiol	

*All: Not recommended in smokers. Increases risk of thromboembolism, CVA, MI, hepatic neoplasia, and gallbladder disease. Nausea, breast tenderness, headache and breakthrough bleeding are common transient side effects. Effectiveness reduced by hepatic enzyme-inducing drugs such as certain anticonvulsants and barbiturates, rifampin, rifabutin, griseofulvin, and protease inhibitors. Coadministration with St. John's wort may decrease efficacy. Vomiting or diarrhea may also increase the risk of contraceptive failure. Consider an additional form of birth control in above circumstances. See product insert for instructions on missing doses.

Progestin only: Must be taken at the same time every day. Because much of the literature regarding OC adverse effects pertains mainly to estrogen/progestin combinations, the extent to which progestin-only contraceptives cause these effects is unclear. No significant interaction has been found with broad-spectrum antibiotics. The effect of St. John's wort is unclear. No placebo days, start new pack immediately after finishing current one. Available in 28-day packs. Readers may find the following website useful: www.managingcontraception.com.

[†]Approved for continuous use without a "pill-free" period.
[††]84 active pills and 7 ethinyl estradiol only pills.

DRUGS GENERALLY ACCEPTED AS SAFE IN PREGNANCY (SELECTED)

Analgesics	acetaminophen, codeine*, meperidine*, methadone*, oxycodone*
Antimicrobials	azithromycin, cephalosporins, clotrimazole, erythromycins (not estolate), metronidazole, penicillins, permethrin, nitrofurantoin***, nystatin
Antivirals	acyclovir, famciclovir, valacyclovir
CV	hydralazine*, labetalol, methyldopa, nifedipine
Derm	benzoyl peroxide, clindamycin, erythromycin
Endo	insulin, levothyroxine, liothyronine
ENT	chlorpheniramine, diphenhydramine, dextromethorphan, guaifenesin, nasal steroids, nasal cromolyn
GI	antacids*, bisacodyl, cimetidine, docusate, doxylamine, famotidine, lactulose, loperamide, meclizine, metoclopramide, nizatidine, ondansetron, psyllium, ranitidine, simethicone, trimethobenzamide
Heme	Heparin, low molecular wt heparins
Psych	bupropion, buspirone, desipramine, doxepin
Pulmonary	beclomethasone, budesonide, cromolyn, montelukast, nedocromil, prednisone**, short-acting inhaled beta-2 agonists, theophylline

*Except if used long-term or in high dose at term.
**Except 1st trimester.
***Contraindicated at term and during labor and delivery.

OB/GYN: Contraceptives—Oral Monophasic

NOTE: Not recommended in women greater than 35 yo who smoke or have complex migraine headaches. Increased risk of thromboembolism, CVA, MI, hepatic neoplasia, cervical cancer and gallbladder disease. Increased risk of breast cancer in current and recent users. Nausea, breast tenderness, and breakthrough bleeding are common transient side effects. Nighttime dosing may minimize nausea. Effectiveness is reduced by hepatic enzyme-inducing drugs such as certain anticonvulsants and barbiturates, rifampin, rifabutin, griseofulvin, and protease inhibitors. Additionally, products that contain St John's wort may decrease efficacy. Vomiting or diarrhea may also increase the risk of contraceptive failure. An additional form of birth control may be advisable. Advise patients to take at the same time every day. See PI for instructions on missing doses. Most available in 21 and 28 day packs. Although not approved by the FDA, combined OCPs are used for dysfunctional uterine bleeding, emergency contraception, dysmenorrhea, pelvic pain, and hirsutism (with spironolactone): 1 tab PO daily. Wait 6 weeks postpartum to initiate combination OCPs to decrease the risk of thromboembolism and to support lactation.

AVIANE (ethinyl estradiol + levonorgestrel, *Falmina, Lessina, Orsythia, *Alesse*) ▶L ♀X ▶– $$
ADULT — Contraception: 1 tab PO daily.
PEDS — Not approved in children.
UNAPPROVED ADULT — Emergency contraception: See table.
FORMS — Generic/Trade: Tabs 20 mcg ethinyl estradiol/0.1 mg levonorgestrel.
NOTES — May cause less nausea and breast tenderness and may increase breakthrough bleeding due to lower estrogen content.
MOA — Contraceptive steroid combination.
ADVERSE EFFECTS — Serious: DVT/PE, stroke, MI, hepatic neoplasia, and gallbladder disease. Frequent: Nausea, breast tenderness, and breakthrough bleeding.

AMETHYST (ethinyl estradiol + levonorgestrel) ▶L - ♀X ▶–
ADULT — Contraception: 1 tab PO daily
PEDS — Not approved in children
FORMS — Generic only: Tabs 20 mcg ethinyl estradiol/90 mcg levonorgestrel
NOTES — Approved for continuous use without a "pill-free" period. May cause breakthrough bleeding.
MOA — Contraceptive steroid combination
ADVERSE EFFECTS — Serious: DVT/PE, stroke, MI, hepatic neoplasia, and gallbladder disease. Frequent: Nausea, breast tenderness, and breakthrough bleeding

BEYAZ (ethinyl estradiol + drospirenone + levomefolate calcium) ▶L - ♀X ▶– $$$
ADULT — Contraception, premenstrual dysphoric disorder, acne, folate supplementation. 1 tab PO daily.
PEDS — Not approved in children.
FORMS — Trade only: Tabs 0.02 mg ethinyl estradiol, 2 mg drospirenone, 0.451 mg levomefolate calcium. 24 active pills followed by 4 inert pills.
NOTES — May cause hyperkalemia due to antimineralcorticoid activity of drospirenone (equal to 25 mg spironolactone). Monitor potassium in patients on ACE inhibitors, ARBs. potassium-sparing diuretics, heparin, aldosterone antagonists, and NSAIDs.
MOA — Contraceptive steroid combination.
ADVERSE EFFECTS — Serious: DVT/PE, stroke, MI, hepatic neoplasia, and gallbladder disease. Frequent: Nausea, HA, breast tenderness, and breakthrough bleeding.

FEMCON FE (ethinyl estradiol + norethindrone + ferrous fumarate) ▶L ♀X ▶– $$$
ADULT — Contraception: 1 tab PO daily.
PEDS — Not approved in children.
FORMS — Trade only: Chewable tabs 35 mcg ethinyl estradiol/0.4 mg norethindrone. Placebo tabs are ferrous fumarate 75 mg.
NOTES — Chewable formulation may be swallowed whole or chewed. If chewed, follow with 8 ounces liquid.
MOA — Contraceptive steroid combination.
ADVERSE EFFECTS — Serious: DVT/PE, stroke, MI, hepatic neoplasia, and gallbladder disease. Frequent: Nausea, breast tenderness, and breakthrough bleeding.

GENERESS FE (ethinyl estradiol + norethindrone + ferrous fumarate) ▶L - ♀X ▶–
ADULT — Contraception: 1 tab PO daily.
PEDS — Not approved in children
FORMS — Generic only: Tabs 0.8 mg norethindrone and 25 mcg ethinyl estradiol with 4 days 75 mg ferrous fumarate.
MOA — Contraceptive steroid combination
ADVERSE EFFECTS — Serious: DVT/PE, stroke, MI, hepatic neoplasia, and gallbladder disease. Frequent: Nausea, headache, breast tenderness, dysmenorrhea, wt gain.

LO LOESTRIN FE (norethindrone + ethinyl estradiol + ferrous fumarate, *Lo Minastrin Fe*) ▶L - ♀X ▶–
ADULT — Contraception: 1 tab PO daily.
PEDS — Not approved in children.
FORMS — Trade only: Lo Minastrin Fe is chewable tabs (24) 1 mg norethindrone/10 mcg ethinyl estradiol, tabs (2) 10 mcg ethinyl estradiol and tabs (2) 70 mg ferrous fumarate. Lo Loestrin is same, but not chewable.
MOA — Contraceptive steroid combination.
ADVERSE EFFECTS — Serious: DVT/PE, stroke, MI, hepatic neoplasia and gallbladder disease. Frequent: Nausea, breast tenderness, headache and breakthrough bleeding.

LO/OVRAL-28 (ethinyl estradiol + norgestrel, *Cryselle, Elinest*) ▶L ♀X ▶– $$
ADULT — Contraception: 1 tab PO daily.
PEDS — Not approved in children.
UNAPPROVED ADULT — Emergency contraception: See table.

LO/OVRAL-28 (*cont.*)

FORMS — Generic/Trade: Tabs: 30 mcg ethinyl estradiol/0.3 mg norgestrel.

MOA — Contraceptive steroid combination.

ADVERSE EFFECTS — Serious: DVT/PE, stroke, MI, hepatic neoplasia, and gallbladder disease. Frequent: Nausea, breast tenderness, and breakthrough bleeding.

LOESTRIN 24 FE (ethinyl estradiol + norethindrone + ferrous fumarate) ▶L ♀X ▶– $$$

ADULT — Contraception: 1 tab PO daily.

PEDS — Not approved in children.

FORMS — Generic/Trade: Tabs 1 mg norethindrone/20 mcg ethinyl estradiol (24 days) with 4 days 75 mg ferrous fumarate.

NOTES — Loestrin 24 Fe 1/20 may cause less nausea and breast tenderness and may increase breakthrough bleeding due to lower estrogen content.

MOA — Contraceptive steroid combination.

ADVERSE EFFECTS — Serious: DVT/PE, stroke, MI, hepatic neoplasia, and gallbladder disease. Frequent: Nausea, breast tenderness, and breakthrough bleeding.

LOESTRIN FE (ethinyl estradiol + norethindrone + ferrous fumarate, *Larin Fe 1/20, Gildess Fe 1/20, Junel Fe 1/20, Microgestin Fe 1/20*) ▶L ♀X ▶– $$$

WARNING — Multiple strengths; see FORMS and write specific product on Rx.

ADULT — Contraception: 1 tab PO daily.

PEDS — Not approved in children.

FORMS — Generic/Trade: Tabs 1 mg norethindrone/20 mcg ethinyl estradiol with 7 days 75 mg ferrous fumarate (1/20); 1.5 mg norethindrone/30 mcg ethinyl estradiol with 7 days 75 mg ferrous fumarate (1.5/30).

NOTES — Loestrin Fe 1/20 may cause less nausea and breast tenderness and may increase breakthrough bleeding due to lower estrogen content. All 28 tabs must be taken.

MOA — Contraceptive steroid combination.

ADVERSE EFFECTS — Serious: DVT/PE, stroke, MI, hepatic neoplasia, and gallbladder disease. Frequent: Nausea, breast tenderness, and breakthrough bleeding.

LOESTRIN (ethinyl estradiol + norethindrone, *Junel,* ✷*Minestrin 1/20*) ▶L ♀X ▶– $$$

WARNING — Multiple strengths; see FORMS and write specific product on Rx.

ADULT — Contraception: 1 tab PO daily.

PEDS — Not approved in children.

FORMS — Generic/Trade: Tabs 1 mg norethindrone/20 mcg ethinyl estradiol (Junel 1/20 or Loestrin 1/20). Tabs 1.5 mg norethindrone/30 mcg ethinyl estradiol (Junel 1.5/30, Loestrin 1.5/30 or Microgestin 1.5/30).

NOTES — Loestrin 1/20 may cause less nausea and breast tenderness and may increase breakthrough bleeding due to lower estrogen content.

MOA — Contraceptive steroid combination.

ADVERSE EFFECTS — Serious: DVT/PE, stroke, MI, hepatic neoplasia, and gallbladder disease. Frequent: Nausea, breast tenderness, and breakthrough bleeding.

LOSEASONIQUE (ethinyl estradiol + levonorgestrel) ▶L ♀X ▶– $$$

ADULT — Contraception: 1 tab PO daily.

PEDS — Not approved in children.

FORMS — Generic/Trade: Tabs 20 mcg ethinyl estradiol/0.1 mg levonorgestrel. 84 orange active pills followed by 7 yellow pills with 10 mcg ethinyl estradiol.

NOTES — Decreases menstrual periods from q month to q 3 months; however, intermenstrual bleeding and spotting is more frequent than with 28-day regimens. All 91 tabs must be taken.

MOA — Contraceptive steroid combination.

ADVERSE EFFECTS — Serious: DVT/PE, stroke, MI, hepatic neoplasia, and gallbladder disease. Frequent: Nausea, breast tenderness, and breakthrough bleeding.

LYBREL (ethinyl estradiol + levonorgestrel) ▶L ♀X ▶– $$$

ADULT — Contraception: 1 tab PO daily.

PEDS — Not approved in children.

FORMS — Generic only: Tabs 20 mcg ethinyl estradiol/90 mcg levonorgestrel.

NOTES — Approved for continuous use without a "pill-free" period. May cause breakthrough bleeding.

MOA — Contraceptive steroid combination.

ADVERSE EFFECTS — Serious: DVT/PE, stroke, MI, hepatic neoplasia, and gallbladder disease. Frequent: Nausea, breast tenderness, and breakthrough bleeding.

MINASTRIN 24 (ethinyl estradiol + norethindrone + ferrous fumarate) ▶L - ♀X ▶– $$$

ADULT — Contraception: 1 cap PO daily.

PEDS — Not approved in children.

FORMS — Trade only. Caps 1 mg norethindrone/20 mcg ethinyl estradiol with 4 days ferrous fumarate.

NOTES — Similar to Microgestin Fe 1/20.

MOA — Contraceptive steroid combination.

ADVERSE EFFECTS — Serious: DVT/PE, stroke, MI, HTN, hepatic neoplasia. Frequent:headache, nausea, spotting, breast tenderness, acne, mood swings, and wt gain.

MODICON (ethinyl estradiol + norethindrone, *Brevicon, Nortrel 0.5/35, Wera*) ▶L ♀X ▶– $$$

ADULT — Contraception: 1 tab PO daily.

PEDS — Not approved in children.

FORMS — Generic/Trade: Tabs 35 mcg ethinyl estradiol/0.5 mg norethindrone.

MOA — Contraceptive steroid combination.

ADVERSE EFFECTS — Serious: DVT/PE, stroke, MI, hepatic neoplasia, and gallbladder disease. Frequent: Nausea, breast tenderness, and breakthrough bleeding.

NORDETTE (ethinyl estradiol + levonorgestrel, *Altavera, Kurvelo, Levora, Marlissa, Portia,* ✷*Min-Ovral*) ▶L ♀X ▶– $$$

ADULT — Contraception: 1 tab PO daily.

PEDS — Not approved in children.

UNAPPROVED ADULT — Emergency contraception: See table.

FORMS — Generic/Trade: Tabs 30 mcg ethinyl estradiol/0.15 mg levonorgestrel.

NORDETTE (*cont.*)

MOA — Contraceptive steroid combination.

ADVERSE EFFECTS — Serious: DVT/PE, stroke, MI, hepatic neoplasia, and gallbladder disease. Frequent: Nausea, breast tenderness, and breakthrough bleeding.

NORETHINDRONE (*Micronor, Nor-Q.D., Camila, Errin, Heather, Jencycla*) ▶L ♀C ▶+

ADULT — Contraception: 1 tab daily

FORMS — Generic/Trade: Tabs 0.35mg

NOTES — Progestin-only pills are often called the "mini-pill."

MOA — Multicausal: Inhibitory cervical mucus, FSH/LH suppression, abnormal ovulation and endometrial changes unfavourable to implantation.

ADVERSE EFFECTS — Frequent: Menstrual irregularity, headache, breast tenderness, nausea, and dizziness.

NORINYL 1+50 (mestranol + norethindrone) ▶L ♀X ▶– $$

ADULT — Contraception: 1 tab PO daily.

PEDS — Not approved in children.

FORMS — Trade only: Tabs 1 mg norethindrone/50 mcg mestranol.

NOTES — 50 mcg estrogen component rarely necessary.

MOA — Contraceptive steroid combination.

ADVERSE EFFECTS — Serious: DVT/PE, stroke, MI, hepatic neoplasia, and gallbladder disease. Frequent: Nausea, breast tenderness, and breakthrough bleeding.

OGESTREL (ethinyl estradiol + norgestrel) ▶L ♀X ▶– $$

ADULT — Contraception: 1 tab PO daily.

PEDS — Not approved in children.

UNAPPROVED ADULT — Emergency contraception : See table.

FORMS — Trade only: Tabs: 50 mcg ethinyl estradiol/0.5 mg norgestrel.

NOTES — 50 mcg estrogen component rarely necessary.

MOA — Contraceptive steroid combination.

ADVERSE EFFECTS — Serious: DVT/PE, stroke, MI, hepatic neoplasia, and gallbladder disease. Frequent: Nausea, breast tenderness, and breakthrough bleeding.

ORTHO CYCLEN (ethinyl estradiol + norgestimate, *Estarylla, Mono-Linyah, Previfem, Sprintec, ✦Cyclen*) ▶L ♀X ▶– $$

ADULT — Contraception: 1 tab PO daily.

PEDS — Not approved in children.

FORMS — Generic/Trade: Tabs 35 mcg ethinyl estradiol/0.25 mg norgestimate.

MOA — Contraceptive steroid combination.

ADVERSE EFFECTS — Serious: DVT/PE, stroke, MI, hepatic neoplasia, and gallbladder disease. Frequent: Nausea, breast tenderness, and breakthrough bleeding.

ORTHO-CEPT (ethinyl estradiol + desogestrel, *Desogen, Emoquette, Enskyce, ✦Marvelon*) ▶L ♀X ▶– $$$

ADULT — Contraception: 1 tab PO daily.

PEDS — Not approved in children.

FORMS — Generic/Trade: Tabs 30 mcg ethinyl estradiol/0.15 mg desogestrel.

MOA — Contraceptive steroid combination.

ADVERSE EFFECTS — Serious: DVT/PE, stroke, MI, hepatic neoplasia, and gallbladder disease. Frequent: Nausea, breast tenderness, and breakthrough bleeding.

ORTHO-NOVUM 1/35 (ethinyl estradiol + norethindrone, *Alyacen 1/35, Cyclafem 1/35, Dasetta 1/35, Norinyl 1+35, Nortrel 1/35, Pirmella 1/35*) ▶L ♀X ▶– $$$

ADULT — Contraception: 1 tab PO daily.

PEDS — Not approved in children.

FORMS — Generic/Trade: Tabs 1 mg norethindrone/35 mcg ethinyl estradiol.

MOA — Contraceptive steroid combination.

ADVERSE EFFECTS — Serious: DVT/PE, stroke, MI, hepatic neoplasia, and gallbladder disease. Frequent: Nausea, breast tenderness, and breakthrough bleeding.

OVCON-35 (ethinyl estradiol + norethindrone, *Balziva, Briellyn, Gildagia, Philith, Vyfemla*) ▶L ♀X ▶– $$$

ADULT — Contraception: 1 tab PO daily.

PEDS — Not approved in children.

FORMS — Generic/Trade: Tabs 35 mcg ethinyl estradiol/0.4 mg norethindrone.

MOA — Contraceptive steroid combination.

ADVERSE EFFECTS — Serious: DVT/PE, stroke, MI, hepatic neoplasia, and gallbladder disease. Frequent: Nausea, breast tenderness, and breakthrough bleeding.

SAFYRAL (ethinyl estradiol + drospirenone + levomefolate calcium) ▶L - ♀C ▶– ©V

ADULT — Contraception and folate supplementation 1 tab PO daily

PEDS — Not approved in children

FORMS — Trade only: Tabs 0.03 mg ethinyl estradiol, 3 mg drospirenone, 0.451 mg levomefolate calcium. 24 active pills are followed by 4 inert pills.

NOTES — May cause hyperkalemia due to antimineralcorticoid activity of drospirenone (equal to 25 mg spironolactone). Monitor potassium in patients on ACE inhibitors, ARBs, potassium-sparing diuretics, heparin, aldosterone antagonists, and NSAIDs. NOTE: Similar to Yasmin.

MOA — Contraceptive steroid combination

ADVERSE EFFECTS — Serious: DVT/PE, stroke, MI, hepatic neoplasia, and gallbladder disease. Frequent: Nausea, headache, breast tenderness, and breakthrough bleeding.

SEASONALE (ethinyl estradiol + levonorgestrel, *Introvale, Quasense*) ▶L ♀X ▶– $$$

ADULT — Contraception: 1 tab PO daily.

PEDS — Not approved in children.

UNAPPROVED ADULT — Emergency contraception: See table.

FORMS — Generic/Trade: Tabs 30 mcg ethinyl estradiol/0.15 mg levonorgestrel. 84 pink active pills followed by 7 white placebo pills.

SEASONALE (*cont.*)

NOTES — Decreases menstrual periods from q month to q 3 months; however, intermenstrual bleeding and spotting is more frequent than with 28-day regimens.
MOA — Contraceptive steroid combination.
ADVERSE EFFECTS — Serious: DVT/PE, stroke, MI, hepatic neoplasia, and gallbladder disease. Frequent: Nausea, breast tenderness, and breakthrough bleeding.

SEASONIQUE (**ethinyl estradiol + levonorgestrel**, *Daysee*) ▶L ♀X ▶– $$$
ADULT — Contraception: 1 tab PO daily.
PEDS — Not approved in children.
UNAPPROVED ADULT — Emergency contraception: See table.
FORMS — Generic/Trade: Tabs 30 mcg ethinyl estradiol/0.15 mg levonorgestrel. 84 active pills followed by 7 pills with 10 mcg ethinyl estradiol.
NOTES — Decreases menstrual periods from q month to q 3 months; however, intermenstrual bleeding and spotting is more frequent than with 28-day regimens. All 91 tabs must be taken.
MOA — Contraceptive steroid combination.
ADVERSE EFFECTS — Serious: DVT/PE, stroke, MI, hepatic neoplasia, and gallbladder disease. Frequent: Nausea, breast tenderness, and breakthrough bleeding.

YASMIN (**ethinyl estradiol + drospirenone**, *Syeda*) ▶L ♀X ▶– $$$
ADULT — Contraception: 1 tab PO daily.
PEDS — Not approved in children.
FORMS — Generic/Trade: Tabs 30 mcg ethinyl estradiol/3 mg drospirenone.
NOTES — May cause hyperkalemia due to antimineralocorticoid activity of drospirenone (equal to 25 mg spironolactone). Monitor potassium in patients on ACE inhibitors, ARBs, potassium-sparing diuretics, heparin, aldosterone antagonists, and NSAIDs. Safyral also contains levomefolate 0.451mg in all tabs.
MOA — Contraceptive steroid combination.
ADVERSE EFFECTS — Serious: DVT/PE, stroke, MI, hepatic neoplasia, and gallbladder disease. Frequent: Nausea, breast tenderness, and breakthrough bleeding.

YAZ (**ethinyl estradiol + drospirenone**, *Loryna, Nikki*) ▶L ♀X ▶– $$$
ADULT — Contraception, premenstrual dysphoric disorder, acne: 1 tab PO daily.
PEDS — Not approved in children.
FORMS — Generic/Trade: Tabs 20 mcg ethinyl estradiol/3 mg drospirenone. 24 active pills are followed by 4 inert pills.
NOTES — May cause hyperkalemia due to antimineralocorticoid activity of drospirenone (equal to 25 mg spironolactone). Monitor potassium in patients on ACE inhibitors, ARBs, potassium-sparing diuretics, heparin, aldosterone antagonists, and NSAIDs.
MOA — Contraceptive steroid combination.
ADVERSE EFFECTS — Serious: DVT/PE, stroke, MI, hepatic neoplasia, and gallbladder disease. Frequent: Nausea, breast tenderness, and breakthrough bleeding.

ZOVIA 1/35 (**ethinyl estradiol + ethynodiol**, *Kelnor 1/35*) ▶L - ♀X ▶–
WARNING — Multiple strengths; See Forms and write specific product on Rx.
ADULT — Contraception: 1 tab PO daily.
PEDS — Not approved in children.
FORMS — Generic/Trade: Tabs 1 mg ethynodiol/35 mcg ethinyl estradiol. Also available as Zovia 1/50E.
MOA — Contraceptive steroid combination.
ADVERSE EFFECTS — Serious: DVT/PD, stroke, MI, hepatic neoplasia, and gallbladder disease. Frequent: Nausea, breast tenderness, and breakthrough bleeding.

ZOVIA 1/50E (**ethinyl estradiol + ethynodiol**) ▶L ♀X ▶– $$
WARNING — Multiple strengths; see FORMS and write specific product on Rx.
ADULT — Contraception: 1 tab PO daily.
PEDS — Not approved in children.
FORMS — Trade only: Tabs 1 mg ethynodiol/50 mcg ethinyl estradiol. Also available as Zovia 1/35.
NOTES — 50 mcg estrogen component rarely necessary.
MOA — Contraceptive steroid combination.
ADVERSE EFFECTS — Serious: DVT/PE, stroke, MI, hepatic neoplasia, and gallbladder disease. Frequent: Nausea, breast tenderness, and breakthrough bleeding.

OB/GYN: Contraceptives—Oral Biphasic

NOTE: Not recommended in women greater than 35 yo who smoke or have complex migraine headaches. Increased risk of thromboembolism, CVA, MI, hepatic neoplasia, and gallbladder disease. Nausea, breast tenderness, and breakthrough bleeding are common transient side effects. Nighttime dosing may minimize nausea. Effectiveness is reduced by hepatic enzyme-inducing drugs such as certain anticonvulsants and barbiturates, rifampin, rifabutin, griseofulvin and protease inhibitors. Additionally, products that contain St. John's wort may decrease efficacy. Vomiting or diarrhea may also increase the risk of contraceptive failure. An additional form of birth control may be advisable. Advise patients to take at the same time every day. See PI for instructions on missing doses. Most available in 21 and 28 day packs. Although not approved by the FDA, combined OCPs are used for dysfunctional uterine bleeding, dysmenorrhea, pelvic pain, and hirsutism (with spironolactone): 1 tab PO daily. Wait 6 weeks postpartum to initiate combination OCPs to decrease the risk of thromboembolism and to support lactation.

MIRCETTE (ethinyl estradiol + desogestrel, *Kariva, Pimtera, Viorele*) ▶L ♀X ▶– $$$
ADULT — Contraception: 1 tab PO daily.
PEDS — Not approved in children.
FORMS — Generic/Trade: Tabs 20 mcg ethinyl estradiol/0.15 mg desogestrel (21), 10 mcg ethinyl estradiol (5).

NOTES — May have less breakthrough bleeding. All 28 tabs must be taken.
MOA — Contraceptive steroid combination.
ADVERSE EFFECTS — Serious: DVT/PE, stroke, MI, hepatic neoplasia, and gallbladder disease. Frequent: Nausea, breast tenderness, and breakthrough bleeding.

OB/GYN: Contraceptives—Oral Triphasic

NOTE: Not recommended in women greater than 35 yo who smoke. Increased risk of thromboembolism, CVA, MI, hepatic neoplasia, and gallbladder disease. Nausea, breast tenderness, and breakthrough bleeding are common transient side effects. Nighttime dosing may minimize nausea. Effectiveness is reduced by hepatic enzyme-inducing drugs such as certain anticonvulsants and barbiturates, rifampin, rifabutin, griseofulvin, and protease inhibitors. Additionally, products that contain St John's wort may decrease efficacy. Vomiting or diarrhea may also increase the risk of contraceptive failure. An additional form of birth control may be advisable. Advise patients to take at the same time every day. See PI for instructions on missing doses. Most available in 21- and 28-day packs. Although not approved by the FDA, combined OCPs are used for dysfunctional uterine bleeding, emergency contraception, dysmenorrhea, pelvic pain, and hirsutism (with spironolactone): 1 tab PO daily. Wait 6 weeks postpartum to initiate combination OCPs to decrease the risk of thromboembolism and to support lactation.

CYCLESSA (ethinyl estradiol + desogestrel, *Velivet*) ▶L ♀X ▶– $$
ADULT — Contraception: 1 tab PO daily.
PEDS — Not approved in children.
FORMS — Generic/Trade: Tabs 25 mcg ethinyl estradiol/0.100 (7), 0.125 (7), 0.150 mg desogestrel (7).
MOA — Contraceptive steroid combination.
ADVERSE EFFECTS — Serious: DVT/PE, stroke, MI, hepatic neoplasia, and gallbladder disease. Frequent: Nausea, breast tenderness, and breakthrough bleeding.

ESTROSTEP FE (ethinyl estradiol + norethindrone + ferrous fumarate, *Tri-Legest Fe*) ▶L ♀X ▶– $$$
ADULT — Contraception: 1 tab PO daily.
PEDS — Not approved in children.
FORMS — Generic/Trade: Tabs 20, 30, 35 mcg ethinyl estradiol/1 mg norethindrone + "placebo" tabs with 75 mg ferrous fumarate. Packs of 28 only.
NOTES — All 28 tabs must be taken.
MOA — Contraceptive steroid combination.
ADVERSE EFFECTS — Serious: DVT/PE, stroke, MI, hepatic neoplasia, and gallbladder disease. Frequent: Nausea, breast tenderness, and breakthrough bleeding.

ORTHO TRI-CYCLEN LO (ethinyl estradiol + norgestimate) ▶L ♀X ▶– $$$
ADULT — Contraception: 1 tab PO daily.
PEDS — Not approved in children.
FORMS — Generic/Trade: Tabs 25 mcg ethinyl estradiol/0.18 (7), 0.215 (7), 0.25 mg norgestimate (7).
MOA — Contraceptive steroid combination.
ADVERSE EFFECTS — Serious: DVT/PE, stroke, MI, hepatic neoplasia, and gallbladder disease. Frequent: Nausea, breast tenderness, and breakthrough bleeding.

ORTHO TRI-CYCLEN (ethinyl estradiol + norgestimate, *Tri-Estarylla, Tri-Linyah, Tri-Previfem, Tri-Sprintec, ✱Tri-Cyclen*) ▶L ♀X ▶– $$
ADULT — Contraception, adult acne: 1 tab PO daily.
PEDS — Not approved in children.

FORMS — Generic/Trade: Tabs 35 mcg ethinyl estradiol/0.18 (7), 0.215 (7), 0.25 mg norgestimate (7).
MOA — Contraceptive steroid combination.
ADVERSE EFFECTS — Serious: DVT/PE, stroke, MI, hepatic neoplasia, and gallbladder disease. Frequent: Nausea, breast tenderness, and breakthrough bleeding.

ORTHO-NOVUM 7/7/7 (ethinyl estradiol + norethindrone, *Alyacen 7/7/7, Cyclafem 7/7/7, Dasetta 7/7/7, Nortrel 7/7/7, Pirmela 7/7/7*) ▶L ♀X ▶– $$
ADULT — Contraception: 1 tab PO daily.
PEDS — Not approved in children.
FORMS — Generic/Trade: Tabs 35 mcg ethinyl estradiol/0.5, 0.75, 1 mg norethindrone.
MOA — Contraceptive steroid combination.
ADVERSE EFFECTS — Serious: DVT/PE, stroke, MI, hepatic neoplasia, and gallbladder disease. Frequent: Nausea, breast tenderness, and breakthrough bleeding.

TRI-LEGEST (ethinyl estradiol + norethindrone) ▶L ♀X ▶– $$$
ADULT — Contraception: 1 tab PO daily.
PEDS — Not approved in children.
FORMS — Trade only: Tabs 20, 30, 35 mcg ethinyl estradiol/1 mg norethindrone.
MOA — Contraceptive steroid combination.
ADVERSE EFFECTS — Serious: DVT/PE, stroke, MI, hepatic neoplasia, and gallbladder disease. Frequent: Nausea, breast tenderness, and breakthrough bleeding.

TRI-NORINYL (ethinyl estradiol + norethindrone, *Aranelle, ✱Synphasic*) ▶L ♀X ▶– $$
ADULT — Contraception: 1 tab PO daily.
PEDS — Not approved in children.
FORMS — Generic/Trade: Tabs 35 mcg ethinyl estradiol/0.5, 1, 0.5 mg norethindrone.
MOA — Contraceptive steroid combination.
ADVERSE EFFECTS — Serious: DVT/PE, stroke, MI, hepatic neoplasia, and gallbladder disease. Frequent: Nausea, breast tenderness, and breakthrough bleeding.

TRIVORA-28 (ethinyl estradiol + levonorgestrel, *Enpresse, Levonest, Myzilra*) ▶L ♀X ▶– $$
ADULT — Contraception: 1 tab PO daily.
PEDS — Not approved in children.
UNAPPROVED ADULT — Emergency contraception: See table.

FORMS — Generic/Trade: Tabs 30, 40, 30 mcg ethinyl estradiol/0.05, 0.075, 0.125 mg levonorgestrel.
MOA — Contraceptive steroid combination.
ADVERSE EFFECTS — Serious: DVT/PE, stroke, MI, hepatic neoplasia, and gallbladder disease. Frequent: Nausea, breast tenderness, and breakthrough bleeding.

OB/GYN: Contraceptives—Oral 4-Phasic

NATAZIA (estradiol valerate and estradiol valerate + dienogest) ▶L - stomach ♀X ▶–
ADULT — Contraception 1 PO daily, start on day 1 of menstrual cycle. Heavy menstrual bleeding 1 PO daily.
PEDS — Not approved in children.
FORMS — Trade only: Tabs 3 mg estradiol valerate (2), 2 mg estradiol valerate/2 mg dienogest (5), 2 mg estradiol valerate/3 mg dienogest (17), 1 mg estradiol valerate (2), inert (2).
NOTES — Not evaluated in BMI greater than 30. Tablets must be taken as directed on blister pack.
MOA — Contraceptive steroid combination.
ADVERSE EFFECTS — Serious: DVT, MI, hepatic. Frequent: HA, irregular bleeding, breast changes, nausea/vomiting, acne, inc. weight.

QUARTETTE (levonorgestrel + ethinyl estradiol) ▶L - ♀X ▶–
ADULT — Contraception: 1 tab PO daily.
PEDS — Not approved in children.
FORMS — Trade only: 91 tabs per pack. (42) 0.15 mg levonorgestrel/20 mcg ethinyl estradiol, (21) 0.15 mg levonorgestrel/25 mcg ethinyl estradiol, (21) 0.15 levonorgestrel/30 mcg ethinyl estradiol, (7) 10 mcg ethinyl estradiol.
NOTES — All 91 tabs must be taken.
MOA — Contraceptive steroid combination.
ADVERSE EFFECTS — Serious: CVT/PE, stroke, MI, hepatic necrosis, and gallbladder disease. Frequent: nausea, headache, breast tenderness, irregular bleeding.

OB/GYN: Contraceptives—Other

ETONOGESTREL (*Implanon, Nexplanon*) ▶L ♀X ▶+ $$$$$
WARNING — Increased risk of thromboembolism and CVA. Effectiveness may be reduced by hepatic enzyme-inducing drugs such as certain anticonvulsants, barbiturates, griseofulvin, rifampin. Additionally, products that contain St John's wort may decrease efficacy; an additional form of birth control may be advisable.
ADULT — Contraception: 1 subdermal implant q 3 years. Specific timing for implantation after other contraceptive methods.
PEDS — Not approved in children.
FORMS — Trade only: Single rod implant, 68 mg etonogestrel. Nexplanon also contains 15mg Barium Sulfate
NOTES — Not studied in women greater than 130% of ideal body wt; may be less effective if overweight. Implant should be palpable immediately after insertion.
MOA — Contraceptive progestin.
ADVERSE EFFECTS — Serious: DVT/PE, stroke. Common: HA, weight gain, vaginitis, bleeding irregularities, depression, liver disease.
LEVONORGESTREL (*Plan B, Next Choice*) ▶L ♀X ▶+ – $$
ADULT — Emergency contraception: 1 tab PO ASAP but within 72 h of intercourse. 2nd tab 12 h later.
PEDS — Not approved in children.
UNAPPROVED ADULT — 2 tabs (1.5 mg) PO ASAP but within 72 h of intercourse (lesser efficacy at up to 120 h).
FORMS — OTC Trade Only: Kit contains 2 tabs 0.75 mg. Rx: Generic/Trade: Kit contains 2 tabs 0.75mg.

NOTES — OTC if at least 17 yo; Rx if younger. Nausea uncommon; however, if vomiting occurs within 1 h, initial dose must be given again. Consider adding an antiemetic. Patients should be instructed to then contact their healthcare providers. Can be used at any time during the menstrual cycle.
MOA — Gonadal steroid.
ADVERSE EFFECTS — Serious: None. Frequent: Menstrual changes, nausea, abdominal pain, fatigue.
LEVONORGESTREL— INTRAUTERINE (*Skyla,* ✻*Jaydess*) ▶L - ♀X ▶+
WARNING — Increased risk of perforation if inserted into lactating women or post-partum women with fixed retroverted uterus.
ADULT — Contraception: 1 intrauterine system q 3 years.
PEDS — Not approved in children.
FORMS — Trade only: Single intrauterine implant, 13.5 mg levonorgestrel.
NOTES — Skyla can only be scanned by MRI under specific conditions.
MOA — Contraceptive steroid
ADVERSE EFFECTS — Serious: Endometrial perforation, ovarian cysts, sepsis. Frequent: bleeding irregularities, vulvovaginitis, abdominal/pelvic pain, acne/seborrhea, ovarian cyst and headache.
LEVONORGESTREL-SINGLE DOSE (*Plan B One-Step, Next Choice One-Step, Fallback Solo*) ▶L ♀X ▶– $$
ADULT — Emergency contraception: 1 tab PO ASAP but within 72 h of intercourse.
PEDS — Not approved in children.
FORMS — OTC Trade only: Tabs 1.5 mg.

LEVONORGESTREL-SINGLE DOSE (*cont.*)

NOTES — OTC if at least 17 yo; Rx if younger. Nausea uncommon; however, if vomiting occurs within 1 h, initial dose must be given again. Consider adding an antiemetic. Patients should be instructed to then contact their healthcare providers. Can be used at any time during the menstrual cycle. Lesser efficacy at up to 120 h.

MOA — Gonadal steroid.

ADVERSE EFFECTS — Serious: None. Frequent: None.

LEVONORGESTREL—INTRAUTERINE (*Mirena*) ▶L - ♀X ▶+

WARNING — Increased risk of perforation if inserted into lactating women or post-postpartum women with fixed retroverted uterus.

ADULT — Contraception: 1 intrauterine system q 5 years.

PEDS — Not approved in children.

FORMS — Trade only: Single intrauterine implant. 25 mg levonorgestrel.

MOA — Contraceptive steroid.

ADVERSE EFFECTS — Serious: Endometrial perforation, ovarian cysts, sepsis. Frequent: bleeding irregularities, mood changes, abdominal/pelvic pain, acne and headache.

NUVARING (ethinyl estradiol + etonogestrel vaginal ring) ▶L ♀X ▶– $$$

ADULT — Contraception: 1 ring intravaginally for 3 weeks each month.

PEDS — Not approved in children.

FORMS — Trade only: Flexible intravaginal ring, 15 mcg ethinyl estradiol/0.120 mg etonogestrel/day in 1, 3 rings/box.

NOTES — Insert on day 5 of cycle or within 7 days of the last oral contraceptive pill. The ring must remain in place continuously for 3 weeks, including during intercourse. Remove for 1 week, then insert a new ring. May be used continuously for 4 weeks and replaced immediately to skip a withdrawal week. Store at room temperature (59° to 86°F) for up to 4 months. In case of accidental removal, reinsert ASAP after rinsing with cool to lukewarm water. If removal is greater than 3 h, use backup method until ring in place for at least 7 days.

MOA — Contraceptive steroid combination.

ADVERSE EFFECTS — Serious: DVT/PE, stroke, MI, hepatic neoplasia, and gallbladder disease. Frequent: Nausea, breast tenderness, breakthrough bleeding, asymptomatic vaginal discharge.

ORTHO EVRA (ethinyl estradiol + norelgestromin, *Xulane*, *Evra*) ▶L ♀X ▶– $$$

WARNING — Average estrogen concentration 60% higher than common oral contraceptives (ie, 35 mcg ethinyl estradiol), which may further increase the risk of thromboembolism.

ADULT — Contraception: 1 patch q week for 3 weeks, then 1 week patch-free.

PEDS — Not approved in children.

FORMS — Trade only: Transdermal patch: 150 mcg norelgestromin/20 mcg ethinyl estradiol/day in 1, 3 patches/box.

NOTES — May be less effective in women 90 kg or greater (198 lbs). Apply new patch on the same day each week. Do not exceed 7 days between patches. Rotate application sites, avoid the waistline. Do not use earlier than 4 weeks postpartum if not breastfeeding.

MOA — Contraceptive steroid combination.

ADVERSE EFFECTS — Serious: DVT/PE, stroke, MI, hepatic neoplasia, and gallbladder disease. Frequent: Nausea, breast tenderness, breakthrough bleeding.

ULIPRISTAL ACETATE (*Ella*) ▶L ♀X ▶?

ADULT — Emergency contraception. 1 tab PO ASAP within 5 days of intercourse.

PEDS — Safety and efficacy are expected to be the same for postpubertal adolescents less than 18 years as for adults.

FORMS — Trade only: Tabs 30 mg.

NOTES — If vomiting occurs within 3 h of administration, consider repeating the dose. Can be used at any time during menstrual cycle. Canadian-only Fibristal has different indication and dose.

MOA — Progesterone receptor modulator causes delay of ovulation with possible changes to endometrium to affect implantation.

ADVERSE EFFECTS — Headache, nausea, abdominal pain, acne.

OB/GYN: Estrogens

NOTE: See also Hormone Combinations. Unopposed estrogens increase the risk of endometrial cancer in postmenopausal women. Malignancy should be ruled out in cases of persistent or recurrent abnormal vaginal bleeding. In women with an intact uterus, a progestin should be administered daily throughout the month or for the last 10 to 12 days of the month. Do not use during pregnancy. May increase the risk of DVT/PE, gallbladder disease. Interactions with oral anticoagulants, certain anticonvulsants, rifampin, barbiturates, corticosteroids, and St. John's wort. Estrogens should not be used in the prevention of cardiovascular disease. In the Women's Health Initiative, the use of conjugated estrogens (Premarin) caused an increase in the risk of CVA and PE. Additionally, the combination with medroxyprogesterone increased the risk of breast cancer and MI. Women greater than 65 yo with 4 years of therapy had an increased risk of dementia. Estrogens should be prescribed at the lowest effective doses and for the shortest durations. Patients should be counseled regarding the risks/benefits of HRT.

BIEST (*estradiol + estriol*) ▶L ♀X ▶– $$$

WARNING — For topical dosages: Patient should take precautions to ensure that children and pets do not make contact with skin where topical estrogen has been applied.

BIEST (*cont.*)

UNAPPROVED ADULT — Hormone replacement therapy. Once or twice a day dosing.

FORMS — Must be compounded by a pharmacist. Most common estriol/estradiol ratios 80%/20% or 50%/50%. May be formulated as cream, gel, troche, or capsule.

NOTES — Compounded bioidentical hormones are not FDA approved. These products should be considered to have the same safety issues raised by the Women's Health Initiative as those associated with hormone therapy agents that are FDA approved.

MOA — Gonadal steroid

ADVERSE EFFECTS — Serious: Endometrial cancer, DVT/PE, gallbladder disease, breast cancer, MI, CVA. Frequent: Nausea, breast tenderness.

ESTERIFIED ESTROGENS (*Menest*) ▶L ♀X ▶– $$

ADULT — Moderate to severe menopausal vasomotor symptoms: 1.25 mg PO daily. Atrophic vaginitis: 0.3 to 1.25 mg PO daily. Female hypogonadism: 2.5 to 7.5 mg PO daily in divided doses for 20 days followed by a 10-day rest period. Repeat until bleeding occurs. Bilateral oophorectomy and ovarian failure: 1.25 mg PO daily. Prevention of postmenopausal osteoporosis: 0.3 to 1.25 mg PO daily.

PEDS — Not approved in children.

FORMS — Trade only: Tabs 0.3, 0.625, 1.25, 2.5 mg.

NOTES — Typical hormone replacement regimen consists of a daily estrogen dose with a progestin added either daily or for the last 10 to 12 days of the cycle.

MOA — Gonadal steroid.

ADVERSE EFFECTS — Serious: Endometrial cancer, DVT/PE, gallbladder disease, breast cancer, MI, CVA. Frequent: Nausea, breast tenderness.

ESTRADIOL (*Estrace, Gynodiol*) ▶L ♀X ▶– $

ADULT — Moderate to severe menopausal vasomotor symptoms and atrophic vaginitis, female hypogonadism, bilateral oophorectomy and ovarian failure: 1 to 2 mg PO daily. Prevention of postmenopausal osteoporosis: 0.5 mg PO daily.

PEDS — Not approved in children.

FORMS — Generic/Trade: Tabs, micronized 0.5, 1, 2 mg, scored. Trade only: 1.5 mg (Gynodiol).

NOTES — Typical hormone replacement regimen consists of a daily estrogen dose with a progestin added either daily or for the last 10 to 12 days of the cycle.

MOA — Gonadal steroid.

ADVERSE EFFECTS — Serious: Endometrial cancer, DVT/PE, gallbladder disease, breast cancer, MI, CVA. Frequent: Nausea, breast tenderness.

ESTRADIOL ACETATE (*Femtrace*) ▶L ♀X ▶– $$

ADULT — Moderate to severe menopausal vasomotor symptoms: 0.45 to 1.8 mg PO daily.

PEDS — Not approved in children.

FORMS — Trade only: Tabs, 0.45, 0.9, 1.8 mg.

NOTES — Typical hormone replacement regimen consists of a daily estrogen dose with a progestin added either daily or for the last 10 to 12 days of the cycle.

MOA — Gonadal steroid.

ADVERSE EFFECTS — Serious: Endometrial cancer, DVT/PE, gallbladder disease, breast cancer, MI, CVA. Frequent: Nausea, breast tenderness.

ESTRADIOL ACETATE VAGINAL RING (*Femring*) ▶L ♀X ▶– $$$

WARNING — A few cases of toxic shock syndrome have been reported. Bowel obstruction.

ADULT — Menopausal vasomotor symptoms or vaginal atrophy: Insert ring into the vagina and replace after 90 days.

PEDS — Not approved in children.

FORMS — Trade only: 0.05 mg/day and 0.1 mg/day.

NOTES — Should the ring fall out or be removed during the 90-day period, rinse in lukewarm water and re-insert. Ring adhesion to vaginal wall has been reported, making removal difficult.

MOA — Gonadal steroid.

ADVERSE EFFECTS — Serious: Toxic shock, bowel obstruction. Frequent: Breast tenderness, breakthrough bleeding.

ESTRADIOL CYPIONATE (*Depo-Estradiol*) ▶L ♀X ▶– – $

WARNING — When estrogen is prescribed for a woman with a uterus, progestin should also be initiated to reduce the risk of endometrial cancer.

ADULT — Moderate to severe menopausal vasomotor symptoms: 1 to 5 mg IM q 3 to 4 weeks. Female hypogonadism: 1.5 to 2 mg IM q month.

PEDS — Not approved in children.

FORMS — Trade only: Injection 5mg/ml in 5ml vials.

MOA — Gonadal steroid.

ADVERSE EFFECTS — Serious: Endometrial cancer, DVT/PE, gallbladder disease, breast cancer, MI, CVA. Frequent: Nausea, breast tenderness.

ESTRADIOL GEL (*Divigel, Estrogel, Elestrin*) ▶L ♀X ▶– $$$

WARNING — Patient should take precautions to ensure that children and pets do not make contact with skin where topical estradiol has been applied.

ADULT — Moderate to severe menopausal vasomotor symptoms and atrophic vaginitis: Thinly apply contents of 1 complete pump depression to one entire arm, from wrist to shoulder (Estrogel) or upper arm (Elestrin) or contents of 1 foil packet to left or right upper thigh on alternating days. Allow to dry completely before dressing. Wash both hands thoroughly after application.

PEDS — Not approved in children.

FORMS — Trade only: Gel 0.06% in nonaerosol, metered-dose pump with #64 or #32 1.25 g doses (Estrogel), #100 0.87 g doses (Elestrin). Gel 0.1% in single-dose foil packets of 0.25, 0.5, 1.0 g, carton of 30 (Divigel).

NOTES — Depress the pump 2 times to prime. Concomitant sunscreen may increase absorption. Typical hormone replacement regimen consists of a daily estrogen dose with a progestin added either daily or for the last 10 to 12 days of the cycle.

MOA — Gonadal steroid.

ESTRADIOL GEL (*cont.*)

ADVERSE EFFECTS — Serious: Endometrial cancer, DVT/PE, gallbladder disease, breast cancer, MI, CVA. Frequent: Nausea, breast tenderness, rash.

ESTRADIOL TOPICAL EMULSION (*Estrasorb*) ▶L ♀X ▶– $$

WARNING — Patient should take precautions to ensure that children and pets do not make contact with skin where topical estradiol has been applied.

ADULT — Moderate to severe menopausal vasomotor symptoms: Apply entire contents of 1 pouch each to left and right legs (spread over thighs and calves) q am. Rub for 3 min until entirely absorbed. Allow to dry completely before dressing. Wash both hands thoroughly after application. Daily dose is two 1.74 g pouches.

PEDS — Not approved in children.

FORMS — Trade only: Topical emulsion, 56 pouches/carton.

NOTES — Typical hormone replacement regimen consists of a daily estrogen dose with a progestin added either daily or for the last 10 to 12 days of the cycle. Concomitant sunscreen may increase absorption.

MOA — Gonadal steroid.

ADVERSE EFFECTS — Serious: Endometrial cancer, DVT/PE, gallbladder disease, breast cancer, MI, CVA. Frequent: Nausea, breast tenderness.

ESTRADIOL TRANSDERMAL PATCH (*Alora, Climara, Menostar, Vivelle Dot, Minivelle, ✦Estradot, Oesclim*) ▶L ♀X ▶– $$$

ADULT — Moderate to severe menopausal vasomotor symptoms and atrophic vaginitis, female hypogonadism, bilateral oophorectomy and ovarian failure: Initiate with 0.025 to 0.05 mg/day patch once or twice per week, depending on the product (see FORMS). Prevention of postmenopausal osteoporosis: 0.025 to 0.1 mg/day patch.

PEDS — Not approved in children.

FORMS — Generic/Trade: Transdermal patches doses in mg/day: Climara (once a week) 0.025, 0.0375, 0.05, 0.06, 0.075, 0.1. Trade only: Vivelle Dot (twice per week) 0.025, 0.0375, 0.05, 0.075, 0.1. Alora (twice per week) 0.025, 0.05, 0.075, 0.1. Minivelle (twice per week) 0.0375, 0.05, 0.075, 0.1mg/day. Menostar (once a week) 0.014mg

NOTES — Rotate application sites, avoid the waistline. Transdermal may be preferable for women with high triglycerides and chronic liver disease.

MOA — Gonadal steroid.

ADVERSE EFFECTS — Serious: Endometrial cancer, DVT/PE, gallbladder disease, breast cancer, MI, CVA. Frequent: Nausea, breast tenderness.

ESTRADIOL TRANSDERMAL SPRAY (*Evamist*) ▶L ♀X ▶– $$$

WARNING — Patient should take precautions to ensure that children and pets do not make contact with skin where topical estradiol has been applied.

ADULT — Moderate to severe menopausal vasomotor symptoms: Initially 1 spray daily to adjacent nonoverlapping inner surface of the forearm. Allow to dry for 2 min and do not wash for 30 min. Adjust up to 3 sprays daily based on clinical response.

PEDS — Not approved in children.

FORMS — Trade only: 1.53 mg estradiol per 90 mcL spray, 56 sprays per metered-dose pump.

NOTES — Depress the pump 3 times with the cover on to prime each new applicator. Hold upright and vertical for spraying; rest the plastic cone against the skin. Typical hormone replacement regimen consists of a daily estrogen dose with a progestin added either daily or for the last 10 to 12 days of the cycle.

MOA — Gonadal steroid.

ADVERSE EFFECTS — Serious: Endometrial cancer, DVT/PE, gallbladder disease, breast cancer, MI, CVA. Frequent: Nausea, breast tenderness, nipple discoloration, rash, alopecia, chloasma.

ESTRADIOL VAGINAL RING (*Estring*) ▶L ♀X ▶– $$$

WARNING — Do not use during pregnancy. Toxic shock syndrome has been reported.

ADULT — Vaginal atrophy and lower urinary tract atrophy: Insert ring into upper third of the vaginal vault and replace after 90 days.

PEDS — Not approved in children.

FORMS — Trade only: 2 mg ring single pack.

NOTES — Should the ring fall out or be removed during the 90-day period, rinse in lukewarm water, and re-insert. Reports of ring adhesion to the vaginal wall making ring removal difficult. Minimal systemic absorption, probable lower risk of adverse effects than systemic estrogens.

MOA — Gonadal steroid.

ADVERSE EFFECTS — Serious: Toxic shock, bowel obstruction, vaginal wall adhesion. Frequent: None.

ESTRADIOL VAGINAL TAB (*Vagifem*) ▶L ♀X ▶– $$$

WARNING — Do not use during pregnancy.

ADULT — Menopausal atrophic vaginitis: Begin with 1 tab vaginally daily for 2 weeks, maintenance 1 tab vaginally twice per week.

PEDS — Not approved in children.

FORMS — Trade only: Vaginal tab: 10 mcg or 25 mcg in disposable single-use applicators, 8, 18/pack.

MOA — Gonadal steroid.

ADVERSE EFFECTS — Serious: None. Frequent: None.

ESTRADIOL VALERATE (*Delestrogen*) ▶L ♀X ▶– – $$

ADULT — Moderate to severe menopausal vasomotor symptoms and atrophic vaginitis, female hypogonadism, bilateral oophorectomy, and ovarian failure: 10 to 20 mg IM q 4 weeks.

PEDS — Not approved in children.

FORMS — Generic/Trade: IM injection containing 10mg, 20mg or 40mg/ml.

MOA — Gonadal steroid.

ADVERSE EFFECTS — Serious: Endometrial cancer, DVT/PE, gallbladder disease, breast cancer, MI, CVA. Frequent: Nausea, breast tenderness.

ESTROGEN VAGINAL CREAM (*Premarin, Estrace*) ▶L ♀X ▶? $$$$

ADULT — Atrophic vaginitis: Premarin: 0.5 to 2 g intravaginally daily for 1 to 2 weeks, then reduce to 0.5 g twice weekly maintenance. Estrace: 1 to 4 g intravaginally daily for 1 to 2 weeks. Gradually reduce to a maintenance dose of 1 g 1 to 3 times per week.

PEDS — Not approved in children.

FORMS — Trade only: Premarin: 0.625 mg conjugated estrogens/g in 42.5 g with or without calibrated applicator. Estrace: 0.1 mg estradiol/g in 42.5 g with calibrated applicator. Generic only: Cream 0.625 mg synthetic conjugated estrogens/g in 30 g with calibrated applicator.

NOTES — Possibility of absorption through the vaginal mucosa. Uterine bleeding might be provoked by excessive use in menopausal women. Breast tenderness and vaginal discharge due to mucus hypersecretion may result from excessive estrogenic stimulation. Endometrial withdrawal bleeding may occur if use is discontinued.

MOA — Gonadal steroid.

ADVERSE EFFECTS — Serious: Endometrial cancer, DVT/PE, gallbladder disease. Frequent: Nausea, breast tenderness.

ESTROGENS CONJUGATED (*Premarin, C.E.S., Congest*) ▶L ♀X ▶– $$$

ADULT — Moderate to severe menopausal vasomotor symptoms, atrophic vaginitis, and urethritis: 0.3 to 1.25 mg PO daily. Female hypogonadism: 0.3 to 0.625 mg PO daily for 3 weeks with 1 week off q month. Bilateral oophorectomy and ovarian failure: 1.25 mg PO daily for 3 weeks with 1 week off q month. Prevention of postmenopausal osteoporosis: 0.625 mg PO daily. Abnormal uterine bleeding: 25 mg IV/IM. Repeat in 6 to 12 h if needed.

PEDS — Not approved in children.

UNAPPROVED ADULT — Prevention of postmenopausal osteoporosis: 0.3 mg PO daily. Normalizing bleeding time in patients with AV malformations or underlying renal impairment: 30 to 70 mg IV/PO daily until bleeding time normalized.

FORMS — Trade only: Tabs 0.3, 0.45, 0.625, 0.9, 1.25 mg.

MOA — Gonadal steroid.

ADVERSE EFFECTS — Serious: Endometrial cancer, DVT/PE, gallbladder disease, breast cancer, MI, CVA. Frequent: Nausea, breast tenderness.

ESTROGENS SYNTHETIC CONJUGATED A (*Cenestin*) ▶L ♀X ▶– $$$

ADULT — Moderate to severe menopausal vasomotor symptoms: 0.3 to 1.25 mg PO daily.

PEDS — Not approved in children.

FORMS — Trade only: Tabs 0.3, 0.45, 0.625, 0.9, 1.25 mg.

NOTES — The difference between synthetic conjugated estrogens A and B is the additional component of delta-8,9-dehydroestrone sulfate in the B preparation. The clinical significance of this is unknown.

MOA — Gonadal steroid.

ADVERSE EFFECTS — Serious: Endometrial cancer, DVT/PE, gallbladder disease, breast cancer, MI, CVA. Frequent: Nausea, breast tenderness.

ESTROGENS SYNTHETIC CONJUGATED B (*Enjuvia*) ▶L ♀X ▶– $$

ADULT — Moderate to severe menopausal vasomotor symptoms: 0.3 to 1.25 mg PO daily.

PEDS — Not approved in children.

FORMS — Trade only: Tabs 0.3, 0.45, 0.625, 0.9, 1.25 mg.

NOTES — Typical hormone replacement regimen consists of a daily estrogen dose with a progestin either daily or for the last 10 to 12 days of the cycle. The difference between synthetic conjugated estrogens A and B is the additional component of delta-8,9-dehydroestrone sulfate in the B preparation. The clinical significance of this is unknown.

MOA — Gonadal steroid.

ADVERSE EFFECTS — Serious: Endometrial cancer, DVT/PE, gallbladder disease, breast cancer, MI, CVA. Frequent: Nausea, breast tenderness.

ESTROPIPATE (*Ogen, Ortho-Est*) ▶L ♀X ▶– $

ADULT — Moderate to severe menopausal vasomotor symptoms, vulvar and vaginal atrophy: 0.75 to 6 mg PO daily. Female hypogonadism, bilateral oophorectomy, or ovarian failure: 1.5 to 9 mg PO daily. Prevention of osteoporosis: 0.75 mg PO daily.

PEDS — Not approved in children.

FORMS — Generic/Trade: Tabs 0.75, 1.5, 3, 6 mg of estropipate.

NOTES — 6 mg estropipate is 5 mg sodium estrone sulfate.

MOA — Gonadal steroid.

ADVERSE EFFECTS — Serious: Endometrial cancer, DVT/PE, gallbladder disease, breast cancer, MI, CVA. Frequent: Nausea, breast tenderness.

TRIEST (*estradiol + estriol + estrone*) ▶L ♀X ▶– $$$

WARNING — For topical dosages: Patient should take precautions to ensure that children and pets do not make contact with skin where topical hormone has been applied.

UNAPPROVED ADULT — Hormone replacement therapy. Once or twice a day dosing.

FORMS — Must be compounded by a pharmacist. May be formulated as capsule, cream, gel, troche, or vaginal suppository.

NOTES — Compounded bioidentical hormones are not FDA approved. These products should be considered to have the same safety issues as those associated with hormone therapy agents that are FDA approved.

MOA — Gonadal steroid

ADVERSE EFFECTS — Serious: Endometrial cancer, DVT/PE, gallbladder disease, breast cancer, MI, CVA. Frequent: Nausea, breast tenderness.

OB/GYN: GnRH Agents

NOTE: Anaphylaxis has occurred with synthetic GnRH agents.

CETRORELIX ACETATE (*Cetrotide*) ▶Plasma ♀X ▶– $$$$$
ADULT — Infertility: Multiple dose regimen: 0.25 mg SC daily during the early to mid follicular phase. Continue treatment daily until the days of hCG administration. Single-dose regimen: 3 mg SC for 1 usually on stimulation day 7.
PEDS — Not approved in children.
FORMS — Trade only: Injection 0.25 mg and 3 mg vials.
NOTES — Best sites for SC self-injection are on the abdomen around the navel. Storage in original carton: 0.25 mg refrigerated (36–46°F); 3 mg room temperature (77°F). Contraindicated with severe renal impairment.
MOA — GnRH analog.
ADVERSE EFFECTS — Serious: Anaphylaxis, ovarian hyperstimulation syndrome. Frequent: Injection site reaction.

GANIRELIX (✦*Orgalutran*) ▶Plasma ♀X ▶? $$$$$
ADULT — Infertility: 250 mcg SC daily during the early to mid follicular phase. Continue treatment daily until the days of hCG administration.
PEDS — Not approved in children.
FORMS — Generic only: Injection 250 mcg/0.5 mL in prefilled, disposable syringe.
NOTES — Best sites for SC self-injection are on the abdomen around the navel or upper thigh. Store at room temperature (77°F) for up to 3 months. Protect from light. Packaging contains natural rubber latex which may cause allergic reactions.
MOA — GnRH analog.
ADVERSE EFFECTS — Serious: Anaphylaxis, ovarian hyperstimulation syndrome. Frequent: Injection site reaction.

LUPANETA PACK (**leuprolide + norethindrone**) ▶L ♀X ▶–
ADULT — Endometriosis: Leuprolide 3.75 mg IM injection q month. Norethindrone 5 mg PO daily.

FORMS — Trade only: 3.75 mg luprolide acetate IM injection + norethindrone acetate 5 mg PO tabs #30 (1 month kit). 11.25 mg luprolide acetate IM injection and norethindrone acetate 5 mg PO tabs #90 (3 month kit).
NOTES — Do not use longer than 6 months at a time for endometriosis and not more than a total of 12 months.
MOA — Leuprolide: Gonadotropin inhibitor; repeated dosing results in decreased secretion of gonadal steroids. Norethindrone: Induces secretory changes in an estrogen-primed endometrium.
ADVERSE EFFECTS — Serious: Renal calculus, urinary tract infection, depression, bone loss. Frequent: Hot flashes, night sweats, headache, depression, pain, visual changes.

NAFARELIN (*Synarel*) ▶L ♀X ▶– $$$$$
ADULT — Endometriosis: 200 mcg spray into 1 nostril q am and the other nostril q pm. May be increased to one 200 mcg spray into each nostril two times per day. Duration of treatment: 6 months.
PEDS — Central precocious puberty: 2 sprays into each nostril two times per day for a total of 1600 mcg/day. May be increased to 1800 mcg/day. Allow 30 sec to elapse between sprays.
FORMS — Trade only: Nasal soln 2 mg/mL in 8 mL bottle (200 mcg per spray) approximately 80 sprays/bottle.
NOTES — Ovarian cysts have occurred in the first 2 months of therapy. Symptoms of hypoestrogenism may occur. Elevations of phosphorus and eosinophil counts, and decreases in serum calcium and WBC counts have been documented. Consider norethindrone as "add back" therapy to decrease bone loss (see norethindrone).
MOA — GnRH analog.
ADVERSE EFFECTS — Serious: Anaphylaxis. Frequent in Peds: Acne, breast enlargement, vaginal bleeding. Frequent in Adults: Hot flashes, nasal irritation.

OB/GYN: Hormone Combinations

NOTE: See also Estrogens. Unopposed estrogens increase the risk of endometrial cancer in postmenopausal women. Malignancy should be ruled out in cases of persistent or recurrent abnormal vaginal bleeding. Do not use during pregnancy. May increase the risk of DVT/PE, gallbladder disease. Interactions with oral anticoagulants, phenytoin, rifampin, barbiturates, corticosteroids, and St. John's wort. For preparations containing testosterone derivatives, observe women for signs of virilization, and lipid abnormalities. In the Women's Health Initiative, the combination of conjugated estrogens and medroxyprogesterone (PremPro) caused an increase in the risk of breast cancer, MI, CVA, and DVT/PE and did not improve overall quality of life. Women greater than 65 yo with 4 years of therapy had an increased risk of dementia. Estrogen/progestin combinations should be prescribed at the lowest effective doses and for the shortest durations. Patients should be counseled regarding the risks/benefits of hormone replacement.

ACTIVELLA (**estradiol + norethindrone**) ▶L ♀X ▶– $$$
ADULT — Moderate to severe menopausal vasomotor symptoms, vulvar and vaginal atrophy, prevention of postmenopausal osteoporosis: 1 tab PO daily.

PEDS — Not approved in children.
FORMS — Trade only: Tabs 1/0.5 mg and 0.5/0.1 mg estradiol/norethindrone acetate in calendar dial pack dispenser.
MOA — Gonadal steroid combination.

ACTIVELLA (cont.)

ADVERSE EFFECTS — Serious: DVT/PE, gallbladder disease, breast cancer, MI, CVA. Frequent: Nausea, breast tenderness.

ANGELIQ (estradiol + drospirenone) ▶L ♀X ▶– $$$

ADULT — Moderate to severe menopausal vasomotor symptoms, vulvar and vaginal atrophy: 1 tab PO daily.

PEDS — Not approved in children.

FORMS — Trade only: Tabs 1 mg estradiol/0.5 mg drospirenone.

NOTES — May cause hyperkalemia in high-risk patients due to antimineralocorticoid activity of drospirenone. Monitor potassium in patients on ACE inhibitors, ARBs, potassium-sparing diuretics, heparin, aldosterone antagonists, and NSAIDs. Should not be used if renal insufficiency, hepatic dysfunction or adrenal insufficiency.

MOA — Gonadal steroid combination.

ADVERSE EFFECTS — Serious: DVT/PE, gallbladder disease, breast cancer, MI, CVA. Frequent: Nausea, breast tenderness.

CLIMARA PRO (estradiol + levonorgestrel) ▶L ♀X ▶– $$$

ADULT — Moderate to severe menopausal vasomotor symptoms, prevention of postmenopausal osteoporosis: 1 patch weekly.

PEDS — Not approved in children.

FORMS — Trade only: Transdermal 0.045/0.015 estradiol/levonorgestrel in mg/day, 4 patches/box.

NOTES — Rotate application sites; avoid the waistline.

MOA — Gonadal steroid combination.

ADVERSE EFFECTS — Serious: DVT/PE, gallbladder disease, breast cancer, MI, CVA. Frequent: Nausea, breast tenderness.

COMBIPATCH (estradiol + norethindrone, ✳Estalis) ▶L ♀X ▶– $$$

ADULT — Moderate to severe menopausal vasomotor symptoms, vulvar and vaginal atrophy, female hypogonadism, bilateral oophorectomy, and ovarian failure, prevention of postmenopausal osteoporosis: 1 patch twice per week.

PEDS — Not approved in children.

FORMS — Trade only: Transdermal patch 0.05 estradiol/0.14 norethindrone and 0.05 estradiol/0.25 norethindrone in mg/day, 8 patches/box.

NOTES — Rotate application sites, avoid the waistline.

MOA — Gonadal steroid combination.

ADVERSE EFFECTS — Serious: DVT/PE, gallbladder disease, breast cancer, MI, CVA. Frequent: HA, nausea, breast tenderness, irregular bleeding.

FEMHRT (ethinyl estradiol + norethindrone) ▶L ♀X ▶– $$$

WARNING — Multiple strengths; see FORMS and write specific product on Rx.

ADULT — Moderate to severe menopausal vasomotor symptoms, prevention of postmenopausal osteoporosis: 1 tab PO daily.

PEDS — Not approved in children.

FORMS — Trade only: Tabs 5/1, 2.5/0.5 mcg ethinyl estradiol/mg norethindrone, 28/blister card.

MOA — Gonadal steroid combination.

ADVERSE EFFECTS — Serious: DVT/PE, gallbladder disease, breast cancer, MI, CVA. Frequent: Nausea, breast tenderness.

PREFEST (estradiol + norgestimate) ▶L ♀X ▶– $$$

ADULT — Moderate to severe menopausal vasomotor symptoms, vulvar atrophy, atrophic vaginitis, prevention of postmenopausal osteoporosis: 1 pink tab PO daily for 3 days followed by 1 white tab PO daily for 3 days, sequentially throughout the month.

PEDS — Not approved in children.

FORMS — Generic/Trade: Tabs in 30 days blister packs 1 mg estradiol (15 pink), 1 mg estradiol/0.09 mg norgestimate (15 white).

MOA — Gonadal steroid combination.

ADVERSE EFFECTS — Serious: DVT/PE, gallbladder disease, breast cancer, MI, CVA. Frequent: Nausea, breast tenderness.

PREMPHASE (estrogens conjugated + medroxyprogesterone) ▶L ♀X ▶– $$$

ADULT — Moderate to severe menopausal vasomotor symptoms, vulvar/vaginal atrophy, and prevention of postmenopausal osteoporosis: 0.625 mg conjugated estrogens PO daily on days 1 to 14 and 0.625 mg conjugated estrogens/5 mg medroxyprogesterone PO daily on days 15 to 28.

PEDS — Not approved in children.

FORMS — Trade only: Tabs in 28 days EZ-Dial dispensers: 0.625 mg conjugated estrogens (14), 0.625 mg/5 mg conjugated estrogens/medroxyprogesterone (14).

MOA — Gonadal steroid combination.

ADVERSE EFFECTS — Serious: DVT/PE, gallbladder disease, breast cancer, MI, CVA. Frequent: Nausea, breast tenderness.

PREMPRO (estrogens conjugated + medroxyprogesterone, ✳Premplus) ▶L ♀X ▶– $$$

WARNING — Multiple strengths; see FORMS and write specific product on Rx.

ADULT — Moderate to severe menopausal vasomotor symptoms, vulvar/vaginal atrophy, and prevention of postmenopausal osteoporosis: 1 PO daily.

PEDS — Not approved in children.

FORMS — Trade only: Tabs in 28-day EZ-Dial dispensers: 0.625 mg/5 mg, 0.625 mg/2.5 mg, 0.45 mg/1.5 mg (Prempro low dose), or 0.3 mg/1.5 mg conjugated estrogens/medroxyprogesterone.

MOA — Gonadal steroid combination.

ADVERSE EFFECTS — Serious: DVT/PE, gallbladder disease, breast cancer, MI, CVA. Frequent: Nausea, breast tenderness.

OB/GYN: Labor Induction / Cervical Ripening

NOTE: Fetal well-being should be documented prior to use.

DINOPROSTONE (*PGE2, Prepidil, Cervidil, Prostin E2*)
▶Lung ♀C ▶? $$$$$
ADULT — Cervical ripening: Gel: 1 syringe via catheter placed into cervical canal below the internal os. May be repeated q 6 h to a max of 3 doses. Vaginal insert: Place in posterior fornix. Evacuation of uterine contents after fetal death up to 28 weeks or termination of pregnancy 12 to 20th gestational week: 20 mg intravaginal suppository; repeat at 3 to 5 h intervals until abortion occurs. Do not use for more than 2 days.
PEDS — Not approved in children.
FORMS — Trade only: Gel (Prepidil) 0.5 mg/3 g syringe. Vaginal insert (Cervidil) 10 mg. Vaginal supps (Prostin E2) 20 mg.
NOTES — Patient should remain supine for 15 to 30 min after gel and 2 h after vaginal insert. For hospital use only. Monitor for uterine hyperstimulation and abnormal fetal heart rate. Caution with asthma or glaucoma. Contraindicated in prior C-section or major uterine surgery due to potential for uterine rupture.
MOA — Uterine stimulant.
ADVERSE EFFECTS — Serious: Uterine hyperstimulation, uterine rupture. Frequent: N/V, diarrhea. Rare: disseminated intravascular coagulation (DIC)

MISOPROSTOL–OB (*PGE1, Cytotec*) ▶LK ♀X ▶– $$
WARNING — Contraindicated in desired early or preterm pregnancy due to its abortifacient property. Pregnant women should avoid contact/exposure to the tabs. Uterine rupture reported with use for labor induction and medical abortion.
UNAPPROVED ADULT — Cervical ripening and labor induction: 25 mcg intravaginally q 3 to 6 h (or 50 mcg q 6 h). First trimester pregnancy failure: 800 mcg intravaginally, repeat on day 3 if expulsion incomplete. Medical abortion less than 63 days gestation: With mifepristone, see mifepristone; with methotrexate: 800 mcg intravaginally 5 to 7 days after 50 mg/m² PO or IM methotrexate. Preop cervical ripening: 400 mcg intravaginally 3 to 4 h before mechanical cervical dilation. Postpartum hemorrhage: 800 mcg PR for 1 dose. Oral dosing has been used but is controversial. Treatment of duodenal ulcers: 100 mcg PO four times per day.
FORMS — Generic/Trade: Oral tabs 100, 200 mcg.
NOTES — Contraindicated with prior C-section. Oral tabs can be inserted into the vagina for labor induction/cervical ripening. Monitor for uterine hyperstimulation and abnormal fetal heart rate. Risk factors for uterine rupture: Prior uterine surgery and 5 or more previous pregnancies.
MOA — Prostaglandin E1 analog, uterine stimulant.
ADVERSE EFFECTS — Serious: Uterine hyperstimulation, uterine rupture. Frequent: diarrhea, abdominal pain.

OXYTOCIN (*Pitocin*) ▶LK ♀? ▶– $
WARNING — Not approved for elective labor induction, although widely used.
ADULT — Induction/stimulation of labor: 10 units in 1000 mL NS, 1 to 2 milliunits/min IV as a continuous infusion (6 to 12 mL/h). Increase in increments of 1 to 2 milliunits/min q 30 min until a contraction pattern is established, up to a max of 20 milliunits/min. Postpartum bleeding: 10 units IM after delivery of the placenta. 10 to 40 units in 1000 mL NS IV infusion, infuse 20 to 40 milliunits/min.
PEDS — Not approved in children.
UNAPPROVED ADULT — Augmentation of labor: 0.5 to 2 milliunits/min IV as a continuous infusion, increase by 1 to 2 milliunits/min q 30 min until adequate pattern of labor to a max of 40 milliunits/min.
NOTES — Use a pump to accurately control the infusion while patient is under continuous observation. Continuous fetal monitoring is required. Concurrent sympathomimetics may result in postpartum HTN. Anaphylaxis and severe water intoxication have occurred. Caution in patients undergoing a trial of labor after C-section.
MOA — Uterine stimulant.
ADVERSE EFFECTS — Serious: Anaphylaxis, water intoxication. Frequent: N/V.

OB/GYN: Ovulation Stimulants

NOTE: Potentially serious adverse effects include DVT/PE, ovarian hyperstimulation syndrome, adnexal torsion, ovarian enlargement and cysts, and febrile reactions.

CHORIOGONADOTROPIN ALFA (*Ovidrel*) ▶L ♀X ▶? $$$
ADULT — Specialized dosing for ovulation induction as part of ART administered one day following the last dose of the follicle stimulating agent.
PEDS — Not approved in children.
FORMS — Trade only: Prefilled syringe 250 mcg.
NOTES — Best site for SC self-injection is on the abdomen below the navel. Beware of multiple pregnancy and multiple adverse effects. Store in original package and protect from light. Use immediately after reconstitution.
MOA — Ovulation induction.
ADVERSE EFFECTS — Serious: Arterial thromboembolism, PE, ovarian hyperstimulation syndrome, adnexal torsion, ovarian enlargement & cysts, & febrile reactions. Frequent: Injection site reactions.

CHORIONIC GONADOTROPIN (*hCG, Pregnyl*) ▶L ♀X ▶? $$$
ADULT — Specialized IM dosing for ovulation induction as part of ART.r
PEDS — Not approved in children.
FORMS — Generic/Trade: 10,000 USP Units per vial must be reconstituted with bacteriostatic water for injection.

CHORIONIC GONADOTROPIN (cont.)

NOTES — Beware of multiple pregnancy and multiple adverse effects. For IM use only.
MOA — Ovulation induction.
ADVERSE EFFECTS — Serious: Arterial thromboembolism, PE, ovarian hyperstimulation syndrome, ovarian cysts, & ascites. Frequent: Injection site reactions.

CLOMIPHENE CITRATE (*Clomid, Serophene*) ▶L ♀D ▶? $$$$$
ADULT — Specialized dosing for ovulation induction.
PEDS — Not approved in children.
FORMS — Generic/Trade: Tabs 50 mg, scored.
NOTES — Beware of multiple pregnancy and multiple adverse effects.
MOA — Estrogenic ovulation induction.
ADVERSE EFFECTS — Serious: Blurred vision, ovarian hyperstimulation syndrome, ovarian enlargement & cysts. Frequent: hot flashes, abdominal discomfort.

FOLLITROPIN ALFA (*FSH, Gonal-f, Gonal-f RFF vial or redi-ject*) ▶L ♀X ▶? $$$$$
ADULT — Specialized dosing for ovulation induction.
PEDS — Not approved in children.
FORMS — Trade only: Powder for injection, 75 international units FSH activity, multidose vial 450, 1050 international units FSH activity. Prefilled, multiple-dose pen, 300 international units, 450 international units, 900 international units FSH activity with single-use disposable needles.
NOTES — Best site for SC self-injection is on the abdomen below the navel. Beware of multiple gestation pregnancy and multiple adverse effects. Store in original package and protect from light. Use immediately after reconstitution. Pen may be stored at room temperature for up to 1 month or expiration, whichever is first.
MOA — Ovulation induction.
ADVERSE EFFECTS — Serious: Arterial thromboembolism, DVT/PE, ovarian hyperstimulation syndrome, adnexal torsion, ovarian cysts, & febrile reactions. Frequent: Injection site reactions.

FOLLITROPIN BETA (*FSH, Follistim AQ, ✱Puregon*) ▶L ♀X ▶? $$$$$
ADULT — Specialized dosing for ovulation stimulation.
PEDS — Not approved in children.

FORMS — Trade only: AQ Cartridge, for use with the Follistim Pen, 150, 300, 600, 900 international units.
NOTES — Best site for SC self-injection is on the abdomen below the navel. Beware of multiple pregnancy and multiple adverse effects. Store in original package and protect from light. Use powder for injection immediately after reconstitution. Cartridge may be stored for up to 28 days. Store aqueous soln in refrigerator.
MOA — Ovulation induction.
ADVERSE EFFECTS — Serious: Arterial thromboembolism, DVT/PE, ovarian hyperstimulation syndrome, adnexal torsion, ovarian cysts, & febrile reactions. Frequent: Injection site reactions.

GONADOTROPINS (*menotropins, FSH and LH, Menopur, Pergonal, Repronex*) ▶L ♀X ▶– $$$$$
ADULT — Specialized dosing for infertility.
PEDS — Not approved in children.
FORMS — Trade only: Powder for injection, 75 units FSH and 75 units LH activity.
NOTES — Best site for SC self-injection is on the abdomen below the navel. Beware of multiple pregnancy and numerous adverse effects. Use immediately after reconstitution.
MOA — Follicular growth and maturation.
ADVERSE EFFECTS — Serious: Anaphylaxis, arterial thromboembolism, DVT/PE, ovarian hyperstimulation syndrome, adnexal torsion, ovarian cysts, & febrile reactions. Frequent: Injection site reactions.

UROFOLLITROPIN (*Bravelle, FSH, Fertinex*) ▶L ♀X ▶– $$$$$
ADULT — Specialized dosing for infertility and polycystic ovary syndrome.
PEDS — Not approved in children.
FORMS — Trade only: Powder for injection, 75 international units FSH activity.
NOTES — Best site for SC self-injection is on the abdomen below the navel. Beware of multiple pregnancy and numerous adverse effects. Use immediately after reconstitution.
MOA — Ovulation induction.
ADVERSE EFFECTS — Serious: Arterial thromboembolism, DVT/PE, ovarian hyperstimulation syndrome, adnexal torsion, ovarian cysts, & febrile reactions. Frequent: Injection site reactions.

OB/GYN: Progestins

NOTE: Do not use in pregnancy. DVT, PE, cerebrovascular disorders, and retinal thrombosis may occur. Effectiveness may be reduced by hepatic enzyme-inducing drugs such as certain anticonvulsants and barbiturates, rifampin, rifabutin, griseofulvin, and protease inhibitors. The effects of St. John's wort-containing products on progestin-only pills is currently unknown. In the Women's Health Initiative, the combination of conjugated estrogens and medroxyprogesterone (PremPro) caused a statistically significant increase in the risk of breast cancer, MI, CVA, and DVT/PE. Additionally, women greater than 65 yo with 4 years of therapy had an increased risk of dementia. Estrogen/progestin combinations should be prescribed at the lowest effective doses and for the shortest durations. Patients should be counseled regarding the risks/benefits of hormone replacement.

MEDROXYPROGESTERONE (*Provera*) ▶L ♀X ▶+ $
ADULT — Secondary amenorrhea: 5 to 10 mg PO daily for 5 to 10 days. Abnormal uterine bleeding: 5 to 10 mg PO daily for 5 to 10 days beginning on the 16th or 21st day of the cycle (after estrogen priming). Withdrawal bleeding usually occurs 3 to 7 days after therapy ends.
PEDS — Not approved in children.

MEDROXYPROGESTERONE (*cont.*)

UNAPPROVED ADULT — Add to estrogen replacement therapy to prevent endometrial hyperplasia: 10 mg PO daily for 10 to 12 days each month, or 2.5 to 5 mg PO daily. Endometrial hyperplasia: 10 to 30 mg PO daily (long-term); 40 to 100 mg PO daily (short-term) or 500 mg IM twice per week.

FORMS — Generic/Trade: Tabs 2.5, 5, 10 mg, scored.

NOTES — Breakthrough bleeding/spotting may occur. Amenorrhea usually after 6 months of continuous dosing.

MOA — Gonadal steroid.

ADVERSE EFFECTS — Serious: Thrombophlebitis, cerebrovascular disorders, retinal thrombosis, DVT/PE. Frequent: Breakthrough bleeding.

MEDROXYPROGESTERONE—INJECTABLE (*Depo-Provera, depo-subQ provera 104*) ▶L ♀X ▶+ $

WARNING — Risk of significant bone loss (possibly reversible) increases with duration of use. Long-term use (greater than 2 years) only recommended if other methods of birth control are inadequate or symptoms of endometriosis return after discontinuation. It is unknown if use by younger women will reduce peak bone mass.

ADULT — Contraception/endometriosis: 150 mg IM in deltoid or gluteus maximus or 104 mg SC in anterior thigh or abdomen q 13 weeks. Also used for adjunctive therapy in endometrial and renal carcinoma.

PEDS — Not approved in children.

UNAPPROVED ADULT — Dysfunctional uterine bleeding: 150 mg IM in deltoid or gluteus maximus q 13 weeks.

NOTES — Breakthrough bleeding/spotting may occur. Amenorrhea usually after 6 months. Wt gain is common. To be sure that the patient is not pregnant give this injection only during the first 5 days after the onset of a normal menstrual period or after a negative pregnancy test. May be given immediately post-pregnancy termination as well as postpartum, including breastfeeding women. May be given as often as 11 weeks apart. If the time between injections is greater than 14 weeks, exclude pregnancy before administering. Return to fertility can be variably delayed after last injection, with the median time to pregnancy being 10 months. Bone loss may occur with prolonged administration. Evaluate bone mineral density if considering retreatment for endometriosis.

MOA — Progestational agent that inhibits release of LH.

ADVERSE EFFECTS — Serious: Thrombophlebitis, cerebrovascular disorders, retinal thrombosis, DVT/PE, bone loss. Frequent: Injection site reactions, breakthrough bleeding, weight gain.

MEGESTROL (*Megace, Megace ES*) ▶L ♀D ▶? $$$$$

ADULT — AIDS anorexia: 800 mg (20 mL) susp PO daily or 625 mg (5 mL) ES daily. Palliative treatment for advanced breast carcinoma: 40 mg (tabs) PO four times per day. Endometrial carcinoma: 40 to 320 mg/day (tabs) in divided doses.

PEDS — Not approved in children.

UNAPPROVED ADULT — Endometrial hyperplasia: 40 to 160 mg PO daily for 3 to 4 months. Cancer-associated anorexia/cachexia: 80 to 160 mg PO four times per day.

FORMS — Generic/Trade: Tabs 20, 40 mg. Susp 40 mg/mL in 240 mL. Trade only: Megace ES susp 125 mg/mL (150 mL).

NOTES — In HIV-infected women, breakthrough bleeding/spotting may occur.

MOA — Gonadal steroid.

ADVERSE EFFECTS — Serious: Thrombophlebitis, cerebrovascular disorders, retinal thrombosis, DVT/PE. Frequent: Breakthrough bleeding, weight gain.

NORETHINDRONE ACETATE (*Aygestin, ✱Norlutate*) ▶L ♀X ▶ $$

ADULT — Amenorrhea, abnormal uterine bleeding: 2.5 to 10 mg PO daily for 5 to 10 days during the second half of the menstrual cycle. Endometriosis: 5 mg PO daily for 2 weeks. Increase by 2.5 mg q 2 weeks to 15 mg/day.

PEDS — Not approved in children.

UNAPPROVED ADULT — "Add back" therapy with GnRH agonists (eg, leuprolide) to decrease bone loss: 5 mg PO daily.

FORMS — Generic/Trade: Tabs 5 mg scored.

NOTES — Contraceptive doses felt compatible with breast feeding, but not higher doses.

MOA — Gonadal steroid.

ADVERSE EFFECTS — Serious: Thrombophlebitis, cerebrovascular disorders, retinal thrombosis, DVT/PE. Frequent: Nausea, breast tenderness, breakthrough bleeding.

PROGESTERONE GEL (*Crinone, Prochieve*) ▶Plasma ♀– ▶? $$$

ADULT — Secondary amenorrhea: 45 mg (4%) intravaginally every other day up to 6 doses. If no response, use 90 mg (8%) intravaginally every other day up to 6 doses. Specialized dosing for infertility.

PEDS — Not approved in children.

FORMS — Trade only: 4%, 8% single-use, prefilled applicators.

NOTES — An increase in dose from the 4% gel can only be accomplished using the 8% gel; doubling the volume of 4% does not increase absorption.

MOA — Gonadal steroid.

ADVERSE EFFECTS — Serious: Thrombophlebitis, cerebrovascular disorders, retinal thrombosis, DVT/PE. Frequent: Vaginal discharge.

PROGESTERONE IN OIL ▶L ♀X ▶? $$

WARNING — Contraindicated in peanut allergy since some products contain peanut oil.

ADULT — Amenorrhea, uterine bleeding: 5 to 10 mg IM daily for 6 to 8 days.

PEDS — Not approved in children.

NOTES — Discontinue with thrombotic disorders, sudden or partial loss of vision, proptosis, diplopia or migraine.

MOA — Gonadal steroid.

ADVERSE EFFECTS — Serious: Thrombophlebitis, cerebrovascular disorders, retinal thrombosis, DVT/PE. Frequent: Breakthrough bleeding.

PROGESTERONE MICRONIZED (*Prometrium*) ▶L ♀B ▶+ $$

WARNING — Contraindicated in patients allergic to peanuts since caps contain peanut oil.

PROGESTERONE MICRONIZED (*cont.*)

ADULT — Hormone therapy to prevent endometrial hyperplasia: 200 mg PO at bedtime 10 to 12 days/month. Secondary amenorrhea: 400 mg PO at bedtime for 10 days.

PEDS — Not approved in children.

UNAPPROVED ADULT — Hormone therapy to prevent endometrial hyperplasia: 100 mg at bedtime daily.

FORMS — Generic/Trade: Caps 100, 200 mg.

NOTES — Breast tenderness, dizziness, headache and abdominal cramping may occur.

MOA — Gonadal steroid.

ADVERSE EFFECTS — Serious: Thrombophlebitis, cerebrovascular disorders, retinal thrombosis, DVT/PE. Frequent: Breakthrough bleeding.

PROGESTERONE MICRONIZED COMPOUNDED (*Progest*) ▶L ♀B? ▶? $

WARNING — For topical dosages: Patient should take precautions to ensure that children and pets do not make contact with skin where topical hormone has been applied.

UNAPPROVED ADULT — Hormone Replacement Therapy. Once or twice a day dosing.

FORMS — Must be compounded by a pharmacist. May be formulated as capsule, cream, gel, troche, or vaginal suppository.

NOTES — Compounded bioidentical hormones are not FDA approved. These products should be considered to have the same safety issues as those associated with hormone therapy agents that are FDA approved.

MOA — Gonadal steroid

ADVERSE EFFECTS — Serious: Thrombophlebitis, cerebrovascular disorders, retinal thrombosis, DVT/PE. Frequent: Breakthrough bleeding.

PROGESTERONE VAGINAL INSERT (*Endometrin*) ▶Plasma ♀– ▶? $$$$

ADULT — Specialized dosing for infertility.

PEDS — Not approved in children.

FORMS — Trade only: 100 mg vaginal insert.

NOTES — Do not use concomitantly with other vaginal products, such as antifungals, as this may alter absorption.

MOA — Gonadal steroid.

ADVERSE EFFECTS — Serious: Thrombophlebitis, cerebrovascular disorders, retinal thrombosis, DVT/PE. Frequent: Vaginal discharge.

OB/GYN: Selective Estrogen Receptor Modulators

OSPEMIFENE (*Osphena*) ▶L ♀X ▶– $$$$

ADULT — Dyspareunia: 1 tab PO daily with food.

PEDS — Not approved for children.

FORMS — Trade only: Tabs 60 mg.

NOTES — Contraindicated with estrogen-dependent neoplasia, DVT/PE, abnormal genital bleeding, history of stroke or MI, and pregnancy.

MOA — Tissue selective estrogen agonist/antagonist.

ADVERSE EFFECTS — Severe: Endometrial cancer, stroke, and DVT. Frequent: Hot flush, vaginal discharge, muscle spasm, and sweating.

RALOXIFENE (*Evista*) ▶L ♀X ▶– $$$$$

WARNING — Increases the risk of venous thromboembolism and CVA. Do not use during pregnancy.

ADULT — Postmenopausal osteoporosis prevention/treatment, breast cancer prevention: 60 mg PO daily.

PEDS — Not approved in children.

FORMS — Generic/Trade: Tabs 60 mg.

NOTES — Contraindicated with history of venous thromboembolism. Interactions with oral anticoagulants and cholestyramine. May increase risk of DVT/PE. Discontinue use 72 h prior to and during prolonged immobilization because of DVT risk. Does not decrease (and may increase) hot flashes. Leg cramps. Triglyceride levels may increase in women with prior estrogen-associated hypertriglyceridemia (greater than 500 mg/dL).

MOA — Selective Estrogen Receptor Modulator.

ADVERSE EFFECTS — Serious: DVT/PE, hypertriglyceridemia, stroke. Frequent: Hot flashes, leg cramps.

TAMOXIFEN (*Soltamox, Tamone,* ✥*Tamofen*) ▶L ♀D ▶– $$

WARNING — Uterine malignancies, CVA and pulmonary embolism, sometimes fatal. Visual disturbances, cataracts, hypercalcemia, increased LFTs, bone pain, fertility impairment, hot flashes, menstrual irregularities, endometrial hyperplasia and cancer, alopecia. Do not use during pregnancy.

ADULT — Breast cancer prevention in high-risk women: 20 mg PO daily for 5 years. Breast cancer: 10 to 20 mg PO two times per day for 5 years.

PEDS — Not approved in children.

UNAPPROVED ADULT — Mastalgia: 10 mg PO daily for 4 months. Anovulation: 5 to 40 mg PO two times per day for 4 days.

FORMS — Generic/Trade: Tabs 10, 20 mg. Trade only (Soltamox): Sugar-free soln 10 mg/5 mL (150 mL).

NOTES — Reliable contraception is recommended. Monitor CBCs, LFTs. Regular gynecologic and ophthalmologic examinations. Interacts with oral anticoagulants. Does not decrease hot flashes.

MOA — Selective Estrogen Receptor Modulator.

ADVERSE EFFECTS — Serious: DVT/PE, retinal thrombosis, hepatotoxicity, endometrial cancer,. Frequent: Hot flashes, leg cramps, vaginal discharge.

OB/GYN: Uterotonics

CARBOPROST (*Hemabate, 15-methyl-prostaglandin F2 alpha*) ▶LK ♀C ▶? $$$

ADULT — Refractory postpartum uterine bleeding: 250 mcg deep IM. If necessary, may repeat at 15 to 90 min intervals up to a total dose of 2 mg (8 doses).

PEDS — Not approved in children.

CARBOPROST (*cont.*)

NOTES — Caution with asthma. Transient fever, HTN, nausea, bronchoconstriction and flushing. May augment oxytocics.

MOA — Uterotonic.

ADVERSE EFFECTS — Serious: Pulmonary edema. Frequent: Fever, flushing, nausea, diarrhea.

METHYLERGONOVINE (*Methergine*) ▶LK ♀C ▶– $$

ADULT — To increase uterine contractions and decrease postpartum bleeding: 0.2 mg IM after delivery of the placenta, delivery of the anterior shoulder, or during the puerperium. Repeat q 2 to 4 h prn. 0.2 mg PO three to four times per day in the puerperium for a max of 1 week.

PEDS — Not approved in children.

FORMS — Trade only: Tabs 0.2 mg.

NOTES — Contraindicated in pregnancy-induced HTN/preeclampsia. Avoid IV route due to risk of sudden HTN and CVA. If IV absolutely necessary, give slowly over no less than 1 min, monitor BP.

MOA — Uterotonic.

ADVERSE EFFECTS — Serious: CVA, seizure. Frequent: Hypertension, headache, nausea.

OB/GYN: Vaginitis Preparations

NOTE: See also STD/vaginitis table in antimicrobial section. Many experts recommend 7 days antifungal therapy for pregnant women with candida vaginitis. Many of these creams and supps are oil-based and may weaken latex condoms and diaphragms. Do not use latex products for 72 h after last dose.

BORIC ACID ▶Not absorbed ♀? ▶– $

PEDS — Not approved in children.

UNAPPROVED ADULT — Resistant vulvovaginal candidiasis: 600 mg suppository intravaginally at bedtime for 2 weeks.

FORMS — No commercial preparation; must be compounded by pharmacist. Vaginal supps 600 mg in gelatin caps.

NOTES — Reported use for azole-resistant nonalbicans (C glabrata) or recurrent albicans failing azole therapy. Do not use if abdominal pain, fever or foul-smelling vaginal discharge is present. Avoid vaginal intercourse during treatment.

MOA — Antifungal.

ADVERSE EFFECTS — Serious: None. Frequent: Vulvovaginal irritation, erythema, & erosions.

BUTOCONAZOLE (*Gynazole, Mycelex-3*) ▶LK ♀C ▶? $(OTC), $$$(Rx)

ADULT — Local treatment of vulvovaginal candidiasis, nonpregnant patients: Mycelex 3: 1 applicatorful (~5 g) intravaginally at bedtime for 3 days, up to 6 days, if necessary. Pregnant patients: (second and third trimesters only) 1 applicatorful (~5 g) intravaginally at bedtime for 6 days. Gynazole-1: 1 applicatorful (~5 g) intravaginally once daily.

PEDS — Not approved in children.

FORMS — OTC: Trade only (Mycelex 3): 2% vaginal cream in 5 g prefilled applicators (3s), 20 g tube with applicators. Rx: Trade only (Gynazole-1): 2% vaginal cream in 5 g prefilled applicator.

NOTES — Do not use if abdominal pain, fever, or foul-smelling vaginal discharge is present. Since small amount may be absorbed from the vagina, use during the first trimester only when essential. During pregnancy, use of a vaginal applicator may be contraindicated and manual insertion may be preferred. Vulvar/vaginal burning may occur. Avoid vaginal intercourse during treatment.

MOA — Antifungal.

ADVERSE EFFECTS — Serious: None. Frequent: Vulvovaginal irritation.

CLINDAMYCIN—VAGINAL (*Cleocin, Clindesse, ✦Dalacin*) ▶L ♀– ▶+ $$

ADULT — Bacterial vaginosis: Cleocin: 1 applicatorful (~100 mg clindamycin phosphate in 5 g cream) intravaginally at bedtime for 7 days, or 1 suppository at bedtime for 3 days. Clindesse: 1 applicatorful cream single dose.

PEDS — Not approved in children.

FORMS — Generic/Trade: 2% vaginal cream in 40 g tube with 7 disposable applicators (Cleocin). Vag suppository (Cleocin Ovules) 100 mg (3) with applicator. 2% vaginal cream in a single-dose prefilled applicator (Clindesse).

NOTES — Clindesse may degrade latex/rubber condoms and diaphragms for 5 days after the last dose (Cleocin for up to 3 days). Not recommended during pregnancy despite B rating, as it does not prevent the adverse effects of bacterial vaginosis (eg, preterm birth, neonatal infection). Cervicitis, vaginitis, and vulvar irritation may occur. Avoid vaginal intercourse during treatment.

MOA — Antibiotic.

ADVERSE EFFECTS — Serious: None. Frequent: Cervicitis, vaginitis, & vulvar irritation.

CLOTRIMAZOLE—VAGINAL (*Mycelex 7, Gyne-Lotrimin, ✦Canesten, Clotrimaderm*) ▶LK ♀B ▶? $

ADULT — Local treatment of vulvovaginal candidiasis: 1 applicatorful 1% cream at bedtime for 7 days. 1 applicatorful 2% cream at bedtime for 3 days. 100 mg suppository intravaginally at bedtime for 7 days. 200 mg suppository at bedtime for 3 days. Topical cream for external symptoms two times per day for 7 days.

PEDS — Not approved in children.

FORMS — OTC Generic/Trade: 1% vaginal cream with applicator (some prefilled). 2% vaginal cream with applicator and 1% topical cream in some combination packs. OTC Trade only (Gyne-Lotrimin): Vaginal suppository 100 mg (7), 200 mg (3) with applicators.

NOTES — Do not use if abdominal pain, fever, or foul-smelling vaginal discharge is present. Since small

CLOTRIMAZOLE—VAGINAL (*cont.*)

amounts of these drugs may be absorbed from the vagina, use during the 1st trimester only when essential. During pregnancy, use of a vaginal applicator may be contraindicated; manual insertion of tabs may be preferred. Skin rash, lower abdominal cramps, bloating, vulvar irritation may occur. Avoid vaginal intercourse during treatment.

MOA — Antifungal.

ADVERSE EFFECTS — Serious: None. Frequent: Vulvovaginal irritation.

METRONIDAZOLE—VAGINAL (*MetroGel-Vaginal, Vandazole★Nidagel*) ▶LK ♀B ▶? $$

ADULT — Bacterial vaginosis: 1 applicatorful (approximately 5 g containing approximately 37.5 mg metronidazole) intravaginally at bedtime or two times per day for 5 days.

PEDS — Not approved in children.

FORMS — Generic/Trade: 0.75% gel in 70 g tube with applicator.

NOTES — Cure rate same with at bedtime and twice daily dosing. Vaginally applied metronidazole could be absorbed in sufficient amounts to produce systemic effects. Caution in patients with CNS diseases due to rare reports of seizures, neuropathy, and numbness. Do not administer to patients who have taken disulfiram within the last 2 weeks. Interaction with ethanol. Caution with warfarin. Candida cervicitis and vaginitis, and vaginal, perineal, or vulvar itching may occur. Avoid vaginal intercourse during treatment.

MOA — Antibiotic.

ADVERSE EFFECTS — Serious: Seizures. Frequent: Cervicitis, vaginitis, & vulvar irritation.

MICONAZOLE (*Monistat, Femizol-M, M-Zole, Micozole, Monazole*) ▶LK ♀+ ▶? $

ADULT — Local treatment of vulvovaginal candidiasis: 1 applicatorful 2% cream intravaginally at bedtime for 7 days or 4% cream at bedtime for 3 days. 100 mg suppository intravaginally at bedtime for 7 days, 400 mg at bedtime for 3 days, or 1200 mg for 1 dose. Topical cream for external symptoms two times per day for 7 days.

PEDS — Not approved in children.

FORMS — OTC Generic/Trade: 2% vaginal cream in 45 g with 1 applicator or 7 disposable applicators. Vaginal suppository 100 mg (7). OTC Trade only: 400 mg (3), 1200 mg (1) with applicator. Generic/Trade: 4% vaginal cream in 25 g tubes or 3 prefilled applicators. Some in combination packs with 2% miconazole cream for external use.

NOTES — Do not use if abdominal pain, fever, or foul-smelling vaginal discharge is present. Since

small amounts of these drugs may be absorbed from the vagina, use during the 1st trimester only when essential. During pregnancy, use of a vaginal applicator may be contraindicated; manual insertion of suppositories may be preferred. Vulvovaginal burning, itching, irritation, and pelvic cramps may occur. Avoid vaginal intercourse during treatment. May increase warfarin effect.

MOA — Antifungal.

ADVERSE EFFECTS — Serious: None. Frequent: Vulvovaginal irritation.

TERCONAZOLE (*Terazol*) ▶LK ♀C ▶– $$

ADULT — Local treatment of vulvovaginal candidiasis: 1 applicatorful 0.4% cream intravaginally at bedtime for 7 days. 1 applicatorful 0.8% cream intravaginally at bedtime for 3 days. 80 mg suppository intravaginally at bedtime for 3 days.

PEDS — Not approved in children.

FORMS — All forms supplied with applicators: Generic/Trade: Vaginal cream 0.4% (Terazol 7) in 45 g tube, 0.8% (Terazol 3) in 20 g tube. Vaginal suppository (Terazol 3) 80 mg (#3).

NOTES — Do not use if abdominal pain, fever, or foul-smelling vaginal discharge is present. Since small amounts of these drugs may be absorbed from the vagina, use during the 1st trimester only when essential. During pregnancy, use of a vaginal applicator may be contraindicated; manual insertion of supps may be preferred. Avoid vaginal intercourse during treatment. Vulvovaginal irritation, burning, and pruritus may occur.

MOA — Antifungal.

ADVERSE EFFECTS — Serious: Anaphylaxis and toxic epidermal necrolysis. Frequent: Vulvovaginal irritation.

TIOCONAZOLE (*Monistat 1-Day, Vagistat-1*) ▶Not absorbed ♀C ▶– $

ADULT — Local treatment of vulvovaginal candidiasis: 1 applicatorful (~ 4.6 g) intravaginally at bedtime for 1 dose.

PEDS — Not approved in children.

FORMS — OTC Trade only: Vaginal ointment: 6.5% (300 mg) in 4.6 g prefilled single-dose applicator.

NOTES — Do not use if abdominal pain, fever, or foul-smelling vaginal discharge is present. Since small amounts of these drugs may be absorbed from the vagina, use during the first trimester only when essential. During pregnancy, use of a vaginal applicator may be contraindicated. Avoid vaginal intercourse during treatment. Vulvovaginal burning and itching may occur.

MOA — Antifungal.

ADVERSE EFFECTS — Serious: None. Frequent: Vulvovaginal irritation.

OB/GYN: Other OB/GYN Agents

DANAZOL (*★Cyclomen*) ▶L ♀X ▶– $$$$$

ADULT — Endometriosis: Start 400 mg PO two times per day, then titrate downward to a dose sufficient to maintain amenorrhea for 3 to 6 months, up to 9

months. Fibrocystic breast disease: 100 to 200 mg PO two times per day for 4 to 6 months.

PEDS — Not approved in children.

DANAZOL (*cont.*)

UNAPPROVED ADULT — Menorrhagia: 100 to 400 mg PO daily for 3 months. Cyclical mastalgia: 100 to 200 mg PO two times per day for 4 to 6 months.

FORMS — Generic only: Caps 50, 100, 200 mg.

NOTES — Contraindications: Impaired hepatic, renal, or cardiac function. Androgenic effects may not be reversible even after the drug is discontinued. May alter voice. Hepatic dysfunction has occurred. Insulin requirements may increase in diabetics. Prolongation of PT/INR has been reported with concomitant warfarin.

MOA — Androgen.

ADVERSE EFFECTS — Serious: Stroke, intracranial hypertension, hepatic adenoma. Frequent: Acne, edema, hirsutism, deepening voice, emotional lability, depression.

HYDROXYPROGESTERONE CAPROATE (*Makena*) ▶L + glucuronidation ♀B ▶? $$$$$

WARNING — For singleton pregnancy in women who have history of spontaneous preterm birth. Not intended in mutiple gestations or other risk factors for preterm birth.

ADULT — To reduce risk of preterm birth: 250 mg IM once weekly. Begin between gestational age 16 weeks, 0 days and 20 weeks 6 days. Continue through birth or week 37, whichever occurs first.

PEDS — Not approved in children

FORMS — Trade only: 5 mL MDV (250 mg/mL) hydroxyprogesterone caproate in castor oil soln.

NOTES — Unique ruling from FDA that compounding pharmacists can continue to make customized hydroxyprogesterone caproate injection.

MOA — unknown

ADVERSE EFFECTS — Serious: Early membrane rupture, cervical incompetence, miscarriage or stillbirth. Common: Injection site pain and swelling, urticaria.

MIFEPRISTONE (*Mifeprex, RU-486*) ▶L ♀X ▶? $$$$$

WARNING — Rare cases of sepsis and death have occurred. Surgical intervention may be necessary with incomplete abortions. Patients need to be given info on where such services are available and what do in case of an emergency.

ADULT — Termination of pregnancy, up to 49 days: Day 1: 600 mg PO. Day 3: 400 mcg misoprostol (unless abortion confirmed). Day 14: Confirmation of pregnancy termination.

PEDS — Not approved in children.

UNAPPROVED ADULT — Termination of pregnancy, up to 63 days: 200 mg PO followed by 800 mcg misoprostol intravaginally 24 to 72 h later.

FORMS — Trade only: Tabs 200 mg.

NOTES — Bleeding/spotting and cramping most common side effects. Prolonged heavy bleeding may be a sign of incomplete abortion. Contraindications: Ectopic pregnancy, IUD use, adrenal insufficiency and long-term steroid use, use of anticoagulants, hemorrhagic disorders and porphyrias. CYP3A4 inducers may increase metabolism and lower levels. Available through physician offices only.

MOA — Anti-progestational/abortifacient.

ADVERSE EFFECTS — Serious: Sepsis, incomplete abortion. Frequent: Bleeding, spotting, cramping, N/V.

PAROXETINE (*Brisdelle*) ▶LK ♀X ▶?

ADULT — Moderate to severe vasomotor symptoms associated with menopause: 7.5 mg at bedtime.

PEDS — Not indicated

FORMS — Trade only: Caps 7.5 mg

NOTES — Paroxetine is a strong inhibitor of CYP2D6 and is contraindicated with thioridazine, pimozide, MAOIs, linezolid and tryptophan; use caution with barbiturates, cimetidine, phenytoin, tamoxifen, theophylline, TCAs, risperidone, atomoxetine, and warfarin.

MOA — Selective serotonin reuptake inhibitor.

ADVERSE EFFECTS — Serious: Suicidality, serotonin syndrome, abnormal bleeding, hyponatremia, bone fracture risk. Frequent: headache, fatigue/malaise/lethargy, and nausea/vomiting.

Premesis-Rx (pyridoxine + folic acid + cyanocobalamin + calcium carbonate) ▶L ♀A ▶+ $$

ADULT — Treatment of pregnancy-induced nausea: 1 tab PO daily.

PEDS — Unapproved in children.

FORMS — Trade only: Tabs 75 mg vitamin B6 (pyridoxine), sustained-release, 12 mcg vitamin B12 (cyanocobalamin), 1 mg folic acid, and 200 mg calcium carbonate.

NOTES — May be taken in conjunction with prenatal vitamins.

MOA — Vitamin combination.

ADVERSE EFFECTS — Serious: None. Frequent: None.

RHO IMMUNE GLOBULIN (*HyperRHO S/D, MICRhoGAM, RhoGAM, Rhophylac, WinRho SDF*) ▶L ♀C ▶? $$$$$

ADULT — Prevention of hemolytic disease of the newborn if mother Rh– and baby is or might be Rh+: 300 mcg vial IM to mother at 28 weeks gestation followed by a second dose within 72 h of delivery. Doses more than 1 vial may be needed if large fetal-maternal hemorrhage occurs during delivery (see complete prescribing information to determine dose). Following amniocentesis, miscarriage, abortion, or ectopic pregnancy at least 13 weeks gestation: 1 vial (300 mcg) IM. Less than 12 weeks gestation: 1 vial (50 mcg) microdose IM. Immune thrombocytopenic purpura (ITP), nonsplenectomized (WinRho): 250 units/kg/dose (50 mcg/kg/dose) IV for 1 dose if hemoglobin greater than 10 g/dL or 125 to 200 units/kg/dose (25 to 40 mcg/kg/dose) IV for 1 dose if hemoglobin less than 10 g/dL. Additional doses of 125 to 300 units/kg/dose (25 to 60 mcg/kg/dose) IV may be given as determined by patient's response.

PEDS — Immune thrombocytopenic purpura (ITP), nonsplenectomized (WinRho): 250 units/kg/dose (50 mcg/kg/dose) IV for 1 dose if hemoglobin

RHO IMMUNE GLOBULIN (*cont.*)

greater than 10 g/dL or 125 to 200 units/kg/dose (25 to 40 mcg/kg/dose) IV for 1 dose if hemoglobin less than 10 g/dL. Additional doses of 125 to 300 units/kg/dose (25 to 60 mcg/kg/dose) IV may be given as determined by patient's response.

UNAPPROVED ADULT — Rh-incompatible transfusion: Specialized dosing.

NOTES — One 300 mcg vial prevents maternal sensitization to the Rh factor if the fetomaternal hemorrhage is less than 15 mL fetal RBCs (30 mL of whole blood). When the fetomaternal hemorrhage exceeds this (as estimated by Kleihauer-Betke testing), administer more than one 300 mcg vial.

MOA — Immune globulin.

ADVERSE EFFECTS — Serious: None. Frequent: Injection site reactions.

ULIPRISTAL ACETATE (✱*Fibristal*) ▶L ♀X ▶–

ADULT — Canadian indication treatment of moderate-to-severe signs/symptoms of uterine fibroids. 5 mg PO daily x 3 months.

FORMS — Canadian Trade only: Tabs 5 mg.

NOTES — Canadian drug only. Ella Brand product in the US is for a different indication at a different dose.

MOA — Selective progesterone receptor modulator.

ADVERSE EFFECTS — Hot flashes, irregular vaginal bleeding, endometrial thickening, headache.

ONCOLOGY

ONCOLOGY: Alkylating agents

BENDAMUSTINE (*Treanda*) ▶Plasma ♀D ▶– $ varies by therapy
WARNING — Anaphylaxis, bone marrow suppression, nephrotoxicity, Stevens-Johnson syndrome, toxic epidermal necrolysis. Instruct patients to report promptly fever, sore throat, signs of local infection, bleeding from any site, or symptoms suggestive of anemia. Take precautions to avoid extravasation, including monitoring intravenous infusion site during and after administration.
ADULT — Chemotherapy doses vary by indication. CLL, non-Hodgkin's lymphoma.
PEDS — Not approved in children. The effectiveness of bendamustine in pediatric patients has not been established. Bendamustine was evaluated in a single Phase 1/2 trial in pediatric patients with leukemia. The safety profile for bendamustine in pediatric patients was consistent with that seen in adults, and no new safety signals were identified.
UNAPPROVED ADULT — Hodgkin lymphoma, mantle cell lymphoma, multiple myeloma.
NOTES — Reliable contraception is recommended. Monitor CBCs and renal function.
MOA — Alkylating agent.
ADVERSE EFFECTS — Serious: Anaphylaxis, bone marrow suppression, nephrotoxicity, Stevens-Johnson syndrome, toxic epidermal necrolysis. Frequent: Bone marrow suppression, N/V.
BUSULFAN (*Myleran, Busulfex*) ▶LK ♀D ▶– $ varies by therapy
WARNING — Secondary malignancies, bone marrow suppression, adrenal insufficiency, hyperuricemia, pulmonary fibrosis, seizures (must initiate prophylactic anticonvulsant therapy prior to use of busulfan), cellular dysplasia, hepatic veno-occlusive disease, fertility impairment, alopecia. Instruct patients to report promptly fever, sore throat, signs of local infection, bleeding from any site, symptoms suggestive of anemia, or yellow discoloration of the skin or eyes.
ADULT — Chemotherapy doses vary by indication. Tabs: CML. Injection: Conditioning regimen prior to allogeneic hematopoietic progenitor cell transplantation for CML. in combination with cyclophosphamide.
PEDS — Chemotherapy doses vary by indication. Tabs: CML. Safety of the injection has not been established.
UNAPPROVED ADULT — High dose in conjunction with stem cell transplant for leukemia and lymphoma.
FORMS — Trade only (Myleran) Tabs 2 mg. Busulfex injection for hospital/oncology clinic use; not intended for outpatient prescribing.
NOTES — Reliable contraception is recommended. Monitor CBCs and LFTs. Hydration and

allopurinol to decrease adverse effects of uric acid. Acetaminophen and itraconazole decrease busulfan clearance. Phenytoin increases clearance.
MOA — Alkylating agent.
ADVERSE EFFECTS — Serious: Bone marrow suppression, adrenal insufficiency, seizures, pulmonary fibrosis, hepatic veno-occlusive disease, febrile neutropenia, severe bacterial, viral [e.g., cytomegaloviraemia] and fungal infections, and sepsis), tumor lysis syndrome, thrombotic micro angiopathy (TMA), hyperpigmentation.
CARMUSTINE (*BCNU, BiCNU, Gliadel*) ▶Plasma ♀D ▶– $ varies by therapy
WARNING — Secondary malignancies, bone marrow suppression, pulmonary fibrosis, nephrotoxicity, hepatotoxicity, ocular nerve fiber-layer infarcts and retinal hemorrhages, fertility impairment, alopecia. Local soft tissue toxicity/extravasation can occur if carmustine is infused too quickly. Infusions should run over at least 2 h. Wafer: Seizures, brain edema and herniation, intracranial infection. Instruct patients to report promptly fever, sore throat, signs of local infection, bleeding from any site, symptoms suggestive of anemia, or yellow discoloration of the skin or eyes.
ADULT — Chemotherapy doses vary by indication. Injection: Glioblastoma, brainstem glioma, medulloblastoma, astrocytoma, ependymoma and metastatic brain tumors, multiple myeloma with prednisone; Hodgkin's disease and non-Hodgkin's lymphomas, in combination regimens. Wafer: Glioblastoma multiforme, adjunct to surgery. High-grade malignant glioma, adjunct to surgery and radiation.
PEDS — Not approved in children.
UNAPPROVED ADULT — Mycosis fungoides, topical soln.
NOTES — Reliable contraception is recommended. Monitor CBCs, PFTs, LFTs, and renal function. May decrease phenytoin and digoxin levels. Cimetidine may increase myelosuppression. Significant absorption to PVC containers will occur. Carmustine must be dispensed in glass or non-PVC containers.
MOA — Alkylating agent.
ADVERSE EFFECTS — Serious: Bone marrow suppression, pulmonary fibrosis, nephrotoxicity, hepatotoxicity, ocular nerve fiber-layer infarcts and retinal hemorrhages. Wafer: Seizures, brain edema and herniation, intracranial infection. Frequent: Bone marrow suppression, N/V.
CHLORAMBUCIL (*Leukeran*) ▶L ♀D ▶– $ varies by therapy
WARNING — Secondary malignancies, bone marrow suppression, seizures, fertility impairment, alopecia. Instruct patients to report promptly fever, sore throat, signs of local infection, bleeding from any site, or symptoms suggestive of anemia.

CHLORAMBUCIL (*cont.*)

ADULT — Chemotherapy doses vary by indication. CLL. Lymphomas including indolent lymphoma and Hodgkin's disease.

PEDS — Not approved in children.

UNAPPROVED ADULT — Uveitis and meningoencephalitis associated with Behcet's disease. Idiopathic membranous nephropathy. Ovarian carcinoma.

FORMS — Trade only: Tabs 2 mg.

NOTES — Reliable contraception is recommended. Monitor CBCs. Avoid live vaccines.

MOA — Alkylating agent.

ADVERSE EFFECTS — The most common side effect is bone marrow suppression, anemia, leukopenia, neutropenia, thrombocytopenia, or pancytopenia. Seizures.

CYCLOPHOSPHAMIDE ▶L ♀D ▶– $ varies by therapy

WARNING — Secondary malignancies, leukopenia, cardiac toxicity, acute hemorrhagic cystitis, hypersensitivity, fertility impairment, alopecia. Instruct patients to report promptly fever, sore throat, signs of local infection, bleeding from any site, symptoms suggestive of anemia, or yellow discoloration of the skin or eyes.

ADULT — Chemotherapy doses vary by indication. Non-Hodgkin's lymphomas, Hodgkin's disease. Multiple myeloma. Disseminated neuroblastoma. Adenocarcinoma of the ovary. Retinoblastoma. Carcinoma of the breast. CLL. CML. AML. Mycosis fungoides.

PEDS — Chemotherapy doses vary by indication. ALL. "Minimal change" nephrotic syndrome.

UNAPPROVED ADULT — Wegener's granulomatosis, other steroid-resistant vasculitides. Severe progressive RA. Systemic lupus erythematosus. Multiple sclerosis. Polyarteritis nodosa. Lung, testicular and bladder cancer, sarcoma.

FORMS — Generic only: Tabs 25, 50 mg. Injection for hospital/oncology clinic use; not intended for outpatient prescribing.

NOTES — Reliable contraception is recommended. Monitor CBCs, urine for red cells. Allopurinol may increase myelosuppression. Thiazides may prolong leukopenia. May reduce digoxin levels, reduce fluoroquinolone activity. May increase anticoagulant effects. Coadministration with mesna reduces hemorrhagic cystitis when used in high doses.

MOA — Alkylating agent.

ADVERSE EFFECTS — Serious: Leukopenia, cardiac toxicity, acute hemorrhagic cystitis, hypersensitivity. Frequent: Alopecia, leukopenia.

DACARBAZINE (*DTIC-Dome*) ▶L K ♀C ▶– $ varies by therapy

WARNING — Extravasation associated with severe necrosis. Secondary malignancies, bone marrow suppression, hepatotoxicity, anorexia, N/V, anaphylaxis, alopecia. Instruct patients to report promptly fever, sore throat, signs of local infection, bleeding from any site, symptoms suggestive of anemia, or yellow discoloration of the skin or eyes.

ADULT — Chemotherapy doses vary by indication. Metastatic melanoma. Hodgkin's disease, in combination regimens.

PEDS — Not approved in children.

UNAPPROVED ADULT — Malignant pheochromocytoma, in combination regimens. Sarcoma.

NOTES — Monitor CBCs and LFTs.

MOA — Alkylating agent.

ADVERSE EFFECTS — Serious: Bone marrow suppression, hepatotoxicity, anaphylaxis. Frequent: Bone marrow suppression, N/V, anorexia.

IFOSFAMIDE (*Ifex*) ▶L ♀D ▶– $ varies by therapy

WARNING — Secondary malignancies, hemorrhagic cystitis, confusion, coma, bone marrow suppression, hematuria, nephrotoxicity, alopecia. Instruct patients to report promptly fever, sore throat, signs of local infection, bleeding from any site, symptoms suggestive of anemia, or yellow discoloration of the skin or eyes.

ADULT — Chemotherapy doses vary by indication. Germ cell testicular cancer, in combination regimens.

PEDS — Not approved in children.

UNAPPROVED ADULT — Bladder cancer, cervical cancer, ovarian cancer, non-small cell and small cell lung cancers, Hodgkin's and non-Hodgkin's lymphomas, ALL, osteosarcoma and soft tissue sarcomas.

UNAPPROVED PEDS — Ewing's sarcoma, osteosarcoma, soft tissue sarcomas, neuroblastoma.

FORMS — Powder for reconstitution: 1 g and 3 g vials. Sol for injection: 50 mg/mL 20 mL and 60 mL vials.

NOTES — Reliable contraception is recommended. Monitor CBCs, renal function, and urine for red cells. Coadministration with mesna reduces hemorrhagic cystitis. Requires extensive hydration to minimize bladder toxicity.

MOA — Alkylating agent.

ADVERSE EFFECTS — Serious: Hemorrhagic cystitis, coma, bone marrow suppression, hematuria, nephrotoxicity. Frequent: Bone marrow suppression, CNS, N/V, hematuria, alopecia.

LOMUSTINE (*CeeNu, CCNU, gleostine*) ▶L ♀D ▶– $ varies by therapy

WARNING — Secondary malignancies, bone marrow suppression, hepatotoxicity, nephrotoxicity, pulmonary fibrosis, fertility impairment, alopecia. Instruct patients to report promptly fever, sore throat, signs of local infection, bleeding from any site, symptoms suggestive of anemia, or yellow discoloration of the skin or eyes.

ADULT — Chemotherapy doses vary by indication. Brain tumors. Hodgkin's disease, in combination regimens.

PEDS — Chemotherapy doses vary by indication. Brain tumors. Hodgkin's disease, in combination regimens.

FORMS — Trade only: Caps 10, 40, 100 mg.

NOTES — Reliable contraception is recommended. Monitor CBCs, LFTs, PFTs, and renal function. Avoid alcohol.

LOMUSTINE (*cont.*)

MOA — Alkylating agent.

ADVERSE EFFECTS — Serious: Bone marrow suppression, hepatotoxicity, nephrotoxicity, pulmonary fibrosis. Frequent: Bone marrow suppression, N/V.

MECHLORETHAMINE (*Mustargen*) ▸Plasma ♀D ▶– $ varies by therapy

WARNING — Extravasation associated with severe necrosis. Secondary malignancies, bone marrow suppression, amyloidosis, herpes zoster, anaphylaxis, fertility impairment, alopecia. Instruct patients to report promptly fever, sore throat, signs of local infection, bleeding from any site, or symptoms suggestive of anemia.

ADULT — Chemotherapy doses vary by indication. Intravenous: Hodgkin's disease (Stages III and IV). Lymphosarcoma. Chronic myelocytic or chronic lymphocytic leukemia. Polycythemia vera. Mycosis fungoides. Bronchogenic carcinoma. Intrapleurally, intraperitoneally, or intrapericardially: Metastatic carcinoma resulting in effusion.

PEDS — Not approved in children.

UNAPPROVED ADULT — Cutaneous mycosis fungoides: Topical soln or ointment.

UNAPPROVED PEDS — Hodgkin's disease (Stages III and IV), in combination regimens.

NOTES — Reliable contraception is recommended. Monitor CBCs.

MOA — Alkylating agent.

ADVERSE EFFECTS — Serious: Bone marrow suppression, amyloidosis, herpes zoster, anaphylaxis. Frequent: Bone marrow suppression, N/V.

MELPHALAN (*Alkeran*) ▸Plasma ♀D ▶– $ varies by therapy

WARNING — Secondary malignancies, bone marrow suppression, anaphylaxis, fertility impairment, alopecia. Instruct patients to report promptly fever, sore throat, signs of local infection, bleeding from any site, or symptoms suggestive of anemia.

ADULT — Chemotherapy doses vary by indication. Multiple myeloma and nonresectable epithelial ovarian carcinoma.

PEDS — Not approved in children.

UNAPPROVED ADULT — Non-Hodgkin's lymphoma in high doses for stem cell transplant, testicular cancer.

FORMS — Trade only: Tabs 2 mg. Injection for hospital/clinic use; not intended for outpatient prescribing.

NOTES — Reliable contraception is recommended. Monitor CBCs. Avoid live vaccines.

MOA — Alkylating agent.

ADVERSE EFFECTS — Serious: Bone marrow suppression, anaphylaxis. Frequent: Bone marrow suppression, N/V.

PROCARBAZINE (*Matulane*) ▸LK ♀D ▶– $ varies by therapy

WARNING — Secondary malignancies, bone marrow suppression, hemolysis and Heinz-Ehrlich inclusion bodies in erythrocytes, hypersensitivity, fertility impairment, alopecia. Peds: Tremors, convulsions and coma have occurred. Instruct patients to report promptly fever, sore throat, signs of local infection, bleeding from any site, symptoms suggestive of anemia, black tarry stools or vomiting of blood.

ADULT — Chemotherapy doses vary by indication. Hodgkin's disease (Stages III and IV), in combination regimens.

PEDS — Chemotherapy doses vary by indication. Hodgkin's disease (Stages III and IV), in combination regimens.

FORMS — Trade only: Caps 50 mg.

NOTES — Reliable contraception is recommended. Monitor CBCs. Renal/hepatic function impairment may predispose toxicity. UA, LFTs, and BUN weekly. May decrease digoxin levels. May increase effects of opioids, sympathomimetics, TCAs. Ingestion of foods with high tyramine content may result in a potentially fatal hypertensive crisis. Alcohol may cause a disulfiram-like reaction.

MOA — Alkylating agent.

ADVERSE EFFECTS — Serious: Bone marrow suppression, hemolysis and Heinz-Ehrlich inclusion bodies in erythrocytes, hypersensitivity. Frequent: Bone marrow suppression, N/V.

STREPTOZOCIN (*Zanosar*) ▸Plasma ♀C ▶– $ varies by therapy

WARNING — Extravasation associated with severe necrosis. Secondary malignancies, nephrotoxicity, N/V, hepatotoxicity, decrease in hematocrit, hypoglycemia, fertility impairment, alopecia.

ADULT — Chemotherapy doses vary by indication. Metastatic islet cell carcinoma of the pancreas.

PEDS — Not approved in children.

NOTES — Hydration important. Monitor renal function, CBCs and LFTs.

MOA — Alkylating agent.

ADVERSE EFFECTS — Serious: Nephrotoxicity, N/V, hepatotoxicity. Frequent: N/V, hepatotoxicity.

TEMOZOLOMIDE (*Temodar,* ✦*Temodal*) ▸Plasma ♀D ▶– varies by therapy

WARNING — Secondary malignancies, bone marrow suppression, fertility impairment, alopecia. Instruct patients to report promptly fever, sore throat, signs of local infection, bleeding from any site, or symptoms suggestive of anemia. Cases of interstitial pneumonitis, alveolitis, and pulmonary fibrosis have been reported.

ADULT — Chemotherapy doses vary by indication. Anaplastic astrocytoma, glioblastoma multiforme.

PEDS — Not approved in children.

UNAPPROVED ADULT — Metastatic melanoma, renal cell carcinoma. Cutaneous T-cell lymphomas.

FORMS — Generic/Trade: Caps 5, 20, 100, 140, 180, 250 mg.

NOTES — Reliable contraception is recommended. Monitor CBCs. Valproic acid decreases clearance.

MOA — Alkylating agent.

ADVERSE EFFECTS — Serious: Bone marrow suppression, erythema multiforme. Frequent: N/V, fatigue, headache.

THIOTEPA (*Thioplex*) ▶L ♀D ▶– $ varies by therapy
WARNING — Secondary malignancies, bone marrow suppression, hypersensitivity, fertility impairment, alopecia. Instruct patients to report promptly fever, sore throat, signs of local infection, bleeding from any site, symptoms suggestive of anemia, black tarry stools or vomiting of blood.
ADULT — Chemotherapy doses vary by indication. Adenocarcinoma of the breast or ovary. Control of intracavitary malignant effusions. Superficial papillary carcinoma of the urinary bladder. Hodgkin's disease. Lymphosarcoma.
PEDS — Not approved in children.
NOTES — Reliable contraception is recommended. Monitor CBCs.
MOA — Alkylating agent.
ADVERSE EFFECTS — Serious: Bone marrow suppression, hypersensitivity. Frequent: Bone marrow suppression.

ONCOLOGY: Antibiotics

BLEOMYCIN (✲*Blenoxane*) ▶K ♀D ▶– $ varies by therapy
WARNING — Pulmonary fibrosis, skin toxicity, nephro/hepatotoxicity, alopecia, and severe idiosyncratic reaction consisting of hypotension, mental confusion, fever, chills, and wheezing. Because of the possibility of an anaphylactoid reaction, lymphoma patients should be treated with 2 units or less for the first 2 doses. If no acute reaction occurs, then the regular dosage schedule may be followed.
ADULT — Chemotherapy doses vary by indication. Squamous cell carcinoma of the head and neck. Carcinoma of the skin, penis, cervix, and vulva. Hodgkin's and non-Hodgkin's lymphoma. Testicular carcinoma. Malignant pleural effusion: Sclerosing agent.
PEDS — Not approved in children.
UNAPPROVED ADULT — Treatment of ovarian germ cell tumors.
NOTES — Reliable contraception is recommended. Frequent chest x-rays. May decrease digoxin and phenytoin levels. Risk of pulmonary toxicity increases with lifetime cumulative dose greater than 400 units.
MOA — Antibiotic.
ADVERSE EFFECTS — Serious: Pulmonary fibrosis, skin toxicity, nephro/hepatotoxicity, severe idiosyncratic reaction: hypotension, mental confusion, fever, chills, and wheezing. Frequent: Pulmonary fibrosis, stomatitis, vomiting, weight loss, alopecia.
DACTINOMYCIN (*Cosmegen*) ▶Not metabolized ♀C ▶– $ varies by therapy
WARNING — Extravasation associated with severe necrosis. Contraindicated with active chickenpox or herpes zoster. Erythema and vesiculation (with radiation), bone marrow suppression, alopecia. Instruct patients to report promptly fever, sore throat, signs of local infection, bleeding from any site, or symptoms suggestive of anemia.
ADULT — Chemotherapy doses vary by indication. Wilms' tumor. Rhabdomyosarcoma. Metastatic and nonmetastatic choriocarcinoma. Nonseminomatous testicular carcinoma. Ewing's sarcoma. Sarcoma botryoides. Most in combination regimens.
PEDS — Chemotherapy doses vary by indication. See adult. Contraindicated in infants less than 6 mo.
NOTES — Monitor CBCs.
MOA — Antibiotic.
ADVERSE EFFECTS — Serious: Erythema and vesiculation (with radiation), bone marrow suppression. Frequent: Bone marrow suppression, N/V, alopecia.
DOXORUBICIN LIPOSOMAL (*Doxil, Lipodox, Lipodox 50, ✲Caelyx, Myocet*) ▶L ♀D ▶+ $ varies by therapy
WARNING — Extravasation associated with severe necrosis. Cardiac toxicity, more frequent in children. Bone marrow suppression, infusion-associated reactions, necrotizing colitis, mucositis, hyperuricemia, palmar-plantar erythrodysesthesia. Secondary malignancies. Instruct patients to report promptly fever, sore throat, signs of local infection, bleeding from any site, or symptoms suggestive of anemia.
ADULT — Chemotherapy doses vary by indication. Advanced HIV-associated Kaposi's sarcoma, multiple myeloma, ovarian carcinoma.
PEDS — Not approved in children.
UNAPPROVED ADULT — Breast cancer, Hodgkin's Lymphoma, non-Hodgkin's lymphoma, soft tissue sarcomas.
NOTES — Heart failure with cumulative doses. Monitor ejection fraction, CBCs, LFTs, uric acid levels, and renal function (toxicity increased with impaired function). Reliable contraception is recommended. Transient urine discoloration (red).
MOA — Antibiotic.
ADVERSE EFFECTS — Serious: Cardiac toxicity, bone marrow suppression, infusion-associated reactions, necrotizing colitis, palmar-plantar erythrodysesthesia, secondary malignancies. Frequent: Cardiac toxicity, bone marrow suppression, hyperuricemia, fatigue, fever, anorexia, N/V, stomatitis, diarrhea, urine discoloration. Very rare cases of secondary oral cancer have been reported in patients with long-term (more than one year) exposure to DOXIL, or those receiving a cumulative DOXIL dose greater than 720 mg/m2.
DOXORUBICIN NON-LIPOSOMAL (*Adriamycin, Rubex*) ▶L ♀D ▶– $ varies by therapy
WARNING — Extravasation associated with severe necrosis. Cardiac toxicity, more frequent in children. Bone marrow suppression, infusion-associated reactions, necrotizing colitis, mucositis, hyperuricemia, alopecia. Secondary malignancies. Instruct patients to report promptly fever, sore throat, signs of local infection, bleeding from any site, or symptoms suggestive of anemia.

(cont.)

DOXORUBICIN NON-LIPOSOMAL (*cont.*)

ADULT — Chemotherapy doses vary by indication. ALL. AML. Wilms' tumor. Neuroblastoma. Soft tissue and bone sarcomas. Breast carcinoma. Ovarian carcinoma. Transitional cell bladder carcinoma. Thyroid carcinoma. Hodgkin's and non-Hodgkin's lymphomas. Bronchogenic carcinoma. Gastric carcinoma.

PEDS — Chemotherapy doses vary by indication: See adult.

UNAPPROVED ADULT — Sarcoma, small cell lung cancer.

NOTES — Heart failure with cumulative doses. Monitor ejection fraction, CBCs, LFTs, uric acid levels, and renal function (toxicity increased with impaired function). Reliable contraception is recommended. Transient urine discoloration (red).

MOA — Antibiotic.

ADVERSE EFFECTS — Serious: Cardiac toxicity, bone marrow suppression, secondary malignancies, infusion-associated reactions, necrotizing colitis. Frequent: Cardiac toxicity, bone marrow suppression, secondary malignancies, hyperuricemia, alopecia, urine discoloration.

EPIRUBICIN (*Ellence, ✸Pharmorubicin*) ▶L ♀D ▶– $ varies by therapy

WARNING — Extravasation associated with severe necrosis. Cardiac toxicity, bone marrow suppression, secondary malignancy (AML), hyperuricemia, fertility impairment, alopecia. Instruct patients to report promptly fever, sore throat, signs of local infection, bleeding from any site, or symptoms suggestive of anemia.

ADULT — Chemotherapy doses vary by indication. Adjuvant therapy for primary breast cancer.

PEDS — Not approved in children.

UNAPPROVED ADULT — Neoadjuvant and metastatic breast cancer. Cervical cancer, esophageal cancer, gastric cancer, soft tissue sarcomas, uterine sarcoma.

FORMS — 2mg/ml soln for IV injection.

NOTES — Reliable contraception is recommended. Monitor CBCs, cardiac, hepatic and renal function (toxicity increased with impaired function). Cimetidine increase levels. Transient urine discoloration (red).

MOA — Antibiotic.

ADVERSE EFFECTS — Serious: Cardiac toxicity, bone marrow suppression, secondary malignancies. Frequent: Cardiac toxicity, bone marrow suppression, N/V, mucositis, hyperuricemia, alopecia.

IDARUBICIN (*Idamycin*) ▶? ♀D ▶– $ varies by therapy

WARNING — Extravasation associated with severe necrosis. Cardiac toxicity, bone marrow suppression, hyperuricemia, alopecia. Instruct patients to report promptly fever, sore throat, signs of local infection, bleeding from any site, or symptoms suggestive of anemia.

ADULT — Chemotherapy doses vary by indication. AML, in combination regimens.

PEDS — Not approved in children.

UNAPPROVED ADULT — ALL, CML.

NOTES — Reliable contraception is recommended. Monitor CBCs, LFTs, cardiac and renal function (toxicity increased with impaired function).

MOA — Antibiotic.

ADVERSE EFFECTS — Serious: Cardiac toxicity, bone marrow suppression, secondary malignancies. Frequent: Cardiac toxicity, bone marrow suppression, N/V, hyperuricemia, alopecia.

MITOMYCIN (*Mutamycin, Mitomycin-C*) ▶L ♀D ▶– $ varies by therapy

WARNING — Extravasation associated with severe necrosis. Bone marrow suppression, hemolytic uremic syndrome, nephrotoxicity, adult respiratory distress syndrome, alopecia. Instruct patients to report promptly fever, sore throat, signs of local infection, bleeding from any site, or symptoms suggestive of anemia.

ADULT — Chemotherapy doses vary by indication. Disseminated adenocarcinoma of stomach, pancreas, or colorectum, in combination regimens.

PEDS — Not approved in children.

UNAPPROVED ADULT — Superficial bladder cancer, intravesical route; pterygia, adjunct to surgical excision: Ophthalmic soln.

NOTES — Reliable contraception is recommended. Monitor CBCs and renal function.

MOA — Antibiotic.

ADVERSE EFFECTS — Serious: Bone marrow suppression, hemolytic uremic syndrome, nephrotoxicity, adult respiratory distress syndrome. Frequent: Bone marrow suppression, N/V, anorexia.

MITOXANTRONE ▶LK ♀D ▶– $ varies by therapy

WARNING — Secondary malignancies (AML), bone marrow suppression, cardiac toxicity/heart failure, hyperuricemia, increased LFTs. Instruct patients to report promptly fever, sore throat, signs of local infection, bleeding from any site, or symptoms suggestive of anemia.

ADULT — Chemotherapy doses vary by indication. AML, in combination regimens. Symptomatic patients with hormone refractory prostate cancer. Multiple sclerosis (secondary progressive, progressive relapsing, or worsening relapsing-remitting): 12 mg/m2 of BSA IV q 3 months.

PEDS — Not approved in children.

UNAPPROVED ADULT — Breast cancer. Non-Hodgkin's lymphoma. ALL, CML, Ovarian carcinoma. Sclerosing agent for malignant pleural effusions.

NOTES — Reliable contraception is recommended. Monitor CBCs and LFTs. Baseline echocardiogram and repeat echoes prior to each dose are recommended. Transient urine and sclera discoloration (blue-green).

MOA — Antibiotic.

ADVERSE EFFECTS — Serious: Bone marrow suppression, cardiac toxicity, secondary malignancies.

MITOXANTRONE (cont.)

Frequent: Bone marrow suppression, N/V, menstrual disorders, stomatitis, urine and sclera discoloration, alopecia.

VALRUBICIN (*Valstar, ＊Valtaxin*) ▶K ♀C ▶– $ varies by therapy

WARNING — Induces complete responses in only 1 in 5 patients. Delaying cystectomy could lead to development of lethal metastatic bladder cancer. Irritable bladder symptoms, alopecia.

ADULT — Chemotherapy doses vary by indication. Bladder cancer, intravesical therapy of BCG-refractory carcinoma in situ.
PEDS — Not approved in children.
NOTES — Reliable contraception is recommended. Transient urine discoloration (red).
MOA — Antibiotic.
ADVERSE EFFECTS — Serious: None. Frequent: Irritable bladder symptoms.

ONCOLOGY: Antimetabolites

AZACITIDINE (*Vidaza*) ▶K ♀D ▶– $ varies by therapy

WARNING — Contraindicated with malignant hepatic tumors. Bone marrow suppression. Fertility impairment. Instruct patients to report promptly fever, sore throat, or signs of local infection or bleeding from any site.

ADULT — Chemotherapy doses vary by indication. Myelodysplastic syndrome subtypes.
PEDS — Not approved in children.
NOTES — Reliable contraception is recommended. Men should not father children while on this drug. Monitor CBC, renal and hepatic function.
MOA — Antimetabolite.
ADVERSE EFFECTS — Serious: Bone marrow suppression, hepatotoxicity, renal failure. Frequent: N/V, bone marrow suppression, fever, diarrhea, fatigue, constipation.

BELINOSTAT (*BELEODAQ*) ▶L ♀D ▶?

WARNING — Thrombocytopenia, leukopenia (neutropenia and lymphopenia), and anemia: Monitor blood counts and modify dosage for hematologic toxicities. Infection: Serious and fatal infections (e.g., pneumonia and sepsis) Hepatotoxicity: may cause hepatic toxicity and liver function test abnormalities. Monitor liver function tests and omit or modify dosage for hepatic toxicities. Tumor lysis syndrome: Monitor patients with advanced stage disease and/or high tumor burden and take appropriate precautions Embryo-fetal toxicity: Beleodaq may cause fetal harm when administered to a pregnant woman. Advise women of potential harm to the fetus and to avoid pregnancy while receiving Beleodaq

ADULT — Treatment of patients with relapsed or refractory peripheral T-cell lymphoma (PTCL). 1,000 mg/m² once daily on days 1-5 of a 21-day cycle.
PEDS — Not approved in peds.
FORMS — 500mg powder for injection.
MOA — Histone deacetylase (HDAC) inhibitor
ADVERSE EFFECTS — Most common: nausea, fatigue, pyrexia, anemia, and vomiting. Thrombocytopenia was reported in 16% of patients with grade 3 or 4 thrombocytopenia in 7% of patients. Serious: pneumonia, pyrexia, infection, anemia, increased creatinine, thrombocytopenia, and multi-organ failure.

CAPECITABINE (*Xeloda*) ▶L ♀D ▶– $ varies by therapy

WARNING — Increased INR and bleeding with warfarin. Contraindicated in severe renal dysfunction (CrCl less than 30 mL/min). Severe diarrhea, fertility impairment, palmar-plantar erythrodysesthesia or chemotherapy-induced acral erythema, cardiac toxicity, hyperbilirubinemia, neutropenia, alopeci, typhlitis. Instruct patients to report promptly fever, sore throat, or signs of local infection or bleeding from any site.

ADULT — Chemotherapy doses vary by indication. Metastatic breast and colorectal cancer.
PEDS — Not approved in children.
UNAPPROVED ADULT — Gastric cancer, esophageal cancer, pancreatic cancer, hepatocellular carcinoma, ovarian cancer, metastatic renal cell cancer, neuroendocrine tumors, metastatic CNS lesions.
FORMS — Trade only: Tabs 150, 500 mg.
NOTES — Reliable contraception is recommended. Antacids containing aluminum hydroxide and magnesium hydroxide increase levels. May increase phenytoin levels. Contraindicated with known dihydropyrimidine dehydrogenase (DPD) deficiency.
MOA — Antimetabolite.
ADVERSE EFFECTS — Serious: Bleeding with warfarin, severe diarrhea, palmar-plantar erythrodysesthesia, cardiac toxicity, neutropenia. Frequent: Palmar-plantar erythrodysesthesia, N/V, diarrhea, stomatitis, hyperbilirubinemia.

CLADRIBINE (*Leustatin, chlorodeoxyadenosine*) ▶intracellular ♀D ▶– $ varies by therapy

WARNING — Bone marrow suppression, nephrotoxicity, neurotoxicity, fever, fertility impairment, alopecia, headache, rash, infection, prolonged depression of CD4 counts. Instruct patients to report promptly fever, sore throat, or signs of local infection, bleeding from any site, or symptoms suggestive of anemia.

ADULT — Chemotherapy doses vary by indication. Hairy cell leukemia.
PEDS — Not approved in children.
UNAPPROVED ADULT — Advanced cutaneous T-cell lymphomas. Chronic lymphocytic leukemia, non-Hodgkin's lymphomas. AML. Autoimmune hemolytic anemia. Mycosis fungoides. Sezary syndrome. Progressive multiple sclerosis.
NOTES — Reliable contraception is recommended. Monitor CBCs and renal function.
MOA — Antimetabolite.
ADVERSE EFFECTS — Serious: Bone marrow suppression, nephrotoxicity, neurotoxicity, fever. Frequent: Bone marrow suppression, fever, N/V, diarrhea, rash.

CLOFARABINE (*Clolar*) ▶K ♀D ▶– $ varies by therapy
WARNING — Myelodysplastic syndrome, bone marrow suppression, tumor lysis syndrome, hepatotoxicity. Instruct patients to report promptly fever, sore throat, or signs of local infection, bleeding from any site, or symptoms suggestive of anemia.
ADULT — Not approved in adults.
PEDS — Age 1 to 21 yo: Chemotherapy doses vary by indication. Relapsed or refractory acute lymphoblastic leukemia.
FORMS — 20 mg/20 mL (1 mg/mL) single-use vial
NOTES — Reliable contraception is recommended. Monitor CBCs, LFTs, and renal function. Dose reduction is recommended with stable, moderate renal impairment.
MOA — Antimetabolite.
ADVERSE EFFECTS — Serious: Myelodysplastic syndrome, bone marrow suppression, serious infections, tumor lysis syndrome, hepatotoxicity. capillary leak, venous occlusive disease, Stevens-Johnson Syndrome (SJS) and toxic epidermal necrolysis (TEN). GI hemorrhage.
Frequent: Bone marrow suppression, N/V, diarrhea.

CYTARABINE (*Cytosar-U, Tarabine, Depo-Cyt, AraC*) ▶LK ♀D ▶– $ varies by therapy
WARNING — Bone marrow suppression, hepatotoxicity, N/V/D, hyperuricemia, pancreatitis, peripheral neuropathy, "cytarabine syndrome" (fever, myalgia, bone pain, occasional chest pain, maculopapular rash, conjunctivitis, and malaise), alopecia. Neurotoxicity. Chemical arachnoiditis (N/V, headache, and fever) with Depo-Cyt. Instruct patients to report promptly fever, sore throat, or signs of local infection, bleeding from any site, symptoms suggestive of anemia, or yellow discoloration of the skin or eyes.
ADULT — Chemotherapy doses vary by indication. AML. ALL. CML. Prophylaxis and treatment of meningeal leukemia. intrathecal (Cytosar-U, Tarabine). Lymphomatous meningitis, intrathecal (Depo-Cyt).
PEDS — Chemotherapy doses vary by indication. AML. ALL. Chronic myelocytic leukemia. Prophylaxis and treatment of meningeal leukemia, intrathecal (Cytosar-U, Tarabine). Depo-Cyt not approved in children.
NOTES — Reliable contraception is recommended. Monitor CBCs, LFTs, and renal function. Decreases digoxin levels. Chemical arachnoiditis can be reduced by coadministration of dexamethasone. Use dexamethasone eye drops with high doses.
MOA — Antimetabolite.
ADVERSE EFFECTS — Serious: Bone marrow suppression, hepatotoxicity, pancreatitis, peripheral neuropathy, "cytarabine syndrome" (fever, myalgia, bone pain, occasional chest pain, maculopapular rash, conjunctivitis, and malaise). Neurotoxicity. Chemical arachnoiditis (N/V, headache, and fever) with Depo-Cyt. Frequent: Bone marrow suppression, N/V, diarrhea, rash.

DECITABINE (*Dacogen*) ▶L ♀D ▶– $ varies by therapy
WARNING — Bone marrow suppression, pulmonary edema. Instruct patients to report promptly fever, sore throat, or signs of local infection, bleeding from any site, or symptoms suggestive of anemia.
ADULT — Myelodysplastic syndromes. Treatment Regimen: Option 1: Administer at a dose of 15 mg/m^2 by continuous IV infusion over 3 h repeated q 8 h for 3 days. Repeat cycle q 6 weeks. Option 2: Administer at a dose of 20 mg/m^2 by continuous IV infusion over 1 h repeated daily for 5 days. Repeat cycle q 4 weeks.
PEDS — Not approved in children.
NOTES — Reliable contraception is recommended. Men should not father children during and 2 months after therapy. Monitor CBCs, baseline LFTs.
MOA — Antimetabolite.
ADVERSE EFFECTS — Serious: Bone marrow suppression, pulmonary edema. Frequent: Bone marrow suppression, N/V, fatigue, fever, diarrhea, constipation, hyperglycemia, stomatitis.

FLOXURIDINE (*FUDR*) ▶L ♀D ▶– $ varies by therapy
WARNING — Bone marrow suppression, nephrotoxicity, increased LFTs, alopecia. Instruct patients to report promptly fever, sore throat, or signs of local infection, bleeding from any site, or symptoms suggestive of anemia.
ADULT — Chemotherapy doses vary by indication. GI adenocarcinoma metastatic to the liver given by intrahepatic arterial pump.
PEDS — Not approved in children.
NOTES — Reliable contraception is recommended. Monitor CBCs, LFTs, and renal function.
MOA — Antimetabolite.
ADVERSE EFFECTS — Serious: Bone marrow suppression. Frequent: Bone marrow suppression, N/V, stomatitis, alopecia.

FLUDARABINE (*Fludara*) ▶Serum ♀D ▶– $ varies by therapy
WARNING — Neurotoxicity (agitation, blindness, and coma), progressive multifocal leukoencephalopathy and death, bone marrow suppression, hemolytic anemia, thrombocytopenia, ITP, Evan's syndrome, acquired hemophilia, pulmonary toxicity, fertility impairment, hyperuricemia, alopecia. Instruct patients to report promptly fever, sore throat, or signs of local infection, bleeding from any site, or symptoms suggestive of anemia.
ADULT — Chemotherapy doses vary by indication. Chronic lymphocytic leukemia.
PEDS — Not approved in children.
UNAPPROVED ADULT — Non-Hodgkin's lymphoma. Mycosis fungoides. Hairy-cell leukemia. Hodgkin's disease.
NOTES — Reliable contraception is recommended. Monitor CBCs and renal function; watch for hemolysis.
MOA — Antimetabolite.
ADVERSE EFFECTS — Serious: Neurotoxicity (agitation, blindness, coma), progressive multifocal leukoencephalopathy and death, bone marrow

FLUDARABINE (*cont.*)

suppression, hemolytic anemia, pulmonary toxicity. Frequent: Bone marrow suppression, edema, N/V, fever, diarrhea, rash, alopecia.

FLUOROURACIL (*Adrucil, 5-FU*) ▶L ♀D ▶– $ varies by therapy

WARNING — Increased INR and bleeding with warfarin. Bone marrow suppression, angina, fertility impairment, alopecia, diarrhea, mucositis, hand and foot syndrome (palmar plantar erythrodysesthesia). Instruct patients to report promptly fever, sore throat, signs of local infection, bleeding from any site, or symptoms suggestive of anemia.

ADULT — Chemotherapy doses vary by indication. Colon, rectum, breast, stomach, and pancreatic carcinoma. Dukes' stage C colon cancer with irinotecan or leucovorin after surgical resection.

PEDS — Not approved in children.

UNAPPROVED ADULT — Head and neck, renal cell, prostate, ovarian, esophageal, anal and topical to skin for basal and squamous cell carcinoma.

NOTES — Reliable contraception is recommended. Monitor CBCs.

MOA — Antimetabolite.

ADVERSE EFFECTS — Serious: Bone marrow suppression, bleeding with warfarin, palmar-plantar erythrodysesthesia, angina. Frequent: Bone marrow suppression, N/V, diarrhea, stomatitis, alopecia.

GEMCITABINE (*Gemzar*) ▶intracellular ♀D ▶– $ varies by therapy

WARNING — Bone marrow suppression, fever, rash, increased LFTs, proteinuria, hematuria, alopecia. Instruct patients to report promptly fever, sore throat, signs of local infection, bleeding from any site, or symptoms suggestive of anemia.

ADULT — Chemotherapy doses vary by indication. Adenocarcinoma of the pancreas. Non-small-cell lung cancer, in combination regimens. Metastatic breast cancer, in combination regimens. Advanced ovarian cancer.

PEDS — Not approved in children.

FORMS — 200mg and 1000mg vials of soln for IV use.

NOTES — Reliable contraception is recommended. Monitor CBCs, LFTs and renal function.

MOA — Antimetabolite.

ADVERSE EFFECTS — Serious: Bone marrow suppression. Frequent: Bone marrow suppression, fever, rash, proteinuria, hematuria, increased LFTs.

MERCAPTOPURINE (*6-MP, Purinethol, Purixan*) ▶L ♀D ▶– $ varies by therapy

WARNING — Mercaptopurine is mutagenic in animals and humans, carcinogenic in animals, and may increase the patient's risk of neoplasia. Cases of hepatosplenic T-cell lymphoma have been reported in patients treated with mercaptopurine for inflammatory bowel disease. The safety and efficacy of mercaptopurine in patients with inflammatory bowel disease have not been established. Bone marrow suppression, hepatotoxicity, hyperuricemia, alopecia. Instruct patients to report promptly fever, sore throat, signs of local infection, bleeding from any site, symptoms suggestive of anemia, or yellow discoloration of the skin or eyes.

ADULT — Treatment of patients with acute lymphoblastic leukemia (ALL) as part of a combination regimen.

PEDS — Treatment of patients with acute lymphoblastic leukemia (ALL) as part of a combination regimen.

UNAPPROVED ADULT — Inflammatory bowel disease: Start at 50 mg PO daily, titrate to response. Typical dose range 0.5 to 1.5 mg/kg PO daily.

UNAPPROVED PEDS — Inflammatory bowel disease: 1.5 mg/kg PO daily.

FORMS — Generic/Trade: Tabs 50 mg. 20 mg/ml oral suspension.

NOTES — Reliable contraception is recommended. Monitor CBCs, LFTs, and renal function. Consider folate supplementation. Allopurinol and trimethoprim/sulfamethoxazole increase toxicity.

MOA — Antimetabolite.

ADVERSE EFFECTS — Serious: Bone marrow suppression, hepatotoxicity, oligospermia. Frequent: Bone marrow suppression, alopecia, rash, diarrhea.

METHOTREXATE—ONCOLOGY (*Rheumatrex, Trexall*) ▶KL -intestinal flora ♀X ▶–

WARNING — Acute renal failure, third-spacing in ascites/pleural effusions/bone marrow suppression/mucositis/hepatotoxicity/pneumonitis

ADULT — Trophoblastic neoplasms, acute lymphocytic leukemia, meningeal leukemia, breast cancer, head and neck cancer, cutaneous T-cell lymphoma, lung cancer, non-Hodgkin's Lymphoma, osteosarcoma

PEDS — Acute lymphocytic leukemia, meningeal leukemia, non-Hodgkin's lymphoma, nonmetastatic osteosarcoma

UNAPPROVED ADULT — Bladder cancer, CNS tumors, acute promyelocytic leukemia, soft tissue sarcomas, acute graft versus host disease prophylaxis

UNAPPROVED PEDS — Dermatomyositis, juvenile idiopathic arthritis,

FORMS — Injection, powder for reconstitution, 1 gm. Injection soln. 25 mg/mL. Oral tabs, 2.5 mg, 5 mg, 7.5 mg, 10 mg, 15 mg.

MOA — Folate antimetabolite that inhibits DNA synthesis.

ADVERSE EFFECTS — Arachnoiditis, hyperuricemia, mucositis, myelosuppression, renal failure.

NELARABINE (*Arranon⁕Atriance*) ▶LK ♀D ▶– $ varies by therapy

WARNING — Peripheral neuropathy, paralysis, demyelination, severe somnolence, convulsions. Bone marrow suppression.

ADULT — Chemotherapy doses vary by indication. ALL, T-cell lymphoblastic lymphoma .

PEDS — Chemotherapy doses vary by indication. ALL, T-cell lymphoblastic lymphoma.

NOTES — Reliable contraception is recommended. Monitor renal function.

MOA — Antimetabolite.

NELARABINE (cont.)

ADVERSE EFFECTS — Serious: Bone marrow suppression, peripheral neuropathy, paralysis, demyelination, convulsions. Frequent: Bone marrow suppression, fatigue, somnolence, N/V/D.

PEMETREXED (Alimta) ▶K ♀D ▶– $ varies by therapy

WARNING — Bone marrow suppression, rash. Instruct patients to report promptly fever, sore throat, signs of local infection, bleeding from any site, symptoms suggestive of anemia. Dose adjustment is required for patients with hepatic impairment.

ADULT — Chemotherapy doses vary by indication. Malignant pleural mesothelioma, in combination with cisplatin. Nonsquamous non-small-cell lung cancer. Seven days prior to pemetrexed therapy start supplementation with folic acid 400-1000 mcg orally daily until 21 days after last dose and Vitamin B12 1000 mcg IM, every 3 cycles. Give dexamethasone 4mg orally twice daily for 3 days starting the day before treatment to minimize cutaneous reactions.

PEDS — Not approved in children. No efficacy in pediatric patients has been reported. Pharmacokinetics in pediatric patients are comparable to adults.

UNAPPROVED ADULT — Metastatic bladder cancer, cervical cancer, thymic malignancies.

NOTES — Reliable contraception is recommended. Monitor CBCs and renal function. Do not use in patients with CrCl less than 45 mL/min. Avoid NSAIDs around the time of administration Drainage of mild or moderate third space fluid collection prior to ALIMTA treatment should be considered, but is probably not necessary. The effect of severe third space fluid on pharmacokinetics is not known.

MOA — Antimetabolite.

ADVERSE EFFECTS — Serious: Bone marrow suppression, severe rash. Frequent: Bone marrow suppression, fatigue, fever, N/V, stomatitis, dyspnea, rash. Cases of esophagitis were reported in clinical trials.

PENTOSTATIN (Nipent) ▶K ♀D ▶– $ varies by therapy

WARNING — Bone marrow suppression, nephrotoxicity, hepatotoxicity, CNS toxicity, pulmonary toxicity, severe rash, fertility impairment, alopecia. Instruct patients to report promptly fever, sore throat, signs of local infection, bleeding from any site, symptoms suggestive of anemia, or yellow discoloration of the skin or eyes.

ADULT — Chemotherapy doses vary by indication. Hairy cell leukemia, refractory to alpha-interferon.

PEDS — Not approved in children.

UNAPPROVED ADULT — ALL, CLL, non-Hodgkin's lymphoma, Mycosis fungoides.

NOTES — Reliable contraception is recommended. Monitor CBCs and renal function.

MOA — Antimetabolite.

ADVERSE EFFECTS — Serious: Bone marrow suppression, nephrotoxicity, hepatotoxicity, CNS toxicity, pulmonary toxicity, severe rash. Frequent: N/V, fever.

PRALATREXATE (Folotyn) ▶+ intracellular ♀D ▶–

WARNING — Bone marrow suppression, mucositis and hepatotoxicity may require dosage modification. Concomitant administration of drugs that are subject to substantial renal clearance (eg, NSAIDs, trimethoprim/sulfamethoxazole) may result in delayed clearance of pralatrexate. Severe and potentially fatal dermatologic reactions may occur, including toxic epidermal necrolysis (TEN). Skin toxicity may be progressive, with severity increasing with continued treatment. Monitor all dermatologic reactions and discontinue or withhold treatment for severe dermatologic reactions.

ADULT — 30mg/m2 IV once weekly for 6 out of 7 weeks. Treatment of relapsed/refractory peripheral T-cell lymphoma. (PTCL)

PEDS — Not approved in pediatrics

UNAPPROVED ADULT — Treatment of relapsed or refractory cutaneous T-cell lymphoma. (CTCL)

NOTES — Folic Acid and Vitamin B12 supplementation needed to reduce hematologic toxicity and treatment related mucositis. Folic Acid 1-1.25mg p.o. daily should be started within 10 days prior to starting pralatrexate, and continued for 30 days post last pralatrexate dose. Vitamin B12 1000mcg I.M. should be administered within 10 weeks prior to starting pralatrexate, and every 8 to 10 weeks thereafter. B12 may be given same day as pralatrexate after the initial dose.

MOA — Antifolate analog. Inhibits DNA, RNA and protein synthesis by entering cells expressing reduced folate carrier. After polyglutamylation by FPGS (folylpolyglutamate synthetase), competes for DHFR-folate binding site to inhibit DHFR (dihydrofolate reductase).

ADVERSE EFFECTS — Significant: Edema, fatigue, fever, rash, mucositis, nausea, vomiting, diarrhea, constipation, bone marrow suppression, increased LFTs, back and limb pain, cough, epistaxis, night sweats.

THIOGUANINE (Tabloid, ✱Lanvis) ▶L ♀D ▶– $ varies by therapy

WARNING — Bone marrow suppression, hepatotoxicity, hyperuricemia, alopecia. Instruct patients to report promptly fever, sore throat, signs of local infection, bleeding from any site, symptoms suggestive of anemia, or yellow discoloration of the skin or eyes.

ADULT — Chemotherapy doses vary by indication. Acute nonlymphocytic leukemias.

PEDS — Chemotherapy doses vary by indication. Acute nonlymphocytic leukemias.

FORMS — Generic only: Tabs 40 mg, scored.

NOTES — Reliable contraception is recommended. Monitor CBCs and LFTs.

MOA — Antimetabolite.

ADVERSE EFFECTS — Serious: Bone marrow suppression, hepatotoxicity. Frequent: Bone marrow suppression, diarrhea.

ONCOLOGY: Cytoprotective Agents

AMIFOSTINE (*Ethyol*) ▶plasma ♀C ▶– $ varies by therapy
WARNING — Hypotension, hypocalcemia, N/V, hypersensitivity.
ADULT — Doses vary by indication. Reduction of renal toxicity with cisplatin. Reduction of xerostomia and mucositis with radiation.
PEDS — Not approved in children.
NOTES — Monitor calcium and BP.
MOA — Cytoprotective.
ADVERSE EFFECTS — Serious: Hypotension, hypocalcemia. Frequent: N/V.

DENOSUMAB—ONCOLOGY (*Xgeva*) ▶? - ♀C ▶? $$$$$
WARNING — Severe symptomatic hypocalcemia, can occur with the use of denosumab. Symptoms include altered mental status, tetany, seizures and QTc prolongation. Atypical femur fractures have been reported in patients receiving denosumab. Osteonecrosis of the jaw has been reported in patients receiving denosumab. Dermatologic reactions, increased incidence of infection.
ADULT — Prevention of skeletal related events in bone metastases from solid tumors. 120 mg SC q 4 weeks. Treatment to increase bone mass in patients at high risk for fracture receiving androgen deprivation therapy (ADT) for nonmetastatic prostate cancer or adjuvant aromatase inhibitor (AI) therapy for breast cancer. Treatment of adults and skeletally mature adolescents with giant cell tumor of bone (GCTB) that is unresectable or where surgical resection is likely to result in severe morbidity.
PEDS — Not approved in peds
UNAPPROVED ADULT — Prevention of bone loss due to androgen deprivation therapy in nonmetastatic prostate cancer, and due to aromatase inhibitor therapy in nonmetastic breast cancer. Treatment of of bone destruction caused by rheumatoid arthritis.
FORMS — 70 mg/mL injection. 1.7 mL vials (120 mg/vial) Xgeva brand.
MOA — Monoclonal antibody with affinity for nuclear fator-kappa ligand. (RANKL). RANKL is secreted by osteoblasts and activates osteoclast precursors and subsequent osteolyisis which promotes release of bone derived growth factors. Denosumab binds to RANKL, blocks the interaction between RANKL and RANK, and prevents osteoclast formation.
ADVERSE EFFECTS — Fatigue, dermatitis, hypophosphatemia, nausea, diarrhea, limb pain, weakness, dyspnea.

DEXRAZOXANE (*Totect, Zinecard*) ▶plasma ♀D ▶– $ varies by therapy
WARNING — Additive bone marrow suppression, secondary malignancies (in pediatric and adult patients), fertility impairment, N/V.
ADULT — Doses vary by indication. Reduction of cardiac toxicity with doxorubicin. Treatment of anthracycline extravasation; give ASAP within 6 h of extravasation.
PEDS — Not approved in children.

FORMS — Generic/Trade: 250mg/vial, 500mg/vial
NOTES — Monitor CBCs.
MOA — Cytoprotective.
ADVERSE EFFECTS — Serious: Additive bone marrow suppression, secondary malignancies. Frequent: N/V.

GLUCARPIDASE (*Voraxaze*) ▶L ♀C ▶?
ADULT — Treatment of toxic plasma methotrexate concentrations (>1 micromole per liter) in patients with delayed methotrexate clearance due to impaired renal function. Given IV 50units/kg.
PEDS — treatment of toxic plasma methotrexate concentrations (>1 micromole per liter) in patients with delayed methotrexate clearance due to impaired renal function.
UNAPPROVED ADULT — 2000 units delivered intrathecally as soon as possible after intrathecal methotrexate overdose.
FORMS — 1000 unit powder for injection.
MOA — Glucarpidase is a recombinant enzyme that is able to rapidly decrease serum levels of methotrexate and thus reduce its concentration in most patients to below the threshold for serious toxicity. It lowers systemic methotrexate levels by rapidly causing methotrexate to convert to glutamate and 4-deoxy-4-amino-N 10-methylpteroic acid (DAMPA). Compared with methotrexate, DAMPA is 25 to 100 times less potent an inhibitor of dihydrofolate reductase (DHFR) and is significantly less cytotoxic.
ADVERSE EFFECTS — Antiglucarpidase antibody development (17%).
1-10% incidence: flushing, hypotension, headache, nausea/vomiting, parathesias.

MESNA (*Mesnex*, ✻*Uromitexan*) ▶plasma ♀B ▶– $ varies by therapy
WARNING — Hypersensitivity, bad taste in the mouth.
ADULT — Doses vary by indication. Reduction of hemorrhagic cystis with ifosfamide.
PEDS — Not approved in children.
UNAPPROVED ADULT — Doses vary by indication. Reduction of hemorrhagic cystis with high-dose cyclophosphamide.
UNAPPROVED PEDS — Doses vary by indication.
FORMS — Trade only: Tabs 400 mg, scored.
NOTES — False positive test urine ketones.
MOA — Cytoprotective.
ADVERSE EFFECTS — Serious: Hypersensitivity. Frequent: Bad taste in mouth.

PALIFERMIN (*Kepivance*) ▶plasma ♀C ▶? $ varies by therapy
ADULT — Doses vary by indication. Decreases incidence, duration, and severity of severe oral mucositis in patients receiving therapy for hematologic malignancies.
PEDS — Not approved in children. Information on the dosing and safety of palifermin in the pediatric population is limited. However, use of palifermin in pediatric patients ages 1 to 16 years is supported

PALIFERMIN (*cont.*)

by evidence from adequate and well-controlled studies of palifermin in adults and a phase 1 study that included 27 pediatric patients with acute leukemia undergoing hematopoietic stem cell transplant.

MOA — Cytoprotective – human keratinocyte growth factor.

ADVERSE EFFECTS — Serious: Fever. Frequent: Rash, erythema, edema, pruritus, oral/perioral dysesthesia, tongue discoloration or thickening, alteration of taste.

ONCOLOGY: Hormones

ABIRATERONE ACETATE (*Zytiga*) ▶L – ♀X ▶–

WARNING — Significant increases in hepatic enzymes have been reported; may require dose reduction.

ADULT — Indicated in combination with prednisone for the treatment of patients with metastatic castration-resistant prostate cancer. 1000 mg PO daily in combination with Prednisone 5 mg twice daily.

PEDS — Not for use in pediatrics.

FORMS — 250 mg tabs.

NOTES — Increased mineralocorticoid levels due to CYP17 inhibition. Avoid concurrent use with CYP3A4 inhibitors and inducers, as well as CYP2D6 substrates. Abiraterone inhibits the hepatic drug-metabolizing enzyme CYP2C8.

MOA — Binds to CYP17 enzyme, resulting in inhibition of the formation of testerone precursors.

ADVERSE EFFECTS — Joint swelling, hypokalemia, hypophosphatemia, hypertriglyceridemia, edema, muscle discomfort, hot flush, diarrhea, urinary tract infection, cough, hypertension, arrhythmia, urinary frequency, nocturia, dyspepsia and upper respiratory tract infection.

ANASTROZOLE (*Arimidex*) ▶L ♀X ▶– $ varies by therapy

WARNING — Patients with estrogen receptor-negative disease and patients who do not respond to tamoxifen therapy rarely respond to anastrozole. Fertility impairment, vaginal bleeding, hot flashes, alopecia, decrease in bone mineral density, trigger finger. Increase in cardiovascular ischemia in women with preexisting ischemic heart disease.

ADULT — Chemotherapy doses vary by indication. Locally advanced or metastatic breast cancer. Adjuvant early breast cancer.

PEDS — Not approved in children.

FORMS — Generic/Trade: Tabs 1 mg.

NOTES — Reliable contraception is recommended. Monitor CBCs. Contraindicated in premenopausal women.

MOA — Aromatase inhibitor.

ADVERSE EFFECTS — Serious: Cardiovascular ischemia. Frequent: Hot flashes, nausea, vasodilatation, mood disturbance, fatigue, arthralgia, myalgia, pharyngitis.

BICALUTAMIDE (*Casodex*) ▶L ♀X ▶ $ varies by therapy

WARNING — Hypersensitivity, hepatotoxicity, interstitial lung disease, gynecomastia/breast pain, fertility impairment, hot flashes, diarrhea, alopecia. Increased risk for cardiovascular disease and diabetes.

ADULT — Prostate cancer: 50 mg PO daily in combination with a LHRH analog (eg, goserelin or leuprolide). Not indicated in women.

PEDS — Not approved in children.

UNAPPROVED ADULT — Monotherapy for locally advanced prostate cancer at a dose of 150mg PO daily.

FORMS — Generic/Trade: Tabs 50 mg.

NOTES — Monitor PSA levels, CBC, ECG, serum testosterone, luteinizing hormone, and LFTs. Monitor glucose closely in diabetics. Displaces warfarin, possibly increasing anticoagulant effects. Gynecomastia and breast pain occur. Avoid concomitant use with tolvaptan.

MOA — Anti-androgen.

ADVERSE EFFECTS — Serious: Hypersensitivity, hepatotoxicity, chest pain, hypertension,angioedema, urticaria, interstitial lung disease. Frequent: Gynecomastia, breast pain, hot flashes, general pain, impotence, anemia.

CYPROTERONE (✱*Androcur*) ▶L ♀X ▶– $ varies by therapy

ADULT — Prostate cancer.

PEDS — Not approved in children.

FORMS — Generic/Trade: Tabs 50 mg.

NOTES — Dose-related hepatotoxicity has occurred, monitor LFTs at initiation and during treatment. Monitor adrenocortical function periodically. May impair carbohydrate metabolism; monitor blood glucose, especially in diabetics.

MOA — Antiandrogen.

ADVERSE EFFECTS — Serious: Hepatotoxicity, thromboembolism, depression. Frequent: Decreased libido, gynecomastia, impotence, abnormal spermatozoa.

DEGARELIX (*Firmagon*) ▶LK ♀X ▶– $$$$$

WARNING — QT prolongation.

ADULT — Advanced prostate cancer: Initial dose: 240 mg SC; maintenance: 80 mg SC q 28 days.

PEDS — Not approved in children.

FORMS — Trade Only: 80mg, 120mg soln for SC injection.

NOTES — Monitor LFTs and PSA. May prolong QT interval. May decrease bone mineral density.

MOA — Gonadotropin-releasing hormone antagonist that suppresses LH and FSH secretion thus lowering serum testosterone.

ADVERSE EFFECTS — Serious: Allergic reactions, hypersensitivity reactions including rash and uticaria, hepatotoxicity, QT prolongation. Frequent: Hot flashes, wt gain, increased LFTs, night sweats.

ENZALUTAMIDE (*Xtandi*) ▶L – ♀X ▶–

WARNING — Seizure occurred in 0.9% of patients receiving XTANDI. There is no clinical trial experience with XTANDI in patients who have had a

ENZALUTAMIDE (*cont.*)

seizure, in patients with predisposing factors for seizure, or in patients using concomitant medications that may lower the seizure threshold.

ADULT — First line treatment of metastatic castration-resistant prostate cancer (mCRPC). 160 mg orally once daily

PEDS — Not approved in peds.

FORMS — 40mg capsules.

NOTES — Enzalutamide is a strong CYP3A4 inducer and a moderate CYP2C9 and CYP2C19 inducer. At steady state XTANDI reduced the plasma exposure to midazolam (a CYP3A4 substrate), warfarin (a CYP2C9 substrate) and omeprazole (a CYP2C19 substrate) by 86%, 56% and 70%, respectively. Therefore, concomitant use of XTANDI with narrow therapeutic index drugs that are metabolized by CYP3A4, CYP2C9 or CYP2C19 should be avoided. If co-administration with warfarin (a CYP2C9 substrate) is unavoidable, conduct additional INR monitoring. The concomitant use of strong CYP2C8 inhibitors (gemfibrozil) should be avoided.

MOA — Androgen receptor inhibitor that targets steps in the androgen receptor signaling pathway.

ADVERSE EFFECTS — Asthenia/fatigue, back pain, diarrhea, arthralgia, hot flush, peripheral edema, musculoskeletal pain, headache, upper respiratory infection, muscular weakness, dizziness, insomnia, lower respiratory infection, spinal cord compression and cauda equina syndrome, hematuria, paresthesia, anxiety, and hypertension.

ESTRAMUSTINE (*Emcyt*) ▶L ♀X ▶– $ varies by therapy

WARNING — Thrombosis, including MI, glucose intolerance, HTN, fluid retention, increased LFTs, alopecia.

ADULT — Chemotherapy doses vary by indication. Hormone refractory prostate cancer.

PEDS — Not approved in children.

FORMS — Trade only: Caps 140 mg.

NOTES — Reliable contraception is recommended. Monitor LFTs, glucose and BP. Milk, milk products and calcium-rich foods or drugs may impair absorption.

MOA — Alkylating agent.

ADVERSE EFFECTS — Serious: Thrombosis, MI, glucose intolerance, HTN, fluid retention. Frequent: None.

EXEMESTANE (*Aromasin*) ▶L ♀D ▶– $ varies by therapy

WARNING — Lymphocytopenia, alopecia.

ADULT — Chemotherapy doses vary by indication. Breast cancer.

PEDS — Not approved in children.

UNAPPROVED ADULT — Chemotherapy doses vary by indication. Prevention of prostate cancer.

FORMS — Generic/Trade: Tabs 25 mg.

NOTES — Contraindicated in premenopausal women. Reliable contraception is recommended. Monitor CBCs.

MOA — Aromatase inhibitor.

ADVERSE EFFECTS — Serious: Lymphocytopenia. hypersensitivity, urticaria, and pruritis. Frequent: Lymphocytopenia, nausea, hot flashes

FLUTAMIDE (*Eulexin*, *✦Euflex*) ▶L ♀D ▶– $ varies by therapy

WARNING — Hepatic failure, methemoglobinemia, hemolytic anemia, breast neoplasms, gynecomastia, fertility impairment, photosensitivity, alopecia.

ADULT — Prostate cancer: 250 mg PO q 8 h in combination with a LHRH analog (eg, goserelin or leuprolide). Not indicated in women.

PEDS — Not approved in children.

UNAPPROVED ADULT — Hirsutism in women.

FORMS — Generic only: Caps 125 mg.

NOTES — Monitor LFTs, PSA, methemoglobin levels. Transient urine discoloration (amber or yellow-green). Avoid exposure to sunlight/use sunscreen. Increased INR with warfarin. Gynecomastia and breast pain occur.

MOA — Anti-androgen.

ADVERSE EFFECTS — Serious: Hepatic failure, methemoglobinemia, hemolytic anemia. Frequent: Gynecomastia, urine discoloration, hot flashes, diarrhea, photosensitivity, impotence.

FULVESTRANT (*Faslodex*) ▶L ♀D ▶– $ varies by therapy

WARNING — Contraindicated in pregnancy. Hypersensitivity, N/V/D, constipation, abdominal pain, hot flashes. Use with caution in patients with bleeding disorders. Hepatic impairment may require dose adjustment.

Elevation of bilirubin, elevation of gamma GT, hepatitis, and liver failure have been reported infrequently (<1%)

ADULT — Chemotherapy doses vary by indication. Breast cancer. 500mg IM on Days 1,15 and 29, then 500mg monthly thereafter.

PEDS — Not approved in children.

FORMS — 250mg/5ml soln for IM injection.

NOTES — Reliable contraception is recommended. FDA approved only in hormone receptor–positive metastatic breast cancer in postmenopausal women with disease progression following antiestrogen therapy.

MOA — Estrogen receptor antagonist.

ADVERSE EFFECTS — Serious: Hypersensitivity, increased LFTs. Frequent: N/V, diarrhea, abdominal pain, hot flashes, joint disorders.

GOSERELIN (*Zoladex*) ▶LK ♀D/X ▶– $ varies by therapy

WARNING — Transient increases in sex hormones, increases in lipids, hypercalcemia, decreases in bone mineral density, vaginal bleeding, fertility impairment, hot flashes, decreased libido, alopecia.

ADULT — Prostate cancer: 3.6 mg implant SC into upper abdominal wall q 28 days, or 10.8 mg implant SC q 12 weeks. Endometriosis: 3.6 mg implant SC q 28 days or 10.8 mg implant q 12 weeks for 6 months. Specialized dosing for breast cancer.

PEDS — Not approved in children.

UNAPPROVED ADULT — Adjuvant prostate cancer. Palliative treatment of breast cancer. 3.6 mg implant SC q 28 days indefinitely. Endometrial

GOSERELIN (*cont.*)

thinning prior to ablation for dysfunctional uterine bleeding: 3.6 mg SC 4 weeks prior to surgery or 3.6 mg SC q 4 weeks for 2 doses with surgery 2 to 4 weeks after last dose.

FORMS — Trade only: Implants 3.6, 10.8 mg.

NOTES — Transient increases in testosterone and estrogen occur. Hypercalcemia may occur in patients with bone metastases. Vaginal bleeding may occur during the first 2 months of treatment and should stop spontaneously. Reliable contraception is recommended. Consider norethindrone as "add back" therapy to decrease bone loss (see norethindrone).

MOA — Gonadotropin inhibitor.

ADVERSE EFFECTS — Serious: Hypersensitivity, anaphylaxis, antibody formation, pituitary apoplexy, osteoporosis, decreased bone mineral density, angina, thromboembolism, heart failure, hypercalcemia. Frequent: Decrease in bone mineral density, vaginal bleeding, hot flashes, gynecomastia, transient worsening of pain. Observed post-marketing: mood swings, acne, convulsions.

HISTRELIN (*Vantas, Supprelin LA*) ▶Not metabolized ♀X ▶– $ varies by therapy

WARNING — Worsening of symptoms, especially during the 1st weeks of therapy: Increase in bone pain, difficulty urinating. Decreases in bone mineral density. Increased risk of cardiovascular disease and diabetes in men with prostate cancer.

ADULT — Palliative treatment of advanced prostate cancer (Vantas): Insert 1 implant SC in the upper arm surgically q 12 months. May repeat if appropriate after 12 months.

PEDS — Central precocious puberty (Supprelin LA), in age older than 2 yo: Insert 1 implant SC in the inner upper arm surgically. May repeat if appropriate after 12 months.

FORMS — Trade only: 50 mg implant.

NOTES — Causes transient increase of testosterone level during the first weeks of treatment which may create or exacerbate symptoms. Patients with metastatic vertebral lesions and/or urinary tract obstruction should be closely observed during the 1st few weeks of therapy. Avoid wetting arm for 24 h after implant insertion and from heavy lifting or strenuous exertion of the involved arm for 7 days after insertion. Measure testosterone levels and PSA periodically. May decrease bone density. Monitor LH, FSH, estradiol or testosterone, height and bone age in children with central precocious puberty at 1 month post implantation and q 6 months thereafter.

MOA — Gonadotropin releasing hormone agonist

ADVERSE EFFECTS — Serious: Bladder outlet obstruction, hematuria, bone pain, neuropathy, spinal cord compression, seizures. Frequent: Implant site reaction, erectile dysfunction, gynecomastia, hot flashes, testicular atrophy, transient worsening of pain.

LETROZOLE (*Femara*) ▶LK ♀D ▶– $$$

WARNING — Fertility impairment, decreases in lymphocytes, increased LFTs, alopecia.

ADULT — 2.5 mg PO daily. Adjuvant treatment of postmenopausal, hormone receptor positive, early breast cancer. Extended adjuvant treatment of early breast cancer after 5 years of tamoxifen therapy. Advanced breast cancer with disease progression after antiestrogen therapy, hormone receptor positive or hormone receptor unknown, locally advanced or metastatic breast cancer.

PEDS — Not approved in children.

UNAPPROVED ADULT — Ovarian (epithelial) cancer. Endometrial cancer.

FORMS — Generic/Trade: Tabs 2.5 mg.

NOTES — Reliable contraception is recommended. Monitor CBCs, LFTs, and lipids.

MOA — Aromatase inhibitor.

ADVERSE EFFECTS — Serious: Lymphocytopenia, angioedema, anaphylaxis, toxic epidermal necrolysis, erythema multiforme, and hepatitis. Frequent: Lymphocytopenia, nausea, hot flashes, bone pain, fatigue, dizziness, increased cholesterol, decreased bone mineral density. Possible: carpal tunnel syndrome and trigger finger.

LEUPROLIDE (*Eligard, Lupron Depot, Lupron Depot-Ped*) ▶L ♀X ▶– $ varies by therapy

WARNING — Possible increase of diabetes and cardiovascular disease in men receiving leuprolide for prostate cancer. Worsening of symptoms: Increase in bone pain, difficulty urinating. Decreases in bone mineral density. Anaphylaxis, alopecia.

Respiratory, thoracic and mediastinal disorder - Interstitial lung disease.

Possible convulsions.

ADULT — Advanced prostate cancer: Lupron: 1 mg SC daily. Eligard: 7.5 mg SC q month, 22.5 mg SC q 3 months, 30 mg SC q 4 months, or 45 mg SC q 6 months. Lupron depot: 7.5 mg IM q month, 22.5 mg IM q 3 months or 30 mg IM q 4 months. Viadur: 65 mg SC implant q 12 months. Endometriosis or uterine leiomyomata (fibroids): 3.75 mg IM q month or 11.25 mg IM q 3 months for total therapy of 6 months (endometriosis) or 3 months (fibroids). Administer concurrent iron for fibroid-associated anemia.

PEDS — Central precocious puberty: Injection: 50 mcg/kg/day SC. Increase by 10 mcg/kg/day until total down regulation. Depot-Ped: 0.3 mg/kg q 4 weeks IM (minimum dose 7.5 mg). Increase by 3.75 mg q 4 weeks until adequate down regulation.

UNAPPROVED ADULT — Treatment of breast cancer, infertility, menses cessation in patients receiving high dose chemotherapy, prostatic hyperplasia.

NOTES — For prostate cancer, monitor testosterone, prostatic acid phosphatase and PSA levels. Transient increases in testosterone and estrogen occur. For endometriosis, a fractional dose of the 3 month depot preparation is not equivalent to the same dose of the monthly formulation. Rotate the injection site periodically. Consider norethindrone as "add back" therapy to decrease bone loss (see norethindrone).

LEUPROLIDE (*cont.*)

MOA — Gonadotropin inhibitor via agonism of luteinizing hormone releasing hormone.

ADVERSE EFFECTS — Serious: Anaphylaxis, urinary obstruction, erythema multiforme, pituitary apoplexy, convulsions. Hepato-biliary disorder: Serious drug-induced liver injury. Frequent: Decrease in bone mineral density, vaginal bleeding, hot flashes, gynecomastia, transient worsening of pain.

NILUTAMIDE (*Nilandron✲Anandron®*) ▶L ♀C ▶– $ varies by therapy

WARNING — Interstitial pneumonitis, hepatitis, aplastic anemia (isolated cases), delay in adaptation to the dark, hot flashes, alcohol intolerance, alopecia.

ADULT — Prostate cancer: 300 mg PO daily for 30 days, then 150 mg PO daily. Begin therapy on same day as surgical castration.

PEDS — Not approved in children.

FORMS — Trade only: Tabs 150 mg.

NOTES — Monitor CBCs, LFTs, and chest X-rays. Caution patients who experience delayed adaptation to the dark about driving at night or through tunnels; suggest wearing tinted glasses. May increase phenytoin and theophylline levels. Avoid alcohol.

MOA — Anti-androgen.

ADVERSE EFFECTS — Serious: Interstitial pneumonitis, hepatitis, aplastic anemia. Frequent: Delay in adaptation to the dark, hot flashes, gynecomastia, alcohol intolerance, alopecia.

TOREMIFENE (*Fareston*) ▶L ♀D ▶– $ varies by therapy

WARNING — QT prolongation that is dose and concentration dependent. Use is contraindicated in the presence of uncorrected hypokalemia or hypomagnesemia. Hypercalcemia and tumor flare, endometrial hyperplasia, thromboembolism, hot flashes,nausea, increased LFTs, vaginal bleeding, fertility impairment, rare myelosuppression, alopecia.

ADULT — Chemotherapy doses vary by indication. Breast cancer.

PEDS — Not approved in children.

UNAPPROVED ADULT — Treatment of soft tissue sarcoma.

FORMS — Trade only: Tabs 60 mg.

NOTES — Avoid concurrent use with strong CYP3A4 inhibitors and QTc prolonging agents. Reliable contraception is recommended. Monitor CBCs, calcium levels and LFTs. May increase effects of anticoagulants.

MOA — Selective estrogen receptor modulator.

ADVERSE EFFECTS — Serious: DVT/PE, endometrial cancer, visual disturbances, cataracts, hypercalcemia, tumor flare, hepatotoxicity. Frequent: Hot flashes, vaginal bleeding.

TRIPTORELIN (*Trelstar*) ▶tissues – ? ♀X ▶–

WARNING — Anaphylactic shock, hypersensitivity, and angioedema have been reported.

Tumor Flare: Transient increase in serum testosterone levels can occur within the first few weeks of treatment. This may worsen prostate cancer and result in spinal cord compression and urinary tract obstruction.

ADULT — Palliative treatment of advanced prostate cancer. Administered as a single intramuscular injection:
• 3.75 mg every 4 weeks.
• 11.25 mg every 12 weeks.
• 22.5 mg every 24 weeks.

PEDS — Not indicated in pediatrics.

FORMS — Injectable suspension: 3.75 mg, 11.25 mg, 22.5 mg.

NOTES — $ - varies by therapy

MOA — Agonist analog of gonadotropin releasing hormone

ADVERSE EFFECTS — Hot flushes, skeletal pain, impotence, and headache, erectile dysfunction, testicular atrophy, convulsions.

TRIPTORELIN (*Trelstar Depot*) ▶LK ♀X ▶– $ varies by therapy

WARNING — Transient increases in sex hormones, bone pain, neuropathy, hematuria, urethral/bladder outlet obstruction, spinal cord compression, anaphylaxis, hot flashes, impotence, alopecia.

ADULT — Chemotherapy doses vary by indication. Prostate cancer.

PEDS — Not approved in children.

MOA — Gonadotropin inhibitor.

ADVERSE EFFECTS — Serious: Bone pain, neuropathy, hematuria, urethral/bladder outlet obstruction, spinal cord compression, anaphylaxis, convulsions. Frequent: Transient worsening of symptoms, hot flashes, impotence.

ONCOLOGY: Immunomodulators

ALDESLEUKIN (*Proleukin, interleukin-2*) ▶K ♀C ▶– $ varies by therapy

WARNING — Capillary leak syndrome, resulting in hypotension and reduced organ perfusion. Exacerbation of autoimmune diseases and symptoms of CNS metastases, impaired neutrophil function, hepato/nephrotoxicity, mental status changes, decreased thyroid function, anemia, thrombocytopenia, fertility impairment, alopecia.

ADULT — Chemotherapy doses vary by indication. Renal-cell carcinoma.

PEDS — Not approved in children.

UNAPPROVED ADULT — Kaposi's sarcoma. Metastatic melanoma. Colorectal cancer. Non-Hodgkin's lymphoma.

NOTES — Monitor CBCs, electrolytes, LFTs, renal function and chest X-rays. Baseline PFTs. Avoid iodinated contrast media. Antihypertensives potentiate hypotension.

MOA — Aldesleukin stimulates a cytokine cascade involving various interferons, interleukins, and tumor necrosis factors, which induces the

ALDESLEUKIN (cont.)

proliferation and differentiation of B and T-cells, monocytes, macrophages, natural killer cells, and other cytotoxic cells.

ADVERSE EFFECTS — Serious: Capillary leak syndrome, resulting in hypotension and reduced organ perfusion. Exacerbation of autoimmune diseases and of symptoms of CNS metastases, immunosuppression, hepato/nephrotoxicity, decreased thyroid function, anemia, thrombocytopenia. Frequent: Hypotension, tachycardia, mental status changes, anemia, thrombocytopenia, N/V, fever, chills, rigors, pruritus.

ALEMTUZUMAB (Campath, ✱MabCampath) ▶? ♀C ▶– $ varies by therapy

WARNING — Idiopathic thrombocytopenic purpura, bone marrow suppression, hemolytic anemia, hypersensitivity, and immunosuppression.

ADULT — Chemotherapy doses vary by indication. B-cell chronic lymphocytic leukemia.

PEDS — Not approved in children.

NOTES — Monitor CBC.

MOA — The exact mechanism of alemtuzumab is unknown; however, the proposed mechanism involves the binding of alemtuzumab to CD52, a nonmodulating antigen that is present on the surface of essentially all B and T lymphocytes, a majority of monocytes, macrophages, NK cells, and a subpopulation of granulocytes, causing an antibody-dependent lysis of leukemic cells.

ADVERSE EFFECTS — Serious: Idiopathic thrombocytopenic purpura, bone marrow suppression, hemolytic anemia, hypersensitivity, and immunosuppression. Frequent: Hypotension, rigors, fever, shortness of breath, bronchospasm, chills, rash, N/V.

BCG VACCINE FOR BLADDER INSTILLATION—ONCOLOGY (Bacillus of Calmette & Guerin, Pacis, TheraCys, Tice BCG, ✱Oncotice, Immucyst) ▶Not metabolized ♀C ▶? $ varies by therapy

WARNING — Hypersensitivity, hematuria, urinary frequency, dysuria, bacterial UTI, flu-like syndrome, alopecia.

ADULT — Chemotherapy doses vary by indication. Carcinoma in situ of the urinary bladder, intravesical.

PEDS — Not approved in children.

NOTES — Bone marrow depressants, immunosuppressants and antimicrobial therapy may impair response. Increase fluid intake after treatments.

MOA — BCG is an immunostimulant used to stimulate the immune system to produce immunity against tuberculosis or to mount a local inflammation and immune reaction against superficial cancers from the activation of T-lymphocytes, B-lymphocytes, and natural killer cells.

ADVERSE EFFECTS — Serious: Hypersensitivity, hematuria, urinary frequency, dysuria, bacterial urinary tract infection. Frequent: Flu-like syndrome.

BEVACIZUMAB (Avastin) ▶? ♀C ▶– $ varies by therapy

WARNING — CVA, MI, TIA, angina, GI perforation, wound dehiscence, serious hemorrhage, HTN, heart failure, nephrotic syndrome, reversible posterior leukoencephalopathy syndrome (brain capillary leak syndrome), nasal septum perforation. Tracheoesophageal fistula has been reported. Microangiopathic hemolytic anemia (MAHA) in patients on concomitant sunitinib malate. Females of reproductive potential should be informed of increased reproductive failure. Increased risk of venous thromboembolic (VTE) and bleeding events in patients receiving anticoagulation therapy after first VTE event while receiving bevacizumab. May cause moderate to severe proteinuria.

ADULT — Chemotherapy doses vary by indication. Metastatic colorectal carcinoma; unresectable, locally advanced, recurrent or metastatic nonsquamous, non-small-cell lung cancer; glioblastoma;metastatic renal cell cancer. Use in combination with fluoropyrimidine-irinotecan or fluoropyrimidine-oxaliplatin based chemotherapy for the treatment of patients with metastatic colorectal cancer (mCRC) whose disease has progressed on a first-line bevacizumab-containing regimen; persistent, recurrent, or late-stage cervical cancer in combination with chemotherapy.

PEDS — Not approved in children.

UNAPPROVED ADULT — Metastatic breast cancer, recurrent ovarian cancer, recurrent cervical cancer, soft tissue sarcomas, age-related macular degeneration.

NOTES — Monitor BP, and UA for protein. Do not use in combination with sunitinib.

MOA — Bevacizumab is a humanized monoclonal antibody which binds the vascular endothelial growth factor (VEGF) preventing the interaction of VEGF to its receptors. In human cancers, VEGF expression is associated with increased microvascular density, tumor growth, metastasis, and poor prognosis.

ADVERSE EFFECTS — Serious: CVA, MI, TIA, angina, GI perforation, wound dehiscence, serious hemorrhage, HTN, heart failure, nephrotic syndrome, reversible posterior leukoencephalopathy syndrome (brain capillary leak syndrome), microangiopathic hemolytic anemia, nasal septum perforation. Osteonecrosis of the jaw without bisphosphonates. necrotizing fasciitis. Frequent: Headache, HTN, stomatitis, constipation, diarrhea, abdominal pain, N/V, epistaxis, dyspnea, proteinuria.

BRENTUXIMAB VEDOTIN (Adcetris) ▶oxidation - feces ♀D ▶–

WARNING — Peripheral motor neuropathy, infusion reactions, including anaphylaxis, (premedication is required),progressive multifocal leukoencephalopathy. Use of brentuximab is contraindicated with bleomycin due to increased risk for pulmonary toxicity.

ADULT — Treatment of Hodgkin lymphoma after failure of at least 2 prior chemotherapy regimens (in patient ineligible for transplant) or after stem

BRENTUXIMAB VEDOTIN (cont.)

cell transplant failure. Systemic anaplastic large cell lymphoma (sALCL) after failure of at least one prior chemotherapy regimen.

PEDS — Not approved in pediatric patients

FORMS — 50mg powder for injection.

MOA — Antibody drug conjugate directed at CD30.

ADVERSE EFFECTS — Myelosuppression, peripheral sensory neuropathy, fatigue, nausea, pyrexia, rash, cough, upper respiratory infection.

CETUXIMAB (Erbitux) ▶? ♀C ▶– $ varies by therapy

WARNING — Anaphylaxis, cardiopulmonary arrest/sudden death, pulmonary toxicity, rash, sepsis, renal failure, pulmonary embolus, hypomagnesemia.

ADULT — Chemotherapy doses vary by indication. Indicated for the treatment of patients with K-ras mutation-negative (wild-type), EGFR-expressing metastatic colorectal cancer as determined by FDA-approved tests. Cetuximab is not indicated for treatment of K-Ras mutation-positive colorectal cancer. Indicated for use in combination with FOLFIRI (irinotecan, 5-fluorouracil, leucovorin) for first-line treatment of K-Ras mutation-negative (wild-type), EGFR-expressing metastatic colorectal cancer. Treatment of squamous cell cancer of the head and neck.

PEDS — Not approved in children. Safety and effectiveness in children not established. No new safety signals identified in pediatric patients after pharmacokinetic evaluation.

UNAPPROVED ADULT — EGFR-expressing advanced nonsmall cell lung cancer.

NOTES — Monitor renal function and electrolytes including magnesium. Caution with known CAD, heart failure, or arrhythmias. Premedication with a H1 antagonist and a 1-h observation period after infusion is recommended due to potential for anaphylaxis. Use is not recommended in patients with codon 12 or 13 KRAS mutations.

MOA — Cetuximab is a recombinant chimeric monoclonal antibody that binds to and blocks the binding of ligands (eg, epidermal growth factor and tissue growth factor) to the epidermal growth factor receptor (EGFR, HER1, c-ErbB-1) on the surface of normal and tumor cells, resulting in inhibition of cell growth, induction of apoptosis, and decreased vascular endothelial growth factor (VEGF) production.

ADVERSE EFFECTS — Serious: Anaphylaxis, cardiopulmonary arrest/sudden death, pulmonary toxicity, rash, sepsis, renal failure, pulmonary embolus, hypomagnesemia. Use with radiation and cisplatin adds mucosal inflammation. Frequent: Rash, pruritus, nail changes, malaise, diarrhea, abdominal pain, N/V, hypomagnesemia. Dermatologic toxicity: Limit sun exposure. Monitor for inflammatory or infectious sequelae.

DENILEUKIN (Ontak) ▶Plasma ♀C ▶– $ varies by therapy

WARNING — Hypersensitivity, vascular leak syndrome (hypotension, edema, hypoalbuminemia), visual loss, thrombosis, rash, diarrhea, alopecia.

ADULT — Chemotherapy doses vary by indication. Cutaneous T-cell lymphoma.

PEDS — Not approved in children.

UNAPPROVED ADULT — Mycosis fungoides, Sezary syndrome. Second-line treatment for peripheral T-cell lymphoma.

NOTES — Monitor CBCs, LFTs, and renal function. Visual loss is usually persistent.

MOA — Denileukin diftitox is a recombinant DNA-derived cytotoxic protein composed of the amino acid sequences for diphtheria toxin fragments A and B, followed by the sequences for interleukin-2, designed to be cytotoxic to cells that express certain high-affinity interleukin (IL)-2 receptors.

ADVERSE EFFECTS — Serious: Hypersensitivity, vascular leak syndrome (hypotension, edema, hypoalbuminemia), visual loss, infection, DVT/PE. Frequent: Hypersensitivity, vascular leak syndrome (hypotension, edema, hypoalbuminemia), fever, rash, N/V, diarrhea.

EVEROLIMUS (Afinitor, Afinitor Disperz) ▶L ♀D ▶– $$$$$

WARNING — Noninfectious pneumonitis, hyperglycemia, bone marrow suppression. Avoid live vaccines.

ADULT — Chemotherapy doses vary by indication. Advanced renal cell carcinoma. Progressive neuroendocrine tumors of pancreatic origin (PNET) in patients with unresectable, locally advanced or metastatic disease. Subependymal giant cell astrocytoma (SEGA) associated with tuberous sclerosis. Renal angiomyolipoma associated with tuberous sclerosis comples (TSC), who do not require immediate surgery. Treatment of postmenopausal women with advanced hormone receptor-positive, HER2-negative breast cancer in combination with exemestane, after failure of treatment with letrozole or anastrozole.

PEDS — Everolimus tabs for oral susp (Afinitor Disperz) for the treatment of pediatric and adult patients with tuberous sclerosis complex (TSC) who have subependymal giant cell astrocytoma (SEGA) that requires therapeutic intervention but cannot be curatively resected. Dosing for adult and pediatric patients with SEGA is 4.5 mg/m2/day, with subsequent dosing based on therapeutic drug monitoring to achieve and maintain everolimus trough levels of 5 to 15 ng/mL.

UNAPPROVED ADULT — Treatment of relapsed or refractory Waldenstrom's macroglobulinemia (WM).

FORMS — AFINITOR: 2.5 mg, 5 mg, 7.5 mg, and 10 mg tabs AFINITOR DISPERZ (everolimus tabs for oral susp): 2 mg, 3 mg and 5 mg tabs for oral susp

NOTES — Reliable contraception is recommended. Drugs that induce the CYP3A4 system such as phenytoin, phenobarbital, rifampin may decrease concentrations. Inhibitors such as clarithromycin, itraconazole, ketoconazole, and ritonavir may increase concentrations. Avoid live vaccines. Monitor CBC, hepatic and renal function, glucose and lipid profile. Increased risk of proteinuria when used in combination with cyclosporine.

EVEROLIMUS (*cont.*)

MOA — m-TOR inhibitor. Reduces protein synthesis and cellular proliferation by binding to the intracellular protein, FK binding protein-12, to form a complex that inhibits activation of m-TOR (mammalian target of rapamycin.)

ADVERSE EFFECTS — Serious: Immunosuppressant properties leading to serious infection, and development of malignancy including lymphoma and skin cancer. Noninfectious pneumonitis, bone marrow suppression. Acute pancreatitis, impaired wound healing. Frequent: Hyperglycemia, hypertriglyceridemia, rash, mucositis, stomatitis, N/V.

IBRITUMOMAB (*Zevalin*) ▶L ♀D ▶– $ varies by therapy

WARNING — Contraindicated in patients with allergy to murine proteins. Hypersensitivity. Serious Infusion reactions, some fatal, may occur within 24 hs of rituximab infusion. Prolonged and severe cytopenias occur in most patients. Severe cutaneous and mucocutaneous reactions, some fatal, reported with Zevalin therapeutic regimen. Do not exceed 32 mCi (1184 MBq) ofY-90 Zevalin.

ADULT — Chemotherapy doses vary by indication. Non-Hodgkin's lymphoma.

PEDS — Not approved in children.

NOTES — Reliable contraception is recommended. Monitor CBCs.

MOA — Ibritumomab tiuxetan contains a monoclonal antibody linked to an active chelator that accounts for its cytotoxic activity. The antibody moiety contains a murine IgG1 kappa monoclonal antibody directed against the CD20 antigen, once bound, the beta emission from the tiuxetan portion induces cellular damage through the formation of free radicals in the target and neighboring cells.

ADVERSE EFFECTS — Serious: Fatal infusion reactions, erythema multiforme, Stevens-Johnson syndrome, toxic epidermal necrolysis, bullous and exfoliative dermatitis, bone marrow suppression, hypersensitivity. Frequent: Bone marrow suppression, N/V, diarrhea.

INTERFERON ALFA-2A (*Roferon-A*) ▶Plasma ♀C ▶– $ varies by therapy

WARNING — GI hemorrhage, CNS reactions, leukopenia, increased LFTs, anemia, neutralizing antibodies, depression/suicidal behavior, alopecia.

ADULT — Discontinued by manufacturer February 2008. Chemotherapy doses vary by indication. Hairy cell leukemia. AIDS-related Kaposi's sarcoma. CML.

PEDS — Not approved in children.

UNAPPROVED ADULT — Superficial bladder tumors. Carcinoid tumor. Cutaneous T-cell lymphoma. Essential thrombocythemia. Non-Hodgkin's lymphoma.

NOTES — Reliable contraception is recommended. Monitor CBCs and LFTs. Hydration important. Decreases clearance of theophylline.

MOA — Interferons exert their cellular activities by binding to specific membrane receptors on the cell surface. Once bound to the cell membrane, interferons initiate a complex sequence of intracellular events. In vitro studies demonstrated that these include the induction of certain enzymes, suppression of cell proliferation, immunomodulating activities such as enhancement of the phagocytic activity of macrophages and augmentation of the specific cytotoxicity of lymphocytes for target cells, and inhibition of virus replication in virus-infected cells.

ADVERSE EFFECTS — Serious: Depression/suicidal behavior, GI hemorrhage, CNS reactions, leukopenia, increased LFTs, anemia. Frequent: Rash, N/V, diarrhea, flu-like syndrome.

IPILIMUMAB (*Yervoy*) ▶endogenous – ♀C ▶–

WARNING — Severe and fatal immune-mediated adverse reactions due to T-cell activation and proliferation. Interacts with Vitamin K antagonists and cardiac glycosides. Adverse effects were observed in animal reproduction studies. Drug is known to cross the placenta. Other adverse effects include autoimmune central neuropathy (encephalitis), neurosensory hypoacusis, myositis, polymyositis, ocular myositis and sarcoidosis.

ADULT — Unresectable or metastatic melanoma. 3 mg/kg q 3 weeks for 4 doses.

PEDS — Not approved in peds.

FORMS — IV.

NOTES — Scheduled doses will need to be withheld for moderate immune-mediated reactions and symptomatic endocrine disorders. Permanently discontinue drug if cannot complete treatment course within 16 weeks of initial dose. Ipilimumab may increase the levels and side effects of vemurafenib.

MOA — Mab which binds to CTLA-4, allowing for enhanced T-cell activation.

ADVERSE EFFECTS — Fatigue, HA, pruritis, rash, N & V, diarrhea, constipation, abdominal pain.

LENALIDOMIDE (*Revlimid*) ▶K ♀X ▶– $ varies by therapy

WARNING — Potential for human birth defects, potential for an increased risk of developing secondary malignancies, bone marrow suppression, DVT, and PE. Instruct patients to report promptly fever, sore throat, signs of local infection, bleeding from any site, or symptoms suggestive of anemia. Increased mortality seen in patients with CLL.

ADULT — Chemotherapy doses vary by indication. Myelodysplastic syndromes in patients with deletion 5q and transfusion dependent anemia (with or without cytogenetic abnormalities.) Multiple myeloma in combination with dexamethasone in patients who have received at least one prior therapy. Mantle cell lymphoma patients whose disease has relapsed or progressed after two prior therapies, one of which included bortezomib.

PEDS — Not approved in children.

FORMS — Trade only: Caps 5, 10, 15, 25 mg.

NOTES — Analog of thalidomide; can cause birth defects or fetal death. Lenalidomide, a thalidomide analogue, caused limb abnormalities in a developmental monkey study similar to birth defects caused by thalidomide in humans. If lenalidomide is used during pregnancy, it may cause birth defects or death to a developing baby. Pregnancy must be

LENALIDOMIDE (*cont.*)

excluded before start of treatment. Prevent pregnancy during treatment by the use of two reliable methods of contraceptionAvailable only through a restricted distribution program. Reliable contraception is mandated; males must use a latex condom. Monitor CBCs. Do not break, chew or open the caps. Adjust dose for CrCl less than 60 mL/min.

MOA — Immunomodulator and angiogenesis inhibitor.

ADVERSE EFFECTS — Serious: Potential for birth defects, neutropenia and thrombocytopenia, DVT/PE. Frequent: Bone marrow suppression, diarrhea, pruritus, rash, fatigue. Tasigna prolongs the QT interval. Prior to Tasigna administration and periodically, monitor for hypokalemia or hypomagnesemia and correct deficiencies Obtain ECGs to monitor the QTc at baseline, seven days after initiation, and periodically thereafter, and follow any dose adjustments

OFATUMUMAB (*Arzerra*) ▸immune system – ♀C ▸?

WARNING — May cause cause serious infusion reactions. Premedicate with acetaminophen, an antihistamine, and a corticosteroid. May cause prolonged cytopenias. Progressive multifocal leukoencephalopathy (PML) can occur. Risk for reactivation of hepatitis B virus (HBV) infection in patients who once had the virus may occur. Some of the cases of HBV reactivation that have been reported have resulted in fulminant hepatitis, hepatic failure, and death. Intestinal obstruction may occur.

ADULT — 300 mg IV initial dose (dose 1), followed 1 week later by 2000 mg IV weekly for 7 doses (doses 2 through 8), followed 4 weeks later by 2,000 mg IV q 4 weeks for 4 doses (doses 9 through 12). Treatment of patients with chronic lymphocytic leukemia (CLL) refractory to fludarabine and alemtuzumab. Treatment of untreated CLL in combination with chlorambucil when fludarabine-based therapy is inappropriate.

PEDS — Not approved for pediatric use.

NOTES — Premedicate 30 min to 2 h prior to ofatumumab infusion with acetaminopen, antihistamine, and corticosteroid. See product labeling for dose reduction guidelines of corticosteroids.

MOA — Binds specifically to both the small and large extracellular loops of the CD20 molecule on B-lymphocytes resulting in complement dependent cell lysis and antibody-dependent cell mediated toxicity.

ADVERSE EFFECTS — Neutropenia, pneumonia, pyrexia, cough, diarrhea, anemia, fatigue, dyspnea, rash, nausea, bronchitis, and upper respiratory tract infections.

PANITUMUMAB (*Vectibix*) ▸Not metabolized ♀C ▸– $ varies by therapy

WARNING — Skin exfoliation, severe dermatologic reactions complicated by sepsis and death.Derm toxicities reported in 90% of patients, 12% severe. Severe infusion reactions. Anaphylaxis.

ADULT — Chemotherapy doses vary by indication. Indicated for EGFR-expressing refractory metastatic colorectal carcinoma. Not indicated for patients with KRAS mutation positive or unknown metastatic colorectal carcinoma.

PEDS — Not approved in children.

NOTES — Reliable contraception is recommended. Monitor potassium and magnesium.

MOA — Panitumumab is a monoclonal antibody that binds to epidermal growth factor receptor (EGFR) on tumor cells preventing autophosphorylation and activation of receptor-associated kinases, resulting in inhibition of cell growth, induction of apoptosis, decreased proinflammatory cytokine and vascular growth factor production.

ADVERSE EFFECTS — Serious: Infusion-related reactions, anaphylaxis, sepsis, pulmonary fibrosis. Frequent: Hypomagnesemia, acne, pruritus, erythema, rash, skin exfoliation, paronychia, stomatitis, mucositis, diarrhea, photosensitivity.

PEGINTERFERON ALFA-2B (*Sylatron*) ▸K - ♀C ▸?

WARNING — May cause or aggravate severe depression. Suicide or suicidal ideation.

ADULT — Sylatron brand indicated for adjuvant treatment of melanoma. 6mcg/kg/week subcutaneously for 8 doses, followed by 3mg/kg/week up to 5 years.

PEDS — No approved oncology indication in pediatrics.

FORMS — Powder for injection.

NOTES — None

MOA — Inhibits cellular growth, alters the state of cellular differentiation, interferes with oncogene expression, alters cell surface antigen expression, increases phagocytic activity of macrophages, and augments cytotoxicity of lymphocytes for target cells.

ADVERSE EFFECTS — Serious: Bone marrow suppression, colitis, acute hypersensitivity reactions, hypertriglyceridemia. Common: fatigue, fever, headache, depression, rash, anorexia, nausea and vomiting, myalgias.

POMALIDOMIDE (*Pomalyst*) ▸L – ♀X ▸– $$$$$

WARNING — Pomalidomide should not be used in pregnant women because it can cause severe life-threatening birth defects and can cause blood clots

ADULT — The treatment of multiple myeloma for patients who have received at least 2 prior therapies, including lenalidomide and bortezomib, and whose disease did not respond to treatment and progressed within 60 days of the last treatment. 4 mg per day taken orally on days 1-21 of repeated 28-day cycles until disease progression.

PEDS — Not approved in peds.

FORMS — Capsules: 1 mg, 2 mg, 3 mg and 4 mg

MOA — Inhibits proliferation and induces apoptosis of hematopoietic tumor cells. Inhibits the proliferation of lenalidomide-resistant multiple myeloma cell lines and synergized with dexamethasone in both lenalidomide-sensitive and lenalidomide-resistant cell lines to induce tumor cell apoptosis.

POMALIDOMIDE (*cont.*)

Pomalidomide enhanced T cell- and natural killer (NK) cell-mediated immunity and inhibited production of pro-inflammatory cytokines (e.g., TNF-α and IL-6) by monocytes. Pomalidomide demonstrated anti-angiogenic activity in a mouse tumor model and in the in vitro umbilical cord mode

ADVERSE EFFECTS — Severe: embryo-fetal toxicity, venous thromboembolism. Common adverse effects include neutropenia, fatigue and weakness, anemia, constipation, diarrhea, thrombocytopenia, upper respiratory tract infections, back pain, and fever.

SIPULEUCEL-T (*Provenge*) ▶? - ♀▶

WARNING — Acute infusion reactions may occur within 1 day of infusion. Cerebrovascular events, including hemorrhagic and ischemic strokes, were observed in clinical trials.

ADULT — Treatment of metastatic hormone-refractory prostate cancer in patients who are symptomatic or minimally symptomatic. Administer a total of 3 doses at 2-week intervals.

PEDS — Not approved in peds.

FORMS — Infusion, premixed in preservative-free LR. Greater than 50 million autologous CD54+ cells activated with PAP-GM-CSF (250 mL).

NOTES — No pregnancy or lactation data. Not indicated for use in women. Premedication with oral acetaminophen and diphenhydramine is recommended to minimize infusion reactions.

MOA — Autologous cellular immunotherapy, designed to stimulate a patient's own immune system to respond against the cancer. Each dose of sipuleucel-T is manufactured by obtaining a patient's peripheral blood mononuclear cells, via leukapheresis. Antigen presenting cell precursors are isolated from these cells. To enhance their response against the cancer, these cells are then exposed to a recombinant human fusion protein, PAP-GM-CSF composed of an antigen specific for prostate cancer linked to prostatic acid phosphatase, and granulocyte-macrophage colony stimulating factor. After this process, the final product, sipuleucel-T, is reinfused into the patient to induce T-cell immunity towards the prostate cancer cells.

ADVERSE EFFECTS — Chills, fatigue, fever, back pain, nausea, joint ache and headache.

TEMSIROLIMUS (*Torisel*) ▶L ♀C ▶– $ varies by therapy

WARNING — Hypersensitivity, interstitial lung disease, bowel perforation, renal failure, hyperglycemia, bone marrow suppression. Avoid live vaccines.

ADULT — Chemotherapy doses vary by indication. Advanced renal cell carcinoma.

PEDS — Not approved in children.

UNAPPROVED ADULT — Relapsed or refractory mantle cell lymphoma.

NOTES — Reliable contraception is recommended. Drugs that induce the CYP3A4 system such as phenytoin, phenobarbital, rifampin may decrease concentrations. Inhibitors such as clarithromycin, itraconazole, ketoconazole, and ritonavir may increase concentrations. Avoid live vaccines.

Monitor CBC, hepatic, and renal function, glucose and lipid profile. Premedicate with an H1 antagonist 30 minutes prior to infusion to prevent infusion reactions,

MOA — Targeted inhibitor of mTOR (mammalian target of rapamycin) kinase activity, halting the cell cycle at the G1 phase in tumor cells. Also reduces levels of HIF-1 (hypoxia inducible factor) and HIF-2 alpha, and VEGF (vascular endothelial growth factor) thus exhibiting angiogenic activity in renal cell carcinoma.

ADVERSE EFFECTS — Serious: Hypersensitivity, interstitial lung disease, bowel perforation, renal failure, bone marrow suppression. Frequent: Hyperglycemia, hypertriglyceridemia, rash, mucositis, anorexia, N/V.

SIDE EFFECTS — Edema, pain, rash, mucositis, myelosuppression, weakness, hepatic and renal impairment, infection.

THALIDOMIDE (*Thalomid*) ▶Plasma ♀X ▶? $$$$$

WARNING — Pregnancy category X. Has caused severe, life-threatening human birth defects. Available only through special restricted distribution program. Prescribers and pharmacists must be registered in this program in order to prescribe or dispense. During therapy with thalidomide, patients with a history of seizures or with other risk factors for the development of seizures should be monitored closely for clinical changes that could precipitate acute seizure activity.

ADULT — Chemotherapy doses vary by indication. Multiple myeloma, with dexamethasone. Erythema nodosum leprosum: 100 to 400 mg PO at bedtime. Use low end of dose range for initial episodes and if wt less than 50 kg.

PEDS — Not approved in children.

UNAPPROVED ADULT — Graft vs. Host reactions after bone marrow transplant, Crohn's disease, Waldenstrom's macroglobinemia. Langerhans cell histiocytosis, AIDs–related aphthous stomatitis.

UNAPPROVED PEDS — Clinical trials show beneficial effects when combined with dexamethasone in multiple myeloma.

FORMS — Trade only: Caps 50, 100, 150, 200 mg.

MOA — Immunomodulatory agent. Exact mechanism unknown.

ADVERSE EFFECTS — Serious: Birth defects, permanent peripheral neuropathy, bradycardia, Stevens-Johnson syndrome, toxic epidermal necrolysis. Frequent: Somnolence, drowsiness, dizziness, orthostatic hypotension, rash, leukopenia.

TOSITUMOMAB (*Bexxar*) ▶Not metabolized ♀X ▶– $ varies by therapy

WARNING — Contraindicated in patients with allergy to murine proteins. Hypersensitivity, anaphylaxis, infusion reactions, neutropenia, thrombocytopenia, anemia. Hypothyroidism.

ADULT — Chemotherapy doses vary by indication. Relapsed or refractory CD20 positive, low grade,follicular or transformed non-Hodgkin's lymphoma with progression during or following treatment with rituximab.

TOSITUMOMAB (cont.)

PEDS — Not approved in children.

NOTES — This product is a combination of tositumomab + iodine I 131 tositumomab. Reliable contraception is recommended. Monitor CBC, TSH.

MOA — Tositumomab induces cytotoxicity by combining the immunological effects of antibody binding with the preferential targeting of radiation therapy. Tositumomab, an anti-CD20 monoclonal antibody, targets B-lymphocytes and induces complement-mediated cytolysis, antibody-dependent cellular cytotoxicity, apoptosis, and cell death caused by ionizing radiation from the radioisotope.

ADVERSE EFFECTS — Serious: Infusion reactions, hypersensitivity, bone marrow suppression, hypothyroidism. Frequent: Bone marrow suppression, N/V.

TRASTUZUMAB (Herceptin) ▶Not metabolized ♀B ▶– $ varies by therapy

WARNING — Hypersensitivity, including fatal anaphylaxis, fatal infusion-related reactions, pulmonary events including ARDS and death, ventricular dysfunction and heart failure. Anemia, leukopenia, diarrhea, alopecia.

ADULT — Chemotherapy doses vary by indication. Breast cancer with tumors overexpressing the HER2 NEU protein. HER2-overexpressing metastatic gastric or gastroesophageal junction adenocarcinoma with cisplatin and a fluoropyrimidine.

PEDS — Not approved in children.

NOTES — Monitor with ECG, echocardiogram, or MUGA scan. CBCs.

MOA — Trastuzumab is a recombinant DNA-derived humanized monoclonal antibody that selectively binds to the extracellular domain of the human epidermal growth factor receptor 2 protein (HER2). It mediates antibody-dependent cellular cytotoxicity by inhibiting proliferation of cells which overexpress the HER2 protein.

ADVERSE EFFECTS — Serious: Anaphylaxis, fatal infusion-related reactions, ARDS, heart failure, bone marrow suppression. Frequent: Fever, chills, N/V, diarrhea, rash.

ONCOLOGY: Mitotic Inhibitors

CABAZITAXEL (Jevtana) ▶L - ♀D ▶–

WARNING — Neutropenia, febrile neutropenia: Neutropenic deaths have been reported. Severe hypersensitivity reactions can occur. Mortality related to diarrhea has been reported. Renal failure, including cases with fatal outcomes, has been reported. Patients older than 65 yo were more likely to experience fatal outcomes not related to disease. Should not be given to patients with hepatic impairment. QTc interval prolongation.

ADULT — Indicated in combination with prednisone for treatment of patients with hormone-refractory metastatic prostate cancer previously treated with a docetaxel-containing treatment regimen. 25 mg/m² administered IV q 3 weeks in combination with oral prednisone 10 mg administered daily throughout treatment.

PEDS — Not indicated in pediatrics.

FORMS — Single use vial 60 mg/1.5 mL, supplied with diluent (5.7 mL)

NOTES — Premedication regimen required 30 minutes before each dose:
Antihistamine, Corticosteroid (dexamethasone 8 mg or equivalent steroid) and H2 antagonist

MOA — Microtubule inhibitor. Binds to tubulin and promotes its assembly into microtubules while simultaneously inhibiting disassembly. This leads to the stabilization of microtubules, which results in the inhibition of mitotic and interphase cellular functions

ADVERSE EFFECTS — Neutropenia, anemia, leukopenia, thrombocytopenia, diarrhea, fatigue, nausea, vomiting, constipation, asthenia, abdominal pain, hematuria, back pain, anorexia, peripheral neuropathy, pyrexia, dyspnea, dysgeusia, cough, arthralgia, and alopecia.

DOCETAXEL (Taxotere, Docefrez) ▶L ♀D ▶– $ varies by therapy

WARNING — Severe hypersensitivity with anaphylaxis, bone marrow suppression, fluid retention, neutropenia, rash, erythema of the extremities, nail hypo- or hyperpigmentation, hepatotoxicity, treatment related mortality, paresthesia/dysesthesia, asthenia, fertility impairment, alopecia. Instruct patients to report promptly fever, sore throat, or signs of local infection.

ADULT — Chemotherapy doses vary by indication. Breast cancer. Non-small-cell lung cancer. Hormone refractory, metastatic prostate cancer. Advanced gastric adenocarcinoma with cisplatin and fluorouracil. Squamous cell carcinoma of the head and neck.

PEDS — Not approved in children.

UNAPPROVED ADULT — Gastric cancer. Melanoma. Non-Hodgkin's lymphoma. Ovarian cancer. Pancreatic cancer. Prostate cancer. Small-cell lung cancer. Soft-tissue sarcoma. Urothelial cancer. Adjuvant and neoadjuvant breast cancer.

FORMS — Intravenous concentrate: 20mg, 80mg, 140mg, 160mg vials.

NOTES — Reliable contraception is recommended. Monitor CBCs and LFTs. CYP3A4 inhibitors or substrates may lead to significant increases in blood concentrations.

MOA — Mitotic Inhibitor.

ADVERSE EFFECTS — Serious: Hypersensitivity/anaphylaxis, cutaneous events, edema, neutropenia, rash, erythema of the extremities, nail hypo- or hyperpigmentation, hepatotoxicity, paresthesia/dysesthesia. Respiratory: dyspnea, acute pulmonary edema, acute respiratory distress syndrome/pneumonitis, interstitial lung disease, interstitial

DOCETAXEL (*cont.*)

pneumonia, respiratory failure, and pulmonary fibrosis have rarely been reported and may be associated with fatal outcome. Rare cases of radiation pneumonitis have been reported in patients receiving concomitant radiotherapy Frequent: Rash, N/V, diarrhea, bone marrow suppression. Cases of cystoid macular edema (CME) have been reported in patients treated with docetaxel, as well as with other taxanes.

ERIBULIN (*Halaven*) ▶feces – ♀D ▶–

WARNING — Dose reduction may be required in patients with hepatic impairment or renal impairment.

ADULT — Metastatic breast cancer in patients who have previously received at least two chemotherapeutic regimens for the treatment of metastatic disease. Prior therapy should have included an anthracycline and a taxane in either the adjuvant or metastatic setting.

PEDS — Not approved in peds.

FORMS — IV only.

NOTES — Dose is 1.4 mg/m^2 on days 1 and 8 q 21 days.

MOA — Inhibits formation of mitotic spindles; suppresses microtubule polymerization, but does not affect depolymerization.

ADVERSE EFFECTS — Neutropenia, peripheral neuropathy, QT interval prolongation. Pancreatitis. Fatigue, alopecia, nausea.

IXABEPILONE (*Ixempra*) ▶L ♀D ▶– $ varies by therapy

WARNING — Contraindicated in patients with AST or ALT greater than 2.5 ULN or bilirubin more than 1 times ULN upper limit of normal or higher. Contraindicated in patients with hypersensitivity reactions to products containing Cremophor EL (polyoxyethylated castor oil). Neutropenia. Instruct patients to report promptly fever, sore throat, signs of local infection or anemia. Peripheral neuropathy (sensory and motor) occurs commonly. Dose reductions, delays or discontinuations may be necessary. Usually occurs during the first 3 cycles of treatment.

ADULT — Chemotherapy doses vary by indication. Metastatic or locally advanced breast cancer.

PEDS — Not approved in children.

FORMS — 15 mg and 45 mg powder for injection.

NOTES — CYP450 inhibitors such as ketoconazole may increase concentration; inducers such as rifampin, phenytoin or carbamazepine may reduce levels Patients should receive an H1 and H2 blocker one hour prior to ixabepilone infusion to minimize hypersensitivity reactions. If patients experience such a reaction, they should also receive a corticosteroid prior to the next dose.

MOA — Mitotic Inhibitor.

ADVERSE EFFECTS — Serious: Anaphylaxis, bone marrow suppression, peripheral neuropathy, MI, ventricular dysfunction. Frequent: Bone marrow suppression, peripheral neuropathy, N/V/D, palmar-plantar erythrodysesthesia syndrome, myalgias.

PACLITAXEL (*Taxol, Abraxane, Onxol*) ▶L ♀D ▶– $ varies by therapy

WARNING — Anaphylaxis,fatal hypersensitivity reactions, bone marrow suppression, cardiac conduction abnormalities, peripheral neuropathy, fertility impairment, alopecia. Contraindicated in patients with hypersensitivity reactions to products containing Cremophor EL (polyoxyethylated castor oil). Instruct patients to report promptly fever, sore throat, signs of local infection or anemia, pneumonitis, cystoid macular edema. Sepsis and neutropenic sepsis have occurred in clinical trials.

ADULT — Chemotherapy doses vary by indication. Ovarian cancer. Metastatic breast cancer. Non-small cell lung cancer, in combination regimens. AIDS-related Kaposi's sarcoma, ABRAXANE® brand approved for use in combination with carboplatin for the initial treatment of patients with locally advanced or metastatic non-small cell lung cancer (NSCLC) who are not candidates for curative surgery or radiation therapy. ABRAXANE® brand also approved for metastatic adenocarcinoma of the pancreas when used in combination with gemcitabine.

PEDS — Not approved in children.

UNAPPROVED ADULT — Advanced head and neck cancer. Small-cell lung cancer. Adenocarcinoma of the upper GI tract. Gastric, esophageal, and colon adenocarcinoma. Hormone-refractory prostate cancer. Non-Hodgkin's lymphoma. Transitional cell carcinoma of the urothelium. Adenocarcinoma or unknown primary, adjuvant, and neoadjuvant breast cancer, uterine cancer. Pancreatic cancer. Polycystic kidney disease.

NOTES — Abraxane is a form of paclitaxel bound to albumin. Reliable contraception is recommended. Monitor CBCs. Ketoconazole, felodipine, diazepam, and estradiol may increase paclitaxel.

MOA — Mitotic Inhibitor.

ADVERSE EFFECTS — Serious: Anaphylaxis, bone marrow suppression, cardiac conduction abnormalities, peripheral neuropathy. Frequent: Bone marrow suppression, peripheral neuropathy, hypotension, mucositis, N/V, atrioventricular block.

VINBLASTINE (*Velban, VLB*) ▶L ♀D ▶– $ varies by therapy

WARNING — Extravasation associated with severe necrosis. Leukopenia, fertility impairment, bronchospasm, alopecia. Instruct patients to report promptly fever, sore throat, or signs of local infection.

ADULT — Chemotherapy doses vary by indication. Hodgkin's disease. Non-Hodgkin's lymphoma. Histiocytic lymphoma. Mycosis fungoides. Advanced testicular carcinoma. Kaposi's sarcoma. Letterer-Siwe disease (histiocytosis X). Choriocarcinoma. Breast cancer.

PEDS — Not approved in children.

UNAPPROVED ADULT — Non-small-cell lung cancer, renal cancer, CML.

VINBLASTINE *(cont.)*

NOTES — Reliable contraception is recommended. May decrease phenytoin levels. Erythromycin/drugs that inhibit CYP450 enzymes may increase toxicity.

MOA — Mitotic Inhibitor.

ADVERSE EFFECTS — Serious: Leukopenia, fertility impairment, bronchospasm. Frequent: Leukopenia, alopecia.

VINCRISTINE (*Oncovin, Vincasar, VCR*) ▶L ♀D ▶– $ varies by therapy

WARNING — Extravasation associated with severe necrosis. CNS toxicity, hypersensitivity, bone marrow suppression, hyperuricemia, bronchospasm, fertility impairment, alopecia. Instruct patients to report promptly fever, sore throat, signs of local infection, or anemia.

ADULT — Chemotherapy doses vary by indication. ALL. Hodgkin's disease. Non-Hodgkin's lymphomas. Rhabdomyosarcoma. Neuroblastoma. Wilms' tumor. All in combination regimens.

PEDS — Chemotherapy doses vary by indication. Acute leukemia. Sarcoma. multiple myeloma.

UNAPPROVED ADULT — Idiopathic thrombocytopenic purpura. Kaposi's sarcoma. Breast cancer. Bladder cancer.

NOTES — Reliable contraception is recommended. Monitor CBCs. May decrease phenytoin and digoxin levels.

MOA — Mitotic Inhibitor.

ADVERSE EFFECTS — Serious: CNS toxicity, hypersensitivity, bone marrow suppression, uric acid nephropathy, bronchospasm. Frequent: Paresthesias, alopecia.

VINCRISTINE SULFATE LIPOSOME (*Marqibo*) ▶feces - ♀D ▶–

WARNING — For Intravenous Use Only – Fatal if Given by Other Routes.

Death has occurred with intrathecal use. Vincristine sulfate liposome injection has different dosage recommendations than vinCRIStine sulfate injection.

Verify drug name and dose prior to preparation and administration to avoid overdosage.

ADULT — Treatment of Philadelphia chromosome-negative (Ph-) acute lymphoblastic leukemia (ALL) in second or greater relapse or whose disease has progressed following two or more anti-leukemia therapies. 2.25 mg/m2 weekly IV.

PEDS — Not approved in peds

FORMS — Marqibo Kit. Contains VinCRIStine Sulfate Injection 5 mg/5 mL. Vial containing Sphingomyelin/Cholesterol Liposome Injection 103 mg/mL. Vial containing Sodium Phosphate Injection.

MOA — Sphingomyelin/cholesterol liposome-encapsulated formulation of vincristine sulfate, an anti-mitotic agent.

ADVERSE EFFECTS — The most common adverse reactions: constipation, nausea, pyrexia, fatigue, peripheral neuropathy, febrile neutropenia, diarrhea, anemia, decreased appetite, and insomnia.

VINORELBINE (*Navelbine*) ▶L ♀D ▶– $ varies by therapy

WARNING — Extravasation associated with severe necrosis. Granulocytopenia, pulmonary toxicity, bronchospasm, peripheral neuropathy, increased LFTs, alopecia. Instruct patients to report promptly fever, sore throat, or signs of local infection.

ADULT — Chemotherapy doses vary by indication. Non-small-cell lung cancer, alone or in combination regimens.

PEDS — Not approved in children.

UNAPPROVED ADULT — Breast cancer. Cervical carcinoma. Desmoid tumors. Kaposi's sarcoma. Ovarian, Hodgkin's disease, head and neck cancer.

NOTES — Reliable contraception is recommended. Monitor CBCs. Drugs that inhibit CYP450 enzymes may increase toxicity.

MOA — Mitotic Inhibitor.

ADVERSE EFFECTS — Serious: Granulocytopenia, pulmonary toxicity, bronchospasm, peripheral neuropathy, ileus. Frequent: Granulocytopenia, alopecia, peripheral neuropathy, N/V.

ONCOLOGY: Monoclonal Antibodies

ADO-TRASTUZUMAB EMTANSINE (Kadcyla) ▶L – ♀D ▶– $$$$$

WARNING — Hepatotoxicity, cardiac toxicity, embryo-fetal toxicity

ADULT — Indicated, as a single agent, for the treatment of patients with HER2-positive, metastatic breast cancer who previously received trastuzumab and a taxane, separately or in combination. Patients should have either received prior therapy for metastatic disease, or developed disease recurrence during or within six months of completing adjuvant therapy. 3.6 mg/kg given as an IV infusion q 3 weeks

PEDS — Not approved in peds.

FORMS — Lyophilized powder in single-use vials containing 100 mg per vial or 160 mg per vial.

NOTES — Administer KADCYLA as an intravenous infusion only with a 0.22 micron in-line

polyethersulfone (PES) filter. Do not administer as an intravenous push or bolus.

The reconstituted lyophilized vials should be used immediately following reconstitution with Sterile Water for Injection. If not used immediately, the reconstituted KADCYLA vials can be stored for up to 24 hours in a refrigerator at 2 degrees C to 8 degrees C (36°F to 46°F); discard unused KADCYLA after 24 hours. Do not freeze.

The diluted KADCYLA infusion solution should be used immediately. If not used immediately, the solution may be stored in a refrigerator at 2 degrees C to 8 degrees C (36°F to 46°F) for up to 24 hours prior to use. This storage time is additional to the time allowed for the reconstituted vials. Do not freeze or shake.

MOA — HER2-targeted antibody-drug conjugate. The antibody is the humanized anti-HER2 IgG1,

ADO-TRASTUZUMAB EMTANSINE (cont.)

trastuzumab. The small molecule cytotoxin, DM1, is a microtubule inhibitor.

ADVERSE EFFECTS — Common: fatigue, nausea, musculoskeletal pain, thrombocytopenia, headache, increased transaminases, and constipation.

OBINUTUZUMAB (*Gazyva*) ▶? – ♀C ▶?

WARNING — Obinutuzumab is being approved with a boxed warning about hepatitis B virus reactivation. Patients should be assessed for hepatitis B virus and their related reactivation risk. The boxed warning includes another concern: the drug's risk of inducing progressive multifocal leukoencephalopathy.

ADULT — Treatment in combination with chlorambucil of patients with previously untreated chronic lymphocytic leukemia (CLL). Cycle 1: 100 mg intravenously on day 1, 900 mg on day 2, and 1000 mg on days 8 and 15. Cycles 2-6: 1000 mg administered intravenously every 28 days

PEDS — Not approved in pecs.

FORMS — 1000 mg/40mL (25 mg/mL) single use vial.

MOA — Obinutuzumab is a monoclonal antibody that targets the CD20 antigen expressed on the surface of pre B- and mature B-lymphocytes. Upon binding to CD20, obinutuzumab mediates B-cell lysis through (1) engagement of immune effector cells, (2) by directly activating intracellular death signaling pathways and/or (3) activation of the complement cascade. The immune effector cell mechanisms include antibody-dependent cellular cytotoxicity and antibody-dependent cellular phagocytosis.

ADVERSE EFFECTS — Infusion-related reactions, neutropenia, thrombocytopenia, anemia, musculoskeletal pain, and pyrexia.

PEMBROLIZUMAB (*KEYTRUDA*) ▶? ♀D ▶–

WARNING — Immune related adverse reactions: pneumonitis, colitis, hepatitis, hypophysitis, nephritis, hyperthyroidism, hypothyroidism. Embryofetal toxicity.

ADULT — 2 mg/kg IV over 30 minutes every 3 weeks. Treatment of unresectable or metastatic melanoma with disease progression following ipilimumab and, if BRAF V600 mutation positive, a BRAF inhibitor.

PEDS — Not approved in ped

FORMS — 50mg powder for injection.

MOA — Monoclonal antibody which inhibits programmed cell death-1 (PD-1) activity by binding to the PD-1 receptor on T-cells to block PD-L1 and PD-L2 ligands from binding. Blocking the PD-1 pathway inhibits the negative immune regulation caused by PD-1 receptor signaling.

ADVERSE EFFECTS — The most common adverse reactions (>20% of patients): fatigue, cough, nausea, pruritis, rash, decreased appetite, constipation, arthralgia, and diarrhea.

PERTUZUMAB (*Perjeta*) ▶? – ♀D ▶– $$$$$

WARNING — BOXED WARNING regarding embryofetal toxicity and birth defects

ADULT — Use in combination with trastuzumab and docetaxel for the treatment of patients with HER2-positive metastatic breast cancer who have not received prior anti-HER2 therapy or chemotherapy for metastatic disease. Pertuzumab is now specifically indicated for the neoadjuvant treatment of breast cancer, in combination with trastuzumab and docetaxel, for patients with HER2-positive, locally advanced, inflammatory, or early-stage breast cancer (>2 cm in diameter) that is high risk, as part of a complete early breast cancer regimen also containing fluorouracil, epirubicin, and cyclophosphamide or carboplatin. As part of this regimen, patients will receive trastuzumab after surgery to complete 1 year of treatment.Initial dose, 840 mg IV, followed by 420 mg q three weeks thereafter.

PEDS — Not approved in pediatrics

FORMS — Trade Only: 420 mg/14 mL single-use vial.

MOA — Recombinant humanized monoclonal antibody that targets the extracellular dimerization domain of HER2, and thereby blocks ligand-dependent heterodimerization of HER2 with other HER family members, including EGFR, HER3 and HER4.

ADVERSE EFFECTS — Most common:diarrhea, alopecia, neutropenia, nausea, fatigue, rash, and peripheral neuropathy. Most severe: left ventricular dysfunction, infusion-associated reactions, hypersensitivity reactions, and anaphylaxis

RAMUCIRUMAB (*Cyramza*) ▶? ♀C ▶?

WARNING — Increased risk of hemorrhage, including severe and sometimes fatal hemorrhagic events. Should be permanently discontinued in patients who experience severe bleeding. Arterial Thromboembolic Events (ATEs): Serious, sometimes fatal ATEs have been reported in clinical trials. Hypertension: Monitor blood pressure and treat hypertension. Infusion Related Reactions: Monitor for signs and symptoms during infusion. Gastrointestinal perforation. Impaired Wound Healing: Withhold prior to surgery.Clinical Deterioration in Patients with Cirrhosis: New onset o rworsening encephalopathy, ascites, or hepatorenal syndrome can occur in patients with Child-Pugh B or C cirrhosis. Reversible Posterior Leukoencephalopathy Syndrome.

ADULT — 8 mg/kg administered as a 60-minute intravenous infusion every 2 weeks for use as a single agent for the treatment of patients with advanced or metastatic, gastric or gastroesophageal junction (GEJ) adenocarcinoma with disease progression on or after prior treatment with fluoropyrimidine- or platinum-containing chemotherapy.

FORMS — 100 mg/10 mL solution, single-dose vial and 500 mg/50 mL solution, single-dose vial

MOA — Ramucirumab is a recombinant monoclonal antibody of the IgG1 class that binds to vascular endothelial growth factor receptor-2 (VEGFR-2) and blocks the activation of the receptor.

ADVERSE EFFECTS — The most common adverse reactions are hypertension and diarrhea.

ONCOLOGY: Platinum-Containing Agents

CARBOPLATIN (*Paraplatin*) ▶K ♀D ▶– $ varies by therapy
WARNING — Secondary malignancies, bone marrow suppression, increased in patients with renal insufficiency; emesis, anaphylaxis, nephrotoxicity, peripheral neuropathy, increased LFTs, alopecia. Instruct patients to report promptly fever, sore throat, signs of local infection, bleeding from any site, symptoms suggestive of anemia, or yellow discoloration of the skin or eyes.
ADULT — Chemotherapy doses vary by indication. Ovarian carcinoma.
PEDS — Not approved in children.
UNAPPROVED ADULT — Small-cell lung cancer, in combination regimens. Squamous cell carcinoma of the head and neck. Advanced endometrial cancer. Acute leukemia. Seminoma of testicular cancer. Non-small-cell lung cancer. Adenocarcinoma of unknown primary. Cervical cancer. Bladder carcinoma. Breast cancer. Hodgkin's Lymphoma. Mesiothelioma. Melanoma. Neuroendocrine tumors. Non-Hodgkin's Lymphoma. Prostate cancer. Sarcomas. Small cell lung cancer.
NOTES — Reliable contraception is recommended. Monitor CBCs, LFTs, and renal function. May decrease phenytoin levels.
MOA — Alkylating agent.
ADVERSE EFFECTS — Serious: Bone marrow suppression, peripheral neuropathy, anaphylaxis, nephrotoxicity. Frequent: Bone marrow suppression, N/V, increased LFTs. Possible: alopecia, dehydration, mucositis.

CISPLATIN (*Platinol-AQ*) ▶K ♀D ▶– $ varies by therapy
WARNING — Secondary malignancies, nephrotoxicity, bone marrow suppression, N/V, very highly emetogenic, ototoxicity, anaphylaxis, hepatotoxicity, vascular toxicity, hyperuricemia, electrolyte disturbances, optic neuritis, papilledema and cerebral blindness, neuropathies, muscle cramps, alopecia. Amifostine can be used to reduce renal toxicity in patients with advanced ovarian cancer. Instruct patients to report promptly fever, sore throat, signs of local infection, bleeding from any site, symptoms suggestive of anemia, or yellow discoloration of the skin or eyes. An increased risk of cisplatin-induced ototoxicity in children has been associated with variants in the thiopurine S-methyltransferase (TPMT) gene.
ADULT — Chemotherapy doses vary by indication. Metastatic testicular and ovarian tumors, bladder cancer.

PEDS — Not approved in children.
UNAPPROVED ADULT — Esophageal cancer, gastric cancer, non-small-cell lung cancer and small-cell lung cancer, head and neck cancer, endometrial cancer, cervical cancer, neoadjuvant bladder sparing chemotherapy, sarcoma.
NOTES — Reliable contraception is recommended. Monitor CBCs, LFTs, renal function, and electrolytes. Audiometry. Aminoglycosides potentiate renal toxicity. Decreases phenytoin levels. Patients older than 65 yo may be more susceptible to nephrotoxicity, bone marrow suppression, and peripheral neuropathy. Verify any dose of cisplatin exceeding 100 mg/m^2 per course of therapy.
MOA — Alkylating agent.
ADVERSE EFFECTS — Serious: Bone marrow suppression, nephrotoxicity, ototoxicity, anaphylaxis, optic neuritis, papilledema and cerebral blindness, peripheral neuropathy. Frequent: Bone marrow suppression, N/V, nephrotoxicity, ototoxicity, hyperuricemia, muscle cramps.

OXALIPLATIN (*Eloxatin*) ▶LK ♀D ▶– $ varies by therapy
WARNING — Anaphylactic reactions to oxaliplatin have been reported, and may occur within minutes of oxaliplatin administration. Epinephrine, corticosteroids, and antihistamines have been employed to alleviate symptoms. Laryngospasm may occur due to infusion reactions/hypersensitivity. Neuropathy, pulmonary fibrosis, bone marrow suppression, transient vision loss, N/V/D, fertility impairment. Instruct patients to report promptly fever, sore throat, signs of local infection, bleeding from any site, or symptoms suggestive of anemia.
ADULT — Chemotherapy doses vary by indication. Colorectal cancer with 5-FU + leucovorin.
PEDS — Not approved in children.
UNAPPROVED ADULT — Esophageal cancer, gastric cancer, non-Hodgkin's Lymphoma, ovarian cancer, testicular cancer, hepatobiliary cancer, pancreatic cancer.
FORMS — 50 mg, 100 mg, 200 mg vials of sol for injection.
NOTES — Reliable contraception is recommended. Monitor CBCs and renal function.
MOA — Alkylating agent.
ADVERSE EFFECTS — Serious: Bone marrow suppression, anaphylaxis, neuropathy, pulmonary fibrosis. Frequent: N/V, diarrhea. Hypersensitivity reactions may occur.

ONCOLOGY: Radiopharmaceuticals

RADIUM-223 DICHLORIDE FOR INJECTION (*Xofigo*) ▶NA – ♀X ▶–
ADULT — 50 kBq/kg body wt given at 4 week intervals for a total of 6 IV injections. Castration-resistant prostate cancer (CRPC) with symptomatic

bone metastases, and no known visceral metastatic disease.
PEDS — Not approved in peds.
FORMS — Single-use vial at a concentration of 1,000 kBq/mL (27 microcurie/mL) at the reference

RADIUM-223 DICHLORIDE FOR INJECTION (cont.)

date with a total radioactivity of 6,000 kBq/vial (162 microcurie/vial) at the reference date

MOA — Alpha particle-emitting isotope which mimics calcium and forms complexes with the bone mineral hydroxyapatite at areas of increased bone turnover, such as bone metastases. The high linear energy transfer of alpha emitters leads to a high frequency of double-strand DNA breaks in adjacent cells, resulting in an anti-tumor effect on bone metastases.

ADVERSE EFFECTS — Severe: Bone marrow suppression. Discontinue Xofigo if hematologic values do not recover within 6 to 8 weeks after treatment. Monitor patients with compromised bone marrow reserve closely. Discontinue Xofigo in patients who experience life-threatening complications despite supportive care measures. Frequent: diarrhea, nausea, vomiting, and thrombocytopenia.

SAMARIUM 153 (Quadramet) ▶Not metabolized ♀C ▶– $ varies by therapy

WARNING — Bone marrow suppression, flare reactions. Instruct patients to report promptly fever, sore throat, signs of local infection or anemia.

ADULT — Chemotherapy doses vary by indication. Osteoblastic metastatic bone lesions, relief of pain.

PEDS — Not approved in children.

UNAPPROVED ADULT — Ankylosing spondylitis. Paget's disease. RA.

NOTES — Reliable contraception is recommended. Monitor CBCs. Radioactivity in excreted urine for 12 h after dose.

MOA — Radiopharmaceutical.

ADVERSE EFFECTS — Serious: Bone marrow suppression, flare reactions. Frequent: Bone marrow suppression, N/V.

STRONTIUM-89 (Metastron) ▶K ♀D ▶– $ varies by therapy

WARNING — Bone marrow suppression, flare reactions, flushing sensation. Instruct patients to report promptly fever, sore throat, signs of local infection, or anemia.

ADULT — Chemotherapy doses vary by indication. Painful skeletal metastases, relief of bone pain.

PEDS — Not approved in children.

NOTES — Reliable contraception is recommended. Monitor CBCs. Radioactivity in excreted urine for 12 h after dose.

MOA — Radiopharmaceutical.

ADVERSE EFFECTS — Serious: Bone marrow suppression, flare reactions, flushing sensation. Frequent: Bone marrow suppression.

ONCOLOGY: Tyrosine Kinase Inhibitors

AFATINIB (Gilotrif) ▶feces – ♀D ▶– $$$$$

WARNING — Severe and prolonged diarrhea not responsive to antidiarrheal agents. Bullous and Exfoliative Skin Disorders: Severe bullous, blistering, and exfoliating lesions occurred in 0.15% of patients. Discontinue for life-threatening cutaneous reactions. Interstitial lung disease. Hepatic toxicity. Keratitis.

ADULT — 40 mg orally once daily taken at least one hour before or two hours after a meal as a first-line treatment of patients with metastatic non-small cell lung cancer (NSCLC) whose tumors have epidermal growth factor receptor (EGFR) exon 19 deletions or exon 21 (L858R) substitution mutations as detected by an FDA-approved test.

PEDS — Not approved in peds.

FORMS — Trade only: 20, 30, 40 mg tablets.

MOA — Afatinib covalently binds to the kinase domains of EGFR (ErbB1), HER2 (ErbB2), and HER4 (ErbB4) and irreversibly inhibits tyrosine kinase autophosphorylation, resulting in downregulation of ErbB signaling.

ADVERSE EFFECTS — Most common adverse reactions (≥20%) are diarrhea, rash/dermatitis acneiform, stomatitis, paronychia, dry skin, decreased appetite, pruritus

AXITINIB (Inlyta) ▶L – ♀D ▶–

ADULT — 5mg orally twice daily. Advanced renal cell cancer after failure of one prior systemic treatment.

PEDS — Not approved in peds.

FORMS — 1mg and 5mg oral tabs.

MOA — Tyrosine kinase inhibitor which inhibits VEGF (vascular endothelial growth factor) receptors.

ADVERSE EFFECTS — Hypertension, fatigue, hand-foot syndrome, bicarbonate decreased, hypocalcemia, hyperglycemia, hypothyroidism, hypernatremia, hyperkalemia, hypoalbuminemia, hyponatremia, hypophosphatemia, hypoglycemia, diarrhea, pancytopenia, hemorrhage, increased liver function tests, weakness, increased creatinine, cough.

BOSUTINIB (Bosulif) ▶L – ♀D ▶–

WARNING — CYP3A Inhibitors and Inducers: Avoid concurrent use of BOSULIF with strong or moderate CYP3A inhibitors and inducers. Proton Pump Inhibitors: May decrease bosutinib drug levels. Consider short-acting antacids in place of proton pump inhibitors.

ADULT — Treatment of chronic, accelerated, or blast phase Philadelphia chromosome positive (Ph+) chronic myelogenous leukemia (CML) in adult patients with resistance or intolerance to prior therapy. 500 mg orally once daily with food.

PEDS — Not approved in peds.

FORMS — 100 mg and 500 mg tabs.

NOTES — Consider dose escalation to 600 mg daily in patients who do not reach complete hematologic response by week 8 or complete cytogenetic response by week 12 and do not have Grade 3 or greater adverse reactions.

MOA — Inhibits the Bcr-Abl kinase that promotes CML; it is also an inhibitor of Src-family kinases including Src, Lyn, and Hck.

BOSUTINIB (*cont.*)

ADVERSE EFFECTS — Diarrhea, nausea, thrombocytopenia, vomiting, abdominal pain, rash, anemia, pyrexia, and fatigue. Serious adverse reactions reported include anaphylactic shock, myelosuppression, gastrointestinal toxicity (diarrhea), fluid retention, hepatoxicity and rash.

CABOZANTINIB (*Cometriq*) ▶L – ♀D? $$$$$

ADULT — Metastatic medullary thyroid cancer. 140mg orally once daily.

PEDS — Not approved in peds.

FORMS — Trade Only: 140mg Daily–Dose Carton (4 blister cards: Each card contains seven 80mg and twenty-one 20mg capsules); 100mg Daily-Dose Carton (4 blister cards: each card contains seven 80mg and seven 20mg capsules); 60mg Daily-Dose Carton (4 blister cards: each card contains twenty-one 20mg capsules)

MOA — Inhibitor of multiple receptor tyrosine kinases, including RET, MET and vascular endothelial growth factor 2 (VEGFR2).

ADVERSE EFFECTS — Diarrhea, stomatitis, palmar-plantar erythrodysesthesia syndrome (PPES), decreased wt, decreased appetite, nausea, fatigue, oral pain, hair color changes, dysgeusia, hypertension, abdominal pain, and constipation. Increased AST, increased ALT, lymphopenia, increased alkaline phosphatase, hypocalcemia, neutropenia, thrombocytopenia, hypophosphatemia, and hyperbilirubinemia Boxed warning: severe and fatal perforations and fistula in the colon. Severe and fatal hemorrhage.

CERITINIB (*Zykadia*) ▶L ♀D ▶?

WARNING — Severe or persistent gastrointestinal toxicity: diarrhea, nausea, vomiting or abdominal pain. Hepatotoxicity. Interstitial Lung Disease (ILD)/Pneumonitis. QT interval prolongation. Hyperglycemia. Bradycardia. Embryofetal Toxicity

ADULT — 750 mg orally once daily for treatment of patients with anaplastic lymphoma kinase (ALK)-positive, metastatic non-small cell lung cancer (NSCLC) with disease progression on or who are intolerant to crizotinib.

FORMS — 150mg capsules

NOTES — Avoid concurrent use with strong CYP3A inhibitors or inducers. If concurrent use of a strong CYP3A inhibitor is unavoidable, reduce the dose of ceritinib. Avoid concurrent use with CYP3A or CYP2C9 substrates with narrow therapeutic indices. A high fat meal increases AUC by73%.

MOA — Inhibits anaplastic lymphoma kinase (ALK)

ADVERSE EFFECTS — The most common adverse reactions are diarrhea, nausea, elevated transaminases, vomiting, abdominal pain, fatigue, decreased appetite, and constipation

DABRAFENIB (*TAFINLAR*) ▶L – ♀D ▶– $$$$$

WARNING — Advise female patients of reproductive potential to use highly effective contraception during treatment and for 4 weeks after treatment. Counsel patients to use a non-hormonal method of contraception since TAFINLAR can render hormonal contraceptives ineffective. New Primary Cutaneous Malignancies: Perform dermatologic evaluations prior to initiation of therapy, every 2 months while on therapy, and for up to 6 months following discontinuation.

ADULT — 150 mg orally twice daily for treatment of patients with unresectable or metastatic melanoma with BRAF V600E mutation. Not indicated for the treatment of patients with wild-type BRAF melanoma. 150mg orally twice daily in metastatic or unresectable melanoma with BRAF V600E or BRAF V600K mutation in combination with trametinib.

PEDS — Not approved in peds.

FORMS — Trade only: 50mg and 75mg capsules.

NOTES — Confirmation of the presence of BRAF V600E is needed prior to initiation of dabrafenib because of the risks of potential risk of tumor promotion in patients with BRAF wild-type melanoma.

MOA — Inhibits BRAF kinase V600 mutation-positive melanoma cell growth.

ADVERSE EFFECTS — Frequent: hyperkeratosis, headache, pyrexia, arthralgia, papilloma, alopecia, and palmar-plantar erythrodysesthesia syndrome. Serious: development of new primary skin cancers (cutaneous squamous cell carcinoma, new primary melanomas, and keratoacanthomas), febrile drug reactions requiring hospitalization, hyperglycemia, and uveitis/iritis.

IBRUTINIB (*Imbruvica*) ▶L ♀D ▶-

WARNING — Renal Toxicity: Monitor renal function and maintain hydration. Second Primary Malignancies: Other malignancies have occurred in patients, including skin cancers, and other carcinomas. Embryo-Fetal Toxicity: Can cause fetal harm. Advise women of the potential risk to a fetus and to avoid pregnancy while taking the drug. Hemorrhage: Monitor for bleeding. Infections: Monitor patients for fever and infections and evaluate promptly. Myelosuppression: Check complete blood counts monthly

ADULT — 560 mg taken orally once daily for mantle cell lymphoma. A kinase inhibitor indicated for the treatment of patients with mantle cell lymphoma (MCL) who have received at least one prior therapy. 420mg orally once daily for chronic lymphocytic leukemia. Treatment of patients with chronic lymphocytic leukemia (CLL) who have received at least one prior therapy.

FORMS — Trade only: Caps 140mg.

NOTES — CYP3A Inhibitors: Avoid co-administration with strong and moderate CYP3A inhibitors. If a moderate CYP3A inhibitor must be used, reduce IMBRUVICA dose. CYP3A Inducers: Avoid co-administration with strong CYP3A inducers. Hepatic Impairment: Avoid use of Ibrutinib in patients with baseline hepatic impairment

MOA — Ibrutinib is a small-molecule inhibitor of BTK. Ibrutinib forms a covalent bond with a cysteine residue in the BTK active site, leading to inhibition of BTK enzymatic activity. BTK is a signaling

IBRUTINIB (cont.)
molecule of the B-cell antigen receptor (BCR) and cytokine receptor pathways.
ADVERSE EFFECTS — The most common adverse reactions (≥10%) are thrombocytopenia, peripheral edema, hyperuricemia, diarrhea, neutropenia, anemia, fatigue, musculoskeletal pain, peripheral edema, upper respiratory tract infection, nausea, bruising, dyspnea, constipation, rash, abdominal pain, vomiting and decreased appetite.

PONATINIB (Iclusig) ▶L + esterases ♀D ▶? $$$$$
WARNING — Boxed warning: arterial thrombosis and liver toxicity.
ADULT — Chronic myeloid leukemia (CML) and Philadelphia chromosome–positive (Ph+) acute lymphoblastic leukemia (Ph+ ALL) in patients for whom no other tyrosine kinase inhibitor therapy is indicated, or who are T315I positive. 45mg once daily.
FORMS — Trade Only: 15mg and 45mg oral tabs.
NOTES — A risk evaluation and mitigation strategy (REMS) is required, due to the risk of serious adverse reactions of vascular occlusions including loss of vision due to blood clots, and occlusion of mesenteric blood vessels, stroke, myocardial infarction, peripheral vascular disease with ischemic necrosis, and other vascular occlusive events.
MOA — Pan-BCR-ABL tyrosine kinase inhibitor with in vitro activity against cells expressing native or mutant BCR-ABL, including T315I.
ADVERSE EFFECTS — Rash, abdominal pain, headache, dry skin, constipation, fatigue, pyrexia, nausea, arthralgia, and hypertension. Pancreatitis, elevation of pancreatic enzymes (lipase in 19%, amylase 7%), and myelosuppression (thrombocytopenia in 42%, neutropenia in 34%, and anemia in 20%). Life-threatening blood clots and blood-vessel narrowing.

REGORAFENIB (Stivarga) ▶L – ♀D ▶– $
WARNING — Black box warning for hepatotoxicity.
ADULT — Treatment of patients with metastatic colorectal cancer (mCRC) who have been previously treated with fluoropyrimidine-, oxaliplatin-, and irinotecan-based chemotherapy, an anti-VEGF therapy, and, if KRAS wild type, an anti-EGFR therapy. Treatment of gastrointestinal stromal tumors (GIST), for use in patients with tumors that cannot

be surgically removed and no longer respond to imatinib and sunitinib. 160 mg orally once daily for the first 21 days of each 28-day cycle.
PEDS — Not approved in peds.
FORMS — Trade Only: 40mg film coated tabs.
MOA — Inhibits multiple membrane-bound and intracellular kinases involved in normal cellular functions and in pathologic processes, including those in the RET, VEGFR1, VEGFR2, VEGFR3, KIT, PDGFR-alpha, PDGFR-beta, FGFR1, FGFR2, TIE2, DDR2, Trk2A, Eph2A, RAF-1, BRAF, BRAFV600E, SAPK2, PTK5, and Abl pathways.
ADVERSE EFFECTS — Asthenia/fatigue, decreased appetite and food intake, hand-foot skin reaction, diarrhea, mucositis, wt loss, infection, hypertension and dysphonia. The most serious: hepatotoxicity, hemorrhage, and gastrointestinal perforation.

RUXOLITINIB (Jakafi, ✦Jakavi) ▶L – ♀C ▶–
ADULT — Treatment of intermediate or high risk myelofibrosis. Doses based on platelet count.
PEDS — Not approved in peds.
FORMS — 5mg, 10mg, 15mg, 20mg, 25mg tablets.
MOA — Kinase inhibitor which selectively inhibits Janus Associated Kinases, JAK1 and JAK2.
ADVERSE EFFECTS — Dizziness, bruising, increased cholesterol, pancytopenias, increased liver function tests.

TRAMETINIB (MEKINIST) ▶degraded chemically – ♀D ▶– $$$$$
WARNING — Instruct female patients to use highly effective contraception during treatment and for 4 months after treatment.
ADULT — 2 mg orally once daily, as a single agent or in combination with dabrafenib, for treatment of patients with unresectable or metastatic melanoma with BRAF V600E or V600K mutation
PEDS — Not approved in peds.
FORMS — Trade only: 0.5 mg, 1 mg, and 2 mg tablets.
NOTES — Re-assess LVEF after one month of treatment, and evaluate approximately every 2 to 3 months thereafter.
MOA — Inhibits BRAF kinase V600 mutation-positive melanoma cell growth via inhibition of MEK1 and MEK2 kinase activity.
ADVERSE EFFECTS — Frequent: rash, diarrhea and lymphedema. Serious: cardiomyopathy, retinal pigment epithelial detachment, retinal vein occlusion, interstitial lung disease and serious skin toxicity

ONCOLOGY: Miscellaneous

ARSENIC TRIOXIDE (Trisenox) ▶L ♀D ▶– $ varies by therapy
WARNING — APL differentiation syndrome: Fever, dyspnea, wt gain, pulmonary infiltrates and pleural/pericardial effusions, occasionally with impaired myocardial contractility and episodic hypotension, with or without leukocytosis. QT prolongation, AV block, torsade de pointes, N/V/D, hyperglycemia, alopecia.

ADULT — Chemotherapy doses vary by indication. Acute promyelocytic leukemia, refractory.
PEDS — Not approved in children younger than 5 yo. Chemotherapy doses vary by indication. Acute promyelocytic leukemia, refractory.
UNAPPROVED ADULT — Chemotherapy doses vary by indication. Chronic myeloid leukemia. ALL.
NOTES — Reliable contraception is recommended. Monitor ECG, electrolytes, renal function, CBCs and PT.

ARSENIC TRIOXIDE (*cont.*)

MOA — Unknown.

ADVERSE EFFECTS — Serious: APL differentiation syndrome: fever, dyspnea, weight gain, pulmonary infiltrates and pleural/pericardial effusions, with or w/o leukocytosis. QT prolongation, tachycardia, AV block, torsade de pointes, hyperleukocytosis. Frequent: Hypotension, N/V, diarrhea, hyperglycemia, fever, fatigue, dermatitis, nausea, electrolyte abnormalities.

ASPARAGINASE ERWINIA CHRYSANTHEMI (*Erwinaze, ✦Erwinase*) ▶? – ♀C ▶?

ADULT — A component of a multi-agent chemotherapeutic regimen for the treatment of patients with acute lymphoblastic leukemia (ALL) who have developed hypersensitivity to E. coli-derived asparaginase.

PEDS — Approved in adults and children with ALL.

FORMS — Powder for injection.

MOA — Catalyzes the deamidation of asparagine to aspartic acid and ammonia, resulting in a reduction in circulating levels of asparagine. The mechanism of action of ERWINAZE is thought to be based on the inability of leukemic cells to synthesize asparagine due to lack of asparagine synthetase activity, resulting in cytotoxicity specific for leukemic cells that depend on an exogenous source of the amino acid asparagine for their protein metabolism and survival.

ADVERSE EFFECTS — Pancreatitis, abnormal transaminases, coagulopathies, hemorrhage, nausea, vomiting and hyperglycemia. Common adverse reactions were similar in severity and incidence to those attributable to E. coli-derived asparaginase.

BEXAROTENE (*Targretin*) ▶L ♀X ▶– $ varies by therapy

WARNING — Gel: Rash, pruritus, contact dermatitis. Caps: Lipid abnormalities, increased LFTs, pancreatitis, hypothyroidism, leukopenia, cataracts, photosensitivity, alopecia.

ADULT — Chemotherapy doses vary by indication. Cutaneous T-cell lymphoma.

PEDS — Not approved in children.

FORMS — Trade only: 1% gel (60 g). Caps 75 mg.

NOTES — Gel: Do not use with DEET (insect repellant) or occlusive dressings. Caps: Monitor lipids, LFTs, thyroid function tests, CBCs. Multiple drug interactions; consult product insert for info. Reliable contraception is recommended.

MOA — Exact mechanism unknown; binds and activates retinoid X receptor subtypes. These receptors ultimately control cellular proliferation and differentiation.

ADVERSE EFFECTS — Gel- Serious: None. Frequent: Rash, pruritus, contact dermatitis. Caps- Serious: Hyperlipidemia, increased LFTs, pancreatitis, hypothyroidism, leukopenia, cataracts, pseudotumor cerebri. Frequent: Nausea, photosensitivity.

BORTEZOMIB (*Velcade*) ▶L ♀D ▶– $ varies by therapy

WARNING — Peripheral neuropathy, orthostatic hypotension, heart failure, pneumonia, acute respiratory distress syndrome, thrombocytopenia, neutropenia, N/V/D. Instruct patients to report promptly acute onset of dyspnea, cough and low-grade fever, and bleeding from any site. Acute liver failure has been reported rarely. Use with caution in patient's with hepatic dysfunction.

ADULT — Chemotherapy doses vary by indication. Multiple myeloma, mantle cell lymphoma. In the U.S. may given IV or subcutaneously.

PEDS — Not approved in children.

UNAPPROVED ADULT — Waldenstrom's Macroglobulinemia, peripheral T-cell lymphoma, cutaneous T-cell lymphoma, systemic light chain amyloidosis.

FORMS — Single use 3.5mg vials.

NOTES — Reliable contraception is recommended. Monitor CBCs.

MOA — Inhibits 26S proteasome.

ADVERSE EFFECTS — Serious: Peripheral neuropathy. Patients with pre-existing peripheral neuropathy should weigh risk/benefit. Thrombocytopenia, neutropenia, orthostatic hypotension, heart failure, pneumonia, acute respiratory distress syndrome, reversible posterior leukoencephalopathy (RPLS). Progressive multifocal leukoencephalopathy. Frequent: Peripheral neuropathy, thrombocytopenia, fatigue, nausea, diarrhea, anorexia, constipation, anemia, rash. Possible: acute febrile neutrophilic dermatosis (Sweet Syndrome).

CARFILZOMIB (*Kyprolis*) ▶proteolysis – ♀D ▶–

WARNING — Heart failure and ischemia: Monitor for cardiac complications. Pulmonary Hypertension. Pulmonary Complications. Infusion Reactions: Premedicate with dexamethasone to prevent.

ADULT — Treatment of patients with multiple myeloma who have received at least two prior therapies, including bortezomib and an immunomodulatory agent, and have demonstrated disease progression on or within 60 days of the completion of the last therapy. Administered IVly over 2 to 10 minutes on 2 consecutive days weekly for 3 weeks, followed by a 12-day rest period (28 day treatment cycle). Dose is 20 mg/m2 at each dose in cycle 1, and 27 mg/m2 in subsequent cycles.

PEDS — Not approved in pediatrics.

FORMS — Single-use vial: 60 mg sterile lyophilized powder

MOA — Proteasome inhibitor.

ADVERSE EFFECTS — Most common: fatigue, anemia, nausea, thrombocytopenia, dyspnea, diarrhea, and pyrexia. Most serious: pneumonia, acute renal failure, pyrexia, and congestive heart failure.

CRIZOTINIB (*Xalkori*) ▶L – ♀D ▶–

WARNING — Severe, fatal pneumonitis, elevations in liver enzymes, QT prolongation.

ADULT — Locally advanced or metastatic non-small cell lung cancer in patients who express an abnormal ALK (anaplastic lymphoma kinase) gene

PEDS — Not approved in pediatrics

FORMS — 200 mg and 250 mg oral capsules

MOA — Multiple tyrosine kinase inhibitor, including ALK.

CRIZOTINIB (*cont.*)

ADVERSE EFFECTS — Vision disorders, myelosuppression, nausea, diarrhea, vomiting, edema, constipation.Avoid concomitant administration with strong CYP3A4 inhibitors or inducers.

DASATINIB (*Sprycel*) ►L ♀D ►– $ varies by therapy

WARNING — Bone marrow suppression, hemorrhage, prolonged QT interval, pleural effusion, congestive heart failure, and myocardial infarction and left ventricular dysfunction. Dasatinib may increase the risk of a rare but serious condition in which there is abnormally high blood pressure in the arteries of the lungs (pulmonary arterial hypertension [PAH]). Symptoms of PAH may include shortness of breath, fatigue, and swelling of the body (such as the ankles and legs). In reported cases, patients developed PAH after starting dasatinib, including after more than one year of treatment.

ADULT — Chemotherapy doses vary by indication. CML. ALL.

PEDS — Not approved in children.

UNAPPROVED ADULT — Post allogeneic stem cell transplant treatment of CML.

FORMS — Trade only: Tabs 20, 50, 70, 100 mg.

NOTES — Reliable contraception is recommended. Monitor LFTs, CBCs, and wt. Monitor for signs and symptoms of fluid retention. Increased by ketoconazole, erythromycin, itraconazole, clarithromycin, ritonavir, atazanavir, indinavir, nelfinavir, saquinavir and telithromycin. Decreased by rifampin, phenytoin, carbamazepine, phenobarbital and dexamethasone. Increases simvastatin. Antacids should be taken at least 2 h pre or post dose. Avoid H2 blockers and PPIs.

MOA — Protein-tyrosine kinase inhibitor that inhibits the Bcr-Abl tyrosine kinase, the constitutive abnormal tyrosine kinase created by the Philadelphia chromosome abnormality in chronic myeloid leukemia, and the SRC family kinases.

ADVERSE EFFECTS — Serious: Bone marrow suppression, hemorrhage, pleural effusion, pulmonary arterial hypertension. Frequent: Bone marrow suppression, N/V, diarrhea, edema.

ERLOTINIB (*Tarceva*) ►L ♀D ►– $$$$$

WARNING — Interstitial lung disease, acute renal failure, hepatic failure, GI perforations, exfoliative skin disorders, MI, CVA, microangiopathic hemolytic anemia, corneal perforation. Elevated International Normalized Ratio and potential bleeding. Patients taking warfarin or other coumarin-derivative anticoagulants should be monitored regularly for changes in prothrombin time or INR.

ADULT — Chemotherapy doses vary by indication. The first-line treatment of patients with metastatic non-small cell lung cancer (NSCLC) whose tumors have epidermal growth factor receptor (EGFR) exon 19 deletions or exon 21 substitution mutations as detected by an FDA-approved test. The maintenance treatment of patients with locally advanced or metastatic non-small cell lung cancer whose disease has not progressed after four cycles of platinum-based first-line chemotherapy. The treatment of patients with locally advanced or metastatic non-small cell lung cancer after failure of at least one prior chemotherapy regimen. Locally advanced, unresectable or metastatic pancreatic cancer

PEDS — Not approved in children.

FORMS — Trade only: Tabs 25, 100, 150 mg.

NOTES — Reliable contraception is recommended. Hepato-renal syndrome has been reported; monitor LFTs and SCr. CYP3A4 inhibitors such as ketoconazole increase concentrations. CYP3A4 inducers such as rifampin decrease concentrations. Increases INR in patients on warfarin. Monitor LFTs. Avoid concomitant use of erlotinib with H2 blockers and PPIs.

MOA — Inhibits the intracellular phosphorylation of tyrosine kinase associated with epidermal growth factor receptor, which is expressed on the surface of normal cells and cancer cells.

ADVERSE EFFECTS — Serious: Pulmonary toxicity, GI bleeding, acute renal failure due to dehydration, hepatic failure, GI perforations, exfoliative skin disorders, MI, CVA, microangiopathic hemolytic anemia, corneal perforation. Frequent: Diarrhea, anorexia, fatigue, stomatitis, rash, infection, pruritus.

ETOPOSIDE (*VP-16, Etopophos, Toposar, VePesid*) ►K ♀D ►– $ varies by therapy

WARNING — Bone marrow suppression, anaphylaxis, hypotension, CNS depression, alopecia. Instruct patients to report promptly fever, sore throat, or signs of local infection.

ADULT — Chemotherapy doses vary by indication. Testicular cancer. Small-cell lung cancer, in combination regimens.

PEDS — Not approved in children.

UNAPPROVED ADULT — ALL, AML, Hodgkin's disease, non-Hodgkin's lymphomas, Kaposi's sarcoma, neuroblastoma, choriocarcinoma, rhabdomyosarcoma, hepatocellular carcinoma, epithelial ovarian cancer, non-small-cell and small-cell lung cancers, testicular cancer, gastric cancer, endometrial cancer, breast cancer, and soft-issue sarcoma.

FORMS — Generic/Trade: Caps 50 mg. Injection for hospital/clinic use; not intended for outpatient prescribing.

NOTES — Reliable contraception is recommended. Monitor CBCs, LFTs and renal function. May increase INR with warfarin.

MOA — Mitotic inhibitor.

ADVERSE EFFECTS — Serious: Bone marrow suppression, anaphylaxis, hypotension, CNS depression. Frequent: Alopecia, bone marrow suppression, N/V, diarrhea.

GEFITINIB (*Iressa*) ►L ♀D ►– $ varies by therapy

WARNING — Pulmonary toxicity, corneal erosion, N/V. Instruct patients to report promptly acute onset of dyspnea, cough, and low-grade fever.

ADULT — Chemotherapy doses vary by indication. Non-small-cell lung cancer.

PEDS — Not approved in children.

GEFITINIB (*cont.*)

FORMS — Trade only: Tabs 250 mg.

NOTES — Reliable contraception is recommended. Monitor LFTs. Potent inducers of CYP3A4 (eg, rifampin, phenytoin) decrease concentration; use 500 mg. May increase warfarin effect; monitor INR. Potent inhibitors of CYP3A4 (eg, ketoconazole, itraconazole) increase toxicity. Ranitidine increases concentrations.

MOA — Inhibits phosphorylation of tyrosine kinases.

ADVERSE EFFECTS — Serious: Pulmonary toxicity, corneal erosion. Frequent: Increased LFTs, diarrhea, rash, acne, dry skin, N/V.

IDELALISIB (*Zydelig*) ▶L ♀D ▶?

WARNING — Boxed Warning alerting patients and healthcare professionals of the following fatal and serious adverse reactions: hepatotoxicity, severe diarrhea or colitis, pneumonitis, and intestinal perforation.

Severe cutaneous reactions: Monitor patients for the development of severe cutaneous reactions. Anaphylaxis: Monitor patients for anaphylaxis and discontinue. Neutropenia: monitor blood counts. Embryo-fetal toxicity: may cause fetal harm. Advise women of potential risk to a fetus and to avoid pregnancy while taking

ADULT — Treatment of patients with relapsed chronic lymphocytic leukemia (CLL), in combination with rituximab, for whom rituximab alone would be considered appropriate therapy due to other co-morbidities.Treatment of patients with relapsed follicular B-cell non-Hodgkin lymphoma (FL) or relapsed small lymphocytic lymphoma (SLL) who have received at least two prior systemic therapies. 150 mg orally twice daily.

PEDS — Not approved in peds.

FORMS — 100mg, 150mg tablets.

MOA — Idelalisib is an inhibitor of PI3K⊠ kinase, which is expressed in normal and malignant B-cells. Idelalisib inhibits several cell signaling pathways, including B-cell receptor (BCR) signaling and the CXCR4 and CXCR5 signaling, which are involved in trafficking and homing of B-cells to the lymph nodes and bone marrow.

ADVERSE EFFECTS — Themost common adverse reactions (incidence ≥20%) are diarrhea, pyrexia, fatigue, nausea, cough, pneumonia, abdominal pain, chills, and rash. The most common laboratory abnormalities (incidence ≥30%) are neutropenia, hypertriglyceridemia, hyperglycemia, ALT elevations, and AST elevations.

IMATINIB (*Gleevec*) ▶L ♀D ▶– $ varies by therapy

WARNING — Cases of fatal tumor lysis syndrome have been reported. Use caution in patients with high tumor burden, or high tumor proliferative rate. Bone marrow suppression, increased LFTs, hemorrhage, erythema multiforme, Stevens-Johnson syndrome, N/V,fluid retention including pulmonary edema, CHF, muscle cramps, GI irritation, hemorrhage. May cause growth retardation in children. Use caution when driving a car or operating machinery.

ADULT — Chemotherapy doses vary by indication. CML. GI stromal tumors (GISTs), Ph+ ALL, agressive systemic mastocytosis, dermatofibrosarcoma protuberans, hypereosinophillic syndrome, myelodysplastic/myeloproliferative disease associated with platelet-derived growth factor recptor mutations.

PEDS — Chemotherapy doses vary by indication. Newly diagnosed pediatric acute lymphoblastic leukemia (ALL) that is Philadelphia chromosome (Ph) positive.

UNAPPROVED ADULT — Treatment of desmoid tumors, poststem cell transplant follow-up treatment in CML.

FORMS — Trade only: Tabs 100, 400 mg.

NOTES — Reliable contraception is recommended. Monitor LFTs, CBCs, and wt. Monitor for signs and symptoms of fluid retention. Increased by ketoconazole, erythromycin, itraconazole, clarithromycin. Decreased by phenytoin, carbamazepine, rifampin, phenobarbital, St. John's wort. Increases acetaminophen levels and warfarin effects. Monitor INR. Reduce dose with renal insufficiency.

MOA — Imatinib mesylate is a protein-tyrosine kinase inhibitor that inhibits the Bcr-Abl tyrosine kinase, the constitutive abnormal tyrosine kinase created by the Philadelphia chromosome abnormality in chronic myeloid leukemia.

ADVERSE EFFECTS — Serious: Bone marrow suppression, hepatotoxicity, hemorrhage, erythema multiforme, Stevens-Johnson syndrome, pulmonary edema, cardiac tamponade, CHF, increased intracranial pressure and papilledema, subdural hematoma. Frequent: Bone marrow suppression, N/V, diarrhea, edema, muscle cramps, rash, fatigue.

IRINOTECAN (*Camptosar*) ▶L ♀D ▶– $ varies by therapy

WARNING — Diarrhea and dehydration (may be life-threatening), bone marrow suppression (worse with radiation), orthostatic hypotension, colitis, hypersensitivity, pancreatitis. Instruct patients to report promptly diarrhea, fever, sore throat, signs of local infection, bleeding from any site, or symptoms suggestive of anemia.

ADULT — Chemotherapy doses vary by indication. Metastatic carcinoma of the colon or rectum, in combination regimens.

PEDS — Not approved in children.

UNAPPROVED ADULT — Non-small-cell lung cancer and small-cell lung cancer, ovarian and cervical cancer.

NOTES — Enzyme-inducing drugs such as phenytoin, phenobarbital, carbamazepine, rifampin, and St. John's wort decrease concentrations and possibly effectiveness. Ketoconazole is contraindicated during therapy. Atazanavir increases concentrations. Reliable contraception is recommended. Monitor CBCs. May want to withhold diuretics during active N/V. Avoid laxatives. Loperamide/fluids/electrolytes for diarrhea. Consider atropine for cholinergic symptoms during the infusion. Patients who are homozygous for the UGT1A1*28 allele are at

IRINOTECAN (*cont.*)

increased risk for neutropenia. Dosage reductions may be necessary.

MOA — Topoisomerase inhibitor.

ADVERSE EFFECTS — Serious: Severe diarrhea, dehydration, bone marrow suppression, orthostatic hypotension, colitis/ileus, hypersensitivity, pancreatitis. Frequent: Diarrhea, bone marrow suppression, alopecia, N/V, rhinitis, salivation, lacrimation, miosis. Also myocardial ischemic events, elevated serum transaminases, hiccups, and megacolon have occurred.

LAPATINIB (*Tykerb*) ▶L ♀D ▶– $ varies by therapy

WARNING — Hepatotoxicity has been reported with lapatinib. May be severe or fatal. Decreased LVEF, QT prolongation, hepatotoxicity, interstitial lung disease, pneumonitis, severe diarrhea.

ADULT — Chemotherapy doses vary by indication. Treatment of HER2 overexpressing Advanced or metastatic breast cancer.in combination with capecitabine, in patients who have received prior therapy including an anthracycline, a taxane, and trastuzumab. Also indicated in combination with letrozole for the treatment of postmenopausal women with hormone receptor positive metastatic breast cancer that overexpresses the HER2 receptor for whom hormonal therapy is indicated.

PEDS — Not approved in children.

FORMS — Trade only: Tabs 250 mg.

NOTES — Monitor LFTs, CBCs, and wt. Monitor for signs and symptoms of fluid retention. Increased by ketoconazole, erythromycin, itraconazole, clarithromycin. Decreased by phenytoin, carbamazepine, rifampin, phenobarbital, St. John's wort. Increases acetaminophen levels and warfarin effects. Monitor INR. Reduce dose with renal insufficiency. Reliable contraception is recommended. Modify dose for cardiac and other toxicities, severe hepatic impairment, and CYP3A4 drug interactions.

MOA — Lapatinib is a protein-tyrosine kinase inhibitor that inhibits epidermal growth factor receptor and human epidermal receptor type 2 in breast cancer cell lines.

ADVERSE EFFECTS — Serious: Diarrhea, decreased ejection fraction, QT prolongation, hepatotoxicity, interstitial lung disease, pneumonitis. Frequent: N/V, diarrhea, fatigue, plantar-palmar erythrodysesthesia, rash.

LEUCOVORIN (*Wellcovorin, folinic acid*) ▶gut ♀C ▶? $ varies by therapy

WARNING — Allergic sensitization.

ADULT — Doses vary by indication. Reduction of toxicity due to folic acid antagonists (ie, methotrexate). Colorectal cancer with 5-FU. Megaloblastic anemias.

PEDS — Not approved in children.

FORMS — Generic only: Tabs 5, 10, 15, 25 mg. Injection for hospital/oncology clinic use; not intended for outpatient prescribing.

NOTES — Monitor methotrexate concentrations and CBCs.

MOA — Folic acid derivative.

ADVERSE EFFECTS — Serious: Bone marrow suppression (with 5-FU). Frequent: Stomatitis, diarrhea (with 5-FU).

LEVOLEUCOVORIN (*Fusilev*) ▶gut ♀C ▶? $ varies by therapy

WARNING — Allergic sensitization.

ADULT — Doses vary by indication. Reduction of toxicity due to high-dose methotrexate for osteosarcoma. Indicated for use in combination chemotherapy with 5-fluorouracil in the palliative treatment of patients with advanced metastatic colorectal cancer. Antidote for impaired methotrexate elimination and for inadvertent overdosage of folic acid antagonists.

PEDS — Not approved in children.

FORMS — 50 mg powder for injection.

NOTES — Monitor methotrexate concentrations and CBCs.

MOA — Folic acid derivative. Counter acts the toxic effects of folic acid antagonists such as methotrexate.

ADVERSE EFFECTS — Serious: None. Frequent: Vomiting, stomatitis, nausea.

MITOTANE (*Lysodren*) ▶L ♀D ▶– $ varies by therapy

WARNING — Adrenal insufficiency, depression, long term use may lead to brain damage and functional impairment. Prolonged bleeding time. Instruct patients to report promptly if N/V, loss of appetite, diarrhea, mental depression, skin rash or darkening of the skin occurs. N/V/D, alopecia.

ADULT — Chemotherapy doses vary by indication. Adrenal cortical carcinoma, inoperable.

PEDS — Not approved in children.

FORMS — Trade only: Tabs 500 mg.

NOTES — Hold after shock or trauma; give systemic steroids. Behavioral and neurological assessments at regular intervals when continuous treatment more than 2 years. May decrease steroid and warfarin effects. Reliable contraception is recommended.

MOA — Unknown.

ADVERSE EFFECTS — Serious: Adrenal insufficiency, depression. Frequent: Anorexia, N/V, diarrhea.

NILOTINIB (*Tasigna*) ▶L ♀D ▶– $ varies by therapy

WARNING — Prolonged QT interval and sudden death, bone marrow suppression, intracranial hemorrhage, pneumonia, elevated lipase. Progressive peripheral arterial occlusive disease. Must be administered on an empty stomach. Food increases bioavailability which may then cause prolonged QTc.

ADULT — Chemotherapy doses vary by indication. Treatment of newly diagnosed adult patients with Philadelphia chromosome positive chronic myeloid leukemia (Ph+ CML in chronic phase. Treatment of chronic phase (CP) and accelerated phase (AP) Ph+ CML in adult patients resistant to or intolerant to prior therapy that included imatinib.

PEDS — Not approved in children.

FORMS — Trade only: Caps 200 mg and 150mg.

NOTES — Contraindicated with hypokalemia, hypomagnesemia, or long QT syndrome. Reliable

NILOTINIB (cont.)

contraception is recommended. Monitor EKG, LFTs, CBCs, and lipase. Serum levels of nilotinib increased by potent CYP450 inhibitors such as ketoconazole and decreased by CYP450 inducers such as rifampin. Avoid food at least 2 h pre-dose or 1 h post-dose. Food Effects: Food increases blood levels of nilotinib.

MOA — Nilotinib is a protein-tyrosine kinase inhibitor that inhibits the Bcr-Abl tyrosine kinase, the constitutive abnormal tyrosine kinase created by the Philadelphia chromosome abnormality in chronic myeloid leukemia.

ADVERSE EFFECTS — Serious: Bone marrow suppression, intracranial hemorrhage, pneumonia. Frequent: Bone marrow suppression, N/V/D, rash, pruritus.

OMACETAXINE MEPESUCCINATE (Synribo) ▶esterases ♀D ▶? $$$$$

WARNING — Most severe adverse reactions: myelosuppression, bleeding, hyperglycemia.

ADULT — Treatment of adults with chronic myelogenous leukemia (CML), who progress after treatment with at least 2 tyrosine kinase inhibitors. 1.25 mg/m2 subcutaneously injected twice daily for 14 consecutive days over a 28-day cycle until a hematologic response occurs and white blood cell counts normalize. The drug is then administered 1.25 mg/m2 twice daily for 7 consecutive days over a 28-day cycle as long as the patient continues to clinically benefit.

PEDS — Not approved in peds.

FORMS — 3.5mg powder for injection.

MOA — The mechanism of action of SYNRIBO has not been fully elucidated but includes inhibition of protein synthesis. It acts independently of direct Bcr-Abl binding to reduce protein levels of both the Bcr-Abl oncoprotein and Mcl-1 which inhibits apoptosis.

ADVERSE EFFECTS — Most common: thrombocytopenia; anemia; neutropenia and febrile neutropenia; diarrhea; nausea, weakness, and fatigue; injection-site reaction; and lymphopenia.

PAZOPANIB (Votrient) ▶L + ♀D ▶– $$$$$

WARNING — Severe and fatal hepatotoxicty have occurred. Observe LFTs prior to and during treatment. Prolonged QT intervals and torsades des pointes have been observed. Fatal hemorrhagic events have occurred. Arterial thrombotic events have occurred and can be fatal.

ADULT — 800 mg orally once daily without food. Treatment of advanced renal cell carcinoma. Treatment of advanced soft tissue sarcoma in patients who have received prior chemotherapy.

PEDS — Not indicated in pediatrics.

FORMS — Trade only: Tabs 200 mg.

MOA — Multi-tyrosine kinase inhibitor, including VEGFR-1, VEGFR-2, VEGFR-3, PDGFR-alpha and beta, FGFR-1, FGFR-3, cKIT, Itk, Lck, and c-FMS.

ADVERSE EFFECTS — Diarrhea, hypertension, hair color changes (depigmentation), nausea, anorexia,

vomiting, fatigue, tumor pain, skin hypopigmentation, arthralgia and spasms.

PEGASPARGASE (Oncaspar) ▶? ♀C ▶– $ varies by therapy

WARNING — Contraindicated with previous/current pancreatitis. Hypersensitivity, including anaphylaxis. Bone marrow suppression, bleeding, hyperuricemia, hyperglycemia, hepato/nephrotoxicity, CNS toxicity, N/V/D, alopecia.

ADULT — Chemotherapy doses vary by indication. ALL, in combination regimens.

PEDS — Chemotherapy doses vary by indication. ALL, in combination regimens.

NOTES — Monitor CBCs, LFTs, renal function, amylase, glucose, and PT. Bleeding potentiated with warfarin, heparin, dipyridamole, aspiri, or NSAIDs.

MOA — Unknown.

ADVERSE EFFECTS — Serious: Anaphylaxis, bone marrow suppression, bleeding, hyperglycemia, hepato/nephrotoxicity, CNS toxicity. Frequent: N/V, diarrhea, bone marrow suppression, hepatotoxicity.

PORFIMER (Photofrin) ▶? ♀C ▶– $ varies by therapy

WARNING — Photosensitivity, ocular sensitivity, chest pain, respiratory distress, constipation.

ADULT — Chemotherapy doses vary by indication. Esophageal cancer. Endobronchial non-small-cell lung cancer. High-grade dysplasia in Barrett's esophagus. (All with laser therapy).

PEDS — Not approved in children.

NOTES — Avoid concurrent photosensitizing drugs.

MOA — Photosensitizer.

ADVERSE EFFECTS — Serious: Photosensitivity, ocular sensitivity, chest pain, respiratory distress. Frequent: Photosensitivity, ocular sensitivity, constipation.

RASBURICASE (Elitek, ✱Fasturtec) ▶L ♀C ▶– $$$$$

WARNING — May cause hypersensitivity reactions including anaphylaxis, hemolysis (G6PD-deficient patients), methemoglobinemia, interference with uric acid measurements.

ADULT — Uric acid elevation prevention with leukemia, lymphoma, and solid tumor malignancies receiving anticancer therapy: 0.2 mg/kg IV over 30 min daily for up to 5 days.

PEDS — Uric acid elevation prevention in children (1 mo to 17 yo) with leukemia, lymphoma, and solid tumor malignancies receiving anticancer therapy: 0.2 mg/kg IV over 30 min daily for up to 5 days.

NOTES — Safety and efficacy have been established only for one 5-day treatment course. Hydrate IV if at risk for tumor lysis syndrome. Screen for G6PD deficiency in high-risk patients.

MOA — Catalyzes enzymatic oxidation of uric acid into an inactive and soluble metabolite.

ADVERSE EFFECTS — Serious: Anaphylaxis, hemolysis, methemoglobinemia, acute renal failure, arrhythmia, cardiac failure, cardiac arrest, cellulitis, cerebrovascular disorder, chest pain, convulsions, dehydration, ileus, infection, intestinal obstruction, hemorrhage, myocardial infarction,

RASBURICASE (*cont.*)

paresthesia, pancytopenia, pneumonia, pulmonary edema, pulmonary hypertension, retinal hemorrhage, rigors, thrombosis, and thrombophlebitis. Frequent: Fever, neutropenia with fever, respiratory distress, sepsis, neutropenia, mucositis, vomiting, nausea, headache, abdominal pain, constipation, diarrhea, rash.

ROMIDEPSIN (*Istodax*) ▶L – ♀D ▶–

WARNING — QTc prolongation/ECG changes have been observed. High potential for drug interactions. Avoid concomitant use with CYP3A4 inhibitors and inducers. Pancytopenias.

ADULT — 14 mg/m² IV Days 1, 8, and 15 of a 28 day cycle. Treatment of cutaneous T-cell lymphoma in patients who have received at least one prior systemic therapy. Refractory peripheral T-cell lymphoma.

PEDS — Not approved in pediatrics

FORMS — 10mg powder for reconstitution.

MOA — Histone deacetylase inhibitor. Induces arrest in cell cycle at G1 and G2/M phases.

ADVERSE EFFECTS — ST-T wave changes, hypotension, fatigue, fever, pruritis, hyperglycemia, electrolyte changes, nausea, vomiting, anorexia, pancytopenias, transaminitis, weakness, infection.

SORAFENIB (*Nexavar*) ▶L ♀D ▶– $ varies by therapy

WARNING — Increased risk of bleeding, cardiac ischemia/infarction, GI perforation. Sorafenib in combination with carboplatin and paclitaxel is contraindicated in patients with squamous cell lung cancer. Co-administration of oral neomycin causes a decrease in sorafenib exposure. Stevens-Johnson syndrome and toxic epidermal necrolysis, and drug induced hepatitis.

ADULT — Chemotherapy doses vary by indication. Advanced renal cell carcinoma. Unresectable hepatocellular carcinoma. Treatment of locally recurrent or metastatic, progressive, differentiated thyroid carcinoma (DTC) refractory to radioactive iodine treatment.

PEDS — Not approved in children.

UNAPPROVED ADULT — Recurrent or metastatic angiosarcoma, imatinib resistant GIST.

FORMS — Trade only: Tabs 200 mg.

NOTES — Take 1 h before or 2 h after meals for best absorption. Monitor BP. Monitor INR with warfarin. Reliable contraception is recommended. Hepatic impairment may reduce concentrations. Increases docetaxel and doxorubicin.

MOA — Multikinase inhibitor; Angiogenesis inhibitor.

ADVERSE EFFECTS — Serious:Angioedema, hepatitis, hemorrhage, myocardial infarction, bone marrow suppression. Frequent: Hand-foot skin reaction and rash, erythema, HTN, hemorrhage, bone marrow suppression, N/V, diarrhea, increased lipase and amylase, mucositis. Hypokalemia, proteinuria, and nephrotic syndrome seen in clinical trials. Interstitial lung disease-like events and osteonecrosis of the jaw seen post marketing.

SUNITINIB (*Sutent*) ▶L ♀D ▶– $ varies by therapy

WARNING — Hepatotoxicity has been observed in clinical trials and post-marketing experience. This hepatotoxicity may be severe, and deaths have been reported. Prolonged QT intervals and Torsade de Pointes have been observed. Hemorrhagic events including tumor-related hemorrhage have occurred. Decrease in LVEF with possible clinical CHF, adrenal toxicity, serious and fatal GI complications, bone marrow suppression, bleeding, HTN, yellow skin discoloration, depigmentation of hair or skin, thyroid dysfunction. Cases of tumor lysis syndrome, some fatal, have been observed in clinical trials and have been reported in post-marketing experience, primarily in patients with RCC or GIST treated with sunitinib.

ADULT — Chemotherapy doses vary by indication. GI stromal tumors (GIST), advanced renal cell carcinoma. Treatment of progressive, well differentiated pancreatic neuroendocrine tumors (pNET) in patients with unresectable, locally advanced, or metastatic disease.

PEDS — Not approved in children.

UNAPPROVED ADULT — Treatment of advanced thyroid cancer, treatment of pancreatic neuroendocrine tumors, treatment of non-GIST soft tissue sarcomas.

FORMS — Trade only: Caps 12.5, 25, 50 mg.

NOTES — Reliable contraception is recommended. CYP3A4 inhibitors such as ketoconazole increase concentrations. CYP3A4 inducers such as rifampin and St. John's wort can decrease concentrations. Increases INR in patients on warfarin. Monitor CBC.

MOA — Inhibits the intracellular phosphorylation of tyrosine kinase associated with epidermal growth factor receptor, which is expressed on the surface of normal cells and cancer cells.

ADVERSE EFFECTS — Serious: CHF, bone marrow suppression, bleeding, thyroid dysfunction. Frequent: Diarrhea, fatigue, anorexia, stomatitis, vomiting, dyspepsia, yellow skin discoloration, depigmentation of hair or skin.

TENIPOSIDE (*Vumon, VM-26*) ▶K ♀D ▶– $ varies by therapy

WARNING — Bone marrow suppression, anaphylaxis, hypotension, CNS depression, alopecia. Instruct patients to report promptly fever, sore throat, or signs of local infection.

ADULT — Not approved in adult patients.

PEDS — Chemotherapy doses vary by indication. ALL, refractory, in combination regimens.

NOTES — Reliable contraception is recommended. Monitor CBCs, LFTs and renal function.

MOA — Mitotic Inhibitor.

ADVERSE EFFECTS — Serious: Bone marrow suppression, anaphylaxis, hypotension, CNS depression. Frequent: Mucositis, alopecia, bone marrow suppression, N/V, diarrhea.

TOPOTECAN (*Hycamtin*) ▶Plasma ♀D ▶— $ varies by therapy
WARNING — Bone marrow suppression (primary neutropenia), severe bleeding, interstitial lung disease. Instruct patients to report promptly fever, sore throat, signs of local infection, bleeding from any site, or symptoms suggestive of anemia.
ADULT — Chemotherapy doses vary by indication. Ovarian and cervical cancer. Small-cell lung cancer, relapsed.
PEDS — Not approved in children.
FORMS — Trade only: Caps 0.25, 1 mg. Generic/Trade: 4 mg powder for injection.
NOTES — Reliable contraception is recommended. Monitor CBCs.
MOA — Topoisomerase inhibitor.
ADVERSE EFFECTS — Serious: Bone marrow suppression, severe bleeding. Frequent: Bone marrow suppression, N/V, diarrhea, headache.

TRETINOIN—ONCOLOGY (*Vesanoid*) ▶L ♀D ▶— $ varies by therapy
WARNING — Retinoic acid-APL (RA-APL) syndrome: Fever, dyspnea, wt gain, pulmonary edema, pulmonary infiltrates and pleural/pericardial effusions, occasionally with impaired myocardial contractility and episodic hypotension, with or without leukocytosis. Reversible hypercholesterolemia/hypertriglyceridemia, increased LFTs, alopecia. Contraindicated in parabens-sensitive patients.
ADULT — Chemotherapy doses vary by indication. Acute promyelocytic leukemia.
PEDS — Not approved in children.
UNAPPROVED PEDS — Acute promyelocytic leukemia. Limited data.
FORMS — Generic/Trade: Caps 10 mg.
NOTES — Reliable contraception is recommended. Monitor CBCs, coags, LFTs, triglyceride, and cholesterol levels. Ketoconazole increases levels.
MOA — Unknown.
ADVERSE EFFECTS — Serious: APL differentiation syndrome: fever, dyspnea, weight gain, pulmonary infiltrates and pleural/pericardial effusions, with or w/o leukocytosis, pseudotumor cerebri. Frequent: Reversible hyperlipidemia, headache, fever.

VANDETANIB (*Caprelsa*) ▶K – ♀? ▶—
WARNING — QT prolongation, torsades de pointes and sudden death. Intestinal perforation has occurred in clinical trials.
ADULT — Unresectable locally advanced or metastatic medullary thyroid carcinoma.
PEDS — Not approved in peds.
FORMS — 100 mg and 300 mg oral capsules.
MOA — Tyrosine Kinase Inhibitor
ADVERSE EFFECTS — Diarrhea/colitis, heart failure, acneiform rash, nausea, hypertension, QT prolongation. Drug has prolonged half-life: monitor for cardiac toxicities throughout treatment. Hemorrhage, hypothyroidism, ischemic events, pulmonary toxicity, severe skin reactions, reversible posterior leukoencephalopathy syndrome.

VEMURAFENIB (*Zelboraf*) ▶? – ♀D ▶—
WARNING — Cutaneous squamous cell carcinomas were detected in 24% of patients receiving vemurafenib in clinical trials. Non-cutaneous squamous cell carcinoma and toxic epidermal necrolysis have occurred. Hypersensitivity reactions, uveitis, severe dermatologic reactions, QT prolongation and liver enzyme abnormalities. Increased hepatotoxicity associated with concurrent ipilimumab administration. DRESS Syndrome. Progression of pre-existing chronic myelomonocytic leukemia with NRAS mutation.
ADULT — Treatment of unrectable or metastatic melanoma in patients with the BRAFV600E mutation. Dose is 960mg orally twice daily.
PEDS — Not approved in pediatric patients.
FORMS — 240mg oral tabs
NOTES — Multiple potentially significant drug interactions may exist. Avoid use with CYP3A4 inhibitors and inducers.
MOA — BRAF kinase inhibitor, active against BRAFV600E mutated form, thereby blocking cellular proliferation of melanoma cells.
ADVERSE EFFECTS — Arthralgias, rash, alopecia, fatigue, photosensitivity and nausea.

VISMODEGIB (*Erivedge*) ▶oxidation - glucuronidation ♀D ▶—
WARNING — Vismodegib has been approved with a boxed warning stating that use of this drug can result in embryo-fetal death or severe birth defects. Pregnancy status must be verified prior to initiation of treatment, and both male and female patients need to be advised of these risks. Women need to be advised of the need for contraception and men of the potential risk for vismodegib exposure through semen.
ADULT — 150 mg orally once daily for Basal cell carcinoma (BCC) that has metastasized or relapsed after treatment with surgery, or for patients who are not candidates for surgery or radiation.
PEDS — Not approved in pediatrics.
FORMS — 150 mg capsules
MOA — Vismodegib is an oral drug that is designed to selectively inhibit abnormal signaling in the Hedgehog pathway, which is an underlying molecular driver of BCC. It binds to and inhibits Smoothened, a transmembrane protein involved in Hedgehog signal transduction.
ADVERSE EFFECTS — Muscle spasms, alopecia, dysgeusia, weight loss, fatigue, nausea, diarrhea, decreased appetite, constipation, arthralgias, vomiting, and ageusia.

VORINOSTAT (*Zolinza*) ▶L ♀D ▶— $$$$$
WARNING — PE/DVT, anemia, thrombocytopenia, QT prolongation.
ADULT — Chemotherapy doses vary by indication. Cutaneous T-cell lymphoma.
PEDS — Not approved in children.
FORMS — Trade only: Caps 100 mg.
NOTES — Reliable contraception is recommended. Monitor CBCs, electrolytes, renal function, ECG.
MOA — Unknown.

VORINOSTAT (*cont.*)

ADVERSE EFFECTS — Serious: PE/DVT, anemia, thrombocytopenia, QT prolongation. Frequent: N/V/D, hyperglycemia, fatigue, chills.

ZIV-AFLIBERCEPT (Zaltrap) ▶? – ♀C ▶–

WARNING — Severe and sometimes fatal hemorrhages, including gastrointestinal hemorrhages, have been reported in patients receiving ziv-aflibercept

ADULT — Treatment of patients with metastatic colorectal cancer (mCRC) that is resistant to or has progressed following an oxaliplatin-containing regimen. 4 mg/kg administered as a 60-minute IV infusion q 2 weeks in combination with the FOLFIRI regimen.

PEDS — Not approved in peds.

FORMS — 100 mg per 4 mL soln, single-use vial 200 mg per 8 mL soln, single-use vial

MOA — Recombinant fusion protein consisting of vascular endothelial growth factor (VEGF)-binding portions from the extracellular domains of human VEGF receptors 1 and 2 that are fused to the Fc portion of the human IgG1 immunoglobulin. By binding to these endogenous ligands, ziv-aflibercept can inhibit the binding and activation of their cognate receptors. This inhibition can result in decreased neovascularization and decreased vascular permeability.

ADVERSE EFFECTS — Leukopenia, diarrhea, neutropenia, proteinuria, increased AST and ALT, stomatitis, fatigue, thrombocytopenia, hypertension, decreased wt, decreased appetite, epistaxis, abdominal pain, dysphonia, increased serum creatinine, and headache.

OPHTHALMOLOGY

OPHTHALMOLOGY: Antiallergy—Decongestants & Combinations

NOTE: Overuse can cause rebound dilation of blood vessels. Do not administer while wearing soft contact lenses. Wait 10 min after use before inserting contact lenses. On average, each mL of eye drop soln contains approximately 20 gtts. Reserve ointment formulations for bedtime use due to severe vision blurring. Most eye medications can be administered 1 gtt at a time despite common manufacturer recommendations of 1 to 2 gtts concurrently. Even a single gtt is typically more than the eye can hold, and thus a second gtt is wasteful and increases the possibility of systemic toxicity. If 2 gtts of the medication are desired separate single gtts by at least 5 min.

NAPHAZOLINE (*Albalon, All Clear, Naphcon, Clear Eyes*) ▶? ♀C ▶? $
ADULT — Ocular vasoconstrictor/decongestant: 1 to 2 gtts four times per day for up to 3 days.
PEDS — Not approved for age younger than 6 yo. Use adult dose for age 6 yo or older.
FORMS — OTC Generic/Trade: Soln 0.012, 0.025% (15, 30 mL). Rx Generic/Trade: 0.1% (15 mL).
NOTES — Avoid in patients with cardiovascular disease, HTN, narrow-angle glaucoma.
MOA — Alpha-adrenergic agonist decongestant.
ADVERSE EFFECTS — Frequent: Blurred vision, cardiovascular stimulation, dizziness, headache, nervousness, nausea, stinging, mucosal irritation, dryness, rebound dilation.

NAPHCON-A (naphazoline + pheniramine) ▶L ♀C ▶? $
ADULT — Ocular decongestant: 1 gtt four times per day prn for up to 3 days.
PEDS — Not approved for age younger than 6 yo. Use adult dose for age 6 yo or older.
FORMS — OTC Trade only: Soln 0.025% + 0.3% (15 mL).
NOTES — Avoid in patients with cardiovascular disease, HTN, narrow-angle glaucoma, age younger than 6 yo.
MOA — Antihistamine, decongestant.
ADVERSE EFFECTS — Frequent: Dry mouth, anticholinergic effects, rebound congestion, pupillary dilation, increase in intraocular pressure.

VASOCON-A (naphazoline + antazoline) ▶L ♀C ▶? $
ADULT — Ocular decongestant: 1 gtt four times per day prn for up to 3 days.
PEDS — Not approved for children younger than 6 yo. Use adult dose for age 6 yo or older.
FORMS — OTC Trade only: Soln 0.05% + 0.5% (15 mL).
NOTES — Avoid in patients with cardiovascular disease, HTN, narrow-angle glaucoma.
MOA — Decongestant, antihistamine.
ADVERSE EFFECTS — Frequent: Dry mouth, anticholinergic effects, rebound congestion.

OPHTHALMOLOGY: Antiallergy—Dual Antihistamine & Mast Cell Stabilizer

NOTE: Wait at least 10 to 15 min after use before inserting contact lenses. On average, each mL of eye drop soln contains approximately 20 gtts. Reserve ointment formulations for bedtime use due to severe vision blurring. Most eye medications can be administered 1 gtt at a time despite common manufacturer recommendations of 1 to 2 gtts concurrently. Even a single gtt is typically more than the eye can hold and thus a second gtt is both wasteful and increases the possibility of systemic toxicity. If 2 gtts of the medication are desired separate single gtts by at least 5 min.

AZELASTINE—OPHTHALMIC (*Optivar*) ▶L ♀C ▶? $$$
ADULT — Allergic conjunctivitis: 1 gtt two times per day.
PEDS — Not approved for age younger than 3 yo. Use adult dose for age 3 yo or older.
FORMS — Trade/generic: Soln 0.05% (6 mL).
MOA — H-1 receptor antagonist, mast cell stabilizer, inhibitor of other mediators of allergic response (eg, leukotrienes).
ADVERSE EFFECTS — Frequent: Burning, stinging, headache, somnolence, bitter taste.

EPINASTINE (*Elestat*) ▶K ♀C ▶? $$$$
ADULT — Allergic conjunctivitis: 1 gtt two times per day.
PEDS — Not approved for age younger than 2 yo. Use adult dose for age 2 yo or older.
FORMS — Trade only: Soln 0.05% (5 mL).
MOA — H-1 receptor antagonist, mast cell stabilizer.
ADVERSE EFFECTS — Frequent: Burning, pruritus, hyperemia.

KETOTIFEN—OPHTHALMIC (*Alaway, Zaditor*) ▶minimal absorption ♀C ▶? $
ADULT — Allergic conjunctivitis: 1 gtt in each eye q 8 to 12 h.
PEDS — Not approved in children younger than 3 yo. Use adult dose in children older than 3 yo.
FORMS — OTC Generic/Trade: Soln 0.025% (5 mL, 10 mL).
MOA — H-1-receptor antagonist and mast cell stabilizer.
ADVERSE EFFECTS — Frequent: Stinging, burning, dry eyes, photophobia.

OLOPATADINE—OPHTHALMIC (*Pataday, Patanol*) ▶K ♀C ▶? $$$$
ADULT — Allergic conjunctivitis: 1 gtt of 0.1% soln in each eye two times per day (Patanol) or 1 gtt of 0.2% soln in each eye daily (Pataday).
PEDS — Not approved for age younger than 3 yo. Use adult dose for age 3 yo or older.

OLOPATADINE—OPHTHALMIC (cont.)

FORMS — Trade only: Soln 0.1% (5 mL, Patanol), 0.2% (2.5 mL, Pataday).

NOTES — Do not administer while wearing soft contact lenses. Allow 6 to 8 h between doses.
MOA — H-1-receptor antagonist and mast cell stabilizer.
ADVERSE EFFECTS — Ocular: Frequent: Headache.

OPHTHALMOLOGY: Antiallergy—Pure Antihistamines

NOTE: Antihistamines may aggravate dry eye symptoms. Wait 10 min after use before inserting contact lenses. On average, each mL of eye drop soln contains approximately 20 gtts. Reserve ointment formulations for bedtime use due to severe vision blurring. Most eye medications can be administered 1 gtt at a time despite common manufacturer recommendations of 1 to 2 gtts concurrently. Even a single gtt is typically more than the eye can hold and thus a second gtt is both wasteful and increases the possibility of systemic toxicity. If 2 gtts of the medication are desired separate single gtts by at least 5 min.

ALCAFTADINE (Lastacaft) ▶not absorbed ♀B ▶? $$$
ADULT — Allergic conjunctivitis: 1 gtt in each eye daily.
PEDS — Not approved in chidlren younger than 2 years. Use adult dosing in children 2 years or older.
FORMS — Trade: Soln 0.25%, 3 mL.
MOA — H1-receptor blocker.
ADVERSE EFFECTS — Frequent: eye irritation, burning, stinging, reness, pruritis.

BEPOTASTINE (Bepreve) ▶L (but minimal absorption) - ♀C ▶? $$$
ADULT — Allergic conjunctivitis: 1 gtt two times per day.
PEDS — Not studied in children younger than 2 yo.

FORMS — Trade only: Soln 1.5% (2.5, 5, 10 mL)
NOTES — Remove contact lenses prior to instillation.
MOA — Direct histamine-1-receptor antagonist.
ADVERSE EFFECTS — Frequent: Mild taste, irritation, headache.

EMEDASTINE (Emadine) ▶L ♀B ▶? $$$
ADULT — Allergic conjunctivitis: 1 gtt daily to four times per day.
PEDS — Not approved for age younger than 3 yo. Use adult dose for age 3 yo or older.
FORMS — Trade only: Soln 0.05% (5 mL).
MOA — H-1-receptor antagonist.
ADVERSE EFFECTS — Frequent: Headache.

OPHTHALMOLOGY: Antiallergy—Pure Mast Cell Stabilizers

NOTE: Works best as preventative agent; use continually during at risk season. Wait 10 min after use before inserting contact lenses. On average, each mL of eye drop soln contains approximately 20 gtts. Reserve ointment formulations for bedtime use due to severe vision blurring. Most eye medications can be administered 1 gtt at a time despite common manufacturer recommendations of 1 to 2 gtts concurrently. Even a single gtt is typically more than the eye can hold and thus a second gtt is both wasteful and increases the possibility of systemic toxicity. If 2 gtts of the medication are desired separate single gtts by at least 5 min.

CROMOLYN—OPHTHALMIC (Crolom, Opticrom) ▶LK ♀B ▶? $$
ADULT — Allergic conjunctivitis: 1 to 2 gtts 4 to 6 times per day.
PEDS — Not approved for age younger than 4 yo. Use adult dose for age 4 yo or older.
FORMS — Generic/Trade: Soln 4% (10 mL).
NOTES — Response may take up to 6 weeks.
MOA — Prevents mast cell degranulation and release of histamine, leukotrienes and slow-reacting substance of anaphylaxis.
ADVERSE EFFECTS — Frequent: Conjunctival redness, dryness, irritation, hypersensitivity reactions.

LODOXAMIDE (Alomide) ▶K ♀B ▶? $$$
ADULT — Allergic conjunctivitis: 1 to 2 gtts in each eye four times per day for up to 3 months.
PEDS — Not approved for age younger than 2 yo. Use adult dose for age 2 yo or older.

FORMS — Trade only: Soln 0.1% (10 mL).
NOTES — Do not administer while wearing soft contact lenses.
MOA — Mast cell stabilizer.
ADVERSE EFFECTS — Frequent: Blurred vision, eye pain, possible corneal erosion.

NEDOCROMIL—OPHTHALMIC (Alocril) ▶L ♀B ▶? $$$
ADULT — Allergic conjunctivitis: 1 to 2 gtts in each eye two times per day.
PEDS — Not approved for age younger than 3 yo.Use adult dosing in children 3 years or older.
FORMS — Trade only: Soln 2% (5 mL).
NOTES — Soln normally appears slightly yellow.
MOA — Mast cell stabilizer.
ADVERSE EFFECTS — Frequent: Burning, irritation, stinging, conjunctival redness, photophobia.

OPHTHALMOLOGY: Antibacterials—Aminoglycosides

NOTE: On average, each mL of eye drop soln contains approximately 20 gtts. Reserve ointment formulations for bedtime use due to severe vision blurring. Most eye medications can be administered 1 gtt at a time despite common manufacturer recommendations of 1 to 2 gtts concurrently. Even a single gtt is typically more than the eye can hold and thus a second gtt is both wasteful and increases the possibility of systemic toxicity. If 2 gtts of the medication are desired separate single gtts by at least 5 min.

GENTAMICIN—OPHTHALMIC (*Garamycin, Genoptic, Gentak, ★Diogent*) ▶K ♀C ▶? $
ADULT — Ocular infections: 1 to 2 gtts q 2 to 4 h or ½ inch ribbon of ointment two to three times per day.
PEDS — Not approved in children.
UNAPPROVED ADULT — Up to 2 gtts q 1 h have been used for severe infections. 1 gtt under nails TID has been used for subungual Pseudomonas infection presenting as a green nail
UNAPPROVED PEDS — Ocular infections: 1 to 2 gtts q 4 h or ½ inch ribbon of ointment two to three times per day.
FORMS — Generic/Trade: Soln 0.3% (5, 15 mL) Ointment 0.3% (3.5 g tube).
NOTES — For severe infections, use up to 2 gtts q 1 h.
MOA — Inhibits RNA-dependent bacterial protein synthesis.
ADVERSE EFFECTS — Frequent: Edema, rash, pruritus, ocular irritation.

TOBRAMYCIN—OPHTHALMIC (*Tobrex*) ▶K ♀B ▶– $
ADULT — Ocular infections, mild to moderate: 1 to 2 gtts q 4 h or ½ inch ribbon of ointment two to three times per day. Ocular infections, severe: 2 gtts q 1 h, then taper to q 4 h or ½ inch ribbon of ointment q 3 to 4 h, then taper to two to three times per day.
PEDS — Use adult dose for age 2 mo or older.
UNAPPROVED PEDS — Ocular infections, mild to moderate: 1 to 2 gtts q 4 h or ½ inch ribbon of ointment two to three times per day. Ocular infections, severe: 2 gtts q 1 h, then taper to q 4 h or ½ inch ribbon of ointment q 3 to 4 h, then taper to two to three times per day.
FORMS — Generic/Trade: Soln 0.3% (5 mL). Trade only: Ointment 0.3% (3.5 g tube).
MOA — Inhibits RNA-dependent bacterial protein synthesis.
ADVERSE EFFECTS — Frequent: Edema, rash, pruritus, ocular irritation.

OPHTHALMOLOGY: Antibacterials—Fluoroquinolones

NOTE: Avoid the overuse of fluoroquinolones for conjunctivitis. Ocular administration has not been shown to cause arthropathy. On average, each mL of eye drop soln contains approximately 20 gtts. Reserve ointment formulations for bedtime use due to severe vision blurring. Most eye medications can be administered 1 gtt at a time despite common manufacturer recommendations of 1 to 2 gtts concurrently. Even a single gtt is typically more than the eye can hold and thus a second gtt is both wasteful and increases the possibility of systemic toxicity. If 2 gtts of the medication are desired separate single gtts by at least 5 min.

BESIFLOXACIN (*Besivance*) ▶LK ♀C ▶? $$$
ADULT — Bacterial conjunctivitis: 1 gtt three times per day for 7 days.
PEDS — Not approved for age younger than 1 yo. Use adult dose for age 1 yo or older.
FORMS — Trade: Soln 0.6% (5 mL).
NOTES — Do not wear contacts during use.
MOA — Inhibits DNA-gyrase in susceptible bacteria.
ADVERSE EFFECTS — Frequent: Blurred vision, eye pain, eye irritation, eye pruritus and headache.

CIPROFLOXACIN—OPHTHALMIC (*Ciloxan*) ▶LK ♀C ▶? $$
ADULT — Corneal ulcers/ keratitis: 2 gtts q 15 min for 6 h, then 2 gtts q 30 min for 1 day; then 2 gtts q 1 h for 1 day, and 2 gtts q 4 h for 3 to 14 days. Bacterial conjunctivitis: 1 to 2 gtts q 2 h while awake for 2 days, then 1 to 2 gtts q 4 h while awake for 5 days; or ½ inch ribbon ointment three times per day for 2 days, then ½ inch ribbon two times per day for 5 days.
PEDS — Bacterial conjunctivitis: Use adult dose for age 1 yo or older (soln) and age 2 yo or older (ointment). Not approved below these ages.
FORMS — Generic/Trade: Soln 0.3% (2.5, 5, 10 mL). Trade only: Ointment 0.3% (3.5 g tube).
NOTES — May cause white precipitate of active drug at site of epithelial defect that may be confused with a worsening infection. Resolves within 2 weeks and does not necessitate discontinuation.
MOA — Inhibits DNA-gyrase in susceptible bacteria.
ADVERSE EFFECTS — Frequent: Headache, eye discomfort, keratopathy, burning sensation. Severe: Hypersensitivity.

GATIFLOXACIN—OPHTHALMIC (*Zymaxid, ★Zymar*) ▶K ♀C ▶? $$$
ADULT — Bacterial conjunctivitis: 1 to 2 gtts q 2 h while awake (up to 8 times per day on days 1 and 2), then 1 to 2 gtts 4 times per day on days 3 thru 7.
PEDS — Not approved for age younger than 1 yo. Use adult dose for age 1 yo or older.
FORMS — Trade only: Soln 0.5% (5 mL).
MOA — Inhibits DNA-gyrase and topoisomerase IV in susceptible bacteria.
ADVERSE EFFECTS — Frequent: Conjunctival irritation, increased lacrimation, keratitis, papillary conjunctivitis.

LEVOFLOXACIN—OPHTHALMIC (*Iquix, Quixin*) ▶KL ♀C ▶? $$$
ADULT — Bacterial conjunctivitis, Quixin: 1 to 2 gtts q 2 h while awake (up to 8 times per day) on days 1 and 2, then 1 to 2 gtts q 4 h (up to 4 times per day) on days 3 to 7. Corneal ulcers, Iquix: 1 to 2 gtts q 30 min to 2 h while awake and q 4 to 6 h overnight on days 1 to 3, then 1 to 2 gtts q 1 to 4 h while awake on day 4 to completion of therapy.
PEDS — Bacterial conjunctivitis, Quixin: 1 to 2 gtts q 2 h while awake (up to 8 times per day) on days 1 and 2, then 1 to 2 gtts q 4 h (up to 4 times/ day) on days 3 to 7 for age older than 1 yo only. Corneal ulcers, Iquix: 1 to 2 gtts q 30 min to 2 h while awake and q 4 to 6 h overnight on days 1 to 3, then 1 to 2 gtts q 1 to 4 h while awake on day 4 to completion of therapy for age older than 6 yo only.
FORMS — Trade/Generic only: Soln 0.5% (5 mL)
MOA — Inhibits DNA-gyrase in susceptible bacteria.

LEVOFLOXACIN—OPHTHALMIC (*cont.*)
ADVERSE EFFECTS — Frequent: Headache, decreased vision, fever, burning, pharyngitis, photophobia. Severe: Hypersensitivity.

MOXIFLOXACIN—OPHTHALMIC (*Vigamox, Moxeza*) ▶LK ♀C ▶? $$$
ADULT — Bacterial conjunctivitis: 1 gtt in each affected eye three times per day for 7 days (Vigamox) or 1 gtt in each affected eye two times per day for 7 days (Moxeza).
PEDS — Use adult dose for age 1 yo or older.
FORMS — Trade only: Soln 0.5% (3 mL, Vigamox and Moxeza).
MOA — Inhibits DNA-gyrase and topoisomerase IV in susceptible bacteria.

ADVERSE EFFECTS — Frequent: Conjunctival irritation, dry eye, ocular discomfort/pain/pruritus, increased lacrimation, keratitis, conjunctivitis.

OFLOXACIN—OPHTHALMIC (*Ocuflox*) ▶LK ♀C ▶? $$
ADULT — Corneal ulcers/keratitis: 1 to 2 gtts q 30 min while awake and 1 to 2 gtts 4 to 6 h after retiring for 2 days, then 1 to 2 gtts q 1 h while awake for 5 days, then 1 to 2 gtts four times per day for 3 days. Bacterial conjunctivitis: 1 to 2 gtts q 2 to 4 h for 2 days, then 1 to 2 gtts four times per day for 5 days.
PEDS — Bacterial conjunctivitis: Use adult dose for age 1 yo or older, not approved age younger than 1 yo.
FORMS — Generic/Trade: Soln 0.3% (5, 10 mL).
MOA — Inhibits DNA-gyrase in susceptible bacteria.
ADVERSE EFFECTS — Frequent: Ocular burning, eye discomfort. Severe: Chemical conjunctivitis/keratitis, ocular/facial edema, hypersensitivity reaction.

OPHTHALMOLOGY: Antibacterials—Other

NOTE: On average, each mL of eye drop soln contains approximately 20 gtts. Reserve ointment formulations for bedtime use due to severe vision blurring. Most eye medications can be administered 1 gtt at a time despite common manufacturer recommendations of 1 to 2 gtts concurrently. Even a single gtt is typically more than the eye can hold and thus a second gtt is both wasteful and increases the possibility of systemic toxicity. If 2 gtts of the medication are desired separate single gtts by at least 5 min.

AZITHROMYCIN—OPHTHALMIC (*Azasite*) ▶L ♀B ▶? $$$
ADULT — Ocular infections: 1 gtt two times per day for 2 days, then 1 gtt daily for 5 more days.
PEDS — Not approved in children younger than 1 year. Use adult dose for age 1 yo or older.
FORMS — Trade only: Soln 1% (2.5 mL).
MOA — Inhibits RNA-dependent protein synthesis.
ADVERSE EFFECTS — Frequent: Eye irritation.

BACITRACIN—OPHTHALMIC (*AK Tracin*) ▶Minimal absorption ♀C ▶? $
ADULT — Ocular infections: Apply ¼ to ½ inch ribbon of ointment q 3 to 4 h or two to four times per day for 7 to 10 days.
PEDS — Not approved in children.
UNAPPROVED PEDS — Ocular infections: Apply ½ inch ribbon of ointment q 3 to 4 h or two to four times per day for 7 to 10 days.
FORMS — Generic/Trade: Ointment 500 units/g (3.5 g tube).
MOA — Inhibits bacterial cell wall synthesis.
ADVERSE EFFECTS — Frequent: Edema of face, pain, rash, pruritus.

ERYTHROMYCIN—OPHTHALMIC (*Ilotycin, AK-Mycin*) ▶L ♀B ▶+ $
ADULT — Ocular infections, corneal ulceration: ½ inch ribbon of ointment q 3 to 4 h or 2 to 6 times per day. For chlamydial infections: two times per day for 2 months or two times per day for the first 5 days of each month for 6 months.
PEDS — Ophthalmia neonatorum prophylaxis: ½ inch ribbon to both eyes within 1 h of birth.
FORMS — Generic only: Ointment 0.5% (1, 3.5 g tube).
MOA — Inhibits RNA-dependent protein synthesis.
ADVERSE EFFECTS — Frequent: None.

FUSIDIC ACID—OPHTHALMIC (*✽Fucithalmic*) ▶L ♀? ▶? $
ADULT — Canada only. Eye infections: 1 gtt in both eyes q 12 h for 7 days for age 2 yo or older.
PEDS — Not approved in children younger than 2 years. Use adult dose for age 2 yo or older.
FORMS — Canada trade only: gtts 1%. Multidose tubes of 3, 5 g. Single-dose preservative-free tubes of 0.2 g in a box of 12.
MOA — Antibacterial, interferes with bacterial protein synthesis.
ADVERSE EFFECTS — Frequent: Stinging, irritation. Severe: Hypersensitivity.

NEOSPORIN OINTMENT—OPHTHALMIC (neomycin—ophthalmic + bacitracin—ophthalmic + polymyxin—ophthalmic) ▶KL ♀C ▶? $
ADULT — Ocular infections: ½ inch ribbon of ointment q 3 to 4 h for 7 to 10 days or ½ inch ribbon two to three times per day for mild to moderate infection.
PEDS — Not approved in children.
UNAPPROVED PEDS — ½ inch ribbon of ointment q 3 to 4 h for 7 to 10 days.
FORMS — Generic only: Ointment. (3.5 g tube).
NOTES — Contact dermatitis can occur after prolonged use.
MOA — Inhibits RNA-dependent protein synthesis and interferes with cell wall membranes.
ADVERSE EFFECTS — Frequent: Topical hypersensitivity, contact dermatitis.

NEOSPORIN SOLUTION—OPHTHALMIC (neomycin—ophthalmic + polymyxin—ophthalmic + gramicidin) ▶KL ♀C ▶? $$
ADULT — Ocular infections: 1 to 2 gtts q 4 to 6 h for 7 to 10 days.
PEDS — Not approved in children.

NEOSPORIN SOLUTION—OPHTHALMIC (cont.)

UNAPPROVED PEDS — 1 to 2 gtts q 4 to 6 h for 7 to 10 days.
FORMS — Generic/Trade: Soln (10 mL).
NOTES — Contact dermatitis can occur after prolonged use.
MOA — Inhibits RNA-dependent protein synthesis and interferes with cell wall membranes.
ADVERSE EFFECTS — Frequent: Topical hypersensitivity, contact dermatitis, eye irritation, burning, stinging, edema, pruritus, failure to heal.

POLYSPORIN—OPHTHALMIC (polymyxin— ophthalmic + bacitracin—ophthalmic) ▶K ♀C ▶? $$

ADULT — Ocular infections: ½ inch ribbon of ointment q 3 to 4 h for 7 to 10 days or ½ inch ribbon two to three times per day for mild to moderate infection.
PEDS — Not approved in children.
UNAPPROVED PEDS — Ocular infections: ½ inch ribbon of ointment q 3 to 4 h for 7 to 10 days.
FORMS — Generic only: Ointment (3.5 g tube).
MOA — Inhibits synthesis of and interferes with bacterial cell wall membranes.
ADVERSE EFFECTS — Frequent: None.

POLYTRIM—OPHTHALMIC (polymyxin—ophthalmic + trimethoprim—ophthalmic) ▶KL ♀C ▶? $

ADULT — Ocular infections: 1 to 2 gtts q 4 to 6 h (up to 6 gtts per day) for 7 to 10 days.

PEDS — Not approved age younger than 2 mo. Use adult dose for age 2 mo or older.
FORMS — Generic/Trade: Soln (10 mL).
MOA — Interferes with bacterial cell wall membranes, folate reduction.
ADVERSE EFFECTS — Frequent: None.

SULFACETAMIDE—OPHTHALMIC (Bleph-10, Sulf-10) ▶K ♀C ▶– $

ADULT — Ocular infections, corneal ulceration: 1 to 2 gtts q 2 to 3 h initially, then taper by decreasing frequency as condition allows over 7 to 10 days or ½ inch ribbon of ointment q 3 to 4 h initially, then taper 7 to 10 days. Trachoma: 2 gtts q 2 h with systemic antibiotic such as doxycycline or azithromycin.
PEDS — Not approved age younger than 2 mo. Use adult dose for age 2 mo or older.
FORMS — Generic/Trade: Soln 10% (15 mL), Ointment 10% (3.5 g tube). Generic only: Soln 30% (15 mL).
NOTES — Ointment may be used as an adjunct to soln. Caution in sulfa-allergic patients.
MOA — Inhibits bacterial folic acid synthesis.
ADVERSE EFFECTS — Frequent: Irritation, stinging, burning. Severe: Stevens-Johnson syndrome, toxic epidermal necrolysis, hypersensitivity.

OPHTHALMOLOGY: Antiviral Agents

GANCICLOVIR—OPHTHALMIC (Zirgan) ▶minimal absorption ♀C ▶? $$$$

ADULT — Herpetic keratitis: 1 gtt five times per day (approximately q 3 h) until ulcer heals, then 1 gtt three times per day for 7 days.
PEDS — Not approved in children younger than 2 years. Use adult dosing for age 2 yo and older.
FORMS — Trade only: Gel 0.15% (5g).
NOTES — Do not wear contact lenses.
MOA — Inhibits DNA replication.
ADVERSE EFFECTS — Frequent: Blurred vision, eye irritation, punctate keratitis, conjunctival hyperemia.

TRIFLURIDINE (Viroptic) ▶Minimal absorption ♀C ▶– $$$

ADULT — Herpetic keratitis: 1 gtt q 2 h to maximum 9 gtts per days. After re-epithelialization, decrease dose to 1 gtt q 4 to 6 h while awake for 7 to 14 days. Max of 21 days of treatment.
PEDS — Not approved age younger than 6 yo. Use adult dose for age 6 yo or older.
FORMS — Generic/Trade Soln 1% (7.5 mL).
NOTES — Avoid continuous use more than 21 days; may cause keratitis and conjunctival scarring. Urge frequent use of topical lubricants (ie, tear substitutes) to minimize surface damage.
MOA — Inhibits viral DNA replication as thymidine analog.
ADVERSE EFFECTS — Frequent: Burning, stinging.

OPHTHALMOLOGY: Corticosteroid & Antibacterial Combinations

NOTE: Recommend that only ophthalmologists or optometrists prescribe due to infection, cataract, corneal/scleral perforation, and glaucoma risk from prolonged use. Monitor intraocular pressure. Gradually taper when discontinuing. Shake suspensions well before using. On average, each mL of eye drop soln contains approximately 20 gtts. Reserve ointment formulations for bedtime use due to severe vision blurring. Most eye medications can be administered 1 gtt at a time despite common manufacturer recommendations of 1 to 2 gtts concurrently. Even a single gtt is typically more than the eye can hold and thus a second gtt is both wasteful and increases the possibility of systemic toxicity. If 2 gtts of the medication are desired separate single gtts by at least 5 min.

BLEPHAMIDE (prednisolone—ophthalmic + sulfacetamide—ophthalmic) ▶KL ♀C ▶? $

ADULT — Steroid-responsive inflammatory condition with bacterial infection or risk of bacterial infection:

Start 1 to 2 gtts q 1 h during the day and q 2 h during the night, then 1 gtt q 4 h and at bedtime; or ½ inch ribbon to lower conjunctival sac 3 to 4 times/day and 1 to 2 times at night.

BLEPHAMIDE (cont.)

PEDS — Not approved in children younger than 6 yo.
FORMS — Generic/Trade: Soln/Susp (5, 10 mL), Trade only: Ointment (3.5 g tube).
MOA — Inhibits bacterial folic acid synthesis, anti-inflammatory.
ADVERSE EFFECTS — Frequent: Insomnia, nervousness, increased appetite, indigestion, local irritation, burning, stinging. Severe: Cataracts, secondary ocular infections, glaucoma, Stevens-Johnson syndrome, toxic epidermal necrolysis, hypersensitivity.

CORTISPORIN—OPHTHALMIC (neomycin—ophthalmic + polymyxin—ophthalmic + hydrocortisone—ophthalmic) ►LK ♀C ▶? $

ADULT — Steroid-responsive inflammatory condition with bacterial infection or risk of bacterial infection: 1 to 2 gtts or ½ inch ribbon of ointment q 3 to 4 h or more frequently prn.
PEDS — Not approved in children.
UNAPPROVED PEDS — 1 to 2 gtts or ½ inch ribbon of ointment q 3 to 4 h.
FORMS — Generic only: Susp (7.5 mL), Ointment (3.5 g tube).
MOA — Inhibits RNA-dependent protein synthesis, interferes with bacterial cell wall membranes, anti-inflammatory.
ADVERSE EFFECTS — Frequent: None. Severe: Cataracts, secondary ocular infections, glaucoma, Stevens-Johnson syndrome, toxic epidermal necrolysis, hypersensitivity.

FML-S LIQUIFILM (prednisolone—ophthalmic + sulfacetamide—ophthalmic) ►KL ♀C ▶? $$

ADULT — Steroid-responsive inflammatory condition with bacterial infection or risk of bacterial infection: Start 1 to 2 gtts q 1 h during the day and q 2 h during the night, then 1 gtt q 4 to 8 h.
PEDS — Not approved in children.
FORMS — Trade only: Susp (10 mL).
MOA — Anti-inflammatory.
ADVERSE EFFECTS — Frequent: Insomnia, nervousness, increased appetite, indigestion, local irritation, burning, stinging. Severe: Cataracts, secondary ocular infections, glaucoma, Stevens-Johnson syndrome, toxic epidermal necrolysis, hypersensitivity.

MAXITROL (dexamethasone—ophthalmic + neomycin—ophthalmic + polymyxin—ophthalmic) ►KL ♀C ▶? $

ADULT — Steroid-responsive inflammatory condition with bacterial infection or risk of bacterial infection: Ointment: Place a small amount (about ½ inch) in the affected eye 3 to 4 times per day or apply at bedtime as an adjunct with gtts. Susp: Instill 1 to 2 gtts into affected eye(s) 4 to 6 times daily; in severe disease, gtts may be used hourly and tapered to discontinuation.
PEDS — Not approved in children.
FORMS — Generic/Trade: Susp (5 mL), Ointment (3.5 g tube).

MOA — Inhibits RNA-dependent protein synthesis, interferes with bacterial cell wall membranes, anti-inflammatory.
ADVERSE EFFECTS — Frequent: None. Severe: Cataracts, secondary ocular infections, glaucoma, Stevens-Johnson syndrome, toxic epidermal necrolysis, hypersensitivity.

PRED G (prednisolone—ophthalmic + gentamicin—ophthalmic) ►KL ♀C ▶? $$

ADULT — Steroid-responsive inflammatory condition with bacterial infection or risk of bacterial infection: Start 1 to 2 gtts q 1 h during the days and q 2 h during the night, then 1 gtt 2 to 4 times daily or ½ inch ribbon of ointment 1 to 3 times per day.
PEDS — Not approved in children.
FORMS — Trade only: Susp (2, 5, 10 mL), Ointment (3.5 g tube).
MOA — Inhibits RNA-dependent protein synthesis, anti-inflammatory.
ADVERSE EFFECTS — Frequent: None. Severe: Cataracts, secondary ocular infections, glaucoma, Stevens-Johnson syndrome, toxic epidermal necrolysis, hypersensitivity.

TOBRADEX (tobramycin—ophthalmic + dexamethasone—ophthalmic) ►L ♀C ▶? $$$

ADULT — Steroid-responsive inflammatory condition with bacterial infection or risk of bacterial infection: 1 to 2 gtts q 2 h for 1 to 2 days, then 1 to 2 gtts q 4 to 6 h; or ½ inch ribbon of ointment three to four times per day.
PEDS — 1 to 2 gtts q 2 h for 1 to 2 days, then 1 to 2 gtts q 4 to 6 h; or ½ inch ribbon of ointment three to four times per day for age 2 yo or older.
FORMS — Trade/generic: susp (tobramycin 0.3%/dexamethasone 0.1%, 2.5, 5, 10 mL) Trade: ointment (tobramycin 0.3%/dexamethasone 0.1%, 3.5 g tube).
MOA — Inhibits RNA-dependent protein synthesis, anti-inflammatory.
ADVERSE EFFECTS — Frequent: Eyelid itching, swelling, conjunctival erythema. Severe: Cataracts, secondary ocular infections, glaucoma.

TOBRADEX ST (tobramycin—ophthalmic + dexamethasone—ophthalmic) ►L ♀C ▶? $$$

ADULT — Steroid-responsive inflammatory condition with bacterial infection or risk of bacterial infection: 1 gtt q 2 h for 1 to 2 days, then 1 gtt q 4 to 6 h.
PEDS — Not approved in children younge than 2 years. Use adult dose in children 2 yo or older.
FORMS — Trade only: Tobramycin 0.3%/dexamethasone 0.05%: Susp (2.5, 5, 10 mL).
MOA — Inhibits RNA-dependent protein synthesis, anti-inflammatory.
ADVERSE EFFECTS — Frequent: Eyelid itching, swelling, conjunctival erythema. Severe: Cataracts, secondary ocular infections, glaucoma.

VASOCIDIN (prednisolone—ophthalmic + sulfacetamide—ophthalmic) ►KL ♀C ▶? $

ADULT — Steroid-responsive inflammatory condition with bacterial infection or risk of bacterial infection: Start 1 to 2 gtts q 1 h during the days and q 2 h

VASOCIDIN (cont.)

during the night, then 1 gtt q 4 to 8 h; or ½ inch ribbon (ointment) three to four times per day initially, then one to two times per day thereafter.
PEDS — Not approved in children.
FORMS — Generic only: Soln (5, 10 mL).
MOA — Inhibits bacterial folic acid synthesis, anti-inflammatory.
ADVERSE EFFECTS — Frequent: Insomnia, nervousness, increased appetite, indigestion, local irritation, burning, stinging. Severe: Cataracts, secondary ocular infections, Stevens-Johnson syndrome, toxic epidermal necrolysis, hypersensitivity.
ZYLET (loteprednol + tobramycin—ophthalmic) ▶LK ♀C ▶? $$$
ADULT — Steroid-responsive inflammatory condition with bacterial infection or risk of bacterial

infection:1 to 2 gtts q 1 to 2 h for 1 to 2 days then 1 to 2 gtts q 4 to 6 h.
PEDS — Steroid-responsive inflammatory condition with bacterial infection or risk of bacterial infection:1 to 2 gtts q 1 to 2 h for 1 to 2 days then 1 to 2 gtts q 4 to 6 h.
FORMS — Trade only: Susp 0.5% loteprednol + 0.3% tobramycin (2.5, 5, 10 mL).
NOTES — Prescribe a maximum of 20 mL initially, then re-evaluate.
MOA — Anti-inflammatory (loteprednol) and inhibits RNA-dependent bacterial protein synthesis (tobramycin).
ADVERSE EFFECTS — Frequent: Injection, superficial punctate keratitis, ocular burning and stinging, headache. Severe: Cataracts, secondary ocular infections, glaucoma.

OPHTHALMOLOGY: Corticosteroids

NOTE: Recommend that only ophthalmologists or optometrists prescribe due to infection, cataract, corneal/scleral perforation, and glaucoma risk. Monitor intraocular pressure. Gradually taper when discontinuing. Shake susp well before using. On average, each mL of eye drop soln contains approximately 20 gtts. Reserve ointment formulations for bedtime use due to severe vision blurring. Most eye medications can be administered 1 gtt at a time despite common manufacturer recommendations of 1 to 2 gtts concurrently. Even a single gtt is typically more than the eye can hold and thus a second gtt is both wasteful and increases the possibility of systemic toxicity. If 2 gtts of the medication are desired separate single gtts by at least 5 min.

DIFLUPREDNATE (*Durezol*) ▶Not absorbed ♀C ▶? $$$$
ADULT — Inflammation and pain associated with ocular surgery: 1 gtt into affected eye four times per day, beginning 24 h after surgery for 2 weeks, then 1 gtt into affected eye 2 times per day for 1 week, then taper based on response. Endogenous anterior uveitis: 1 gtt into affected eye 4 times daily for 14 days followed by tapering as indicated.
PEDS — Not approved in children. Limited efficacy and safety data in children 0 to 3 yo indicated similar effects as seen with prednisolone acetate susp.
FORMS — Trade only: Ophthalmic emulsion 0.05% (2.5, 5 mL).
NOTES — If used for more than 10 days, monitor IOP.
MOA — Anti-inflammatory.
ADVERSE EFFECTS — Frequent: Corneal edema, ciliary and conjunctival hyperemia, pain, photophobia, posterior capsule opacification, blepharitis. Severe: Cataracts, secondary ocular infections, glaucoma.
FLUOCINOLONE—OPHTHALMIC (*Retisert*) ▶Not absorbed ♀C ▶? $$$$$
PEDS — Not approved in children younger than 12 yo.
FORMS — Implantable tablet 0.59 mg only available from manufacturer.
NOTES — Releases 0.6 mcg/day decreasing over about 1 month, then 0.3 to 0.4 mcg/day over about 30 months. Within 34 weeks 60% require medication to control intraocular pressure and within 2 years nearly all phakic eyes develop cataracts.
MOA — Anti-inflammatory
ADVERSE EFFECTS — Frequent: headache, eye pain, procedural complications including implant

expulsion, injury, migration of implant, wound dehiscence. Severe: cataracts, secondary ocular infections, glaucoma.
FLUOROMETHOLONE (*FML, FML Forte, Flarex*) ▶L ♀C ▶? $$
ADULT — 1 to 2 gtts q 1 to 2 h or ½ inch ribbon of ointment q 4 h for 1 to 2 days, then 1 to 2 gtts two to four times per day or ½ inch of ointment one to three times per day.
PEDS — Not approved age younger than 2 yo. Use adult dose for age 2 yo or older.
FORMS — Trade only: Susp 0.1% (5, 10, 15 mL), 0.25% (2, 5, 10, 15 mL), Ointment 0.1% (3.5 g tube).
NOTES — Fluorometholone acetate (Flarex) is more potent than fluorometholone (FML, FML Forte). Use caution in glaucoma.
MOA — Anti-inflammatory.
ADVERSE EFFECTS — Frequent: Burning, blurred vision. Severe: Cataracts, secondary ocular infections, glaucoma.
LOTEPREDNOL (*Alrex, Lotemax*) ▶L ♀C ▶? $$$
ADULT — 1 to 2 gtts four times per day, may increase to 1 gtt q 1 h during first weeks of therapy prn. Postop inflammation: 1 to 2 gtts four times per day or 1/2 inch four times daily beginning 24 h after surgery.
PEDS — Not approved in children.
FORMS — Trade only: Susp 0.2% (Alrex 5, 10 mL), 0.5% (Lotemax 2.5, 5, 10, 15 mL). Oint 0.5% 3.5 g, Gel drop 0.5% (Lotemax 10 mL).
MOA — Anti-inflammatory.

LOTEPREDNOL (*cont.*)

ADVERSE EFFECTS — Frequent: Headache, rhinitis, pharyngitis, blurring of vision, chemosis, dry eyes, pruritus. Severe: Cataracts, secondary ocular infections, glaucoma.

PREDNISOLONE—OPHTHALMIC (*Pred Forte, Pred Mild, Inflamase Forte, Econopred Plus, ★AK Tate, Diopred*) ▶L ♀C ▶? $$

ADULT — Soln: 1 to 2 gtts (up to q 1 h during day and q 2 h at night), when response observed, then 1 gtt q 4 h, then 1 gtt three to four times per day. Susp: 1 to 2 gtts two to four times per day.

PEDS — Not approved in children.

FORMS — Generic/Trade: Soln, Susp 1% (5, 10, 15 mL). Trade only (Pred Mild): Susp 0.12% (5, 10 mL), Susp (Pred Forte) 1% (1 mL).

NOTES — Prednisolone acetate (Pred Mild, Pred Forte) is more potent than prednisolone sodium phosphate (AK-Pred, Inflamase Forte).

MOA — Anti-inflammatory.

ADVERSE EFFECTS — Frequent: Insomnia, nervousness, indigestion, increased appetite, hirsutism, diabetes mellitus. Severe: Cataracts, secondary ocular infections, glaucoma.

RIMEXOLONE (*Vexol*) ▶L ♀C ▶? $$

ADULT — Postop inflammation: 1 to 2 gtts four times per day for 2 weeks. Uveitis: 1 to 2 gtts q 1 h while awake for 1 week, then 1 gtt q 2 h while awake for 1 week, then taper.

PEDS — Not approved in children.

FORMS — Trade only: Susp 1% (5, 10 mL).

NOTES — Prolonged use associated with corneal/scleral perforation and cataracts.

MOA — Anti-inflammatory.

ADVERSE EFFECTS — Frequent: Blurred vision. Severe: Cataracts, secondary ocular infections, glaucoma.

TRIAMCINOLONE—VITREOUS (*Triesence*) ▶L ♀D ▶? ?

ADULT — Administered intravitreally.

PEDS — Not approved in children.

NOTES — Do not use in patients with systemic fungal infections.

MOA — Anti-inflammatory

ADVERSE EFFECTS — Severe: cataracts, secondary ocular infections, glaucoma

OPHTHALMOLOGY: Glaucoma Agents—Beta-Blockers

NOTE: May be absorbed and cause side effects and drug interactions associated with systemic beta-blocker therapy. Use caution in cardiac conditions and asthma. Advise patients to apply gentle pressure over nasolacrimal duct for 5 min after instillation to minimize systemic absorption. On average, each mL of eye drop soln contains approximately 20 gtts. Reserve ointment formulations for bedtime use due to severe vision blurring. Most eye medications can be administered 1 gtt at a time despite common manufacturer recommendations of 1 to 2 gtts concurrently. Even a single gtt is typically more than the eye can hold and thus a second gtt is both wasteful and increases the possibility of systemic toxicity. If 2 gtts of the medication are desired separate single gtts by at least 5 min.

BETAXOLOL—OPHTHALMIC (*Betoptic, Betoptic S*) ▶LK ♀C ▶? $$

ADULT — Chronic open angle glaucoma or ocular HTN: 1 to 2 gtts two times per day.

PEDS — Chronic open angle glaucoma or ocular HTN: 1 to 2 gtts two times per day.

FORMS — Trade only: Susp 0.25% (10, 15 mL). Generic only: Soln 0.5% (5, 10, 15 mL).

NOTES — Selective beta-1-blocking agent. Shake susp before use.

MOA — Inhibits beta-1 receptors to decrease aqueous fluid production.

ADVERSE EFFECTS — Frequent: Dizziness, erythema, conjunctival hyperemia, anisocoria, keratitis, corneal staining, eye pain, vision disturbances.

CARTEOLOL—OPHTHALMIC (*Ocupress*) ▶KL ♀C ▶? $

ADULT — Chronic open angle glaucoma or ocular HTN: 1 gtt two times per day.

PEDS — Not approved in children.

FORMS — Generic only: Soln 1% (5, 10, 15 mL).

NOTES — Non-selective beta-blocker but has intrinsic sympathomimetic activity.

MOA — Inhibits beta receptors to decrease aqueous fluid production.

ADVERSE EFFECTS — Frequent: Conjunctival hyperemia.

LEVOBUNOLOL (*Betagan*) ▶? ♀C ▶– $$

ADULT — Chronic open angle glaucoma or ocular HTN: 1 to 2 gtts (0.5%) one to two times per day or 1 to 2 gtts (0.25%) two times per day.

PEDS — Not approved in children.

FORMS — Generic/Trade: Soln 0.25% (5, 10 mL), 0.5% (5, 10, 15 mL).

NOTES — Non-selective beta-blocker.

MOA — Inhibits beta receptors to decrease aqueous fluid production.

ADVERSE EFFECTS — Frequent: Stinging, burning eyes.

METIPRANOLOL (*Optipranolol*) ▶? ♀C ▶? $

ADULT — Chronic open angle glaucoma or ocular HTN: 1 gtt two times per day.

PEDS — Not approved in children.

FORMS — Generic/Trade: Soln 0.3% (5, 10 mL).

NOTES — Non-selective beta-blocker.

MOA — Nonselectively inhibits beta receptors to decrease aqueous fluid production.

ADVERSE EFFECTS — Frequent: Transient, local discomfort.

TIMOLOL—OPHTHALMIC (*Betimol, Timoptic, Timoptic XE, Istalol, Timoptic Ocudose*) ▶LK ♀C ▶+ $$

ADULT — Chronic open angle glaucoma or ocular HTN: 1 gtt (0.25 or 0.5%) two times per day or 1 gtt

TIMOLOL—OPHTHALMIC *(cont.)*
of gel-forming soln (0.25 or 0.5% Timoptic XE) daily or 1 gtt (0.5% Istalol soln) daily.
PEDS — Chronic open angle glaucoma or ocular HTN: 1 gtt (0.25 or 0.5%) of gel-forming soln daily.
FORMS — Generic/Trade: Soln 0.25, 0.5% (5, 10, 15 mL), Preservative-free soln (Timoptic Ocudose) 0.25% (0.2 mL), Gel-forming soln (Timoptic XE) 0.25, 0.5% (5 mL).
NOTES — Administer other eye meds at least 10 min before Timoptic XE. Greatest effect if Timoptic XE is administered in the morning. Non-selective beta-blocker.
MOA — Inhibits beta receptors to decrease aqueous fluid production.
ADVERSE EFFECTS — Frequent: Conjunctival hyperemia.

OPHTHALMOLOGY: Glaucoma Agents—Carbonic Anhydrase Inhibitors

NOTE: Sulfonamide derivatives; verify absence of sulfa allergy before prescribing. On average, each mL of eye drop soln contains approximately 20 gtts. Reserve ointment formulations for bedtime use due to severe vision blurring. Most eye medications can be administered 1 gtt at a time despite common manufacturer recommendations of 1 to 2 gtts concurrently. Even a single gtt is typically more than the eye can hold and thus a second gtt is both wasteful and increases the possibility of systemic toxicity. If 2 gtts of the medication is desired separate single gtts by at least 5 min.

BRINZOLAMIDE *(Azopt)* ▶LK ♀C ▶? $$$
ADULT — Chronic open angle glaucoma or ocular HTN: 1 gtt three times per day.
PEDS — Not approved in children.
FORMS — Trade only: Susp 1% (10, 15 mL).
NOTES — Do not administer while wearing soft contact lenses. Wait 10 min after use before inserting contact lenses.
MOA — Inhibition of carbonic anhydrase to decrease aqueous fluid production.
ADVERSE EFFECTS — Frequent: Dermatitis, taste disturbances, transient blurred vision.

DORZOLAMIDE *(Trusopt)* ▶KL ♀C ▶– $$$
ADULT — Chronic open angle glaucoma or ocular HTN: 1 gtt three times per day.
PEDS — Chronic open angle glaucoma or ocular HTN: 1 gtt three times per day.
FORMS — Generic/Trade: Soln 2% (10 mL).
NOTES — Do not administer while wearing soft contact lenses. Keep bottle tightly capped to avoid crystal formation. Wait 10 min after use before inserting contact lenses.

MOA — Inhibition of carbonic anhydrase to decrease aqueous fluid production.
ADVERSE EFFECTS — Frequent: Bitter taste, ocular burning and stinging. Severe: Corneal edema in patients with low endothelial cell counts, Stevens-Johnson syndrome, and toxic epidermal necrolysis.

METHAZOLAMIDE ▶LK ♀C ▶? $$
ADULT — Glaucoma: 100 to 200 mg PO initially, then 100 mg PO q 12 h until desired response. Maintenance dose: 25 to 50 mg PO (up to three times per day).
PEDS — Not approved in children.
FORMS — Generic only: Tabs 25, 50 mg.
NOTES — Mostly metabolized in the liver thus less chance of renal calculi than with acetazolamide.
MOA — Inhibition of carbonic anhydrase to decrease aqueous fluid production.
ADVERSE EFFECTS — Frequent: Malaise, anorexia, diarrhea, metallic taste, polyuria, muscular weakness.

OPHTHALMOLOGY: Glaucoma Agents—Combinations and Other

NOTE: On average, each mL of eye drop soln contains approximately 20 gtts. Reserve ointment formulations for bedtime use due to severe vision blurring. Most eye medications can be administered 1 gtt at a time despite common manufacturer recommendations of 1 to 2 gtts concurrently. Even a single gtt is typically more than the eye can hold and thus a second gtt is both wasteful and increases the possibility of systemic toxicity. If 2 gtts of the medication are desired separate single gtts by at least 5 min.

COMBIGAN (brimonidine + timolol—ophthalmic) ▶LK ♀C ▶– $$$
ADULT — Chronic open angle glaucoma or ocular HTN: 1 gtt twice a day.
PEDS — Contraindicated in age younger than 2 yo. Use adult dosing in 2 yo or older.
FORMS — Trade only: Soln brimonidine 0.2% + timolol 0.5% (5, 10 mL).
NOTES — Do not administer while wearing soft contact lenses. Wait 10 min after use before inserting contact lenses. Contraindicated with MAOIs. See beta-blocker warnings.

MOA — Stimulation of alpha-2 receptors and inhibition of beta-1 receptors to decrease aqueous fluid production.
ADVERSE EFFECTS — Ocular: Frequent: Headache, drowsiness, fatigue, xerostomia, hyperemia, burning, stinging, blurring, foreign body sensation, hypersensitivity.

COSOPT (dorzolamide + timolol—ophthalmic) ▶LK ♀D ▶– $$$
ADULT — Chronic open angle glaucoma or ocular HTN: 1 gtt two times per day.

COSOPT (cont.)

PEDS — Not approved in children younger than 2 yo. Children older than 2 yo, use adult dose.

FORMS — Generic/Trade: Soln dorzolamide 2% + timolol 0.5% (5, 10 mL). Trade only: Soln preservative free dorzolamide 2% + timolol 0.5% (30 single use containers).

NOTES — Do not administer while wearing soft contact lenses. Wait 10 min after use before inserting contact lenses. Not recommended if severe renal or hepatic dysfunction. Use caution in sulfa allergy. See beta-blocker warnings.

MOA — Inhibition of carbonic anhydrase and beta-1 receptors to decrease aqueous fluid production.

ADVERSE EFFECTS — Ocular: Frequent: Bitter taste, burning, stinging in eyes, allergic reaction, conjunctivitis, lid reactions. Severe: Corneal edema in patients with low endothelial cell counts, Stevens-Johnson syndrome, and toxic epidermal necrolysis.

SIMBRINZA (brinzolamide + brimonidine) ▶LK - ♀C ▶? $$$$

ADULT — Open-angle glaucoma, ocular hypertension: 1 gtt in each affected eye three times per day.

PEDS — Contraindicated in younger than 2 yo.

FORMS — Trade: brinzolamide 1% and brimonidine 0.2% 8 mL.

MOA — See components.

ADVERSE EFFECTS — See components.

UNOPROSTONE (*Rescula*) ▶esterases ♀C ▶? $$$

ADULT — Glaucoma: 1 gtt in each affected eye two times a day.

PEDS — Not approved in children.

FORMS — Trade: 0.15% (5 mL).

MOA — unknown

ADVERSE EFFECTS — Frequent: hyperpigmentation of iris, burning, stinging, dry eyes, itching, increased length of eyelashes

OPHTHALMOLOGY: Glaucoma Agents—Miotics

NOTE: Observe for cholinergic systemic effects (eg, salivation, lacrimation, urination, diarrhea, GI upset, excessive sweating). On average, each mL of eye drop soln contains approximately 20 gtts. Reserve ointment formulations for bedtime use due to severe vision blurring. Most eye medications can be administered 1 gtt at a time despite common manufacturer recommendations of 1 to 2 gtts concurrently. Even a single gtt is typically more than the eye can hold and thus a second gtt is both wasteful and increases the possibility of systemic toxicity. If 2 gtts of the medication are desired separate single gtts by at least 5 min.

ACETYLCHOLINE (*Miochol-E*) ▶Acetylcholinesterases ♀? ▶? $$

ADULT — Intraoperative miosis or pressure lowering: 0.5 mL to 2 mL injected intraocularly.

PEDS — Not approved in children.

MOA — Stimulates cholinergic receptors to increase aqueous fluid outflow.

ADVERSE EFFECTS — Frequent: Blurred vision, miosis, headache.

CARBACHOL (*Isopto Carbachol, Miostat*) ▶? ♀C ▶? $$

ADULT — Glaucoma: 1 gtt three times per day. Intraoperative miosis or pressure lowering: 0.5 mL injected intraocularly.

PEDS — Not approved in children.

FORMS — Trade only: Soln (Isopto Carbachol) 1.5, 3% (15 mL). Intraocular soln (Miostat) 0.01%.

MOA — Inhibits acetylcholinesterase resulting in cholineric stimulation to increase aqueous fluid outflow.

ADVERSE EFFECTS — Frequent: Blurred vision, miosis, headache.

ECHOTHIOPHATE IODIDE (*Phospholine Iodide*) ▶? ♀C ▶? $$$

ADULT — Glaucoma: 1 gtt two times per day.

PEDS — Accommodative esotropia: 1 gtt daily (0.06%) or 1 gtt every other day (0.125%).

FORMS — Trade only: Soln 0.125% (5 mL).

NOTES — Use lowest effective dose strength. Use extreme caution if asthma, spastic GI diseases, GI ulcers, bradycardia, hypotension, recent MI, epilepsy, Parkinson's disease, history of retinal detachment. Stop 3 weeks before general anesthesia as may cause prolonged succinylcholine paralysis. Discontinue if cardiac effects noted.

MOA — Inhibits acetylcholinesterase resulting in cholineric stimulation to increase aqueous fluid outflow.

ADVERSE EFFECTS — Frequent: Blurred vision, miosis, headache. Infrequent: Iris cysts, cataracts, ocular surface scarring.

PILOCARPINE—OPHTHALMIC (*Isopto Carpine, ❋Diocarpine, Akarpine*) ▶plasma ♀C ▶? $

ADULT — Reduction of IOP with open-angle glaucoma, acute angle-closure glaucoma, prevention of postoperative elevated IOP associated with laser surgery, induction of miosis: 1 gtt up to four times per day.

PEDS — Glaucoma: 1 gtt up to four times per day.

FORMS — Generic/Trade: Soln 0.5% (15 mL), 1% (2 mL, 15 mL), 2% (2 mL, 15 mL), 4% (2 mL, 15 mL), 6% (15 mL).

NOTES — Do not administer while wearing soft contact lenses. Wait at least 15 min after use before inserting contact lenses. Causes miosis. May cause blurred vision and difficulty with night vision.

MOA — Stimulates cholinergic receptors to increase aqueous fluid outflow.

ADVERSE EFFECTS — Ocular: Frequent: Blurred vision, miosis.

OPHTHALMOLOGY: Glaucoma Agents—Prostaglandin Analogs

NOTE: Do not administer while wearing soft contact lenses. Wait 10 min after use before inserting contact lenses. May aggravate intraocular inflammation. On average, each mL of eye drop soln contains approximately 20 gtts. Reserve ointment formulations for bedtime use due to severe vision blurring. Most eye medications can be administered 1 gtt at a time despite common manufacturer recommendations of 1 to 2 gtts concurrently. Even a single gtt is typically more than the eye can hold and thus a second gtt is both wasteful and increases the possibility of systemic toxicity. If 2 gtts of the medication are desired separate single gtts by at least 5 min.

BIMATOPROST (*Lumigan, Latisse*) ▶LK ♀C ▶? $$$
ADULT — Chronic open angle glaucoma or ocular HTN: 1 gtt to affected eyes at bedtime. Hypotrichosis of the eyelashes (Latisse): Apply at bedtime to the skin of the upper eyelid margin at the base of the eyelashes.
PEDS — Not approved in children.
FORMS — Trade only: Soln 0.01%, 0.03% (Lumigan, 2.5, 5, 7.5 mL), (Latisse, 3 mL with 60 sterile, disposable applicators).
NOTES — Concurrent administration of bimatoprost for hypotrichosis and IOP-lowering prostaglandin analogs in ocular hypertensive patients may decrease the IOP-lowering effect. Monitor closely for changes in intraocular pressure.
MOA — Prostaglandin F-2 analog increases aqueous fluid outflow.
ADVERSE EFFECTS — Ocular: Frequent: Blurred vision, burning, stinging, ocular hyperemia, increased pigmentation of iris and eyelid skin, growth of eyelashes, ocular pruritus.

LATANOPROST (*Xalatan*) ▶LK ♀C ▶? $
ADULT — Chronic open angle glaucoma or ocular HTN: 1 gtt at bedtime.
PEDS — Not approved in children.
FORMS — Generic/Trade: Soln 0.005% (2.5 mL).
MOA — Prostaglandin F-2 analog increases aqueous fluid outflow.
ADVERSE EFFECTS — Ocular: Frequent: Blurred vision, burning, stinging, ocular hyperemia, increased pigmentation of iris and eyelid skin, growth of eyelashes, ocular pruritus, headache, dizziness.

TAFLUPROST (*Zioptan*) ▶L ♀C ▶? $$$
ADULT — Chronic open angle glaucome or ocular HTN: 1 gtt in each affect eye q pm.
PEDS — Not approved in children.
FORMS — Trade: Soln 0.0015%
NOTES — Can cause pigmentation of iris, periorbital tissue and eyelashes.
MOA — Prostaglandin analog.
ADVERSE EFFECTS — Frequent: conjunctival hyperemia. Severe: uveitis and iritis

TRAVOPROST (*Travatan Z*) ▶L ♀C ▶? $$$$
ADULT — Chronic open angle glaucoma or ocular HTN: 1 gtt at bedtime.
PEDS — Not approved in children.
FORMS — Trade only: benzalkonium chloride-free (Travatan Z) 0.004% (2.5, 5 mL). Generic only: travoprost 0.004% (2.5 mL, 5 mL)
NOTES — Wait 10 min after use before inserting contact lenses. Avoid if prior or current intraocular inflammation.
MOA — Prostaglandin F-2 analog increases aqueous fluid outflow.
ADVERSE EFFECTS — Ocular: Frequent: Conjunctival hyperemia, ocular hyperemia, increased pigmentation of iris and eyelid skin, growth of eyelashes, decreased visual acuity, eye discomfort, foreign body sensation, pain, and pruritus. Severe: Contraindicated in pregnancy, pigmentation changes.

OPHTHALMOLOGY: Glaucoma Agents—Sympathomimetics

NOTE: Do not administer while wearing soft contact lenses. Wait 10 min after use before inserting contact lenses. On average, each mL of eye drop soln contains approximately 20 gtts. Reserve ointment formulations for bedtime use due to severe vision blurring. Most eye medications can be administered 1 gtt at a time despite common manufacturer recommendations of 1 to 2 gtts concurrently. Even a single gtt is typically more than the eye can hold and thus a second gtt is both wasteful and increases the possibility of systemic toxicity. If 2 gtts of the medication are desired separate single gtts by at least 5 min.

APRACLONIDINE (*Iopidine*) ▶KL ♀C ▶? $$$$
ADULT — Perioperative IOP elevation: 1 gtt (1%) 1 h prior to surgery, then 1 gtt immediately after surgery.
PEDS — Not approved in children.
FORMS — Generic/Trade: Soln 0.5% (5, 10 mL). Trade only: Soln 1% (0.1 mL).
NOTES — Rapid tachyphylaxis may occur. Do not use long term.
MOA — Alpha-2-agonist decreases aqueous fluid production.
ADVERSE EFFECTS — Frequent: Decreases night vision, distance vision alterations, lethargy, xerostomia, burning and itching eyes.

BRIMONIDINE (*Alphagan P, ✦Alphagan*) ▶L ♀B ▶? $$
ADULT — Chronic open angle glaucoma or ocular HTN: 1 gtt three times per day.
PEDS — Glaucoma: 1 gtt three times per day for age older than 2 yo.
FORMS — Trade only: Soln 0.1% (5, 10, 15 mL). Generic/Trade: Soln 0.15% (5, 10, 15 mL). Generic only: Soln 0.2% (5, 10, 15 mL).

BRIMONIDINE (cont.)

NOTES — Contraindicated in patients receiving MAOIs. Twice daily dosing may have similar efficacy.
MOA — Alpha-2-agonist decreases aqueous fluid production.
ADVERSE EFFECTS — Frequent: Headache, drowsiness, fatigue, xerostomia, hyperemia, burning, stinging, blurring, foreign body sensation.

DIPIVEFRIN (Propine) ▶Eye/plasma/L ♀B ▶? $

ADULT — Chronic open angle glaucoma or ocular HTN: 1 gtt two times per day.
PEDS — Glaucoma: 1 gtt two times per day.
FORMS — Generic/Trade: Soln 0.1% (5, 10, 15 mL).
MOA — Prodrug of epinephrine which stimulates alpha and beta adrenergic receptors to increase aqueous fluid outflow and decrease production.
ADVERSE EFFECTS — Frequent: Headache, stinging, blurred vision, ocular pain, photophobia, conjunctivitis, local dermatitis.

OPHTHALMOLOGY: Macular Degeneration

PEGAPTANIB (Macugen) ▶Minimal absorption ♀B ▶? $$$$$

ADULT — "Wet" macular degeneration: 0.3 mg intravitreal injection q 6 weeks.
PEDS — Not approved in children.
MOA — Selective antagonist of vascular endothelial growth factor.
ADVERSE EFFECTS — Ocular: Chamber inflammation, blurred vision, cataracts, corneal edema, reduced visual acuity, visual changes. Injection-related adverse events include: Endophthalmitis, retinal detachment, iatrogenic traumatic cataract, subconjunctival hemorrhage, and increased intraocular pressure. Severe: Anaphylaxis/anaphylactoid, angioedema.

RANIBIZUMAB (Lucentis) ▶Intravitreal ♀C ▶? $$$$$

ADULT — Treatment of neovascular (wet) macular degeneration: 0.5 mg intravitreal injection q 28 days. If monthly injections not feasible, can administer q 3 months or 3 monthly doses followed by less frequent dosing with regular assessment, but these regimens are less effective. Macular edema following retinal vein occlusion: 0.5 mg intravitreal injection q 28 days.

PEDS — Not approved in children.
NOTES — Increased CVA risk noted with higher doses (0.5 mg) and with prior CVA.
MOA — Binds to the receptor of VEGF-A.
ADVERSE EFFECTS — Severe: Stroke. Frequent: Eye pain, vitreous floaters, intraocular inflammation, blurred vision. Injection-related adverse events include: Endophthalmitis, retinal detachment, iatrogenic traumatic cataract, subconjunctival hemorrhage, and increased intraocular pressure.

VERTEPORFIN (Visudyne) ▶L/plasma ♀C ▶– $$$$$

ADULT — Treatment of exudative age-related macular degeneration: 6 mg/m² IV over 10 min; laser light therapy 15 min after start of infusion.
PEDS — Not approved in children.
NOTES — Severe risk of photosensitivity for 5 days; must avoid exposure to sunlight.
MOA — Laser-induced free radicals cause occlusion of abnormal vessels.
ADVERSE EFFECTS — Frequent: Injection-site irritation, blurred vision, visual field defects, decreased visual acuity (sometimes severe).

OPHTHALMOLOGY: Mydriatics & Cycloplegics

NOTE: Use caution in infants. On average, each mL of eye drop soln contains approximately 20 gtts. Reserve ointment formulations for bedtime use due to severe vision blurring. Most eye medications can be administered 1 gtt at a time despite common manufacturer recommendations of 1 to 2 gtts concurrently. Even a single gtt is typically more than the eye can hold and thus a second gtt is both wasteful and increases the possibility of systemic toxicity. If 2 gtts of the medication are desired separate single gtts by at least 5 min.

ATROPINE—OPHTHALMIC (Isopto Atropine, Atropine Care) ▶L ♀C ▶+ $

ADULT — Uveitis: 1 to 2 gtts of 0.5% or 1% soln daily to four times per day, or 1/8 to 1/4 inch ribbon (1% ointment) daily (up to three times per day). Refraction: 1 to 2 gtts of 1% soln 1 h before procedure or 1/8 to 1/4 inch ribbon one to three times per day.
PEDS — Uveitis: 1 to 2 gtts of 0.5% soln one to three times per day) or 1/8 to 1/4 inch ribbon one to three times per day. Refraction: 1 to 2 gtts (0.5%) two times per day for 1 to 3 days before procedure or 1/8 inch ribbon (1% ointment) for 1 to 3 days before procedure.
UNAPPROVED PEDS — Amblyopia: 1 gtt in good eye daily.

FORMS — Generic/Trade: Soln 1% (2, 5, 15 mL). Generic only: Ointment 1% (3.5 g tube).
NOTES — Cycloplegia may last up to 5 to 10 days and mydriasis may last up to 7 to 14 days. Each drop of a 1% soln contains 0.5 mg atropine. Treat atropine overdose with physostigmine 0.25 mg every 15 min until symptoms resolve.
MOA — Anticholinergic blockage of ciliary body and iris muscles to produce loss of accommodation and pupil dilation.
ADVERSE EFFECTS — Frequent: Dry, hot skin, impaired GI motility, dry throat, xerostomia, dry eyes, blurred vision, especially reading vision, photophobia.

CYCLOPENTOLATE (*AK-Pentolate, Cyclogyl, Pentolair*) ▶? ♀C ▶? $
ADULT — Refraction: 1 to 2 gtts (1% or 2%), repeat in 5 to 10 min prn. Give 45 min before procedure.
PEDS — May cause CNS disturbances in children. Refraction: 1 to 2 gtts (0.5%, 1%, or 2%), repeat in 5 to 10 min prn. Give 45 min before procedure.
FORMS — Generic/Trade: Soln 1% (2, 15 mL). Trade only (Cyclogyl): 0.5% (15 mL), 1% (5 mL), 2% (2, 5, 15 mL).
NOTES — Cycloplegia may last 6 to 24 h; mydriasis may last 1 day.
MOA — Anticholinergic blockage of ciliary body and iris muscles to produce loss of accommodation and pupil dilation.
ADVERSE EFFECTS — Frequent: Tachycardia, CNS effects, blurred vision, especially reading vision, increased sensitivity to light, photophobia.

HOMATROPINE—OPHTHALMIC (*Isopto Homatropine*) ▶? ♀C ▶? $
ADULT — Refraction: 1 to 2 gtts (2%) or 1 gtt (5%) in eye(s) immediately before procedure, repeat q 5 to 10 min prn. Max 3 doses. Uveitis: 1 to 2 gtts (2 to 5%) two to three times per day or as often as q 3 to 4 h.
PEDS — Refraction: 1 gtt (2%) in eye(s) immediately before procedure, repeat q 10 min prn. Uveitis: 1 gtt (2%) two to three times per day.
FORMS — Trade only: Soln 2% (5 mL), 5% (15 mL). Generic/Trade: Soln 5% (5 mL).
NOTES — Cycloplegia and mydriasis last 1 to 3 days.
MOA — Anticholinergic blockage of ciliary body and iris muscles to produce loss of accommodation and pupil dilation.
ADVERSE EFFECTS — Ocular: Frequent: Blurred vision, especially reading vision, photophobia.

PHENYLEPHRINE—OPHTHALMIC (*AK-Dilate, Altafrin, Mydfrin, Refresh*) ▶plasma L ♀C ▶? $
ADULT — Ophthalmologic exams: 1 to 2 gtts (2.5%, 10%) before procedure. Ocular surgery: 1 to 2 gtts (2.5%, 10%) before surgery. Red eyes: 1 or 2 gtts (0.12%) in affected eyes up to four times daily.
PEDS — Not routinely used in children.
UNAPPROVED PEDS — Ophthalmologic exams: 1 gtt (2.5%) before procedure. Ocular surgery: 1 gtt (2.5%) before surgery.
FORMS — Rx Generic/Trade: Soln 2.5% (2, 3, 5, 15 mL), 10% (5 mL). OTC Trade only (Altafrin and Refresh): Soln 0.12% (15 mL).
NOTES — Overuse can cause rebound dilation of blood vessels. No cycloplegia; mydriasis may last up to 5 h. Systemic absorption, especially with 10% soln, may be associated with sympathetic stimulation (eg, increased BP).
MOA — Alpha-adrenergic and (weak) beta-adrenergic agonist to stimulate iris dilator and cause mydriasis.
ADVERSE EFFECTS — Frequent: Reflex bradycardia, excitability, restlessness, photophobia.

TROPICAMIDE (*Mydriacyl, Tropicacyl*) ▶? ♀C ▶? $
ADULT — Dilated eye exam: 1 to 2 gtts (0.5%) in eye(s) 15 to 20 min before exam, repeat q 30 min prn.
PEDS — Not approved in children.
FORMS — Generic/Trade: Soln 0.5% (15 mL), 1% (3, 15 mL). Generic only: Soln 1% (2 mL).
NOTES — Mydriasis may last 6 h and has weak cycloplegic effects.
MOA — Anticholinergic blockage of iris sphincter muscle to produce pupil dilation.
ADVERSE EFFECTS — Frequent: Tachycardia, CNS effects, blurred vision, photophobia, possible increased intraocular pressure.

OPHTHALMOLOGY: Non-Steroidal Anti-Inflammatories

NOTE: On average, each mL of eye drop soln contains approximately 20 gtts. Reserve ointment formulations for bedtime use due to severe vision blurring. Most eye medications can be administered 1 gtt at a time despite common manufacturer recommendations of 1 to 2 gtts concurrently. Even a single gtt is typically more than the eye can hold and thus a second gtt is both wasteful and increases the possibility of systemic toxicity. If 2 gtts of the medication are desired separate single gtts by at least 5 min.

BROMFENAC—OPHTHALMIC (*Bromday, Prolensa*) ▶minimal absorption ♀C, D (3rd trimester) ▶? $$$$$
ADULT — Postop inflammation and pain following cataract surgery: 1 gtt in each affected eye once daily beginning 1 day prior to surgery and continuing for 14 days after surgery (Bromday, Prolensa) or twice daily (generic).
PEDS — Not approved in children.
FORMS — Trade only: Soln 0.09% (Bromday) 1.7 mL, 3.4 mL(two x 1.7ml twin pack), Soln 0.07% (Prolensa) 1.6 mL, 3 mL. Generic Only: Soln 0.09% (twice-daily soln 2.5 mL, 5 mL)
NOTES — Not for use with soft contact lenses. Contains sodium sulfite and may cause allergic reactions.

MOA — Blocks prostaglandin synthesis by inhibiting cyclooxygenase.
ADVERSE EFFECTS — Frequent: Abnormal eye sensation, conjunctival hyperemia, eye irritation, pain, pruritus, redness, headache, iritis. Severe: Keratitis, corneal thinning, erosion, ulceration, perforation.

DICLOFENAC—OPHTHALMIC (*Voltaren, ✦Voltaren Ophtha*) ▶L ♀C ▶? $$$
ADULT — Postop inflammation following cataract surgery: 1 gtt four times per day for 1 to 2 weeks. Ocular photophobia and pain associated with corneal refractive surgery: 1 to 2 gtt to operative eye(s) 1 h prior to surgery and 1 to 2 gtt within 15 min after surgery, then 1 gtt four times per day prn for no more than 3 days.

DICLOFENAC—OPHTHALMIC (cont.)

PEDS — Not approved in children.

FORMS — Generic/Trade: Soln 0.1% (2.5, 5 mL).

NOTES — Contraindicated for use with soft contact lenses.

MOA — Blocks prostaglandin synthesis by inhibiting cyclooxygenase.

ADVERSE EFFECTS — Frequent: Lacrimation, keratitis, eye pain, increased intraocular pressure, burning, stinging. Severe: Keratitis, corneal thinning, erosion, ulceration, perforation.

FLURBIPROFEN—OPHTHALMIC (Ocufen) ▶L ♀C ▶? $

ADULT — Inhibition of intraoperative miosis: 1 gtt q 30 min beginning 2 h prior to surgery (total of 4 gtts).

PEDS — Not approved in children.

UNAPPROVED ADULT — Treatment of cystoid macular edema, inflammation after glaucoma or cataract laser surgery, uveitis syndromes.

FORMS — Generic/Trade: Soln 0.03% (2.5 mL).

MOA — Blocks prostaglandin synthesis by inhibiting cyclooxygenase.

ADVERSE EFFECTS — Frequent: Transient stinging/burning. Severe: Keratitis, corneal thinning, erosion, ulceration, perforation.

KETOROLAC—OPHTHALMIC (Acular, Acular LS, Acuvail) ▶L ♀C ▶? $$$$

ADULT — Allergic conjunctivitis: 1 gtt (0.5%) four times per day (Acular). Postop inflammation following cataract surgery: 1 gtt (0.5%) four times per day beginning 24 h after surgery for 1 to 2 weeks (Acular). 1 gtt in each affected eye twice daily (Aculvail). Postop corneal refractive surgery:1 gtt (0.4%) prn for up to 4 days (Acular LS).

PEDS — Not approved age younger than 3 yo. Use adult dose for age 3 yo or older.

FORMS — Generic/Trade: Soln (Acular LS) 0.4% (5 mL). Trade only: Acular 0.5% (3, 5, 10 mL), preservative-free Acuvail 0.45% unit dose (0.4 mL).

NOTES — Do not administer while wearing soft contact lenses. Wait 10 min after use before inserting contact lenses. Avoid use in late pregnancy.

MOA — Blocks prostaglandin synthesis by inhibiting cyclooxygenase.

ADVERSE EFFECTS — Frequent: Transient stinging/burning. Severe: Keratitis, corneal thinning, erosion, ulceration, perforation.

NEPAFENAC (Nevanac, Ilevro) ▶minimal absorption ♀C, D in third trimester ▶? $$$$

ADULT — Postop inflammation following cataract surgery: 1 gtt three times per day beginning 24 h before cataract surgery and continued for 2 weeks after surgery.

PEDS — Not approved in children.

FORMS — Trade only: Susp 0.1% (Nevanac-3 mL). Susp 0.3% (Ilevro-1.7 mL)

NOTES — Not for use with contact lenses. Caution if previous allergy to aspirin or other NSAIDs.

MOA — A prodrug that is converted by ocular tissues to amfenac, which blocks prostaglandin synthesis by inhibiting cyclooxygenase.

ADVERSE EFFECTS — Frequent: Abnormal eye sensation, conjunctival hyperemia, eye irritation, pain, photophobia, dry eye, pruritus, redness, headache, iritis. Severe: Increased bleeding time, keratitis, corneal thinning, erosion, ulceration, perforation.

OPHTHALMOLOGY: Other Ophthalmologic Agents

AFLIBERCEPT (Eylea) ▶minimal absorption - ♀C ▶– $$$$$

ADULT — Wet macular degeneration, macular edema after central retinal vein occlusion: 2 mg (0.05 mL) intravitreal injection q 4 weeks x 3 mo, then 2 mg (0.05 mL) intravitreal injection q 8 weeks.

PEDS — Not approved for us in children.

FORMS — Sterile powder for reconstitution.

NOTES — Endophthalmitis and retinal detachments may occur. Can increases intraocular pressure. Potential risk of arterial thromboembolic events following intravitreal use.

MOA — Inhibits binding and activation of vascular endothelial growth factor-A (VEGF-A) and placental growth factor (PIGF) receptors

ADVERSE EFFECTS — Frequent: conjunctival hemorrhage, eye pain, cataract, vitreous detachment, vitreous floaters, and increased intraocular pressure. Severe: Endophthalmitis, retinal detachments, arterial thromboembolic events.

ARTIFICIAL TEARS (Tears Naturale, Hypotears, Refresh Tears, GenTeal, Systane) ▶Minimal absorption ♀A ▶+ $

ADULT — Ophthalmic lubricant: 1 to 2 gtts prn.

PEDS — Ophthalmic lubricant: 1 to 2 gtts prn.

FORMS — OTC Generic/Trade: Soln (15, 30 mL, among others).

MOA — Lubricant.

ADVERSE EFFECTS — Frequent: Mild stinging, temporary blurred vision.

CYCLOSPORINE—OPHTHALMIC (Restasis) ▶Minimal absorption ♀C ▶? $$$$

ADULT — Keratoconjunctivitis sicca (chronic dry eye disease): 1 gtt in each eye q 12 h.

PEDS — Not approved in children.

FORMS — Trade only: Emulsion 0.05% (0.4 mL single-use vials).

NOTES — Wait 10 min after use before inserting contact lenses. May take 1 month to note clinical improvement.

MOA — Immunomodulator and anti-inflammatory.

ADVERSE EFFECTS — Frequent: Ocular burning.

CYSTEAMINE (Cystaran) ▶minimal absorption – ♀C ▶? $$$$$

ADULT — Corneal cysteine crystal accumulation: 1 gtt in each eye q waking h.

PEDS — Not approved in children.

FORMS — Trade: 0.44% soln, 15mL.

CYSTEAMINE (*cont.*)

NOTES — Insert contact lenses 15 min after administration.

MOA — converts cystine to cysteine and cysteine-cysteamine mixed disulfides thereby reducing corneal cystine crystal accumulation

ADVERSE EFFECTS — Frequent" sensitivity to light, erythema/itching/irritation of eyes, headache, visual field defects.

FLUORESCEIN (*Fluor-I-Strip, Fluor-I-Strip AT, Ful-Glo*) ▶Minimal absorption ♀? ▶? $

ADULT — Following ocular anesthetic: Apply enough stain to bulbar conjunctiva to assess integrity of cornea.

PEDS — Following ocular anesthetic: Apply enough stain to bulbar conjunctiva to assess integrity of cornea.

FORMS — Trade only (Fluor-I-Strip AT): Fluorescein 1 mg in sterile ophthalmic strip. (Fluor-I-Strip): Fluorescein 9 mg in sterile ophthalmic strip.

NOTES — Do not use with soft contact lenses

MOA — Dye

ADVERSE EFFECTS — Frequent: local irritation.

HYDROXYPROPYL CELLULOSE (*Lacrisert*) ▶minimal absorption ♀+ ▶+ $$$

ADULT — Moderate to severe dry eyes: 1 insert in each eye daily. Some patients may require twice daily use.

PEDS — Not approved in children.

FORMS — Trade only: Ocular insert 5 mg.

NOTES — Do not use with soft contact lenses.

MOA — Lubricant.

ADVERSE EFFECTS — Frequent: Blurred vision, ocular discomfort, matting of eyelashes.

LIDOCAINE—OPHTHALMIC ▶L ♀B ▶? $

ADULT — Do not prescribe for unsupervised use. Corneal toxicity may occur with repeated use. Local anesthetic: 2 gtts before procedure, repeat prn.

PEDS — Not approved in children.

FORMS — Generic only: Gel 3.5% (5 mL).

MOA — Ester-type local anesthetic that prevents nerve impulse initiation and potentiation through blockage of sodium ion channels.

ADVERSE EFFECTS — Ocular: Frequent: Hyperemia, corneal epithelial changes, headache, and burning.

OCRIPLASMIN (*Jetrea*) ▶minimal absorption – ♀C ▶? $$$$$

ADULT — Symptomatic vitreomacular adhesion: 0.125 mg (0.1 mL) intravitreal injection as a single dose.

PEDS — Not approved in children.

FORMS — Sterile solution of 0.5mg in 0.2ml. Dilution required with 0.2ml of normal saline (0.5mg/0.4ml). Final concentration 0.125mg/0.1ml

MOA — Proteolytic enzyme

ADVERSE EFFECTS — Severe: decreased vision, intravitreal injection procedure effects, lens sublxation, retinal breaks

PETROLATUM (*Lacri-lube, Dry Eyes, Refresh PM, ✦Duolube*) ▶minimal absorption ♀A ▶+ $

ADULT — Ophthalmic lubricant: Apply ¼ to ½ inch ointment to inside of lower lid prn.

PEDS — Ophthalmic lubricant: Apply ¼ to ½ inch ointment to inside of lower lid prn.

FORMS — OTC Trade only: Ointment (3.5, 7 g) tube.

MOA — Lubricates dry eyes.

ADVERSE EFFECTS — Frequent: Blurred vision.

PROPARACAINE (*Ophthaine, Ophthetic, ✦Alcaine*) ▶L ♀C ▶? $

ADULT — Do not prescribe for unsupervised use. Corneal toxicity may occur with repeated use. Local anesthetic: 1 to 2 gtts before procedure. Repeat q 5 to 10 min for 1 to 3 doses (suture or foreign body removal) or for 5 to 7 doses (ocular surgery).

PEDS — Not approved in children.

FORMS — Generic/Trade: Soln 0.5% (15 mL).

MOA — Amide-type local anesthetic that prevents nerve impulse initiation and potentiation through blockage of sodium ion channels.

ADVERSE EFFECTS — Ocular: Frequent: Burning, stinging.

TETRACAINE—OPHTHALMIC (*Pontocaine*) ▶plasma ♀C ▶? $

ADULT — Do not prescribe for unsupervised use. Corneal toxicity may occur with repeated use. Local anesthetic: 1 to 2 gtts before procedure.

PEDS — Not approved in children.

FORMS — Generic only: Soln 0.5% (15 mL), unit-dose vials (0.7, 2 mL).

MOA — Ester-type local anesthetic that prevents nerve impulse initiation and potentiation through blockage of sodium ion channels.

ADVERSE EFFECTS — Ocular: Frequent: Burning, stinging, angioedema, contact dermatitis, chemosis, lacrimation, photophobia, transient stinging.

TRYPAN BLUE (*Vision Blue, Membrane Blue*) ▶Not absorbed ♀C ▶? $$

ADULT — Aid during ophthalmic surgery by staining anterior cap: Inject into anterior chamber of eye.

PEDS — Not approved in children.

FORMS — Trade only: 0.06% (Vision Blue) Ophthalmic soln (0.5 mL), 0.15% (Membrane Blue) Ophthalmic soln (0.5 mL).

MOA — Acid di-azo group dye.

ADVERSE EFFECTS — Inadvertent staining of posterior lens capsule and vitreous face.

PSYCHIATRY

BODY MASS INDEX

BMI	Class	4' 10"	5' 0"	5' 4"	5' 8"	6' 0"	6' 4"
< 19	Underweight	< 91	< 97	< 110	< 125	< 140	< 156
19–24	Healthy weight	91–119	97–127	110–144	125–163	140–183	156–204
25–29	Overweight	120–143	128–152	145–173	164–196	184–220	205–245
30–40	Obese	144–191	153–204	174–233	197–262	221–293	246–328
> 40	Very Obese	> 191	> 204	174–233	> 262	> 293	> 328

*BMI = kg/m^2 = (wt in pounds)(703)/(height in inches)^2. Anorectants appropriate if BMI ≥30 (with comoribidities ≥27); surgery an option if BMI > 40 (with comorbidities 35–40). www.nhlbi.nih.gov

PSYCHIATRY: Antidepressants—Heterocyclic Compounds

NOTE: Gradually taper when discontinuing cyclic antidepressants to avoid withdrawal symptoms. Seizures, orthostatic hypotension, arrhythmias, and anticholinergic side effects may occur. Don't use with MAOIs. Avoid use during treatment with linezolid or IV methylene blue. Antidepressants increase the risk of suicidal thinking and behavior in children, adolescents, and young adults; carefully weigh the risks and benefits before starting and monitor patients closely.

AMITRIPTYLINE ▶L ♀D ▶– $$

ADULT — Depression: Start 25 to 100 mg PO at bedtime; gradually increase to usual effective dose of 50 to 300 mg/day.

PEDS — Depression, adolescents: Use adult dosing. Not approved in children younger than 12 yo.

UNAPPROVED ADULT — Migraine prophylaxis and/or chronic pain: 10 to 100 mg/day. Fibromyalgia: 25 to 50 mg/day.

UNAPPROVED PEDS — Depression, age younger than 12 yo: Start 1 mg/kg/day PO divided three times per day for 3 days, then increase to 1.5 mg/kg/day. Max 5 mg/kg/day.

FORMS — Generic: Tabs 10, 25, 50, 75, 100, 150 mg. Elavil brand name no longer available; has been retained in this entry for name recognition purposes only.

NOTES — Tricyclic, tertiary amine; primarily inhibits serotonin reuptake. Demethylated to nortriptyline, which primarily inhibits norepinephrine reuptake. Usual therapeutic range is 150 to 300 ng/mL (amitriptyline + nortriptyline).

MOA — Serotonin/norepinephrine reuptake inhibitor.

ADVERSE EFFECTS — Serious: Atrial/ventricular arrhythmias, seizures, MI, CHF, stroke. Frequent: Drowsiness, dry mouth, constipation, nausea, orthostatic hypotension, dizziness, confusion, urinary retention, sexual dysfunction.

AMOXAPINE ▶L ♀C ▶– $$$

ADULT — Rarely used; other drugs preferred. Depression: Start 25 to 50 mg PO two to three times per day; increase by 50 to 100 mg two to three times per day after 1 week. Usual effective dose is 150 to 400 mg/day. Max 600 mg/day.

PEDS — Not approved in children younger than 16 yo.

FORMS — Generic only: Tabs 25, 50, 100, 150 mg.

NOTES — Tetracyclic; primarily inhibits norepinephrine reuptake. Dose 300 mg/day or less may be given once daily at bed time.

MOA — Norepinephrine/serotonin reuptake inhibitor. Active metabolite is a partial dopamine receptor antagonist.

ADVERSE EFFECTS — Serious: Atrial/ventricular arrhythmias, seizures, MI, CHF, stroke, neuroleptic malignant syndrome, tardive dyskinesia. Frequent: Drowsiness, dry mouth, constipation, nausea, orthostatic hypotension, dizziness, confusion, urinary retention, sexual dysfunction, extrapyramidal side effects.

CLOMIPRAMINE (*Anafranil***)** ▶L ♀C ▶+ $$$

ADULT — OCD: Start 25 mg PO at bedtime; gradually increase over 2 weeks to usual effective dose of 150 to 250 mg/day. Max 250 mg/day.

PEDS — OCD, age 10 yo or older: Start 25 mg PO at bedtime, then increase gradually over 2 weeks to 3 mg/kg/day or 100 mg/day, max 200 mg/day. Not approved for age younger than 10 yo.

UNAPPROVED ADULT — Depression: 100 to 250 mg/day. Panic disorder: 12.5 to 150 mg/day. Chronic pain: 100 to 250 mg/day.

FORMS — Generic/Trade: Caps 25, 50, 75 mg.

NOTES — Tricyclic, tertiary amine; primarily inhibits serotonin reuptake.

MOA — Serotonin/norepinephrine reuptake inhibitor.

ADVERSE EFFECTS — Serious: Atrial/ventricular arrhythmias, seizures, MI, CHF, stroke. Frequent: Drowsiness, dry mouth, constipation, nausea, orthostatic hypotension, dizziness, confusion, urinary retention, sexual dysfunction.

DESIPRAMINE (*Norpramin***)** ▶L ♀C ▶+ $$

ADULT — Depression: Start 25 to 100 mg PO given once daily or in divided doses. Gradually increase to usual effective dose of 100 to 200 mg/day, max 300 mg/day.

DESIPRAMINE (cont.)

PEDS — Depression, adolescents: 25 to 100 mg/day. Not approved in children.

FORMS — Generic/Trade: Tabs 10, 25, 50, 75, 100, 150 mg.

NOTES — Tricyclic, secondary amine; primarily inhibits norepinephrine reuptake. Usual therapeutic range is 125 to 300 ng/mL. May cause fewer anticholinergic side effects than tertiary amines. Use lower doses in adolescents or elderly.

MOA — Norepinephrine/serotonin reuptake inhibitor.

ADVERSE EFFECTS — Serious: Atrial/ventricular arrhythmias, seizures, MI, CHF, stroke. Frequent: Drowsiness, dry mouth, constipation, nausea, orthostatic hypotension, dizziness, confusion, urinary retention, sexual dysfunction.

DOXEPIN (Silenor) ▶L ♀C ▶– $$

ADULT — Depression and/or anxiety: Start 75 mg PO at bedtime. Gradually increase to usual effective dose of 75 to 150 mg/day, max 300 mg/day. Insomnia (Silenor): 6 mg PO 30 min before bedtime, 3 mg in age 65 yo or older.

PEDS — Adolescents: Use adult dosing. Not approved in children younger than 12 yo.

UNAPPROVED ADULT — Chronic pain: 50 to 300 mg/day. Pruritus: Start 10 to 25 mg at bedtime. Usual effective dose is 10 to 100 mg/day.

FORMS — Generic only: Caps 10, 25, 50, 75, 100, 150 mg. Oral concentrate 10 mg/mL. Trade only: Tabs 3, 6 mg (Silenor)

NOTES — Tricyclic, tertiary amine; primarily inhibits norepinephrine reuptake. Do not mix oral concentrate with carbonated beverages. Some patients with mild symptoms may respond to 25 to 50 mg/day. Brand name Sinequan no longer available.

MOA — Norepinephrine/serotonin reuptake inhibitor.

ADVERSE EFFECTS — Serious: Atrial/ventricular arrhythmias, seizures, MI, CHF, stroke. Frequent: Drowsiness, dry mouth, constipation, nausea, orthostatic hypotension, dizziness, confusion, urinary retention, sexual dysfunction.

IMIPRAMINE (Tofranil, Tofranil PM) ▶L ♀D ▶– $$$

ADULT — Depression: Start 75 to 100 mg PO at bedtime or in divided doses; gradually increase to max 300 mg/day.

PEDS — Enuresis age 6 yo or older: 10 to 25 mg/day PO given 1 h before bedtime, then increase in increments of 10 to 25 mg at 1 to 2 week intervals not to exceed 50 mg/day in 6 to 12 yo or 75 mg/day in children age older than 12 yo. Do not exceed 2.5 mg/kg/day.

UNAPPROVED ADULT — Panic disorder: Start 10 mg PO at bedtime, titrate to usual effective dose of 50 to 300 mg/day. Enuresis: 25 to 75 mg PO at bedtime.

UNAPPROVED PEDS — Depression, children: Start 1.5 mg/kg/day PO divided three times per day; increase by 1 to 1.5 mg/kg/day q 3 to 4 days to max 5 mg/kg/day.

FORMS — Generic/Trade: Tabs 10, 25, 50 mg. Caps 75, 100, 125, 150 mg (as pamoate salt).

NOTES — Tricyclic, tertiary amine; inhibits serotonin and norepinephrine reuptake. Demethylated to desipramine, which primarily inhibits norepinephrine reuptake.

MOA — Serotonin/norepinephrine reuptake inhibitor.

ADVERSE EFFECTS — Serious: Atrial/ventricular arrhythmias, seizures, MI, CHF, orthostatic hypotension, stroke, agranulocytosis. Frequent: Drowsiness, dry mouth, constipation, nausea, dizziness, confusion, urinary retention, sexual dysfunction.

MAPROTILINE (Ludiomil) ▶KL ♀B ▶? $$$

ADULT — Rarely used; other drugs preferred. Depression: Start 25 mg PO daily, then gradually increase by 25 mg q 2 weeks to max 225 mg/day. Usual effective dose is 150 to 225 mg/day. Max 200 mg/day for chronic use.

PEDS — Not approved in children.

FORMS — Generic only: Tabs 25, 50, 75 mg.

NOTES — Tetracyclic—primarily inhibits norepinephrine reuptake.

MOA — Norepinephrine reuptake inhibitor

ADVERSE EFFECTS — Serious: atrial/ventricular arrhythmias, seizures, MI, CHF, stroke. Frequent: drowsiness, dry mouth, constipation, nausea, orthostatic hypotension, dizziness, confusion, urinary retention, sexual dysfunction

NORTRIPTYLINE (Aventyl, Pamelor) ▶L ♀D ▶+ $$$

ADULT — Depression: Start 25 mg PO given once daily or divided two to four times per day. Gradually increase to usual effective dose of 75 to 100 mg/day, max 150 mg/day.

PEDS — Not approved in children.

UNAPPROVED ADULT — Panic disorder: Start 25 mg PO at bedtime, titrate to usual effective dose of 50 to 150 mg/day. Smoking cessation: Start 25 mg PO daily 14 days prior to quit date. Titrate to 75 mg/day as tolerated. Continue for 6 weeks or more after quit date. Chronic pain: Start 10 to 25 mg PO q am or at bedtime. Max 150 mg/day.

UNAPPROVED PEDS — Depression age 6 to 12 yo: 1 to 3 mg/kg/day PO divided three to four times per day or 10 to 20 mg/day PO divided three to four times per day.

FORMS — Generic/Trade: Caps 10, 25, 50, 75 mg. Oral soln 10 mg/5 mL.

NOTES — Tricyclic, secondary amine; primarily inhibits norepinephrine reuptake. Usual therapeutic range is 50 to 150 ng/mL. May cause fewer anticholinergic side effects than tertiary amines. May be used in combination with nicotine replacement for smoking cessation.

MOA — Norepinephrine/serotonin reuptake inhibitor.

ADVERSE EFFECTS — Serious: Atrial/ventricular arrhythmias, seizures, MI, CHF, stroke. Frequent: Drowsiness, dry mouth, constipation, nausea, orthostatic hypotension, dizziness, confusion, urinary retention, sexual dysfunction.

PROTRIPTYLINE (Vivactil) ▶L ♀C ▶+ $$$$

ADULT — Depression: 15 to 40 mg/day PO divided three to four times per day. Maximum dose is 60 mg/day.

PEDS — Not approved in children.

FORMS — Generic/Trade: Tabs 5, 10 mg.

PROTRIPTYLINE (*cont.*)

NOTES — Tricyclic, secondary amine; primarily inhibits norepinephrine reuptake. May cause fewer anticholinergic side effects than tertiary amines. Dose increases should be made in the morning.

MOA — Serotonin/norepinephrine reuptake inhibitor.

ADVERSE EFFECTS — Serious: Atrial/ventricular arrhythmias, seizures, MI, CHF, stroke. Frequent: Drowsiness, dry mouth, constipation, nausea, orthostatic hypotension, dizziness, confusion, urinary retention, sexual dysfunction.

TRIMIPRAMINE (*Surmontil*) ▶L ♀C ▶? $$$

ADULT — Depression: Start 25 mg PO at bedtime; gradually increase to 75 to 150 mg/day. Max 300 mg/day.

PEDS — Not approved in children.

FORMS — Generic/Trade: Caps 25, 50, 100 mg.

NOTES — Tricyclic, tertiary amine—primarily inhibits norepinephrine reuptake.

MOA — Serotonin/norepinephrine reuptake inhibitor

ADVERSE EFFECTS — Serious: atrial/ventricular arrhythmias, seizures, MI, CHF, stroke. Frequent: drowsiness, dry mouth, constipation, nausea, orthostatic hypotension, dizziness, confusion, urinary retention, sexual dysfunction

PSYCHIATRY: Antidepressants—Monoamine Oxidase Inhibitors (MAOIs)

NOTE: May interfere with sleep; avoid at bedtime dosing. Must be on tyramine-free diet throughout treatment, and for 2 weeks after discontinuation. Numerous drug interactions; risk of hypertensive crisis and serotonin syndrome with many medications, including OTC. Allow ≥2 weeks wash-out when converting from an MAOI to an SSRI (6 weeks after fluoxetine), TCA, or other antidepressant. Contraindicated with carbamazepine or oxcarbazepine. Antidepressants increase the risk of suicidal thinking and behavior in children, adolescents, and young adults; carefully weigh the risks and benefits before starting and monitor patients closely.

ISOCARBOXAZID (*Marplan*) ▶L ♀C ▶? $$$

ADULT — Depression: Start 10 mg PO two times per day; increase by 10 mg q 2 to 4 days. Usual effective dose is 20 to 40 mg/day. Max 60 mg/day divided two to four times per day.

PEDS — Not approved in children younger than 16 yo.

FORMS — Trade only: Tabs 10 mg.

NOTES — Requires MAOI diet.

MOA — Irreversible, nonselective monoamine oxidase inhibitor.

ADVERSE EFFECTS — Serious: Hypertensive crisis with food/drug interactions, serotonin syndrome, seizures, hepatotoxicity, agranulocytosis. Frequent: Dizziness, dry mouth, constipation, urinary retention, headache, confusion, blurred vision, weight gain.

MOCLOBEMIDE ▶L ♀C ▶− $$

ADULT — Canada only. Depression: Start 300 mg/day PO divided two times per day after meals. May increase after 1 week to max 600 mg/day.

PEDS — Not approved in children.

FORMS — Generic/Trade: Tabs 150, 300 mg. Generic only: Tabs 100 mg.

NOTES — No dietary restrictions. Do not use with TCAs; use caution with conventional MAOIs, other antidepressants, epinephrine, thioridazine, sympathomimetics, dextromethorphan, meperidine, and other opiates. Reduce dose in severe hepatic dysfunction.

MOA — Short-acting, reversible MAOI (preferentially affects MAO-A).

ADVERSE EFFECTS — Serious: Hypertensive crisis with drug or food interactions (theoretical risk), hypotension, bradycardia. Frequent: Sleep disturbance, tremor.

PHENELZINE (*Nardil*) ▶L ♀C ▶? $$$

ADULT — Depression: Start 15 mg PO three times per day. Usual effective dose is 60 to 90 mg/day in divided doses.

PEDS — Not approved in children younger than 16 yo.

FORMS — Trade only: Tabs 15 mg.

NOTES — Requires MAOI diet. May increase insulin sensitivity. Contraindicated with meperidine.

MOA — Irreversible, nonselective monoamine oxidase inhibitor.

ADVERSE EFFECTS — Serious: Hypertensive crisis with food/drug interactions, serotonin syndrome, hepatotoxicity, agranulocytosis. Frequent: Dizziness, dry mouth, constipation, urinary retention, headache, confusion, blurred vision, weight gain.

SELEGILINE—TRANSDERMALL (*Emsam*) ▶L ♀C ▶? $$$$$

ADULT — Depression: Start 6 mg/24 h patch q 24 h. Adjust dose in 2-week intervals or more to max 12 mg/24 h.

PEDS — Not approved in children.

FORMS — Trade only: Transdermal patch 6 mg/day, 9 mg/24 h, 12 mg/24 h.

NOTES — MAOI diet is required for doses 9 mg/day or higher. Intense urges (gambling and sexual for example) have been reported. Consider discontinuing the medication or reducing the dose if these occur.

MOA — Irreversible inhibitor of MAO-B; also inhibits MAO-A when doses at least 9 mg/day are used.

ADVERSE EFFECTS — Serious: Hypertensive crisis with food/drug interactions, serotonin syndrome, orthostatic hypotension, mania/hypomania, impulse control disorders. Frequent: Application site reactions, headache, insomnia, dry mouth.

TRANYLCYPROMINE (*Parnate*) ▶L ♀C ▶− $$

ADULT — Depression: Start 10 mg PO q am; increase by 10 mg/day at 1- to 3-week intervals to usual effective dose of 10 to 40 mg/day divided two times per day. Max 60 mg/day.

PEDS — Not approved in children younger than 16 yo.

(cont.)

TRANYLCYPROMINE (cont.)

FORMS — Generic/Trade: Tabs 10 mg.
NOTES — Requires MAOI diet.
MOA — Reversible, nonselective monoamine oxidase inhibitor.

ADVERSE EFFECTS — Serious: Hypertensive crisis with food/drug interactions, serotonin syndrome, seizures, hepatotoxicity, agranulocytosis. Frequent: Dizziness, dry mouth, constipation, urinary retention, headache, confusion, blurred vision, weight gain.

PSYCHIATRY: Antidepressants—Selective Serotonin Reuptake Inhibitors (SSRIs)

NOTE: Gradually taper when discontinuing SSRIs to avoid withdrawal symptoms. Observe patients for worsening depression or the emergence of suicidality, anxiety, agitation, panic attacks, insomnia, irritability, hostility, impulsivity, akathisia, mania, or hypomania, particularly early in therapy or after increases in dose. Antidepressants increase the risk of suicidal thinking and behavior in children, adolescents, and young adults; carefully weigh the risks and benefits before starting treatment and then monitor patients closely. Use of SSRIs during the third trimester of pregnancy has been associated with neonatal complications including respiratory (including persistent pulmonary HTN), GI, and feeding problems, as well as seizures and withdrawal symptoms. Balance these risks against those of withdrawal and depression for the mother. Paroxetine should be avoided throughout pregnancy. Don't use sibutramine with SSRIs. Increased risk of abnormal bleeding; use caution when combined with NSAIDs or aspirin. SSRIs have been associated with serotonin syndrome and neuroleptic malignant syndrome. Use cautiously and observe closely for serotonin syndrome if SSRI is used with a triptan or other serotonergic drugs. SSRIs and SNRIs have been associated with hyponatremia, which is often associated with SIADH. The elderly and those taking diuretics may be at increased risk. Avoid use with MAOIs used for psychiatric conditions or during active treatment wtih linezolid or IV methylene blue.

CITALOPRAM (*Celexa*) ▶LK ♀C but − in third trimester ▶− $$$
ADULT — Depression: Start 20 mg PO daily. May increase after 1 or more weeks to max 40 mg PO daily or 20 mg daily if > 60 yo.
PEDS — Not approved in children.
FORMS — Generic/Trade: Tabs 10, 20, 40 mg. Generic only: Oral disintegrating tab 10, 20, 40 mg, oral soln 10 mg/5 mL.
NOTES — Do not use with MAOIs or tryptophan.
MOA — Selective serotonin reuptake inhibitor.
ADVERSE EFFECTS — Serious: Suicidality, serotonin syndrome, neuroleptic malignant syndrome, abnormal bleeding, withdrawal reactions, increased QTc interval. Frequent: N/V, diarrhea, insomnia, drowsiness, headache, sexual dysfunction, dry mouth, anorexia, anxiety, nervousness.

ESCITALOPRAM (*Lexapro*, ✦*Cipralex*) ▶LK ♀C but − in 3rd trimester ▶− $$$$
ADULT — Depression, generalized anxiety disorder: Start 10 mg PO daily; may increase to max 20 mg PO daily after 1st week.
PEDS — Depression, adults and age 12 yo and older: Start 10 mg PO daily. May increase to max 20 mg/day.
UNAPPROVED ADULT — Social anxiety disorder: 5 to 20 mg PO daily.
FORMS — Generic/Trade: Tabs 5, 10, 20 mg. Oral soln 1 mg/mL.
NOTES — Do not use with MAOIs. Doses greater than 20 mg daily have not been shown to be superior to 10 mg daily. Escitalopram is the active isomer of citalopram.
MOA — Selective serotonin reuptake inhibitor.
ADVERSE EFFECTS — Serious: Suicidality, serotonin syndrome, abnormal bleeding, withdrawal reactions. Frequent: Insomnia, ejaculatory disorders, nausea, sweating, fatigue, somnolence.

FLUOXETINE (*Prozac, Prozac Weekly, Sarafem*) ▶L ♀C but − in 3rd trimester ▶− $$$
ADULT — Depression, OCD: Start 20 mg PO q am; may increase after several weeks to usual effective dose of 20 to 40 mg/day, max 80 mg/day. Depression, maintenance therapy: 20 to 40 mg/day (standard-release) or 90 mg PO once weekly (Prozac Weekly) starting 7 days after last standard-release dose. Bulimia: 60 mg PO q am; may need to titrate up to this dose slowly over several days. Panic disorder: Start 10 mg PO q am; titrate to 20 mg/day after 1 week, max 60 mg/day. Premenstrual dysphoric disorder (Sarafem): 20 mg PO daily given continuously throughout the menstrual cycle (continuous dosing) or 20 mg PO daily for 14 days prior to menses (intermittent dosing); max 80 mg daily. Doses greater than 20 mg/day can be divided two times per day (in morning and at noon). Bipolar depression, olanzapine + fluoxetine: Start 5 mg olanzapine + 20 mg fluoxetine daily in the evening. Increase to usual range of 5 to 12.5 mg olanzapine plus 20 to 50 mg fluoxetine as tolerated. Treatment-resistant depression, olanzapine + fluoxetine: Start 5 mg olanzapine + 20 mg fluoxetine daily in the evening. Increase to usual range of 5 to 20 mg olanzapine plus 20 to 50 mg fluoxetine as tolerated.
PEDS — Depression, age 7 to 17 yo: 10 to 20 mg PO q am (10 mg for smaller children), max 20 mg/day. OCD: Start 10 mg PO q am; max 60 mg/day (30 mg/day for smaller children).
UNAPPROVED ADULT — Hot flashes: 20 mg PO daily. Posttraumatic stress disorder: 20 to 80 mg PO daily. Social anxiety disorder: 10 to 60 mg PO daily.
FORMS — Generic/Trade: Tabs 10 mg. Caps 10, 20, 40 mg. Oral soln 20 mg/5 mL. Caps (Sarafem) 10, 20 mg. Trade only: Tabs (Sarafem) 10, 15, 20

FLUOXETINE (*cont.*)

mg. Caps delayed-release (Prozac Weekly) 90 mg. Generic only: Tabs 20, 40 mg.

NOTES — Half-life of parent is 1 to 3 days and for active metabolite norfluoxetine is 6 to 14 days. Do not use with thioridazine, pimozide, MAOIs, cisapride, or tryptophan; use caution with lithium, phenytoin, TCAs, and warfarin. Pregnancy exposure has been associated with premature delivery, low birth wt, and lower Apgar scores. Decrease dose with liver disease. Increases risk of mania with bipolar disorder.

MOA — Selective serotonin reuptake inhibitor.

ADVERSE EFFECTS — Serious: Suicidality, serotonin syndrome, neuroleptic malignant syndrome, SIADH, abnormal bleeding, withdrawal reactions, hypoglycemia. Frequent: N/V, diarrhea, insomnia, drowsiness, headache, sexual dysfunction, dry mouth, anorexia, anxiety, nervousness.

FLUVOXAMINE (*Luvox, Luvox CR*) ▶L ♀C but – in third trimester ▶– $$$$

ADULT — OCD: Start 50 mg PO at bedtime, then increase by 50 mg/day q 4 to 7 days to usual effective dose of 100 to 300 mg/day divided two times per day. Max 300 mg/day.

PEDS — OCD (children age 8 yo or older): Start 25 mg PO at bedtime; increase by 25 mg/day q 4 to 7 days to usual effective dose of 50 to 200 mg/day divided two times per day. Max 200 mg/day (8 to 11 yo) or 300 mg/day (older than 11 yo). Therapeutic effect may be seen with lower doses in girls.

FORMS — Generic/Trade: Tabs 25, 50, 100 mg. Caps, extended-release 100, 150 mg.

NOTES — Do not use with thioridazine, alosetron, cisapride, tizanidine, tryptophan, or MAOIs; use caution with benzodiazepines, theophylline, TCAs, and warfarin. Luvox brand not currently on US market.

MOA — Selective serotonin reuptake inhibitor.

ADVERSE EFFECTS — Serious: Suicidality, serotonin syndrome, neuroleptic malignant syndrome, SIADH, seizures, abnormal bleeding, withdrawal reactions. Frequent: N/V, diarrhea, insomnia, drowsiness, headache, sexual dysfunction, dry mouth, anorexia, anxiety, nervousness.

PAROXETINE (*Paxil, Paxil CR, Pexeva*) ▶LK ♀D ▶? $$$

ADULT — Depression: Start 20 mg PO q am; increase by 10 mg/day at intervals of 1 week or more to usual effective dose of 20 to 50 mg/day, max 50 mg/day. Depression, controlled-release tabs: Start 25 mg PO q am; may increase by 12.5 mg/day at intervals of 1 week or more to usual effective dose of 25 to 62.5 mg/day; max 62.5 mg/day. OCD: Start 20 mg PO q am; increase by 10 mg/day at intervals of 1 week or more to usual recommended dose of 40 mg/day; max 60 mg/day. Panic disorder: Start 10 mg PO q am; increase by 10 mg/day at intervals of 1 week or more to target dose of 40 mg/day; max 60 mg/day. Panic disorder, controlled-release tabs: Start 12.5 mg/day; increase by 12.5 mg/day at intervals of 1 week or more to

usual effective dose of 12.5 to 75 mg/day; max 75 mg/day. Social anxiety disorder: Start 20 mg PO q am (which is the usual effective dose); max 60 mg/day. Social anxiety disorder, controlled-release tabs: Start 12.5 mg PO q am; may increase at intervals of 1 week or more to max 37.5 mg/day. Generalized anxiety disorder: Start 20 mg PO q am (which is the usual effective dose); max 50 mg/day. Posttraumatic stress disorder: Start 20 mg PO q am; usual effective dose is 20 to 40 mg/day; max 50 mg/day. Premenstrual dysphoric disorder (PMDD), continuous dosing: Start 12.5 mg PO q am (controlled-release tabs); may increase dose after 1 week to max 25 mg q am. PMDD, intermittent dosing (given for 2 weeks prior to menses): Start 12.5 mg PO q am (controlled-release tabs), max 25 mg/day.

PEDS — Not recommended for use in children or adolescents due to increased risk of suicidality.

UNAPPROVED ADULT — Hot flashes related to menopause or breast cancer: 20 mg PO daily (tabs), or 12.5 to 25 mg PO daily (controlled-release tabs).

FORMS — Generic/Trade: Tabs 10, 20, 30, 40 mg. Oral susp 10 mg/5 mL. Controlled-release tabs 12.5, 25 mg. Trade only: (Paxil CR) 37.5 mg.

NOTES — Start at 10 mg/day and do not exceed 40 mg/day in elderly or debilitated patients or those with renal or hepatic impairment. Paroxetine is an inhibitor of CYP2D6, and is contraindicated with thioridazine, pimozide, MAOIs, linezolid, and tryptophan; use caution with barbiturates, cimetidine, phenytoin, theophylline, TCAs, risperidone, atomoxetine, and warfarin. Taper gradually after long-term use; reduce by 10 mg/day q week to 20 mg/day; continue for 1 week at this dose, and then stop. If withdrawal symptoms develop, then restart at prior dose and taper more slowly. Pexeva is paroxetine mesylate and is a generic equivalent for paroxetine HCl. Some data suggest paroxetine may reduce the efficacy of tamoxifen. Avoid the combination if possible.

MOA — Selective serotonin reuptake inhibitor.

ADVERSE EFFECTS — Serious: Suicidality, serotonin syndrome, SIADH, hyponatremia, abnormal bleeding, withdrawal reactions. Frequent: Asthenia, nausea, diarrhea, constipation, insomnia, drowsiness, sexual dysfunction, dry mouth, anorexia, nervousness, sweating, dizziness, tremor.

SERTRALINE (*Zoloft*) ▶LK ♀C but – in third trimester ▶+ $$$

ADULT — Depression, OCD: Start 50 mg PO daily; may increase after 1 week. Usual effective dose is 50 to 200 mg/day, max 200 mg/day. Panic disorder, posttraumatic stress disorder, social anxiety disorder: Start 25 mg PO daily; may increase after 1 week to 50 mg PO daily. Usual effective dose is 50 to 200 mg/day; max 200 mg/day. PMDD, continuous dosing: Start 50 mg PO daily; max 150 mg/day. PMDD, intermittent dosing (given for 14 days prior to menses): Start

(cont.)

SERTRALINE (*cont.*)
50 mg PO daily for 3 days, then increase to max 100 mg/day.
PEDS — OCD, age 6 to 12 yo: Start 25 mg PO daily, max 200 mg/day. OCD, age 13 yo or older: Use adult dosing.
UNAPPROVED PEDS — Major depressive disorder: Start 25 mg PO daily; usual effective dose is 50 to 200 mg/day.
FORMS — Generic/Trade: Tabs 25, 50, 100 mg. Oral concentrate 20 mg/mL (60 mL).
NOTES — Do not use with cisapride, tryptophan, or MAOIs; use caution with cimetidine, warfarin, pimozide, or TCAs. Must dilute oral concentrate before administration. Administration during pregnancy has been associated with premature delivery, low birth wt, and lower Apgar scores.
MOA — Selective serotonin reuptake inhibitor.
ADVERSE EFFECTS — Serious: Suicidality, serotonin syndrome, neuroleptic malignant syndrome, SIADH, hyponatremia, abnormal bleeding, withdrawal symptoms. Frequent: N/V, diarrhea, insomnia, drowsiness, headache, sexual dysfunction, dry mouth, anorexia, anxiety, nervousness.

VORTIOXETINE (*Brintellix*) ▶L - ♀C ▶? $$$$$
ADULT — Depression: Start 10 mg PO daily. Increase to recommended dose of 20 mg daily as tolerated. Max 20 mg/day.
PEDS — Not approved for use in children.
FORMS — Trade only: Tabs 5, 10, 15, 20 mg
NOTES — Reduce dose by half when using with strong CYP2D6 inhibitors such as bupropion, fluoxetine, and paroxetine, or in CYP2D6 poor metabolizers..
MOA — Serotonin reuptake inhibitor, 5-HT3 antagonist, 5-HT1 agonist
ADVERSE EFFECTS — Serious: serotonin syndrome, hyponatremia, bleeding, suicidal thoughts and behaviors, activation of mania. Frequent: nausea, vomiting, constipation.

PSYCHIATRY: Antidepressants—Serotonin-Norepinephrine Reuptake Inhibitors (SNRIs)

NOTE: Monitor for the emergence of anxiety, agitation, panic attacks, insomnia, irritability, hostility, impulsivity, akathisia, mania, or hypomania, and for worsening depression or the emergence of suicidality, particularly early in therapy or after increases in dose. Antidepressants increase the risk of suicidal thinking and behavior in children, adolescents, and young adults; carefully weigh the risks and benefits before starting treatment, and then monitor closely. SSRIs and SNRIs have been associated with hyponatremia, which is often associated with SIADH. The elderly and those taking diuretics may be at increased risk. Do not use with MAOIs. SNRIs have been associated with serotonin syndrome and neuroleptic malignant syndrome when used alone and especially in combination with other serotonergic drugs.

DESVENLAFAXINE (*Pristiq, Khedezla*) ▶LK ♀C ▶? $$$$
ADULT — Depression: 50 mg PO daily. Max 400 mg/day.
PEDS — Not approved for use in children.
FORMS — Trade only: Tabs (Pristiq, Khedezla) extended-release 50, 100 mg. Generic only: Extended release tabs 50, 100 mg tabs
NOTES — There is no evidence that doses greater than 50 mg/day offer additional benefit. Reduce dose to 50 mg PO every other day in severe renal impairment (CrCl less than 30 mL/min). Caution in cardiovascular, cerebrovascular, or lipid disorders. Gradually taper when discontinuing therapy to avoid withdrawal symptoms after prolonged use. Exposure to SSRIs or SNRIs during the 3rd trimester of pregnancy has been associated with neonatal complications including respiratory, GI, and feeding problems, as well as seizures and withdrawal symptoms. Balance these risks against those of withdrawal and depression for the mother.
MOA — Selective inhibitor of serotonin and norepinephrine reuptake.
ADVERSE EFFECTS — Serious: Hypersensitivity, suicidality, serotonin syndrome, neuroleptic malignant syndrome, hypertension, hyperlipidemia, abnormal bleeding, hyponatremia, mania, seizures, narrow angle glaucoma. Frequent: Nausea, vomiting, dry mouth, constipation, diarrhea, fatigue, decreased appetite, insomnia, hyperhidrosis, headache, dizziness.

DULOXETINE (*Cymbalta*) ▶L ♀C ▶? $$$$
ADULT — Depression: 20 mg PO two times per day; max 60 mg/day given once daily or divided two times per day. Generalized anxiety disorder: Start 30 to 60 mg PO daily, max 120 mg/day. Diabetic peripheral neuropathic pain: 60 mg PO daily, max 60 mg/day. Fibromyalgia: Start 30 to 60 mg PO daily, max 60 mg/day.
PEDS — Not approved in children.
FORMS — Generic/Trade: Caps 20, 30, 60 mg.
NOTES — Avoid in renal insufficiency (CrCl less than 30 mL/min), hepatic insufficiency, or substantial alcohol use. Do not use with thioridazine, MAOIs, or potent inhibitors of CYP1A2; use caution with inhibitors of CYP2D6. Small BP increases have been observed. Exposure during the 3rd trimester of pregnancy has been associated with neonatal complications including respiratory, GI, and feeding problems, as well as seizures, and withdrawal symptoms; balance these risks against those of withdrawal and depression for the mother.
MOA — Serotonin and norepinephrine reuptake inhibitor; also a weak inhibitor of dopamine reuptake.
ADVERSE EFFECTS — Serious: Suicidality, hypertension, seizures, hepatitis, cholestatic jaundice, serotonin syndrome, abnormal bleeding, orthostatic

DULOXETINE (*cont.*)

hypotension, hyponatremia. Frequent: N/V, dry mouth, constipation, decreased appetite, fatigue, somnolence, insomnia, sweating, dizziness, headache.

LEVOMILNACIPRAN (*Fetzima*) ▶KL ♀C ▶?

ADULT — Major depressive disorder: Start 20 mg PO once daily. Increase after 2 days to 40 mg PO once daily. May increase in increments of 40 mg/day at intervals of 2 or more days to max of 120mg/day based on response.

PEDS — Not approved for use in children or adolescents.

FORMS — Trade only: Caps 20, 40, 80, 120 mg.

NOTES — Reduce max dose to 80 mg/day for moderate renal insufficiency and 40 mg/day for severe.

MOA — Serotonin-norepinephrine reuptake inhibitor

ADVERSE EFFECTS — Serious: suicidal thoughts and behaviors, hypertension, serotonin syndrome, bleeding, mania/hypomania, hypersensitivity, angle closure glaucoma. Frequent: nausea, constipation, vomiting, hyperhidrosis, tachycardia, palpitations, erectile dysfunction.

VENLAFAXINE (*Effexor XR*) ▶LK ♀C but – in 3rd trimester ▶? $$$$

ADULT — Depression: Start 37.5 to 75 mg PO daily (Effexor XR) or 75 mg/day divided two to three times per day (Effexor). Increase in 75 mg increments q 4 days to usual effective dose of 150 to 225 mg/day, max 225 mg/day (Effexor XR) or 375 mg/day (Effexor). Generalized anxiety disorder: Start 37.5 to 75 mg PO daily (Effexor XR); increase in 75 mg increments q 4 days to max 225 mg/day. Social anxiety disorder: 75 mg PO daily (Effexor XR). Panic disorder: Start 37.5 mg PO daily (Effexor XR), may titrate by 75 mg/day at weekly intervals to max 225 mg/day.

PEDS — Not approved in children. May increase the risk of suicidality in children and teenagers.

UNAPPROVED ADULT — Hot flashes (primarily in cancer patients): 37.5 to 75 mg/day of the extended-release form.

FORMS — Generic/Trade: Caps, extended-release 37.5, 75, 150 mg. Tabs 25, 37.5, 50, 75, 100 mg. Generic only: Tabs extended-release 37.5, 75, 150, 225 mg.

NOTES — Noncyclic, serotonin-norepinephrine reuptake inhibitor (SNRI). Decrease dose in renal or hepatic impairment. Monitor for increases in BP. Do not give with MAOIs; use caution with cimetidine and haloperidol. Use caution and monitor for serotonin syndrome if used with triptans. Gradually taper when discontinuing therapy to avoid withdrawal symptoms after prolonged use. Hostility, suicidal ideation, and self-harm have been reported when used in children. Exposure during the 3rd trimester of pregnancy has been associated with neonatal complications including respiratory, GI, and feeding problems, as well as seizures and withdrawal symptoms. Balance these risks against those of withdrawal and depression for the mother. Mydriasis and increased intraocular pressure can occur; use caution in glaucoma.

MOA — Serotonin and norepinephrine reuptake inhibitor; also a weak inhibitor of dopamine reuptake.

ADVERSE EFFECTS — Serious: Suicidality, mania/hypomania, seizures, hypertension, withdrawal symptoms, serotonin syndrome, neuroleptic malignant syndrome, interstitial lung disease and eosinophilic pneumonia, toxic epidermal necrolysis. Frequent: Drowsiness, dizziness, sexual dysfunction, anorexia, N/V, asthenia, nervousness, insomnia, diaphoresis, constipation, dry mouth, abnormal vision.

PSYCHIATRY: Antidepressants—Other

NOTE: Monitor for the emergence of anxiety, agitation, panic attacks, insomnia, irritability, hostility, impulsivity, akathisia, mania, or hypomania, and for worsening depression or the emergence of suicidality, particularly early in therapy or after increases in dose. Antidepressants increase the risk of suicidal thinking and behavior in children, adolescents, and young adults; carefully weigh the risks and benefits before starting treatment, and then monitor closely. Avoid use with MAOIs and don't use during treatment with linezolid or IV methylene blue.

BUPROPION (*Wellbutrin, Wellbutrin SR, Wellbutrin XL, Aplenzin, Zyban, Buproban, Forfivo XL*) ▶LK ♀C ▶– $$

ADULT — Depression: Start 100 mg PO two times per day (immediate-release tabs); can increase to 100 mg three times per day after 4 to 7 days. Usual effective dose is 300 to 450 mg/day, max 150 mg/dose and 450 mg/day. Depression, sustained-release tabs (Wellbutrin SR): Start 150 mg PO q am; may increase to 150 mg two times per day after 4 to 7 days, max 400 mg/day. Give the last dose no later than 5 pm. Depression, extended-release tabs (Wellbutrin XL): Start 150 mg PO q am; may increase to 300 mg q am after 4 days, max 450 mg q am. Depression, extended-release

(Aplenzin): Start 174 mg PO q am; increase to target dose of 348 mg/day after 4 days or more. May increase to max dose of 522 mg/day after 4 weeks or more. Extended-release (Forfivo XL): Do not use to initiate therapy. If standard tabs tolerated and pateint requires more than 300 mg/day may use 450 mg PO daily, max 450 mg/day. Seasonal affective disorder, extended-release tabs (Wellbutrin XL): Start 150 mg PO q am in autumn; may increase after 1 week to target dose of 300 mg q am, max 300 mg/day. In the spring, decrease to 150 mg/day for 2 weeks and then discontinue. Extended-release (Aplenzin): Start 174 mg PO each morning. Increase to

BUPROPION (*cont.*)

348 mg/day after 7 days. Smoking cessation (Zyban, Buproban): Start 150 mg PO q am for 3 days, then increase to 150 mg PO two times per day for 7 to 12 weeks. Allow 8 h between doses, with the last dose given no later than 5 pm. Max 150 mg PO two times per day. Target quit date should be after at least 1 week of therapy. Stop if there is no progress toward abstinence by the 7th week. Write "dispense behavioral modification kit" on first script.

PEDS — Not approved in children.

UNAPPROVED ADULT — Insomnia: 150 to 450 mg/day PO.

UNAPPROVED PEDS — ADHD: 1.4 to 5.7 mg/kg/day PO.

FORMS — Generic/Trade (for depression, bupropion HCl): Tabs 75, 100 mg. Sustained-release tabs 100, 150, 200 mg. Extended-release tabs 150, 300 mg (Wellbutrin XL). Generic/Trade (Smoking cessation): Sustained-release tabs 150 mg (Zyban, Buproban). Trade only: Extended-release (Aplenzin, bupropion hydrobromide) tabs 174, 348, 522 mg. Extended-release (Forfivo XL) tab 450 mg.

NOTES — Weak inhibitor of dopamine reuptake. Do not use with MAOIs. Seizures occur in 0.4% of patients taking 300 to 450 mg/day. Contraindicated in seizure disorders, eating disorders, or with abrupt alcohol or sedative withdrawal. Wellbutrin SR, Zyban, and Buproban are all the same formulation. Equivalent doses: 174 HBr = 150 mg HCl, 348 mg HBr = 300 mg HCl, 522 mg HBr = 450 mg HCl. Consider dose reductions for hepatic and renal impairment. Has been associated with false positive urine test results for amphetamines when using immunoassay procedures.

MOA — Norepinephrine and dopamine reuptake inhibitor.

ADVERSE EFFECTS — Serious: Suicidality, seizures, psychosis, HTN, Stevens-Johnson syndrome, rhabdomyolysis, hallucinations. Frequent: Headache, tremor, agitation, insomnia, diaphoresis, weight loss, dry mouth, nausea, constipation, dizziness.

MIRTAZAPINE (*Remeron, Remeron SolTab*) ▶LK ♀C ▶? $$

ADULT — Depression: Start 15 mg PO at bedtime, increase after 1 to 2 weeks to usual effective dose of 15 to 45 mg/day.

PEDS — Not approved in children.

FORMS — Generic/Trade: Tabs 15, 30, 45 mg. Tabs orally disintegrating (SolTab) 15, 30, 45 mg. Generic only: Tabs 7.5 mg.

NOTES — 0.1% risk of agranulocytosis. May cause drowsiness, increased appetite, and wt gain. Don't use with MAOIs.

MOA — Presynaptic alpha-2 receptor antagonist; 5-HT2A, 5-HT-2C, and 5-HT-3 receptor antagonist; enhances norepinephrine and serotonin release.

ADVERSE EFFECTS — Serious: Suicidality, agranulocytosis, dyslipidemia, serotonin syndrome, hyponatremia. Frequent: Drowsiness, increased appetite, weight gain, dizziness, dry mouth, constipation.

NEFAZODONE ▶L ♀C ▶? $$$

WARNING — Rare reports of life-threatening liver failure. Discontinue if signs or symptoms of liver dysfunction develop. Brand name product withdrawn from the market in the United States and Canada.

ADULT — Depression: Start 100 mg PO two times per day. Increase by 100 to 200 mg/day at 1-week intervals or longer to usual effective dose of 150 to 300 mg PO two times per day, max 600 mg/day. Start 50 mg PO two times per day in elderly or debilitated patients.

PEDS — Not approved in children.

FORMS — Generic only: Tabs 50, 100, 150, 200, 250 mg.

NOTES — Do not use with MAOIs, pimozide, or triazolam; use caution with alprazolam. Many other drug interactions.

MOA — Serotonin reuptake inhibitor and 5-HT2 receptor antagonist.

ADVERSE EFFECTS — Serious: Suicidality, hepatotoxicity, liver failure. Frequent: N/V, dry mouth, constipation, drowsiness, dizziness, asthenia.

TRAZODONE (*Oleptro*) ▶L ♀C ▶– $

ADULT — Depression: Start 50 to 150 mg/day PO in divided doses, increase by 50 mg/day q 3 to 4 days. Usual effective dose is 400 to 600 mg/day. Extended release: Start 150 mg PO at bedtime. May increase by 75 mg/day q 3 days to max 375 mg/day.

PEDS — Not approved in children.

UNAPPROVED ADULT — Insomnia: 50 to 100 mg PO at bedtime, max 150 mg/day.

UNAPPROVED PEDS — Depression, 6 to 18 yo: Start 1.5 to 2 mg/kg/day PO divided two to three times per day; may increase q 3 to 4 days to max 6 mg/kg/day.

FORMS — Trade only: Extended-release tabs (Oleptro) 150, 300 mg. Generic only: Tabs 50, 100, 150, 300 mg.

NOTES — May cause priapism. Rarely used as monotherapy for depression; most often used as a sleep aid and adjunct to another antidepressant. Use caution with CYP3A4 inhibitors or inducers. Brand name Desyrel no longer available.

MOA — Serotonin reuptake inhibitor and 5-HT2A receptor antagonist.

ADVERSE EFFECTS — Serious: Orthostatic hypotension, priapism, syncope. Frequent: Drowsiness, dizziness, nervousness, headache, tremor, fatigue, dry mouth, blurred vision.

TRYPTOPHAN ▶K ♀? ▶? $$

ADULT — Canada only. Adjunct to antidepressant treatment for affective disorders: 8 to 12 g/day in 3 to 4 divided doses.

PEDS — Not indicated.

TRYPTOPHAN (*cont.*)

FORMS — Trade only: L-tryptophan tabs 250, 500, 750, 1000 mg.

NOTES — Caution in diabetics; may worsen glycemic control.

MOA — An essential amino acid that increases serotonin synthesis in the CNS.

ADVERSE EFFECTS — Serious: Serotonin syndrome. Frequent: Drowsiness, dizziness, nausea, dry mouth.

VILAZODONE (*Viibryd*) ▶L – ♀C ▶?

ADULT — Major depressive disorder: Start 10 mg PO once daily for 7 days. Then increase to 20 mg/day for another 7 days then increase to target dose of 40 mg/day.

PEDS — Not approved for use in children.

FORMS — Trade only: Tabs 10, 20, and 40 mg.

NOTES — Give this medication with food. Bioavailability is reduced up to 50% if taken on empty stomach. Metabolized primarily by CYP3A4. Refer to package insert for dosing with stong CYP3A4 inhibitors or inducers.

MOA — Inhibition of serotonin reuptake and 5-HT1A partial agonist

ADVERSE EFFECTS — Severe: serotonin syndrome, bleeding, seizures, mania, hyponatremia. Frequent: nausea, diarrhea, vomiting, dry mouth, insomnia, dizziness.

PSYCHIATRY: Antimanic (Bipolar) Agents

LAMOTRIGINE (*Lamictal, Lamictal CD, Lamictal ODT, Lamictal XR*) ▶LK ♀C (see notes) ▶– $$$$

WARNING — Potentially life-threatening rashes (eg, Stevens-Johnson syndrome, toxic epidermal necrolysis) have been reported in 0.3% of adults and 0.8% of children, usually within 2 to 8 weeks of initiation; discontinue at first sign of rash. Drug reaction with eosinophilia and systemic symptoms (DRESS) has also been reported. Drug interaction with valproate; see adjusted dosing guidelines. Recent data suggest an increased risk of suicidal ideation or behaviors with antiepileptic drugs. Monitor closely for signs of depression, anxiety, hostility, and hypomania/mania. Symptoms may develop within 1 week of initiation and risk continues through at least 24 weeks.

ADULT — Bipolar disorder (maintenance): Start 25 mg PO daily, 50 mg PO daily if on carbamazepine or other enzyme-inducing drugs, or 25 mg PO every other day if on valproate. Increase for week 3 to 4 to 50 mg/day, 50 mg twice per day if on enzyme-inducing drugs, or 25 mg/day if on valproate, then adjust over weeks 5 to 7 to target doses of 200 mg/day, 400 mg/day divided twice per day if on enzyme-inducing drugs, or 100 mg/day if on valproate. See neurology section for epilepsy dosing.

PEDS — Not approved in children.

FORMS — Generic/Trade: Chewable dispersible tabs (Lamictal CD) 5, 25 mg. Tabs 25, 100, 150, 200 mg.Extended-release tabs (XR) 25, 50, 100, 200, 250, 300 mg. Trade only: Orally disintegrating tabs (ODT) 25, 50, 100, 200 mg. Chewable dispersible tab 2mg.

NOTES — Drug interactions with valproate and enzyme-inducing antiepileptic drugs (ie, carbamazepine, phenobarbital, phenytoin, primidone); may need to adjust dose. May increase carbamazepine toxicity. Preliminary evidence suggests that exposure during the 1st trimester of pregnancy is associated with a risk for cleft palate and/or cleft lip. Please report all fetal exposure to the Lamotrigine Pregnancy Registry (800-336-2176) and the North American Antiepileptic Drug Pregnancy Registry (888-233-2334). The extended release product has not been FDA approved for use in bipolar disorder.

MOA — Unknown in bipolar.

ADVERSE EFFECTS — Serious: Rash (including Stevens-Johnson syndrome and toxic epidermal necrolysis), hypersensitivity reactions, drug reaction with eosinophilia and systemic symptoms (DRESS), blood dyscrasias, multiorgan failure, aseptic meningitis. Frequent: N/V, insomnia, back pain, fatigue, rhinitis, abdominal pain, dry mouth, constipation, exacerbation of cough, pharyngitis.

LITHIUM (*Lithobid, ✦Lithane*) ▶K ♀D ▶– $

WARNING — Lithium toxicity can occur at therapeutic levels.

ADULT — Acute mania: Start 300 to 600 mg PO two to three times per day; usual effective dose is 900 to 1800 mg/day. Bipolar maintenance usually 900 to 1200 mg/day titrated to therapeutic trough level of 0.6 to 1.2 mEq/L.

PEDS — Age 12 yo or older: Use adult dosing.

UNAPPROVED PEDS — Mania (age younger than 12 yo): Start 15 to 60 mg/kg/day PO divided three to four times per day. Adjust weekly to achieve therapeutic levels.

FORMS — Generic/Trade: Caps 300, Extended-release tabs 300, 450 mg. Generic only: Caps 150, 600 mg, Tabs 300 mg, Syrup 300 mg/5 mL.

NOTES — Steady state levels occur in 5 days (later in elderly or renally impaired patients). Usual therapeutic trough levels are 1.0 to 1.5 mEq/L (acute mania) or 0.6 to 1.2 mEq/L (maintenance). 300 mg = 8 mEq or mmol. A dose increase of 300 mg/day will increase the level by approx 0.2 mEq/L. Monitor renal and thyroid function, avoid dehydration or salt restriction, and watch closely for polydipsia or polyuria. Diuretics, ACE inhibitors, angiotensin receptor blockers, and NSAIDs may increase lithium levels (aspirin and sulindac OK). Dose-related side effects (eg, tremor, GI upset) may improve by dividing doses three to four times per day or using extended-release tabs. Monitor renal function and electrolytes. Brand name Eskalith no longer available.

LITHIUM (*cont.*)

MOA — Unknown, may increase synthesis and release of serotonin and inhibit its reuptake.

ADVERSE EFFECTS — Serious: Seizures, ventricular arrhythmias, leukocytosis, hypothyroidism, renal failure, nephrogenic diabetes insipidus, coma, drug-induced parkinsonism. Frequent: Tremor, N/V, diarrhea, cramps, polyuria, polydipsia, rash, fatigue.

TOPIRAMATE (*Topamax*) ▶K ♀D ▶? $$$$$

WARNING — Recent data suggest an increased risk of suicidal ideation or behaviors with antiepileptic drugs. Monitor closely for signs of depression, anxiety, hostility, and hypomania/mania. Symptoms may develop within 1 week of initiation and risk continues through at least 24 weeks.

ADULT — See entry in neurology section.

PEDS — Not approved for psychiatric use in children; see Neurology section.

UNAPPROVED ADULT — Bipolar disorder: Start 25 to 50 mg/day PO; titrate prn to max 400 mg/day divided bid. Alcohol dependence: Start 25 mg/day PO; titrate weekly to max 150 mg bid.

FORMS — Generic/Trade: Tabs 25, 50, 100, 200 mg. Sprinkle Caps 15, 25 mg.

NOTES — Give ½ usual adult dose to patients with renal impairment (CrCl < 70 mL/min). Cognitive symptoms, confusion, renal stones, glaucoma, and wt loss may occur. Risk of oligohidrosis and hyperthermia, particularly in children; use caution in warm ambient temperatures and/or with vigorous physical activity. Hyperchloremic, nonanion gap metabolic acidosis may occur; monitor serum bicarbonate and reduce dose or taper off if this occurs. Report fetal exposure to North American Antiepileptic Drug Pregnancy Registry (888-233-2334). May increase the risk of hyperammonemia if used with valproic acid.

MOA — Unknown, but may modulate sodium channels and enhance GABA action. Weak carbonic anhydrase inhibitor.

ADVERSE EFFECTS — Serious: Angle closure glaucoma, visual field defects, nephrolithiasis, oligohidrosis, hyperthermia, metabolic acidosis. Frequent: Sedation, ataxia, psychomotor slowing, cognitive symptoms, confusion, diplopia, nystagmus, dizziness, depression, nervousness, weight loss, paresthesia.

VALPROIC ACID (*Depakote, Depakote ER, Stavzor, divalproex, ✱Epival*) ▶L ♀D ▶+ $$$$

WARNING — Fatal hepatic failure has occurred, especially in children younger than 2 yo with multiple anticonvulsants and comorbidities. Monitor LFTs frequently during first 6 months. Life-threatening pancreatitis has been reported after initial or prolonged use. Evaluate for abdominal pain, N/V, and/or anorexia and discontinue if pancreatitis occurs. May be more teratogenic than other anticonvulsants (eg, carbamazepine, lamotrigine, and phenytoin). Hepatic failure and clotting disorders have also occurred when used during pregnancy. Recent data suggest an increased risk of suicidal ideation or behaviors with antiepileptic drugs. Monitor closely for signs of depression, anxiety, hostility, and hypomania/mania. Symptoms may develop within 1 week of initiation and risk continues through at least 24 weeks. Life-threatening pancreatitis has been reported.

ADULT — Mania: Start 250 mg PO three times per day (Depakote or Stavzor) or 25 mg/kg once daily (Depakote ER); titrate to therapeutic level. Max 60 mg/kg/day.

PEDS — Not approved for mania in children.

UNAPPROVED PEDS — Bipolar disorder, manic or mixed phase (age older than 2 yo): Start 125 to 250 mg PO two times per day or 15 mg/kg/day in divided doses. Titrate to therapeutic trough level of 45 to 125 mcg/mL, max 60 mg/kg/day.

FORMS — Generic only: Syrup (Valproic acid) 250 mg/5 mL. Generic/Trade: Delayed-release tabs (Depakote) 125, 250, 500 mg. Extended-release tabs (Depakote ER) 250, 500 mg. Delayed-release sprinkle caps (Depakote) 125 mg. Trade only (Stavzor): Delayed-release caps 125, 250, 500 mg.

NOTES — Contraindicated in urea cycle disorders or hepatic dysfunction. Reduce dose in the elderly. Recommended therapeutic trough level is 50 to 125 mcg/mL for Depakote and 85 to 125 mcg/mL for Depakote ER, though higher levels have been used. Many drug interactions. Hyperammonemia, GI irritation, or thrombocytopenia may occur. Depakote ER is approximately 10% less bioavailable than Depakote. Depakote-releases divalproex sodium over 8 to 12 h (one to four times per day dosing) and Depakote ER-releases divalproex sodium over 18 to 24 h (daily dosing). Concurrent use of topiramate may increase risk of hyperammonemia. Contraindicated for use in patients with genetic mutations in mitochondrial DNA polymerase gamma.

MOA — Anticonvulsant; may increase GABA levels and modulate sodium channels.

ADVERSE EFFECTS — Serious: Hepatotoxicity, anaphylaxis, polycystic ovarian syndrome, bone marrow suppression, thrombocytopenia, pancreatitis, Stevens-Johnson syndrome, hyperammonemia, drug-induced parkinsonism. Frequent: N/V, diarrhea, dyspepsia, weight gain, CNS depression, drowsiness, dizziness, tremor, alopecia, rash, nystagmus.

PSYCHIATRY: Antipsychotics—First Generation (Typical)

ANTIPSYCHOTIC RELATIVE ADVERSE EFFECTS[a]

Gene-ration	Antipsychotic	Anti-cholinergic	Sedation	Hypo-tension	EPS	Weight Gain	Diabetes/Hyper-glycemia	Dyslipi-demia
1st	chlorpromazine	+++	+++	++	++	++	?	?
1st	fluphenazine	++	+	+	++++	++	?	?
1st	haloperidol	+	+	+	++++	++	0	?
1st	loxapine	++	+	+	++	+	?	?
1st	molindone	++	++	+	++	+	?	?
1st	perphenazine	++	++	+	++	+	+/?	?
1st	pimozide	+	+	+	+++	?	?	?
1st	thioridazine	++++	+++	+++	+	+++	+/?	?
1st	thiothixene	+	++	++	+++	++	?	/
1st	trifluoperazine	++	+	+	+++	++	?	?
2nd	aripiprazole	++	+	0	0	0/+	0	0
2nd	asenapine	+	+	++	++	+	?	?
2nd	clozapine	++++	+++	+++	0	+++	+	+
2nd	lurasidone	+	+	+	+	=/-	?	?
2nd	iloperidone	++	+	+++	+	++	?	?
2nd	olanzapine	+++	++	+	0[b]	+++	+	+
2nd	paliperidone	+	+	++	++	++	?	?
2nd	risperidone	+	++	+	+[b]	++	?	?
2nd	quetiapine	+	+++	++	0	++	?	?
2nd	ziprasidone	+	+	0	0	/0	0	0

[a]Risk of specific adverse effects is graded from 0 (absent) to ++++ (high). ? = Limited or inconsistent comparative data.

NOTE: Antipsychotic potency is determined by affinity for D2 receptors. Extrapyramidal side effects (EPS) including tardive dyskinesia and dystonia may occur with antipsychotics. Use cautiously in patients with Parkinson’s disease. High-potency agents are more likely to cause EPS and hyperprolactinemia. Can be given at bedtime, but may be divided initially to decrease side effects and daytime sedation. Antipsychotics have been associated with an increased risk of venous thromboembolism, especially early in therapy. Assess for other risk factors and monitor carefully. Off-label use for dementia-related psychosis in the elderly has been associated with increased mortality. Newborns exposed during the third trimester are at increased risk for abnormal muscle movements (EPS) and withdrawal symptoms.

CHLORPROMAZINE ▶LK ♀C ▶– $$$
ADULT — Psychotic disorders: 10 to 50 mg PO two to three times per day or 25 to 50 mg IM, can repeat in 1 h. Severe cases may require 400 mg IM q 4 to 6 h up to maximum of 2000 mg/day IM. Intractable Hiccups: 25 to 50 mg PO/IM three to four times per day. Persistent hiccups may require 25 to 50 mg in 0.5 to 1 liter NS by slow IV infusion.
PEDS — Severe behavioral problems/psychotic disorders age 6 mo to 12 yo: 0.5 mg/kg PO q 4 to 6 h prn or 1 mg/kg PR q 6 to 8 h prn or 0.5 mg/kg IM q 6 to 8 h prn.

FORMS — Generic only: Tabs 10, 25, 50, 100, 200 mg. Generic/Trade: Oral concentrate 30 mg/mL, 100 mg/mL. Trade only: Syrup 10 mg/5 mL, Supps 25, 100 mg.
NOTES — Monitor for hypotension with IM or IV use. Brand name Thorazine no longer available.
MOA — Low-potency dopamine antagonist.
ADVERSE EFFECTS — Serious: Seizures, neuroleptic malignant syndrome, extrapyramidal side effects, tardive dyskinesia, QT prolongation, jaundice. Frequent: Drowsiness, nausea, dry mouth, constipation, urinary retention, hypotension, headache, hyperprolactinemia.

FLUPENTHIXOL (*flupenthixol, ❋Fluanxol, Fluanxol Depot*) ▶? ♀? ▶– $$
ADULT — Canada only. Schizophrenia/psychosis: Tabs initial dose: 3 mg PO daily in divided doses, maintenance 3 to 12 mg daily in divided doses. IM initial dose 5 to 20 mg IM q 2 to 4 weeks, maintenance 20 to 40 mg q 2 to 4 weeks. Higher doses may be necessary in some patients.
PEDS — Not approved in children.
FORMS — Trade only: Tabs 0.5, 3 mg.
NOTES — Relatively nonsedating antipsychotic.
MOA — High-potency dopamine receptor antagonist.
ADVERSE EFFECTS — Serious: NMS, tardive dyskinesia. Frequent: Extrapyramidal reactions, restlessness, agitation.

FLUPHENAZINE (❋Modecate) ▶LK ♀C ▶? $$$
ADULT — Psychotic disorders: Start 0.5 to 10 mg/day PO divided q 6 to 8 h. Usual effective dose 1 to 20 mg/day. Maximum dose is 40 mg/day PO or 1.25 to 10 mg/day IM divided q 6 to 8 h. Maximum dose is 10 mg/day IM. May use long-acting formulations (enanthate/decanoate) when patients are stabilized on a fixed daily dose. Approximate conversion ratio: 12.5 to 25 mg IM/SC (depot) q 3-6 weeks is equivalent to 10 to 20 mg/day PO.
PEDS — Not approved in children.
FORMS — Generic/Trade: Tabs 1, 2.5, 5, 10 mg. Elixir 2.5 mg/5 mL. Oral concentrate 5 mg/mL.
NOTES — Do not mix oral concentrate with coffee, tea, cola, or apple juice. Brand name Prolixin no longer available .
MOA — High-potency dopamine antagonist.
ADVERSE EFFECTS — Serious: Seizures, neuroleptic malignant syndrome, agranulocytosis, aplastic anemia, extrapyramidal side effects, tardive dyskinesia, QT prolongation. Frequent: Drowsiness, nausea, dry mouth, constipation, urinary retention, hypotension, headache, hyperprolactinemia.

HALOPERIDOL (*Haldol*) ▶LK ♀C ▶– $$
ADULT — Psychotic disorders/Tourette syndrome: 0.5 to 5 mg PO two to three times per day. Usual effective dose is 6 to 20 mg/day, maximum dose is 100 mg/day or 2 to 5 mg IM q 1 to 8 h prn. May use long-acting (depot) formulation when patients are stabilized on a fixed daily dose. Approximate conversion ratio: 100 to 200 mg IM (depot) q 4 weeks is equivalent to 10 mg/day PO haloperidol.
PEDS — Psychotic disorders age 3 to 12 yo: 0.05 to 0.15 mg/kg/day PO divided two to three times per day. Tourette syndrome or nonpsychotic behavior disorders age 3 to 12 yo: 0.05 to 0.075 mg/kg/day PO divided two to three times per day. Increase dose by 0.5 mg q week to maximum dose of 6 mg/day. Not approved for IM administration in children.
UNAPPROVED ADULT — Acute psychosis and combative behavior: 5 to 10 mg IV/IM, repeat prn in 10 to 30 min. IV route associated with QT prolongation, torsades de pointes, and sudden death; use ECG monitoring.
UNAPPROVED PEDS — Psychosis age 6 to 12 yo: 1 to 3 mg/dose IM (as lactate) q 4 to 8 h, max 0.15 mg/kg/day.

FORMS — Generic only: Tabs 0.5, 1, 2, 5, 10, 20 mg. Oral concentrate 2 mg/mL.
NOTES — Therapeutic range is 2 to 15 ng/mL.
MOA — High-potency dopamine antagonist.
ADVERSE EFFECTS — Serious: Seizures, neuroleptic malignant syndrome, extrapyramidal side effects, tardive dyskinesia, QT prolongation, sudden death, jaundice. Frequent: Drowsiness, nausea, dry mouth, constipation, urinary retention, hypotension, headache, hyperprolactinemia.

LOXAPINE (*Loxitane, ❋Loxapac*) ▶LK ♀C ▶– $$$$
ADULT — Psychotic disorders: Start 10 mg PO two times per day, usual effective dose is 60 to 100 mg/day divided two to four times per day. Maximum dose is 250 mg/day.
PEDS — Not approved in children.
FORMS — Generic/Trade: Caps 5, 10, 25, 50 mg.
MOA — Mid-potency dopamine antagonist.
ADVERSE EFFECTS — Serious: Seizures, neuroleptic malignant syndrome, extrapyramidal side effects, tardive dyskinesia, QT prolongation, jaundice. Frequent: Drowsiness, nausea, dry mouth, constipation, urinary retention, hypotension, headache, hyperprolactinemia.

METHOTRIMEPRAZINE ▶L ♀? ▶? $
ADULT — Canada only. Anxiety/analgesia: 6 to 25 mg PO per day given three times per day. Sedation: 10 to 25 mg bedtime. Psychoses/intense pain: Start 50 to 75 mg PO per day given in 2 to 3 doses, max 1000 mg/day. Postop pain: 20 to 40 mg PO or 10 to 25 mg IM q 8 h. Anesthesia premedication: 10 to 25 mg IM or 20 to 40 mg PO q 8 h with last dose of 25 to 50 mg IM 1 h before surgery. Limit therapy to less than 30 days.
PEDS — Canada only. 0.25 mg/kg/day given in 2 to 3 doses, max 40 mg/day for child age younger than 12 yo.
FORMS — Canada only: Generic/Trade: Tabs 2, 5, 25, 50 mg.
MOA — Mid-potency dopamine antagonist.
ADVERSE EFFECTS — Serious: QT interval prolongation, neuroleptic malignant syndrome, tardive dyskinesia, orthostatic hypotension, agranulocytosis, jaundice. Frequent: Drowsiness, dry mouth, nausea, constipation, urinary retention, tachycardia, weight gain.

PERPHENAZINE ▶LK ♀C ▶? $$$
ADULT — Psychotic disorders: Start 4 to 8 mg PO three times per day or 8 to 16 mg PO two to four times per day (hospitalized patients), maximum PO dose is 64 mg/day. Can give 5 to 10 mg IM q 6 h, maximum IM dose is 30 mg/day.
PEDS — Not approved in children.
FORMS — Generic only: Tabs 2, 4, 8, 16 mg. Oral concentrate 16 mg/5 mL.
NOTES — Do not mix oral concentrate with coffee, tea, cola, or apple juice.
MOA — High-potency dopamine antagonist.
ADVERSE EFFECTS — Serious: Seizures, neuroleptic malignant syndrome, extrapyramidal side effects, tardive dyskinesia, QT prolongation, jaundice. Frequent: Drowsiness, nausea, dry mouth, constipation, urinary retention, hypotension, headache, hyperprolactinemia.

PIMOZIDE (*Orap*) ▶L ♀C ▶– $$$

ADULT — Tourette syndrome: Start 1 to 2 mg/day PO in divided doses, increase q 2 days to usual effective dose of 1 to 10 mg/day. Maximum dose is 0.2 mg/kg/day up to 10 mg/day.

PEDS — Tourette syndrome: older than 12 yo: 0.05 mg/kg PO at bedtime, increase q 3 days to maximum of 0.2 mg/kg/day up to 10 mg/day.

FORMS — Trade only: Tabs 1, 2 mg.

NOTES — QT prolongation may occur. Monitor ECG at baseline and periodically throughout therapy. Contraindicated with macrolide antibiotics, nefazodone, sertraline, citalopram, and escitalopram. Use caution with inhibitors of CYP3A4 and contraindicated with strong inhibitors.

MOA — High-potency dopamine antagonist.

ADVERSE EFFECTS — Serious: Seizures, neuroleptic malignant syndrome, extrapyramidal side effects, tardive dyskinesia, QT prolongation, jaundice. Frequent: Drowsiness, nausea, dry mouth, constipation, urinary retention, hypotension, headache, hyperprolactinemia.

THIORIDAZINE ▶LK ♀C ▶? $$

WARNING — Can cause QTc prolongation, torsade de pointes–type arrhythmias, and sudden death.

ADULT — Psychotic disorders: Start 50 to 100 mg PO three times per day, usual effective dose is 200 to 800 mg/day divided two to four times per day. Maximum dose is 800 mg/day.

PEDS — Behavioral disorders 2 to 12 yo: 10 to 25 mg PO two to three times per day, maximum dose is 3 mg/kg/day.

FORMS — Generic only: Tabs 10, 15, 25, 50, 100, 150, 200 mg. Oral concentrate 30, 100 mg/mL.

NOTES — Not recommended as 1st-line therapy. Contraindicated in patients with a history of cardiac arrhythmias, congenital long QT syndrome, or those taking fluvoxamine, propranolol, pindolol, drugs that inhibit CYP2D6 (eg, fluoxetine, paroxetine), and other drugs that prolong the QTc interval. Only use for patients with schizophrenia who do not respond to other antipsychotics. Monitor baseline ECG and potassium. Pigmentary retinopathy with doses greater than 800 mg/day. Brand name Mellaril no longer available.

MOA — Low-potency dopamine antagonist.

ADVERSE EFFECTS — Serious: Seizures, neuroleptic malignant syndrome, extrapyramidal side effects, tardive dyskinesia, QT prolongation, jaundice. Frequent: Drowsiness, nausea, dry mouth, constipation, urinary retention, hypotension, headache, hyperprolactinemia.

THIOTHIXENE ▶LK ♀C ▶? $$$

ADULT — Psychotic disorders: Start 2 mg PO three times per day. Usual effective dose is 20 to 30 mg/day, maximum dose is 60 mg/day PO.

PEDS — Adolescents: Adult dosing. Not approved in children younger than 12 yo.

FORMS — Generic/Trade: Caps 1, 2, 5, 10. Oral concentrate 5 mg/mL. Trade only: Caps 20 mg.

NOTES — Brand name Navane no longer available.

MOA — High-potency dopamine antagonist.

ADVERSE EFFECTS — Serious: Seizures, neuroleptic malignant syndrome, orthostatic hypotension, hyperglycemia, dysphagia, jaundice, dystonia. Frequent: Headache, anxiety, insomnia, N/V, lightheadedness, somnolence, akathisia, constipation, weight gain.

TRIFLUOPERAZINE ▶LK ♀C ▶– $$$

ADULT — Psychotic disorders: Start 2 to 5 mg PO two times per day. Usual effective dose is 15 to 20 mg/day, some patients may require 40 mg/day or more. Anxiety: 1 to 2 mg PO two times per day for up to 12 weeks. Maximum dose is 6 mg/day.

PEDS — Psychotic disorders age 6 to 12 yo: 1 mg PO one to two times per day, gradually increase to maximum dose of 15 mg/day.

FORMS — Generic/Trade: Tabs 1, 2, 5, 10 mg. Trade only: Oral concentrate 10 mg/mL.

NOTES — Dilute oral concentrate just before giving.

MOA — High-potency dopamine antagonist.

ADVERSE EFFECTS — Serious: Seizures, neuroleptic malignant syndrome, extrapyramidal side effects, tardive dyskinesia, QT prolongation, jaundice. Frequent: Drowsiness, nausea, dry mouth, constipation, urinary retention, hypotension, headache, hyperprolactinemia.

ZUCLOPENTHIXOL (✱ *Clopixol, Clopixol Depot, Clopixol Accuphase*) ▶L ♀? ▶? $$$$

ADULT — Canada only. Antipsychotic. Tabs: Start 10 to 50 mg PO daily, maintenance 20 to 60 mg daily. Injectable: Accuphase (acetate) 50 to 150 mg IM q 2 to 3 days, Depot (decanoate) 150 to 300 mg IM q 2 to 4 weeks.

PEDS — Not approved in children.

FORMS — Trade, Canada-only: Tabs 10, 20 mg (Clopixol).

MOA — Low-potency dopamine antagonist.

ADVERSE EFFECTS — Serious: NMS, tardive dyskinesia. Frequent: Extrapyramidal reactions, drowsiness, dizziness.

PSYCHIATRY: Antipsychotics—Second Generation (Atypical)

NOTE: Tardive dyskinesia, neuroleptic malignant syndrome, drug-induced parkinsonism, dystonia, and other extrapyramidal side effects may occur with antipsychotic medications. Atypical antipsychotics have been associated with wt gain, dyslipidemia, hyperglycemia, and diabetes mellitus; monitor closely. Off-label use for dementia-related psychosis in the elderly has been associated with increased mortality. Antipsychotics have been associated with an increased risk of venous thromboembolism, particularly early in therapy; assess for other risk factors and monitor carefully. Antipsychotics when used for schizophrenia or bipolar disorder have been associated with an increased risk of suicidal thinking and behavior. Monitor closely.

ARIPIPRAZOLE (*Abilify, Abilify Discmelt, Abilify Maintena*) ▶L ♀C ▷? $$$$$
WARNING — Antipsychotics when used for schizophrenia or bipolar disorder have been associated with an increased risk of suicidal thinking and behavior. Monitor closely.
ADULT — Schizophrenia: Start 10 to 15 mg PO daily. Max 30 mg daily. Schizophrenia, maintenance (Maintena): Start 400 mg IM monthly. May reduce to 300 mg IM monthly if adverse reactions to higher dose. Bipolar disorder (acute and maintenance for manic or mixed episodes): Start 30 mg PO daily; reduce dose to 15 mg/day if higher dose poorly tolerated. May increase to 30 mg/day based on response and tolerability. Agitation associated with schizophrenia or bipolar disorder: 9.75 mg IM recommended. May consider 5.25 to 15 mg if indicated. May repeat after 2 h up to max 30 mg/day. Depression, adjunctive therapy: Start 2 to 5 mg PO daily. Increase by 5 mg/day at intervals 1 week or more to max of 15 mg/day.
PEDS — Schizophrenia, 13 to 17 yo: Start 2 mg PO daily. May increase to 5 mg/day after 2 days, and to target dose of 10 mg/day after 2 more days. Max 30 mg/day. Bipolar disorder (acute and maintenance for manic or mixed episodes, monotherapy or adjunctive to lithium or valproate), 10 to 17 yo: Start 2 mg PO daily. May increase to 5 mg/day after 2 days, and to target dose of 10 mg/day after 2 more days. Increase by 5 mg/day to max 30 mg/day. Irritability associated with autism: Start 2 mg PO daily. Increase by 5 mg/day prn at weekly intervals up to max 15 mg/day.
FORMS — Trade only: Tabs 2, 5, 10, 15, 20, 30 mg. Oral soln 1 mg/mL (150 mL). Orally disintegrating tabs (Discmelt) 10 and 15 mg. Sol for injection 9.75 mg/1.3 mL. Susp extended release for Injection (Abilify Maintena) 300 mg and 400 mg/vial.
NOTES — Low EPS and tardive dyskinesia risk. Increase dose when used with CYP3A4 inducers such as carbamazepine. Decrease usual dose by at least half when used with CYP3A4 or CYP2D6 inhibitors such as ketoconazole, fluoxetine, or paroxetine. Increase dose by ½ to 20 to 30 mg/day when used with CYP3A4 inducers such as carbamazepine. Reduce when inducer is stopped. Establish tolerability to oral aripiprazole prior to initiating long-acting IM formulation. Continue oral aripiprazole for 14 days after first dose of long-acting IM form and then discontinue. Avoid use of CYP3A4 inducers for more than 14 days with long-acting IM form. Dose adjustments required when used with CYP2D6 or 3A4 inhibitors. See PI.
MOA — Dopamine-2 partial agonist, serotonin-1A partial agonist, serotoin-2A antagonist.
ADVERSE EFFECTS — Serious: Seizures, neuroleptic malignant syndrome, orthostatic hypotension, hyperglycemia, dysphagia, jaundice, suicidal thinking/behavior. Frequent: Headache, anxiety, insomnia, N/V, lightheadedness, somnolence, akathisia, constipation, weight gain.

ASENAPINE (*Saphris*) ▶L ♀C ▷–
WARNING — Antipsychotics when used for schizophrenia or bipolar disorder have been associated with an increased risk of suicidal thinking and behavior. Monitor closely.
ADULT — Schizophrenia: Initial and maintenance, 5 mg sublingual two times per day. Max 20 mg/day. Bipolar disorder, acute manic or mixed episodes: Start 5 mg sublingual two times per day (adjunctive) or 10 mg sublingual two times per day (monotherapy). Max 20 mg/day.
PEDS — Not approved for use in children
FORMS — Trade: Sublingual tabs 5, 10 mg
NOTES — Must be used sublingually and not chewed or crushed.
MOA — Serotonin and dopamine receptor antagonist.
ADVERSE EFFECTS — Serious: Neuroleptic malignant syndrome, tardive dyskinesia, hyperglycemia/diabetes, syncope, orthostatic hypotension, leukopenia, neutropenia, agranulocytosis, seizures. Frequent: Akathisia, EPS, oral hypoesthesia, somnolence, dizziness, weight gain.

CLOZAPINE (*Clozaril, FazaClo ODT, Versacloz*) ▶L ♀B ▷– $$$$$
WARNING — Risk of agranulocytosis is 1 to 2%, monitor WBC and ANC counts q week for 6 months, then q 2 weeks thereafter, and weekly for 4 weeks after discontinuation. Contraindicated if WBC less than 3500 or ANC less than 2000/mm³. Discontinue if WBC less than 3000/mm³. May decrease monitoring to q 4 weeks after 12 months if WBC greater than 3500/mm³ and ANC greater than 2000/mm³. See prescribing information for more details. Risk of myocarditis (particularly during the first month), seizures, orthostatic hypotension, and cardiopulmonary arrest. Antipsychotics when used for schizophrenia or bipolar disorder have been associated with an increased risk of suicidal thinking and behavior. Monitor closely.
ADULT — Severe, medically refractory schizophrenia or schizophrenia/schizoaffective disorder with suicidal behavior: Start 12.5 mg PO one or two times per day; increase by 25 to 50 mg/day to usual effective dose of 300 to 450 mg/day, max 900 mg/day. Retitrate if stopped for more than 3 to 4 days.
PEDS — Not approved in children.
FORMS — Generic/Trade: Tabs 25, 100 mg. Generic only: Tabs 12.5, 50, 200 mg. Oral disintegrating tabs 12.5, 25, 100 mg Trade only: Orally disintegrating tab (Fazaclo ODT) 12.5, 25, 100, 150, 200 mg (scored). Susp (Versacloz): 50 mg/mL.
NOTES — Patients rechallenged with clozapine after an episode of leukopenia are at increased risk of agranulocytosis, and must undergo weekly monitoring for 12 months. Register all occurrences of leukopenia, discontinuation, and/or rechallenge to the Clozaril National Registry at 1-800-448-5938. Much lower risk of EPS and tardive dyskinesia than other neuroleptics. May be effective for treatment-resistant patients who have not responded to conventional agents. May cause significant wt gain, dyslipidemia, hyperglycemia, or new onset diabetes; monitor wt, fasting blood glucose, and triglycerides before initiation and at regular intervals during treatment. Excessive sedation or respiratory

CLOZAPINE (*cont.*)

depression may occur when used with CNS depressants, particularly benzodiazepines. If an orally disintegrating tab is split, then discard the remaining portion.
MOA — Dopamine receptor antagonist; 5-HT2A receptor antagonist.
ADVERSE EFFECTS — Serious: Agranulocytosis, leukopenia, seizures, hyperglycemia, diabetes, dyslipidemia, neuroleptic malignant syndrome, hepatotoxicity, QT prolongation, orthostatic hypotension, syncope, cardiopulmonary arrest, myocarditis, cardiomyopathy. Frequent: Drowsiness, weight gain, N/V, dry mouth, constipation, tachycardia, hypersalivation.

ILOPERIDONE (*Fanapt*) ▶L ♀C ▶– ?

ADULT — Schizophrenia, acute: Start 1 mg PO two times per day. Increase to 2 mg PO two times per day on day 2, then increase total daily dose by 2 mg/dose each day to usual effective range of 6 to 12 mg PO two times per day. Max 24 mg/day.
PEDS — Not approved in children.
FORMS — Trade: Tabs 1, 2, 4, 6, 8, 10, 12 mg.
NOTES — Dose must be titrated slowly to avoid orthostatic hypotension. Retitrate the dose if off the drug more than 3 days. Reduce dose by 50% if given with strong inhibitors of CYP2D6 or CYP3A4. Avoid use with other drugs that prolong the QT interval. Fanapt is not recommended for patients with severe hepatic impairment.
MOA — Receptor antagonist; 5-HT2A receptor antagonist.
ADVERSE EFFECTS — Serious: Neuroleptic malignant syndrome, ventricular arrhythmias, tardive dyskinesia, hyperglycemia/diabetes, lipid abnormalities, seizures, orthostatic hypotension. Frequent: Dizziness, dry mouth, fatigue, nasal congestion, somnolence, tachycardia, weight gain.

LURASIDONE (*Latuda*) ▶K – ♀B ▶?

ADULT — Schizophrenia: Start 40 mg PO daily. Effective dose range 40-160 mg/day, max 160 mg/day. Reduce starting dose to 20 mg PO daily if moderate to severe renal or hepatic insufficiency or use with moderate CYP3A4 inhibitors, max 80 mg/day unless severe hepatic insufficiency which is 40 mg/day. Depression associated with bipolar I disorder (monotherapy or adjunctive with lithium or valproate): Start 20 mg PO daily. Usual range 20-120 mg/day. Doses greater than 20-60 mg/day did not provide further efficacy as monotherapy.
PEDS — Not approved for use in children.
FORMS — Trade only: Tabs 20, 40, 60, 80, 120 mg.
NOTES — Take with a meal of at least 350 Cal. Do not use with strong CYP3A4 inhibitors or inducers. Reduce dose if used with moderate inhibitors.
MOA — Dopamine-2/serotonin 2A antagonist
ADVERSE EFFECTS — Serious: Neuroleptic malignant syndrome, hyperglycemia, diabetes, tardive dyskinesia, hyperlipidemia, hyperprolactinemia, leukopenia, neutropenia, agranulocytosis, orthostatic hypotension, syncope. Frequent: Parkinsonism, akathisia, somnolence, nausea, agitation.

OLANZAPINE (*Zyprexa, Zyprexa Zydis, Zyprexa Relprevv*) ▶L ♀C ▶– $$$$$

WARNING — Antipsychotics when used for schizophrenia or bipolar disorder have been associated with an increased risk of suicidal thinking and behavior. Monitor closely.
ADULT — Agitation in acute bipolar mania or schizophrenia: Start 10 mg IM (2.5 to 5 mg in elderly or debilitated patients); may repeat after 2 h to max 30 mg/day. Schizophrenia, oral therapy: Start 5 to 10 mg PO daily. Increase weekly to usual effective dose of 10 to 15 mg/day, max 20 mg/day. Schizophrenia, extended release injection: Dose based on prior oral dose and ranges from 150 mg to 300 mg deep IM (gluteal) q 2 weeks or 300 mg to 405 mg q 4 weeks. See prescribing information. Bipolar disorder, maintenance treatment or monotherapy for acute manic or mixed episodes: Start 10 to 15 mg PO daily. Increase by 5 mg/day at intervals after 24 h. Clinical efficacy seen at doses of 5 to 20 mg/day, max 20 mg/day. Bipolar disorder, adjunctive therapy for acute mixed or manic episodes: Start 10 mg PO daily; usual effective dose is 5 to 20 mg/day, max 20 mg/day. Bipolar depression, olanzapine + fluoxetine: Start 5 mg olanzapine + 20 mg fluoxetine daily in the evening. Increase to usual range of 5 to 12.5 mg olanzapine plus 20 to 50 mg fluoxetine as tolerated. Treatment-resistant depression, olanzapine + fluoxetine: Start 5 mg olanzapine + 20 mg fluoxetine daily in the evening. Increase to usual range of 5 to 20 mg olanzapine plus 20 to 50 mg fluoxetine as tolerated.
PEDS — Schizophrenia and bipolar manic or mixed episodes (13 to 17 yo): Start 2.5 to 5 mg PO once daily. Increase to target of 10 mg/day. Max 20 mg/day. Bipolar depression, olanzapine + fluoxetine (Symbyax): Start 3mg/25 mg (olanzapine/fluoxetine) and increase as needed or tolerated to max 12 mg/50 mg.
UNAPPROVED ADULT — Augmentation of SSRI therapy for OCD: Start 2.5 to 5 mg PO daily, max 20 mg/day. Posttraumatic stress disorder, adjunctive therapy: Start 5 mg PO daily, max 20 mg/day.
UNAPPROVED PEDS — Bipolar disorder, manic or mixed phase: Start 2.5 mg PO daily; increase by 2.5 mg/day q 3 days to max 20 mg/day.
FORMS — Generic/Trade: Tabs 2.5, 5, 7.5, 10, 15, 20 mg. Tabs orally disintegrating (Zyprexa Zydis) 5, 10, 15, 20 mg. Trade only: Long-acting injection (Zyprexa Relprevv) 210, 300, 405 mg/vial.
NOTES — Use for acute manic episodes associated with bipolar disorder. Must be given with meals of at least 500 kcal. May cause significant wt gain, dyslipidemia, hyperglycemia, or new onset diabetes; monitor wt, fasting blood glucose, and triglycerides before initiation and at regular intervals during treatment. Monitor for orthostatic hypotension, particularly when given IM. IM injection can also be associated with bradycardia and hypoventilation especially if used with other drugs that have these

OLANZAPINE (*cont.*)

effects. Use lower initial doses of the combination of olanzapine plus fluoxetine in patients predisposed to hypotension or those with liver disease. Use caution with benzodiazepines. Use of Zyprexa Relprevv requires registration in the Zyprexa Relprevv Patient Care Program 1-877-772-9390.

MOA — Dopamine receptor antagonist; 5-HT2A receptor antagonist.

ADVERSE EFFECTS — Serious: Seizures, orthostatic hypotension, syncope, hyperglycemia, diabetes, dyslipidemia, neuroleptic malignant syndrome, extrapyramidal side effects, QT prolongation, hepatitis, suicidal thinking/behavior. Frequent: Drowsiness, weight gain, nausea, dry mouth, constipation, dizziness.

PALIPERIDONE (*Invega, Invega Sustenna*) ▶KL ♀C ▶– $$$$$

WARNING — Antipsychotics when used for schizophrenia or bipolar disorder have been associated with an increased risk of suicidal thinking and behavior. Monitor closely.

ADULT — Schizophrenia and schizoaffective disorder (adjunctive and monotherapy): Start 6 mg PO q am. 3 mg/day may be sufficient in some. Max 12 mg/day. Extended-release injection: Start 234 mg IM (deltoid) and then 156 mg IM 1 week later. Recommended monthly dose 117 mg IM (deltoid or gluteal) or within range of 39 to 234 mg based on response.

PEDS — Schizophrenia: adolescents (12-17 yrs): Start 3 mg PO once daily. Max 6 mg/day (weight less than 51 kg) or 12 mg/day (51 kg and greater). Not approved in children under 12 yrs.

FORMS — Trade only: Extended-release tabs 1.5, 3, 6, 9 mg.

NOTES — Active metabolite of risperidone. For CrCl 50 to 79 mL/min start 3 mg/day with a max of 6 mg/day. For CrCl 10 to 50 mL/min start 1.5 mg/day with a max of 3 mg/day. Refer to PI for instructions if injections of the long-acting form are missed.

MOA — Dopamine receptor antagonist; 5-HT2A receptor antagonist.

ADVERSE EFFECTS — Serious: Orthostatic hypotension, syncope, QT prolongation, neuroleptic malignant syndrome, tardive dyskinesia, hyperglycemia, diabetes, stroke, extrapyramidal symptoms, suicidal thinking/behavior. Frequent: Drowsiness, salivary hypersecretion, tachycardia, akathisia, dystonia, hypertonia, parkinsonism, weight gain, dyspepsia, dizziness, headache, anxiety.

QUETIAPINE (*Seroquel, Seroquel XR*) ▶LK ♀C ▶– $$$$

WARNING — Antipsychotics when used for schizophrenia or bipolar disorder have been associated with an increased risk of suicidal thinking and behavior. Monitor closely.

ADULT — Schizophrenia: Start 25 mg PO two times per day (regular tabs); increase by 25 to 50 mg two to three times per day on days 2 and 3, and then to target dose of 300 to 400 mg/day divided two to three times per day on day 4. Usual effective dose is 150 to 750 mg/day, max 800 mg/day. Schizophrenia, extended-release tabs: Start 300

mg PO daily in evening, increase by up to 300 mg/day at intervals of more than 1 day to usual effective range of 400 to 800 mg/day. Acute bipolar mania, monotherapy or adjunctive: Start 50 mg PO two times per day on day 1, then increase to no higher than 100 mg two times per day on day 2, 150 mg two times per day on day 3, and 200 mg two times per day on day 4. May increase prn to 300 mg two times per day on day 5 and 400 mg two times per day thereafter. Usual effective dose is 400 to 800 mg/day. Acute bipolar mania, monotherapy or adjunctive, extended-release: Start 300 mg PO in evening on day 1, 600 mg day 2, and 400 to 800 mg/day thereafter. Bipolar depression, regular and extended release: 50 mg, 100 mg, 200 mg and 300 mg per day for days 1 to 4 respectively, administered at bedtime. May increase prn to 400 mg at bedtime on day 5 and 600 mg at bedtime on day 8. Bipolar maintenance: Use dose required to maintain remission of symptoms. Major depressive disorder, adjunctive to antidepressants, extended release: Start 50 mg evening of day 1, may increase to 150 mg on day 3. Max 300 mg/day.

PEDS — Schizophrenia (13 to 17 yo): Start 50 mg PO day 1, 100 mg day 2, 200 mg day 3, 300 mg day 4, and 400 mg day 5, all given two to three times per day. Recommended range 400 to 800 mg/day. Max 800 mg/day. Acute bipolar mania (10 to 17 yo): Start 50 mg PO day 1, 100 mg day 2, 200 mg day 3, 300 mg day 4, 400 mg day 5, all given two to three times per day. Recommended range 400 to 600 mg/day. Bipolar maintenance: Use dose required to maintain remission of symptoms.

UNAPPROVED ADULT — Augmentation of SSRI therapy for OCD: Start 25 mg PO two times per day, max 300 mg/day. Adjunctive for posttraumatic stress disorder: Start 25 mg daily, max 300 mg/day.

UNAPPROVED PEDS — Bipolar disorder (manic or mixed phase): Start 12.5 mg PO two times per day (children) or 25 mg PO two times per day (adolescents); max 150 mg PO three times per day.

FORMS — Generic/Trade: Tabs 25, 50, 100, 200, 300, 400 mg. Trade only: Extended-release tabs 50, 150, 200, 300, 400 mg.

NOTES — Eye exam for cataracts recommended q 6 months. Low risk of EPS and tardive dyskinesia. May cause significant wt gain, dyslipidemia, hyperglycemia, or new onset diabetes; monitor wt, fasting blood glucose, and triglycerides before initiation and at regular intervals during treatment. Use lower doses and slower titration in elderly patients or hepatic dysfunction. Extended-release tabs should be taken without food or after light meal.

MOA — Dopamine receptor antagonist; 5-HT2A receptor antagonist.

ADVERSE EFFECTS — Serious: Seizures, orthostatic hypotension, syncope, hyperglycemia, diabetes, dyslipidemia, neuroleptic malignant syndrome, QT prolongation, suicidal thinking/behavior. Frequent: Drowsiness, weight gain, nausea, dry mouth, constipation, dizziness.

RISPERIDONE (*Risperdal, Risperdal Consta, Risperdal M-Tab*) ►LK ♀C ▶– $$$$

WARNING — Antipsychotics when used for schizophrenia or bipolar disorder have been associated with an increased risk of suicidal thinking and behavior. Monitor closely.

ADULT — Schizophrenia: Start 2 mg/day PO given once daily or divided two times per day; increase by 1 to 2 mg/day at intervals of 24 h or more. Start 0.5 mg/dose and titrate by no more than 0.5 mg two times per day in elderly, debilitated, hypotensive, or renally or hepatically impaired patients; increases to doses greater than 1.5 mg two times per day should occur at intervals 1 week or more. Usual effective dose is 4 to 8 mg/day given once daily or divided two times per day; max 16 mg/day. Schizophrenia (long-acting injection, Consta): Start 25 mg IM q 2 weeks while continuing oral dose for 3 weeks. May increase q 4 weeks to max 50 mg q 2 weeks. Bipolar mania: Start 2 to 3 mg PO daily; may adjust by 1 mg/day at 24 h intervals to max 6 mg/day.

PEDS — Autistic disorder irritability (5 to 16 yo): Start 0.25 mg (wt less than 20 kg) or 0.5 mg (wt 20 kg or greater) PO daily. May increase after 4 days to 0.5 mg/day (wt less than 20 kg) or 1.0 mg/day (wt 20 kg or greater). Maintain at least 14 days. May then increase at 14-day intervals or more by increments of 0.25 mg/day (wt less than 20 kg) or 0.5 mg/day (wt 20 kg or greater) to max 1.0 mg/day for wt less than 20 kg, max 2.5 mg/day for wt 20 to 44 kg or max 3.0 mg/day for wt 45 kg or greater. Schizophrenia (13 to 17 yo): Start 0.5 mg PO daily; increase by 0.5 to 1 mg/day at intervals of 24 h or more to target dose of 3 mg/day. Max 6 mg/day. Bipolar mania (10 to 17 yo): Start 0.5 mg PO daily; increase by 0.5 to 1 mg/day at intervals of 24 h or more to recommended dose of 2.5 mg/day. Max 6 mg/day.

UNAPPROVED ADULT — Augmentation of SSRI therapy for OCD: Start 1 mg/day PO, max 6 mg/day. Adjunctive therapy for posttraumatic stress disorder: Start 0.5 mg PO at bedtime, max 3 mg/day.

UNAPPROVED PEDS — Psychotic disorders, mania, aggression: 0.5 to 1.5 mg/day PO.

FORMS — Generic/Trade: Tabs 0.25, 0.5, 1, 2, 3, 4 mg. Oral soln 1 mg/mL (30 mL). Orally disintegrating tabs 0.5, 1, 2, 3, 4 mg. Generic only: Orally disintegrating tabs 0.25 mg. Trade only: IM Injection (Risperdal Consta) 12.5, 25, 37.5, 50 mg

NOTES — Has a greater tendency to produce extrapyramidal side effects (EPS) than other atypical antipsychotics. EPS reported in neonates following use in third trimester of pregnancy. May cause wt gain, hyperglycemia, or new onset diabetes; monitor closely. Patients with Parkinson's disease and dementia have increased sensitivity to side effects such as EPS, confusion, falls, and neuroleptic malignant syndrome. Soln is compatible with water, coffee, orange juice, and low-fat milk; is not compatible with cola or tea. Place orally disintegrating tabs on tongue and do not chew. Establish tolerability with oral form before starting long-acting injection. Alternate injections between buttocks. May also give in deltoid.

MOA — Dopamine receptor antagonist; 5-HT2A receptor antagonist.

ADVERSE EFFECTS — Serious: Seizures, orthostatic hypotension, syncope, hyperglycemia, diabetes, neuroleptic malignant syndrome, tardive dyskinesia, extrapyramidal symptoms, QT prolongation, stroke, transient ischemic attack, suicidal thinking/behavior. Frequent: Drowsiness, insomnia, weight gain, N/V, dyspepsia, dry mouth, constipation, dizziness, orthostatic hypotension, agitation, anxiety, akathisia, tachycardia.

ZIPRASIDONE (*Geodon, ✦Zeldox*) ►L ♀C ▶– $$$$$

WARNING — May prolong QTc. Avoid with drugs that prolong QTc or in those with long QT syndrome or cardiac arrhythmias. Antipsychotics when used for schizophrenia or bipolar disorder have been associated with an increased risk of suicidal thinking and behavior. Monitor closely.

ADULT — Schizophrenia: Start 20 mg PO two times per day with food; may increase at greater than 2-day intervals to max 80 mg PO two times per day. Acute agitation in schizophrenia: 10 to 20 mg IM. May repeat 10 mg dose q 2 h or 20 mg dose q 4 h, to max 40 mg/day. Bipolar mania: Start 40 mg PO two times per day with food; may increase to 60 to 80 mg two times per day on day 2. Usual effective dose is 40 to 80 mg two times per day.

PEDS — Not approved in children.

FORMS — Trade/generic Caps 20, 40, 60, 80 mg Trade only: 20 mg/mL injection

NOTES — Drug interactions with carbamazepine and ketoconazole. Olanzapine may be used in combination with fluoxetine in bipolar depression. Refer to Symbyax monograph for details.

MOA — Dopamine receptor antagonist; 5-HT2A receptor antagonist.

ADVERSE EFFECTS — Serious: Seizures, orthostatic hypotension, syncope, hyperglycemia, diabetes, dyslipidemia, neuroleptic malignant syndrome, tardive dyskinesia, extrapyramidal side effects, QT prolongation, suicidal thinking/behavior. Frequent: Drowsiness, weight gain, nausea, dry mouth, constipation, dizziness.

PSYCHIATRY: Anxiolytics / Hypnotics - Barbiturates

BUTABARBITAL (*Butisol*) ►LK ♀D ▶? ©III $$$

ADULT — Rarely used; other drugs preferred. Sedative: 15 to 30 mg PO three to four times per day. Hypnotic: 50 to 100 mg PO at bedtime for up to 2 weeks.

PEDS — Preop sedation: 2 to 6 mg/kg PO before procedure, maximum 100 mg.

FORMS — Trade only: Tabs 30, 50 mg. Elixir 30 mg/5 mL.

MOA — Nonselective CNS depressant

BUTABARBITAL (*cont.*)

ADVERSE EFFECTS — Serious: Respiratory depression, blood dyscrasias, anemia, thrombocytopenia, Stevens-Johnson syndrome, angioedema, dependence, withdrawal reactions, "sleep driving". Frequent: drowsiness, fatigue, N/V bradycardia, paradoxical CNS excitation

SECOBARBITAL (*Seconal*) ▶LK ♀D ▶+ ©II $

ADULT — Rarely used; other drugs preferred. Hypnotic: 100 mg PO at bedtime for up to 2 weeks.

PEDS — Pre-anesthetic: 2 to 6 mg/kg PO up to 100 mg.

FORMS — Trade only: Caps 100 mg.

MOA — Nonselective CNS depressant

ADVERSE EFFECTS — Serious: Respiratory depression, blood dyscrasias, anemia, thrombocytopenia, Stevens-Johnson syndrome, angioedema, dependence, withdrawal reactions. Frequent: drowsiness, fatigue, N/V bradycardia, paradoxical CNS excitation

PSYCHIATRY: Anxiolytics/Hypnotics—Benzodiazepines—Long Half-Life (25-100 h)

NOTE: To avoid withdrawal, gradually taper when discontinuing after prolonged use. Use cautiously in the elderly; may accumulate and lead to side effects, psychomotor impairment. Sedative-hypnotics have been associated with severe allergic reactions and complex sleep behaviors including sleep driving. Use caution and discuss with patients.

BROMAZEPAM (✱*Lectopam*) ▶L ♀D ▶– $

ADULT — Canada only. 6 to 18 mg/day PO in equally divided doses.

PEDS — Not approved in children.

FORMS — Generic/Trade: Tabs 1.5, 3, 6 mg.

NOTES — Do not exceed 3 mg/day initially in the elderly or debilitated. Gradually taper when discontinuing after prolonged use. Half-life approximately 20 h in adults but increased in elderly. Cimetidine may prolong elimination.

MOA — Benzodiazepine; enhances actions of GABA.

ADVERSE EFFECTS — Serious: Respiratory depression, dependence, withdrawal reactions. Frequent: Sedation, ataxia, depression, confusion, tinnitus, N/V.

CHLORDIAZEPOXIDE ▶LK ♀D ▶– ©IV $$

ADULT — Anxiety: 5 to 25 mg PO three to four times per day or 25 to 50 mg IM/IV three to four times per day (acute/severe anxiety). Acute alcohol withdrawal: 50 to 100 mg PO/IM/IV, repeat q 3 to 4 h prn up to 300 mg/day.

PEDS — Anxiety, age older than 6 yo: 5 to 10 mg PO two to four times per day.

FORMS — Generic/Trade: Caps 5, 10, 25 mg.

NOTES — Half-life 5 to 30 h. Brand product Librium no longer available.

MOA — Enhances actions of GABA.

ADVERSE EFFECTS — Serious: Respiratory depression, dependence, withdrawal reactions, seizures. Frequent: Sedation, fatigue, ataxia, memory impairment, depression, confusion, nausea, constipation, dry mouth, rash.

CLONAZEPAM (*Klonopin, Klonopin Wafer, ✱Rivotril, Clonapam*) ▶LK ♀D ▶– ©IV $

ADULT — Panic disorder: 0.25 mg PO two times per day, increase by 0.125 to 0.25 mg q 3 days to maximum dose of 4 mg/day. Akinetic or myoclonic seizures: Start 0.5 mg PO three times per day. Increase by 0.5 to 1 mg q 3 days prn. Max 20 mg/day.

PEDS — Akinetic or myoclonic seizures, Lennox-Gastaut syndrome (petit mal variant), or absence seizures (10 yo or younger or 30 kg or less): 0.01 to 0.03 mg/kg/day PO divided two to three times per day. Increase by 0.25 to 0.5 mg q 3 days prn. Max 0.1 to 0.2 mg/kg/day divided three times per day.

UNAPPROVED ADULT — Neuralgias: 2 to 4 mg PO daily. Restless legs syndrome: Start 0.25 mg PO at bedtime. Max 2 mg at bedtime. REM sleep behavior disorder: 1 to 2 mg PO at bedtime.

FORMS — Generic/Trade: Tabs 0.5, 1, 2 mg. Orally disintegrating tabs (approved for panic disorder only) 0.125, 0.25, 0.5, 1, 2 mg.

NOTES — Half-life 18 to 50 h. Usual therapeutic range is 20 to 80 ng/mL. Contraindicated in hepatic failure or acute narrow angle glaucoma.

MOA — Enhances actions of GABA.

ADVERSE EFFECTS — Serious: Respiratory depression, CNS depression, dependence, withdrawal reactions, seizures. Frequent: Sedation, fatigue, ataxia, memory impairment, depression, confusion, nausea, constipation, dry mouth, rash.

CLORAZEPATE (*Tranxene*) ▶LK ♀D ▶– ©IV $$$$

ADULT — Anxiety: Start 7.5 to 15 mg PO at bedtime or two to three times per day, usual effective dose is 15 to 60 mg/day. Partial seizures, adjunctive: 13 yo and older start 7.5 mg PO three times daily. May increase by no more than 7.5 mg per week to max 90 mg/day. Acute alcohol withdrawal: 60 to 90 mg/day on 1st day divided two to three times per day, gradually reduce dose to 7.5 to 15 mg/day over 5 days. Maximum dose is 90 mg/day. May transfer patients to single-dose Tabs (Tranxene-SD) when dose stabilized.

PEDS — Partial seizures, adjunctive: Ages 9-12 yo start 7.5 mg PO twice daily. May increase by no more than 7.5 mg per week to max of 60 mg/day.

FORMS — Generic/Trade: Tabs 3.75, 7.5, 15 mg.

NOTES — Half-life 40 to 50 h.

MOA — Enhances actions of GABA.

ADVERSE EFFECTS — Serious: Respiratory depression, dependence, withdrawal reactions, seizures. Frequent: Sedation, fatigue, ataxia, memory impairment, depression, confusion, nausea, constipation, dry mouth, rash.

DIAZEPAM (*Valium, Diastat, Diastat AcuDial, Diazemuls*) ▶LK ♀D ▶– ©IV $

ADULT — Status epilepticus: 5 to 10 mg IV. Repeat q 10 to 15 min prn to max 30 mg. Epilepsy, adjunctive therapy: 2 to 10 mg PO two to four times per day. Increased seizure activity: 0.2 to 0.5 mg/kg

DIAZEPAM (*cont.*)

PR (rectal gel) to max 20 mg/day. Skeletal muscle spasm, spasticity related to cerebral palsy, paraplegia, athetosis, "stiff man syndrome": 2 to 10 mg PO/PR three to four times per day. 5 to 10 mg IM/IV initially, then 5 to 10 mg q 3 to 4 h prn. Decrease dose in elderly. Anxiety: 2 to 10 mg PO two to four times per day or 2 to 20 mg IM/IV, repeat dose in 3 to 4 h prn. Alcohol withdrawal: 10 mg PO three to four times per day for 24 h then 5 mg PO three to four times per day prn.

PEDS — Skeletal muscle spasm: 0.04 to 0.2 mg/kg/dose IV/IM q 2 to 4 h. Max dose 0.6 mg/kg within 8 h. Status epilepticus, age 1 mo to 5 yo: 0.2 to 0.5 mg IV slowly q 2 to 5 min to max 5 mg. Status epilepticus, age older than 5 yo: 1 mg IV slowly q 2 to 5 min to max 10 mg. Repeat q 2 to 4 h prn. Epilepsy, adjunctive therapy, muscle spasm, and anxiety disorders, age older than 6 mo: 1 to 2.5 mg PO three to four times per day; gradually increase as tolerated and needed. Increased seizure activity (rectal gel, age older than 2 yo): 0.5 mg/kg PR (2 to 5 yo), 0.3 mg/kg PR (6 to 11 yo), or 0.2 mg/kg PR (age older than 12 yo). Max 20 mg. May repeat in 4 to 12 h prn.

UNAPPROVED ADULT — Loading dose strategy for alcohol withdrawal: 10 to 20 mg PO or 10 mg slow IV in closely monitored setting, then repeat similar or lower doses q 1 to 2 h prn until sedated. Further doses should be unnecessary due to long half-life. Restless legs syndrome: 0.5 to 4 mg PO at bedtime.

FORMS — Generic/Trade: Tabs 2, 5, 10 mg. Rectal gel 2.5 mg ($$$$$). Generic only: Oral soln 5 mg/5 mL. Oral concentrate (Intensol) 5 mg/mL. Rectal gel 10, 20 mg ($$$$$). Trade only: Rectal gel (Diastat AcuDial-$$$$$) 10, 20 mg syringes. Available doses from 10 mg AcuDial syringe 5, 7.5, 10 mg. Available doses from 20 mg AcuDial syringe 12.5, 15, 17.5, 20 mg.

NOTES — Half-life 20 to 80 h. Respiratory and CNS depression may occur. Caution in liver disease. Abuse potential. Long half-life may increase the risk of adverse effects in the elderly. Cimetidine, oral contraceptives, disulfiram, fluoxetine, isoniazid, ketoconazole, metoprolol, propoxyphene, propranolol, and valproic acid may increase diazepam concentrations. Diazepam may increase digoxin and phenytoin concentrations. Rifampin may increase the metabolism of diazepam. Avoid combination with protease inhibitors. Diastat AcuDial is for home use and allows dosing from 5 to 20 mg in 2.5 mg increments.

MOA — Enhances actions of GABA, skeletal muscle relaxant.

ADVERSE EFFECTS — Serious: Respiratory depression, oversedation, dependence, withdrawal reactions, cardiovascular collapse (parenteral), vascular impairment or venous thrombosis (IV only), seizures. Frequent: Sedation, ataxia, CNS stimulation, depression, N/V, constipation or diarrhea, confusion, tinnitus, blurred vision.

FLURAZEPAM ▶LK ♀X ▶– ©IV $

ADULT — Insomnia: 15 to 30 mg PO at bedtime.

PEDS — Not approved in children age younger than 15 yo.

FORMS — Generic/Trade: Caps 15, 30 mg.

NOTES — Half-life 70 to 90 h. For short-term treatment of insomnia. Brand name discontinued.

MOA — Enhances actions of GABA.

ADVERSE EFFECTS — Serious: Respiratory depression, dependence, withdrawal reactions, seizures. Frequent: Sedation, fatigue, ataxia, memory impairment, depression, confusion, nausea, constipation, dry mouth, rash.

QUAZEPAM (*Doral*) ▶L ♀C ▶? ©IV

ADULT — Insomnia:Start 7.5 mg PO at bedtime. May increase to max 15 mg if needed.

PEDS — Not approved for use by children or adolescents.

FORMS — Trade: Tabs 15 mg

MOA — Enhances actions of GABA.

ADVERSE EFFECTS — Serious: Resiratory depression, dependence, withdrawal reactions including seizures, worsening depression. Frequent: Sedation, fatigue, ataxia, memory impairment, confusion, nausea.

PSYCHIATRY: Anxiolytics/Hypnotics—Benzodiazepines—Medium Half-Life (10 to 15 h)

NOTE: To avoid withdrawal, gradually taper when discontinuing after prolonged use. Sedative-hypnotics have been associated with severe allergic reactions and complex sleep behaviors including sleep driving. Use caution and discuss with patients.

ESTAZOLAM (*ProSom*) ▶LK ♀X ▶– ©IV $$

ADULT — Insomnia: 1 to 2 mg PO at bedtime for up to 12 weeks. Reduce dose to 0.5 mg in elderly, small, or debilitated patients.

PEDS — Not approved in children.

FORMS — Generic/Trade: Tabs 1, 2 mg.

NOTES — For short-term treatment of insomnia. Avoid with ketoconazole or itraconazole; caution with less potent inhibitors of CYP3A4. Brand name Prosom no longer available.

MOA — Enhances actions of GABA.

ADVERSE EFFECTS — Serious: Respiratory depression, dependence, withdrawal reactions, seizures. Frequent: Sedation, fatigue, ataxia, memory impairment, depression, confusion, nausea, constipation, dry mouth, rash.

LORAZEPAM (*Ativan*) ▶LK ♀D ▶– ©IV $

ADULT — Anxiety: Start 0.5 to 1 mg PO two to three times per day, usual effective dose is 2 to 6 mg/day. Maximum dose is 10 mg/day PO. Anxiolytic/

(cont.)

LORAZEPAM (*cont.*)

sedation: 0.04 to 0.05 mg/kg IV/IM; usual dose 2 mg, max 4 mg. Insomnia: 2 to 4 mg PO at bedtime. Status epilepticus: 4 mg IV over 2 min. May repeat in 10 to 15 min.

PEDS — Not approved in children.

UNAPPROVED ADULT — Alcohol withdrawal: 1 to 2 mg PO/IM/IV q 2 to 4 h prn or 2 mg PO/IM/IV q 6 h for 24 h then 1 mg q 6 h for 8 doses. Chemotherapy-induced N/V: 1 to 2 mg PO/SL/IV/IM q 6 h.

UNAPPROVED PEDS — Status epilepticus: 0.05 to 0.1 mg/kg IV over 2 to 5 min. May repeat 0.05 mg/kg for 1 dose in 10 to 15 min. Do not exceed 4 mg as single dose. Anxiolytic/Sedation: 0.05 mg/kg/dose q 4 to 8 h PO/IV, max 2 mg/dose. Chemotherapy-induced N/V: 0.05 mg/kg PO/IV q 8 to 12 h prn, max 3 mg/dose; or 0.02 to 0.05 mg/kg IV q 6 h prn, max 2 mg/dose.

FORMS — Generic/Trade: Tabs 0.5, 1, 2 mg. Generic only: Oral concentrate 2 mg/mL.

NOTES — Half-life 10 to 20 h. No active metabolites. For short-term treatment of insomnia.

MOA — Enhances actions of GABA.

ADVERSE EFFECTS — Serious: Cardiovascular collapse, hypotension, apnea (parenteral), respiratory depression, dependence, withdrawal syndrome.

Frequent: Drowsiness, dizziness, ataxia, headache, confusion, memory problems, depression, paradoxical CNS stimulation.

NITRAZEPAM (✱*Mogadan*) ▶L ♀C ▶– $

ADULT — Canada only. Insomnia: 5 to 10 mg PO at bedtime.

PEDS — Canada only. Myoclonic seizures: 0.3 to 1 mg/kg/day in 3 divided doses.

FORMS — Generic/Trade: Tabs 5, 10 mg.

NOTES — Use lower doses in elderly/debilitated patients.

MOA — Benzodiazepine with an intermediate half life.

ADVERSE EFFECTS — Serious: Dependence. Frequent: Dizziness, drowsiness, fatigue.

TEMAZEPAM (*Restoril*) ▶LK ♀X ▶– ©IV $

ADULT — Insomnia: 7.5 to 30 mg PO at bedtime for 7 to 10 days.

PEDS — Not approved in children.

FORMS — Generic/Trade: Caps 7.5, 15, 22.5, 30 mg.

NOTES — Half-life 8 to 25 h. For short-term treatment of insomnia.

MOA — Enhances actions of GABA.

ADVERSE EFFECTS — Serious: Respiratory depression, dependence, withdrawal reactions, seizures. Frequent: Sedation, fatigue, ataxia, memory impairment, depression, confusion, nausea, constipation, dry mouth, rash.

PSYCHIATRY: Anxiolytics/Hypnotics—Benzodiazepines—Short Half-Life (< 12 h)

ALPRAZOLAM (*Xanax, Xanax XR, Niravam*) ▶LK ♀D ▶– ©IV $

ADULT — Anxiety: Start 0.25 to 0.5 mg PO three times per day, may increase q 3 to 4 days to a maximum dose of 4 mg/day. Use 0.25 mg PO two times per day in elderly or debilitated patients. Panic disorder: Start 0.5 mg PO three times per day (or 0.5 to 1 mg PO daily of Xanax XR), may increase by up to 1 mg/day q 3 to 4 days to usual effective dose of 5 to 6 mg/day (3 to 6 mg/day for Xanax XR), maximum dose is 10 mg/day.

PEDS — Not approved in children.

FORMS — Generic/Trade: Tabs 0.25, 0.5, 1, 2 mg. Tabs, extended-release 0.5, 1, 2, 3 mg. Orally disintegrating tab (Niravam) 0.25, 0.5, 1, 2 mg. Generic only: Oral concentrate (Intensol) 1 mg/mL.

NOTES — Half-life 12 h, but need to give three times per day. Divide administration time evenly during waking hours to avoid interdose symptoms. Do not give with antifungals (ie, ketoconazole, itraconazole); use caution with macrolides, propoxyphene, oral contraceptives, TCAs, cimetidine, antidepressants, anticonvulsants, paroxetine, sertraline, and others that inhibit CYP3A4.

MOA — Enhances actions of GABA.

ADVERSE EFFECTS — Serious: Respiratory depression, dependence, withdrawal reactions, seizures. Frequent: Sedation, fatigue, ataxia, memory impairment, depression, confusion, nausea, constipation, dry mouth, rash.

OXAZEPAM ▶LK ♀D ▶– ©IV $$$

ADULT — Anxiety: 10 to 30 mg PO three to four times per day. Acute alcohol withdrawal: 15 to 30 mg PO three to four times per day.

PEDS — Not approved in children younger than 6 yo.

UNAPPROVED ADULT — Restless legs syndrome: Start 10 mg PO at bedtime. Max 40 mg at bedtime.

FORMS — Generic/Trade: Caps 10, 15, 30 mg. Trade only: Tabs 15 mg.

NOTES — Half-life 8 h. Brand name discontinued.

MOA — Enhances actions of GABA.

ADVERSE EFFECTS — Serious: Respiratory depression, dependence, withdrawal reactions, seizures. Frequent: Sedation, fatigue, ataxia, memory impairment, depression, confusion, nausea, constipation, dry mouth, rash.

TRIAZOLAM (*Halcion*) ▶LK ♀X ▶– ©IV $

ADULT — Hypnotic: 0.125 to 0.25 mg PO at bedtime for 7 to 10 days, maximum dose is 0.5 mg/day. Start 0.125 mg/day in elderly or debilitated patients.

PEDS — Not approved in children.

UNAPPROVED ADULT — Restless legs syndrome: Start 0.125 mg PO at bedtime. Max 0.5 mg at bedtime.

FORMS — Generic/Trade: Tabs 0.25 mg. Generic only: Tabs 0.125 mg

NOTES — Half-life 2 to 3 h. Anterograde amnesia may occur. Do not use with protease inhibitors, ketoconazole, itraconazole, or nefazodone; use caution with macrolides, cimetidine, and other CYP3A4 inhibitors.

TRIAZOLAM *(cont.)*

MOA — Enhances actions of GABA.
ADVERSE EFFECTS — Serious: Respiratory depression, dependence, withdrawal reactions, seizures.

Frequent: Sedation, fatigue, ataxia, memory impairment, depression, confusion, nausea, constipation, dry mouth, rash.

PSYCHIATRY: Anxiolytics/Hypnotics—Other

NOTE: Sedative-hypnotics have been associated with severe allergic reactions and complex sleep behaviors including sleep driving. Use caution and discuss with patients.

BUSPIRONE ▶K ♀B ▶– $$$
ADULT — Anxiety: Start 15 mg "dividose" daily (7.5 mg PO two times per day), increase by 5 mg/day q 2 to 3 days to usual effective dose of 30 mg/day, maximum dose is 60 mg/day.
PEDS — Not approved in children.
FORMS — Generic/Trade: Tabs 5, 10, Dividose Tabs 15, 30 mg (scored to be easily bisected or trisected). Generic only: Tabs 7.5 mg.
NOTES — Slower onset than benzodiazepines; optimum effect requires 3 to 4 weeks of therapy. Do not use with MAOIs; caution with itraconazole, cimetidine, nefazodone, erythromycin, and other CYP3A4 inhibitors. Brand name no longer available.
MOA — Serotonin 5-HT1A partial agonist.
ADVERSE EFFECTS — Serious: Parkinsonism, akathisia, dystonia, restless legs syndrome. Frequent: Drowsiness, dizziness, nausea, headache, nervousness.

ESZOPICLONE *(Lunesta)* ▶L ♀C ▶? ©IV $$$$$
ADULT — Insomnia: 2 mg PO at bedtime prn, max 3 mg. Elderly: 1 mg PO at bedtime prn, max 2 mg.
PEDS — Not approved for children.
FORMS — Generic/Trade: Tabs 1, 2, 3 mg.
NOTES — Half-life is approximately 6 h. Take immediately before bedtime.
MOA — Binds to GABA-A receptors.
ADVERSE EFFECTS — Serious: chest pain. Frequent: Headache, unpleasant taste, dry mouth, dizziness, nervousness, dyspepsia, sleepdriving and other complex sleep behaviors.

RAMELTEON *(Rozerem)* ▶L ♀C ▶? $$$$
ADULT — Insomnia: 8 mg PO at bedtime.
PEDS — Not approved for children.
FORMS — Trade only: Tabs 8 mg.
NOTES — Do not take with/after high-fat meal. No evidence of dependence or abuse liability. Inhibitors or CYP1A2, 3A4, and 2C9 may increase serum level and effect. Avoid with severe liver disease. May decrease testosterone and increase prolactin.
MOA — Melatonin receptor agonist.
ADVERSE EFFECTS — Serious: None. Frequent: Headache, somnolence, fatigue, dizziness.

TASIMELTEON *(Hetlioz)* ▶L ♀C ▶?
ADULT — Non 24-hour sleep/wake disorder:20 mg before bedtime. Take on empty stomach.
PEDS — Not approved for use in children and adolescents.
FORMS — Trade only: Caps 20 mg.
NOTES — Avoid use with strong CYP1A2 inhibitors or CYP3A4 inducers.

MOA — Agonist of melatonin MT1 and MT2 receptors.
ADVERSE EFFECTS — Serious: none. Frequent: headache, somnolence, increased ALT, nightmares, abnormal dreams, upper respiratory infections, urinary tract infection.

ZALEPLON *(Sonata)* ▶L ♀C ▶– ©IV $$$$
ADULT — Insomnia: 5 to 10 mg PO at bedtime prn, maximum 20 mg.
PEDS — Not approved in children.
FORMS — Generic/Trade: Caps 5, 10 mg.
NOTES — Half-life is approximately 1 h. Useful if problems with sleep initiation or morning grogginess. For short-term treatment of insomnia. Take immediately before bedtime or after going to bed and experiencing difficulty falling asleep. Use 5 mg dose in patients with mild to moderate hepatic impairment, elderly patients, and in patients taking cimetidine. Possible drug interactions with rifampin, phenytoin, carbamazepine, and phenobarbital. Do not use for benzodiazepine or alcohol withdrawal.
MOA — Selective GABA-benzodiazepine omega-1 agonist.
ADVERSE EFFECTS — Serious: Rebound insomnia, nightmares, seizures, sleepdriving, anaphylactic reactions. Frequent: Drowsiness, abdominal pain, chest pain, headache, asthenia, fatigue, photosensitivity.

ZOLPIDEM *(Ambien, Ambien CR, Zolpimist, Intermezzo, Edluar✦Sublinox)* ▶L ♀C ▶+ ©IV $$$$
ADULT — Adult: Insomnia: Standard tabs:women 5 mg and men 5-10 mg PO at bedtime. May increase the 5 mg dose to 10 mg if needed. Age older than 65 yo or debilitated: 5 mg PO at bedtime. Oral spray: women 5 mg and men 5-10 mg PO at bedtime. May increase the 5 mg dose to 10 mg if needed. Age older than 65 yo or debilitated: 5 mg PO at bedtime. Control-release tabs: women 6.25 mg and men 6.25-12.5 mg PO at bedtime. May increase the 6.25 mg dose to 12.5 mg if needed. Age older than 65 yo or debilitated: 6.25 mg PO at bedtime. Sublingual tabs (Edluar): women 5 mg and men 5-10 mg SL at bedtime. May increase the 5 mg dose to 10 mg if needed. Age older than 65 yo or debilitated: 5 mg SL at bedtime. Middle of the night awakening: Sublingual tabs (Intermezzo): Women 1.75 mg and men 3.5 mg SL once nightly with at least 4 hours of sleep remaining.
PEDS — Not approved in children.
FORMS — Generic/Trade: Tabs 5, 10 mg. Controlled-release tabs 6.25, 12.5 mg. Trade only:

(cont.)

ZOLPIDEM (*cont.*)

oral spray 5 mg/actuation (Zolpimist), sublingual tab 5, 10 mg (Edluar) sublingual tab 1.75, 3.5 mg (Intermezzo).

NOTES — Half-life is 2.5 h. Ambien regular-release is for short-term treatment of insomnia characterized by problems with sleep initiation. CR is useful for problems with sleep initiation and maintenance, and has been studied for up to 24 weeks. Do not use for benzodiazepine or alcohol withdrawal. Oral spray is sprayed into the mouth over the tongue. Device must be primed with 5 pumps prior to first use or if not used for 14 days.

MOA — Selective GABA-benzodiazepine omega-1 agonist.

ADVERSE EFFECTS — Serious: Sleepdriving, abnormal thinking, behavioral changes, depression, suicidal ideation, hallucinations, anaphylaxis.

Frequent: Drowsiness, dizziness, nausea, headache, nervousness, decreased daytime recall.

ZOPICLONE (✦*Imovane*) ▶L ♀D ▶− $

ADULT — Canada only. Short-term treatment of insomnia: 5 to 7.5 mg PO at bedtime. In elderly or debilitated, use 3.75 mg at bedtime initially, and increase prn to 5 to 7.5 mg at bedtime. Maximum 7.5 mg at bedtime.

PEDS — Not approved in children.

FORMS — Generic/Trade: Tabs 5, 7.5 mg. Generic only: Tabs 3.75 mg.

NOTES — Treatment should usually not exceed 7 to 10 days without re-evaluation.

MOA — Short-acting hypnotic; structurally unrelated to benzodiazepines but shares a similar pharmacological profile to many of the benzodiazepines.

ADVERSE EFFECTS — Frequent: Taste alteration (bitter taste), anterograde amnesia, confusion, N/V, anorexia.

PSYCHIATRY: Combination Drugs

LIMBITROL (**chlordiazepoxide + amitriptyline**) ▶LK ♀D ▶− ©IV $$$

ADULT — Rarely used; other drugs preferred. Depression/anxiety: 1 tab PO three to four times per day, may increase up to 6 tabs/day.

PEDS — Not approved in children younger than 12 yo.

FORMS — Generic/Trade: Tabs 5/12.5, 10/25 mg chlordiazepoxide/amitriptyline.

MOA — Antidepressant- benzodiazepine combination.

ADVERSE EFFECTS — Serious: Seizures, arrhythmias, hypotension, agranulocytosis, dependence, withdrawal reactions, respiratory depression. Frequent: Drowsiness, dizziness, dry mouth, constipation, urinary retention, confusion, memory problems.

SYMBYAX (**olanzapine + fluoxetine**) ▶LK ♀C ▶− $$$$$

WARNING — Observe patients started on SSRIs for worsening depression or emergence of suicidal thoughts or behaviors in children, adolescents, and young adults, especially early in therapy or after increases in dose. Monitor for emergence of anxiety, agitation, panic attacks, insomnia, irritability, hostility, impulsivity, akathisia, mania and hypomania. Carefully weigh risks and benefits before starting and then monitor such individuals closely. The use of atypical antipsychotics to treat behavioral problems in patients with dementia has been associated with higher mortality rates. Atypical antipsychotics have been associated with wt gain, dyslipidemia, hyperglycemia, and diabetes mellitus; monitor closely.

ADULT — Bipolar type 1 with depression and treatment-resistant depression: Start 6/25 mg PO at bedtime. Max 18/75 mg/day.

PEDS — Depression associated with bipolar disorder type I (10 to 17 years old): Start 3/25 mg PO at bedtime. Max 12/50 mg/day.

FORMS — Generic/Trade: Caps (olanzapine/fluoxetine) 3/25, 6/25, 6/50, 12/25, 12/50 mg.

NOTES — Efficacy beyond 8 weeks not established. Monitor wt, fasting glucose, and triglycerides before initiation and periodically during treatment. Contraindicated with thioridazine; do not use with cisapride, thioridazine, tryptophan, or MAOIs; caution with lithium, phenytoin, TCAs, aspirin, NSAIDs and warfarin. Do not use during active therapy with linezolid or IV methylene blue. Pregnancy exposure to fluoxetine associated with premature delivery, low birth wt, and lower Apgar scores. Decrease dose with liver disease or patients predisposed to hypotension.

MOA — Olanzapine: Dopamine antagonist, serotonin 2A antagonist. Fluoxetine: Inhibits serotonin reuptake.

ADVERSE EFFECTS — Serious: Serotonin syndrome, neuroleptic malignant syndrome, hyponatremia, SIADH, seizures, hypotension, hyperglycemia/diabetes, QT prolongation, hepatitis, abnormal bleeding. Frequent: Asthenia, edema, increased appetite, peripheral edema, pharyngitis, somnolence, abnormal thinking, tremor, weight gain.

PSYCHIATRY: Drug Dependence Therapy

ACAMPROSATE (*Campral*) ▶K ♀C ▶? $$$$$

ADULT — Maintenance of abstinence from alcohol: 666 mg (2 tabs) PO three times per day. Start after alcohol withdrawal and when patient is abstinent.

PEDS — Not approved in children.

FORMS — Generic/Trade: Tabs, delayed-release 333 mg.

NOTES — Reduce dose to 333 mg if CrCl 30 to 50 mL/min. Contraindicated if CrCl less than 30 mL/min.

MOA — Unknown. Structural analogue of GABA and may restore balance to that system.

ACAMPROSATE (cont.)

ADVERSE EFFECTS — Serious: Depression, suicidality. Frequent: Asthenia, diarrhea, anxiety, insomnia.

DISULFIRAM (Antabuse) ▶L ♀C ▶? $$

WARNING — Never give to an intoxicated patient.

ADULT — Maintenance of abstinence from alcohol: 125 to 500 mg PO daily.

PEDS — Not approved in children.

FORMS — Generic/Trade: Tabs 250, 500 mg.

NOTES — Patient must abstain from any alcohol for at least 12 h before using. Disulfiram-alcohol reaction may occur for up to 2 weeks after discontinuing disulfiram. Metronidazole and alcohol in any form (e.g., cough syrups, tonics) contraindicated. Hepatotoxicity.

MOA — Inhibits aldehyde dehydrogenase.

ADVERSE EFFECTS — Serious: Angina, MI, hypotension, tachycardia, heart failure, syncope, seizures. Frequent: Rash, drowsiness, headache, impotence, rash, optic neuropathy.

NALTREXONE (ReVia, Depade, Vivitrol) ▶LK ♀C ▶? $$$$

WARNING — Naltrexone has been associated with hepatotoxicity. Monitor for signs and symptoms.

ADULT — Alcohol dependence: 50 mg PO daily. Extended-release injectable susp: 380 mg IM q 4 weeks or monthly. Opioid dependence following detoxification: Start 25 mg PO daily, increase to 50 mg PO daily if no signs of withdrawal. Extended-release injectable susp: 380 mg IM q 4 weeks or monthly.

PEDS — Not approved in children.

FORMS — Generic/Trade: Tabs 50 mg. Trade only (Vivitrol): Extended-release injectable susp kits 380 mg.

NOTES — Avoid if recent (past 7 to 10 days) ingestion of opioids. Conflicting evidence of efficacy for chronic, severe alcoholism. Extended release injectable suspension (Vivitrol) should be given in the gluteal muscle and use alternate side each month.

MOA — Opiate antagonist.

ADVERSE EFFECTS — Serious: Suicidal ideation, paranoia, depression, hepatotoxicity. Frequent: Insomnia, nervousness, headache, dizziness, N/V.

NICOTINE GUM (Nicorette, Nicorette DS) ▶LK ♀C ▶- $$$$

ADULT — Smoking cessation: Gradually taper 1 piece (2 mg) q 1 to 2 h for 6 weeks, 1 piece (2 mg) q 2 to 4 h for 3 weeks, then 1 piece (2 mg) q 4 to 8 h for 3 weeks. Max 30 pieces/day of 2 mg gum or 24 pieces/day of 4 mg gum. Use 4 mg pieces (Nicorette DS) for high cigarette use (more than 24 cigarettes/day).

PEDS — Not approved in children.

FORMS — OTC/Generic/Trade: Gum 2, 4 mg.

NOTES — Chew slowly and park between cheek and gum periodically. May cause N/V, hiccups. Coffee, juices, wine, and soft drinks may reduce absorption. Avoid eating/drinking for 15 min before/during gum use. Available in original, orange, or mint flavor. Do not use beyond 6 months.

MOA — Nicotine receptor agonist.

ADVERSE EFFECTS — Serious: Atrial and ventricular arrhythmias. Frequent: Local reactions, burning, stinging, headache, insomnia, nausea, diarrhea, tachycardia, chest pain, hypertension.

NICOTINE INHALATION SYSTEM (Nicotrol Inhaler, *Nicorette inhaler) ▶LK ♀D ▶- $$$$$

ADULT — Smoking cessation: 6 to 16 cartridges/day for 12 weeks.

PEDS — Not approved in children.

FORMS — Trade only: Oral inhaler 10 mg/cartridge (4 mg nicotine delivered), 42 cartridges/box.

MOA — Nicotine receptor agonist.

ADVERSE EFFECTS — Serious: Atrial and ventricular arrhythmias. Frequent: Local reactions, burning, stinging, headache, insomnia, nausea, diarrhea, tachycardia, chest pain, hypertension.

NICOTINE LOZENGE (Commit, Nicorette) ▶LK ♀D ▶- $$$$$

ADULT — Smoking cessation: In those who smoke within 30 min of waking use 4 mg lozenge; others use 2 mg. Take 1 to 2 lozenges q 1 to 2 h for 6 weeks, then q 2 to 4 h in week 7 to 9, then q 4 to 8 h in week 10 to 12. Length of therapy 12 weeks.

PEDS — Not approved in children.

FORMS — OTC Generic/Trade: Lozenge 2, 4 mg.

NOTES — Allow lozenge to dissolve and do not chew. Do not eat or drink within 15 min before use. Avoid concurrent use with other sources of nicotine.

MOA — Nicotine receptor agonist.

ADVERSE EFFECTS — Serious: Atrial and ventricular arrhythmias. Frequent: Local reactions, headache, insomnia, nausea, diarrhea, tachycardia, chest pain, hypertension.

NICOTINE NASAL SPRAY (Nicotrol NS) ▶LK ♀D ▶- $$$$$

ADULT — Smoking cessation: 1 to 2 doses each h, each dose is 2 sprays, 1 in each nostril (1 spray contains 0.5 mg nicotine). Minimum recommended: 8 doses/day, max 40 doses/day.

PEDS — Not approved in children.

FORMS — Trade only: Nasal soln 10 mg/mL (0.5 mg/inhalation); 10 mL bottles.

MOA — Nicotine receptor agonist.

ADVERSE EFFECTS — Serious: Atrial and ventricular arrhythmias. Frequent: Local reactions, burning, stinging, headache, insomnia, nausea, diarrhea, tachycardia, chest pain, hypertension.

NICOTINE PATCHES (Habitrol, NicoDerm CQ, Nicotrol) ▶LK ♀D ▶- $$$$

ADULT — Smoking cessation: Start 1 patch (14 to 22 mg) daily and taper after 6 weeks. Total duration of therapy is 12 weeks.

PEDS — Not approved in children.

FORMS — OTC/Rx/Generic/Trade: Patches 11, 22 mg/24 h. 7, 14, 21 mg/24 h (Habitrol and NicoDerm). OTC/Trade: 15 mg/16 h (Nicotrol).

NOTES — Ensure patient has stopped smoking. Dispose of patches safely; can be toxic to kids, pets. Remove opaque NicoDerm CQ patch prior to MRI procedures to avoid possible burns.

MOA — Nicotine receptor agonist.

NICOTINE PATCHES (cont.)

ADVERSE EFFECTS — Serious: Atrial and ventricular arrhythmias. Frequent: Local reactions, burning, stinging, headache, insomnia, nausea, diarrhea, tachycardia, chest pain, hypertension.

SUBOXONE (buprenorphine + naloxone, Zubsolv) ▶L ♀C ▶– ©III $$$$$

ADULT — Treatment of opioid dependence: Induction (SL film): Day 1 start with 2 mg/0.5 mg SL or 4 mg/1 mg SL and titrate upwards in increments of 2 or 4 mg of buprenorphine at approximately 2 hour intervals to 8 mg/2 mg total dose. Day 2 a dose of up to 16 mg/4 mg is recommended. Maintenance (SL tab or film): 16 mg SL daily. Can individualize to range of 4 to 24 mg SL daily. Maintenance (Zubsolv): 11.4mg/2.8 mg SL daily. Can individualize to range of 2.8/0.72 to 17.1/4.2 mg SL daily.

PEDS — Not approved in children.

FORMS — Generic only: SL tabs 2/0.5 mg and 8/2 mg buprenorphine/naloxone. Trade only: SL film 2/0.5 mg, 4/1mg, 8/2 mg, and 12/3 mg buprenorphine/naloxone, SL tabs (Zubsolv) 1.4/0.36 mg and 5.7/1.4 mg.

NOTES — Suboxone preferred over Subutex for unsupervised administration. Titrate in 2 to 4 mg increments/decrements to maintain therapy compliance and prevent withdrawal. Prescribers must complete training and apply for special DEA number. See www.suboxone.com. Zubsolv 5.7/1.4 mg tablet is equivalent to Suboxone 8/2 mg tablet. During induction, therapy should be started when objective signs of moderate withdrawal appear.

MOA — Partial opiate agonist/antagonist.

ADVERSE EFFECTS — Serious: Respiratory/CNS depression, hepatitis, dependence. Frequent: Headache, N/V, constipation, abdominal pain, sweating.

VARENICLINE (Chantix, ✣Champix) ▶K ♀C ▶? $$$$

WARNING — Has been associated with the development of suicidal ideation, changes in behavior, depressed mood and attempted/completed suicides, both during treatment and after withdrawal. Unclear safety in serious psychiatric conditions.

ADULT — Smoking cessation: Start 0.5 mg PO daily for days 1 to 3, then 0.5 mg two times per day days 4 to 7, then 1 mg two times per day thereafter. Take after meals with full glass of water. Start 1 week prior to cessation and continue for 12 weeks or patient may start the drug and stop smoking between days 8-35 of treatment.

PEDS — Not approved in children.

FORMS — Trade only: Tabs 0.5, 1 mg.

NOTES — For severe renal dysfunction reduce max dose to 0.5 mg two times per day. For renal failure on hemodialysis may use 0.5 mg once daily if tolerated. May worsen underlying neuropsychiatric symptoms in patients with pre-existing psychiatric conditions.

MOA — Nicotinic acetylcholine receptor agonist.

ADVERSE EFFECTS — Serious: Depression, suicidal thoughts, aggression, erratic behavior, MI, stroke, angina. Frequent: N/V, drowsiness, dreaming disturbances, insomnia, headache, abnormal dreams, constipation.

PSYCHIATRY: Stimulants/ADHD/Anorexiants

NOTE: Sudden cardiac death has been reported with stimulants and atomoxetine at usual ADHD doses; carefully assess prior to treatment and avoid if cardiac conditions or structural abnormalities. Amphetamines are associated with high abuse potential and dependence with prolonged administration. Stimulants may also cause or worsen underlying psychosis or induce a manic or mixed episode in bipolar disorder. Problems with visual accommodation have also been reported with stimulants.

ADDERALL XR (dextroamphetamine + amphetamine, Adderall) ▶L ♀C ▶– ©II $$$$

ADULT — Narcolepsy, standard-release: Start 10 mg PO q am, increase by 10 mg q week, maximum dose is 60 mg/day divided two to three times per day at 4- to 6-h intervals. ADHD, extended-release caps (Adderall XR): 20 mg PO daily.

PEDS — ADHD, standard-release tabs: Start 2.5 mg (3 to 5 yo) or 5 mg (age 6 yo or older) PO one to two times per day, increase by 2.5 to 5 mg q week, max 40 mg/day. ADHD, extended-release caps (Adderall XR): If age 6 to 12 yo, then start 5 to 10 mg PO daily to a max of 30 mg/day. If 13 to 17 yo, then start 10 mg PO daily to a max of 20 mg/day. Not recommended age younger than 3 yo. Narcolepsy, standard-release: Age 6 to 12 yo: Start 5 mg PO daily, increase by 5 mg q week. Age older than 12 yo: Start 10 mg PO q am, increase by 10 mg q week, maximum dose is 60 mg/day divided two to three times per day at 4 to 6 h intervals.

FORMS — Generic/Trade: Tabs 5, 7.5, 10, 12.5, 15, 20, 30 mg. Caps, extended-release (Adderall XR) 5, 10, 15, 20, 25, 30 mg.

NOTES — Caps may be opened and the beads sprinkled on applesauce; do not chew beads. Adderall XR should be given upon awakening. Avoid evening doses. Monitor growth and use drug holidays when appropriate. May increase pulse and BP. May exacerbate bipolar or psychotic conditions.

MOA — CNS stimulant, increases norepinephrine and dopamine.

ADVERSE EFFECTS — Serious: Sudden death, seizures, psychosis, hypertension, priapism, Raynaud's phenomenon, vasculopathy. Frequent: Appetite suppression, weight loss, insomnia, nervousness, N/V, dizziness, palpitations, tachycardia, headache.

ARMODAFINIL (Nuvigil) ▶L ♀C ▶? ©IV $$$$$

ADULT — Obstructive sleep apnea/hypopnea syndrome and narcolepsy: 150 to 250 mg PO q am. Inconsistent evidence for improved efficacy of 250 mg/day dose.

ARMODAFINIL (cont.)

Shift work sleep disorder: 150 mg PO 1 h prior to start of shift.

PEDS — Not approved in children.

FORMS — Trade only: Tabs 50, 100, 150, 200, 250 mg.

NOTES — Weak inducer for substrates of CYP3A4/5 (eg, carbamazepine, cyclosporine) which may require dose adjustments. May inhibit metabolism of substrates of CYP2C19 (eg, omeprazole, diazepam, phenytoin). May reduce efficacy of oral contraceptives; consider alternatives during treatment. Reduce dose with severe liver impairment.

MOA — R-enantiomer of modafinil. Wake promoting agent – CNS stimulant.

ADVERSE EFFECTS — Serious: Rash, Stevens-Johnson syndrome, multi-organ hypersensitivity reactions, mania, psychosis, suicidal ideation, aggression. Frequent: Headache, nausea, dizziness, insomnia.

ATOMOXETINE (Strattera) ▶K ♀C ▶? $$$$$

WARNING — Severe liver injury and failure have been reported; discontinue if jaundice or elevated LFTs. Increases risk of suicidal thinking and behavior in children and adolescents; carefully weigh risks/benefits before starting and then monitor such individuals closely for worsening depression or emergence of suicidal thoughts or behaviors especially early in therapy or after increases in dose. Monitor for emergence of anxiety, agitation, panic attacks, insomnia, irritability, hostility, impulsivity, akathisia, mania and hypomania.

ADULT — ADHD: Start 40 mg PO daily, then increase after more than 3 days to target of 80 mg/day divided one to two times per day. Max dose 100 mg/day.

PEDS — ADHD: Children/adolescents wt 70 kg or less: Start 0.5 mg/kg daily, then increase after more than 3 days to target dose of 1.2 mg/kg/day divided one to two times per day. Max dose 1.4 mg/kg or 100 mg/day, whichever is less. If wt greater than 70 kg use adult dose.

FORMS — Trade only: Caps 10, 18, 25, 40, 60, 80, 100 mg.

NOTES — If taking strong CYP2D6 inhibitors (eg, paroxetine or fluoxetine), use same starting dose but only increase if well tolerated at 4 weeks and symptoms unimproved. Caution when coadministered with oral or parenteral albuterol or other beta-2 agonists, as increases in heart rate and BP may occur. May be stopped without tapering. Monitor growth. Give "Patient Medication Guide" when dispensed. Does not appear to exacerbate tics.

MOA — Selective norepinephrine reuptake inhibitor.

ADVERSE EFFECTS — Serious: Sudden death, increased blood pressure and heart rate, liver injury and failure, psychosis, mania, aggression, priapism. Frequent: N/V, dyspepsia, fatigue, decreased appetite, weight loss, dizziness, mood swings, constipation, dry mouth, insomnia, sexual dysfunction, urinary hesitancy/retention, hot flushes, dysuria, dysmenorrhea.

BENZPHETAMINE (Didrex) ▶K ♀X ▶? ©III $$$

WARNING — Chronic overuse/abuse can lead to marked tolerance and psychic dependence; caution with prolonged use.

ADULT — Obesity (short-term): Start with 25 to 50 mg once daily in the morning and increase if needed to 1 to 3 times daily.

PEDS — Not approved for children younger than 12 yo.

FORMS — Generic/Trade: Tabs 50 mg.

NOTES — Tolerance to anorectic effect develops within week and cross-tolerance to other drugs in class common.

MOA — CNS stimulant, increases dopamine and norepinephrine.

ADVERSE EFFECTS — Serious: Seizures, psychosis, hypertension, dependence. Frequent: Appetite suppression, weight loss, insomnia, nervousness, N/V, dizziness, palpitations, tachycardia, headache.

CAFFEINE (NoDoz, Vivarin, Caffedrine, Stay Awake, Quick-Pep, Cafcit) ▶L ♀B/C ▶? $

ADULT — Fatigue: 100 to 200 mg PO q 3 to 4 h prn.

PEDS — Not approved in children younger than 12 yo, except apnea of prematurity in infants between 28 and less than 33 weeks gestational age (Cafcit): Load 20 mg/kg IV over 30 min. Maintenance 5 mg/kg PO q 24 h. Monitor for necrotizing enterocolitis.

FORMS — OTC Generic/Trade: Tabs/Caps 200 mg. Oral soln caffeine citrate (Cafcit) 20 mg/mL. OTC Trade only: Tabs, extended-release 200 mg. Lozenges 75 mg.

NOTES — 2 mg caffeine citrate = 1 mg caffeine base.

MOA — CNS and cardiovascular stimulant.

ADVERSE EFFECTS — Serious: Arrhythmias, delirium, seizures, necrotizing enterocolitis. Frequent: Tremor, anxiety, twitches, headache, insomnia, N/V.

DEXMETHYLPHENIDATE (Focalin, Focalin XR) ▶LK ♀C ▶? ©II $$$

ADULT — ADHD (not already on stimulants): Start 10 mg PO q am (extended-release) or 2.5 mg PO two times per day (immediate-release). Max 20 mg/day for immediate release and 40 mg/day for extended-release. If taking racemic methylphenidate use conversion of 2.5 mg for each 5 mg of methylphenidate.

PEDS — ADHD (age 6 yo or older and not already on stimulants): Start 5 mg PO q am (extended-release) or 2.5 mg PO two times per day (immediate-release), max 20 mg/day (immediate-release) or 30 mg/day (extended-release). If already on racemic methylphenidate, use conversion of 2.5 mg for each 5 mg of methylphenidate.

FORMS — Generic/Trade: Tabs, immediate-release 2.5, 5, 10 mg. Extended-release caps (generic) 10, 15, 20, 30, 40 mg. Trade Only: Extended-release caps (Focalin XR-$$$$$) 5, 10, 15, 20, 25, 30, 35, 40 mg.

DEXMETHYLPHENIDATE (*cont.*)

NOTES — Avoid evening doses. Monitor growth and use drug holidays when appropriate. May increase pulse and BP. 2.5 mg is equivalent to 5 mg racemic methylphenidate. Focalin XR caps may be opened and sprinkled on applesauce, but beads must not be chewed. May exacerbate bipolar or psychotic conditions. Avoid in patients allergic to methylphenidate.

MOA — CNS stimulant, increases norepinephrine and dopamine.

ADVERSE EFFECTS — Serious: Sudden death, seizures, psychosis, hypertension, priapism, peripheral vasculopathy, Raynaud's phenomenon. Frequent: Appetite suppression, weight loss, insomnia, nervousness, N/V, dizziness, palpitations, tachycardia, headache.

DEXTROAMPHETAMINE (*Dexedrine, Procentra, Zenzedi*) ▶L ♀C ▶– ©II $$$$$

ADULT — Narcolepsy: Start 10 mg PO q am, increase by 10 mg/day q week, max 60 mg/day divided daily (sustained-release) or two to three times per day at 4- to 6-h intervals.

PEDS — Narcolepsy: Age 6 to 12 yo: Start 5 mg PO q am, increase by 5 mg/day q week. Age older than 12 yo: Start 10 mg PO q am, increase by 10 mg/day q week, max 60 mg/day divided daily (sustained-release) or two to three times per day at 4- to 6-h intervals. ADHD: Age 3 to 5 yo: Start 2.5 mg PO daily, increase by 2.5 mg q week. Age 6 yo or older: Start 5 mg PO one to two times per day, increase by 5 mg q week, usual max 40 mg/day divided one to three times per day at 4- to 6-h intervals. Not recommended for patients younger than 3 yo. Extended-release caps not recommended for age younger than 6 yo.

FORMS — Generic/Trade: Caps, extended-release 5, 10, 15 mg. Tabs 5, 10 mg. Oral soln 5 mg/5 mL. Trade only: Tabs 2.5, 7.5 mg (Zenzedi)

NOTES — Avoid evening doses. Monitor growth and use drug holidays when appropriate. May exacerbate bipolar or psychotic conditions.

MOA — CNS stimulant, increases norepinephrine and dopamine.

ADVERSE EFFECTS — Serious: Sudden death, seizures, psychosis, hypertension, priapism, peripheral vasculopathy, Raynaud's phenomenon. Frequent: Appetite suppression, weight loss, insomnia, nervousness, N/V, dizziness, palpitations, tachycardia, headache.

DIETHYLPROPION (*Tenuate, Tenuate Dospan*) ▶K ♀B ▶? ©IV $

WARNING — Chronic overuse/abuse can lead to marked tolerance and psychic dependence; caution with prolonged use.

ADULT — Obesity (short term): 25 mg PO three times per day 1 h before meals and mid evening if needed or 75 mg sustained-release daily at midmorning.

PEDS — Not approved for children younger than 12 yo.

FORMS — Generic/Trade: Tabs 25 mg, Tabs, extended-release 75 mg.

NOTES — Tolerance to anorectic effect develops within week and cross-tolerance to other drugs in class common.

MOA — CNS stimulant, increases dopamine and norepinephrine.

ADVERSE EFFECTS — Serious: Seizures, psychosis, hypertension, dependence. Frequent: Appetite suppression, weight loss, insomnia, nervousness, N/V, dizziness, palpitations, tachycardia, headache.

GUANFACINE (*Intuniv*) ▶LK – ♀B ▶?

ADULT — ADHD: Start 1 mg PO once daily in the morning or evening. Increase by 1 mg/ week to max 4 mg/day.

PEDS — ADHD (6 yrs and above): Start 1 mg PO once daily in the morning or evening. Increase by 1 mg/ week to max 4 mg/day.

FORMS — Trade only: Tabs 1, 2, 3, 4 mg.

NOTES — Taper when discontinuing. Use cautiously with strong CYP3A4 inhibitors.

MOA — Selective alpha-2A adrenergic agonist.

ADVERSE EFFECTS — Serious: Hypotension, bradycardia, syncope. Frequent: Somnolence/sedation, abdominal pain, dizziness, hypotension, dry mouth, constipation, headache.

LISDEXAMFETAMINE (*Vyvanse*) ▶L ♀C ▶– ©II $$$$

ADULT — ADHD: Start 30 mg PO q am. May increase weekly by 10 to 20 mg/day to max 70 mg/day.

PEDS — ADHD children and adolescents ages 6 yo and above: Start 30 mg PO q am. May increase weekly by 10 to 20 mg/day to max 70 mg/day.

FORMS — Trade: Caps 20, 30, 40, 50, 60, 70 mg.

NOTES — May open cap and place contents in water for administration. Avoid evening doses. Monitor growth and use drug holidays when appropriate.

MOA — Prodrug of dextroamphetamine. CNS stimulant, increases norepinephrine and dopamine.

ADVERSE EFFECTS — Serious: Sudden death, seizures, psychosis, hypertension, priapism, peripheral vasculopathy, Raynaud's phenomonon. Frequent: Appetite suppression, weight loss, insomnia, nervousness, N/V, dizziness, palpitations, tachycardia, headache, irritability, dry mouth.

METHYLPHENIDATE (*Ritalin, Ritalin LA, Ritalin SR, Methylin, Methylin ER, Metadate ER, Metadate CD, Concerta, Daytrana, Quillivant XR, ✦Biphentin*) ▶LK ♀C ▶? ©II $$

ADULT — Narcolepsy: 10 mg PO two to three times per day before meals. Usual effective dose is 20 to 30 mg/day, max 60 mg/day. Use sustained-release tabs when the 8 h dosage corresponds to the titrated 8 h dosage of the conventional tabs. ADHD (Concerta): Start 18 to 36 mg PO q am, usual dose range 18 to 72 mg/day. Sustained-release suspension: Start 20 mg PO in the morning. May increase weekly by 10-20 mg daily to max 60 mg/day.

PEDS — ADHD age 6 yo or older: Start 5 mg PO two times per day before breakfast and lunch, increase gradually by 5 to 10 mg/day at weekly intervals to

METHYLPHENIDATE (*cont.*)

max 60 mg/day. Sustained and extended-release: Start 20 mg PO daily, max 60 mg daily. Concerta (extended-release) start 18 mg PO q am; titrate in 9 to 18 mg increments at weekly intervals to max 54 mg/day (age 6 to 12 yo) or 72 mg/day (13 to 17 yo). Consult product labeling for dose conversion from other methylphenidate regimens. Discontinue after 1 month if no improvement observed. Transdermal patch age 6 to 17 yo: Start 10 mg/9 h, may increase at weekly intervals to max dose of 30 mg/9 h. Apply 2 h prior to desired onset and remove 9 h later. Effect may last up to 12 h after application. Must alternate sites daily. Sustained-release suspension (6 yo and older): Start 20 mg PO in the morning. May increase weekly by 10-20 mg daily to max 60 mg/day.

FORMS — Trade only: Tabs chewable 2.5, 5, 10 mg (Methylin). Tabs extended-release 10, 20 mg (Methylin ER, Metadate ER). Tabs sustained-release 20 mg (Ritalin SR). Transdermal patch (Daytrana) 10 mg/9 h, 15 mg/9 h, 20 mg/9 h, 30 mg/9 h. Susp extended release 5 mg/mL (Quillivant XR). Generic/Trade: Tabs, 5, 10, 20 mg (Ritalin). Tabs extended-release 18, 27, 36, 54 mg (Concerta). Caps, extended-release 10, 20, 30, 40, 50, 60 mg (Metadate CD) may be sprinkled on food. Caps extended-release 10, 20, 30, 40 mg (Ritalin LA). Oral soln 5 mg/5 mL, 10 mg/5 mL. Generic only: Tabs 5, 10, 20 mg, tabs extended-release 10, 20 mg, tabs sustained-release 20 mg.

NOTES — Avoid evening doses. Avoid use with severe anxiety, tension, or agitation. Monitor growth and use drug holidays when appropriate. May increase pulse and BP. Ritalin LA may be opened and sprinkled on applesauce. Avoid alcohol ingestion with Ritalin LA , Concerta, and Metadate CD as it may change release patterns. Apply transdermal patch to hip below beltline to avoid rubbing it off. May exacerbate bipolar, psychotic, or seizure conditions.

MOA — CNS stimulant, increases norepinephrine and dopamine.

ADVERSE EFFECTS — Serious: Sudden death, seizures, psychosis, hypertension, priapism, peripheral valsculopathy, Raynaud's phenomenon, contact sensitization (Daytrana). Frequent: Appetite suppression, weight loss, insomnia, nervousness, N/V, dizziness, palpitations, tachycardia, headache.

MODAFINIL (*Provigil, ✦Alertec*) ▶L ♀C ▶? ©IV $$$$$

WARNING — Associated with serious, life-threatening rashes in adults and children; discontinue immediately if unexplained rash.

ADULT — Narcolepsy and sleep apnea/hypopnea: 200 mg PO q am. Shift work sleep disorder: 200 mg PO 1 h before shift.

PEDS — Not approved in children younger than 16 yo.

FORMS — Generic/Trade: Tabs 100, 200 mg.

NOTES — May increase levels of diazepam, phenytoin, TCAs, warfarin, or propranolol; may decrease levels of cyclosporine, oral contraceptives, or theophylline. Reduce dose in severe liver impairment.

MOA — Wake-promoting agent; CNS stimulant.

ADVERSE EFFECTS — Serious: Rash, Stevens-Johnson syndrome, multi-organ hypersensitivity, leukopenia, psychosis, mania, suicidal ideation, aggression. Frequent: Insomnia, nausea, headache, nervousness, anxiety.

PHENTERMINE (*Adipex-P, Suprenza*) ▶KL ♀C ▶– ©IV $

WARNING — Chronic overuse/abuse can lead to marked tolerance and psychic dependence; caution with prolonged use.

ADULT — Obesity: 8 mg PO three times per day before meals or 1 to 2 h after meals. May give 15 to 37.5 mg PO q am or 10 to 14 h before bedtime.

PEDS — Not approved in children younger than 16 yo.

FORMS — Generic/Trade: Caps 15, 30, 37.5 mg. Tabs 37.5 mg. Trade only: Orally disintegrating tables (Suprenza) 15, 30 mg. Generic only: Caps extended-release 15, 30 mg (Ionamin)

NOTES — Indicated for short-term (8 to 12 weeks) use only. Contraindicated for use during or within 14 days of MAOIs (hypertensive crisis). Brand name Ionamin discontinued.

MOA — CNS stimulant, increases norepinephrine and dopamine.

ADVERSE EFFECTS — Serious: Seizures, psychosis, hypertension. Frequent: Appetite suppression, weight loss, insomnia, nervousness, N/V, dizziness, palpitations, tachycardia, headache.

PULMONARY

INHALED STEROIDS: ESTIMATED COMPARATIVE DAILY DOSES*

Adults and Children older than 12 yo				
Drug	**Form**	**Low dose**	**Medium dose**	**High dose**
beclomethasone HFA MDI	40 mcg/puff 80 mcg/puff	2–6 puffs/day 1–3 puffs/day	6–12 puffs/day 3–6 puffs/day	> 12 puffs/day > 6 puffs/day
budesonide DPI	90 mcg/dose 180 mcg/dose	2–6 inhalations/day 1–3 inhalations/day	6–13 inhalations/day 3–7 inhalations/day	> 13 inhalations/day > 7 inhalations/day
budesonide	soln for nebs	—	—	—
flunisolide HFA MDI	80 mcg/puff	4 puffs/day	5–8 puffs/day	> 8 puffs/day
fluticasone HFA MDI	44 mcg/puff 110 mcg/puff 220 mcg/puff	2–6 puffs/day 1–2 puffs/day 1 puff/day	6–10 puffs/day 2–4 puffs/day 1–2 puffs/day	> 10 puffs/day > 4 puffs/day > 2 puffs/day
Buticasone DPI	50 mcg/dose 100 mcg/dose 250 mcg/dose	2–6 inhalations/day 1–3 inhalations/day 1 inhalation/day	6–10 inhalations/day 3–5 inhalations/day 2 inhalations/day	> 10 inhalations/day > 5 inhalations/day > 2 inhalations/day
mometasone DPI	220 mcg/dose	1 inhalation/day	2 inhalations/day	> 2 inhalations/day
CHILDREN (age 5 to 11 yo)				
Drug	**Form**	**Low dose**	**Medium dose**	**High dose**
beclomethasone HFA MDI	40 mcg/puff 80 mcg/puff	2–4 puffs/day 1–2 puffs/day	4–8 puffs/day 2–4 puffs/day	> 8 puffs/day > 4 puffs/day
budesonide DPI	90 mcg/dose 180 mcg/dose	2–4 inhalations/day 1–2 inhalations/day	4–9 inhalations/day 2–4 inhalations/day	> 9 inhalations/day > 4 inhalations/day
budesonide	soln for nebs	0.5 mg 0.25–0.5 mg (0–4 yo)	1 mg > 0.5–1 mg (0–4 yo)	2 mg > 1 mg (0–4 yo)
flunisolide HFA MDI	80 mcg/puff	2 puffs/day	4 puffs/day	≥ 8 puffs/day
fluticasone HFA MDI (0–11 yo)	44 mcg/puff 110 mcg/puff 220 mcg/puff	2–4 puffs/day 1–2 puff/day n/a	4–8 puffs/day 2–3 puffs/day 1–2 puffs/day	> 8 puffs/day > 4 puffs/day > 2 puffs/day
fluticasone DPI	50 mcg/dose 100 mcg/dose 250 mcg/dose	2–4 inhalations/day 1–2 inhalations/day n/a	4–8 inhalations/day 2–4 inhalations/day 1 inhalation/day	> 8 inhalations/day > 4 inhalations/day > 1 inhalation/day
mometasone DPI	220 mcg/dose	n/a	n/a	n/a

*HFA = Hydrofluororalkane (propellant). MDI = metered dose inhaler. DPI = dry powder inhaler.
Reference: http://www.nhlbi.nih.gov/guidelines/asthma/asthsumm.pdf

INHALER COLORS (Body then cap–Generics may differ)

Inhaler	Colors
Advair	purple
Advair HFA	purple/light purple
Aerobid-M	grey/green
Aerospan	purple/grey
Alupent	clear/blue
Alvesco 80 mcg 160 mcg	brown/red red/red
Asmanex	white/pink
Atrovent HFA	clear/green
Combivent	clear/orange
Flovent HFA	orange/peach
Foradil	grey/beige
Maxair Autohaler	white/white
ProAir HFA	red/white
Proventil HFA	yellow/orange
Pulmicort	white/brown
QVAR 40 mcg 80 mcg	beige/grey mauve/grey
Serevent Diskus	green
Spiriva	grey
Ventolin HFA	light blue/navy
Xopenex HFA	blue/red

PREDICTED PEAK EXPIRATORY FLOW (liters/min)

Age (yo)	Women (height in inches)					Men (height in inches)					Child (height in inches)
	55"	60"	65"	70"	75"	60"	65"	70"	75"	80"	
20	390	423	460	496	529	554	602	649	693	740	44" – 160
30	380	413	448	483	516	532	577	622	664	710	46" – 187
40	370	402	436	470	502	509	552	596	636	680	48" – 214
50	360	391	424	457	488	486	527	569	607	649	50" – 240
60	350	380	412	445	475	463	502	542	578	618	52" – 267
70	340	369	400	432	461	440	477	515	550	587	54" – 293

Am Rev Resp Dis 1963;88:644.

PULMONARY: Beta Agonists—Long-Acting

NOTE: Long-acting beta-agonists may increase the risk of asthma-related death. Use only as a second agent if inadequate control with an optimal dose of inhaled corticosteroids. Do not use for rescue therapy. Palpitations, tachycardia, tremor, lightheadedness, nervousness, headache, and nausea may occur. Decreases in serum potassium can occur, rarely leading to adverse cardiovascular effects; monitor accordingly.

ARFORMOTEROL (*Brovana*) ▶L ♀C ▶? $$$$$
ADULT — COPD: 15 mcg nebulized two times per day.
PEDS — Not approved in children.
FORMS — Trade only: Soln for inhalation 15 mcg in 2 mL vial.
NOTES — Not for acute COPD exacerbations.
MOA — Long-acting beta agonist bronchodilator.
ADVERSE EFFECTS — Serious: Hypersensitivity, paradoxical bronchospasm. Frequent: Palpitations, tachycardia, hypokalemia, tremor, lightheadedness, nervousness, headache, and nausea.

FORMOTEROL (*Foradil, Perforomist, ❋Oxeze Turbuhaler*) ▶L ♀C ▶? $$$
ADULT — Chronic asthma, COPD: 1 puff two times per day. Prevention of exercise-induced bronchospasm: 1 puff 15 min prior to exercise. COPD: 20 mcg nebulized q 12 h.
PEDS — Chronic asthma, age 5 yo or older: 1 puff two times per day. Prevention of exercise-induced bronchospasm age 12 yo or older: Use adult dose.
FORMS — Trade only: DPI 12 mcg, 12, 60 blisters/pack (Foradil). To be used only with Aerolizer device. Soln for inhalation: 20 mcg in 2 mL vial (Perforomist). Canada only (Oxeze): DPI 6, 12 mcg 60 blisters/pack.
NOTES — For asthma, must use in combination with inhaled steroid. Do not use additional doses for exercise if on maintenance.
MOA — Long-acting beta agonist bronchodilator.
ADVERSE EFFECTS — Serious: Hypersensitivity, paradoxical bronchospasm. Frequent: Palpitations, tachycardia, hypokalemia, tremor, insomnia, lightheadedness, nervousness, headache, and nausea.

INDACATEROL (*Arcapta, ❋Onbrez Breezhaler*) ▶L - ♀C ▶?
ADULT — COPD: DPI: 75 mcg inhaled once daily.
PEDS — Not approved for children.
FORMS — Trade only: DPI: 75 mcg caps for inhalation, 30 blisters. To be used only with Neohaler device. Contains lactose.
MOA — Long-acting beta agonist bronchodilator.
ADVERSE EFFECTS — Serious: Hypersensitivity. Frequent: Palpitations, tachycardia, hypokalemia, tremor, lightheadedness, nervousness, headache, pharyngitis, and nausea.

SALMETEROL (*Serevent Diskus*) ▶L ♀C ▶? $$$$
ADULT — Chronic asthma/COPD: 1 puff two times per day. Prevention of exercise-induced bronchospasm: 1 puff 30 min before exercise.
PEDS — Chronic asthma age 4 yo or older: 1 puff two times per day. Prevention of exercise-induced bronchospasm: 1 puff 30 min before exercise.
FORMS — Trade only: DPI (Diskus): 50 mcg, 60 blisters.
NOTES — For asthma, must use in combination with inhaled steroid. Do not use additional doses for exercise if on maintenance. Concomitant ketoconazole increases levels and prolongs QT interval. Do not use with strong CYP3A4 inhibitors such as ritonavir, itraconazole, clarithromycin, nefazodone, etc.
MOA — Long-acting beta agonist bronchodilator.
ADVERSE EFFECTS — Serious: Hypersensitivity. Frequent: Palpitations, tachycardia, hypokalemia, tremor, lightheadedness, nervousness, headache, pharyngitis, and nausea.

PULMONARY: Beta Agonists—Short-Acting

NOTE: Palpitations, tachycardia, tremor, lightheadedness, nervousness, headache, and nausea may occur; these effects may be more pronounced with systemic administration. Hypokalemia can occur from the transient shift of potassium into cells, rarely leading to adverse cardiovascular effects; monitor accordingly. Potential for tolerance with continued use of short-acting beta-agonists.

ALBUTEROL (*AccuNeb, Ventolin HFA, Proventil HFA, ProAir HFA, VoSpire ER, ❋Airomir, salbutamol*) ▶L ♀C ▶? $$
ADULT — Acute asthma: MDI: 2 puffs q 4 to 6 h prn. Soln for inhalation: 2.5 mg nebulized three to four times per day. Dilute 0.5 mL 0.5% soln with 2.5 mL NS. Deliver over 5 to 15 min. One 3 mL unit dose (0.083%) nebulized three to four times per day. Caps for inhalation: 200 to 400 mcg inhaled q 4 to 6 h via a Rotahaler device. Prevention of exercise-induced bronchospasm: MDI: 2 puffs 10 to 30 min before exercise. Chronic asthma: 2 to 4 mg PO three times per day to four times per day or extended-release 4 to 8 mg PO q 12 h up to 16 mg PO q 12 h.

PEDS — Acute asthma: MDI: Age 4 yo or older: 1 to 2 puffs q 4 to 6 h prn. Soln for inhalation (0.5%): 2 to 12 yo: 0.1 to 0.15 mg/kg/dose not to exceed 2.5 mg three to four times per day, diluted with NS to 3 mL. Caps for inhalation: Age 4 yo or older 200 to 400 mcg inhaled q 4 to 6 h via a Rotahaler device. Chronic asthma: Tabs, syrup 6 to 12 yo: 2 to 4 mg PO three to four times per day, max dose 24 mg/day in divided doses or extended-release 4 mg PO q 12 h. Syrup 2 to 5 yo: 0.1 to 0.2 mg/kg/dose PO three times per day up to 4 mg three times per day. Prevention of exercise-induced bronchospasm age 4 yo or older: 2 puffs 10 to 30 min before exercise.

ALBUTEROL (*cont.*)

UNAPPROVED ADULT — COPD: MDI, soln for inhalation: Use asthma dose. Acute asthma: MDI, soln for inhalation: Dose as above q 20 min × 3 or until improvement. Continuous nebulization: 10 to 15 mg/h until improvement. Emergency hyperkalemia: 10 to 20 mg via MDI or soln for inhalation.

UNAPPROVED PEDS — Acute asthma: Soln for inhalation: 0.15 mg/kg (minimum dose is 2.5 mg) q 20 min for 3 doses then 0.15 to 0.3 mg/kg up to 10 mg q 1 to 4 h prn, or 0.5 mg/kg/h continuous nebulization. MDI: 4 to 8 puffs q 20 min for 3 doses then q 1 to 4 h prn. Soln for inhalation (0.5%): Age younger than 2 yo: 0.05 to 0.15 mg/kg/dose q 4 to 6 h. Syrup age younger than 2 yo: 0.3 mg/kg/24 h PO divided three times per day, max dose 12 mg/24 h. Prevention of exercise-induced bronchospasm: MDI: Age 4 yo or older 2 puffs 10 to 30 min before exercise.

FORMS — Trade only: MDI 90 mcg/actuation, 200 metered doses/canister. "HFA" inhalers use hydrofluoroalkane propellant instead of CFCs but are otherwise equivalent. Generic/Trade: Soln for inhalation 0.021% (AccuNeb), 0.042% (AccuNeb), and 0.083% in 3 mL vials, 0.5% (5 mg/mL) in 20 mL with dropper. Tabs extended-release 4, 8 mg (VoSpire ER). Generic only: Syrup 2 mg/5 mL. Tabs immediate-release 2, 4 mg.

NOTES — Do not crush or chew extended-release tabs. Use with caution in patients on MAOIs or cyclic antidepressants: May increase cardiovascular side effects.

MOA — Short-acting beta agonist bronchodilator.

ADVERSE EFFECTS — Serious: Hypersensitivity, paradoxical bronchospasm. Frequent: Palpitations, tachycardia, hypokalemia, tremor, lightheadedness, nervousness, headache, and nausea.

LEVALBUTEROL (*Xopenex, Xopenex HFA*) ▶L ♀C ▶? $$$

ADULT — Acute asthma: MDI 2 puffs q 4 to 6 h prn. Soln for inhalation: 0.63 to 1.25 mg nebulized q 6 to 8 h.

PEDS — Acute asthma: MDI age 4 yo or older: 2 puffs q 4 to 6 h prn. Soln for inhalation age 12 yo or older: Use adult dose. For age 6 to 11 yo: 0.31 mg nebulized three times per day.

FORMS — Generic/Trade: Soln for inhalation 0.31, 0.63, 1.25 mg in 3 mL and 1.25 mg in 0.5 mL unit-dose vials. Trade only: HFA MDI 45 mcg/actuation, 15 g 200/canister. "HFA" inhalers use hydrofluoroalkane propellant.

NOTES — R-isomer of albuterol. Dyspepsia may occur. Use with caution in patients on MAOIs or cyclic antidepressants; may increase cardiovascular side effects.

MOA — Short-acting beta agonist bronchodilator.

ADVERSE EFFECTS — Serious: Hypersensitivity, paradoxical bronchospasm, arrhythmias. Frequent: Palpitations, tachycardia, hypokalemia, tremor, lightheadedness, nervousness, headache, and nausea.

METAPROTERENOL (*Alupent, ✦orciprenaline*) ▶L ♀C ▶? $$

ADULT — Acute asthma: MDI: 2 to 3 puffs q 3 to 4 h; max dose 12 puffs/day. Soln for inhalation: 0.2 to 0.3 mL of the 5% soln in 2.5 mL NS. 20 mg PO three to four times per day.

PEDS — Acute asthma: Soln for inhalation: 0.1 to 0.3 mL of the 5% soln in 2.5 mL NS for age older than 6 yo. Tabs or syrup: 1.3 to 2.6 mg/kg/day PO in divided doses three to four times per day for age 2 to 5 yo. 10 mg PO three to four times per day for age 6 to 9 yo or wt less than 60 lbs, 20 mg PO three to four times per day for age older than 9 yo or wt 60 lbs or greater.

UNAPPROVED PEDS — Acute asthma: MDI: 2 to 3 puffs q 3 to 4 h (up to 12 puffs/day) for age older than 6 yo. Soln for inhalation: 0.1 to 0.3 mL of the 5% soln in 2.5 mL NS q 4 to 6 h prn or q 20 min until improvement. Tabs or syrup age younger than 2 yo: 0.4 mg/kg/dose PO three to four times per day.

FORMS — Trade only: MDI 0.65 mg/actuation, 14 g 200/canister. Generic/Trade: Soln for inhalation 0.4%, 0.6% in 2.5 mL unit-dose vials. Generic only: Syrup 10 mg/5 mL, Tabs 10, 20 mg.

MOA — Short-acting beta agonist bronchodilator.

ADVERSE EFFECTS — Serious: Hypersensitivity, paradoxical bronchospasm. Frequent: Palpitations, tachycardia, hypokalemia, tremor, lightheadedness, nervousness, headache, and nausea.

PIRBUTEROL (*Maxair Autohaler*) ▶L ♀C ▶? $$$$

ADULT — Acute asthma: MDI: 1 to 2 puffs q 4 to 6 h. Max dose 12 puffs/day.

PEDS — Not approved in children.

UNAPPROVED PEDS — Acute asthma age 12 yo or older: Use adult dose.

FORMS — Trade only: MDI 200 mcg/actuation, 14 g 400/canister.

NOTES — Breath-actuated autohaler.

MOA — Short-acting beta agonist bronchodilator.

ADVERSE EFFECTS — Serious: Hypersensitivity. Frequent: Palpitations, tachycardia, hypokalemia, tremor, lightheadedness, nervousness, headache, and nausea.

TERBUTALINE (*Brethine, ✦Bricanyl Turbuhaler*) ▶L ♀B ▶– $$$

ADULT — Asthma: 2.5 to 5 mg PO q 6 h while awake. Max dose 15 mg/24 h. Acute asthma: 0.25 mg SC into lateral deltoid area; may repeat once within 15 to 30 min. Max dose 0.5 mg/4 h.

PEDS — Not approved in children.

UNAPPROVED ADULT — Preterm labor: 0.25 mg SC q 30 min up to 1 mg in 4 h. Infusion: 2.5 to 10 mcg/min IV, gradually increased to effective max doses of 17.5 to 30 mcg/min.

UNAPPROVED PEDS — Asthma: 0.05 mg/kg/dose PO three times per day, increase to max of 0.15 mg/kg/dose three times per day, max 5 mg/day for age 12 yo or younger, use adult dose for age older than 12 yo up to max 7.5 mg/ 24 h. Acute asthma: 0.01 mg/kg SC q 20 min for 3 doses then q 2 to 6 h prn.

FORMS — Generic Only: Tabs 2.5, 5 mg. Injectable 1 mg/1 mL.

MOA — Short-acting beta agonist bronchodilator; tocolytic.

PULMONARY: Combinations

ADVAIR (fluticasone—inhaled + salmeterol) ▶L ♀C ▶? $$$$$

WARNING — Long-acting beta-agonists may increase the risk of asthma-related death; use as an adjunct only if inadequate control with an optimal dose of inhaled corticosteroids. Avoid in significantly worsening or acute asthma. Do not use for rescue therapy. Do not stop abruptly.

ADULT — Chronic asthma: DPI: 1 puff two times per day (all strengths). MDI: 2 puffs two times per day (all strengths). COPD maintenance: DPI: 1 puff two times per day (250/50 only).

PEDS — Chronic asthma: DPI: 1 puff two times per day (100/50 only) for age 4 to 11 yo. Use adult dose for 12 yo or older.

UNAPPROVED ADULT — COPD: 500/50, 1 puff two times per day.

FORMS — Trade only: DPI: 100/50, 250/50, 500/50 mcg fluticasone/salmeterol per actuation; 60 doses/ DPI. Trade only (Advair HFA): MDI 45/21, 115/21, 230/21 mcg fluticasone/salmeterol per actuation; 120 doses/canister.

NOTES — See individual components for additional information. Ritonavir and other CYP3A4 inhibitors such as ketoconazole significantly increase both salmeterol and fluticasone concentrations, resulting in prolongation of QT interval (salmeterol) and systemic effects, including adrenal suppression (fluticasone). Very rare anaphylactic reaction in patients with severe milk protein allergy. Increased risk of pneumonia in COPD.

MOA — Anti-inflammatory/long-acting beta agonist bronchodilator combination.

ADVERSE EFFECTS — Serious: Hypersensitivity, anaphylaxis, paradoxical bronchospasm, Churg-Strauss syndrome. Frequent: Thrush, dysphonia, pharyngitis, palpitations, tachycardia, tremor, lightheadedness, nervousness, headache, nausea.

BREO ELLIPTA (fluticasone—inhaled + vilanterol) ▶L - ♀C ▶? $$$$$

WARNING — Long-acting beta-agonists may increase the risk of asthma-related death; use as an adjunct only if inadequate control with an optimal dose of inhaled corticosteroids. Avoid in significantly worsening or acute asthma. Do not use for rescue therapy. Do not stop abruptly.

ADULT — COPD maintenance: 1 inhalation once daily.

PEDS — Not approved in children.

UNAPPROVED ADULT — Chronic asthma: 1 inhalation once daily.

FORMS — Trade only: DPI: 100/25 mcg fluticasone/ vilanterol per actuation; 30 doses/DPI.

NOTES — See individual components for additional information. Ritonavir and other CYP3A4 inhibitors such as ketoconazole significantly increase both vilanterol and fluticasone concentrations, resulting in prolongation of QT interval (vilanterol) and systemic effects, including adrenal suppression (fluticasone). Very rare anaphylactic reaction in patients

with severe milk protein allergy. Increased risk of pneumonia in COPD.

MOA — Anti-inflammatory/long-acting beta agonist bronchodilator combination.

ADVERSE EFFECTS — Serious: Hypersensitivity, anaphylaxis, paradoxical bronchospasm, Churg-Strauss syndrome. Frequent: Thrush, dysphonia, pharyngitis, palpitations, tachycardia, tremor, lightheadedness, nervousness, headache, nausea.

COMBIVENT (albuterol-—inhaled + ipratropium-— inhaled Combivent Respimat) ▶L ♀C ▶? $$$$

ADULT — COPD: MDI: 2 puffs four times per day. Max dose 12 puffs/24 h. Respimat: 1 puff four times per day. Max dose 6 inhalations/24 h.

PEDS — Not approved in children.

FORMS — Trade only: MDI: 90 mcg albuterol/18 mcg ipratropium per actuation, 200/canister. Respimat: 100 mcg albuterol/20 mcg ipratroprium per inhalation, 120/canister.

NOTES — MDI contraindicated with soy or peanut allergy. Refer to components.

MOA — Short-acting beta agonist/anticholinergic bronchodilator combination.

ADVERSE EFFECTS — Serious: Paradoxical broncho-spasm. Frequent: Palpitations, tachycardia, tremor, lightheadedness, nervousness, headache, and nausea.

DULERA (mometasone—inhaled + formoterol, ✱Zenhale) ▶L – ♀C ▶? $$$$$

WARNING — Long-acting beta-agonists may increase the risk of asthma-related death; use as an adjunct only if inadequate control with an optimal dose of inhaled corticosteroids. Avoid in significantly worsening or acute asthma. Do not use for rescue therapy. Do not stop abruptly.

ADULT — Chronic asthma: 2 inhalations two times per day (all strengths).

PEDS — Chronic asthma: use adult dose for 12 yo or older.

UNAPPROVED ADULT — COPD: 2 puffs two times per day (all strengths).

FORMS — Trade only: MDI 100/5, 200/5 mcg mometasone/formoterol per actuation; 120 doses/canister.

NOTES — See individual components for additional information. Ritonavir and other CYP3A4 inhibitors such as ketoconazole significantly increase mometasone concentration resulting in systemic effects including adrenal suppression. Canister comes with 124 doses; patient must prime before first use and after more than 5 days of disuse by spraying 4 doses in air away from face, shaking canister after each spray.

MOA — Anti-inflammatory/long-acting beta agonist bronchodilator combination.

ADVERSE EFFECTS — Serious: Hypersensitivity, anaphylaxis, paradoxical bronchospasm, Churg-Strauss syndrome. Frequent: Thrush, dysphonia, pharyngitis, palpitations, tachycardia, tremor, lightheadedness, nervousness, headache, nausea.

DUONEB (albuterol-—inhaled + ipratropium-— inhaled, ✲*Combivent inhalation soln*) ▶L ♀C ▶? $$$$$
ADULT — COPD: 1 unit dose nebulized four times per day; may add 2 doses/day prn to max of 6 doses/day.
PEDS — Not approved in children.
FORMS — Generic/Trade: Unit dose: 2.5 mg albuterol/0.5 mg ipratropium per 3 mL vial, premixed; 30, 60 vials/carton.
NOTES — Refer to components; 3.0 mg albuterol is equivalent to 2.5 mg albuterol base.
MOA — Short-acting beta agonist/anticholinergic bronchodilator combination.
ADVERSE EFFECTS — Serious: None. Frequent: Palpitations, tachycardia, tremor, lightheadedness, nervousness, headache, nausea, dry mouth, blurred vision.

DUOVENT UDV (ipratropium-—inhaled + fenoterol) ▶L ♀? ▶? $$$$$
ADULT — Canada only. Bronchospasm associated with asthma/COPD: 1 vial (via nebulizer) q 6 h prn.
PEDS — Canada only. Children age 12 yo or older: 1 vial (via nebulizer) q 6 h prn.
FORMS — Canada trade only: Unit dose vial (for nebulization) 0.5 mg ipratropium, 1.25 mg fenoterol in 4 mL of saline.
MOA — Anticholinergic and short-acting beta agonist bronchodilator.
ADVERSE EFFECTS — Serious: Hypokalemia, bronchospasm. Frequent: Dry mouth or throat, tremor.

SYMBICORT (budesonide-—inhaled + formoterol, ✲*Symbicort Turbuhaler*) ▶L ♀C ▶? $$$$
WARNING — Long-acting beta-agonists may increase the risk of asthma-related death; use as an adjunct only if inadequate control with an optimal dose of inhaled corticosteroids. Avoid in significantly worsening or acute asthma. Do not use for rescue therapy. Do not stop abruptly.
ADULT — Chronic asthma: 2 puffs two times per day (both strengths). COPD: 2 puffs two times per day (160/4.5).
PEDS — Chronic asthma age 12 yo or older: Use adult dose.
FORMS — Trade only: MDI: 80/4.5, 160/4.5 mcg budesonide/formoterol per actuation; 120 doses/canister.
NOTES — See individual components for additional information. Ritonavir and other CYP3A4 inhibitors such as ketoconazole significantly increase budesonide concentrations, resulting in systemic effects, including adrenal suppression.
MOA — Anti-inflammatory/long-acting beta agonist bronchodilator combination.
ADVERSE EFFECTS — Serious: Hypersensitivity, anaphylaxis, paradoxical bronchospasm, Churg-Strauss syndrome. Frequent: Thrush, dysphonia, pharyngitis, palpitations, tachycardia, tremor, lightheadedness, nervousness, headache, nausea.

PULMONARY: Inhaled Steroids

NOTE: See Endocrine-Corticosteroids when oral steroids necessary. Beware of adrenal suppression when changing from systemic to inhaled steroids. Inhaled steroids are not for treatment of acute asthma; higher doses may be needed for severe asthma and exacerbations. Adjust to lowest effective dose for maintenance. Use of a DPI, a spacing device, and rinsing the mouth with water after each use may decrease the incidence of thrush and dysphonia. Pharyngitis and cough may occur with all products. Use with caution in patients with active or quiescent TB, untreated systemic fungal, bacterial, viral or parasitic infections or in patients with ocular HSV. Inhaled steroids produce small, transient reductions in growth velocity in children. Prolonged use may lead to decreases in bone mineral density and osteoporosis, thereby increasing fracture risk.

BECLOMETHASONE—INHALED (*QVAR*) ▶L ♀C ▶? $$$
ADULT — Chronic asthma: 40 mcg: 1 to 4 puffs two times per day. 80 mcg: 1 to 2 puffs two times per day.
PEDS — Chronic asthma in 5 to 11 yo: 40 mcg 1 to 2 puffs two times per day.
UNAPPROVED ADULT — Chronic asthma: NHLBI dosing schedule (puffs/day divided two times per day): Low dose: 2 to 6 puffs of 40 mcg or 1 to 3 puffs of 80 mcg. Medium dose: 6 to 12 puffs of 40 mcg or 3 to 6 puffs of 80 mcg. High dose: More than 12 puffs of 40 mcg or more than 6 puffs 80 mcg.
UNAPPROVED PEDS — Chronic asthma (5 to 11 yo): NHLBI dosing schedule (puffs/day divided two times per day): Low dose: 2 to 4 puffs of 40 mcg or 1 to 2 puffs of 80 mcg. Medium dose: 4 to 8 puffs of 40 mcg or 2 to 4 puffs of 80 mcg. High dose: More than 8 puffs of 40 mcg or more than 4 puffs of 80 mcg.

FORMS — Trade only: HFA MDI: 40, 80 mcg/actuation, 7.3 g 100 actuations/canister.
MOA — Steroidal anti-inflammatory.
ADVERSE EFFECTS — Serious: Adrenal suppression (high dose), hypersensitivity, bronchospasm. Frequent: Thrush, dysphonia.

BUDESONIDE—INHALED (*Pulmicort Respules, Pulmicort Flexhaler*✲*Pulmicort Turbuhaler*) ▶L ♀B ▶? $$$$
ADULT — Chronic asthma: DPI: 1 to 2 puffs daily to two times per day up to 4 puffs two times per day.
PEDS — Chronic asthma 6 to 12 yo: DPI: 1 to 2 puffs daily to two times per day. 12 mo to 8 yo: Susp for inhalation (Respules): 0.5 mg to 1 mg daily or divided two times per day.
UNAPPROVED ADULT — Chronic asthma: NHLBI dosing schedule (puffs/day daily or divided two times per day): DPI: Low dose is in the range of 1 to 3 puffs of 180 mcg or 2 to 6 puffs of 90 mcg. Medium

BUDESONIDE—INHALED (*cont.*)

dose is in the range of 3 to 7 puffs of 180 mcg or 6 to 13 puffs of 90 mcg. High dose more than 7 puffs of 180 mcg or more than 13 puffs of 90 mcg.

UNAPPROVED PEDS — Chronic asthma (5 to 11 yo): NHLBI dosing schedule (puffs/day daily or divided two times per day) DPI: Low dose: 1 to 2 puffs of 180 mcg or 2 to 4 puffs of 90 mcg. Medium dose: 2 to 4 puffs of 180 mcg or 4 to 9 puffs of 90 mcg. High dose more than 4 puffs of 180 mcg or more than 9 puffs of 90 mcg. Susp for inhalation (daily or divided two times per day): Low dose is in the range of 0.25 to 0.5 mg for age 4 yo or younger and about 0.5 mg for age 5 to 11 yo. Medium dose more than 0.5 to 1 mg for age 4 yo or younger and 1 mg for age 5 to 11 yo. High dose more than 1 mg for age 4 yo or younger and 2 mg for age 5 to 11 yo. Some doses may be outside the package labeling.

FORMS — Trade only: DPI (Flexhaler) 90, 180 mcg powder/actuation 60, 120 doses respectively/canister, Respules 1 mg/2 mL unit dose. Generic/Trade: Respules 0.25, 0.5 mg/2 mL unit dose.

NOTES — Respules should be delivered via a jet nebulizer with a mouthpiece or face mask. CYP3A4 inhibitors such as ketoconazole, erythromycin, ritonavir, etc., may significantly increase systemic concentrations, possibly causing adrenal suppression. Flexhaler contains trace amounts of milk proteins; caution with severe milk protein hypersensitivity.

MOA — Steroidal anti-inflammatory.

ADVERSE EFFECTS — Serious: Adrenal suppression (high dose), hypersensitivity, bronchospasm. Frequent: Thrush, dysphonia, headache, nausea.

CICLESONIDE—INHALED (*Alvesco*) ▶L ♀C ▶? $$$$

ADULT — Chronic asthma: MDI: 80 mcg/puff: 1 to 4 puffs two times per day. 160 mcg/puff: 1 to 2 puffs two times per day.

PEDS — Chronic asthma, age 12 yo or older: Use adult dose.

FORMS — Trade only: 80 mcg/actuation, 60 per canister. 160 mcg/actuation, 60, 120 per canister.

NOTES — CYP3A4 inhibitors such as ketoconazole may significantly increase systemic concentrations, possibly causing adrenal suppression.

MOA — Steroidal anti-inflammatory.

ADVERSE EFFECTS — Serious: Adrenal suppression (high dose), hypersensitivity, bronchospasm. Frequent: Thrush, dysphonia, headache, nausea.

FLUNISOLIDE—INHALED (*AeroBid, AeroBid-M, Aerospan*) ▶L ♀C ▶? $$$

ADULT — Chronic asthma: MDI: 2 puffs two times per day up to 4 puffs two times per day.

PEDS — Chronic asthma, age: 6 to 15 yo: MDI: 2 puffs two times per day.

UNAPPROVED ADULT — Chronic asthma: NHLBI dosing schedule (puffs/day divided two times per day): Low dose: 2 to 4 puffs. Medium dose: 4 to 8 puffs. High dose: More than 8 puffs.

UNAPPROVED PEDS — Chronic asthma (5 to 11 yo): NHLBI dosing schedule (puffs/day divided two times per day): Low dose: 2 to 3 puffs. Medium dose: 4 to 5 puffs. High dose: More than 5 puffs (8 puffs or more for 80 mcg HFA).

FORMS — Trade only: MDI: 250 mcg/actuation, 100 metered doses/canister. AeroBid-M (AeroBid + menthol flavor). Aerospan HFA MDI: 80 mcg/actuation, 60, 120 metered doses/canister.

MOA — Steroidal anti-inflammatory.

ADVERSE EFFECTS — Serious: Adrenal suppression (high dose), bronchospasm. Frequent: Thrush, dysphonia.

FLUTICASONE—INHALED (*Flovent HFA, Flovent Diskus*) ▶L ♀C ▶? $$$$

ADULT — Chronic asthma: MDI: 2 puffs two times per day up to 4 puffs two times per day. Max dose 880 mcg two times per day.

PEDS — Chronic asthma: 2 puffs two times per day of 44 mcg/puff for age 4 to 11 yo, Use adult dose for age 12 yo or older.

UNAPPROVED ADULT — Chronic asthma: NHLBI dosing schedule (puffs/day divided two times per day): Low dose: 2 to 6 puffs of 44 mcg MDI. Medium dose: 2 to 4 puffs of 110 mcg MDI or 2 puffs of 220 mcg MDI. High dose: More than 4 puffs 110 mcg MDI or more than 2 puffs 220 mcg MDI.

UNAPPROVED PEDS — Chronic asthma, age 11 yo or younger: NHLBI dosing schedule (puffs/day divided two times per day): Low dose: 2 to 4 puffs of 44 mcg MDI. Medium dose: 4 to 8 puffs of 44 mcg MDI. 2 to 3 puffs of 110 mcg MDI. 1 to 2 puffs of 220 mcg MDI. High dose: 4 puffs or more 110 mcg MDI. 2 puffs or more 220 mcg MDI.

FORMS — Trade only: HFA MDI: 44, 110, 220 mcg/actuation 120/canister. DPI (Diskus): 50, 100, 250 mcg/actuation delivering 44, 88, 220 mcg respectively.

NOTES — Ritonavir and other CYP3A4 inhibitors such as ketoconazole significantly increase fluticasone concentrations, resulting in systemic effects, including adrenal suppression. Increased risk of pneumonia in COPD.

MOA — Steroidal anti-inflammatory.

ADVERSE EFFECTS — Serious: Adrenal suppression (high dose), anaphylaxis, Churg-Strauss syndrome, bronchospasm. Frequent: Thrush, dysphonia, pharyngitis, headache.

MOMETASONE—INHALED (*Asmanex Twisthaler*) ▶L ♀C ▶? $$$$

ADULT — Chronic asthma: 1 to 2 puffs q pm or 1 puff two times per day. If prior oral corticosteroid therapy: 2 puffs two times per day.

PEDS — Chronic asthma: Age 12 yo or older: Use adult dose.

UNAPPROVED ADULT — Chronic asthma: NHLBI dosing schedule (puffs/day divided two times per day): Low dose: 1 puff. Medium dose: 2 puffs. High dose: More than 2 puffs.

FORMS — Trade only: DPI: 110 mcg/actuation with #30 dosage units, 220 mcg/actuation with #30, 60, 120 dosage units.

MOMETASONE—INHALED (cont.)

NOTES — CYP3A4 inhibitors such as ketoconazole may significantly increase concentrations.

MOA — Steroidal anti-inflammatory.

ADVERSE EFFECTS — Serious: Adrenal suppression (high dose). Frequent: Thrush, dysphonia.

TRIAMCINOLONE—INHALED (Azmacort) ▶L ♀C ▶? $$$$

ADULT — Chronic asthma: MDI: 2 puffs three to four times per day or 4 puffs two times per day. Max dose 16 puffs/day. Severe asthma: 12 to 16 puffs/day and adjust downward.

PEDS — Chronic asthma, children older than 12 yo: Use adult dose. 6 to 12 yo: 1 to 2 puffs three to four times per day or 2 to 4 puffs two times per day. Max dose 12 puffs/day.

UNAPPROVED ADULT — Chronic asthma for age 5 to 11 yo: NHLBI dosing schedule (puffs/day divided two times per day): Low dose: 4 to 10 puffs. Medium dose: 10 to 20 puffs. High dose: More than 20 puffs.

UNAPPROVED PEDS — Chronic asthma: NHLBI dosing schedule (puffs/day divided two times per day): Low dose: 4 to 8 puffs. Medium dose: 8 to 12 puffs. High dose: More than 12 puffs.

FORMS — Trade only: MDI: 75 mcg/actuation, 240/canister. Built-in spacer.

MOA — Steroidal anti-inflammatory.

ADVERSE EFFECTS — Serious: Adrenal suppression (high dose), anaphylaxis, angioedema. Frequent: Thrush, dysphonia.

PULMONARY: Leukotriene Inhibitors

NOTE: Not for treatment of acute asthma. Abrupt substitution for corticosteroids may precipitate Churg-Strauss syndrome. Postmarket cases of agitation, aggression, anxiousness, dream abnormalities and hallucinations, depression, insomnia, irritability, restlessness, suicidal thinking and behavior (including suicide), and tremor have been reported.

MONTELUKAST (Singulair) ▶L ♀B ▶? $$$$

ADULT — Chronic asthma, allergic rhinitis: 10 mg PO daily. Administer in evening for asthma. Prevention of exercise-induced bronchoconstriction: 10 mg PO 2 h before exercise.

PEDS — Chronic asthma, allergic rhinitis: Give 5 mg PO daily for age 6 to 14 yo, give 4 mg (chew tab or oral granules) PO daily for age 2 to 5 yo. Asthma age 12 to 23 mo: 4 mg (oral granules) PO daily. Allergic rhinitis age 6 to 23 mo: 4 mg (oral granules) PO daily. Prevention of exercise-induced bronchoconstriction: Age 6 yo or older: Use adult dose.

FORMS — Generic/Trade only: Tabs 10 mg. Oral granules 4 mg packet, 30/box. Chewable tabs (cherry flavored) 4, 5 mg.

NOTES — Chewable tabs contain phenylalanine. Oral granules may be placed directly into the mouth or mixed with a spoonful of breast milk, baby formula, applesauce, carrots, rice or ice cream. If mixed with food, must be taken within 15 min. Do not mix with other liquids. Levels decreased by phenobarbital and rifampin. Dyspepsia may occur. Do not take an additional dose for exercise-induced bronchospasm if already taking other doses chronically.

MOA — Leukotriene receptor antagonist.

ADVERSE EFFECTS — Serious: Churg-Strauss syndrome, hepatitis, anaphylaxis, angioedema, erythema nodosum, suicidal thinking, pancreatitis. Frequent: Headache, dyspepsia.

ZAFIRLUKAST (Accolate) ▶L ♀B ▶– $$$$

WARNING — Hepatic failure has been reported.

ADULT — Chronic asthma: 20 mg PO two times per day, 1 h before meals or 2 h after meals.

PEDS — Chronic asthma age 5 to 11 yo: 10 mg PO two times per day, 1 h before meals or 2 h after meals. Use adult dose for age 12 yo or older.

UNAPPROVED ADULT — Allergic rhinitis: 20 mg PO two times per day, 1 h before meals or 2 h after meals.

FORMS — Trade only: Tabs 10, 20 mg.

NOTES — Potentiates warfarin and theophylline. Levels decreased by erythromycin and increased by high-dose aspirin. Nausea may occur. If liver dysfunction is suspected, discontinue drug and manage accordingly. Consider monitoring LFTs.

MOA — Leukotriene receptor antagonist.

ADVERSE EFFECTS — Serious: Churg-Strauss syndrome, hypersensitivity, hepatotoxicity, anaphylaxis, angioedema. Frequent: Headache, dyspepsia.

ZILEUTON (Zyflo CR) ▶L ♀C ▶? $$$$$

WARNING — Contraindicated in active liver disease.

ADULT — Chronic asthma: 1200 mg PO two times per day.

PEDS — Chronic asthma age 12 yo or older: Use adult dose.

FORMS — Trade only: Tabs extended-release 600 mg.

NOTES — Monitor LFTs for elevation. Potentiates warfarin, theophylline, and propranolol. Dyspepsia and nausea may occur.

MOA — Leukotriene formation inhibitor.

ADVERSE EFFECTS — Serious: Hepatotoxicity, leukopenia. Frequent: Headache, dyspepsia.

PULMONARY: Other Pulmonary Medications

ACETYLCYSTEINE—INHALED (Mucomyst) ▶L ♀B ▶? $

ADULT — Mucolytic nebulization: 3 to 5 mL of the 20% soln or 6 to 10 mL of the 10% soln three to four times per day. Instillation, direct or via tracheostomy: 1 to 2 mL of a 10% to 20% soln q 1 to 4 h; via percutaneous intratracheal catheter: 1 to 2

(cont.)

ACETYLCYSTEINE—INHALED (*cont.*)
mL of the 20% soln or 2 to 4 mL of the 10% soln q 1 to 4 h.
PEDS — Mucolytic nebulization: Use adult dosing.
FORMS — Generic/Trade: Soln for inhalation 10, 20% in 4, 10, 30 mL vials.
NOTES — Increased volume of liquefied bronchial secretions may occur; maintain an open airway. Watch for bronchospasm in asthmatics. Stomatitis, N/V, fever, and rhinorrhea may occur. A slight disagreeable odor may occur and should soon disappear. A face mask may cause stickiness on the face after nebulization; wash with water. The 20% soln may be diluted with NaCl or sterile water.
MOA — Mucolytic.
ADVERSE EFFECTS — Serious: Bronchospasm (asthmatics), anaphylaxis. Frequent: Stomatitis, N/V, fever, and rhinorrhea.

ACLIDINIUM (*Tudorza*) ▶L − ♀C ▶? $$$$$
ADULT — COPD: Pressair: 400 mcg two times per day.
PEDS — Not approved in children.
FORMS — Trade only: Sealed aluminum pouches 400 mcg per actuation. To be used with "Pressair" device only. Packages of 60 with Pressair device.
NOTES — Not for acute bronchospasm. Use with caution in narrow-angle glaucoma, myasthenia gravis, BPH, or bladder-neck obstruction. Paradoxical bronchospasm may occur. Eye pain or blurred vision may occur if powder enters eyes. Avoid if severe lactose allergy.
MOA — Long-acting anticholinergic bronchodilator.
ADVERSE EFFECTS — Serious: anaphylaxis, paradoxical bronchospasm. Common: headache, nasopharyngitis, cough.

ALPHA-1 PROTEINASE INHIBITOR (*alpha-1 antitrypsin, Aralast, Prolastin, Zemaira*) ▶Plasma ♀C ▶? $
WARNING — Possible transmission of viruses and Creutzfeldt-Jakob disease.
ADULT — Congenital alpha-1 proteinase inhibitor deficiency with emphysema: 60 mg/kg IV once per week.
PEDS — Not approved in children.
NOTES — Contraindicated in selected IgA deficiencies with known antibody to IgA. Hepatitis B vaccine recommended in preparation for Prolastin use.
MOA — Alpha-1 proteinase inhibitor.
ADVERSE EFFECTS — Serious: Anaphylaxis, increased LFTs. Frequent: Headache, somnolence, flu-like symptoms.

AMINOPHYLLINE ▶L ♀C ▶? $
ADULT — Acute asthma: Loading dose if currently not receiving theophylline: 6 mg/kg IV over 20 to 30 min. Maintenance IV infusion: Dose 0.5 to 0.7 mg/kg/h, mix 1 g in 250 mL D5W (4 mg/mL) set at rate 11 mL/h delivers 0.7 mg/kg/h for wt 70 kg patient. In patients with cor pulmonale, heart failure, liver failure, use 0.25 mg/kg/h. If currently on theophylline, each 0.6 mg/kg aminophylline will increase the serum theophylline concentration by approximately 1 mcg/mL. Maintenance: 200 mg PO two to four times per day.

PEDS — Acute asthma: Loading dose if currently not receiving theophylline: 6 mg/kg IV over 20 to 30 min. Maintenance oral route age older than 1 yo: 3 to 4 mg/kg/dose PO q 6 h. Maintenance IV route for age older than 6 mo: 0.8 to 1 mg/kg/hr IV infusion.
UNAPPROVED PEDS — Neonatal apnea of prematurity: Loading dose 5 to 6 mg/kg IV/PO, maintenance: 1 to 2 mg/kg/dose q 6 to 8 h IV/PO.
NOTES — Aminophylline is 79% theophylline. Administer IV infusion no faster than 25 mg/min. Multiple drug interactions (especially ketoconazole, rifampin, carbamazepine, isoniazid, phenytoin, macrolides, zafirlukast, and cimetidine). Review meds before initiating treatment. Irritability, nausea, palpitations, and tachycardia may occur. Overdose may be life-threatening.
MOA — Bronchodilator.
ADVERSE EFFECTS — Serious: Arrhythmias, seizures. Frequent: Irritability, nausea, palpitations, tachycardia.

BERACTANT (*Survanta*) ▶Lung ♀? ▶? $$$$$
PEDS — RDS (hyaline membrane disease) in premature infants: Specialized dosing.
MOA — Lung surfactant.
ADVERSE EFFECTS — Serious: Bradycardia, nosocomial sepsis. Frequent: Bradycardia, oxygen desaturation.

CALFACTANT (*Infasurf*) ▶Lung ♀? ▶? $$$$$
PEDS — RDS (hyaline membrane disease) in premature infants: Specialized dosing.
FORMS — Trade only: Oral susp: 35 mg/mL in 3, 6 mL vials. Preservative-free.
MOA — Lung surfactant.
ADVERSE EFFECTS — Serious: Bradycardia, cyanosis. Frequent: Cyanosis, bradycardia, airway obstruction.

CROMOLYN—INHALED (*Intal, Gastrocrom, ✹Nalcrom*) ▶LK ♀B ▶? $
ADULT — Chronic asthma: MDI: 2 to 4 puffs four times per day. Soln for inhalation: 20 mg four times per day. Prevention of exercise-induced bronchospasm: MDI: 2 puffs 10 to 15 min prior to exercise. Soln for nebulization: 20 mg 10 to 15 min prior. Mastocytosis: 200 mg PO four times per day, 30 min before meals and at bedtime.
PEDS — Chronic asthma for age older than 5 yo using MDI: 2 puffs four times per day; for age older than 2 yo using soln for nebulization 20 mg four times per day. Prevention of exercise-induced bronchospasm for age older than 5 yo using MDI: 2 puffs 10 to 15 min prior to exercise, using soln for nebulization for age older than 2 yo: 20 mg 10 to 15 min prior. Mastocytosis: Age 2 to 12 yo: 100 mg PO four times per day 30 min before meals and at bedtime.
FORMS — Generic only: Soln for nebs: 20 mg/2 mL. Generic/Trade: Oral concentrate 100 mg/5 mL in individual amps
NOTES — Not for treatment of acute asthma. Pharyngitis may occur. Directions for oral concentrate: 1) Break open and squeeze liquid contents of ampule(s) into a glass of water. 2) Stir soln. 3) Drink all of the liquid.

CROMOLYN—INHALED (cont.)

MOA — Mast cell stabilizer.

ADVERSE EFFECTS — Serious: Paradoxical broncho-spasm, anaphylaxis. Frequent: Cough, pharyngitis.

DORNASE ALFA (Pulmozyme) ▶L ♀B ▶? $$$$$

ADULT — Cystic fibrosis: 2.5 mg nebulized one to two times per day.

PEDS — Cystic fibrosis age 6 yo or older: 2.5 mg nebulized one to two times per day.

UNAPPROVED PEDS — Has been used in a small number of children as young as 3 mo with similar efficacy and side effects.

FORMS — Trade only: Soln for inhalation: 1 mg/mL in 2.5 mL vials.

NOTES — Voice alteration, pharyngitis, laryngitis, and rash may occur. Do not dilute or mix with other drugs.

MOA — Mucolytic.

ADVERSE EFFECTS — Serious: None. Frequent: Voice alteration, pharyngitis, laryngitis, and rash.

DOXAPRAM (Dopram) ▶L ♀B ▶? $$$

ADULT — Acute hypercapnia due to COPD: 1 to 2 mg/min IV, max 3 mg/min. Maximum infusion time: 2 h.

PEDS — Not approved in children.

UNAPPROVED PEDS — Apnea of prematurity unre-sponsive to methylxanthines: Load 2.5 to 3 mg/kg over 15 min, then 1 mg/kg/h titrated to lowest effective dose. Max: 2.5 mg/kg/h. Contains benzyl alcohol; caution in neonates.

NOTES — Monitor arterial blood gases at baseline and q 30 min during infusion. Do not use with mechanical ventilation. Contraindicated with sei-zure disorder, severe HTN, CVA, head injury, CAD and severe heart failure.

MOA — Respiratory stimulant.

ADVERSE EFFECTS — Serious: None. Frequent: Hypertension, N/V, diarrhea, cough, dyspnea, tachy-pnea, tachycardia, arrhythmias, seizure, fever, and sweating.

EPINEPHRINE RACEMIC (S-2, ✱Vaponefrin) ▶Plasma ♀C ▶– $

ADULT — See cardiovascular section.

PEDS — Severe croup: Soln for inhalation: 0.05 mL/kg/dose diluted to 3 mL with NS over 15 min prn not to exceed q 1 to 2 h dosing. Max dose 0.5 mL.

FORMS — Trade only: Soln for inhalation: 2.25% epi-nephrine in 15, 30 mL.

NOTES — Cardiac arrhythmias and HTN may occur.

MOA — Bronchodilator.

ADVERSE EFFECTS — Serious: Arrhythmias, cerebral hemorrhage, hypertension. Frequent: Palpitations, tachycardia, tremor, lightheadedness, nervousness, headache, and nausea.

IPRATROPIUM—INHALED (Atrovent, Atrovent HFA) ▶Lung ♀B ▶? $$$$

ADULT — COPD: MDI (Atrovent, Atrovent HFA): 2 puffs four times per day; may use additional inhalations not to exceed 12 puffs/day. Soln for inhalation: 500 mcg nebulized three to four times per day.

PEDS — Not approved in children younger than 12 yo.

UNAPPROVED PEDS — Acute asthma: MDI (Atrovent, Atrovent HFA): 1 to 2 puffs three to four times per day for age 12 yo or younger. Soln for inhalation: Give 250 mcg/dose three to four times per day for age 12 yo or younger: Give 250 to 500 mcg/dose three to four times per day for age older than 12 yo. Acute asthma: Age 2 to 18 yo: 500 mcg nebulized with 2nd and 3rd doses of albuterol.

FORMS — Trade only: Atrovent HFA MDI: 17 mcg/actuation, 200/canister. Generic/Trade: Soln for nebulization: 0.02% (500 mcg/vial) in unit dose vials.

NOTES — Atrovent MDI is contraindicated with soy or peanut allergy; HFA not contraindicated. Caution with glaucoma, myasthenia gravis, BPH, or blad-der neck obstruction. Cough, dry mouth, and blurred vision may occur.

MOA — Short-acting anticholinergic bronchodilator.

ADVERSE EFFECTS — Serious: Anaphylaxis, angio-edema. Frequent: Dry mouth, blurred vision.

KETOTIFEN (✱Zaditen) ▶L ♀C ▶– $$

ADULT — Not approved.

PEDS — Canada only. Chronic asthma: 6 mo to 3 yo: 0.05 mg/kg PO two times per day. Children older than 3 yo: 1 mg PO two times per day.

FORMS — Generic/Trade: Tabs 1 mg. Syrup 1 mg/5 mL.

NOTES — Several weeks may be necessary before therapeutic effect. Full clinical effectiveness is generally reached after 10 weeks.

MOA — Non-bronchodilator antihistamine.

ADVERSE EFFECTS — Serious: Seizures, thrombocy-topenia. Frequent: Drowsiness, weight gain.

METHACHOLINE (Provocholine) ▶Plasma ♀C ▶? $$

WARNING — Life-threatening bronchoconstric-tion can result; have resuscitation capability available.

ADULT — Diagnosis of bronchial airway hyperre-activity in nonwheezing patients with suspected asthma: 5 breaths each of ascending serial con-centrations, 0.025 mg/mL to 25 mg/mL, via nebu-lization. The procedure ends when there is more than 20% reduction in the FEV1 compared with baseline.

PEDS — Diagnosis of bronchial airway hyperreactiv-ity: Use adult dose.

NOTES — Avoid with epilepsy, bradycardia, peptic ulcer disease, thyroid disease, urinary tract obstruc-tion, or other conditions that could be adversely affected by a cholinergic agent. Hold beta-blockers. Do not inhale powder.

MOA — Bronchoconstrictor.

ADVERSE EFFECTS — Serious: Respiratory/cardiac arrest, syncope. Frequent: Wheezing.

NEDOCROMIL—INHALED (Tilade) ▶L ♀B ▶? $$$

ADULT — Chronic asthma: MDI: 2 puffs four times per day. Reduce dose to two to three times per day as tolerated.

PEDS — Chronic asthma age older than 6 yo: MDI: 2 puffs four times per day.

NEDOCROMIL—INHALED (cont.)

FORMS — Trade only: MDI: 1.75 mg/actuation, 112/ canister.

NOTES — Product to be discontinued when supplies run out. Not for treatment of acute asthma. Unpleasant taste and dysphonia may occur.

MOA — Mast cell stabilizer.

ADVERSE EFFECTS — Serious: None. Frequent: Cough, pharyngitis, bad taste.

OMALIZUMAB (*Xolair*) ▶Plasma, L ♀B ▶? $$$$$

WARNING — Anaphylaxis may occur; monitor closely and be prepared to treat. Anaphylaxis most commonly occurs within 1 hr of administration; 78% of cases occur within 12 hrs.

ADULT — Moderate to severe asthma with perennial allergy when symptoms not controlled by inhaled steroids: 150 to 375 mg SC q 2 to 4 weeks, based on pretreatment serum total IgE level and body wt.

PEDS — Moderate to severe asthma with perennial allergy: Age 12 yo or older: Use adult dose.

NOTES — Not for treatment of acute asthma. Divide doses greater than 150 mg over more than 1 injection site. Monitor for signs of anaphylaxis including bronchospasm, hypotension, syncope, urticaria, angioedema.

MOA — Monoclonal antibody that inhibits IgE binding to mast cells and basophils.

ADVERSE EFFECTS — Serious: Anaphylaxis, malignancy. Frequent: Injection site reactions.

PORACTANT (*Curosurf*) ▶Lung ♀? ▶? $$$$$

PEDS — RDS (hyaline membrane disease) in premature infants: Specialized dosing.

MOA — Lung surfactant.

ADVERSE EFFECTS — Serious: Bradycardia, hypotension. Frequent: Bradycardia, hypotension, oxygen desaturation.

ROFLUMILAST (*Daliresp*, *♣Daxas*) ▶L – ♀C ▶– $$$$$

ADULT — Severe COPD due to chronic bronchitis: 500 mcg PO daily with or without food.

PEDS — Not approved for use in children.

FORMS — Trade only: Tabs 500 mcg.

NOTES — Contraindicated in moderate-to-severe liver disease. Inhibitors of CYP3A4 or dual CYP3A4 and 1A2 (erythromycin, ketoconazole, cimetidine) may increase concentrations. Not recommended for use with strong CYP inducers (rifampin, carbamazepine, phenobarbital, phenytoin). Not for relief of acute bronchospasm. Main effect is decreased exacerbations.

MOA — Phosphodiesterase-4 inhibitor. Exact mechanism in COPD is unknown but believed to be related to the increase in intracellular cyclic AMP in lung cells.

ADVERSE EFFECTS — Serious: psychiatric events including suicidality, depression, anxiety. Frequent: diarrhea, weight loss, nausea, headache, insomnia.

THEOPHYLLINE (*Elixophyllin, Uniphyl, Theo-24, T-Phyl, ♣Theo-Dur, Theolair*) ▶L ♀C ▶+ $

ADULT — Chronic asthma: 5 to 13 mg/kg/day PO in divided doses. Max dose 900 mg/day.

PEDS — Chronic asthma: Initial: Age older than 1 yo and wt less than 45 kg: 12 to 14 mg/kg/day PO divided q 4 to 6 h to max of 300 mg/24 h. Maintenance: 16 to 20 mg/kg/day PO divided q 4 to 6 h to max of 600 mg/24 h. for age older than 1 yo and wt 45 kg or more: Initial: 300 mg/24 h PO divided q 6 to 8 h. Maintenance: 400 to 600 mg/24 h PO divided q 6 to 8 h. Infants age 6 to 52 weeks: [(0.2 × age in weeks) + 5] × kg = 24 h dose in mg PO divided q 6 to 8 h.

UNAPPROVED ADULT — COPD: 10 mg/kg/day PO in divided doses.

UNAPPROVED PEDS — Apnea and bradycardia of prematurity: 3 to 6 mg/kg/day PO divided q 6 to 8 h. Maintain serum concentrations 3 to 5 mcg/mL.

FORMS — Generic/Trade: Elixir 80 mg/15 mL. Trade only: Caps: Theo-24: 100, 200, 300, 400 mg. T-Phyl: 12 hr SR tabs 200 mg. Theolair: Tabs 125, 250 mg. Generic only: 12 hr tabs 100, 200, 300, 450 mg, 12 hr caps 125, 200, 300 mg.

NOTES — Multiple drug interactions (especially ketoconazole, rifampin, carbamazepine, isoniazid, phenytoin, macrolides, zafirlukast, and cimetidine). Review meds before initiating treatment. Overdose may be life-threatening.

MOA — Bronchodilator.

ADVERSE EFFECTS — Serious: Arrhythmias, seizures. Frequent: Irritability, nausea, palpitations, tachycardia.

TIOTROPIUM (*Spiriva*) ▶K ♀C ▶– $$$$

WARNING — QT prolongation has been reported.

ADULT — COPD: HandiHaler: 18 mcg inhaled daily.

PEDS — Not approved in children.

FORMS — Trade only: Caps for oral inhalation 18 mcg. To be used with "HandiHaler" device only. Packages of 5, 30, 90 caps with HandiHaler device.

NOTES — Not for acute bronchospasm. Administer at the same time each day. Use with caution in narrow-angle glaucoma, myasthenia gravis, BPH, or bladder-neck obstruction. Avoid touching opened cap. Glaucoma, eye pain, or blurred vision may occur if powder enters eyes. May increase dosing interval in patients with CrCl less than 50 mL/min. Avoid if severe lactose allergy.

MOA — Long-acting anticholinergic bronchodilator.

ADVERSE EFFECTS — Serious: Anaphylaxis, angioedema, paradoxical bronchospasm, QT prolongation. Frequent: Dry mouth, cough.

RHEUMATOLOGY

INITIAL TREATMENT OF RHEUMATOID ARTHRITIS (RA): AMERICAN COLLEGE OF RHEUMATOLOGY RECOMMENDATIONS

Disease activity	No poor prognostic factors*	Poor prognostic factors present*
Early disease (duration <6 months)		
Low	DMARD monotherapy[†]	DMARD monotherapy[†]
Moderate	DMARD monotherapy[†]	DMARD combination[‡]
High	DMARD monotherapy[†] OR MTX + HCQ	DMARD combination[‡] OR TNF-blocker ± MTX[¶]
Established disease (duration ≥6 months)		
Low	DMARD monotherapy[†]	MTX monotherapy OR DMARD combination[‡]
Moderate/High	MTX monotherapy OR DMARD combination[‡]	MTX monotherapy OR DMARD combination[‡]

Adapted from: Arthritis Care Res 2012;64:625-39. Available online at: http://www.rheumatology.org.

DMARD = disease-modifying anti-rheumatic drug; HCQ=hydroxychloroquine; LEF=leflunomide; MTX=methotrexate; TNF = tumor necrosis factor.

*Poor prognostic factors: Functional limitation; extraarticular disease (e.g. rheumatoid nodules; RA vasculitis; Felty's syndrome); positive rheumatoid factor or anti-cyclic citrullinated peptide antibodies; bony erosions by radiograph.

[†]DMARD monotherapy: HCQ, LEF, MTX, minocycline (usually only for early RA), or sulfasalazine. Reassess after 3 months of therapy.

[‡]DMARD combination: MTX + HCQ; MTX + LEF; MTX + sulfasalazine; sulfasalazine + HCQ; sulfasalazine + HCQ + MTX. Reassess after 3 months of therapy.

[¶]TNF-blocker regimens include: adalimumab ± MTX; certolizumab ± MTX; etanercept ± MTX; golimumab ± MTX; infliximab + MTX. Reassess after 3 months of therapy.

RHEUMATOLOGY: Biologic Response Modifiers—TNF-Blockers

NOTE: TNF-blockers increase the risk of serious infections, including TB, sepsis, invasive fungal and opportunistic infections; discontinue if a serious infection occurs. Test all patients for latent TB before starting a TNF-blocker; if present, treat TB for at least 1 month before starting a TNF-blocker. Monitor for signs and symptoms of active TB. Hold TNF-blockers for at least 1 week before and after surgery. Lymphoma and other malignancies have been reported in children and adolescents. Other adverse effects include new onset or exacerbation of demyelinating disorders and heart failure (avoid if NYHA Class III/IV heart failure), reactivation of hepatitis B virus infection, a lupus-like syndrome, and serious hypersensitivity reactions including anaphylaxis. Avoid live vaccines. Do not coadminister with abatacept or anakinra. Refer to American College of Rheumatology RA guidelines (www.rheumatology.org) for advice on TB screening, vaccine administration, and other safety issues. Monitor CBC, hepatic transaminases, and serum creatinine.

ADALIMUMAB (*Humira*) ▶proteolysis ♀B ▶? Use with caution but no significant risks have been identified $$$$$
WARNING — Increased risk of serious infections, including TB, sepsis, invasive fungal and opportunistic infections; discontinue if a serious infection occurs. Test for latent TB before starting a TNF-blocker; if present, treat TB before starting a TNF-blocker. Monitor for signs and symptoms of active TB. Lymphoma

ADALIMUMAB (cont.)

and other malignancies have been reported with TNF-blockers in children and adolescents. Hepatosplenic T-cell lymphoma has been reported in adolescents and young adults with inflammatory bowel disease.

ADULT — RA, psoriatic arthritis, ankylosing spondylitis: 40 mg SC q 2 weeks, alone or in combination with methotrexate or other DMARD. May increase frequency to q week if not receiving methotrexate. Plaque psoriasis: 80 mg SC at week 0, 40 mg SC at week 1, then 40 mg SC q 2 weeks. Crohn's disease, ulcerative colitis: 160 mg SC at week 0, 80 mg at week 2, then 40 mg q 2 weeks starting at week 4. Only continue treatment in ulcerative colitis patients with evidence of clinical remission by week 8. Inject SC into thigh or abdomen, rotating injection sites.

PEDS — JIA: 20 mg SC q 2 weeks for 15 to <30 kg; 40 mg SC q 2 weeks for 30 kg and greater. Inject SC into thigh or abdomen, rotating injection sites.

FORMS — Trade only: Single-use injection pen (2 per pack) or vial: 40 mg/0.8 mL. Crohn's disease/ulcerative colitis starter pack: six 40 mg pens. Psoriasis starter pack: four 40 mg pens. Pediatric single-use syringe (2 per pack): 20 mg/0.4 mL.

NOTES — Do not coadminister with other biologic DMARDs. Refrigerate and protect from light. Onset of response in RA in 2 to 4 weeks; effects may last up to 4 months after discontinuation.

MOA — Human IgG1 monoclonal antibody against TNF-α. Blockade of TNF inhibits production of pro-inflammatory cytokines.

ADVERSE EFFECTS — Serious: Increased risk of serious infections, including sepsis, TB, opportunistic, and invasive fungal infections. Reactivation of hepatitis B infection. Increased risk of malignancies, esp lymphoma, in young people. New onset and exacerbation of heart failure and demyelinating disorders. Hematologic cytopenias. Serious hypersensitivity reactions. Increased transaminases. Autoantibodies and lupus-like syndrome. Frequent: Injection site reaction.

CERTOLIZUMAB (Cimzia) ▶K proteolysis ♀B ▶? $$$$$

WARNING — Increased risk of serious infections, including TB, sepsis, invasive fungal and opportunistic infections; discontinue if a serious infection occurs. Test for latent TB before starting a TNF-blocker; if present, treat TB before starting a TNF-blocker. Monitor for signs and symptoms of active TB. Lymphoma and other malignancies have been reported with TNF-blockers in children and adolescents.

ADULT — Crohn's disease: 400 mg SC at 0, 2, and 4 weeks. Maintain with 400 mg SC q 4 weeks if response. RA, psoriatic arthritis: 400 mg SC at 0, 2, and 4 weeks. Maintain with 200 mg SC q 2 weeks; can consider 400 mg SC q 4 weeks. Ankylosing spondylitis: 400 mg at 0, 2 and 4 weeks, then 200

mg q 2 weeks or 400 mg q 4 weeks. Divide 400 mg dose into 2 separate 200 mg SC injections at different sites on thigh or abdomen. Rotate injection sites.

PEDS — Not approved for use in children.

FORMS — Trade only: Packs containing 2 vials for reconstitution or 2 prefilled syringes, 200 mg/1 mL each. Starter pack of 6 syringes.

NOTES — Do not coadminister with rituximab or natalizumab. Store SC syringes in refrigerator. Onset of response in RA in 2 to 4 weeks. Effects may last up to 5 months after discontinuation.

MOA — Fab antibody fragment against humanTNF-α that is PEG-conjugated. Blockade of TNF inhibits production of pro-inflammatory cytokines.

ADVERSE EFFECTS — Serious: Increased risk of serious infections, including sepsis, TB, opportunistic, and invasive fungal infections. Reactivation of hepatitis B infection. Increased risk of malignancies, esp lymphoma, in young people. New onset and exacerbation of heart failure and demyelinating disorders. Hematologic cytopenias. Serious hypersensitivity reactions. Autoantibodies and lupus-like syndrome. Frequent: Rash, UTI, upper respiratory infection.

ETANERCEPT (Enbrel) ▶proteolysis ♀B ▶? $$$$$

WARNING — Combination use with other immunomodulators increases the risk of serious infections. Rare nervous system disorders (e.g., multiple sclerosis, myelitis, optic neuritis) have been reported. May worsen heart failure; monitor closely.

ADULT — RA, psoriatic arthritis, ankylosing spondylitis: 50 mg SC q week. Can be used alone or with methotrexate for RA and psoriatic arthritis. Plaque psoriasis: 50 mg SC twice per week for 3 months, then 50 mg SC q week. Initial doses of 25 or 50 mg SC q week can also be used. Inject into thigh, abdomen, or outter upper arm. Rotate injection sites.

PEDS — JIA, age 2 yo and older: 0.8 mg/kg SC q week for wt less than 63 kg; 50 mg SC q week for wt of 63 kg or greater. Inject into thigh, abdomen, or outer upper arm. Rotate injection sites. Use 50 mg autoinjector only in children with wt of 63 kg or greater.

UNAPPROVED PEDS — Plaque psoriasis, age 4 to 17 yo: 0.8 mg/kg (max dose 50 mg) SC q week. Inject into thigh, abdomen, or outer upper arm. Rotate injection sites.

FORMS — Trade only: Single-use prefilled syringe or autoinjector 50 mg/1 mL. Single-use prefilled syringe 25 mg/0.5 mL. Multidose vial 25 mg.

NOTES — Warn latex-sensitive patients that the needle cover contains latex. Refrigerate and protect from light; leave at room temperature for 15 to 30 minutes before injecting. In the US, autoinjector or syringes can be stored at room temperature for up to 14 days; discard after 14 days at room temperature.

(cont.)

ETANERCEPT (*cont.*)

MOA — Fusion protein of human p75 TNF-α receptor linked to Fc portion of human IgG1. Blockade of TNF inhibits production of pro-inflammatory cytokines.

ADVERSE EFFECTS — Serious: Increased risk of serious infections, including sepsis, TB, opportunistic, and invasive fungal infections. Reactivation of hepatitis B infection. Increased risk of malignancies, esp. lymphoma, in young people. New onset and exacerbation of heart failure and demyelinating disorders. Hematologic cytopenias. Serious hypersensitivity reactions. Autoantibodies and lupus-like syndrome. Frequent: Infections; injection site reactions.

GOLIMUMAB (*Simponi, Simponi Aria*) ▶? ♀B ▶– $$$$$

WARNING — Increased risk of serious infections, including TB, sepsis, invasive fungal and opportunistic infections; discontinue if a serious infection occurs. Test for latent TB before starting a TNF-blocker; if present, treat TB before starting a TNF-blocker. Monitor for signs and symptoms of active TB. Lymphoma and other malignancies have been reported with TNF-blockers in children and adolescents.

ADULT — RA, psoriatic arthritis, ankylosing spondylitis: 50 mg SC q month. IV regimen (Simponi Aria) for RA: 2 mg/kg IV infused over 30 minutes at weeks 0 and 4, then q 8 weeks thereafter. Use IV/SC golimumab with methotrexate to treat RA. Ulcerative colitis: 200 mg SC at week 0, 100 mg SC at week 2, then 100 mg SC q 4 weeks. Give SC injection in thigh, abdomen, or upper outer arm. Rotate injection sites. Give at separate sites if a dose requires more than 1 injection.

PEDS — Not approved for use in children.

FORMS — Trade only: Single-dose autoinjector or prefilled syringe: 50 mg/0.5 mL, 100 mg/1 mL.

NOTES — Do not use with other biologics to treat RA, psoriatic arthritis, or ankylosing spondylitis. Warn latex-sensitive patients that needle cover contains latex. Refrigerate for storage; leave at room temperature for 30 minutes before injection. Clinical response to golimumab is usually achieved within 14 to 16 weeks.

MOA — Monoclonal antibody against human TNF-α. Blockade of TNF inhibits production of pro-inflammatory cytokines.

ADVERSE EFFECTS — Serious: Increased risk of serious infections, including sepsis, TB, opportunistic, and invasive fungal infections. Reactivation of hepatitis B infection. Increased risk of malignancies, esp lymphoma, in young people. New onset and exacerbation of heart failure and demyelinating disorders. Hematologic cytopenias. Serious hypersensitivity reactions. Increased transaminases. Autoantibodies and lupus-like syndrome. Frequent: upper respiratory infections, nasopharyngitis, injection site reactions.

INFLIXIMAB (*Remicade*) ▶proteolysis ♀B ▶? $$$$$

WARNING — Increased risk of serious infections, including TB, sepsis, invasive fungal and opportunistic infections; discontinue if a serious infection occurs. Test for latent TB before starting a TNF-blocker; if present, treat TB before starting a TNF-blocker. Monitor for signs and symptoms of active TB. Lymphoma and other malignancies have been reported with TNF-blockers in children and adolescents. Hepatosplenic T-cell lymphoma has been reported in adolescents and young adults with inflammatory bowel disease.

ADULT — RA, with methotrexate: 3 mg/kg IV at weeks 0, 2, and 6. Maintain with 3 mg/kg IV q 8 weeks. For incomplete response, can increase dose to max of 10 mg/kg or reduce dosing interval to as short as q 4 weeks. Ankylosing spondylitis: 5 mg/kg IV at weeks 0, 2, and 6. Maintain with 5 mg/kg IV q 6 weeks. Plaque psoriasis, psoriatic arthritis: 5 mg/kg IV at weeks 0, 2, and 6. Maintain with 5 mg/kg IV q 8 weeks. Crohn's disease, moderate to severe or fistulizing; ulcerative colitis: 5 mg/kg IV at weeks 0, 2, and 6. Maintain with 5 mg/kg IV q 8 weeks. For Crohn's disease: Consider discontinuing if no response by week 14; consider increasing to 10 mg/kg in patients who respond and then lose response. Infuse IV over 2 h or more.

PEDS — Ulcerative colitis, Crohn's disease, age 6 yo or older: 5 mg/kg IV infusion at weeks 0, 2 and 6. Maintain with 5 mg/kg IV q 8 weeks. Infuse IV over 2 h or more.

UNAPPROVED PEDS — JIA, with methotrexate, age 4 yo or older: 3 to 6 mg/kg IV at weeks 0, 2, and 6. Maintain with 3 to 6 mg/kg IV q 8 weeks. Infuse IV over 2 h or more.

NOTES — Consider antihistamines, acetaminophen, and/or corticosteroids to prevent infusion reactions. Three cases of toxic optic neuropathy reported. Hepatotoxicity (rare); discontinue if LFTs more than 5 times upper limit of normal.

MOA — Chimeric mouse-human monoclonal antibody against human TNF. Blockade of TNF inhibits production of pro-inflammatory cytokines.

ADVERSE EFFECTS — Serious: Increased risk of serious infections, including sepsis, TB, opportunistic, and invasive fungal infections. Reactivation of hepatitis B infection. Increased risk of malignancies, esp lymphoma, in young people. New onset and exacerbation of heart failure and demyelinating disorders. Hematologic cytopenias. Serious hypersensitivity reactions. Increased transaminases. Autoantibodies and lupus-like syndrome. Hepatotoxicity. Optic neuropathy (rare). Frequent: Upper respiratory infections, sinusitis, pharyngitis, infusion-related reactions, headache, abdominal pain.

RHEUMATOLOGY: Biologic Response Modifiers—Other

ABATACEPT (*Orencia*) ▶serum ♀C ▐– $$$$$
ADULT — RA, moderate to severe. IV regimen: Infuse IV over 30 minutes with weight-based doses of 500 mg for wt less than 60 kg, 750 mg for 60 to 100 kg, 1000 mg for greater than 100 kg. Give additional IV doses at weeks 2 and 4, and q 4 weeks thereafter. SC regimen: 125 mg SC once weekly with or without an initial IV dose. If patient receives first dose IV, give first SC dose within 1 day of IV infusion. Give SC injection in thigh, abdomen, or upper outer arm. Rotate injection sites.
PEDS — JIA, moderate to severe, age 6 yo or older: 10 mg/kg IV infused over 30 minutes. Give additional IV doses at weeks 2 and 4, and q 4 weeks thereafter. Use adult dose if weight 75 kg or greater.
FORMS — Trade only: Prefilled single-dose syringe 125 mg/1 mL.
NOTES — Do not coadminister with TNF-blockers, other biologic DMARDs, or tofacitinib. May increase risk of infection in patients at risk for recurrent infections. Discontinue if serious infection occurs. Test for latent TB before treatment; if present, treat TB before starting abatacept. Do not give live vaccines during or for 3 months after treatment. Bring immunizations up to date before starting abatacept. Adverse events more frequent in patients with COPD; monitor for exacerbation and pulmonary infections. Maltose in IV abatacept can cause falsely high blood glucose readings on the day of infusion with glucose monitoring systems that use test strips containing glucose dehydrogenase pyrroloquinolinequinone (GDH-PQQ). Store SC syringes in the refrigerator.
MOA — Soluble fusion protein composed of extracellular domain of T-lymphocyte-associated antigen 4 linked to Fc portion of human IgG1. A selective costimulation modulator that inhibits T-cell activation.
ADVERSE EFFECTS — Serious: Increased risk of infection. More frequent respiratory adverse events in patients with COPD. Hypersensitivity (reported with IV infusion). Frequent: Headache, nausea, pharyngitis, upper respiratory infection.

ANAKINRA (*Kineret*) ▶K ♀B ▐? $$$$$
ADULT — RA: 100 mg SC daily, alone or in combination with other DMARDs, except TNF blockers. Neonatal-onset multisystem inflammatory disease: 1 to 2 mg/kg SC daily, adjusted in 0.5 to 1 mg/kg increments to max of 8 mg/kg/day. Inject SC into thigh, abdomen, outer upper arm, or upper outer area of buttocks. Rotate injection sites.
PEDS — Neonatal-onset multisystem inflammatory disease: 1 to 2 mg/kg SC daily, adjusted in 0.5 to 1 mg/kg increments to max of 8 mg/kg/day. Inject SC into thigh, abdomen, outer upper arm, or upper outer area of buttocks. Rotate injection sites.
UNAPPROVED PEDS — JIA: Initial dose of 1 to 2 mg/ kg (max 100 mg) SC once daily. Inject SC into thigh,

abdomen, outer upper arm, or upper outer area of buttocks.
FORMS — Trade only: Prefilled graduated syringe 100 mg/0.67 mL.
NOTES — Contraindicated if hypersensitivity to E coli-derived proteins. Increased incidence of serious infections. Do not use in active infection or with TNF-blockers. Can cause neutropenia; monitor neutrophil counts q month for 3 months, then q 3 months for up to 1 year. Avoid live vaccines. Graduated syringes can provide doses between 20 and 100 mg. Refrigerate and protect from light. Dosage adjustment for CrCl <30 mL/min: Consider giving every other day.
MOA — Recombinant interleukin-1 receptor antagonist (IL-1 ra).
ADVERSE EFFECTS — Serious: Increased risk of serious infection; neutropenia,hypersensitivity reactions. Frequent: Injection site reaction.

CANAKINUMAB (*Ilaris*) ▶? ♀C ▐? $$$$$
ADULT — Cryopyrin-associated periodic syndromes (familial cold autoinflammatory syndrome, Muckle-Wells syndrome): 150 mg SC q 8 weeks.
PEDS — Systemic JIA, age 2 yo and older and wt 7.5 kg and greater: 4 mg/kg (max 300 mg) SC q 4 weeks. Cryopyrin-associated periodic syndromes (familial cold autoinflammatory syndrome, Muckle-Wells syndrome), age 4 years old and older: 150 mg SC q 8 weeks for wt greater than 40 kg; 2 mg/kg SC q 8 weeks, increasing to 3 mg/kg q 8 weeks if inadequate response for wt 15 to 40 kg.
NOTES — Increased risk of serious infections; do not use during treatment of active infection. Do not coadminister TNF-blockers due to increased risk of serious infections. May increase the risk of TB; evaluate for active and latent TB before starting canakinumab. If positive, treat TB before starting canakinumab. Avoid live vaccines. Monitor for macrophage activation syndrome, especially in systemic JIA.
MOA — Recombinant monoclonal antibody against interleukin-1 beta (IL1β), a pro-inflammatory cytokine.
ADVERSE EFFECTS — Serious: Increased risk of serious infections, including upper respiratory and opportunistic infections, and possibly TB. Possible increased risk of malignancy due to immunosuppression. Frequent: nasopharyngitis, diarrhea, influenza, headache, nausea, abdominal pain, injection site reactions. Decreased WBC, increased transaminases and slightly increased bilirubin.

RITUXIMAB (*Rituxan*) ▶? ♀C ▐– $$$$$
WARNING — Life-threatening infusion reactions, especially with first infusion. Monitor closely. Discontinue if severe reaction and treat grade 3/4 infusion reactions. Can cause life-threatening mucocutaneous reactions and progressive multifocal leukoencephalopathy; discontinue if these occur. Can cause life-threatening hepatitis

RITUXIMAB (*cont.*)

B reactivation. Screen for hepatitis B infection before treatment. Monitor during and after treatment; discontinue rituximab and concominant chemotherapy if hepatitis B reactivation occurs. Can cause tumor lysis syndrome in NHL; use IV hydration and anti-hyperuricemic drugs in high-risk patients.

ADULT — RA, in combination with methotrexate: 1000 mg IV infusion weekly for 2 doses q 24 weeks. Premedicate with acetaminophen and antihistamine. Give methylprednisolone 100 mg IV 30 minutes before infusion. Granulomatosis with polyangiitis (Wegener's), microscopic polyangitis, in combination with corticosteroids: 375 mg/m^2 q week for 4 weeks. Chemotherapy doses vary by indication. Non-Hodgkin's lymphoma (NHL). A 90-minute infusion can be used starting at Cycle 2 for patients with NHL who did not experience a grade 3 or 4 infusion-related adverse reaction during Cycle 1. Do not use faster infusion in patients with clinically significant cardiovascular disease and high circulating lymphocyte counts (>5000/mcL). Chronic lymphocytic leukemia (CLL), previously untreated and previously treated CD20-positive CLL, in combination with fludarabine and cyclophosphamide (FC).

PEDS — Not approved for use in children.

UNAPPROVED ADULT — Immune thrombocytopenic purpura (ITP), thrombotic thrombocytopenic purpura (TTP), multiple sclerosis, Hodgkin's lymphoma, systemic autoimmune diseases other than RA, steroid-refractory chronic graft-versus-host disease.

UNAPPROVED PEDS — Autoimmune hemolytic anemia.

NOTES — Can cause serious bacterial, fungal, and new or reactivated viral infections. If serious infection occurs, discontinue rituximab and treat infection. Monitor CBC q 2 to 4 months in patients with RA or granulomatosis/ microscopic polyangitis. Avoid live vaccines. Give non-live vaccines at least 4 weeks before rituximab in RA/polyangiitis patients.

MOA — Chimeric murine-human monoclonal antibody that binds to the CD20 antigen on the surface of B-cell precursors and mature B-lymphocytes.

ADVERSE EFFECTS — Serious: Life-threatening infusion reactions, hepatitis, hepatic failure, tumor lysis syndrome in non-Hodgkin's lymphoma (NHL), severe mucocutaneous reactions, progressive multifocal leukoencephalopathy, hepatitis B reactivation, cardiac arrhythmias during or after infusion, nephrotoxicity in NHL, bowel obstruction and perforation (rituximab with chemotherapy), hypersensitivity, bone marrow suppression, infection. Frequent: Bone marrow suppression, infection, infusion reactions.

SILTUXIMAB (*Sylvant*) ▶unknown ♀C ▶– $$$$$
ADULT — Multicentric Castleman's disease, HIV-negative and herpesvirus-8 negative: 11 mg/kg

infused IV over 1 hour every 3 weeks until treatment failure. Can cause serious infusion reactions; administer in a facility with resuscitation equipment, drugs, and personnel trained to provide resuscitation. Discontinue if patient develops signs/symptoms of anaphylaxis. Stop infusion if patient experiences mild/moderate infusion reaction. Consider restarting infusion at a slower rate if reaction resolves. Consider giving antihistamines, corticosteroids, and acetaminophen. Discontinue if the patient does not tolerate infusion after these interventions.

PEDS — Safety and efficacy not established in children.

NOTES — Monitor hematologic indices before each dose for the first year and every 3 doses thereafter. Consider delaying treatment if ANC is <1 X 10^9/L, platelet count <75 X 10^9/L, or Hg >17 g/L. May mask signs and symptoms of inflammation; monitor for signs of infection and hold if severe infection develops. Discontinue if patient experiences severe infusion reaction, anaphylaxis, severe allergic reation, or cytokine release syndrome. Avoid live vaccines. May cause GI perforation; use with caution in at-risk patients. May increase CYP450 activity; monitor INR with warfarin, cyclosporine levels, and use oral contraceptives with caution.

MOA — Mouse-human monoclonal antibody that binds to human interleukin-6 (IL-6).

ADVERSE EFFECTS — Serious: Infusion reactions (back/chest pain, N/V, flushing, erythema, palpitations). Anaphylaxis. May cause GI perforation. Frequent: pruritus, weight gain, rash, hyperuricemia, upper respiratory infection.

TOCILIZUMAB (*Actemra*) ▶? ♀C ▶– $$$$$
WARNING — Increased risk of serious infections, including TB, and other bacterial, viral, invasive fungal, and opportunistic infections. Hold tocilizumab if serious infection occurs. Screen for latent TB before starting tocilizumab. If positive, start TB treatment before starting tocilizumab. Monitor all tocilizumab-treated patients for TB.

ADULT — RA, moderate to severe with inadequate response to DMARD: 162 mg SC q 2 weeks titrated to q week based on clinical response for wt less than 100 kg; 162 mg SC q week for wt 100 kg or greater. IV regimen: 4 mg/kg IV q 4 weeks, increasing to 8 mg/ kg IV q 4 weeks based on clinical response. Infuse over 1 h with not more than 800 mg/infusion. Can be used alone or with other non-biologic DMARDs. See product labeling for dosage adjustments for elevated liver enzymes, low ANC, or low platelet count.

PEDS — Polyarticular JIA, age 2 yo or older: 10 mg/ kg IV q 4 weeks for wt less than 30 kg; 8 mg/kg IV q 4 weeks for wt 30 kg or greater. Infuse over 1 hour. Can be used alone or with methotrexate. Systemic JIA, age 2 yo or older: 12 mg/kg q 2 weeks for wt less than 30 kg; 8 mg/kg q 2 weeks for wt 30 kg or greater. Infuse over 1 hour. Can be used alone or

TOCILIZUMAB (*cont.*)

with methotrexate. See product labeling for managing elevated liver enzymes, low ANC, or low platelet count.

FORMS — Trade only: 162 mg/0.9 mL prefilled single-use syringe.

NOTES — Can cause neutropenia, thrombocytopenia, and increased AST/ALT. Do not start tocilizumab if baseline ANC less than 2000, platelet count less than 100,000, or ALT/AST greater than 1.5 times upper limit of normal. In adults with RA, monitor neutrophils, platelets, AST/ALT after 4 to 8 weeks of treatment, then q 3 months. For children, monitor neutrophils, platelets, ALT/AST at second dose, then q 4 to 8 weeks for polyarticular JIA and q 2 to 4 weeks for systemic JIA. Can cause hyperlipidemia; monitor lipids after 4 to 8 weeks of treatment, then q 6 months in all patients. Monitor for signs of infection; do not give during active infection. May increase risk of GI perforation (esp RA patients with history of diverticulitis). Do not coadminister with biologic DMARDs. Avoid live vaccines during treatment with tocilizumab. Not for use in active liver disease or impaired liver function.

MOA — Monoclonal antibody that is an interleukin-6 receptor antagonist.

ADVERSE EFFECTS — Serious: Neutropenia, thrombocytopenia, serious infections (TB, bacterial, viral, invasive fungal, opportunistic), anaphylaxis (rare). Reactivation of viral infections like herpes zoster. GI perforation, primarily as complication of diverticulitis in RA patients. May increase risk of malignancy. Possible risk of demyelinating disorders like multiple sclerosis. Frequent: upper respiratory tract infection, nasopharyngitis, headache, HTN, increased ALT, injection site reactions.

TOFACITINIB (*Xeljanz*) ▸LK ♀C ▸— $$$$$

WARNING — Increased risk of serious infections, including TB. If serious infection occurs, hold tofacitinib until infection is controlled. Screen for latent TB before starting tofacitinib. If positive, start TB treatment before starting tofacitinib. Monitor all tofacitinib-treated patients for active TB. May increase the risk of lymphoma and other malignancies. Increased rate of Epstein Barr Virus-associated post-transplant lymphoproliferative disorder in renal transplant patients treated with both tofacitinib and immunosuppressive drugs.

ADULT — RA: 5 mg PO two times per day. Reduce to 5 mg PO once daily if given with fluconazole, strong CYP3A4 inhibitor, or combination of moderate CYP3A4 inhibitor and strong CYP2C19 inhibitor (see P450 isozyme table). Dosage adjustments for lymphopenia, neutropenia, and anemia in product labeling. Indicated for moderate to severe RA with inadequate response or intolerance to methotrexate. For use as monotherapy or in combination with methotrexate or another non-biologic DMARD.

PEDS — Not approved in children.

FORMS — Trade only: Tabs 5 mg.

NOTES — Can cause lymphopenia, neutropenia, anemia, increased LFTs, hyperlipidemia, and may increase risk of GI perforation (esp if history of diverticulitis). Do not start tofacitinib if baseline ANC less than 1000, absolute lymphocyte count less than 500, or Hg less than 9 mg/dL. Monitor lymphocyte count at baseline and q 3 months. Monitor ANC and hemoglobin at baseline, after 4 to 8 weeks of treatment, then q 3 months. Monitor LFTs routinely. Monitor lipids after 4 to 8 weeks of treatment. Refer to product labeling for dosage adjustments for lymphopenia, neutropenia, or anemia. Do not coadminister biologic DMARDs or potent immunosuppressants like cyclosporine or azathioprine. Avoid live vaccines during treatment with tofacitinib. Do not coadminister strong CYP3A4 inducers (carbamazepine, phenobarbital, phenytoin, rifampin, rifapentine, St John's wort). Dosage reduction for moderate/severe renal impairment or moderate hepatic impairment: 5 mg PO once daily.

MOA — Janus kinase (JAK) inhibitor. JAKs activate Signal Transducers and Activators of Transcription (STATs) in an intracellular cytokine signaling pathway. Inhibition of JAK 1 and 3 by tofacitinib blocks production of inflammatory mediators and suppresses STAT1-dependent genes in joint tissue.

ADVERSE EFFECTS — Serious: Serious infections, including TB and reactivation of viral infections like herpes zoster. May increase risk of lymphoma, other malignancies, and non-melanoma skin cancers. Increased rate of Epstein Barr Virus-associated post-transplant lymphoproliferative disorder in renal transplant patients treated with both tofacitinib and immunosuppressive drugs. May increase risk of GI perforation (esp if history of diverticulitis). Lymphocytopenia, neutropenia, anemia, hyperlipidemia, and increased LFTs. Frequent: Upper respiratory tract infections, headache, diarrhea, nasopharyngitis.

RHEUMATOLOGY: Disease-Modifying Antirheumatic Drugs (DMARDs)

AURANOFIN (*Ridaura*) ▸K ♀C ▸+ $$$$$

WARNING — Gold toxicity may manifest as marrow suppression, proteinuria, hematuria, pruritus, rash, stomatitis, or persistent diarrhea. Monitor CBC and urine protein q 4 to 12 weeks.

ADULT — RA: Initial 3 mg PO two times per day or 6 mg PO daily. May increase to 3 mg PO three times per day after 6 months.

PEDS — Safety and efficacy not established in children.

AURANOFIN (*cont.*)

UNAPPROVED ADULT — Psoriatic arthritis: 3 mg PO two times per day or 6 mg PO daily.

FORMS — Trade only: Caps 3 mg.

NOTES — Contraindicated in patients with a history of any of the following gold-induced disorders: Anaphylactic reactions, necrotizing enterocolitis, pulmonary fibrosis, exfoliative dermatitis, bone marrow suppression. Not recommended in pregnancy. Proteinuria reported in 3% to 9% of patients. Diarrhea, rash, stomatitis, chrysiasis (gray-to-blue pigmentation of skin) may occur. Minimize exposure to sunlight or artificial UV light. Auranofin may increase phenytoin levels.

MOA — Decreases synovial inflammation; slows cartilage/bone destruction.

ADVERSE EFFECTS — Serious: Anaphylaxis, bone marrow suppression, proteinuria, chrysiasis (see NOTES). Frequent: Diarrhea, dermatitis, stomatitis.

AZATHIOPRINE (*Azasan, Imuran, AZA*) ▶LK ♀D ▶– $$$

WARNING — Chronic immunosuppression with azathioprine increases the risk of neoplasia, including lymphoma and skin malignancies. May cause marrow suppression or GI hypersensitivity reaction characterized by severe N/V.

ADULT — Severe RA: Initial dose 1 mg/kg (50 to 100 mg) PO daily or divided two times per day. Increase by 0.5 mg/kg/day at 6 to 8 weeks; if no serious toxicity and if initial response is unsatisfactory can then increase thereafter at 4-week intervals. Max dose 2.5 mg/kg/day. In patients with clinical response, use the lowest effective dose for maintenance therapy. Prevention of rejection after renal transplant: Individualized dosing with initial dose of 3 to 5 mg/kg IV/PO daily; usual maintenance dose of 1 to 3 mg/kg PO daily.

PEDS — Not approved in children.

UNAPPROVED ADULT — Crohn's disease: 50 to 100 mg PO daily or 2 to 3 mg/kg/day PO. Myasthenia gravis, multiple sclerosis: 2 to 3 mg/kg/day PO. Behcet's syndrome: 2.5 mg/kg/day PO. Vasculitis: 2 mg/kg/day PO. Ulcerative colitis: 1.5 to 2.5 mg/kg/day PO. Lupus nephritis: 2 mg/kg/day PO.

UNAPPROVED PEDS — Prevention of rejection after renal transplant: Individualized dosing with usual doses ranging from 1 to 3 mg/kg/day PO.

FORMS — Generic/Trade: Tabs 50 mg, scored. Trade only (Azasan): 75, 100 mg, scored.

NOTES — Monitor CBC q 1 to 2 weeks with dose changes, then q 1 to 3 months. Can cause severe myelosuppression in TPMT-deficient patients; consider TPMT testing, esp. if cytopenia does not respond to azathioprine dosage reduction. Dosage adjustments based on TPMT testing available at www.pharmgkb.org. ACE inhibitors, allopurinol (dosage reduction required), and methotrexate may increase activity and toxicity.

Azathioprine may decrease the activity of anticoagulants, cyclosporine, and neuromuscular blockers.

MOA — Immunosuppressant. Metabolized to 6-mercaptopruine.

ADVERSE EFFECTS — Serious: Bone marrow depression. Increased risk of serious infections. Increased risk of malignancy. GI hypersensitivity. Progressive multifocal leukencephalopathy. Frequent: Malaise, skin rash.

HYDROXYCHLOROQUINE (*Plaquenil, HCQ*) ▶K ♀C ▶+ $

WARNING — Clinicians should be knowledgeable about hydroxychloroquine product labeling before prescribing.

ADULT — Doses as hydroxychloroquine sulfate. RA: 400 to 600 mg PO daily to start, taken with food or milk. After clinical response, decrease to 200 to 400 mg PO daily. Discontinue if no objective improvement within 6 months. SLE: 400 mg PO one to two times per day to start. Decrease to 200 to 400 PO daily for prolonged maintenance. Malaria prophylaxis, chloroquine-sensitive areas: 400 mg PO q week from 1 to 2 weeks before exposure until 4 weeks after. Malaria treatment, chloroquine-sensitive areas: 800 mg PO once, then 400 mg at 6, 24, and 48 h (total dose of 2 g).

PEDS — Doses as hydroxychloroquine base (200 mg hydroxychloroquine sulfate = 155 mg base). Malaria prophylaxis, chloroquine-sensitive areas: 5 mg/kg to max of 310 mg base PO q week from 1 to 2 weeks before exposure until 4 weeks after. Malaria treatment, chloroquine-sensitive areas: 10 mg/kg base PO once, then 5 mg/kg base at 6, 24, and 48 h.

UNAPPROVED PEDS — JIA or SLE: 3 to 5 mg/kg/day, up to a max of 400 mg/day PO daily or divided two times per day. Max dose 7 mg/kg/day. Take with food or milk.

FORMS — Generic/Trade: Tabs 200 mg hydroxychloroquine sulfate (200 mg sulfate equivalent to 155 mg base), scored.

NOTES — May exacerbate psoriasis or porphyria. Retinal toxicity (rare); American Academy of Ophthalmology recommends baseline ophthalmic exam within first year of treatment for all patients followed by annual screening after 5 years of use; annual exam from the start of therapy for high-risk patients. Risk factors for retinal toxicity include cumulative dose of 1000 g; treatment for >7 years; obesity; significant liver/kidney disease or advanced age; pre-existing retinal, macular disease or cataracts. See www.aao.org for details. Anorexia, nausea, and vomiting may occur. May increase digoxin and metoprolol levels.

MOA — Unclear in the treatment of RA.

ADVERSE EFFECTS — Serious: Retinopathy, angioedema, bronchospasm. Frequent: Anorexia, nausea.

LEFLUNOMIDE (*LEF, Arava*) ▶LK ♀X ▶– $$$$$
WARNING — Hepatotoxicity, interstitial lung disease. Rare reports of lymphoma, pancytopenia, agranulocytosis, thrombocytopenia, Stevens-Johnson syndrome, cutaneous necrotizing vasculitis, and severe HTN. Exclude pregnancy before starting. Women of childbearing potential must use reliable contraception.
ADULT — RA: Loading dose: 100 mg PO daily for 3 days. Maintenance dose: 10 to 20 mg PO daily.
PEDS — Not approved in children.
UNAPPROVED ADULT — Psoriatic arthritis: Initial: 100 mg PO daily for 3 days. Maintenance: 10 to 20 mg PO daily.
FORMS — Generic/Trade: Tabs 10, 20 mg. Trade only: Tabs 100 mg.
NOTES — Elimination of loading dose may reduce risk of hematologic and hepatic toxicity. Avoid in hepatic or renal insufficiency, severe immunodeficiency, bone marrow dysplasia, or severe infections. Consider interruption of therapy if serious infection occurs and administer cholestyramine (see below). Monitor LFTs, CBC, and creatinine monthly until stable, then q 1 to 2 months. Avoid in men wishing to father children. Avoid live vaccines. May increase INR with warfarin; check INR within 1 to 2 days of initiation, then weekly for 2 to 3 weeks and adjust the dose accordingly. Rifampin increases and cholestyramine decreases leflunomide levels. Give charcoal or cholestyramine in cases of overdose or drug toxicity. Cholestyramine: 8 g PO three times per day for up to 11 days. Activated charcoal: 50 g PO or NG q 6 h for 24 h. Administration on consecutive days is not necessary unless rapid elimination desired.
MOA — Immunosuppressant that inhibits pyrimidine synthesis.
ADVERSE EFFECTS — Serious: Lymphoma, pancytopenia, Stevens-Johnson Syndrome, hepatotoxicity, interstitial lung disease, cutaneous necrotizing vasculitis. Frequent: Diarrhea.

METHOTREXATE— RHEUMATOLOGY (*Otrexup, Rasuvo, Rheumatrex, Trexall, MTX*) ▶LK ♀X ▶– $$
WARNING — Deaths have occurred from hepatotoxicity, pulmonary disease, intestinal perforation, and marrow suppression. According to the manufacturer, use is restricted to patients with severe, recalcitrant, disabling rheumatic disease unresponsive to other therapy. Contraindicated in pregnancy due to risk of fetal harm. Use with extreme caution in renal insufficiency. Folate deficiency may increase toxicity. The ACR recommends supplementation with 1 mg/day of folic acid.
ADULT — Severe RA: Initial dose of 7.5 mg PO/SC once weekly. Alternative regimen: 2.5 mg PO q 12 h for 3 doses given as a course once weekly. May increase dose gradually to max of 20 mg/week. After clinical response, reduce to lowest effective dose. Severe psoriasis: 10 to 25 mg PO/SC/IV/IM once weekly until response, then decrease to lowest effective dose. Max usual dose is 30 mg/week. Supplement with 1 mg/day of folic acid. When converting between PO and SC administration, consider that SC administration has higher bioavailability. Give SC injection in abdomen or thigh.
PEDS — Severe JIA: 10 mg/m^2 PO/SC q week. When converting between PO and SC administration, consider that SC administration has higher bioavailability. Give SC injection in abdomen or thigh.
UNAPPROVED ADULT — Severe RA, psoriasis: 25 mg PO q week. After clinical response, reduce to lowest effective dose. Supplement with 1 mg/day of folic acid. Early ectopic pregnancy: 50 mg/m^2 IM single dose.
FORMS — Trade only (Trexall): Tabs 5, 7.5, 10, 15 mg. Dose Pak (Rheumatrex) 2.5 mg (# 8, 12, 16, 20, 24). Generic/Trade: Tabs 2.5 mg, scored. Trade only: Single-dose SC auto-injector. Otrexup: 10, 15, 20, 25 mg/0.4 mL. Rasuvo: 7.5, 10, 12.5, 15, 17.5, 20, 22.5, 25, 27.5, 30 mg (volume ranges from 0.15 to 0.6 mL).
NOTES — Contraindicated in pregnant and lactating women, alcoholism, liver disease, immunodeficiency, blood dyscrasias. Monitor CBC q month, liver and renal function q 1 to 3 months. Beware of medication errors in which intended weekly doses of methotrexate are given daily. Can cause dizziness and fatigue which can impair driving ability.
MOA — Immunosuppressant, antimetabolite.
ADVERSE EFFECTS — Serious: Hepatotoxicity, pulmonary disease, lymphoma, bone marrow suppression, intestinal perforation. Frequent: Increased LFTs, diarrhea, stomatitis, bone marrow suppression.

SULFASALAZINE—RHEUMATOLOGY (*Azulfidine, Azulfidine EN-tabs, ✱Salazopyrin EN-tabs*) ▶L ♀B ▶? $$
WARNING — Beware of hypersensitivity, marrow suppression, renal and liver damage, central nervous system effects, irreversible neuromuscular and CNS changes, fibrosing alveolitis.
ADULT — RA: 500 mg PO two times per day after meals to start. Increase to 1 g PO two times per day.
PEDS — JIA, age 6 yo or older: Initial dose of 10 mg/kg/day, increasing to 30 to 50 mg/kg/day (EN-tabs) PO divided two times per day to max of 2 g/day. Safety and efficacy not established for age less than 2 yo.
UNAPPROVED ADULT — Ankylosing spondylitis with peripheral arthritis: 500 mg PO once daily for first week, 500 mg PO two times per day for second week, then slowly titrated to max of 3 g/day. Psoriasis: Initial dose of 500 mg PO two times per day increased up to 3 to 4 g/day as tolerated. Psoriatic arthritis: 1 g PO two times per day.
FORMS — Generic/Trade: Tabs 500 mg, scored. Enteric-coated, delayed-release (EN-tabs) 500 mg.

SULFASALAZINE—RHEUMATOLOGY (cont.)

NOTES — Avoid with hepatic or renal dysfunction, intestinal or urinary obstruction, porphyria, or sulfonamide or salicylate sensitivity. Monitor CBC q 2 to 4 weeks for 3 months then q 3 months. Monitor LFTs and renal function. Oligospermia and infertility, and photosensitivity may occur. May decrease folic acid, digoxin, cyclosporine, and iron levels. May turn body fluids, contact lenses, or skin orange-yellow. Enteric-coated (Azulfidine EN, Salazopyrin EN) tabs may cause fewer GI adverse effects. Supplement with folic acid during pregnancy. Reports of bloody stools or diarrhea in breast-fed infants of mothers taking sulfasalazine.

ADVERSE EFFECTS — Serious: Agranulocytosis, hemolytic anemia, nephro/hepatotoxicity, hepatic failure, drug rash and other severe skin reactions, hypersensitivity, anaphylaxis, angioedema, neural tube defect, reversible male infertility. Frequent: Nausea, dyspepsia, rash.

RHEUMATOLOGY: Gout-Related—Xanthine Oxidase Inhibitors

ALLOPURINOL (Aloprim, Zyloprim) ▶K ♀C ▶+ $

ADULT — Mild gout, recurrent calcium oxalate stones: 200 to 300 mg PO daily (start with 100 mg PO daily). Moderate gout: 400 to 600 mg PO daily. Prevention of tumor lysis syndrome: 600 to 800 mg PO daily with hydration. Doses in excess of 300 mg should be divided. Max 800 mg/day. Prevention of tumor lysis syndrome in patients unable to tolerate PO: 200 to 400 mg/m²/day IV as single infusion or in equally divided infusions q 6 to 12 h. Max 600 mg/day. Initiate 24 to 48 h before chemotherapy. To improve tolerability, take PO allopurinol after meals.

PEDS — Prevention of tumor lysis syndrome: 150 mg PO daily for age younger than 6 yo; 300 mg PO daily for age 6 to 10 yo. Evaluate response after 48 h and adjust dose. Prevention of tumor lysis syndrome in patients unable to tolerate PO: Initial dose of 200 mg/m²/day IV as single infusion or in equally divided infusions q 6 to 12 h. Initiate 24 to 48 h before chemotherapy. To improve tolerability, take PO allopurinol after meals.

UNAPPROVED PEDS — Prevention of tumor lysis syndrome: 50 to 100 mg/m²/dose PO q 8 h (max 300 mg/m²/day) or 10 mg/kg/day PO divided q 8 h (max 800 mg/day). Prevention of tumor lysis syndrome in patients unable to tolerate PO: 200 to 400 mg/m²/day IV in 1 to 3 divided doses (max 600 mg/day).

FORMS — Generic/Trade: Tabs 100, 300 mg.

NOTES — May precipitate acute gout; consider using NSAIDs or colchicine prophylactically. Start with 100 mg PO daily and increase weekly to target serum uric acid of less than 6 mg/dL. Renal impairment increases risk of rash and allopurinol hypersensitivity syndrome. Discontinue if rash or allergic symptoms; do not restart after severe rash. Allopurinol increases risk of rash with amoxicillin/ampicillin. Drug interactions with warfarin, mercaptopurine, azathioprine. Normal serum uric acid levels are usually achieved after 1 to 3 weeks of therapy. Ensure hydration before IV administration. Dosage reduction of PO/IV allopurinol for renal insufficiency: 200 mg/day for CrCl 10 to 20 mL/min; 100 mg/day for CrCl 3 to 10 mL/min; 100 mg/day at extended intervals for CrCl less than 3 mL/min.

MOA — Inhibits xanthine oxidase, decreasing uric acid production.

ADVERSE EFFECTS — Serious: Hepatotoxicity, hypersensitivity reaction, severe rash, renal failure, mobilization gout, bone marrow depression. Frequent: Headache, peripheral neuropathy, rash, neuritis, somnolence, N/V, diarrhea, dyspepsia, abdominal pain, fever, myopathy.

FEBUXOSTAT (Uloric) ▶LK ♀C ▶? $$$$

ADULT — Hyperuricemia with gout: Start 40 mg PO daily. After 2 weeks, if uric acid greater than 6 mg/dL may increase to 80 mg daily.

PEDS — Not approved in children.

FORMS — Trade only: Tabs 40, 80 mg.

NOTES — May precipitate acute gout; consider using NSAIDs or colchicine prophylactically for up to 6 months. Monitor LFTs at baseline and periodically, transaminase elevations reported. Do not use with azathioprine, mercaptopurine or theophylline. May increase risk of thromboembolic events, monitor for cardiovascular events (MI, CVA). Caution in severe renal or hepatic impairment.

MOA — Inhibits xanthine oxidase, decreasing uric acid production.

ADVERSE EFFECTS — Serious: Thromboembolism, anaphylaxis, Stevens Johnson syndrome, rhabdomyolysis. aggressive psychotic behavior, interstitial nephritis, hepatic failure. Frequent: Transaminase elevations, nausea, arthralgia, rash, gout flare.

RHEUMATOLOGY: Gout-Related—Other

COLCHICINE: DOSAGE REDUCTIONS FOR COADMINISTRATION WITH INHIBITORS OF COLCHICINE METABOLISM

Usual colchicine dose	Colchicine dosage reduction for...		
	Strong CYP3A4 inhibitors*	Moderate CYP3A4 inhibitors[†]	P-glycoprotein inhibitors[‡]
Prevention of gout flares: 0.6 mg PO two times per day	0.3 mg PO once daily	0.3 mg PO two times per day or 0.6 mg PO once daily	0.3 mg PO once daily
Prevention of gout flares: 0.6 mg PO once daily	0.3 mg PO once every other day	0.3 mg PO once daily	0.3 mg PO once every other day
Treatment of gout flares: 1.2 mg PO followed by 0.6 mg 1 hour later	0.6 mg PO followed by 0.3 mg 1 hour later	1.2 mg PO in a single dose	0.6 mg PO in a single dose
Familial Mediterranean Fever: Up to 1.2 to 2.4 mg/day PO	Up to 0.6 mg/day PO (can be given as 0.3 mg two times per day)	Up to 1.2 mg/day PO (can be given as 0.6 mg two times per day)	Up to 0.6 mg/day PO (can be given as 0.3 mg two times per day)

Notes: Do not give colchicine to patients with renal or hepatic impairment who are taking a strong CYP3A4 or P-glycoprotein inhibitor. Do not treat gout flares with colchicine in patients already receiving colchicine for prevention of gout flares and who are also receiving a CYP3A4 inhibitor. Dosage reductions of colchicine are recommended for patients who are currently taking or have discontinued a CYP3A4 or P-glycoprotein inhibitor within the past 14 days. Be aware that this table may not list all possible CYP3A4 and P-glycoprotein inhibitors that increase the risk of colchicine toxicity via inhibition of colchicine metabolism.

* **Strong CYP 3A4 inhibitors**: atazanavir, boceprevir, clarithromycin, cobicistat (in Stribild), conivaptan, darunavir-ritonavir, fosamprenavir-ritonavir, indinavir, itraconazole, ketoconazole, lopinavir-ritonavir, nefazodone, nelfinavir, posaconazole, ritonavir, saquinavir-ritonavir, telithromycin, tipranavir-ritonavir, voriconazole.

[†]**Moderate CYP 3A4 inhibitors**: aprepitant, ciprofloxacin, crizotinib, diltiazem, dronedarone, erythromycin, fluconazole, fosamprenavir (unboosted), grapefruit juice, imatinib, verapamil.

[‡]**P-glycoprotein inhibitors**: cyclosporine, ranolazine.

COLCHICINE (*Colcrys*) ▶L ♀C ▶? $$$$
ADULT — Treatment of gout flares: 1.2 mg (2 tabs) PO at signs of attack then 0.6 mg (1 tab) 1 h later. Do not repeat this regimen earlier than 3 days. In patients already receiving colchicine for prevention of gout flares, give this regimen and resume prophylactic dose 12 h later. Prevention of gout flares: 0.6 mg PO one or two times per day. Max dose of 1.2 mg/day. Familial Mediterranean Fever: 1.2 to 2.4 mg PO daily or divided two times per day, with dose titrated up or down in 0.3 mg/day increments. See table for colchicine dose reduction when given with strong/moderate CYP3A4 inhibitors or P-glycoprotein inhibitors.
PEDS — Familial Mediterranean Fever: 0.3 to 1.8 mg PO daily or divided two times per day for age 4 to 6 yo; 0.9 to 1.8 mg daily or divided two times per day for age 6 to 12 yo; see adult dosage for age 12 yo or older. Prevention of gout flares, greater than 16 yo: 0.6 mg PO one or two times per day. Max dose of 1.2 mg/day.
UNAPPROVED ADULT — Primary biliary cirrhosis: 0.6 mg PO two times per day. Acute pericarditis: 0.6 mg PO once daily for wt 70 kg or less; 0.6 mg PO two times per day for wt greater than 70 kg. Treat for 3 months in combination with ibuprofen or aspirin.
FORMS — Trade only: Tabs 0.6 mg.
NOTES — Coadministration of colchicine and P-glycoprotein or strong CYP3A4 inhibitors (including all HIV protease inhibitors, except unboosted fosamprenavir) is contraindicated in renal or hepatic impairment. Dosage reductions required for coadministration with strong or moderate CYP

(cont.)

COLCHICINE (*cont.*)

3A4 inhibitors or P-glycoprotein inhibitors (see table). Most effective when initiated on the 1st day of gouty arthritis. Do not treat gout flares with colchicine in patients with renal impairment who are already receiving colchicine for prevention of gout flares. Dosage adjustment for renal dysfunction. Treatment of gout flares: Usual dose given no more frequently than q 2 weeks for CrCl less than 30 mL/min; 0.6 mg PO single dose given no more frequently than q 2 weeks for dialysis. Prevention of gout flares: 0.3 mg PO once daily initially with any dosage increase closely monitored for CrCl less than 30 mL/min; 0.3 mg PO two times per week with close monitoring for dialysis. Familial Mediterranean Fever: 0.3 mg PO once daily initially with close monitoring for any dosage increase for CrCl <30 mL/min or dialysis.

MOA — Reduces the inflammatory response to deposited crystals, and diminishes phagocytosis.

ADVERSE EFFECTS — Serious: Peripheral neuritis, hepatotoxicity, renal failure, bone marrow depression, leukocytopenia, granulocytopenia, aplastic anemia, thrombocytopenia, purpura, myopathy, rhabdomyolysis, hypersensitivity. Frequent: Diarrhea, N/V, abdominal pain, dermatoses, hair loss.

COLCHICINE + PROBENECID ▶KL ♀C ▶? $

ADULT —Chronic gouty arthritis: Start 1 tab PO daily for 1 week, then 1 tab PO two times per day.

PEDS — Not approved in children.

FORMS — Generic only: Tabs 0.5 mg colchicine + 500 mg probenecid.

NOTES — Maintain alkaline urine. Probenecid ineffective if CrCl less than 30 ml/min.

MOA — Combination product that reduces the inflammatory response to deposited crystals, diminishes phagocytosis and inhibits tubular reabsorption of uric acid.

ADVERSE EFFECTS — Serious: Peripheral neuritis, hepatotoxicity, renal failure, bone marrow depression with aplastic anemia, thrombocytopenia, purpura, myopathy, hypersensitivity, nephrotic syndrome, hemolytic anemia, mobilization gout. Frequent: Diarrhea, N/V, abdominal pain, dermatoses, hair loss, headache, anorexia, urinary frequency, sore gums, dizziness

PEGLOTICASE (*Krystexxa*) ▶? ♀C ▶? $$$$$

WARNING — Anaphylaxis and infusion reactions reported. Premedicate with antihistamines and corticosteroids and administer in a healthcare setting. Anaphylaxis and infusion reactions more common if loss of therapeutic response. Monitor uric acid levels before infusion and discontinue if greater than 6 mg/dL, especially if two consecutive levels greater than 6.

ADULT —Chronic gout (refractory): 8 mg IV infusion q 2 weeks. Administer over 120 minutes or longer.

NOTES — Gout flares frequent upon initiation. Recommend gout flare prophylaxis with NSAID or colchicine to start 1 week prior to therapy and continue for 6 months. Discontinue urate lowering therapy. Contraindicated in G6PD deficiency due to risk of hemolysis and methemoglobinemia; screen those at high risk including those of African and Mediterranean ancestry.

MOA — Recombinant uricase which causes oxidation of uric acid

ADVERSE EFFECTS — Serious: anaphylaxis, delayed-type hypersensitivity, heart failure exacerbation, chest pain. Frequent: infusion reactions, gout flare, nausea, vomiting, constipation, bruising, nasopharyngitis.

PROBENECID ▶KL ♀B ▶? $

ADULT — Gout: 250 mg PO two times per day for 7 days, then 500 mg PO two times per day. May increase by 500 mg/day q 4 weeks not to exceed 2 g/day. Adjunct to penicillin: 2 g/day PO in divided doses.

PEDS — Adjunct to penicillin: In children 2 to 14 yo use 25 mg/kg PO initially, then 40 mg/kg/day divided four times per day. For wt greater than 50 kg, use adult dose. Contraindicated in children age younger than 2 yo.

FORMS — Generic only: Tabs 500 mg.

NOTES — Decrease dose if GI intolerance occurs. Maintain alkaline urine. Begin therapy 2 to 3 weeks after acute gouty attack subsides. Ineffective if CrCl less than 30 ml/min. Not recommended in combination with penicillin if renal impairment.

MOA — Inhibits tubular reabsorption of uric acid.

ADVERSE EFFECTS — Serious: Hepatotoxicity, nephrotic syndrome, hemolytic anemia, hypersensitivity, mobilization gout. Frequent: Headache, anorexia, N/V, urinary frequency, sore gums, dizziness.

RHEUMATOLOGY: Other

APREMILAST (*Otezla*) ▶L ♀C ▶? $$$$$

ADULT — Psoriatic arthritis, moderate to severe plaque psoriasis : Give PO 10 mg in am on day 1, 10 mg two times per day on day 2, 10 mg in am and 20 mg in pm on day 3, 20 mg two times per day on day 4, 20 mg in am and 30 mg in pm on day 5, 30 mg two times per day on day 6 and thereafter. Do not crush, split, or chew tabs.

PEDS — Safety and efficacy not established in children.

FORMS — Trade only: Tabs 30 mg. Two-week starter pack of 10, 20, and 30 mg tabs.

NOTES — May cause or worsen depression; monitor symptoms. May cause weight loss; monitor weight. Do not coadminister strong CYP450 inducers (e.g., carbamazepine phenobarbital, phenytoin, rifampin, St. John's wort). Dosage adjustment for CrCl <30 mL/min: Give PO 10 mg q am for 3 days, then 20 mg q am for 2 days, then 30 mg q am thereafter.

MOA — Phosphodiesterase 4 inhibitor; mechanism of action in psoriatic arthritis unclear.

ADVERSE EFFECTS — Serious: May cause or worsen depression. Weight loss (up to 10% of body weight). Frequent: Diarrhea, nausea, headache, weight loss.

BELIMUMAB (*Benlysta*) ▶? – ♀C ▶? $$$$$
ADULT — Systemic lupus erythematosus (SLE): 10 mg/kg IV infusion q 2 weeks for first 3 doses. Then, 10 mg/kg IV infusion q 4 weeks. Infuse over 1 h. Slow or hold infusion if symptoms of infusion reaction. Consider premedication to prevent reactions.
PEDS — Not approved in children.
NOTES — Use for autoantibody positive SLE in patients on standard therapy. Do not give live vaccines during therapy. More deaths reported with belimumab than placebo during clinical trials. Use with caution in patients with chronic infections and consider stopping therapy if new serious infection develops; reports of serious or fatal infections. Reports of progressive multifocal leukoencephalopathy. Suicide and depression reported. Do not combine with biologic therapies or IV cyclophosphamide.
MOA — Human 1gG1 monoclonal antibody that is a B-lymphocyte stimulator-specific inhibitor (inhibits survival of B cells and the autoimmune response).
ADVERSE EFFECTS — Serious: Progressive multifocal leukoencephalopathy; acute hypersensitivity including anaphylaxis; non-acute hypersensitivity or infusion reactions. Frequent: nausea, diarrhea, itching, nasopharyngitis, pharyngitis, bronchitis, insomnia, pain in extremity, depression, migraine.

HYALURONATE (*Hyalgan, Supartz, Euflexxa, Orthovisc★Neovisc*) ▶KL ♀? ▶? $$$$$
WARNING — Do not inject extra-articularly; avoid the synovial tissues and cap. Do not use disinfectants containing benzalkonium chloride for skin preparation.
ADULT — OA (knee): Hyalgan: 2 mL intra-articular injection q week for 3 to 5 weeks. Supartz: 2.5 mL intra-articular injection q week for 5 weeks. Orthovisc and Neovisc (Canada): 2 mL intra-articular injection q week for 3 weeks. Inject a local anesthetic SC prior to injections.
PEDS — Not approved in children.
FORMS — Trade only: Hyalgan: 2 mL (10 mg/mL) vial, prefilled syringe. Supartz: 2.5 mL (10 mg/mL) prefilled syringe. Euflexxa: 2 mL (10mg/ml) prefilled syringe. Orthovisc: 2 mL (15 mg/mL) prefilled syringe.
NOTES — For those who have failed conservative therapy. Caution in allergy to eggs, avian proteins, or feathers (except Neovisc—synthetic). Remove synovial fluid or effusion before each injection. Knee pain and swelling most common side effects.
MOA — Improves viscosity/elasticity of synovial fluid.
ADVERSE EFFECTS — Serious: Anaphylactoid reactions. Frequent: Knee pain and swelling, joint pain, back pain, injection site pain.

HYLAN GF-20 (*Synvisc*) ▶KL ♀? ▶? $$$$$
WARNING — Do not inject extra-articularly; avoid the synovial tissues and cap. Do not use disinfectants containing benzalkonium chloride for skin preparation.
ADULT — OA (knee): 2 mL intra-articular injection q week for 3 weeks.
PEDS — Not approved in children.
FORMS — Trade only: Synvisc: 2 mL (8 mg/mL) in glass syringe; 3/pack. Synvisc-One: 6 mL (8 mg/mL) in single syringe.
NOTES — For those who have failed conservative therapy. Caution in allergy to eggs, avian proteins, or feathers. Remove synovial fluid or effusion before each injection. Knee pain and swelling most common side effects.
MOA — Improves viscosity/elasticity of synovial fluid.
ADVERSE EFFECTS — Serious: Anaphylactoid reactions. Frequent: Knee pain and swelling.

TOXICOLOGY

ANTIDOTES

Toxin	Antidote/Treatment
acetaminophen	N-acetylcysteine
TCAs	sodium bicarbonate
arsenic, mercury	dimercaprol (BAL)
benzodiazepine	flumazenil
beta-blockers	glucagon
calcium channel blockers	calcium chloride, glucagon
cyanide	cyanide antidote kit, Cyanokit (hydroxocobalamin)
digoxin	dig immune Fab
ethylene glycol	fomepizole
heparin	protamine
iron	deferoxamine
lead	BAL, EDTA, succimer
methanol	fomepizole
methemoglobin	methylene blue
opioids/opiates	naloxone
organophosphates	atropine + pralidoxime
warfarin	vitamin K, FFP

ACETYLCYSTEINE (*N-acetylcysteine, Mucomyst, Acetadote, ✱Parvolex*) ▶L ♀B ▶? $$$$
ADULT — Acetaminophen toxicity: Mucomyst: Loading dose 140 mg/kg PO or NG, then 70 mg/kg q 4 h for 17 doses. May be mixed in water or soft drink diluted to a 5% soln. Acetadote (IV): Loading dose 150 mg/kg in 200 mL of D5W infused over 60 min; maintenance dose 50 mg/kg in 500 mL of D5W infused over 4 h followed by 100 mg/kg in 1000 mL of D5W infused over 16 h.
PEDS — Acetaminophen toxicity: Same as adult dosing.
UNAPPROVED ADULT — Prevention of contrast-induced nephropathy: 600 to 1200 mg PO two times per day for 2 doses before procedure and 2 doses after procedure.
FORMS — Generic/Trade: Soln 10%, 20%. Intravenous (Acetadote).
NOTES — May be diluted with water or soft drink to a 5% soln; use diluted soln within 1 h. Repeat loading dose if vomited within 1 h. Critical ingestion-treatment interval for maximal protection against severe hepatic injury is between 0 to 8 h. Efficacy diminishes after 8 h and treatment initiation between 15 and 24 h post-ingestion yields limited efficacy. However, treatment should not be withheld, since the reported time of ingestion may not be correct. Anaphylactoid reactions usually occur 30 to 60 min after initiating infusion. Stop infusion, administer antihistamine or epinephrine, restart infusion slowly. If anaphylactoid reactions return or severity increases, then stop treatment.
MOA — Directly combines with the toxic acetaminophen metabolite as a glutathione substitute. Antioxidant believed to attenuate ischemic renal failure.
ADVERSE EFFECTS — Serious: Hypersensitivity, anaphylaxis, angioedema, bronchoconstriction, chest tightness. Frequent: Nausea, vomiting, disagreeable odor, generalized urticaria, rash, stomatitis, fever, rhinorrhea, drowsiness, clamminess, pruritus, tachycardia, hypertension, hypotension.

CHARCOAL (*activated charcoal, Actidose-Aqua, CharcoAid, EZ-Char, ✤Charcodate*) ▶Not absorbed ♀+ ▶+ $

ADULT — Gut decontamination: 25 to 100 g (1 to 2 g/kg or 10× the amount of poison ingested) PO or NG as soon as possible. May repeat q 1 to 4 h prn at doses equivalent to 12.5 g/h. When sorbitol is coadministered, use only with the first dose if repeated doses are to be given.

PEDS — Gut decontamination: 1 g/kg for age younger than 1 yo; 15 to 30 g or 1 to 2 g/kg for age 1 to 12 yo PO or NG as soon as possible. Repeat doses in children have not been established, but half the initial dose is recommended. Repeat q 2 to 6 h prn. When sorbitol is coadministered, use only with the first dose if repeated doses are to be given.

FORMS — OTC/Generic/Trade: Powder 15, 30, 40, 120, 240 g. Soln 12.5 g/60 mL, 15 g/75 mL, 15 g/120 mL, 25 g/120 mL, 30 g/120 mL, 50 g/240 mL. Susp 15 g/120 mL, 25 g/120 mL, 30 g/150 mL, 50 g/240 mL. Granules 15 g/120 mL.

NOTES — Some products may contain sorbitol to improve taste and reduce GI transit time. Chocolate milk/powder may enhance palatability for pediatric use. Not usually effective for toxic alcohols (methanol, ethylene glycol, isopropanol), heavy metals (lead, iron, bromide), arsenic, lithium, potassium, hydrocarbons, and caustic ingestions (acids, alkalis). Mix powder with 8 oz water. Greatest effect when administered within 1 h of ingestion.

MOA — Adsorbs substances therefore inhibiting GI absorption.

ADVERSE EFFECTS — Serious: Bronchiolitis obliterans, aspiration. Frequent: Vomiting, constipation, diarrhea, black stools, hypokalemia, hypernatremia.

DEFERIPRONE (*Ferriprox, ✤Ferriprox*) ▶glucuronidation – ♀D ▶– ©V $$$$$

WARNING — Ferriprox can cause agranulocytosis and neutropenia may precede this development. Measure the ANC before starting and monitor weekly. Interrupt Ferriprox if infection develops and monitor the ANC more frequently.

ADULT — Transfusional iron overload due to thalassemia syndromes when current chelation therapy is inadequate: 25 mg/kg, orally, three times per day for a total of 75 mg/kg/day. The maximum dose is 33 mg/kg, three times per day for a total of 99 mg/kg/day

PEDS — Not approved

FORMS — 500 mg film-coated tabs with a functional score

NOTES — Contraindicated with pre-existing agranulocytosis or neutropenia. Advise patients taking Ferriprox to report immediately any symptoms indicative of infection. Inform patients that their urine might show a reddish/brown discoloration due to the excretion of the iron-deferiprone complex.

MOA — Binds with ferric ions(iron III) to form neutral 3:1 (deferiprone:iron) and has a lower affinity for copper, aluminum and zinc.

ADVERSE EFFECTS — Serious: agranulocytosis. Common: chromaturia, nausea, vomiting, abdominal pain, LFT increase, arthralgia and neutropenia.

DEFEROXAMINE (*Desferal*) ▶K ♀C ▶? $$$$$

ADULT — Chronic iron overload: 500 to 1000 mg IM daily and 2 g IV infusion (no faster than 15 mg/kg/h) with each unit of blood or 1 to 2 g SC daily (20 to 40 mg/kg/day) over 8 to 24 h via continuous infusion pump. Acute iron toxicity: IV infusion up to 15 mg/kg/h (consult poison center).

PEDS — Acute iron toxicity: IV infusion up to 15 mg/kg/h (consult poison center).

NOTES — Contraindicated in renal failure/anuria unless undergoing dialysis.

MOA — Chelates iron in serum, ferritin, and hemosiderin.

ADVERSE EFFECTS — Serious: Cataracts, neurotoxicity-related hearing loss, hypersensitivity, hypotension, ARDS. Frequent: Visual changes (decreased acuity; impaired peripheral, night, and color vision), red urine, generalized erythema, dysuria, abdominal pain, leg cramps, tachycardia, fever, skin rash.

DIMERCAPROL (*BAL in oil*) ▶KL ♀C ▶? $$$$$

ADULT — Specialized dosing for arsenic, mercury, gold, and lead toxicity. Consult poison center. Mild arsenic or gold toxicity: 2.5 mg/kg IM four times per day for 2 days, then two times per day for 1 day, then daily for 10 days. Severe arsenic or gold toxicity: 3 mg/kg IM q 4 h for 2 days, then four times per day for 1 day, then two times per day for 10 days. Mercury toxicity: 5 mg/kg IM initially, then 2.5 mg/kg daily to two times per day for 10 days. Begin therapy within 1 to 2 h of toxicity. Acute lead encephalopathy: 4 mg/kg IM initially, then q 4 h in combination (separate syringe) with calcium edetate for 2 to 7 days. May reduce dose to 3 mg/kg IM for less severe toxicity. Deep IM injection needed.

PEDS — Not approved in children.

UNAPPROVED PEDS — Same as adult dosing. Consult poison center.

MOA — Chelates arsenic, gold, and mercury to promote fecal and urinary excretion of the complex.

ADVERSE EFFECTS — Serious: Hemolytic anemia, HTN, tachycardia, hypersensitivity. Frequent: N/V, headache, perioral burning sensation, feeling of constriction or pain (in throat, chest or hands), conjunctivitis, blepharospasm, rhinorrhea, salivation, burning penis sensation, sweating, abdominal pain, injection-site irritation, painful sterile abscess, anxiety, weakness.

DUODOTE (*atropine + pralidoxime*) ▶K ♀C ▶? $

ADULT — Organophosphate insecticide/nerve agent poisoning, mild symptoms: 1 injection in thigh. Severe symptoms: 3 injections in rapid succession (may administer through clothes).

PEDS — Not approved in children.

FORMS — Each auto-injector dose delivers atropine 2.1 mg + pralidoxime 600 mg.

MOA — Atropine is to reverse muscarinic toxicity. Pralidoxime reactives acetylcholinesterase deactivated by organophosphate nerve agents or insecticide.

DUODOTE (cont.)

ADVERSE EFFECTS — Serious: Hyperthermia, anticholinergic syndrome, myocardial ischemia. Frequent: Anticholinergic syndrome, hypertension, diplopia, dizziness.

EDETATE (*EDTA, Endrate, versenate*) ▶K ♀C ▶– $$$

WARNING — Beware of elevated intracranial pressure in lead encephalopathy.

ADULT — Consult poison center. Use calcium disodium form only for lead indications. Noncalcium form (e.g., Endrate) is not interchangeable and is rarely used anymore. Lead toxicity: 1000 mg/m^2/day IM (divided into equal doses q 8 to 12 h) or IV (infuse total dose over 8 to 12 h) for 5 days. Interrupt therapy for 2 to 4 days, then repeat same regimen. Two courses of therapy are usually necessary. Acute lead encephalopathy: Edetate alone or in combination with dimercaprol. Lead nephropathy: 500 mg/m^2/dose q 24 h for 5 doses (if creatinine 2 to 3 mg/dL), q 48 h for 3 doses (if creatinine 3 to 4 mg/dL), or once per week (if creatinine greater than 4 mg/dL). May repeat at 1 month intervals.

PEDS — Specialized dosing for lead toxicity; same as adult dosing also using calcium form. Consult poison center.

FORMS — Calcium disodium formulation used for lead poisoning, other form without calcium (e.g., Endrate) is not interchangeable and rarely used anymore.

MOA — Chelates heavy metals to form complexes that undergo urinary excretion.

ADVERSE EFFECTS — Serious: Arrhythmia, renal toxicity (proteinuria, hematuria, acute tubular necrosis), hypersensitivity, transient bone marrow suppression. Frequent: Hypotension, tremor, headache, numbness, tingling, cheilosis, vomiting, anorexia, thirst, glycosuria, pain at injection site, hypercalcemia, zinc deficiency, nasal congestion, rash, increased serum transaminases, fever, chills, fatigue, malaise, myalgia, arthralgia.

ETHANOL (*alcohol*) ▶L ♀D ▶+ $

PEDS — Not approved in children.

UNAPPROVED ADULT — Consult poison center. Specialized dosing for methanol, ethylene glycol toxicity if fomepizole is unavailable or delayed: 1000 mg/kg (10 mL/kg) of 10% ethanol (100 mg/mL) IV over 1 to 2 h then 100 mg/kg/h (1 mL/kg/h) to keep ethanol level approximately 100 mg/dL.

MOA — Prevents formation of toxic methanol metabolite formic acid by saturating alcohol dehydrogenase.

ADVERSE EFFECTS — Serious: Multiple reports with chronic use. Frequent: Acute intoxication, dehydration, numerous others with chronic use.

FLUMAZENIL (*Romazicon*) ▶LK ♀C ▶? $$$$

WARNING — Do not administer in chronic benzodiazepine use or acute overdose with TCAs due to seizure risk.

ADULT — Benzodiazepine sedation reversal: 0.2 mg IV over 15 sec, then 0.2 mg q 1 min prn up to 1 mg total dose. Usual dose is 0.6 to 1 mg. Benzodiazepine overdose reversal: 0.2 mg IV over 30 sec, then 0.3 to 0.5 mg q 30 sec prn up to 3 mg total dose.

PEDS — Benzodiazepine sedation reversal: 0.01 mg/kg up to 0.2 mg IV over 15 sec; repeat q min to max 4 additional doses.

UNAPPROVED PEDS — Benzodiazepine overdose reversal: 0.01 mg/kg IV. Benzodiazepine sedation reversal: 0.01 mg/kg IV initially (max 0.2 mg), then 0.005 to 0.01 mg/kg (max 0.2 mg) q 1 min to max total dose 1 mg. May repeat doses in 20 min, max 3 mg in 1 h.

NOTES — Onset of action 1 to 3 min, peak effect 6 to 10 min. For IV use only, preferably through an IV infusion line into a large vein. Local irritation may occur following extravasation.

MOA — Benzodiazepine receptor antagonist.

ADVERSE EFFECTS — Serious: Seizures, arrhythmia, chest pain. Frequent: Injection-site irritation, sweating, hot flashes, flushing, hypotension, hypertension, bradycardia, tachycardia, dizziness, agitation, dry mouth, tremor, insomnia, dyspnea, hyperventilation, emotional lability, confusion, dysphonia, glossitis, N/V, hiccups, visual changes, paresthesia, abnormal hearing, rigors, shivering.

FOMEPIZOLE (*Antizol*) ▶L ♀C ▶? $$$$$

ADULT — Consult poison center. Ethylene glycol or methanol toxicity: 15 mg/kg IV (load), then 10 mg/kg IV q 12 h for 4 doses, then 15 mg/kg IV q 12 h until ethylene glycol or methanol level is below 20 mg/dL. Administer doses as slow IV infusions over 30 min. Increase frequency to q 4 h during hemodialysis.

PEDS — Not approved in children.

MOA — Inhibits alcohol dehydrogenase.

ADVERSE EFFECTS — Serious: Hypersensitivity, seizure, shock, hypotension, disseminated intravascular coagulation, multiorgan system failure. Frequent: Injection-site irritation, rash, eosinophilia, tachycardia, sinus bradycardia/tachycardia, phlebitis, phlebosclerosis, lightheadedness, nystagmus, agitation, flushing, anxiety, feeling of decreased environmental awareness, abdominal pain, diarrhea, dyspepsia, anorexia, heartburn, increases serum transaminases, anemia, pharyngitis, lymphangitis, hiccups, speech/visual disturbance, abnormal smell, blurred vision, N/V.

HYDROXOCOBALAMIN (*Cyanokit*) ▶K ♀C ▶? $$$$$

ADULT — Cyanide poisoning: 5 g IV over 15 min; may repeat prn.

PEDS — Not approved in children.

MOA — Binds cyanide.

ADVERSE EFFECTS — Serious: Anaphylaxis, allergy, hypertension. Frequent: None.

IPECAC SYRUP ▶Gut ♀C ▶? $

ADULT — Induction of emesis: 15 to 30 mL PO, then 3 to 4 glasses of water.

PEDS — AAP no longer recommends home ipecac for poisoning. Emesis, age younger than 1 yo: 5 to 10 mL, then ½ to 1 glass of water (controversial in children younger than 1 yo). Emesis, age 1 to 12 yo: 15 mL, then 1 to 2 glasses of water. May repeat dose (15 mL) if vomiting does not occur within 20 to 30 min.

(cont.)

IPECAC SYRUP (*cont.*)

FORMS — OTC Generic only: Syrup 30 mL.

NOTES — Many believe ipecac to be contraindicated in infants age younger than 6 mo. Do not use if any potential for altered mental status (eg, seizure, neurotoxicity), strychnine, beta-blocker, calcium channel blocker, clonidine, digitalis glycoside, corrosive, petroleum distillate ingestions, or if at risk for GI bleeding (coagulopathy).

MOA — Locally irritates the GI mucosa and stimulates the chemoreceptor trigger zone in the central medullary to produce vomiting.

ADVERSE EFFECTS — Serious: Cardiomyopathy (after prolonged use). Frequent: Diarrhea, coughing, choking, drowsiness, dyspepsia.

METHYLENE BLUE (*Urolene blue*) ▶K ♀C ▶? $

ADULT — Methemoglobinemia: 1 to 2 mg/kg IV over 5 min. Dysuria: 65 to 130 mg PO three times per day after meals with liberal water.

PEDS — Not approved in children.

UNAPPROVED PEDS — Methemoglobinemia: 1 to 2 mg/kg/dose IV over 5 min; may repeat in 1 h prn.

FORMS — Trade only: Tabs 65 mg.

NOTES — Avoid in G6PD deficiency. May turn urine, stool, skin, contact lenses, and undergarments blue-green. Can interact with serotonergic drugs due to its MAOI properties (e.g., SSRIs, SNRIs, clomipramine). Generally avoid coadministration with serotonergic drugs; monitor for signs/symptoms of serotonin syndrome if coadministration is unavoidable.

MOA — Converts methemoglobin to hemoglobin by reducing the ferric iron form of oxidized hemoglobin to ferrous form. Converts methemoglobin (Fe3+) to hemoglobin (Fe2+) by enhancing the activity of NADPH-methemoglobin reductase. Also genitourinary antiseptic and germicidal agent.

ADVERSE EFFECTS — Serious: Hypersensitivity, hemolytic anemia, cyanosis, cardiovascular abnormalities. Frequent: Photosensitivity, N/V, diarrhea, fever, bladder irritation, blue-green urine and/or stool.

PENICILLAMINE (*Cuprimine, Depen*) ▶K ♀D ▶– $$$$$

WARNING — Fatal drug-related adverse events have occurred, caution if penicillin allergy.

ADULT — Consult poison center: Specialized dosing for copper toxicity. 750 mg to 1.5 g/day PO for 3 months based on 24 h urinary copper excretion, max 2 g/day. May start 250 mg/day PO in patients unable to tolerate.

PEDS — Specialized dosing for copper toxicity. Consult poison center.

FORMS — Trade only: Caps 125, 250 mg; Tabs 250 mg.

NOTES — Patients may require supplemental pyridoxine 25 to 50 mg/day PO. Promotes excretion of heavy metals in urine.

MOA — Chelates excess copper.

ADVERSE EFFECTS — Serious: Proteinuria, hematuria, aplastic anemia, hepatotoxicity, pancreatitis, agranulocytosis, production of insulin antibodies, thrombocytopenia, sideroblastic anemia, leukopenia, autoimmune syndromes (Goodpasture's syndrome, myasthenia gravis, pemphigus vulgaris, drug-induced lupus), hypoglycemia, hypersensitivity.

Frequent: Increased serum transaminases, oral ulcers, metallic taste, rash, fever, tinnitus, neuropathy, muscle weakness, anorexia, epigastric pain.

PHYSOSTIGMINE (*Antilirium*) ▶LK ♀D ▶? $

WARNING — Discontinue if excessive salivation, emesis, frequent urination, or diarrhea. Rapid administration can cause bradycardia, hypersalivation, respiratory difficulties and seizures. Atropine should be available as an antagonist.

ADULT — Life-threatening anticholinergic toxicity: 2 mg IV/IM, administer IV no faster than 1 mg/min. May repeat q 10 to 30 min for severe toxicity.

PEDS — Life-threatening anticholinergic toxicity: 0.02 mg/kg IM/IV injection, administer IV no faster than, 0.5 mg/min. May repeat q 15 to 30 min until a therapeutic effect or max 2 mg dose.

UNAPPROVED ADULT — Postanesthesia reversal of neuromuscular blockade: 0.5 to 1 mg IV/IM, administer IV no faster than 1 mg/min. May repeat q 10 to 30 min prn.

FORMS — Generic/Trade: 1 mg/mL in 2 mL ampules.

MOA — Reversible anticholinesterase agent, acts as substrate for acetylcholinesterase.

ADVERSE EFFECTS — Serious: cardiac arrest, bradycardia, hypersalivation leading to respiratory problems or convulsions. Frequent: salivation, N/V, miosis, sweating, lacrimation, bronchospasm, abdominal pain

PRALIDOXIME (*Protopam, 2-PAM*) ▶K ♀C ▶? $$$$

ADULT — Consult poison center: Specialized dosing for organophosphate toxicity: 1 to 2 g IV infusion over 15 to 30 min or slow IV injection over 5 min or longer (max rate 200 mg/min). May repeat dose after 1 h if muscle weakness persists.

PEDS — Not approved in children.

UNAPPROVED ADULT — Consult poison center: 20 to 40 mg/kg/dose IV infusion over 15 to 30 min.

UNAPPROVED PEDS — Consult poison center. 25 mg/kg load then 10 to 20 mg/kg/h or 25 to 50 mg/kg load followed by repeat dose in 1 to 2 h then q 10 to 12 h.

NOTES — Administer within 36 h of exposure when possible. Rapid administration may worsen cholinergic symptoms. Give in conjunction with atropine. IM or SC may be used if IV access is not available.

MOA — Reactivates cholinesterase (primarily peripherally).

ADVERSE EFFECTS — Serious: Myasthenia gravis exacerbation. Frequent: Pain at injection site, transient increase in serum transaminases, increased CK, dizziness, visual changes (blurred, diplopia, decreased accommodation), headache, drowsiness, nausea, tachycardia, increased blood pressure, hyperventilation, muscular weakness.

PRUSSIAN BLUE (*Radiogardase*) ▶Fecal ♀C ▶+ $$$$$

ADULT — Internal contamination with radioactive cesium/thallium: 3 g PO three times per day.

PEDS — Internal contamination with radioactive cesium/thallium, 2 to 12 yo: 1 g PO three times per day.

FORMS — Trade only: Caps 500 mg.

MOA — Enhances excretion of cesium and thallium through ion exchange, adsorption, and mechanical trapping.

PRUSSIAN BLUE (*cont.*)

ADVERSE EFFECTS — Serious: Hypokalemia. Frequent: Constipation.

SUCCIMER (*Chemet*) ▶K ♀C ▶? $$$$$

PEDS — Lead toxicity 1 yo or older: Start 10 mg/kg PO or 350 mg/m2 q 8 h for 5 days, then reduce the frequency to q 12 h for 2 weeks. Not approved in children younger than 1 yo.

FORMS — Trade only: Caps 100 mg.

NOTES — Manufacturer recommends doses of 100 mg (wt 8 to 15 kg), 200 mg (wt 16 to 23 kg), 300 mg (wt 24 to 34 kg), 400 mg (wt 35 to 44 kg), and 500 mg (wt 45 kg or greater). Can open cap and sprinkle medicated beads over food, or give them in a spoon and follow with fruit drink. Indicated for blood lead levels greater than 45 mcg/dL. Allow at least 4 weeks between edetate disodium and succimer treatment.

MOA — Chelates lead to increase urinary excretion.

ADVERSE EFFECTS — Serious: Hypersensitivity, arrhythmia. Frequent: Rash, increased serum transaminases (transient), N/V, anorexia, hemorrhoids, loose stools, metallic taste, body pain, abdominal cramps, fever, flu-like syndrome, drowsiness, dizziness, paresthesia, sensorimotor neuropathy, headache, moniliasis.

UROLOGY

UROLOGY: Benign Prostatic Hyperplasia

ALFUZOSIN (*UroXatral*, ✱*Xatral*) ▶KL ♀B ▶– $

WARNING — Postural hypotension with or without symptoms may develop within a few hours after administration. Avoid in moderate or severe hepatic insufficiency. Avoid coadministration with potent CYP3A4 inhibitors.

ADULT — BPH: 10 mg PO daily after a meal.

PEDS — Not approved in children.

UNAPPROVED ADULT — Promotes spontaneous passage of ureteral calculi: 10 mg PO daily usually combined with an NSAID, antiemetic and opioid of choice.

FORMS — Generic/Trade: Tab extended-release 10 mg.

NOTES — Caution in congenital or acquired QT prolongation, and severe renal insufficiency. Intraoperative floppy iris syndrome has been observed during cataract surgery.

MOA — Selective alpha-1 receptor antagonist that increases urinary flow rate.

ADVERSE EFFECTS — Serious: Postural hypotension, chest pain, priapism, angioedema. Frequent: Dizziness, headache.

DUTASTERIDE (*Avodart*) ▶L ♀X ▶– $$$$

ADULT — BPH: 0.5 mg PO daily with/without tamsulosin 0.4 mg PO daily.

PEDS — Not approved in children.

FORMS — Trade only: Caps 0.5 mg.

NOTES — 6 months therapy may be needed to assess effectiveness. Pregnant or potentially pregnant women should not handle caps due to fetal risk from absorption. Caution in hepatic insufficiency. Dutasteride will decrease PSA by 50%; new baseline PSA should be established after 3 to 6 months to assess potentially cancer-related PSA changes. Cap should be swallowed whole and not chewed or opened to avoid oropharyngeal irritation.

MOA — 5-alpha reductase inhibitor that decreases conversion of testosterone into dihydrotestosterone.

ADVERSE EFFECTS — Serious: Angioedema. Frequent: Impotence, decreased libido, ejaculatory dysfunction.

FINASTERIDE (*Proscar, Propecia*) ▶L ♀X ▶– $

ADULT — Proscar: 5 mg PO daily alone or in combination with doxazosin to reduce the risk of symptomatic progression of BPH. Propecia: Androgenetic alopecia in men: 1 mg PO daily.

PEDS — Not approved in children.

UNAPPROVED ADULT — Cancer prevention in "at-risk" men older than 55 yo: 5 mg daily. Androgenetic alopecia in postmenopausal women (no evidence of efficacy): 1 mg PO daily.

FORMS — Generic/Trade: Tabs 1 mg (Propecia), 5 mg (Proscar).

NOTES — Therapy for 6 to 12 months may be needed to assess effectiveness for BPH and at least 3 months for alopecia. Pregnant or potentially pregnant women should not handle crushed tabs because of possible absorption and fetal risk. Use with caution in hepatic insufficiency. Monitor PSA before therapy; finasteride will decrease PSA by 50% in patients with BPH, even with prostate cancer. Does not appear to alter detection of prostate cancer.

MOA — 5-alpha reductase inhibitor that decreases conversion of testosterone into dihydrotestosterone.

ADVERSE EFFECTS — Serious: Hypersensitivity, swelling of lips and face, breast cancer (long-term treatment), depression. Frequent: Impotence, decreased libido, decreased ejaculatory volume, testicular pain, rash, pruritus.

JALYN (**dutasteride + tamsulosin**) ▶LK – ♀X ▶– $$$$

ADULT — BPH: 0.5 mg dutasteride + 0.4 mg tamsulosin daily 30 minutes after a meal.

PEDS — Not approved in children.

FORMS — Trade only: Caps 0.5 mg dutasteride + 0.4 mg tamsulosin.

NOTES — Refer to components.

MOA — Combination 5-alpha reductase inhibitor and selective alpha-1 antagonist.

ADVERSE EFFECTS — Serious: Angioedema, arrhythmia, orthostatic hypotension, chest pain. Frequent: impotence, breast enlargement and pain, decreased libido, dizziness, ejaculatory dysfunction.

SILODOSIN (*RAPAFLO*) ▶LK – ♀B ▶– $$$$

ADULT — BPH: 8 mg daily with a meal.

PEDS — Not approved in children.

FORMS — Trade: Caps 8 mg.

NOTES — Dizziness, headache, abnormal ejaculation. Alpha-blockers are generally considered to be first-line treatment in men with more than minimal obstructive urinary symptoms. Intraoperative floppy iris syndrome with cataract surgery reported. Avoid administration with strong inhibitors of CYP3A4 (ketoconazole, clarithromycin, itraconazole, ritonavir).

MOA — Selective alpha-1 receptor antagonist that increases urinary flow rate.

ADVERSE EFFECTS — Serious: orthostatic hypotension. Frequent: dizziness, headache, nasal congestion, diarrhea, abnormal ejaculation.

TAMSULOSIN (*Flomax*) ▶LK ♀B ▶– $$$$

ADULT — BPH: 0.4 mg PO daily 30 min after the same meal each days. If an adequate response is not seen after 2 to 4 weeks, may increase dose to 0.8 mg PO daily. If therapy is interrupted for several days, restart at the 0.4 mg dose.

PEDS — Not approved in children.

UNAPPROVED ADULT — Promotes spontaneous passage of ureteral calculi: 0.4 mg PO daily usually combined with an NSAID, antiemetic and opioid of choice.

TAMSULOSIN (*cont.*)

FORMS — Generic/Trade: Caps 0.4 mg.

NOTES — Dizziness, headache, abnormal ejaculation. Alpha-blockers are generally considered to be first-line treatment in men with more than minimal obstructive urinary symptoms. Caution in serious sulfa allergy: rare allergic reactions reported. Intraoperative floppy iris syndrome with cataract surgery reported. Caution with strong inhibitors of CYP450 2D6 (fluoxetine) or 3A4 (ketoconazole).

MOA — Selective alpha-1 receptor antagonist that increases urinary flow rate.

ADVERSE EFFECTS — Serious: Arrhythmia, orthostatic hypotension, chest pain. Frequent: Dizziness, headache, fatigue, somnolence, edema, dyspnea, asthenia, diarrhea, dyspepsia, dry mouth, nausea, palpitations, blurred vision, abnormal ejaculation.

UROLOGY: Bladder Agents—Anticholinergics and Combinations

B&O supprettes (**belladonna + opium**) ▶L ♀C ▶? ☺II $$$$

ADULT — Bladder spasm: 1 suppository PR once or twice daily, max 4 doses/day.

PEDS — Not approved in children younger than 12 yo.

FORMS — Trade only: Supps 30 mg opium (15A), 60 mg opium (16A).

NOTES — Store at room temperature. Contraindicated in narrow-angle glaucoma, obstructive conditions (eg, pyloric, duodenal or other intestinal obstructive lesions, ileus, achalasia, and obstructive uropathies).

MOA — Belladonna: Inhibits the muscarinic action of acetylcholine to decrease motility in the urinary tract. Opium: Opioid agonist analgesic.

ADVERSE EFFECTS — Serious: Hypersensitivity, respiratory coma, bradycardia, hallucinations. Frequent: Dizziness, drowsiness, sedation, N/V, lightheadedness, euphoria, constipation, dry mouth, blurred vision, urinary retention, decreased sweating.

DARIFENACIN (*Enablex*) ▶LK ♀C ▶– $$$$

ADULT — Overactive bladder with symptoms of urinary urgency, frequency and urge incontinence: 7.5 mg PO daily. May increase to max dose 15 mg PO daily in 2 weeks. Max dose 7.5 mg PO daily with moderate liver impairment or when coadministered with potent CYP3A4 inhibitors (ketoconazole, itraconazole, ritonavir, nelfinavir, clarithromycin and nefazodone).

PEDS — Not approved in children.

FORMS — Trade only: Tabs extended-release 7.5, 15 mg.

NOTES — Contraindicated with uncontrolled narrow-angle glaucoma, urinary and gastric retention. Avoid use in severe hepatic impairment. May increase concentration of medications metabolized by CYP2D6.

MOA — Muscarinic receptor antagonist, inhibiting detrusor muscle contractions.

ADVERSE EFFECTS — Serious: Hypersensitivity, angioedema, hallucinations. Frequent: Dry mouth, constipation, blurred vision, dyspepsia.

FESOTERODINE (*Toviaz*) ▶plasma ♀C ▶– $$$$

ADULT — Overactive bladder: 4 mg PO daily. Increase to 8 mg if needed. Do not exceed 4 mg daily with renal insufficiency (CrCl less than 30 mL/min) or specific coadministered drugs (see Notes).

PEDS — Not approved in children.

FORMS — Trade only: Tabs extended-release 4, 8 mg.

NOTES — Contraindicated with urinary or gastric retention, or uncontrolled glaucoma. 4 mg daily max dose in renal dysfunction or with concomitant use of CYP3A4 inhibitors (eg, erythromycin, ketoconazole, itraconazole).

MOA — Muscarinic receptor antagonist to decrease bladder spasm.

ADVERSE EFFECTS — Serious: QT prolongation, angioedema. Frequent: Dry mouth, constipation, headache, vertigo/dizziness, abdominal pain.

FLAVOXATE (*Urispas*) ▶K ♀B ▶? $$$$

ADULT — Bladder spasm: 100 or 200 mg PO three to four times per day. Reduce dose when improved.

PEDS — Not approved in children younger than 12 yo.

FORMS — Generic/Trade: Tabs 100 mg.

NOTES — May cause dizziness, drowsiness, blurred vision, dry mouth, N/V, urinary retention. Contraindicated in glaucoma, obstructive conditions (eg, pyloric, duodenal or other intestinal obstructive lesions, ileus, achalasia, GI hemorrhage, and obstructive uropathies).

MOA — Anticholinergic that directly counteracts urinary smooth muscle contraction.

ADVERSE EFFECTS — Serious: Increased ocular pressure, eosinophilia, leukopenia. Frequent: N/V, dry mouth, nervousness, vertigo, headache, drowsiness, mental confusion, fever, blurred vision, rash, dysuria, tachycardia, disturbed eye accommodation.

OXYBUTYNIN (*Ditropan, Ditropan XL, Gelnique, Oxytrol, ✻Oxybutyn, Uromax*) ▶LK ♀B ▶? $$

ADULT — Bladder instability: 2.5 to 5 mg PO two to three times per day, max 5 mg PO four times per day. Extended-release tabs: 5 to 10 mg PO daily same time each day, increase 5 mg/day q week to 30 mg/day. Oxytrol: 1 patch twice per week on abdomen, hips or buttocks. Gelnique: Apply contents of 1 sachet once daily to abdomen, upper arms/shoulders, or thighs. Rotate application sites.

PEDS — Bladder instability older than 5 yo: 5 mg PO four times per day, max dose: 5 mg PO three times per day. Extended-release, older than 6 yo: 5 mg PO daily, max 20 mg/day. Transdermal patch not approved in children.

UNAPPROVED ADULT — Case reports of use for hyperhidrosis.

UNAPPROVED PEDS — Bladder instability for age younger than 6 yo: 0.2 mg/kg/dose PO two to four times per day.

OXYBUTYNIN (*cont.*)

FORMS — Generic/Trade: Tabs 5 mg. Syrup 5 mg/5 mL. Tabs extended-release 5, 10, 15 mg. Trade only: OTC Transdermal patch (Oxytrol) 3.9 mg/day. Gelnique 3%, 10% gel, 1 g unit dose.

NOTES — May cause dizziness, drowsiness, blurred vision, dry mouth, urinary retention. Contraindicated with glaucoma, urinary retention, obstructive GU or GI disease, unstable cardiovascular status, and myasthenia gravis. Transdermal patch causes less dry mouth than oral form; avoid dose reduction by cutting. Wash hands immediately after applying Gelnique.

MOA — Anticholinergic that exerts direct antispasmodic effects and inhibits muscarinic effects on smooth muscle.

ADVERSE EFFECTS — Serious: Heat stroke, hallucinations, QT prolongation, angioedema. Frequent: Somnolence, headache, dizziness, agitation, confusion, dry mouth, constipation, diarrhea, nausea, dyspepsia, blurred vision, dry eyes, asthenia, pain, rhinitis, urinary tract infection, application site reaction.

PROSED/DS (methylene + phenyl salicylate + methylene blue + benzoic acid + hyoscyamine) ▶KL ♀C ▶? $$

ADULT — Bladder spasm: 1 tab PO four times per day with liberal fluids.

PEDS — Not approved in children.

FORMS — Trade only: Tabs (methenamine 81.6 mg/phenyl salicylate 36.2 mg/methylene blue 10.8 mg/benzoic acid 9.0 mg/hyoscyamine sulfate 0.12 mg).

NOTES — May cause dizziness, drowsiness, blurred vision, dry mouth, N/V, urinary retention. May turn urine/contact lenses blue.

MOA — Combination product that decreases bladder spasm and has mild antiseptic and analgesic activity.

ADVERSE EFFECTS — Serious: Respiratory depression. Frequent: Blue urine, rash, dry mouth, flushing, urinary retention, tachycardia, dizziness, blurred vision.

SOLIFENACIN (*VESIcare*) ▶LK ♀C ▶– $$$$

ADULT — Overactive bladder with symptoms of urinary urgency, frequency or urge incontinence: 5 mg PO daily. Max dose: 10 mg PO daily (5 mg PO daily if CrCl less than 30 mL/min, moderate hepatic impairment, or concurrent ketoconazole or other potent CYP3A4 inhibitors).

PEDS — Not approved in children.

FORMS — Trade only: Tabs 5, 10 mg.

NOTES — Contraindicated with uncontrolled narrowangle glaucoma, urinary and gastric retention. Avoid use in severe hepatic impairment. Hallucinations have been reported.

MOA — Muscarinic receptor antagonist, inhibiting detrusor muscle contractions.

ADVERSE EFFECTS — Serious: Fecal impaction, intestinal obstruction, angioedema, hallucinations, QT prolongation, torsade de pointes. Frequent: Dry mouth, constipation, blurred vision.

TOLTERODINE (*Detrol, Detrol LA*) ▶L ♀C ▶– $$$$$

ADULT — Overactive bladder: 2 mg PO two times per day (Detrol) or 4 mg PO daily (Detrol LA). Decrease dose to 1 mg PO two times per day (Detrol) or 2 mg PO daily (Detrol LA) if adverse symptoms, hepatic insufficiency, or specific coadministered drugs (see notes).

PEDS — Not approved in children.

FORMS — Generic/Trade: Tabs 1, 2 mg. Caps extended-release 2, 4 mg.

NOTES — Contraindicated with urinary or gastric retention, or uncontrolled glaucoma. High doses may prolong the QT interval. Decrease dose to 1 mg PO two times per day or 2 mg PO daily (Detrol LA) in severe hepatic or renal dysfunction or with concomitant use of CYP3A4 inhibitors (eg, erythromycin, ketoconazole, itraconazole).

MOA — Muscarinic receptor antagonist to decrease bladder spasm.

ADVERSE EFFECTS — Serious: Angioedema, QT prolongation. Frequent: Dry mouth, constipation, headache, vertigo/dizziness, abdominal pain.

TROSPIUM (*Sanctura, Sanctura XR, ✦Trosec*) ▶LK ♀C ▶? $$$$

ADULT — Overactive bladder with urge incontinence: 20 mg PO two times per day; give 20 mg at bedtime if CrCl less than 30 mL/min. If age 75 yo or older may taper down to 20 mg daily. Extended-release: 60 mg PO q am, 1 h before food; this form not recommended with CrCl less than 30 mL/min.

PEDS — Not approved in children.

FORMS — Generic/Trade: Tabs 20 mg, Caps extended-release 60 mg.

NOTES — Contraindicated with uncontrolled narrowangle glaucoma, urinary retention, gastroparesis. May cause heat stroke due to decreased sweating. Take on an empty stomach. Improvement in signs and symptoms may be seen in a week.

MOA — Acetylcholine antagonist that reduces bladder smooth muscle tone and spasms.

ADVERSE EFFECTS — Serious: Supraventricular tachycardia, Stevens-Johnson syndrome, anaphylaxis, angioedema, hypertensive crisis, rhabdomyolysis, hallucinations, delirium, heat stroke. Frequent: Dry mouth, constipation, headache, dizziness, blurred vision.

URISED (methenamine + phenyl salicylate + atropine + hyoscyamine + benzoic acid + methylene blue) ▶K ♀C ▶? $

ADULT — Dysuria: 2 Tabs PO four times per day.

PEDS — Dysuria, age 6 yo or older: Reduce dose based on age and wt. Not recommended for children younger than 6 yo.

FORMS — Trade only: Tabs (methenamine 40.8 mg/phenyl salicylate 18.1 mg/atropine 0.03 mg/hyoscyamine 0.03 mg/4.5 mg benzoic acid/5.4 mg methylene blue).

NOTES — Take with food to minimize GI upset. May precipitate urate crystals in urine. Avoid use with sulfonamides. May turn urine/contact lenses blue.

URISED (cont.)

MOA — Combination product that decreases bladder spasm and has mild antiseptic and analgesic activity.

ADVERSE EFFECTS — Serious: Respiratory depression. Frequent: Blue urine, rash, dry mouth, flushing, urinary retention, tachycardia, dizziness, blurred vision.

UTA (methenamine + sodium phosphate + phenyl salicylate + methylene blue + hyoscyamine) ▶KL ♀C ▶? $

ADULT — Treatment of irritative voiding/relief of inflammation, hypermotility and pain with lower UTI/relief of urinary tract symptoms caused by diagnostic procedures: 1 cap PO four times per day with liberal fluids.

PEDS — Not recommended age younger than 6 yo. Dosing must be individualized by physician for age older than 6 yo.

FORMS — Trade only: Caps (methenamine 120 mg/sodium phosphate 40.8 mg/phenyl salicylate 36 mg/methylene blue 10 mg/hyoscyamine 0.12 mg).

NOTES — May turn urine/feces blue to blue-green. Take 2 h apart from ketoconazole. May decrease absorption of thiazide diuretics. Antacids and antidiarrheals may decrease effectiveness of methenamine.

MOA — Combination product that decreases bladder spasms and has mild antiseptic and analgesic activity.

ADVERSE EFFECTS — Serious: respiratory depression. Frequent: blue to blue-green urine/feces, tachycardia, blurred vision, dizziness, urinary retention, dry mouth, N/V.

UTIRA-C (methenamine + sodium phosphate + phenyl salicylate + methylene blue + hyoscyamine) ▶KL ♀C ▶? $$

ADULT — Treatment of irritative voiding/relief of inflammation, hypermotility and pain with lower UTI/relief of urinary tract symptoms caused by diagnostic procedures: 1 cap PO four times per day with liberal fluids.

PEDS — Not recommended age younger than 6 yo. Dosing must be individualized by physician for age older than 6 yo.

FORMS — Trade only: Tabs (methenamine 81.6 mg/sodium phosphate 40.8 mg/phenyl salicylate 36.2 mg/methylene blue 10.8 mg/hyoscyamine 0.12 mg).

NOTES — May turn urine/feces blue to blue-green. Take 2 h apart from ketoconazole. May decrease absorption of thiazide diuretics. Antacids and antidiarrheals may decrease effectiveness of methenamine.

MOA — Combination product that decreases bladder spasms and has mild antiseptic and analgesic activity.

ADVERSE EFFECTS — Serious: Respiratory depression. Frequent: Blue to blue-green urine/feces, tachycardia, blurred vision, dizziness, urinary retention, dry mouth, N/V.

UROLOGY: Bladder Agents—Other

BETHANECHOL (*Urecholine, Duvoid, ✦Myotonachol*) ▶L ♀C ▶? $$$$

ADULT — Urinary retention: 10 to 50 mg PO three to four times per day or 2.5 to 5 mg SC three to four times per day. Take 1 h before or 2 h after meals to avoid N/V. Determine the minimum effective dose by giving 5 to 10 mg PO initially and repeat at hourly intervals until response or to a maximum of 50 mg.

PEDS — Not approved in children.

UNAPPROVED PEDS — Urinary retention/abdominal distention: 0.6 mg/kg/day PO divided q 6 to 8 h or 0.12 to 0.2 mg/kg/day SC divided q 6 to 8 h.

FORMS — Generic/Trade: Tabs 5, 10, 25, 50 mg.

NOTES — May cause drowsiness, lightheadedness, and fainting. Not for obstructive urinary retention. Avoid with cardiac disease, hyperthyroidism, parkinsonism, peptic ulcer disease, and epilepsy.

MOA — Cholinergic agent that stimulates the parasympathetic nervous system to increase the strength of detrusor muscle contraction.

ADVERSE EFFECTS — Serious: Hypersensitivity, hypotension with tachycardia, bronchoconstriction. Frequent: Flushing, sense of warmth, sweating, abdominal pain, nausea, belching, diarrhea, salivation, borborygmi, lacrimation, myosis, urinary urgency, headache, malaise.

DIMETHYL SULFOXIDE (*DMSO, Rimso-50*) ▶KL ♀C ▶? $$$

ADULT — Interstitial cystitis: Instill 50 mL soln into bladder by catheter and allow to remain for 15 min; expelled by spontaneous voiding. Repeat q 2 weeks until symptomatic relief is obtained; thereafter, may increase time intervals between treatments.

PEDS — Not approved in children.

NOTES — Apply analgesic lubricant gel to urethra prior to inserting the catheter to avoid spasm. May administer oral analgesics or supps containing belladonna and opium prior to instillation to reduce spasms. May give anesthesia in patients with severe interstitial cystitis and very sensitive bladders during the first, second and third treatment. May cause lens opacities and changes in refractive index; perform eye exams before and periodically during treatment. May cause a hypersensitivity reaction by liberating histamine. Monitor liver and renal function tests and CBC q 6 months. May be harmful in patients with urinary tract malignancy; can cause DMSO-induced vasodilation. Peripheral neuropathy may occur when used with sulindac. Garlic-like taste may occur within a few min of administration; odor on breath and skin may be present and remain for up to 72 h.

DIMETHYL SULFOXIDE (*cont.*)

MOA — Has broad pharmacological properties: anti-inflammatory, antifungal activity cryoprotective effects for living cells and tissues, dissolution of collagen, nerve blockade, diuresis, cholinesterase inhibition, vasodilation, and muscle relaxation.

ADVERSE EFFECTS — Serious: Hypersensitivity, transient chemical cystitis. Frequent: Sedation, N/V, headache, dizziness, garlic-like breath, burning on urination, diarrhea, transient disturbance of color perception, photophobia, burning or aching eyes, weight loss/gain, flu syndrome, discomfort during administration.

MIRABEGRON (*Myrbetriq*) ▶LK - ♀C ▶?

ADULT — Overactive bladder with symptoms of urge urinary incontinence, urgency, and urinary frequency: 25 mg PO daily. May increase to 50 mg unless severe renal impairment (CrCl less than 30 mL/min) or moderate hepatic impairment (Child-Pugh Class B). Not recommended in ESRD or Child-Pugh Class C liver disease.

PEDS — Not approved in children.

FORMS — Trade only: Extended-release tabs: 25, 50 mg.

NOTES — Do not chew, crush, or split tablets. May increase blood pressure; not recommended in patients with severe uncontrolled hypertension. Moderate CYP2D6 inhibitor; may increase concentrations of CYP2D6 substrates such as metoprolol.

MOA — Beta-3 adrenergic agonist.

ADVERSE EFFECTS — Common: Hyppertension, nasopharyngitis, urinary tract infection, headache.

PENTOSAN (*Elmiron*) ▶LK ♀B ▶? $$$$$

ADULT — Interstitial cystitis: 100 mg PO three times per day 1 h before or 2 h after a meal.

PEDS — Not approved in children.

FORMS — Trade only: Caps 100 mg.

NOTES — Pain relief usually occurs at 2 to 4 months and decreased urinary frequency takes 6 months. May increase risk of bleeding, especially with NSAID use. Use with caution in hepatic or splenic dysfunction.

MOA — Heparin-like molecule that adheres to bladder wall mucosa and exerts anticoagulant and fibrinolytic effects and prevents irritation by buffering cell permeability.

ADVERSE EFFECTS — Serious: Thrombocytopenia, bleeding. Frequent: Alopecia, headache, rash, nausea, abdominal pain.

PHENAZOPYRIDINE (*Pyridium, Azo-Standard, Urogesic, Prodium, Pyridiate, Urodol, Baridium, UTI Relief*) ▶K ♀B ▶? $

ADULT — Dysuria: 200 mg PO three times per day after meals for 2 days.

PEDS — Dysuria in children 6 to 12 yo: 12 mg/kg/day PO divided three times per day for 2 days.

FORMS — OTC Generic/Trade: Tabs 95, 97.2 mg. Rx Generic/Trade: Tabs 100, 200 mg.

NOTES — May turn urine/contact lenses orange. Contraindicated with hepatitis or renal insufficiency.

MOA — Produces a topical analgesic effect on the urinary mucosa.

ADVERSE EFFECTS — Serious: Hypersensitivity, hemolytic anemia, methemoglobinemia, nephrotoxicity, hepatotoxicity. Frequent: Headache, rash, pruritus, dyspepsia, contact lens staining, urine discoloration, yellowish tinge on sclera or skin.

UROQUID-ACID NO. 2 (methenamine + sodium phosphate) ▶K ♀C ▶? $

ADULT — Chronic/recurrent UTIs: Initial: 2 tabs PO four times per day with full glass of water. Maintenance: 2 to 4 tabs PO daily, in divided doses with full glass of water.

PEDS — Not approved in children.

FORMS — Trade only: Tabs methenamine mandelate 500 mg/sodium acid phosphate 500 mg.

NOTES — 83 mg sodium/tab. Thiazide diuretics, carbonic anhydrase inhibitors, antacids and urinary alkalinizing agents may decrease effectiveness. Caution with concurrent salicylates, may increase levels.

MOA — Antibacterial/urinary acidifier.

ADVERSE EFFECTS — Serious: Hematuria. Frequent: N/D/V, rash, headache, dizziness.

UROLOGY: Erectile Dysfunction

ALPROSTADIL (*Muse, Caverject, Caverject Impulse, Edex, Prostin VR Pediatric, prostaglandin E1, ✦Prostin VR*) ▶L ♀- ▶- $$$$

ADULT — Erectile dysfunction: 1.25 to 2.5 mcg intracavernosal injection over 5 to 10 sec initially using a ½ in, 27 or 30 gauge needle. If no response, may give next higher dose after 1 h, max 2 doses/day. May increase by 2.5 mcg and then 5 to 10 mcg incrementally on separate occasions. Dose range is 1 to 40 mcg. Alternative: 125 to 250 mcg intraurethral pellet (Muse). Increase or decrease dose on separate occasions until erection achieved. Maximum intraurethral dose 2 pellets/24 h. The lowest possible dose to produce an acceptable erection should be used.

PEDS — Temporary maintenance of patent ductus arteriosus in neonates: Start 0.1 mcg/kg/min IV infusion. Reduce dose to minimal amount that maintains therapeutic response. Max dose 0.4 mcg/kg/min.

UNAPPROVED ADULT — Erectile dysfunction intracorporeal injection: Specially formulated mixtures of alprostadil, papaverine and phentolamine. 0.10 to 0.50 mL injection.

FORMS — Trade only: Syringe system (Edex) 10, 20, 40 mcg. (Caverject) 5, 10, 20, 40 mcg. (Caverject Impulse) 10, 20 mcg. Pellet (Muse) 125, 250, 500, 1000 mcg. Intracorporeal injection of locally compounded combination agents (many variations): "Bi-mix" can be 30 mg/mL papaverine + 0.5 to 1 mg/mL phentolamine, or 30 mg/mL papaverine + 20 mcg/mL alprostadil in 10 mL vials. "Tri-mix" can

(cont.)

ALPROSTADIL (*cont.*)

be 30 mg/mL papaverine + 1 mg/mL phentolamine + 10 mcg/mL alprostadil in 5, 10, or 20 mL vials.

NOTES — Contraindicated in patients at risk for priapism, with penile fibrosis (Peyronie's disease), with penile implants, in women or children, in men for whom sexual activity is inadvisable, and for intercourse with a pregnant woman. Onset of effect is 5 to 20 min.

MOA — Relaxes trabecular smooth muscles and dilates cavernosal arteries to produce erection. Relaxes smooth muscle of the ductus arteriosus.

ADVERSE EFFECTS — Serious: Priapism, hypotension. Frequent: Penile and testicular pain, urethral discomfort (pain, burning, bleeding/spotting).

AVANAFIL (*Stendra*) ▶L – ♀C ▶? $$$$

ADULT — Erectile dysfunction: 100 mg PO 30 minutes prior to sexual activity. Maximum 1 dose/day. Use lower dose (50 mg) if taking certain coadministered drugs (see notes).

PEDS — Not approved in children.

FORMS — Trade only (Stendra): Tabs 50, 100, 200 mg.

NOTES — For patients taking strong CYP3A4 inhibitors (ketoconazole, ritonavir, atazanavir, clarithromycin, indinavir, itraconazole, nefazodone, nelfinavir, saquinavir and telithromycin), do not use. For patients taking moderate CYP3A4 inhibitors (erythromycin, amprenavir, aprepitant, diltiazem, fluconazole, fosamprenavir, and verapamil), use 50 mg dose. For patients taking alpha blocker, start at 50 mg. Do not initiate alpha blocker and avanafil at same time. Not recommended for patients within 6 months of MI, CVA, life-threatening arrhythmia, or coronary revascularization, resting BP < 90/50 or > 170/100, or unstable angina, angina with sexual intercourse, or NYHA Class 2 or greater.

MOA — Selectively inhibits phosphodiesterase-5 resulting in enhanced relaxation of penile arteries & corpus cavernosal smooth muscle; enhances erectile function by increasing penile blood flow. Relaxes pulmonary vascular smooth muscle cells resulting in vasodilation of the pulmonary vascular bed.

ADVERSE EFFECTS — Serious: Priapism, hypotension, syncope, vision loss (nonarteritic ischemic optic neuropathy). Frequent: Headache, flushing, nasal congestion.

SILDENAFIL (*Viagra*) ▶LK ♀B ▶– $$$$

ADULT — Erectile dysfunction: 50 mg PO approximately 1 h (range 0.5–4 h) before sexual activity. Usual effective dose range: 25 to 100 mg. Maximum 1 dose/day. Use lower dose (25 mg) if older than 65 yo, hepatic/renal impairment, or certain coadministered drugs (see notes).

PEDS — Not approved in children.

UNAPPROVED ADULT — Antidepressant-associated sexual dysfunction: Same dosing as above.

FORMS — Trade only (Viagra): Tabs 25, 50, 100 mg. Unscored tab but can be cut in half.

NOTES — Drug interactions with cimetidine, erythromycin, ketoconazole, itraconazole, saquinavir,

ritonavir and other CYP3A4 inhibitors; use 25 mg dose. Do not exceed 25 mg/48 h with ritonavir. Doses > 25 mg should not be taken less than 4 h after an alpha-blocker. Caution if CVA, MI or other cardiovascular event within last 6 months. Do not use with itraconazole, ketoconazole, ritonavir or pulmonary veno-occlusive disease. Coadministration with CYP3A4 inducers (i.e., bosentan; barbiturates, carbamazepine, phenytoin, efavirenz, nevirapine, rifampin, rifabutin) may change levels of either medication; adjust doses as needed. Use caution with CVA, MI or life-threatening arrhythmia in last 6 months; unstable angina; BP > 170/110; or retinitis pigmentosa. Contraindicated in patients taking nitrates within prior/subsequent 24 h. Caution with alpha blockers due to potential for symptomatic hypotension. There have been a few reports of sudden vision loss due to nonarteritic ischemic optic neuropathy (NAION). Patients with prior NAION are at higher risk. Sudden hearing loss, with or without tinnitus, vertigo or dizziness, has been reported. Transient global amnesia has also been reported.

MOA — Selectively inhibits phosphodiesterase-5 resulting in enhanced relaxation of penile arteries & corpus cavernosal smooth muscle; enhances erectile function by increasing penile blood flow. Relaxes pulmonary vascular smooth muscle cells resulting in vasodilation of the pulmonary vascular bed.

ADVERSE EFFECTS — Serious: MI, CVA, hypotension, syncope, cerebral thrombosis, retinal hemorrhage, vision loss (nonarteritic ischemic optic neuropathy). Frequent: Headache, flushing, dyspepsia, abnormal vision.

TADALAFIL (*Cialis*) ▶L ♀B ▶– $$$$

WARNING — Contraindicated with nitrates. Caution with alpha-blockers due to potential for symptomatic hypotension. There have been a few reports of sudden vision loss due to nonarteritic ischemic optic neuropathy (NAION). Patients with prior NAION are at higher risk. Retinal artery occlusion has been reported. Sudden hearing loss, with or without tinnitus, vertigo, or dizziness, has been reported. Transient global amnesia.

ADULT — Erectile dysfunction: 2.5 to 5 mg PO daily without regard to timing of sexual activity. As needed dosing: 10 mg PO prn prior to sexual activity. Optimal timing of administration unclear, but should be at least 30 to 45 min before sexual activity. May increase to 20 mg or decrease to 5 mg. Max 1 dose/day. Start 5 mg (max 1 dose/day) if CrCl 31 to 50 mL/min. Max 5 mg/day if CrCl > 30 mL/min on dialysis. Max 10 mg/day if mild to moderate hepatic impairment; avoid in severe hepatic impairment. Max 10 mg once in 72 h if concurrent potent CYP3A4 inhibitors. BPH with or without erectile dysfunction: 5 mg PO daily. Caution with ritonavir, see prescribing information for specific dose adjustments.

PEDS — Not approved in children.

FORMS — Trade only (Cialis): Tabs 2.5, 5, 10, 20 mg.

NOTES — If nitrates needed give at least 48 h after the last tadalafil dose. Improves erectile function

(cont.)

TADALAFIL (*cont.*)

for up to 36 h. Not FDA-approved for women. Not recommended if MI in prior 90 days, angina during sexual activity, NYHA Class II or greater in prior 6 months, hypotension (< 90/50), HTN (> 170/100) or CVA in prior 6 months. Rare reports of prolonged erections. Do not use with ketoconazole or itraconazole.

MOA — Selectively inhibits phosphodiesterase-5 resulting in enhanced relaxation of penile arteries & corpus cavernosal smooth muscle; enhances erectile function by increasing penile blood flow.

ADVERSE EFFECTS — Serious: Priapism, hypotension, myocardial infarction, vision loss (nonarteritic ischemic optic neuropathy), retinal artery occlusion. Frequent: Headache, flushing, dyspepsia, back pain.

VARDENAFIL (*Levitra, Staxyn*) ▶LK ♀B ▶– $$$$$

WARNING — Contraindicated with nitrates (time interval for safe administration unknown). Caution with alpha blockers due to potential for symptomatic hypotension. There have been a few reports of sudden vision loss due to nonarteritic ischemic optic neuropathy (NAION). Patients with prior NAION are at higher risk. Sudden hearing loss, with or without tinnitus, vertigo or dizziness, has been reported. Seizures and seizure recurrence have been reported.

ADULT — Erectile dysfunction: 10 mg PO 1 h before sexual activity. Usual effective dose range: 5 to 20 mg. Maximum 1 dose/day. Use lower dose (5 mg) if age 65 yo or older or moderate hepatic impairment (max 10 mg); 2.5 mg when coadministered with certain drugs (see notes). Not FDA-approved in women.

PEDS — Not approved in children.

FORMS — Trade only: Tabs 2.5, 5, 10, 20 mg. Oral disintegrating tab 10 mg (Staxyn)

NOTES — See the following parenthetical vardenafil dose adjustments when taken with ritonavir (max 2.5 mg/72 h); indinavir, saquinavir, atazanavir,

clarithromycin, ketoconazole 400 mg daily, or itraconazole 400 mg daily (max 2.5 mg/24 h); ketoconazole 200 mg daily, itraconazole 200 mg daily, or erythromycin (max 5 mg/24 h). Avoid with alpha-blockers and antiarrhythmics, and in congenital QT prolongation. Caution if CVA, MI or other cardiovascular event within last 6 months, unstable angina, severe liver impairment, end stage renal disease or retinitis pigmentosa.

MOA — Selectively inhibits phosphodiesterase-5 resulting in enhanced relaxation of penile arteries & corpus cavernosal smooth muscle; enhances erectile function by increasing penile blood flow.

ADVERSE EFFECTS — Serious: Hypotension, syncope, myocardial infarction, priapism, vision loss (nonarteritic ischemic optic neuropathy), seizures, transient global amnesia. Frequent: Headache, flushing, rhinitis, dyspepsia.

YOHIMBINE (*Yocon, Yohimex*) ▶L ♀– ▶– $

ADULT — No approved indications.

PEDS — No approved indications.

UNAPPROVED ADULT — Erectile dysfunction: 1 tab PO three times per day. If side effects (e.g., tremor, tachycardia, nervousness) occur, reduce to ½ tab three times per day, followed by gradual increases to 1 tab three times per day.

FORMS — Generic/Trade: Tabs 5.4 mg.

NOTES — Prescription yohimbine and yohimbine bark extract (see Herbal section) are not interchangeable. Contraindicated with renal disease. Avoid with antidepressant use, psychiatric disorders, the elderly, women, or ulcer history. Efficacy of therapy longer than 10 weeks unclear. American Urological Association does not recommend as a standard treatment due to unproven efficacy.

MOA — An alpha-2-adrenergic receptor blocker.

ADVERSE EFFECTS — Serious: Respiratory paralysis with overdose. Frequent: HTN, tachycardia, nervousness, irritability, tremor and increased motor activity.

UROLOGY: Nephrolithiasis

ACETOHYDROXAMIC ACID (*Lithostat*) ▶K ♀X ▶? $$$$

ADULT — Chronic UTI, adjunctive therapy: 250 mg PO three to four times per day for a total dose of 10 to 15 mg/kg/day. Maximum dose is 1.5 g/day. Decrease dose in patients with renal impairment to no more than 1 g/day.

PEDS — Adjunctive therapy in chronic urea-splitting UTI (eg, Proteus): 10 mg/kg/day PO divided two to three times per day.

FORMS — Trade only: Tabs 250 mg.

NOTES — Do not use if CrCl less than 20 mL/min. Administer on an empty stomach.

MOA — Inhibits urease and the production of ammonia by urea-splitting urinary organisms (eg, Proteus).

ADVERSE EFFECTS — Serious: Bone marrow suppression, hemolytic anemia. Frequent: Headache, rash, malaise, nervousness, anxiety, depression, vomiting, anorexia, phlebitis.

AMINOHIPPURATE (*PAH*) ▶K ♀C ▶? $

ADULT — Estimation of effective renal plasma flow and measurement of functional capacity of renal tubular secretory mechanism: Specialized infusion dosing available.

PEDS — Not approved in children.

NOTES — May precipitate heart failure. Patients receiving sulfonamides, procaine or thiazolsulfone may interfere with chemical color development essential for analysis. Concomitant use of probenecid my result in erroneously low effective renal plasma flow.

MOA — Chemical filtered by the glomeruli and actively secreted by the proximal tubules.

ADVERSE EFFECTS — Serious: Hypersensitivity, anaphylaxis. Frequent: Sensation of warmth or the desire to defecate or urinate during or shortly following initiation of infusion.

CELLULOSE SODIUM PHOSPHATE (*Calcibind*) ▶Fecal ♀C ▶+ $$$$
WARNING — Avoid in heart failure or ascites due to high sodium content.
ADULT — Absorptive hypercalciuria Type 1 (age older than 16 yo): Initial dose with urinary calcium greater than 300 mg/day (on moderate calcium-restricted diet): 5 g with each meal. Decrease dose to 5 g with supper, 2.5 g with each remaining meal when calcium declines to less than 150 mg/day. Initial dose with urinary calcium 200 to 300 mg/day (controlled calcium-restricted diet): 5 g with supper, 2.5 g with each remaining meal. Mix with water, soft drink, or fruit juice. Ingest within 30 min of meal.
PEDS — Do not use if younger than 16 yo.
FORMS — Trade only: Bulk powder 300 mg.
NOTES — Give concomitant supplement of 1.5 g magnesium gluconate with 15 g/day. 1 g magnesium gluconate with 10 g/day. Take magnesium supplement at least 1 h before or after each dose to avoid binding. May cause hyperparathyroidism. Long-term use may cause hypomagnesemia, hyperoxaluria, hypomagnesiuria, depletion of trace metals (copper, zinc, iron); monitor calcium, magnesium, trace metals, and CBC q 3 to 6 months; monitor parathyroid hormone once between the first 2 weeks and 3 months, then q 3 to 6 months thereafter. Adjust or stop treatment if PTH rises above normal. Stop when inadequate hypocalciuric response (urinary calcium of less than 30 mg/5 g of cellulose sodium phosphate) occurs while patient is on moderate calcium restriction. Avoid vitamin C supplementation since metabolized to oxalate.
MOA — Nonabsorbable ion-exchange resin. Binds to divalent cations.
ADVERSE EFFECTS — Serious: Hyperoxaluria. Frequent: Diarrhea, dyspepsia, altered taste, hypomagnesemia, hyperparathyroidism.

CITRATE (*Polycitra-K, Urocit-K, Bicitra, Oracit, Polycitra, Polycitra-LC*) ▶K ♀C ▶? $$$
ADULT — Prevention of calcium and urate kidney stones: 1 packet in water/juice PO three to four times per day with meals. 15 to 30 mL PO soln three to four times per day with meals. Tabs 10 to 20 mEq PO three to four times per day with meals. Max 100 mEq/day.
PEDS — Urinary alkalinization: 5 to 15 mL PO four times per day with meals.
FORMS — Generic/Trade: Polycitra-K packet 3300 mg potassium citrate/ea, Polycitra-K oral soln (1100 mg potassium citrate/5 mL, 480 mL). Oracit oral soln (490 mg sodium citrate/5 mL, 15, 30, 480 mL). Bicitra oral soln (500 mg sodium citrate/5 mL, 480 mL). Urocit-K wax (potassium citrate) Tabs 5, 10 mEq. Polycitra-LC oral soln (550 mg potassium citrate/500 mg sodium citrate per 5 mL, 480 mL). Polycitra oral syrup (550 mg potassium citrate/500 mg sodium citrate per 5 mL, 480 mL.
NOTES — Contraindicated in renal insufficiency, PUD, UTI, and hyperkalemia.
MOA — Increases urinary-free bases thereby increasing pH.
ADVERSE EFFECTS — Serious: Hyperkalemia. Frequent: N/V, diarrhea, dyspepsia.

APPENDIX

ADULT EMERGENCY DRUGS (selected)

ALLERGY

diphenhydramine (*Benadryl*): 25 to 50 mg IV/IM/PO.
epinephrine: 0.1 to 0.5 mg IM/SC (1:1000 solution), may repeat after 20 minutes.
methylprednisolone (*Solu-Medrol*): 125 mg IV/IM.

HYPERTENSION

esmolol (*Brevibloc*): 500 mcg/kg IV over 1 minute, then titrate 50 to 200 mcg/kg/min.
fenoldopam (*Corlopam.*): Start 0.1 mcg/kg/min, titrate up to 1.6 mcg/kg/min.
labetalol: Start 20 mg slow IV, then 40 to 80 mg IV q10 min prn up to 300 mg total cumulative dose.
nitroglycerin: Start 10 to 20 mcg/min IV infusion, then titrate prn up to 100 mcg/min.
nitroprusside (*Nitropress*): Start 0.3 mcg/kg/min IV infusion, then titrate prn up to 10 mcg/kg/min.

DYSRHYTHMIAS / ARREST

adenosine (*Adenocard*): PSVT (not A-fib): 6 mg rapid IV & flush, preferably through a central line or proximal IV. If no response after 1-2 minutes, then 12 mg. A third dose of 12mg may be given prn.
amiodarone: V-fib or pulseless V-tach: 300 mg IV/IO; may repeat 150 mg just once. Life-threatening ventricular arrhythmia: Load 150 mg IV over 10 min, then 1 mg/min × 6 h, then 0.5 mg/min × 18 h.
atropine: 0.5 to 1 mg IV, repeat q 3-5 minutes prn to maximum of 3 mg.
diltiazem (*Cardizem*): Rapid A-fib: bolus 0.25 mg/kg or 20 mg IV over 2 min. May repeat 0.35 mg/kg or 25 mg 15 min after 1st dose. Infusion 5-15 mg/h.
epinephrine: 1 mg IV/IO q 3-5 minutes for cardiac arrest. [1:10,000 solution].
lidocaine (Xylocaine): Load 1 mg/kg IV, then 0.5 mg/kg q 8-10 min prn to max 3 mg/kg. Maintenance 2 g in 250 mL D5W (8 mg/mL) at 1 to 4 mg/min drip (7-30 mL/h).

PRESSORS

dobutamine: 2 to 20 mcg/kg/min. 70 kg: 5 mcg/kg/min with 1 mg/mL concentration (eg, 250 mg in 250 mL D5W) = 21 mL/h.
dopamine: Pressor: Start at 5 mcg/kg/min, increase prn by 5 to 10 mcg/kg/min increments at 10 min intervals, max 50 mcg/kg/min. 70 kg: 5 mcg/kg/min with 1600 mcg/mL concentration (eg, 400 mg in 250 mL D5W) = 13 mL/h. Doses in mcg/kg/min: *2-4* = (traditional renal dose, apparently ineffective) dopaminergic receptors; 5-10= (cardiac dose) dopaminergic and beta1 receptors; >10 = dopaminergic, beta1, and alpha1 receptors.
norepinephrine (*Levophed*): 4 mg in 500 mL D5W (8 mcg/mL), start 8 to 12 mcg/min (1 to 1.5 mL/h), usual dose once BP is stabilized 2 to 4 mcg/min. 22.5 mL/h = 3 mcg/min.
phenylephrine: 20 mg in 250 mL D5W (80 mcg/mL), start 100 to 180 mcg/min (75 to 135 mL/h), usual dose once BP is stabilized 40 to 60 mcg/min (30 to 45 mL/h).

INTUBATION

etomidate (*Amidate*): 0.3 mg/kg IV.
methohexital (*Brevital*): 1 to 1.5 mg/kg IV.
propofol (*Diprivan*): 2.0 to 2.5 mg/kg IV.
rocuronium (*Zemuron*): 0.6 to 1.2 mg/kg IV.
succinylcholine (*Anectine, Quelicin*): 0.6 to 1.1 mg/kg IV. Peds (<5 yo): 2 mg/kg IV.
thiopental: 3 to 5 mg/kg IV.

SEIZURES

diazepam (*Valium*): 5 to 10 mg IV, or 0.2 to 0.5 mg/kg rectal gel up to 20 mg PR.
fosphenytoin (*Cerebyx*): Load 15 to 20 mg "phenytoin equivalents" (PE)/ kg IV, no faster than 100 to 150 mg PE/min.
lorazepam (Ativan): Status epilepticus: 4 mg IV over 2 min, may repeat in 10-15 min. Anxiolytic/ sedation: 0.04 to 0.05 mg/kg IV/IM; usual dose 2 mg, max 4 mg.
phenobarbital: Status epilepticus: 15 to 20 mg/kg IV load; may give additional 5 mg/kg doses q 15-30 mins to max total dose of 30 mg/kg.
phenytoin (*Dilantin*): 15 to 20 mg/kg up to 1000mg IV no faster than 50 mg/min.

CARDIAC DYSRHYTHMIA PROTOCOLS (for adults and adolescents)

Chest compressions ~100/min. Ventilations 8-10/min if intubated; otherwise 30:2 compression/ventilation ratio. Drugs that can be administered down ET tube (use 2–2.5 × usual dose): epinephrine, atropine, lidocaine, naloxone, vasopressin*.

V-Fib, Pulseless V-Tach
Airway, oxygen, CPR until defibrillator ready
Defibrillate 360 J (old monophasic), 120–200 J (biphasic), or with AED
Resume CPR × 2 min (5 cycles)
Repeat defibrillation if no response
Vasopressor during CPR:
- Epinephrine 1 mg IV/IO q 3–5 minutes, or
- Vasopressin* 40 units IV to replace 1st or 2nd dose of epinephrine
Rhythm/pulse check every ~2 minutes
Consider antiarrhythmic during CPR:
- Amiodarone 300 mg IV/IO; may repeat 150 mg just once
- Lidocaine 1.0–1.5 mg/kg IV/IO, then repeat 0.5–0.75 mg/kg to max 3 doses or 3 mg/kg
- Magnesium sulfate 1–2 g IV/IO if suspect torsades de pointes

Asystole or Pulseless Electrical Activity (PEA)
Airway, oxygen, CPR
Vasopressor (when IV/IO access):
- Epinephrine 1 mg IV/IO q 3–5 min, or
- Vasopressin* 40 units IV/IO to replace 1st or 2nd dose of epinephrine
Consider atropine 1 mg IV/IO for asystole or slow PEA. Repeat q 3–5 min up to 3 doses.
Rhythm/pulse check every ~2 minutes
Consider 6 H's: hypovolemia, hypoxia, H+acidosis, hyper/ hypokalemia, hypoglycemia, hypothermia
Consider 5 T's: Toxins, tamponade-cardiac, tension pneumothorax, thrombosis (coronary or pulmonary), trauma

Bradycardia, <60 bpm and Inadequate Perfusion
Airway, oxygen, IV
Prepare for transcutaneous pacing; don't delay if advanced heart block
Consider atropine 0.5 mg IV; may repeat q 3–5 min to max 3 mg
Consider epinephrine (2–10 mcg/min) or dopamine(2–10 mcg/kg/min)
Prepare for transvenous pacing

Tachycardia with Pulses
Airway, oxygen, IV
If unstable and heart rate >150 bpm, then synchronized cardioversion
If stable narrow-QRS (<120 ms):
- Regular: Attempt vagal maneuvers, If no success, adenosine 6 mg IV, then 12 mg prn (may repeat x 1),
- Irregular: Control rate with diltiazem or beta blocker (caution in CHF or severe obstructive disease).
If stable wide-QRS (>120 ms):
- Regular and suspect V-tach: Amiodarone 150 mg IV over 10 min; repeat prn to max 2.2 g/24 h. Prepare for elective synchronized cardioversion.
- Regular and suspect SVT with aberrancy: adenosine as per narrow-QRS above.
- Irregular and A-fib: Control rate with diltiazem or beta blocker (caution in CHF/ severe obstructive pulmonary disease).
- Irregular and A-fib with pre-excitation (WPW): Avoid AV nodal blocking agents; consider amiodarone 150 mg IV over 10 min,
- Irregular and torsades de pointes: magnesium 1–2 g IV load over 5–60 min, then infusion.

bpm=beats per minute; CPR=cardiopulmonary resuscitation; ET=endotracheal; IO=intraosseous; J=Joules; ms=milliseconds; WPW=Wolff-Parkinson-White. Sources: *Circulation* 2005; 112, suppl IV; *NEJM* 2008;359:21–30 (demonstrated no benefit over epinephrine and worse long-term neurological outcomes).

INDEX

B

tinidazole, 30, 32, 33, 50
tioconazole, 30, 345
tiotropium, 435
tipranavir, 64–65
tipranavir-ritonavir, 445
tirofiban, 135
Tirosint, 208
Tivicay, 55
tizanidine, 2–3, 108
TMP- SMX, 94–95
TNKase, 152
Tobi, 34
Tobradex, 388
Tobradex ST, 388
tobramycin, 34
tobramycin—ophthalmic,
385, 388, 389
Tobrex, 385
tocilizumab, 440–441
tocopherol, 215
Toctino, 175
tofacitinib, 441
Tofranil, 399
Tofranil PM, 399
tolazamide, 196
tolbutamide, 196
tolcapone, 318
Tolectin, 9
tolmetin, 6, 9
tolnaftate, 166
Toloxin, 115
tolterodine, 108, 455
tolvaptan, 219–220
Topamax, 311, 407
Topicort, 58, 158, 172
Topicort LP, 172
Topilene Glycol, 171
topiramate, 262, 311,
407
Toposar, 376
topotecan, 381
Toprol-XL, 137–138
Topsyn, 173
Toradol, 8
toremifene, 361
Torisel, 366
torsades, 108
torsemide, 143
tositumomab, 366–367
Totect, 357
Toviaz, 454
tpa, 151
TPV, 64–65
Tracleer, 148–149
Tracrium, 21
Tradjenta, 192–193
Trajenta, 192–193
Tramacet, 4
tramadol, 4, 17
trametinib, 374
Trandate, 137
trandolapril, 104, 111,
130
tranexamic acid, 275
Transderm-Nitro, 146
Transderm-Scop, 246
Transderm-V, 246
transdermal fentanyl, 10
Tranxene, 415
tranylcypromine, 400–401
trastuzumab, 367

traumatic, 108
Travatan Z, 393
travoprost, 393
trazodone, 405
Treanda, 348
trefoil, 287–288
Trelstar, 361
Trelstar Depot, 361
Trental, 153
treprostinil sodium—
injectable, 150–151
treprostinil—inhaled
solution, 151
treprostinil—oral, 151
tretinoin, 162, 179
tretinoin—oncology, 381
tretinoin—topical,
161–162
Trexall, 355, 443
Treximet, 314
Tri- Linyah, 326
Tri-Cyclen, 332
Tri-Estarylla, 326, 332
Tri-Legest, 326, 332
Tri-Legest Fe, 326, 332
Tri-Linyah, 332
Tri-Luma, 179
Tri-Nasal, 239
Tri-Norinyl, 326, 332
Tri-Previfem, 326, 332
Tri-Sprintec, 326, 332
Triaderm, 174–175
triamcinolone, 158, 180,
188
triamcinolone—inhaled,
432
triamcinolone—nasal, 239
triamcinolone—topical,
171, 174–175
triamcinolone—vitreous,
390
Triaminic Chest and Nasal
Congestion, 227
Triaminic Cold and Allergy,
221, 227
Triaminic Cough and Sore
Throat, 227
Triaminic Day Time Cold
and Cough, 228
Triaminic Flu Cough and
Fever, 228
Triaminic Night Time Cold
and Cough, 228
Triaminic Oral Infant
Drops, 235
triamterene, 129–130,
143
Trianal, 3
Trianal C-1/2, 14
Trianal C-1/4, 14
Trianex, 174–175
Triazide, 105, 129–130
triazolam, 417–418
Tribenzor, 105, 130–131
TriCor, 121
Tridesilon, 158, 172
Tridural, 17
Triesence, 390
triest, 337
trifluoperazine, 408, 410
trifluridine, 387

Trifolium pratense,
287–288
Triglide, 121
Trigonelle foenum-grae-
cum, 281
trihexyphenidyl, 318
Trileptal, 309
TriLipix, 121
Trilisate, 5, 6
TriLyte, 255
trimethobenzamide, 246,
327
trimethoprim, 103
trimethoprim-sulfamethox-
azole, 94–95
trimethoprim—ophthalmic,
387
trimipramine, 400
Trinipatch, 146
Trinovin, 287–288
Triostat, 208
Tripacel, 292–293
triprolidine, 221, 225
triptans, 313–314
triptorelin, 361
Trisenox, 374–375
Trivaris, 188
Trivora, 325
Trivora-28, 326, 333
Trizivir, 53–54
Trokendi XR, 311
Tropicacyl, 395
tropicamide, 395
Trosec, 455
trospium, 455
Trusopt, 391
Truvada, 54
trypan blue, 397
tryptophan, 405–406
tuberculin PPD, 302
Tubersol, 302
Tucks, 175
Tucks Hemorrhoidal
Ointment,
175
Tucks Suppositories, 175
Tudorza, 433
Tums, 200–201
Tuss-HC, 234
Tussicaps, 234
Tussionex, 235
Tussionex II, 222
Twinrix, 297
292 tab, 14
2-PAM, 451
Twynsta, 105, 131
Tygacil, 102–103
Tykerb, 378
Tylenol, 16
Tylenol #1, 15
Tylenol # 2, 15
Tylenol # 3, 15
Tylenol # 4, 15
Tylenol with Codeine, 15
Typherix, 297
Typhim Vi, 297
typhoid vaccine—
inactivated injection,
297
typhoid vaccine—live oral,
297
Tysabri, 316–317

Tyvaso, 151
Tyzeka, 74

U

ubiquinone, 279
Uceris, 259
Ulesfia, 166
ulipristal acetate, 334,
347
Uloric, 444
Ultane, 19
Ultiva, 19
Ultracet, 4
Ultram, 17
Ultram ER, 17
Ultrathon, 176
Ultravate, 158, 173
Ultravist, 156
Ultresa, 261–262
Uniphyl, 435
Uniretic, 105, 131
Unisom Nighttime Sleep
Aid, 244
Unithroid, 208
Univasc, 104, 110
unoprostone, 392
urea, 178
Urecholine, 456
Urex, 100
Urised, 455–456
Urispas, 454
Urocit-K, 460
Urodol, 457
urofollitropin, 341
Urogesic, 457
urokinase, 152
Urolene blue, 451
Uromax, 454–455
Uromitexan, 357
Uroquid-Acid No. 2,
457
UroXatral, 453
URSO, 262
URSO Forte, 262
ursodiol, 262
Urtica dioica radix, 286
ustekinumab, 168–169
UTA, 456
uterotonics, 343–344
UTI Relief, 457
Utira-C, 456
Uvadex, 168

V

vaccinia vaccine, 296
Vaccinium macrocarpon,
279
Vaccinium myrtillus, 277
Vagifem, 336
Vagistat-1, 345
valacyclovir, 31, 66, 327
Valcyte, 51
valerian, 290
Valeriana officinalis, 290
valganciclovir, 51
Valium, 415–416, 461

NOTES

NOTES

NOTES

NOTES

Stay Connected with Tarascon Publishing!

Monthly Dose eNewsletter
—Tarascon's Monthly eNewsletter

Stay up-to-date and subscribe today at: www.tarascon.com

Written specifically with **Tarascon** customers in mind, the Tarascon Monthly Dose will provide you with new drug information, tips and tricks, updates on our print, mobile and online products as well as some extra topics that are interesting and entertaining.

Sign up to receive the Tarascon Monthly Dose Today! Simply register at www.tarascon.com.

You can also stay up-to-date with **Tarascon** news, new product releases, and relevant medical news and information on Facebook, Twitter page, and our Blog.

STAY CONNECTED

Facebook: www.facebook.com/tarascon
Twitter: @JBL_Medicine
Blog: blogs.jblearning.com/medicine